Targeted Therapies in Rheumatology

Targeted Therapies in Rheumatology

Josef S Smolen MD

Professor of Medicine
Chairman, Division of Rheumatology
Department of Internal Medicine III
University of Vienna
Vienna, Austria

Peter E Lipsky MD

Director, Intramural Research Program
National Institute for Arthritis and
Musculoskeletal and Skin Diseases
Bethesda MD
USA

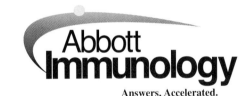

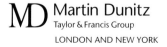 Martin Dunitz
Taylor & Francis Group
LONDON AND NEW YORK

First published in the United Kingdom in 2003
by Martin Dunitz, Taylor & Francis Group plc, 11 New Fetter Lane,
London EC4P 4EE

Tel.:	44 (0) 20 7583 9855
Fax.:	+44 (0) 20 7842 2298
E-mail:	info.dunitz@tandf.co.uk
Website:	http://www.dunitz.co.uk

A CIP record for this book is available from the British Library.

ISBN 1-84184-157-9

Distributed in the USA by
Fulfilment Center
Taylor & Francis
10650 Tobben Drive
Independence, KY 41051, USA
Toll Free Tel.: +1 800 634 7064
E-mail: taylorandfrancis@thomsonlearning.com

Distributed in Canada by
Taylor & Francis
74 Rolark Drive
Scarborough, Ontario M1R 4G2, Canada
Toll Free Tel.: +1 877 226 2237
E-mail: tal_fran@istar.ca

Distributed in the rest of the world by
Thomson Publishing Services
Cheriton House
North Way
Andover, Hampshire SP10 5BE, UK
Tel.: +44 (0)1264 332424
E-mail: salesorder.tandf@thomsonpublishingservices.co.uk

Composition by Scribe Design, Gillingham, Kent
Printed and bound in Spain by Grafos S.A. Arte Sobre Papel

Contents

Section II. Cytokines, chemokines and other effector molecules

Section III. Transcription factors and signalling molecules

Section IV. Inflammatory mediators

Section V. Matrix molecules

Section VI. Targeted therapies in human and experimental rheumatic diseases

Section VII. Immunoglobulin manipulation

Section VIII. Ethics and study design

Contributors

Steven B Abramson MD
Department of Rheumatology/Medicine
Hospital for Joint Diseases
New York University School of Medicine
New York NY, USA

Christian Antoni MD
Department of Medicine III
Friedrich Alexander University
Erlangen-Nuremberg, Erlangen
Germany

William P Arend MD
Division of Rheumatology
University of Colorado Health Sciences Center
Denver CO, USA

Martin Aringer MD
Department of Rheumatology
Internal Medicine III
University of Vienna, Vienna
Austria

John P Atkinson MD
Professor of Medicine and Microbiology
Department of Internal Medicine
Rheumatology Division
Washington University School of Medicine
St Louis MO, USA

Roberto G Baccala PhD
Assistant Professor of Immunology
Department of Immunology
The Scripps Research Institute
La Jolla CA, USA

Jürgen Braun MD
Professor of Medicine and Consultant in
Rheumatology
Department of Medicine/Rheumatology
University Hospital Benjamin Franklin, Berlin
and Rheumazentrum Ruhrgebiet, Herne
Germany

Ferdinand C Breedveld MD
Professor of Rheumatology
Leiden University
Department of Rheumatology
Leiden University Medical Center, Leiden
The Netherlands

Keith Brown BSc MSc PhD
Staff Scientist
Laboratory of Immunoregulation
National Institute of Allergy and Infectious Diseases
National Institutes of Health
Bethesda MD, USA

Danielle Burger PhD
Division of Immunology and Allergy
Clinical Immunology Unit (Hans Wilsdorf
Laboratory)
University Hospital, Geneva
Switzerland

Gerd R Burmester MD
Department of Rheumatology
Charite Humboldt University, Berlin
Germany

Leonard H Calabrese DO
Director, Center for Vasculitis Care and Research
Cleveland Clinic Foundation A50
Cleveland OH, USA

Naresh Chauhan MB BS MD MRCP
Rheumatology Fellow
National Institutes of Arthritis and Musculoskeletal
and Skin Diseases
National Institutes of Health
Bethesda MD, USA

Estefania Claudio PhD
Research Fellow
Laboratory of Immunoregulation
National Institute of Allergy and Infectious Diseases
National Institutes of Health
Bethesda MD, USA

Leslie J Crofford MD
Associate Professor of Internal Medicine
Division of Rheumatology
Department of Internal Medicine
University of Michigan
Ann Arbor MI, USA

John J Cush MD
Chief, Rheumatology and Immunology
Presbytarian Hospital of Dallas
and Clinical Professor of Medicine
The University of Texas Southwestern Medical
School
Dallas TX, USA

Anne Davidson MBBS
Professor of Medicine
Microbiology and Immunology Albert Einstein
College of Medicine
Bronx NY, USA

Jean-Michel Dayer MD
Professor of Medicine
Head, Division of Immunology & Allergy
University Hospital, Geneva
Switzerland

Betty Diamond MD
Weinstck Chair in Immunology
Microbiology and Immunology and Medicine
Albert Einstein College of Medicine
Bronx NY, USA

Charles A Dinarello MD
Professor of Medicine
University of Colorado Health Sciences Center
Division Infectious Diseases
Denver CO, USA

Paul Emery MA MD FRCP
ARC Professor of Rheumatology
Head of Academic Unit of Musculoskeletal Disease
Department of Rheumatology
Leeds General Infirmary
Leeds, UK

Marc Feldmann MB BS PhD FRCP DRCPath
FMedSci
Professor of Cellular Immunology and Head
Kennedy Institute of Rheumatology Division, Faculty
of Medicine
Imperial College School of Medicine
London, UK

Alison Finnegan PhD
Professor of Medicine, Section of Rheumatology
Professor of Immunology/Microbiology
Rush Presbyterian-St. Luke's-Medical Center
Chicago IL, USA

Gary S Firestein MD
Professor of Medicine
Chief, Division of Rheumatology, Allergy and
Immunology
UCSD School of Medicine
La Jolla CA, USA

Judah Folkman MD
Surgeon-in-Chief Emeritus
Director, Surgical Research Laboratory
Departments of Surgery and Cellular Biology
Harvard Medical School and Children's Hospital
Boston MA, USA

David M Frucht MD
Principal Investigator
Center for Biologics Evaluation and Research
Food and Drug Administration
Bethesda MD, USA

Cem Gabay MD
Associate Professor of Medicine
Division of Rheumatology
University Hospital of Geneva, Geneva
Switzerland

Massimo Gadina PhD
Staff Scientist
Molecular Immunology and Inflammation Branch
NIAMS
National Institutes of Health
Bethesda MD, USA

Steffen Gay MD
Center of Experimental Rheumatology
Department of Rheumatology
University Hospital Zurich, Zurich
Switzerland

Winfried Graninger MD
Associate Professor of Medicine
Division of Rheumatology
Department of Internal Medicine III
Vienna General Hospital
University of Vienna, Vienna
Austria

Ellen M Gravallese MD
Director of Molecular Pathology
Harvard Institutes of Medicine
New England Baptist Bone and Joint Institute
Boston MA, USA

Bevra H Hahn MD
Chief of Rheumatology
UCLA School of Medicine
Los Angeles CA, USA

Gary S Hoffman MD
Harold C Schott Chair for Rheumatic and
Immunologic Diseases
Director, Center for Vasculitis Care and Research
Cleveland Clinic Foundation A50
Cleveland OH, USA

V Michael Holers MD
Professor of Rheumatology
University of Colorado
Denver CO, USA

Hui-Chen Hsu PhD
Assistant Professor
Department of Medicine
The University of Alabama at Birmingham
Birmingham AL, USA

Joachim R Kalden MD PhD
Professor of Internal Medicine
Head, Department for Internal Medicine III
Institute for Clinical Immunology
Friedrich-Alexander-Universität
Erlangen-Nuremberg, Erlangen
Germany

George A Karpouzas MD
UCLA Rehab Center
Los Angeles CA, USA

Arthur Kavanaugh MD
Center for Innovative Therapy
UCSD
Division of Rheumatology, Allergy and Immunology
La Jolla CA, USA

Hans-Peter Kiener MD
Faculty Member
Division of Rheumatology
Department of Internal Medicine III
Vienna General Hospital
University of Vienna, Vienna
Austria

Joon Kim MD PhD
Department of Medicine, Section of Arthritis and
Connective Tissue Diseases
Northwestern University Medical School
Chicago IL, USA

Tadamitsu Kishimoto MD
Department of Molecular Medicine
Graduate School of Medicine
and President, Osaka University
Osaka, Japan

Alisa Erika Koch MD
Gallagher Research Professor of Medicine
Northwestern University Medical School
Chicago IL, USA

Dwight H Kono MD
Assistant Professor of Immunology
Department of Immunology
The Scripps Research Institute
La Jolla CA, USA

Konstantin Konstantinov MD
Fellow in Rheumatology, Department of Medicine
Albert Einstein College of Medicine
Bronx NY, USA

Eswar Krishnan MD MPhil
Division of Rheumatology and Immunology
Department of Medicine
Stanford Univeristy
Stanford CA, USA

Sang-Heon Lee MD PhD
Assistant Professor
St. Mary's Hospital
Department of Internal Medicine
Seoul, Korea

Iris Leinhase MSc
Department of Rheumatology
Charite Humboldt University, Berlin
Germany

Patrick Liang MD
Director, Center for Vasculitis Care and Research
Cleveland Clinic Foundation A50
Cleveland OH, USA

Foo Y Liew BSc (Hons) PhD DSc FRSE FRCPath
Head, Division of Immunology, Infection and
Inflammation
University of Glasgow
Glasgow, UK

M Kathryn Liszewski BA
Research Scientist of Medicine
Department of Internal Medicine
Washington University School of Medicine
St Louis MO, USA

Ravinder N Maini BA MB BCh FRCP FRCPE
FMedSci
Professor of Rheumatology and, Former Head
Kennedy Institute of Rheumatology Division
Imperial College School of Medicine
London, UK

Iain B McInnes BSc (Hons) MBChB (Hons)
MRCP(UK) PhD
Professor/Honorary Consultant Rheumatologist
Centre for Rheumatic Diseases
Department of Medicine
Royal Infirmary
Glasgow, UK

Ela Martin BSc (Hons) PhD
Centre for Immunology and Cancer Research
University of Queensland
Princess Alexandra Hospital, Brisbane
Australia

Andrea Matucci MD
Department of Internal Medicine and Immunology
University of Florence, Florence
Italy

Philip J Mease MD
Seattle Rheumatology Associates
Swedish Hospital Medical Center Division of Clinical
Research
Clinical Professor, Department of Medicine
University of Washington
Seattle WA, USA

Frederick W Miller MD PhD
Chief, Environmental Autoimmunity Group
Office of Clinical Research
National Institute of Environmental Health Sciences,
NIH
Bethesda MD, USA

Masato Moriguchi MD PhD
Research Fellow of Molecular Immunology and
Inflammation Branch
National Institute of Arthritis, Musculoskeletal and
Skin Diseases
National Institutes of Health
Bethesda MD, USA

John D Mountz MD PhD
Professor of Medicine
JW & Virginia Goodwin-Warren D Blackburn Jr
Professor of Medicine
Division of Clinical Immunology and Rheumatology
Department of Medicine
University of Alabama at Birmingham
Birmingham AL, USA

Norihiro Nishimoto MD PhD
Associate Professor
Department of Medical Science I
School of Health and Sport Sciences
Osaka University, Osaka
Japan

John J O'Shea MD
Chief, Lymphocyte Cell Biology Section
Arthritis and Rheumatism Branch
National Institute of Arthritis and Musculoskeletal
and Skin Diseases
National Institutes of Health
Bethesda MD, USA

Brendan John O'Sullivan BSc (Hons) PhD
Centre for Immunology and Cancer Research
University of Queensland
Princess Alexandra Hospital, Brisbane
Australia

Thomas Pap MD
Division of Experimental Rheumatology
Center of Internal Medicine
University Hospital Magdeburg, Magdeburg
Germany

Richard S Panush MD
Professor and Chair Deparment of Med
St. Barnabas Medical Center
Livingston NJ, USA

Alison R Pettit PhD
New England Baptist Bone and Joint Institute
Harvard Institutes of Medicine
Beth Israel Deaconess Medical Center
Boston MA, USA

Sergio Romagnani MD
Department of Internal Medicine and Immunology
University of Florence, Florence
Italy

Paul L Romain MD
Department of Rheumatology
Cambridge Health Alliance
Cambridge Hospital
Cambridge MA, USA

Oliviero Rossi MD
Department of Internal Medicine and Immunology
University of Florence, Florence
Italy

Jane Salmon MD
Attending Physician
Hospital for Special Surgery and
Professor of Medicine
Weill Medical College of Cornell University
New York NY, USA

Georg Schett MD
Division of Rheumatology
Department of Internal Medicine III
University of Vienna Medical School
Vienna, Austria

Hendrik Schulze-Koops MD PhD
Nikolaus-Fiebiger-Zentrum für Molekulare Medizin
Erlangen
Germany

Yaniv Sherer MD
Center for Autoimmune Diseases
Department of Medicine B
Sheba Medical Center
Tel Hashomer & Sackler Faculty of Medicine
Tel-Aviv, Israel

Yehuda Shoenfeld MD
Head, Department of Medicine B
Research Unit of Autoimmune Diseases
Chaim Sheba Medical Center
Sackler Faculty of Medicine
Tel-Aviv University
Tel-Aviv, Israel

Ulrich K Siebenlist PhD
Section Head, Immune Activation
Laboratory of Immunoregulation
NIAID
National Institutes of Health
Bethesda MD, USA

Joachim Sieper MD
Professor of Medicine and Consultant in
Rheumatology
Department of Medicine/Rheumatology
University Hospital Benjamin Franklin, Berlin
Germany

Jeffrey Siegel MD
Immunology and Infectious Disease Branch
Division of Clinical Trial Design and Analysis
Food and Drug Administration
Rockville MD, USA

Lee S Simon MD
Associate Professor of Medicine
Harvard Medical School
Boston MA, USA
and Division Director
Division of Analgesic, Anti-inflammatory and
Ophthalmogic Drug Products
Center for Drug Evaluation and Research
Food and Drug Administration
Rockville MD, USA

Gurkipal Singh MD
Division of Rheumatology and Immunology
Department of Medicine
Stanford Univeristy
Stanford CA, USA

Michael Sittinger PhD
Associate Professor of Experimental Medicine
Charite Humboldt University, Berlin
Germany

Vibeke Strand MD
Biopharmaceutical Consultant
Clinical Professor, Division of Immunology,
Stanford University
Portola Valley CA, USA

Warren Strober MD
Mucosal Immunity Section
NIAID
NIH
Bethesda MD, USA

Zoltan Szekanecz MD PhD
Associate Professor of
Medicine, Immunology and Rheumatology
3rd Department of Medicine
University Medical School, Debrecen
Hungary

Argyrios N Theofilopoulos MD
Professor of Immunology
Department of Immunology
The Scripps Research Institute
La Jolla CA, USA

Ranjeny Thomas MBBS MD FRACP
Associate Professor of Rheumatology
Deputy Director Centre for Immunology and Cancer
Research
University of Queensland
Princess Alexandra Hospital, Brisbane
Australia

Angus Thompson BSc (Hons)
Centre for Immunology and Cancer Research
University of Queensland
Princess Alexandra Hospital, Brisbane
Australia

Peter Tugwell MD
Director
Center for Global Health
Institute of Population Health
University of Ottawa, Ottawa, Ontario
Canada

Peter Valent MD
Department of Internal Medicine I
Division of Hematology and Haemostaseology
University of Vienna, Vienna
Austria

Wim B van den Berg PhD
Professor of Experimental Rheumaology
Rheumatol Research and Advanced Therapeutics
University Medical Center Nijmegen, Nijmegen
The Netherlands

Peter LEM van Lent PhD
Professor of Experimental Rheumatology
Rheumatology Research and Advanced Therapeutics
University Medical Center Nijmegen, Nijmegen
The Netherlands

Wendy Watford PhD
Molecular Immunology and Inflammation Branch
National Institute of Arthritis and Musculoskeletal
and Skin Diseases
National Institutes of Health
Bethesda MD, USA

Patricia Woo PhD FRCP FRCPCH
Professor of Pediatric Rheumatology
Royal Free and University College Medical School
Department of Immunology and Molecular
Pathology
London, UK

Kazuyaki Yoshizaki MD PhD
Professor
Department of Medical Science I
School of Health and Sport Sciences
Osaka University, Osaka
Japan

Huang-Ge Zhang MD PhD DVM
Assistant Professor of Medicine
Department of Medicine, Division of Rheumatology
Birmingham AL, USA

Preface

Recent dramatic advances in immunology, cell biology, genetics and molecular biology have made it possible to consider truly targeted therapies in rheumatic diseases for the first time. Traditionally, treatment of rheumatic diseases has involved the use of agents with poorly understood or non-specific effects. The use of these agents was frequently empiric and the outcome unpredictable. As the understanding of the pathophysiology of rheumatic diseases increased, it became possible to consider specific events in the immunologic/inflammatory cascade as targets of specific therapy. In parallel, new technologies to produce specific targeted therapies enabled the validity of these targets to be tested. With the success of the first targeted agents, especially blockers of the cytokine TNF, the validity of this approach was dramatically confirmed. The idea of interfering specifically with a process known to be centrally involved in disease pathogenesis developed credibility.

Since these early days of targeted therapies in rheumatology, many additional potential targets have been identified, some of which have already been proven to be important.

The future of rheumatology will include the development of an even more precise knowledge of the pathogenesis of rheumatic diseases and the development of additional targeted therapies. Some of these targeted therapies may demonstrate even better efficacy than the currently available agents, whereas others may surprisingly fail to be of significant value in initial trials. However, each will provide important new information about the pathogenesis of rheumatic disease. Even agents that fail in initial trials may eventually be demonstrated to be efficacious in other disease situations or in combination with additional agents.

The optimal development of these agents will not only depend upon basic science and technology, but also upon the creativity and clinical judgment of translational researchers who will be essential to find the appropriate diseases or disease situations for these remedies.

This book focuses on newly emerging pathophysiologic targets in specific rheumatic diseases and novel emerging targeted therapies. The goal of this book is to stimulate a dialogue between basic science, metrology, clinical investigation and biotechnology to foster the development of an appropriate use for the emerging targeted treatment modalities and search for new pathophysiological targets. Each of the contributions in this volume come from leading experts in their field who focus their chapters to address these concepts.

The dialogue will not end with this book, since this is a dynamic and rapidly changing field. This volume presents the first chapter in this story. Subsequent volumes, already in the planning stage, will not only update current insights, but also focus on new targets as they emerge and thus contribute to this continuing dialogue.

The editors have been privileged to work with the authors and the publisher of this novel initiative and hope that in some small way our efforts contribute to the development of better therapies for our patients.

Josef S Smolen
Peter L Lipsky

Abbreviations

Where there are several subtypes of an abbreviation (e.g. IL-1 interleukin-1, IL-2 interleukin-2 etc.) only the basic abbreviation is given (e.g. IL inteleukin)

AA	adjuvant arthritis
ACR	American College of Rheumatology
ADAM	a disintegrin and a metalloproteinase
ADAMT	a disintegrin and a metalloproteinase with thrombospondin motif
ADCC	antibody-dependent cellular cytotoxicity
aFGF	acidic fibroblast growth factor
AIA	antigen-induced arthritis
AICD	activation-induced cell death
AIMS/AIMS 2	Arthritis Impact Measurement Scale
ANA	anti-nuclear antibody
ANCAs	anti-neutrophil cytoplasmic antibodies
AP	alternative pathway
APC	antigen-presenting cell
ARAMIS-PMS	Arthritis Rheumatism and Aging Information System - Post Marketing Surveillance Program
ARDS	adult respiratory distress syndrome
AS	ankylosing spondylitis
ATTRACT	Anti-TNF Trial in Rheumatoid Arthritis with Concomitant Therapy
BASDAI	Bath Ankylosing Spondylitis Disease Activity Index
BCMA	B-cell maturation antigen
BCR	B-cell receptor
bFGF	basic fibroblast growth factor
BILAG	British Isles Lupus Assessment Group

BLyS	B-lymphocyte stimulator
BMD	bone mineral density
BMP	bone morphogenic protein
BPI	bacteriocidal permeability increasing protein
BPTI	bovine pancreatic trypsin inhibitor
βTG	β-thromboglobulin
BTK	Bruton's tyrosine kinase
C1-INH	complement 1 inhibitor
CA	cofactor activity
CAB	complement activation blocker
CAML	calcium modulator and cyclophilin ligand
CBP	cardiopulmonary bypass
CCR2	chemokine receptor-2
CHAQ	Childhood Health Assessment Questionnaire
CIA	collagen-induced arthritis
CII	collagen II
CIS	cytokine inducible SH2-containing proteins
CK	creatine kinase
CLASS	celecoxib long-term safety study
CME	continuing medical education
CMV	cytomegalovirus
CNTF	ciliary neurotrophic factor
COMP	cartilage oligometric protein
COX	cyclooxygenase
COXIB	cyclooxygenase-2 inhibitor
CP	cyclophosphamide *or* classical pathway of complement system
CR1	complement receptor type1
CRP	C-reactive protein
CS	corticosteroids

CSA	cyclosporin A	Fc-OPG	Fc-osteoprotegerin
CSAIDs	cytokine-suppressing anti-inflammatory drugs	FDA	US Food and Drug Administration
CSS	Churg–Strauss syndrome	FDC	follicular dendritic cell
CTLA-4	cytotoxic T-lymphocyte antigen 4	FGF	fibroblast growth factor
CT-1	cardiotrophin-1	FLAP	5-lipoxygenase activating protein
CX3CL1	fractalkine	FLIP	Fas-associated death domain-like
DAA	decay-accelerating activity		IL-1-converting enzyme-inhibitory protein
DAS	Disease Activity Score		
DBPCRCT	double-blind placebo-controlled randomized clinical trial	FLS	fibroblast-like synoviocytes
		GAG	glycosaminoglycans
DC	dendritic cell	GCA	giant cell arteritis
DEXA	dual energy X-ray absorptiometry	G-CSF	granulocyte colony-stimulating factor
DHODH	dihydroorotate dehydrogenase		
DM	dermatomyositis	*gld*	generalized lymphoproliferation gene
DMARDs	disease-modifying anti-rheumatic drugs		
		GM-CSF	granulocyte–macrophage colony-stimulating factor
DN	dominant negative		
dsDNA	double-stranded DNA	GP	glycoproteins
DSS	dextran sodium sulfate	GPCR	G-protein-coupled receptor
EAE	experimental allergic encephalomyelitis	GPI	glucose-6-phosphate isomerase, glucose phosphate isomerase
EBV	Epstein–Barr virus	GuBP	Gu/RNA helicase II binding protein
ECLAM	European Consensus Lupus Activity Measure		
		GVHD	graft-versus-host disease
ECM	extracellular matrix	GVHR	graft-versus-host response
EDA-ID	anhydrotic ectodermal dysplasia associated with immunodeficiency	HAE	hereditary angiodema
		HAQ	Health Assessment Questionnaire
		HAQ-DI	Health Assessment Questionnaire Disability Index
EDRF	endothelium-derived relaxation factor		
		HBV	hepatitis B virus
EGF	endothelial growth factor, epidermal growth factor	HCV	hepatitis C virus
		HCV-MC	hepatitis C virus-associated mixed cryoglobulinemia
EMEA	The European Agency for the Evaluation of Medicinal Products		
		HDL	high density lipoprotein
e-NOS	endothelial nitric oxide synthase	HEV	high endothelial venule
EPBI3	Epstein–Barr virus-induced gene 3	HGF	hepatocyte growth factor
EPO	erythropoietin	HGFA	hepatocyte growth factor activator
EQ5D	EuroQOL 5 Dimensional		
ESAF	endothelial cell stimulating angiogenesis factor	HIF	hypoxia inducible factor
		hILP	inhibitor of apoptosis-like protein
ESR	erythrocyte sedimentation rate	HIV-1	human immunodeficiency virus-type 1
ET	endothelin		
FACIT	fibril-associated collagen with interrupted triple helix	HLA	human leukocyte antigen
		HMG	high mobility globin
FACS	fluorescence-activated cell sorting	HNE	human neutrophil elastase
FasL	Fas ligand	HUVEC	human umbilical vein epithelial cells
FcγR	Fcγ receptors		

IAP	inhibitor of apoptosis, inhibitor of apoptosis protein	L-NMMA	*N*-monomethyl-L-arginine
IBM	inclusion body myositis	*lpr*	lymphoproliferation gene
IC	immune complex	LPS	lipopolysaccharide
ICAM	intercellular adhesion molecule	LSP	long signaling peptide
ICE	interleukin-converting enzyme	mAbs	monoclonal antibodies
IDO	indoleamine-2,3-dioxygenase	MAC	membrane attack complex
IFN	interferon	MACTAR	McMaster Toronto Arthritis patient preference questionnaire
IGF	insulin-like growth factor	MAPEG	membrane-associated proteins involved in eicosanoid and glutathione metabolism
IIM	idiopathic inflammatory myopathies		
IKK	IκB kinase	MAPK	mitogen-activated protein kinase
IL	interleukin	MASP	mannose-binding lectin-associated serum protease
ILAR	International League of Associations of Rheumatology		
IL-1R AcP	interleukin-1 receptor accessory protein	MBL	mannan/mannose-binding lectin
		mBSA	methylated bovine serum albumin
IL-1ra	interleukin-1 receptor antagonist	MC	mast cell
IL-1RII	decoy interleukin-1 receptor II	MCAF	monocyte chemotactic protein
IL-1sRII	soluble interleukin-1 receptor II	MCID	minimal clinically important differences
IL-18BP	interleukin-18 binding protein		
IND	investigational new drug	MCMV	murine cytomegalovirus
INH	isoniazide	MCP-1	monocyte chemoattractant 1
i-NOS	inducible nitric oxide synthase	M-CSF	macrophage colony-stimulating factor
IRAD	International Rheumatoid Arthritis Database		
		Mφ	monocyte–macrophages
IRAK	interleukin-1 receptor-associated kinase	mFasL	murine Fas ligand
		MGST	microsomal glutathione transferase
IRB	institutional review board		
ITAM	immunoreceptor tyrosine-based activation motif	MGUS	monoclonal gammopathies of undetermined origin
ITIM	immunoreceptor tyrosine-based inhibition motif	MHAQ	Modified Health Assessment Questionnaire
		MHC	major histocompatibility complex
JAK	Janus kinase	MIF	macrophage inhibitory factor
JCA	juvenile chronic arthritis	MIP	macrophage inflammatory protein
JDM	juvenile dermatomyositis	MMP	matrix metalloproteinase
JIA	juvenile idiopathic arthritis	MPA	microscopic polyangiitis
JNK	c-Jun N-terminal kinase	mPGES	microsomal PGE synthase
JRA	juvenile rheumatoid arthritis	MPO	myeloperoxidase
KIR	killer cell immunoglobulin-like receptor	MRA	humanized anti-human inter-leukin-6 mAb
LC	Langerhans cell	MRI	magnetic resonance imaging
LF	lactoferrin	MS	multiple sclerosis
LFA	leukocyte function-associated antigen	MTD	maximally tolerated doses
		MTX	methotrexate
LGL	large granular lymphocyte	NAP-2	neutrophil-activating protein-2
LIF	leukemia inhibitory factor	NCGN	necrotizing crescentic glomeru-lonephritis
L-NIL	*N*-iminoethyl-lysine		

NES	nuclear export signal	POBs	perforations, obstructions and bleeds
NF-κB	nuclear factor κB		
NGF	nerve growth factor	PPAR	peroxisome proliferator-activated receptor
NIH	National Institutes of Health		
NK	natural killer	PPD	purified protein derivative
NK cells	natural killer cells	PPI	proton pump inhibitor
NLS	nuclear localization	PR3	proteinase 3
n-NOS	neuronal nitric oxide synthase	PsA	psoriatic arthritis
NO	nitric oxide	PsARC	Psoriatic Arthritis Response Criteria
NOD	non-obese diabetic		
NOS	nitric oxide synthase	PTH	parathyroid hormone
NSAIDs	non-steroidal anti-inflammatory drugs	PTHrP	parathyroid hormone related peptide
OASF	osteoarthritic synovial fibroblast	PUBs	perforations, symptomatic ulcers and ulcer-related bleeds
OB	osteoblast		
OC	osteoclast	PUVA	psoralen plus ultraviolet A
ODAR	osteoclast differentiation/ activation receptor	RA	rheumatoid arthritis
		RANK	receptor activator of nuclear factor kappaB
ODF	osteoclast differentiation factor		
ODN	antisense oligonucleotide	RANKL	receptor activator of nuclear factor kappaB ligand
OMERACT	Outcome Measures in Rheumatology Clinical Trials		
		RANTES	regulated upon activation, normal T cell expressed and secreted
OPG	osteoprotegerin		
OPGL	osteoprotegerin ligand	RAPOLO	Rheumatoid Arthritis Prospective Observational Longitudinal Outcomes Study
OSM	oncostatin M		
PAMP	pathogen-associated molecular pattern		
		RASF	rheumatoid arthritis synovial fibroblast
PAN	polyarteritis nodosa		
PASI	Psoriasis Area and Severity Index	RCT	randomized controlled trial
PB	peripheral blood	ReA	reactive arthritis
PBL	peripheral blood lymphocytes	RHD	Rel homology domain
PBMC	peripheral blood mononuclear cells	RIFLE	Responder Index for Lupus Erythematosus
PDGF	platelet-derived growth factor	RNI	reactive nitrogen intermediate
PEA	*Pseudomonas aeruginosa* exotoxin A	RNP	ribonucleoprotein
PG	prostaglandin	SAA	serum amyloid A
Pg	proteoglycan	SAE	serious adverse event
PGA	Physician's Global Assessment	SAP	serum amyloid P protein
PGES	prostaglandin E synthase	SAPK	stress-activated protein kinase
PgH	prostaglandin H	SCF	stem cell factor
PHA	phytohemagglutinin	SCID	severe combined immunodeficiency
PIAS	protein inhibitors of activated STATs		
		SCORE	standarized calculator for risk events
PKA	protein kinase A		
PM	polymyositis	sCR1	soluble complement receptor type 1
PMA	phorbol myristate acetate		
PMN	polymorphonuclear leucocyte, neutrophil granulocyte	SCW	streptococcal cell wall
		SDF-1	stromal-derived factor-1

SEER	Surveillance Epidemiology and End Results	TCR	T-cell antigen receptor, T-cell receptors
SF	synovial fluid	TES	*Toxocara canis* excretory/secretory
SF-36	Medical Outcomes Survey Short Form-36	TGF	transforming growth factor
sIL-6Ra	soluble interleukin-6 receptor	Th	T-helper
SLAM	systemic lupus activity measure	TIMPs	tissue inhibitors of metalloproteinases
SLE	systemic lupus erythematosus	TLR	Toll-like receptor
SLEDAI	Systemic Lupus Erythematosus Disease Activity Index	TNBS	trinitrobenzene sulfonate
SLICC	Systemic Lupus International Collaborating Clinics	TNF	tumor necrosis factor
		t-PA	tissue-type plasminogen activator
Sm	Smith	TRAF6	TNF receptor-associated factor 6
SMC	smooth muscle cell	TRAIL	TNF-related apoptosis-inducing ligand
SOCS	suppressor(s) of cytokine signaling	TRANCE	TNF-related activation-induced cytokine (RANKL, OPG ligand)
SP	surfactant protein	TRANCER	TRANCE receptor
SpA	ankylosing spondylitis, spondyloarthropathies or spondylarthritides	TRAP	tartrate-resistant acid phosphatase
		TX	thromboxane
		TYK	tyrosine kinase
SRP	signal recognition particle	UMP	uridine monophosphate
SS	Sjogren's syndrome	uSpA	undifferentiated spondyloarthropathies
SSP	short signaling peptide	VAS	visual analog scale
STAT	signal transducer and activator of transcription	VCAM	vascular cell adhesion molecule
		VEGF	vascular endothelial growth factor
sTNFR	soluble tumor necrosis factor receptor	VIGOR	VIOXX GI outcome research
SUMO	small ubiquitin-like modifier	VIP	vasointestinal peptide
TA	Takayasu's arteritis	VLA-4	very late antigen-4
TACE	tumor necrosis factor alpha converting enzyme	VNTR	variable numbers of 86-bp tandem repeats
TACI	transmembrane activator and calcium modulator and cyclophilin ligand interactor	VPF	vascular permeability factor
		WG	Wegener's granulomatosis
		WGET	WG Etanercept Trial
		XCL1	lymphoactin
TB	tuberculosis	X-SCID	X chromosome-linked SCID

Section I

Cells and cell surface receptors

1

T cells

Hendrik Schulze-Koops and Joachim R Kalden

INTRODUCTION

Sustained specific immunity against self-antigens is the pathogenetic basis of many rheumatic diseases. As a consequence of persistent autoimmune responses, local inflammation and cellular infiltration occur and, subsequently, tissue damage results. Whereas the specific autoantigen(s) eliciting the detrimental immune reactions have rarely been defined, it has become clear that the mechanisms resulting in the destruction of tissue and the loss of organ function during the course of an autoimmune disease are essentially the same as in protective immunity against invasive microorganisms. Of fundamental importance in initiating, controlling and driving these specific immune responses are CD4+ T cells. CD4+ T cells are activated by an antigen, i.e. peptide, recognized specifically by their T-cell receptor if presented in the context of a specific MHC class II molecule on the surface of an antigen-presenting cell. Once activated, CD4+ T cells become the central regulators of specific immune responses and determine to a large extent the outcome of immune reactions by activating different effector functions of the immune system. It is no surprise, therefore, that activated CD4+ T cells can be found in inflammatory infiltrates in many human rheumatic diseases, and it is generally agreed that CD4+ T cells play a pivotal role in initiating and maintaining autoimmunity. The induction of tissue-damaging autoimmunity in animal models of autoimmune diseases by transfer of CD4+ T cells from sick animals into healthy syngeneic recipients can be regarded as further evidence of the importance of CD4+ T cells in autoimmunity.

T-CELL-DIRECTED THERAPY BY DEPLETION

Based on the concept that activated T cells are the key mediators of chronic autoimmune inflammation, T-cell-directed therapeutic interventions, such as total lymphoid irradiation[1] or thoracic duct drainage,[2] have been introduced for the treatment of rheumatic diseases in an attempt to control disease progression by means of reducing the number or the activation of T cells (Table 1.1). These approaches, however, have provided only modest and inconsistent clinical benefit and have been associated with a number of side-effects.

Table 1.1 T-cell-targeted approaches in rheumatic diseases.

Reduction of T-cell number and/or function
  Total lymphoid irradiation
  Thoracic duct drainage
Immunosuppressive drugs
  Glucocorticoids
  Methotrexate
  Leflunomide
  Cyclosporine
  FK506 (tacrolimus)
  Rapamycine (sirolimus)
Biologicals
  TCR vaccination
  mAbs to T-cell surface receptors
  mAbs to surface receptors on cells interacting
  with T cells
  Cytokines

mAb, monoclonal antibody.

T-CELL-DIRECTED THERAPY WITH IMMUNOSUPPRESSIVE DRUGS

Significant advances in the understanding of T-cell biology in recent years have led to the development of novel compounds designed to specifically interfere with T-cell activation. Cyclosporin A and FK506 (tacrolimus), for example, inhibit T-cell activation by interfering with calcineurin-mediated transcriptional activation of a number of cytokine genes, such as interleukin (IL)-2, IL-3, IL-4, IL-8 and interferon (IFN)-γ. Leflunomide, which has recently been approved for the treatment of rheumatoid arthritis (RA), is a potent non-cytotoxic inhibitor of the enzyme dihydroorotate dehydrogenase (DHODH), a key enzyme in the de novo synthesis of uridine monophosphate (UMP).[3] In contrast to resting cells, activated T lymphocytes depend on pyrimidine de novo synthesis to fulfill their metabolic needs for clonal expansion and terminal differentiation into effector cells. Thus, by limiting de novo pyrimidine biosynthesis, leflunomide inhibits the activation and proliferation of T cells that are important in the inflammation and degradation of synovial tissues.

Whereas cyclosporin, FK506 and leflunomide exert their anti-inflammatory activity by inhibiting T-cell activation, the precise mechanisms of action of other disease-modifying anti-rheumatic drugs (DMARDs) are not completely understood. Interestingly, several recent studies have indicated that DMARDs might be effective in rheumatic diseases at least in part because of their immunomodulatory effects on T-cell subsets. Evidence has emerged that RA may reflect ongoing inflammation largely mediated by activated proinflammatory T-helper (Th)-1 cells without the sufficient differentiation of immuno-regulatory Th2 cells to downmodulate inflammation.[4–7] Importantly, Th1 and Th2 cells antagonize each other by blocking the generation of the antipodic cell type and by blocking each other's effector functions. Thus, a shift in the balance of Th1/Th2 effector cells toward anti-inflammatory Th2 cells can be expected to induce clinical benefit. The concept of modulating the Th1/Th2 balance as a treatment for chronic autoimmunity has been successfully applied in a number of animal models of autoimmune disease.[8,9] It is therefore of great interest to note that DMARDs appear to be able to modulate the Th1/Th2 balance. For example, leflunomide selectively decreases the activation of proinflammatory Th1 cells while promoting Th2 cell differentiation from naive precursors.[10] Sulfasalazine potently inhibits the production of IL-12 in a dose-dependent manner in mouse macrophages stimulated with lipopolysaccharide. Importantly, pretreatment of macrophages with sulfasalazine either in vitro or in vivo reduces their ability to induce the Th1 cytokine IFN-γ and increases their ability to induce the Th2 cytokine IL-4 in antigen-primed CD4+ T cells.[11] Methotrexate (MTX) significantly decreases the production of IFN-γ and IL-2 in in vitro stimulated PBMC while increasing the concentration of IL-4 and IL-10.[12] Likewise, the clinical efficacy of cyclosporin is associated with decreased serum levels of IFN-γ, IL-2 and IL-12 and with significant increases in IL-10.[13]

Bucillamine decreases the frequency of IFN-γ-producing CD4[+] T cells among generated CD4[+] T cells after priming culture of peripheral blood mononuclear cells (PBMC).[14] Recent reports have suggested that glucocorticoids inhibit cytokine expression indirectly through promotion of a Th2 cytokine secretion profile, presumably through their action on monocyte activation.[15] Together, the data suggest that a number of current treatment modalities in RA exert their anti-inflammatory effects by inhibiting Th1 cell activation and/or differentiation and by favoring Th2 differentiation, thereby shifting the Th1/Th2 balance toward the Th2 direction.

T-CELL-DIRECTED THERAPY WITH CYTOKINES

Few studies have been performed with the goal of ameliorating human autoimmune diseases by directly modulating the Th1/Th2 balance. Intravenous application of IL-4 was not associated with clinical benefit, however, at the doses required to attain trough levels that were thought to be sufficient to induce Th2 differentiation in the lymph nodes, IL-4 was associated with significant side-effects. IL-10 was inefficient in RA, which is probably related to the fact that IL-10 in humans is not a Th2 cytokine and does not have prominent Th2-inducing effects. Gene therapy has only been performed in selected RA patients, and no controlled attempts have been made to modify T-cell functions in humans. Thus, although extremely successful in animals, T-cell-directed therapy by means of modulating T-cell effector functions with exogenous cytokines has not resulted in consistent clinical benefit in humans.

T-CELL-DIRECTED THERAPIES WITH BIOLOGICALS

Notwithstanding the immense progress that has been made in recent years in the treatment of rheumatic diseases, current therapy with immunosuppressive drugs is still associated with a number of side-effects related to general immunosuppression. Therefore, it cannot be considered optimal therapy. An ideal form of therapy would be one that specifically targeted only those cells perpetuating the chronic inflammation and had minimal effects on other aspects of the immune or inflammatory systems. The substantial progress in our understanding of molecular and cellular biology has allowed us to specifically design therapeutic tools ('biologicals') with defined targets and effector functions. Based on the increased knowledge of pathogenetic mechanisms of rheumatic diseases, biologicals have been developed that are intended to selectively target only those cells mediating the disease process, with few or no side-effects, while maintaining the integrity of the remainder of the immune system. As CD4[+] T cells are central in initiating and perpetuating the chronic autoimmune response in rheumatic diseases, a huge number of biologicals have been designed with the aim of interfering with T-cell activation and/or migration.

Biologicals, such as monoclonal antibodies (mAbs), have greatly contributed to the substantial increase in our knowledge of pathogenetic mechanisms of RA. Moreover, some biologicals have been extremely successful in treating the symptoms of chronic inflammation. However, although the concept of T-cell-directed immunotherapy with biologicals is evidence based and intriguing and has been successfully employed in animal models of autoimmune diseases, T-cell-directed biologicals have generally failed to induce sustained clinical improvement in patients with RA.[16,17] A number of reasons, such as the selection of the targeted molecules, the design of the biologicals, and the selection of patients at advanced stages of their disease, might have contributed to the unfavorable results of some T-cell-directed therapies with biologicals in humans. A further problem in targeting specifically the disease-promoting T cells in human autoimmune rheumatic diseases is the fact that neither the eliciting (auto)antigens nor the specific disease-initiating or perpetuating T cells are known. Therefore, the most rational approach to the treatment of human autoimmune diseases is to interfere with the activation of CD4[+] T cells in a rather non-antigen-specific manner. Nevertheless, despite those difficulties, the studies have clearly established a potential utility of interfering with the activation of CD4[+] T cells as a treatment of human

Table 1.2 Target structures for biological therapy in rheumatic diseases.

Target molecule	Biochemistry	Main cellular distribution	Ligand	Biological	Possible modes of action
CD2	m gp45–58	T cells NK cells	CD58	sCD58–IgG1 fusion protein[a]	Prevention of T-cell costimulation
CD4	m gp55	T-helper cells Monocytes Macrophages	MHC class II	mAb (mu, mu/hu, hu)	Inhibition of CD4/MHC class II interaction Negative signal for CD4 T cells Killing of CD4 T cells Switch from Th1 to Th2 immune response
CD5	m gp67	T cells Memory B-cell subsets	Unknown	mAb–ricin-A conjugate (mu)	Depletion of CD5 lymphocytes
CD7	m gp40	T cells NK cells	Unknown	mAb (mu, mu/hu)	Depletion of CD7 lymphocytes
CD25	m gp55	Activated T cells B cells Monocytes	IL-2	mAb (mu) IL-2–diphtheria toxin conjugate[b]	Depletion of activated T cells Prevention of T-cell activation
CD52	m gp21–28	Lymphocytes Monocytes	Unknown	mAb (mu, hu)	Depletion of lymphocytes

Target molecule	Biochemistry	Main cellular distribution	Ligand	Biological	Possible modes of action
CD54	m gp85–110	Activated endothelial cells Leukocytes	CD11a/CD18 CD11b/CD18 CD11c/CD18	mAb (mu)	Inhibition of T-cell migration Inhibition of T-cell costimulation
CD80	m gp80	Activated B cells Activated T cells Activated monocytes Activated dendritic cells	CD28 CD152 (CTLA-4)	CTLA-4-Ig[c]	Inhibition of T-cell costimulation
CD86	m gp70	Activated B cells Activated T cells Activated monocytes Activated dendritic cells	CD28 CD152 (CTLA-4)	CTLA-4-Ig[d]	Inhibition of T-cell costimulation

[a]Used for plaque psoriasis and psoriatic arthritis.
[b]mAbs to CD25 in clinical trials for organ transplantation and severe psoriasis.
[c]mAbs to CD80 in clinical trials for solid organ transplantation, graft-versus-host diseases and mild-to-severe plaque psoriasis.
[d]mAbs to CD86 in clinical trials for solid organ transplantation and graft-versus-host diseases.
m, monomer; gp, glycoprotein; mu, murine; hu, human.

autoimmune rheumatic diseases under appropriate critical application using suitably designed mAbs.

Different approaches have been pursued to prevent the continuous activation of T cells by their specific autoantigens in rheumatic diseases (Table 1.2). T-cell-directed therapies can be performed with biologicals that directly target T-cell surface receptors or disrupt the cell–cell interactions that are important for the recruitment of T cells to sites of inflammation and/or for T-cell costimulation. Excellent reviews have been published on the treatment of experimental autoimmune diseases in animals with biologicals, and the results from those studies will not be the focus of this chapter. In humans, direct comparison of the individual studies is difficult because of differences in study design, different definitions of a clinical response, and the use of different biologicals that are directed against distinct epitopes of the targeted molecule and are associated with diverse effector functions. Nevertheless, some common principles have arisen that will be presented.

Apart from the treatment principles described in more detail in this chapter, other innovative therapeutic strategies have been defined, some of which have already entered clinical trials. However, to date, few concise data exist on these interesting approaches with regard to their value as treatment principles in rheumatic diseases. For example, the induction of oral tolerance, which has been successfully used in a number of animal models of autoimmune diseases,[18] was not confirmed in RA. In RA, it appeared that a subgroup of patients might have responded to this type of treatment, as shown in a double-blind, placebo-controlled randomized trial of 90 patients.[19] In this study, an increased clinical response was observed in the type II collagen-treated group compared to placebo-treated patients; however, no significant difference was noted. Further investigations, including placebo-controlled double-blind trials, are necessary to substantiate the reported treatment effects. In a different protocol, the cartilage glycoprotein, gp39, was administered intranasally to patients with active RA who were under concomitant treatment with MTX. At present, the clinical data are still blinded, but it appears from the preliminary data that no clinical response was achieved. Further studies are required for a precise evaluation of the feasibility and the role of T-cell-directed therapy by induction of oral tolerance in rheumatic diseases.

An interesting approach has involved a vaccination strategy, using peptides from the variable region from T-cell receptors that are overexpressed in autoimmune inflammation and that were therefore implicated in the perpetuation of inflammation. It was reasoned that if it were possible to induce immunomodulatory Th2 cells specific for portions of the T-cell receptor of clonally expanded pathogenic Th1 cells, those regulatory Th2 cells, once they were specifically activated, might inhibit inflammatory Th1 cells through a non-specific bystander mechanism. The preliminary data from more than 800 patients with autoimmune diseases suggest that TCR peptide vaccination is safe and well tolerated, and can produce significant clinical improvement in a subset of patients who respond to immunization.[20,21] Additional clinical trials are planned to confirm and extend these observations.

T-CELL-DIRECTED THERAPIES IN RHEUMATIC DISEASES WITH MABS TO CELL SURFACE RECEPTORS

As the vast majority of treatment trials employing biologicals in rheumatic diseases has been conducted in patients with RA, we will concentrate on the data obtained in RA and only briefly comment on the experiences with biologicals in other autoimmune diseases. RA is a chronic systemic inflammatory disease characterized by persistent intense immunologic activity, local destruction of bone and cartilage, the accumulation of activated leukocytes within the inflamed synovium, and a variety of systemic manifestations.[22–24] Although the present understanding of the pathogenesis of RA is incomplete, there is convincing evidence supporting the conclusion that CD4+ T cells play a central role in initiating and perpetuating the chronic autoimmune response characteristic of rheumatoid inflammation.[25,26] Apart from the observations of a dense infiltration of the rheumatoid synovium with activated CD4[+] memory T cells[26] and the clinical efficacy of T-cell-directed therapeutic interventions,[1,2,27] the most compelling finding implying a central role for CD4[+] T cells in propagating rheumatoid inflammation remains the association of aggressive forms of the disease with particular HLA-DR alleles, such as subtypes of DR4, that contain similar amino acid motifs in the third hypervariable region of the DRβ-chain.[28,29] Although the exact meaning of this association has not been resolved, all interpretations imply that CD4[+] T cells orchestrate the local inflammation and cellular infiltration, following which many subsequent inflammatory events are unleashed. Moreover, recent evidence suggests that the role of T cells in RA seems not to be restricted to the synovium, and their pathogenic role may extend beyond antigen recognition in the joint. Consequently, a vast array of biologicals has been employed in patients with RA in an attempt to prevent the continuous activation of pathogenic CD4[+] T cells.

TARGETING CD2

The CD2 molecule is a monomeric membrane glycoprotein that is expressed in the peripheral circulation predominantly by mature T cells and natural killer (NK) cells.[30] The extracellular region of CD2 is composed of two immunoglobulin (Ig)-like domains, and the α-terminal domain is responsible for binding to its ligand.[31] In humans, CD2 binds to CD58 (leukocyte function-associated antigen-3, LFA-3), another member of the immunoglobulin superfamily. Engagement of CD2 and CD58 causes a costimulatory signal in T cells that amplifies the primary signal generated by interaction between the T-cell receptor and the antigen presented on the MHC. Inhibition of CD2–CD58 interactions therefore reduces T-cell stimulation by preventing costimulatory signals.

A soluble fully human recombinant fusion protein comprising the first extracellular domain of CD58 and the hinge, CH2 and CH3 sequences of human IgG1 (LFA-3–IgG$_1$, alefacept) has been engineered and has been shown to block LFA-3–CD2 interactions. Alefacept has been employed in patients with moderate-to-severe plaque psoriasis, with substantial clinical response. Interestingly, alefacept selectively binds to and reduces circulating levels of the memory T-cell population, while spanning the naive T-cell subset.[32] Fourteen of 339 patients who received LFA-3–IgG$_1$ tested positive for anti-alefacept antibodies; however, the overall titers were low and transient in 8 of the 14 patients. Of particular interest for rheumatic diseases, the clinical effect and changes in the synovium were tested in 11 patients with psoriatic arthritis undergoing treatment with alefacept. Patients with chronic plaque psoriasis for ≥ 12 months underwent a 28-day washout phase, after which they received 7.5 mg alefacept weekly via a 30-s intravenous bolus for 12 weeks, followed by 12 weeks of treatment follow-up. No concomitant treatment was allowed, with the exception of non-steroidal anti-inflammatory drugs (NSAIDs). Significant reductions in CD4 T cells, CD8 T cells and activated macrophages in sequential synovial biopsies were noted, as well as an improvement in tender and swollen joint counts.[33] The data suggest that prevention of T-cell activation can be achieved by targeting CD2–CD58 interactions and, moreover, that reduced T-cell activity results in reduced synovial cellularity in psoriatic arthritis with concomitant clinical improvement. Thus, T-cell-directed therapy by means of LFA-3–IgG$_1$ is feasible and clinically successful in autoimmune joint inflammation.

TARGETING CD4

The CD4 molecule is a single-chain 55-kDa plasma membrane glycoprotein.[34,35] It is a member of the immunoglobulin superfamily and is the characteristic surface receptor of all helper T cells.[36] In humans, monocytes/macrophages, dendritic cells, eosinophils and reticuloendothelial cells may also express CD4, although at a much lower density compared to T-helper cells.[36,37] The CD4 molecule comprises four extra-cellular immunoglobulin-like domains, a transmembrane portion, and a cytoplasmic tail that is highly conserved across mammalian species.[35,38] The natural ligands for CD4 are MHC class II molecules on antigen-presenting cells, where CD4 binds to a non-polymorphic region through areas on its first two extracellular domains.[38,39] The physiologic function of CD4 on non-T cells is unknown. On T cells, CD4 provides a site of anchorage between the antigen-presenting cell and the T-cell during antigen presentation and T-cell activation and stabilizes the MHC class II–antigen–T-cell receptor interaction by binding to the same MHC class II molecule engaged by the T-cell receptor.[36,38,39] Moreover, the intracellular part of the CD4 molecule is associated with the cytoplasmic protein tyrosine kinase $p56^{lck}$.[38,40–42] During antigen recognition, CD4 and the T-cell receptor–CD3 complex, which is associated with the protein tyrosine kinase $p59^{fyn}$, come into close proximity, and, as a result, their intracellular domains and their associated protein tyrosine kinases can act synergistically in generating activation signals.[38,42,43] In particular, $p56^{lck}$ and $p59^{fyn}$ phosphorylate tyrosine residues on the ϵ- and the ζ-chain of the CD3 complex, and this in turn results in binding and activation of the tyrosine kinase, ZAP-70, a key mediator of T-cell activation signals.[38,42] Consequently, co-aggregation of the T-cell receptor and CD4 dramatically decreases the threshold for MHC class II–T-cell receptor interactions to result in antigen-specific T-cell activation. In vitro, mAbs to CD4 have been shown to interfere with antigen recognition by T-helper cells,[36,44] to block physiologic stimulation of resting T cells,[44] and to inhibit the mixed lymphocyte reaction.[45,46]

In a variety of experimental autoimmune diseases in animals, monoclonal antibodies (mAbs) to the CD4 receptor on the T-cell surface have been successfully used to prevent the induction of the disease.[47,48] Of relevance to human disease, mAbs to CD4 were also able to inhibit further progression when given after the initial inflammation has already become manifest.[48–52] Moreover, antigen-specific unresponsiveness (tolerance) to soluble antigens or tissue allografts could be induced by anti-CD4 mAbs in animals.[53,54] As activation of CD4+ T cells in the absence of appropriate costimulation results in anergy of the specific CD4+ T cells,[55–57] it was reasoned that coating CD4 molecules with mAbs might prevent costimulation through the CD4 molecule during T-cell activation and thus might permanently silence those CD4+ T cells that were activated under the 'umbrella' of the anti-CD4 mAb.[58,59] This is of particular interest in autoimmune diseases, where it can be surmised that CD4+ T cells are continuously activated by their specific autoantigen(s) presented by antigen-presenting cells expressing MHC class II molecules. In fact, tolerance could be induced in animal models of human autoimmune diseases,[53,60–62] and the hypothesis was generated that short-term treatment of human autoimmune diseases with mAbs to CD4 might induce long-term or even permanent clinical and immunological remission. Consequently, anti-CD4 mAbs were administered to patients with several different autoimmune diseases.

At least 10 different anti-CD4 mAbs have been investigated in the treatment of RA. Direct comparison of the results is difficult, as study design, and definitions of a clinical response varied greatly. Moreover, the initial trials were of open, uncontrolled design with the primary aim of assessing safety and objective biological effects. Nevertheless, without exception, all open-label studies applying multiple doses of anti-CD4 mAbs reported a direct amelioration of arthritis activity lasting for several months. In most studies, however, this was not accompanied by a consistent improvement in laboratory measures of disease activity such as acute-phase proteins.

One of the most impressive immediate effects seen during the first trials of anti-CD4 mAb administration is the clearance of CD4+ T cells from the circulation. After application of several murine CD4 mAbs, the number of CD4+ T cells reached pretreatment levels within 24 h, but others, such as Max.16H5[63] and, in particular, the chimeric cMT 412,[64] induced a prolonged depletion of CD4+ T cells that lasted for several years in some patients. To date, the mechanisms responsible for the prolonged depletion of circulating CD4+ T cells have not been elucidated. It is of great interest that no correlation between the clinical response and the changes in circulating CD4+ T cells was found. On the other hand, despite the low number of circulating T-helper cells induced during several studies, no overt clinical signs of immunosuppression have been observed.[64] Thus, it appears that depletion of CD4+ T cells does not result in any form of suppression of T-cell-mediated immune responses.

Several placebo-controlled double-blind trials with chimerized depleting mAbs to CD4 have shown no clinical efficacy despite significant peripheral CD4+ T-cell depletion[65,66] and a marked but transient reduction in synovial cellular infiltration.[67] This observation is consistent with results from animal models of autoimmune diseases indicating that depletion of CD4+ T cells is not the mechanism underlying the efficacy of anti-CD4 mAb therapy.[68,69] In this regard, there are numerous reports documenting the immunosuppressive actions of non-depleting mAbs to CD4 in animals.[69–72] Moreover, non-depleting mAbs to CD4, which modulate and/or block T-cell functions, were found to be more effective than depleting mAbs in inducing tolerance in different experimental situations in the mouse, such as transfer of β-cells into NOD mice[61] or allogeneic skin grafting.[72] Finally, sustained suppression of autoimmunity in NZB/NZW F1 mice was shown to depend on continuous inhibition, but not depletion, of CD4+ T cells.[49,68] Taken together, these observations are all consistent with the hypothesis that successful treatment of RA in humans with mAbs to CD4 by means of inducing tolerance to putative autoantigens might require long-term inhibition of peripheral T-cell functions by non-depleting mAbs to CD4 rather than depletion of CD4+ T cells. In this regard, it is interesting to note that several studies reported that the percentage of peripheral blood and synovial fluid lymphocytes coated with anti-CD4 mAbs correlated with the clinical response seen in patients.[66,73]

A possible explanation for the lack of clinical efficacy of the depleting mAb cMT 412 derives from studies with this mAb in patients with multiple sclerosis. Treatment with the anti-CD4 mAb cMT 412 in these patients resulted in a long-lasting depletion of CD4+ T cells but did not affect CD8+ T-cell numbers.[74] Analysis of CD4+ T-cell subpopulations showed that unprimed CD45RA cells were approximately three times more sensitive to the mAb than primed CD45RO cells. Remarkably, while a decrease in the number of IL-4-producing Th2 cells in the anti-CD4-treated group was observed, the number of IFN-γ-producing Th1 cells remained stable, resulting in a significant increase in the Th1/Th2 ratio. As outlined above, it is speculated that a chronic Th1-cell-mediated immune response might drive rheumatoid inflammation. Therefore, the data provide evidence that treatment with depleting mAbs to CD4 does not eliminate the cells most strongly involved in the disease process, i.e. primed, IFN-γ-producing Th1-type cells.[74]

Most recently, different mAbs to CD4 were tested as therapy for RA that were genetically engineered by engrafting the complementary determining regions of the parental mAb to CD4 onto a human immunoglobulin to reduce their immunogenicity. In a double-blind, placebo-controlled multicenter study with a humanized anti-CD4 mAb, hIgG1–CD4, patients received either 300 mg of the mAb daily for 5 days or placebo.[75] In a dose-escalating manner, three cohorts of 16 patients each were treated for one, two or three cycles of mAb/placebo treatment in 4-weekly intervals. There were frequent adverse effects during the administration of hIgG1–CD4, such as pruritic rashes (62%), nausea and vomiting (62%), temperature-regulation disturbances (53%) or headache (44%). Although the clinical efficacy, as measured by patient global assessment, physician global assessment, joint swelling and a modified health assessment questionnaire, following mAb treatment was significant, it was of limited magnitude and duration. Of importance was the fact that a significant and protracted depletion of peripheral blood CD4+ T cells was associated with repeated administrations of the anti-CD4 mAb. Because of the unexpected and unacceptable degree of lymphopenia and the limiting effects of the cutaneous rash, which included one case of biopsy-confirmed cutaneous vasculitis, treatment with hIgG1–CD4 was halted.

A different mAb to CD4, OKTcdr4a, was derived from the murine mAb to CD4, OKT4a, by engrafting its CDR regions onto a human IgG$_4$/κ immunoglobulin.[76] The humanized mAb retained the immunosuppressive activities of the murine parental mAb, and both mAbs were equally effective in blocking mixed lymphocyte reactions in vitro or prolonging renal allograft survival in cynomolgus monkeys.[76,77] A multi-center, placebo-controlled, randomized, double-blind study was initiated in patients with RA refractory to standard therapy with DMARD.[78] The patients were randomized into one of two treatment groups receiving placebo or ≥ 450 mg OKTcdr4a per week for two treatment cycles with a 6-week interval. For the third cycle, patients who had received anti-CD4 mAb during the first two courses were given placebo, whereas the patients who were originally given placebo received the anti-CD4 mAb. Based on dose-finding studies, the concentration of the mAb administered could be expected to result in saturation of all peripheral CD4$^+$ T cells for up to 2 weeks.

Clinical response as assessed by modified Paulus criteria[79] was achieved after the first treatment week in 67% of the patients who received the anti-CD4 mAb, compared to 25% of the placebo-treated group. Six weeks after treatment, the clinical effect had waned; however, 1 week after the second treatment cycle, all patients who had received the mAb had a clinical response, compared to 25% of the patients from the placebo group. Again, the clinical effect was transient. After crossover, 75% of the patients from the initial placebo group responded to anti-CD4 mAb at the third treatment cycle, compared to 17% from the initial treatment group who were given placebo. There was a significant decrease in C-reactive protein (CRP) levels in all patients 1 week after mAb administration. By contrast, no significant changes were observed after placebo. Remarkably, the administration of OKTcdr4a was not associated with a drop in the numbers of total white blood cells, lymphocytes, neutrophils, monocytes, or CD4$^+$ T cells (Figure 1.1). In fact, the numbers of CD4$^+$ T cells increased during the first treatment week in the anti-CD4 mAb-treated patient group and the placebo group. Similarly, the numbers of CD8$^+$ T cells and, consequently, the CD4/CD8 ratio were not affected by OKTcdr4a.[78]

To evaluate the impact of OKTcdr4a on T-cell functions, cytokine production by mitogen-stimulated peripheral blood T cells was monitored

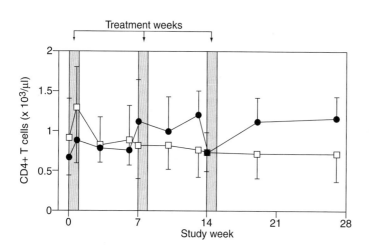

Figure 1.1 CD4$^+$ T-cell counts in the peripheral circulation of RA patients receiving the anti-CD4 mAb OKTcdr4a. Treatment weeks were weeks 0, 7 and 14. Data represent mean ± SD of patients receiving ≥ 450 mg OKTcdr4a (open squares, n = 6; week 3, n = 5; weeks 19 and 27, n = 4) or placebo (filled circles, n = 4; week 19, n = 2; week 27, n = 3) at weeks 0 and 7. At week 14, patients who had received OKTcdr4a during the first two treatment cycles received placebo, and patients who were on placebo during weeks 0 and 7 received the active anti-CD4 mAb. (Reproduced with permission from Schulze-Koops H et al. *J Rheum* 1998; **25**: 2065–76.[78])

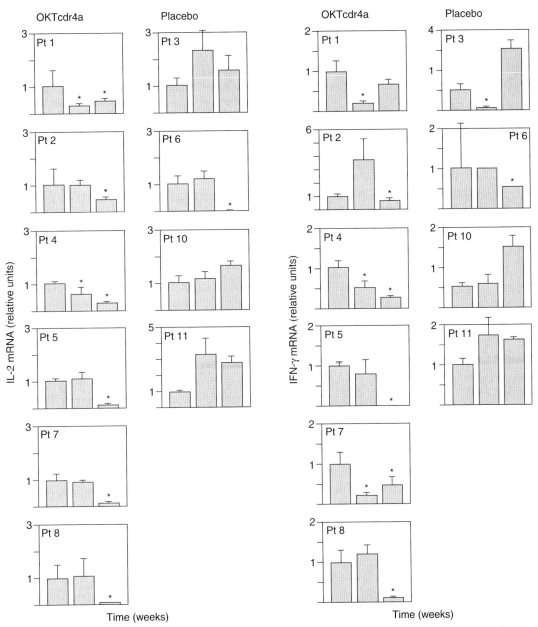

Figure 1.2   IL-2 and IFN-γ mRNA levels in PBMC of RA patients treated with anti-CD4 mAb OKTcdr4a after mitogen-induced activation in vitro. PBMC were isolated from the patients immediately before the first, second and third treatment cycles (weeks 0, 7 and 14, respectively). mRNA was extracted from the cells after overnight stimulation with 10 μg/ml soluble mAb to CD3 (OKT3). Cytokine mRNA levels were assessed by semiquantitative PCR. The amount of target DNA was calculated using positive controls and corrected for glyceraldehyde-3-phosphatedehydrogenase (G3PDH). For each individual patient, cytokine mRNA levels at different time points were normalized for a given individual's pretreatment mRNA level, which was defined as one relative unit. Bars represent the mean ± SEM of triplicate determinations. Pt, patient; *a significant decrease in cytokine mRNA level from week 0. (Reproduced with permission from Schulze-Koops H et al. *J Rheum* 1998; **25**: 2065–76.[78])

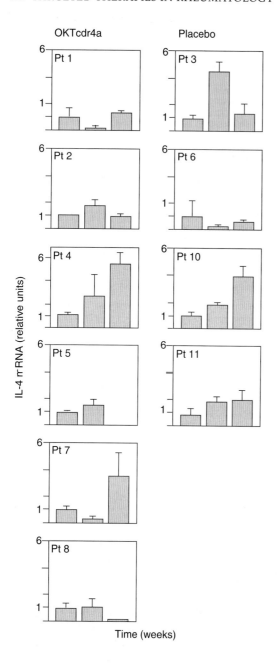

OKTcdr4a   Placebo

IL-4 mRNA (relative units)

Time (weeks)

Figure 1.3 IL-4 mRNA levels in PBMC of RA patients treated with anti-CD4 mAb OKTcdr4a after mitogen-induced activation in vitro. PBMC were isolated from the patients immediately before the first, second and third treatment cycles (weeks 0, 7 and 14, respectively). Cytokine mRNA levels at different time points were determined as described in the legend to Figure 1.2. Any given individual's pretreatment mRNA level was defined as one relative unit. Bars represent the mean ± SEM of triplicate determinations. Pt, patient; *a significant decrease in cytokine mRNA level from week 0. (Reproduced with permission from Schulze-Koops H et al. *J Rheum* 1998; **25**: 2065–76.[78])

to anti-CD3 mAb stimulation in vitro and a significant reduction in anti-CD3-induced IFN-γ production as determined by ELISA.[78] The reduced capacity of the anti-CD4 mAb-treated patients' peripheral blood T cells to secrete IL-2 and IFN-γ in response to anti-CD3 mAb stimulation was confirmed by decreased mRNA levels as determined by semiquantitative PCR (Figure 1.2). By contrast, IL-4 mRNA levels were inconsistently altered by anti-CD4 mAb treatment (Figure 1.3) and no difference was seen between the anti-CD4 mAb- and the placebo-treated groups. These data suggest that clinical improvement in patients with RA treated with a non-depleting mAb to CD4 may be related to a decrease in the function of IL-2- and IFN-γ-producing Th1 cells.

In summary, following the disappointing results of controlled studies with the chimeric mAb cMT 412 in RA, favorable results with high dosages of a non-depleting CD4 mAb were recently presented. It is not yet clear which characteristics of the mAbs are important to achieve this clinical effect. Variations of the antigen-binding characteristics, the constant regions of the immunoglobulin, as well as variations in the dose and timing of CD4 mAb, may be essential to obtain clinical efficacy. Future studies with non-depleting mAbs to CD4 are necessary to delineate precisely the dosing requirements for clinical benefit and to elucidate the mode of actions of anti-CD4 mAbs. Whereas depletion of CD4+ T cells cannot explain clinical efficacy, exciting new data have emerged that are indicative of a modulation of the detrimental

during treatment and follow-up, and cytokine mRNA levels were assessed in stimulated PBMC by semiquantitative polymerase chain reaction (PCR).[78] Administration of OKTcdr4a was associated with a substantially decreased potential of peripheral blood T cells to secrete IL-2 in response

Th1-dominated immune response.[78] However, these results require further confirmation.

TARGETING CD5

CD5 is present on more than 90% of human mature T cells and in up to 10% of circulating B cells, which represent a subset of activated memory-type B cells potentially important for the production of autoantibodies.[80] The rationale for targeting CD5 was, therefore, to deplete T cells and simultaneously memory B cells potentially involved in autoimmunity by using a mAb to CD5 coupled to an immunotoxin, the A-chain of ricin, which inhibits ribosomes and thereby kills cells.[81] In pilot trials with the anti-CD5 immunoconjugate CD5–IC, administration of the anti-CD5 mAb led to depletion of CD5+ T cells which was accompanied by a clinical improvement in nearly half of the patients.[82] The initial trial showing both clinical efficacy and only minor toxicity, led to a phase II trial.[83] Fifty-five per cent of the patients improved during the first week of treatment; however, there was a rapid decline thereafter, dropping to 15% after 12 months. Of note, approximately one-third of the patients showed a 50% reduction in erythrocyte sedimentation rate (ESR), CRP and rheumatoid factor levels. The clinical benefit was associated with a marked lymphopenia and a median depletion of CD4+ T cells to 21% of the initial value between days 2 and 5 of the infusion period. Subsequently, a multicenter double-blind placebo-controlled trial was performed.[84] In this trial, there was no marked prolonged T-cell depletion; however, treatment was not more effective than placebo. Of special interest, in this study a very high placebo response was noted in 48% of the patients. The conclusion was drawn from this study that the dose chosen was ineffective. Similar to the data presented for anti-CD4 mAbs, there was no correlation between T-cell depletion and clinical response. In summary, despite the intriguing approach of combining an anti-T-cell reagent with a toxin that addresses not only T lymphocytes but also a subset of B cells, the trials with CD5–IC have been disappointing. The initial hypothesis that a maximum depletion of T cells would result in an induction of tolerance was not supported by the subsequent clinical data, which demonstrated that there was no correlation between depletion and clinical success and that no sustained benefits could be achieved even in those patients reaching maximum T-cell depletion.

TARGETING CD7

The CD7 molecule is a monomeric transmembrane glycoprotein that is expressed on a major subset of peripheral blood T and NK cells. Its function is unknown, but it was chosen as a target for T-cell-directed therapy for its characteristic expression on the T-cell lineage. A rather limited number of patients were treated in open-label trials with a murine anti-CD7 mAb or the chimeric version of the reagent. Despite a decrease in T-cell numbers, only 2/6 patients responded to the murine mAb for a limited time. The chimeric mAb was associated with a somewhat higher efficacy; however, there were frequent adverse effects, such as fever, nausea and malaise.[85,86] No further developments of the anti-CD7 mAb for future trials in RA have been reported.

TARGETING CD25

Three patients were treated with a murine mAb to CD25, the α-chain of the IL-2 receptor. Despite excellent clinical responses[87] for extended periods of time, no further studies have been reported with anti-CD25 mAbs. Recently, two genetically engineered anti-CD25 mAbs have been tested, with good clinical response, in the prevention of acute rejection in renal transplant recipients with delayed graft function and in severe psoriasis.[88] Clinical data from treatment trials in rheumatic disease are, however, not available.

A different approach to targeting the IL-2 receptor involved coupling recombinant human IL-2 to the toxic region of diphtheria toxin. Thus, activated lymphocytes were effectively killed by these agents at low concentrations.[89] After encouraging results from open-label, uncontrolled dose-escalation studies, subsequent double-blind placebo-controlled studies have been performed. Forty-five RA patients were enrolled in the trial, and were randomized, after a 3–4-week DMARD washout, to receive a daily intravenous dose of either DAB486–IL-2 or placebo (saline) for 5 days. Adverse events included transient fever/chills (45%), nausea/vomiting (50%), elevated transaminases (55%), and increased joint pain (45%). Clinical responses were noted in 18% of the patients treated with DAB486–IL-2 compared with none of the placebo controls.[90] It appears that a clinical response occurred in a minority of patients, and striking clinical benefits were rarely noted. The results published so far are not encouraging, at least in patients with long-standing and treatment-refractory disease.

TARGETING CD28

CD28 is a 44-kDa glycoprotein that was originally identified as a molecule providing non-antigen-driven costimulatory signals to complement T-cell receptor-derived signals during T-cell responses for optimal T-cell activation. CD28 is the most pivotal and effective costimulatory molecule on T cells. In fact, ligation of the T-cell receptor in the absence of sufficient costimulation via CD28 results in antigen-specific anergy of T cells.[91] CD28 is engaged by binding to one of two ligands, CD80 (B7-1) and CD86 (B7-2). Expression of CD80 and CD86 on antigen-presenting cells is tightly regulated to ensure that the costimulatory signaling initiated via CD28 takes place in a controlled fashion. Preventing the CD28-mediated costimulatory signal has potent immunosuppressive effects; it can be achieved by blocking either CD28 or CD80 and CD86. Currently, humanized anti-B7 mAbs are in phase II clinical trials for solid organ transplantation, graft-versus-host disease and mild-to-severe plaque psoriasis. An alternative approach to block CD28 costimulation is by coating CD80 and CD86 with a soluble Ig fusion protein of the extracellular domain of CD152 (cytotoxic T-lymphocyte antigen 4, CTLA-4). CTLA-4 is a homolog of CD28 and is expressed by activated T cells. It can bind both CD80 and CD86 with higher affinity than CD28. Because CD152 has a high affinity for CD80 and CD86, soluble forms of CTLA-4 inhibit the interaction of CD28 with its ligands.

Forty-three patients with stable psoriasis vulgaris received four infusions of the CTLA-4–Ig. Forty-six per cent of all study patients achieved a 50% or greater sustained improvement in clinical disease activity, and this was associated with quantitative reductions in epidermal hyperplasia.[92] Results from a phase II study in patients with RA showed that CTLA-4–Ig was well tolerated and produced significant clinical benefit. In a subsequent multicenter placebo-controlled trial, CTLA4-Ig and LEA29Y, a second generation molecule, that expresses increased avidity to CD86 due to two amino acid residue exchanges, were administered intravenously in different concentrations (0.5, 2, or 10 mg/kg) to 214 patients with RA who had been treated unsuccessfully with at least one DMARD. Patients received 4 infusions of the study medication (days 1, 15, 29, and 57) and were evaluated on day 85. Both compounds were safe and well-tolerated at all dose levels. Clinical efficacy (ACR20 responses) was related to the treatment dose as indicated by the fact that 23%, 44% and 53% of the CTLA4-Ig treated patients, and 34%, 45% and 61% of the LEA29Y-treated patients met the ACR20 criteria in the 0.5, 2 and 10 mg/kg treatment groups, respectively. It should be noted, however, that the placebo response was 31%, and less than 20% of the patients met the ACR50 criteria at day 85.[93] Whereas the study demonstrated a favorable clinical effect of both compounds, further studies will have to be conducted to establish blockade of costimulation via CD28 as a valuable treatment principle in RA.

It should be kept in mind, however, that it has recently begun to be appreciated that T cells might be activated in vitro and in vivo through conventional 'costimulatory' ligands, such as CD28, in a T-cell receptor-independent, and hence antigen-independent, manner. For example, T-cell proliferation[94–96] and increases of cytokine mRNA levels[94,97] could be induced by

CD28 without the further requirement for T-cell receptor ligation. Moreover, recent findings indicate that CD28 is not only a stimulatory molecule but also plays a central role in regulating T-cell differentiation. Naive and memory T cells are biased toward a Th1 phenotype in the absence of CD28 ligation and will only generate IL-4-producing Th2 effectors if CD28 is engaged.[98,99] Consequently, CD28-knockout mice have preserved Th1-mediated cytotoxic T-lymphocyte and cellular immunity, but impaired Th2-dependent immunoglobulin production.[100] Conversely, it has been demonstrated that the extent of stimulation through CD28 regulates the extent of Th2 effector generation.[99,101] For example, as a result of unopposed signaling through CD28, there is a massive polyclonal expansion of Th2 cells in CTLA-4-knockout mice.[102] Taken together, the data indicate that CD28 is a key regulatory molecule in T-cell differentiation. Moreover, recent data also demonstrate that CD28 may be sufficient to induce Th2-cell differentiation from memory T cells in the absence of T-cell receptor-mediated signals to induce Th2 differentiation.[7,96] Inhibition of CD28-mediated signals by CTLA-4–Ig might therefore not only inhibit activation of proinflammatory Th1 cells but also prevent the differentiation of immunomodulatory Th2 effectors. The consequences of such a blockade in Th1-mediated autoimmune disease, such as RA, need to be carefully documented in future studies.

TARGETING CD52

CD52 is expressed at high levels on all human T and B cells in high density, but is not expressed on other myeloid cell types or CD34+ pluripotent stem cells.[103] Thus, although the function of CD52 is currently unknown, it provides an excellent target for lymphocyte-directed therapies. A humanized antibody to CD52, CAMPATH-1H, has been used in a variety of treatment trials in RA. CAMPATH-1H has a human IgG$_1$ constant region and is efficient at complement- and cell-mediated lysis of human lymphocytes. Intravenous as well as subcuta-

neous application leads to a rapid fall in peripheral blood lymphocytes, affecting predominantly the CD4+ T-cell subset, within a few hours. This suppression of peripheral blood lymphocyte numbers lasts for at least 20 months following a single infusion and for at least 84 months after multiple infusions.[104,105] However, despite the occurrence of profound and long-lasting lymphopenia following treatment with CAMPATH-1H therapy for RA, this therapy is not associated with a large excess of mortality or with an unusual spectrum of infections, at least during a medium-term period of follow-up (283 patient years).[105] In addition to the severe lymphocyte depletion, a significant clinical improvement was noted in initial trials and several phase I studies. It became clear from those trials, however, that increased doses did not increase clinical benefit, but were rather associated with a higher incidence and more severe adverse effects. Moreover, no correlation of peripheral blood lymphocyte counts and clinical effect was noted. In contrast to the profound lymphocytopenia, the CRP fell modestly and the ESR did not change at all. Nevertheless, the relatively good clinical responses to anti-CD52 mAb treatment were bought at the expense of marked side-effects: severe headache, fever, chills, nausea, and vomiting, indicative of a severe cytokine release syndrome were frequently observed and occurred shortly after the infusion. Moreover, the favorable clinical results could not be confirmed in phase II studies, and therefore most investigators believe that CAMPATH-1H, although an interesting agent with a potent biological action, will not be a preferential tool in treating autoimmune disease.

TARGETING CD54

One of the hallmarks of RA is the continuous entry of large numbers of mononuclear cells into the synovial tissue and fluid. Activation of these cells initiates the pathogenic events characteristic of the disease.[24] The processes that control the entry into and accumulation of mononuclear cells in the tissues are, therefore, critical for the perpetuation of the inflammation. Thus, it was reasoned that inhibition of recruitment of mononuclear cells into the tissue may attenuate the inflammatory manifestations of RA. Several lines of evidence suggest that interactions between the endothelial cells of post-capillary venules and mononuclear cells in the circulation, mediated by a variety of adhesion molecules, govern the entry of inflammatory cells into the tissues.[106,107] Interference with these interactions, therefore, might be effective in the therapy of RA.

Given the key role played by T cells in RA,[24,108] one possible target for adhesion receptor-directed therapy in this disease would be the adhesion receptor/counter receptor pair, leukocyte function associated antigen-1 (LFA-1, CD11α/CD18) and intercellular adhesion molecule-1 (ICAM-1, CD54). It has been shown that the interaction of these receptors is critical for transendothelial migration of T cells and their subsequent activation.[109–111] Therefore, a study was designed to test the hypothesis that amelioration of the signs and symptoms of RA could be achieved by blocking migration of T cells into the synovium and their subsequent stimulation by locally expressed antigenic peptides in vivo.[112]

The initial study population consisted of 32 patients with long-standing (> 4 years) RA who met the ACR criteria for the diagnosis.[113] All patients were required to have failed therapy with at least two DMARDs. A second subsequent trial examined patients with earlier disease (median from diagnosis: 3 months) who had not received more than one DMARD previously.[114] The studies were of open-label design. Thus, the primary objectives were to evaluate safety, biological impact and pharmacokinetics, with efficacy as a secondary endpoint.

Administration of the anti-ICAM-1 mAb was immediately followed by a peripheral blood lymphocytosis that persisted throughout therapy. Analysis with fluorescence-activated cell sorting (FACS) indicated that there was a significant increase in the number of circulating CD3+ T cells. Thus, the mAb appeared to block the ability of T lymphocytes to enter inflammatory sites. In

contrast, there were no significant changes in circulating B-cell numbers or either neutrophils or monocytes. Further analysis revealed that the increase in T-cell numbers primarily reflected an increase in CD4+ T cells, with no preferential effect on naive or memory cells. Of note, there was an increase in the numbers of activated, circulating T cells (increased expression of HLA-DR and CD25). The data are consistent with the conclusion that the T-cell lymphocytosis occurred because these cells were blocked from leaving the circulation by the anti-ICAM-1 mAb. It is interesting to note that almost all patients were found to be anergic during mAb therapy to delayed-type hypersensitivity skin testing, whereas, 1 month following therapy, most of the responses had returned. Thus, it seems likely that the administration of anti-ICAM-1 blocked the entry of lymphocytes into inflammatory sites, and presumably into the synovium, and also that it diminished the signs and symptoms of inflammation.[115]

Although the studies were not especially designed to test clinical efficacy, they provided encouraging clinical data. Using modified composite criteria for the evaluation of the clinical response,[79] 57% of the patients who received five daily infusions of the mAb to ICAM-1 had a marked or moderate response to treatment from days 8 to 29 of follow-up which lasted for up to 90 days in some individuals. Moreover, the responses of patients with early disease appeared to be somewhat better than those obtained in the refractory group. Seven of the 10 patients achieved a clinical response up to 29 days of follow-up, and five sustained their response up to day 60. Three had long-term clinical benefit, including one who met the ACR criteria for a complete remission[116] for almost a year after treatment. Of interest, 6/7 patients with clinical benefit also manifested > 30% decreases of ESR and/or CRP.

In summary, the data are consistent with the conclusion that ICAM-1 plays a central role in rheumatoid inflammation and is, therefore, an important target in the treatment of RA. Anti-ICAM-1 effectively inhibited T-cell entry into sites of inflammation and, in particular, altered the circulatory pattern of activated Th1 cells in patients who responded to therapy.[6] However, as the mAb employed was of murine origin, it was of considerable immunogenicity. When patients were retreated with this agent, immune complex-mediated side-effects, including urticaria, angioedema, and serum complement protein consumption, were noted.[117] Therefore, if this type of treatment is to provide any beneficial effect in autoimmune diseases, it has to be substantiated by further double-blind placebo-controlled studies using agents with lower immunogenicity.

CONCLUSION

Based on increasing knowledge of pathogenetic mechanisms of rheumatic diseases and the immense progress in the understanding of cellular and molecular biology, several treatment trials were performed with specifically designed therapeutic tools that interfered with particular pathogenetic mechanisms of human rheumatic disease. In particular, because of the dominant role of CD4+ T cells in the pathogenesis of rheumatic disease, biologicals were designed to interfere with continuous T-cell activation by blocking T-cell stimulation and/or T-cell migration. Although controlled clinical trials with T-cell-directed biologicals have largely failed to confirm the promising results from animal models of autoimmune diseases, the first-generation biologicals were invaluable in testing hypotheses of pathogenicity. It should be kept in mind, when interpreting the clinical efficacy, that the doses of mAbs used in the human studies were much below the equivalent concentrations of the mAbs that had been shown to be the minimum required amount in animal models to achieve clinical efficacy. It should also be emphasized that the patients selected for the initial studies were patients with long-standing diseases, which have been shown in animal models to be less likely to respond to T-cell-directed therapies than early disease. Owing to the exploding advances in the knowledge of molecular biology, however, we will have compounds at hand in the future that will allow specific interference with a given immunopathogenic mechanism. Exciting concepts are being currently tested in animal models or in patients with non-rheumatic immunologic diseases and will soon enter clinical trials for rheumatic diseases. Those biologicals include mAbs to adhesion receptors, such as VLA-4 or LFA-1, mAbs to costimulatory molecules, such as CD154, or mAbs to chemokine receptors, such as CCR5.

Because of the chronic nature of autoimmune diseases, parenteral delivery of biologicals is associated with several problems related to patients' compliance and convenience of application. Moreover, production of macromolecules, in particular recombinant proteins, on a large scale is very expensive. Thus, the next generation of biologicals will be orally bioavailable formulations that can be produced effectively by sources other than eukaryotic hybridomas in sufficient amounts and high quantities. One possible way to meet these goals is to focus on the development of low-molecular-weight compounds that interfere with T-cell activation not by blocking costimulatory receptors but by inhibiting the signal transduction cascade downstream of the receptors. It can be anticipated that some of these novel therapeutic interventions, in particular those directed to autoantigen-specific pathogenic T cells, will soon enter clinical use and will have the power to permanently stop chronic inflammation in rheumatic diseases without imposing intolerable side-effects.

ACKNOWLEDGMENT

The work of H.S.K. is supported in part by the Deutsche Forschungsgemeinschaft (Schu 786/2-3), the Fritz Bender Foundation, the German Ministry for Education and Science (Network for Competence Rheumatology, Project C2-5) and the Interdisciplinary Center for Clinical Research in Erlangen (Project B27).

REFERENCES

1. Strober S, Tanay A, Field E et al. Efficacy of total lymphoid irradiation in intractable rheumatoid arthritis. A double-blind, randomized trial. *Ann Intern Med* 1985; **102**: 441–9.
2. Paulus HE, Machleder HI, Levine S, Yu DT, MacDonald NS. Lymphocyte involvement in rheumatoid arthritis. Studies during thoracic duct drainage. *Arthritis Rheum* 1977; **20**: 1249–62.
3. Bruneau JM, Yea CM, Spinella-Jaegle S et al. Purification of human dihydro-orotate dehydrogenase and its inhibition by A77 1726, the active metabolite of leflunomide. *Biochem J* 1998; **336**: 299–303.
4. Miltenburg AM, van Laar JM, de Kuiper R, Daha MR, Breedveld FC. T cells cloned from human rheumatoid synovial membrane functionally represent the Th1 subset. *Scand J Immunol* 1992; **35**: 603–10.
5. Simon AK, Seipelt E, Sieper J. Divergent T-cell cytokine patterns in inflammatory arthritis. *Proc Natl Acad Sci USA* 1994; **91**: 8562–6.
6. Schulze-Koops H, Lipsky PE, Kavanaugh AF, Davis LS. Elevated Th1- or Th0-like cytokine mRNA in peripheral circulation of patients with rheumatoid arthritis: modulation by treatment with anti-ICAM-1 correlates with clinical benefit. *J Immunol* 1999; **155**: 5029–37.
7. Skapenko A, Wendler J, Lipsky PE, Kalden JR, Schulze-Koops H. Altered memory T-cell differentiation in patients with early rheumatoid arthritis. *J Immunol* 1999; **163**: 491–9.
8. Joosten LA, Lubberts E, Helsen MM et al. Protection against cartilage and bone destruction by systemic interleukin-4 treatment in established murine type II collagen-induced arthritis. *Arthritis Res* 1999; **1**: 81–91.
9. Bessis N, Boissier MC, Ferrara P, Blankenstein T, Fradelizi B, Fournier C. Attenuation of collagen-induced arthritis in mice by treatment with vector cells engineered to secrete interleukin-13. *Eur J Immunol* 1996; **26**: 2399–403.
10. Dimitrova P, Skapenko A, Herrmann M, Schleyerbach R, Kalden JR, Schulze-Koops H. Restriction of de novo pyrimidine biosynthesis inhibits Th1 cell activation and promotes Th2 cell differentiation. *J Immunol* 2002; **169**: 3392–9.
11. Kang BY, Chung SW, Im SY, Choe YK, Kim TS. Sulfasalazine prevents T-helper 1 immune response by suppressing interleukin-12 production in macrophages. *Immunology* 1999; **98**: 98–103.
12. Constantin A, Loubet-Lescoulie P, Lambert N et al. Antiinflammatory and immunoregulatory action of methotrexate in the treatment of rheumatoid arthritis: evidence of increased interleukin-4 and interleukin-10 gene expression demonstrated in vitro by competitive reverse transcriptase–polymerase chain reaction. *Arthritis Rheum* 1998; **41**: 48–57.
13. Kim WU, Cho ML, Kim SI et al. Divergent effect of cyclosporine on Th1/Th2 type cytokines in patients with severe, refractory rheumatoid arthritis. *J Rheumatol* 2000; **27**: 324–31.
14. Morinobu A, Wang Z, Kumagai S. Bucillamine suppresses human Th1 cell development by a hydrogen peroxide-independent mechanism. *J Rheumatol* 2000; **27**: 851–8.
15. Almawi WY, Melemedjian OK, Rieder MJ. An alternate mechanism of glucocorticoid antiproliferative effect: promotion of a Th2 cytokine-secreting profile. *Clin Transplant* 1999; **13**: 365–74.
16. Kalden JR, Breedveld FC, Burkhardt H, Burmester GR. Immunological treatment of autoimmune diseases. *Adv Immunol* 1998; **68**: 333–418.
17. Schulze-Koops H, Lipsky PE. Anti-CD4 monoclonal antibody therapy in human autoimmune diseases. *Curr Dir Autoimmun* 2000; **2**: 24–49.
18. Hafler DA, Weiner HL. Oral tolerance for the treatment of autoimmune diseases. In: Strand V, Scott DL, Simon LS, eds, *Novel Therapeutic Agents for the Treatment of Autoimmune Diseases* (Dekker: New York, 1997) 210–20.
19. Sieper J, Kary S, Sorensen H et al. Oral type II collagen treatment in early rheumatoid arthritis. A double-blind, placebo-controlled, randomized trial. *Arthritis Rheum* 1996; **39**: 41–51.
20. Vandenbark AA, Morgan E, Bartholomew R et al. TCR peptide therapy in human autoimmune diseases. *Neurochem Res* 2001; **26**: 713–30.
21. Moreland LW, Morgan EE, Adamson III TC et al. T-cell receptor peptide vaccination in rheumatoid arthritis: a placebo-controlled trial using a combination of Vbeta3, Vbeta14, and Vbeta17 peptides. *Arthritis Rheum* 1998; **41**: 1919–29.
22. Cush JJ, Lipsky PE. Cellular basis for rheumatoid inflammation. *Clin Orthop* 1991; **265**: 9–22.
23. Cush JJ, Lipsky PE. The immunopathogenesis of rheumatoid arthritis: the role of cytokines in chronic inflammation. *Clin Aspects Autoimmun* 1987; **1**: 2–12.

24. Harris ED. Rheumatoid arthritis: pathophysiology and implications for treatment. *N Engl J Med* 1990; **322**: 1277–89.

25. Cush JJ, Lipsky PE. Phenotypic analysis of synovial tissue and peripheral blood lymphocytes isolated from patients with rheumatoid arthritis. *Arthritis Rheum* 1988; **31**: 1230–8.

26. Van Boxel JA, Paget SA. Predominantly T-cell infiltrate in rheumatoid synovial membranes. *N Engl J Med* 1975; **293**: 517–20.

27. Panayi GS, Tugwell P. The use of cyclosporin A in rheumatoid arthritis: conclusions of an international review. *Br J Rheumatol* 1994; **33**: 967–9.

28. Calin A, Elswood J, Klouda PT. Destructive arthritis, rheumatoid factor, and HLA-DR4. Susceptibility versus severity, a case-control study. *Arthritis Rheum* 1989; **32**: 1221–5.

29. Winchester R. The molecular basis of susceptibility to rheumatoid arthritis. *Adv Immunol* 1994; **56**: 389–466.

30. Moingeon P, Chang HC, Sayre PH et al. The structural biology of CD2. *Immunol Rev* 1989; **111**: 111–44.

31. Richardson NE, Chang HC, Brown NR, Hussey RE, Sayre PH, Reinherz EL. Adhesion domain of human T11 (CD2) is encoded by a single exon. *Proc Natl Acad Sci USA* 1988; **85**: 5176–80.

32. Ellis CN, Krueger GG. Treatment of chronic plaque psoriasis by selective targeting of memory effector T lymphocytes. *N Engl J Med* 2001; **345**: 248–55.

33. Patel S, Veale D, FitzGerald O, McHugh NJ. Psoriatic arthritis – emerging concepts. *Rheumatology* 2001; **40**: 243–6.

34. Reinherz EL, Schlossman SF. The differentiation and function of human T lymphocytes. *Cell* 1980; **19**: 821–7.

35. Maddon PJ, Littman DR, Godfrey M, Maddon DE, Chess L, Axel R. The isolation and nucleotide sequence of a cDNA encoding the T-cell surface protein T4: a new member of the immunoglobulin gene family. *Cell* 1985; **42**: 93–104.

36. Parnes JR. Molecular biology and function of CD4 and CD8. *Adv Immunol* 1989; **44**: 265–311.

37. Scoazec JY, Feldmann G. Both macrophages and endothelial cells of the human hepatic sinusoid express the CD4 molecule, a receptor for the human immunodeficiency virus. *Hepatology* 1990; **12**: 505–10.

38. Littman DR. The CD4 molecule. Roles in T lymphocytes and in HIV disease. Introduction. *Curr Top Microbiol Immunol* 1996; **205**: v–x.

39. Sakihama T, Smolyar A, Reinherz EL. Molecular recognition of antigen involves lattice formation between CD4, MHC class II and TCR molecules. *Immunol Today* 1995; **16**: 581–7.

40. Rudd CE, Trevillyan JM, Dasgupta JD, Wong LL, Schlossman SF. The CD4 receptor is complexed in detergent lysates to a protein-tyrosine kinase (pp58) from human T lymphocytes. *Proc Natl Acad Sci USA* 1988; **85**: 5190–4.

41. Veillette A, Bookman MA, Horak EM, Bolen JB. The CD4 and CD8 T-cell surface antigens are associated with the internal membrane tyrosine-protein kinase p56lck. *Cell* 1988; **55**: 301–8.

42. Zamoyska R. The CD8 coreceptor revisited: one chain good, two chains better. *Immunity* 1994; **1**: 243–6.

43. Owens T, Fazekas de St Groth B, Miller JF. Coaggregation of the T-cell receptor with CD4 and other T-cell surface molecules enhances T-cell activation. *Proc Natl Acad Sci USA* 1987; **84**: 9209–13.

44. Biddison WE, Rao PE, Talle MA, Goldstein G, Shaw S. Possible involvement of the OKT4 molecule in T-cell recognition of class II HLA antigens. Evidence from studies of cytotoxic T lymphocytes specific for SB antigens. *J Exp Med* 1982; **156**: 1065–76.

45. Fournel S, Vincent C, Assossou O et al. CD4 mAbs prevent progression of alloactivated CD4+ T cells into the S phase of the cell cycle without interfering with early activation signals. *Transplantation* 1999; **62**: 1136–43.

46. Sakane T, Takada S. Possible involvement of the CD4 molecule in a late activation event on CD4+ T-cell proliferation in the human autologous mixed lymphocyte reaction. *Clin Exp Immunol* 1989; **75**: 269–74.

47. Ranges GE, Sriram S, Cooper SM. Prevention of type II collagen-induced arthritis by in vivo treatment with anti-L3T4. *J Exp Med* 1985; **162**: 1105–10.

48. Waldor MK, Sriram R, Hardy R et al. Reversal of experimental allergic encephalomyelitis with monoclonal antibody to a T-cell subset marker. *Science* 1985; **227**: 415–17.

49. Wofsy D, Seaman WE. Successful treatment of autoimmunity in NZB/NZW F1 mice with monoclonal antibody to L3T4. *J Exp Med* 1985; **161**: 378–91.

50. Shizuru JA, Taylor-Edwards C, Banks BA, Gregory AK, Fathman CG. Immunotherapy of the nonobese diabetic mouse: treatment with an

antibody to T-helper lymphocytes. *Science* 1988; **240**: 659–62.

51. Brinkman CJ, Ter Laak HJ, Hommes OR. Modulation of experimental allergic encephalomyelitis in Lewis rats by monoclonal anti-T-cell antibodies. *J Neuroimmunol* 1985; **7**: 231–8.

52. Wofsy D, Seaman WE. Reversal of advanced murine lupus in NZB/NZW F1 mice by treatment with monoclonal antibody to L3T4. *J Immunol* 1999; **138**: 3247–53.

53. Benjamin RJ, Waldmann H. Induction of tolerance by monoclonal antibody therapy. *Nature* 1986; **320**: 449–51.

54. Shizuru JA, Alters SE, Fathman CG. Anti-CD4 monoclonal antibodies in therapy: creation of nonclassical tolerance in the adult. *Immunol Rev* 1992; **129**: 105–30.

55. Bretscher P, Cohn M. A theory of self-nonself discrimination. *Science* 1970; **169**: 1042–9.

56. Jenkins MK, Pardoll DM, Mizuguchi J, Quill H, Schwartz RH. T-cell unresponsiveness in vivo and in vitro: fine specificity of induction and molecular characterization of the unresponsive state. *Immunol Rev* 1987; **95**: 113–35.

57. Schwartz RH. A cell culture model for T lymphocyte clonal anergy. *Science* 1999; **248**: 1349–56.

58. Waldmann H. Manipulation of T-cell responses with monoclonal antibodies. *Annu Rev Immunol* 1989; **7**: 407–44.

59. Cobbold SP, Qin SX, Waldmann H. Reprogramming the immune system for tolerance with monoclonal antibodies. *Semin Immunol* 1990; **2**: 377–87.

60. Gutstein NL, Seaman WE, Scott JH, Wofsy D. Induction of immune tolerance by administration of monoclonal antibody to L3T4. *J Immunol* 1986; **137**: 1127–32.

61. Hutchings PL, O'Reilly L, Parish NM, Waldmann H, Cooke A. The use of a non-depleting anti-CD4 monoclonal antibody to re-establish tolerance to beta cells in NOD mice. *Eur J Immunol* 1992; **22**: 1913–18.

62. Van den Broek MF, Van de Langerijt LG, Van Bruggen MC, Billingham ME, van den Berg WB. Treatment of rats with monoclonal anti-CD4 induces long-term resistance to streptococcal cell wall-induced arthritis. *Eur J Immunol* 1992; **22**: 57–61.

63. Horneff G, Burmester GR, Emmrich F, Kalden JR. Treatment of rheumatoid arthritis with an anti-CD4 monoclonal antibody. *Arthritis Rheum* 1991; **34**: 129–40.

64. Moreland LW, Bucy PR, Jackson B, James T, Koopman WJ. Longterm (5 years) follow-up of rheumatoid arthritis patients treated with a depleting anti-CD4 monoclonal antibody, cM-T412. *Arthritis Rheum* 1996; **39**: S244.

65. Moreland LW, Pratt PW, Mayes MD et al. Double-blind, placebo-controlled multicenter trial using chimeric monoclonal anti-CD4 antibody, cM-T412, in rheumatoid arthritis patients receiving concomitant methotrexate. *Arthritis Rheum* 1995; **38**: 1581–8.

66. van der Lubbe PA, Dijkmans BA, Markusse HM, Nassander U, Breedveld FC. A randomized, double-blind, placebo-controlled study of CD4 monoclonal antibody therapy in early rheumatoid arthritis. *Arthritis Rheum* 1995; **38**: 1097–106.

67. Tak PP, van der Lubbe PA, Cauli A et al. Reduction of synovial inflammation after anti-CD4 monoclonal antibody treatment in early rheumatoid arthritis. *Arthritis Rheum* 1995; **38**: 1457–65.

68. Gutstein NL, Wofsy D. Administration of F(ab')2 fragments of monoclonal antibody to L3T4 inhibits humoral immunity in mice without depleting L3T4+ cells. *J Immunol* 1986; **137**: 3414–19.

69. Carteron NL, Wofsy D, Seaman WE. Induction of immune tolerance during administration of monoclonal antibody to L3T4 does not depend on depletion of L3T4+ cells. *J Immunol* 1988; **140**: 713–16.

70. Brostoff SW, Mason DW. Experimental allergic encephalomyelitis: successful treatment in vivo with a monoclonal antibody that recognizes T helper cells. *J Immunol* 1984; **133**: 1938–42.

71. Burkhardt K, Charlton B, Mandel TE. An increase in the survival of murine H-2-mismatched cultured fetal pancreas allografts using depleting or nondepleting anti-CD4 monoclonal antibodies, and a further increase with the addition of cyclosporine. *Transplantation* 1989; **47**: 771–5.

72. Qin SX, Wise M, Cobbold SP et al. Induction of tolerance in peripheral T cells with monoclonal antibodies. *Eur J Immunol* 1990; **20**: 2737–45.

73. Choy EH, Pitzalis C, Cauli A et al. Percentage of anti-CD4 monoclonal antibody-coated lymphocytes in the rheumatoid joint is associated with clinical improvement. Implications for the development of immunotherapeutic dosing regimens. *Arthritis Rheum* 1996; **39**: 52–6.

74. Rep MH, van Oosten BW, Roos MT, Ader HJ, Polman CH, Van Lier. RA. Treatment with

depleting CD4 monoclonal antibody results in a preferential loss of circulating naive T cells but does not affect IFN-gamma secreting TH1 cells in humans. *J Clin Invest* 1997; **99**: 2225–31.

75. Panayi GS, Choy EHS, Emery P et al. Repeat-cycle study of high-dose intravenous (iv) 4162W94 anti-CD4 monocloncal antibody (mAb) in rheumatoid arthritis (RA). *Arthritis Rheum* 1998; **41**: S56.

76. Pulito VL, Roberts VA, Adair JR et al. Humanization and molecular modeling of the anti-CD4 monoclonal antibody, OKT4A. *J Immunol* 1996; **156**: 2840 50.

77. Delmonico FL, Cosimi AB, Kawai T et al. Nonhuman primate responses to murine and humanized OKT4A. *Transplantation* 1993; **55**: 722–8.

78. Schulze-Koops H, Davis LS, Haverty TP, Wacholtz MC, Lipsky PE. 1998. Reduction of Th1 cell activity in the peripheral circulation of patients with rheumatoid arthritis after treatment with a non-depleting humanized monoclonal antibody to CD4. *J Rheumatol* 1998; **25**: 2065–76.

79. Paulus HE, Egger MJ, Ward JR, Williams HJ, the Cooperative Systemic Studies of Rheumatic Diseases Group. Analysis of improvement in individual rheumatoid arthritis patients treated with disease-modifying antirheumatic drugs, based on the findings in patients treated with placebo. *Arthritis Rheum* 1990; **33**: 477–84.

80. Lydyard PM, Lamour A, MacKenzie LE, Jamin C, Mageed RA, Youinou P. CD5+ B cells and the immune system. *Immunol Lett* 1993; **38**: 159–66.

81. Cush JJ. Anti-CD5/Ricin A chain immunoconjugate therapy in rheumatoid arthritis. In: Strand V, Scott DL, Simon LS, eds. *Novel Therapeutic Agents for the Treatment of Autoimmune Diseases.* (Dekker: New York, 1997) pp. 11–24.

82. Byers BS, Caperton E, Ackerman S, Shephard J, Scannon PJ. Modification of the immune system in patients with rheumatoid arthritis treated with anti-CD5 ricin A chain immunotoxin. *FASEB J* 1989; **3**: A1122.

83. Strand V, Lipsky PE, Cannon GW et al. Effects of administration of an anti-CD5 plus immunoconjugate in rheumatoid arthritis. Results of two phase II studies. The CD5 Plus Rheumatoid Arthritis Investigators Group. *Arthritis Rheum* 1993; **36**: 620–30.

84. Olsen NJ, Brooks RH, Cush JJ et al. A double-blind, placebo-controlled study of anti-CD5 immunoconjugate in patients with rheumatoid arthritis. The Xoma RA Investigator Group. *Arthritis Rheum* 1996; **39**: 1102–8.

85. Kirkham BW, Pitzalis C, Kingsley GH et al. Monoclonal antibody treatment in rheumatoid arthritis: the clinical and immunological effects of a CD7 monoclonal antibody. *Br J Rheumatol* 1991; **30**: 459–63.

86. Kirkham BW, Thien F, Pelton BK et al. Chimeric CD7 monoclonal antibody therapy in rheumatoid arthritis. *J Rheumatol* 1992; **19**: 1348–52.

87. Kyle V, Coughlan RJ, Tighe H et al. Beneficial effect of monoclonal antibody to interleukin 2 receptor on activated T cells in rheumatoid arthritis. *Ann Rheum Dis* 1989; **48**: 428–9.

88. Bumgardner GL, Ramos E, Lin A, Vincenti F. Daclizumab (humanized anti-IL2Ralpha mAb) prophylaxis for prevention of acute rejection in renal transplant recipients with delayed graft function. *Transplantation* 2000; **72**: 642–7.

89. Thasia G, Woodworth TG, Parker K. Early clinical studies of IL-2-fusion toxin in patients with severe rheumatoid arthritis, recent-onset insulin-dependent diabetes mellitus, and psoriasis. In: Strand V, Scott DL, Simon LS, eds. *Novel Therapeutic Agents for the Treatment of Autoimmune Diseases.* (Dekker: New York, 1997) pp. 25–39.

90. Moreland LW, Sewell KL, Trentham DE et al. Interleukin-2 diphtheria fusion protein (DAB486IL-2) in refractory rheumatoid arthritis. A double-blind, placebo-controlled trial with open-label extension. *Arthritis Rheum* 1995; **38**: 1177–86.

91. Mueller DL, Jenkins MK, Schwartz RH. Clonal expansion versus functional clonal inactivation: a costimulatory signalling pathway determines the outcome of T-cell antigen receptor occupancy. *Annu Rev Immunol* 1989; **7**: 445–80.

92. Abrams JR, Lebwohl MG, Guzzo CA et al. CTLA4Ig-mediated blockade of T-cell costimulation in patients with psoriasis vulgaris. *J Clin Invest* 1999; **103**: 1243–52.

93. Moreland LW, Alten R, Van Den Bosch et al. Costimulatory blockade in patients with rheumatoid arthritis: a pilot, dose-finding, double-blind, placebo-controlled clinical trial evaluating CTLA-4Ig and LEA29Y eighty-five days after the first infusion. *Arthritis Rheum* 2002; **46**: 1470–9.

94. Siefken R, Klein-Hessling S, Serfling E, Kurrle R, Schwinzer R. A CD28-associated signaling pathway leading to cytokine gene transcription and T-cell proliferation without TCR engagement. *J Immunol* 1998; **161**: 1645–51.

95. Schafer PH, Wadsworth SA, Wang L, Siekierka JJ. p38 alpha mitogen-activated protein kinase is activated by CD28-mediated signaling and is required for IL-4 production by human CD4+CD45RO+ T cells and Th2 effector cells. *J Immunol* 1999; **162**: 7110–19.

96. Schulze-Koops H, Lipsky PE, Davis LS. Human memory T-cell differentiation into Th2-like effector cells is dependent on IL-4 and CD28 and inhibited by TCR ligation. *Eur J Immunol* 1998; **28**: 2517–29.

97. Li-Weber M, Giasi M, Krammer PH. Involvement of Jun and Rel proteins in up-regulation of interleukin-4 gene activity by the T-cell accessory molecule CD28. *J Biol Chem* 1998; **273**: 32460–6.

98. Webb LM, Feldmann M. Critical role of CD28/B7 costimulation in the development of human Th2 cytokine-producing cells. *Blood* 1995; **86**: 3479–86.

99. King CL, Stupi RJ, Craighead N, June CH, Thyphronitis G. CD28 activation promotes Th2 subset differentiation by human CD4+ cells. *Eur J Immunol* 1995; **25**: 587–95.

100. Shahinian A, Pfeffer K, Lee KP et al. Differential T-cell costimulatory requirements in CD28-deficient mice. *Science* 1993; **261**: 609–12.

101. Rulifson IC, Sperling AI, Fields PE, Fitch FW, Bluestone JA. CD28 costimulation promotes the production of Th2 cytokines. *J Immunol* 1997; **158**: 658–65.

102. Khattri R, Auger JA, Griffin MD, Sharpe AH, Bluestone JA. Lymphoproliferative disorder in CTLA-4 knockout mice is characterized by CD28–regulated activation of Th2 responses. *J Immunol* 1999; **162**: 5784–91.

103. Hale G, Xia MQ, Tighe HP, Dyer MJ, Waldmann H. The CAMPATH-1 antigen (CDw52). *Tissue Antigens* 1990; **35**: 118–27.

104. Brett S, Baxter G, Cooper H, Johnston JM, Tite J, Rapson N. Repopulation of blood lymphocyte sub-populations in rheumatoid arthritis patients treated with the depleting humanized monoclonal antibody, CAMPATH-1H. *Immunology* 1996; **88**: 13–19.

105. Issacs JD, Greer S, Sharma S et al. Morbidity and mortality in rheumatoid arthritis patients with prolonged and profound therapy-induced lymphopenia. *Arthritis Rheum* 2001; **44**: 1998–2008.

106. Springer TA. Adhesion receptors of the immune system. *Nature* 1990; **346**: 425–34.

107. Carlos TM, Harlan JM. Membrane proteins involved in phagocyte adherence to endothelium. *Immunol Rev* 1990; **114**: 5–28.

108. Strober S, Holoshitz J. Mechanisms of immune injury in rheumatoid arthritis: evidence for the involvement of T-cells and heat-shock protein. *Immunol Rev* 1990; **118**: 233–55.

109. Kavanaugh AF, Lightfoot E, Lipsky PE, Oppenheimer-Marks N. The role of CD11/CD18 in adhesion and transendothelial migration of T cells: analysis utilizing CD18 deficient T-cell clones. *J Immunol* 1991; **146**: 4149–56.

110. Oppenheimer-Marks N, Davis LS, Bogue DT, Ramberg J, Lipsky PE. Differential utilization of ICAM-1 and VCAM-1 during the adhesion and transendothelial migration of human T lymphocytes. *J Immunol* 1991; **147**: 2913–21.

111. Wacholtz MC, Patel SS, Lipsky PE. Leukocyte function-associated antigen 1 is an activation molecule for human T cells. *J Exp Med* 1989; **170**: 431–48.

112. Kavanaugh AF, Davis LS, Nichols LA et al. Treatment of refractory rheumatoid arthritis with a monoclonal antibody to intercellular adhesion molecule 1. *Arthritis Rheum* 1994; **37**: 992–9.

113. Arnett FC, Edworthy SM, Bloch DA et al. The American Rheumatism Association 1987 revised criteria for the classification of rheumatoid arthritis. *Arthritis Rheum* 1988; **31**: 315–24.

114. Kavanaugh AF, Davis LS, Jain RI, Nichols LA, Norris SH, Lipsky PE. A phase I/II open label study of the safety and efficacy of an anti-ICAM-1 (intercellular adhesion molecule-1; CD54) monoclonal antibody in early rheumatoid arthritis. *J Rheumatol* 1996; **23**: 1338–44.

115. Lipsky PE, Kavanaugh AF, Schulze-Koops H, Davis LS. Adhesion molecules as targets for therapy in rheumatoid arthritis. In: Bazan N, Bottig J, Van SJ, eds. *New Targets in Inflammation. Inhibitors of COX-2 or Adhesion Molecules.* (Kluwer Academic Publishers: Dordrecht, 1996) 139–44.

116. Pinals RS, Masi AT, Larsen RA. Preliminary criteria for clinical remission in rheumatoid arthritis. *Arthritis Rheum* 1981; **24**: 1308–15.

117. Kavanaugh AF, Schulze-Koops H, Davis LS, Lipsky PE. Repeat treatment of rheumatoid arthritis patients with a murine anti-intercellular adhesion molecule 1 monoclonal antibody. *Arthritis Rheum* 1997; **40**: 849–53.

2

B cells

Anne Davidson, Konstantin Konstantinov and Betty Diamond

Introduction • B-cell development • B-cell receptor activation and signaling • B-cell subsets • Mechanisms that regulate autoreactivity • B-cell costimulation pathways • Genetic determinants of autoreactivity • Novel therapeutic strategies • Opportunities for new therapeutic strategies • Conclusions • Acknowledgment • References

INTRODUCTION

B cells play a major role in host defenses against infection. Their most obvious function is the production of high-affinity antibodies that target pathogens for elimination or destruction during the adaptive immune response. However, they also act as antigen-presenting cells to diversify the epitopes of microbial antigens that are recognized by T cells, and they produce cytokines involved both in lymphoid regulation and in inflammatory processes. In genetically predisposed individuals, B cells can produce autoantibodies that mediate tissue injury by a variety of mechanisms. Once activated, such cells function as antigen-presenting cells that take up autoantigen through their antigen receptor and diversify the epitopes of self-antigen presented to autoreactive T cells. Thus, the autoreactive B cell may play a role in both the inductive and the effector arm of autoimmune disease, and contribute to an expansion of autoreactive T- and B-cell specificities.[1] To learn how to target B cells to alter the induction or pathogenesis of rheumatologic disease, it is necessary to review aspects of B-cell biology.

B-CELL DEVELOPMENT

Naive B-cell development is a highly regulated process, which progresses through a series of critical stages involving B-lineage commitment and initial generation of an antibody molecule (B-cell receptor, BCR). B-cell repertoire selection is then based on BCR affinity and specificity and exposure to antigen. Finally, maturation occurs into distinct functional subsets. The critical B-cell subsets are the B1 cells, or the B2 cells, which include both marginal zone cells and follicular cells.[2,3]

The early stages of B-cell lymphopoiesis take place in primary lymphoid tissues (fetal liver and bone marrow). Final maturation, encounter with microbial antigen and further differentiation into cells that release antibodies or persist as long-lived memory cells occur in secondary or peripheral lymphoid tissues (spleen, lymph nodes, tonsils, gut).

B cells acquire their BCR in the fetal liver and bone marrow in the absence of any knowledge of foreign antigen or self-antigen. Random rearrangements of V, D and J (heavy chain) and V and J (light chain) immunoglobulin gene

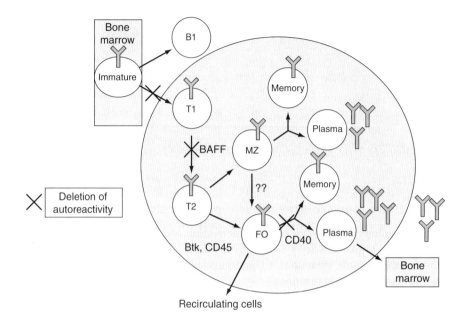

Figure 2.1 B-cell development in the spleen: B cells exit from the bone marrow and enter the spleen as transitional type 1 (T1) cells that are sensitive to apoptotic signals upon exposure to autoantigen. These cells then develop into T2 cells that can either become marginal zone cells, in part under the influence of BAFF, or follicular cells. Both Btk and CD45 are needed for follicular cell development. Marginal zone cells respond to T-independent type II antigens and can become short-lived plasma cells. Follicular cells respond to T-dependent antigens and enter germinal centers, where they undergo class switching and somatic mutation. Autoreactivity is regulated both at the T1 stage and within germinal centers. B1 cells constitute a separate lineage that predominantly populates the peritoneal and pleural cavities.

segments occur to form the complete immunoglobulin variable region genes in developing B cells. These random gene rearrangements, together with the insertion of non-template-encoded nucleotides at V–D and D–J junctions and random combinations of heavy and light chain genes, are responsible for the generation of a vast repertoire of antibody specificities, including autospecificities (reviews: Nemazee[4] and Tonegawa[5]). Thus, there needs to be a process of selection whereby autoreactive B cells are eliminated from the naive B-cell repertoire. Those cells that survive initial selection in the bone marrow migrate to the spleen as transitional-stage T1 B cells which express membrane

IgM.[6,7] Over half of the naive B cells that are made are lost during the transition from the bone marrow to the secondary lymphoid organs, presumably due to deletion following exposure to autoantigen (Figure 2.1).[8,9]

The signaling apparatus of transitional B cells is such that they undergo apoptosis upon BCR engagement,[10] although they are fully capable of undergoing a proliferative response to a mitogenic stimulus such as lipopolysaccharide (LPS).[11] Within the spleen, T1 cells differentiate to a second transitional stage (T2) marked by acquisition of IgD expression and of expression of the C3d receptor CD21 and the low-affinity IgE Fc receptor CD23. This differentiation stage is highly dependent on a recently described molecule BAFF (also called BLyS, TALL or THANK), a member of the tumor necrosis factor (TNF) family of molecules.[12,13] Maturation of B cells past the T1 stage is almost completely blocked in mice deficient in either BAFF or its receptor BAFF-R.[13,14] Survival of T2 B cells, which are found in splenic primary follicles, depends on signals generated through the BCR during the process of differentiation into mature B cells.[6,15] Once full maturation into naive resting B cells has occurred, signaling through the BCR will induce cell activation and proliferation, rather than apoptosis.[16,17]

B-CELL RECEPTOR ACTIVATION AND SIGNALING

The B-cell receptor is a complex of surface immunoglobulin and the accessory molecules Igα and Igβ (CD79a and CD79b; Figure 2.2).[18] The ligand-binding portion of this receptor, the membrane immunoglobulin, is a tetrameric complex of two Ig heavy (H) and two light (L)

chains. BCR aggregation, induced by multivalent antigen, leads to signaling through tyrosine phosphorylation of the BCR transducer elements (Igα/(β), which occurs within motifs known as immunoreceptor tyrosine-based activation motifs (ITAMs).[19] The ITAM sequence contains two tyrosine residues that are critical for signaling. These are phosphorylated by intracellular kinases Blk, Lyn and Fyn, and, once phosphorylated, recruit Syk to the complex. Syk phosphorylation triggers the activation of BLNK, phospholipase C, phosphatidylinositol-3-kinase, and Ras pathways.[10,20–22]

BCR crosslinking leads also to tyrosine phosphorylation of Btk and activation of its kinase activity, which appears critical for phospholipase activation. A mutation in the Btk gene has been identified in patients with X-linked agammaglobulinemia, a disease characterized by reduced numbers of mature B cells and poor antibody responses.[23] Tyrosine phosphorylation of other BCR-associated transmembrane glycoproteins such as CD19[24] creates docking sites for

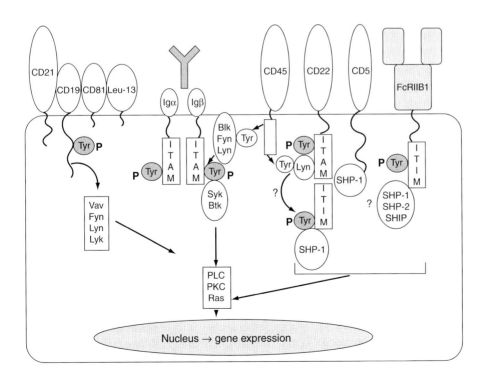

Figure 2.2 B-cell signaling. The membrane Ig associates with CD79α and CD79β. These are phosphorylated by blk, lyn and fyn following BCR crosslinking. These in turn activate downstream kinases. Co-receptor molecules CD19 or CD22 serve to enhance or diminish the signal.

downstream effector and adapter proteins, which enhance the initial signal.

Negative regulation is achieved by an emerging group of 'inhibitory co-receptors', all of which have a similar immunoreceptor tyrosine-based inhibitory motif (ITIM). These inhibitory receptors recruit SH-2-containing tyrosine phosphatases (SHP-1 and SHIP) to the BCR complex.[25,26] Thus, the BCR plays a central role in B-cell biology, transducing signals that are required for cell fate decisions that include both negative selection and initiation of the immune response. The strength of BCR signaling is dependent not only on interaction with antigen but also on the level of expression of associated enhancers or inhibitors of BCR signaling.

B-CELL SUBSETS

There are several B lymphocyte subsets that appear to be regulated differently with respect to their migration patterns, their threshold for activation and their antigenic specificity. B1 B cells are produced early in ontogeny and appear to be relatively independent of BAFF stimulation, as they are present in BAFF-deficient mice.[13] Most B1 cells (B1a cells) constitutively express the CD5 surface antigen. A small population of B1 cells (B1b cells) does not express CD5. The B1 population is thought to be self-renewing, because it does not appear to be replenished by lymphopoiesis in the bone marrow. B1 cells are the predominant source of 'natural' low-affinity IgM autoantibodies, which are polyspecific, germline encoded, and display limited V gene usage.[3] It has also recently been shown that the expression of the B-cell chemokine CXCL13 by cells in the pleural and peritoneal cavities is essential for accumulation of B1 cells in these areas.[27] The relative restriction of the B1 lymphocytes to these cavities implies that these cells may also have specialized functions that are associated with the niche that they occupy in the immune system. The activation threshold of B1 cells is increased compared with mature follicular B cells, but it is still not known what triggers the activation of B1 cells in physiologic situations. Recent data using B- and T-cell transgenic mice show that non-cognate help from self-reactive γδ T

cells can assist in the activation of B1 cells and induce their migration to mesenteric lymph nodes and their differentiation into antibody-secreting cells.[28,29]

Differentiation of B cells into B1 cells is controlled not only by the nature of the antigen, but also by the strength of the signal transmitted through the BCR.[30] CD19 decreases the threshold for stimulation of the B cell through the BCR; deficiency of CD19 results in a decrease in size of the B1 compartment. Conversely, deficiency of the negative regulator CD22 results in an increase in B1 cells. Altered expression of these molecules has also been shown to alter transition of transgenic autoreactive anti-Sm B cells to the B1 compartment. In mice transgenic for an anti-Sm antibody, B cells are found predominantly in the B1 compartment, where they are present in a non-activated state. Increasing the signal to these cells by overexpressing CD19 breaks tolerance and leads to autoantibody production. Decreasing the signal delivered to these cells by eliminating CD19 will allow them to traffic to the B2 compartment.[31] Finally, decreasing the signal affinity even further will result in differentiation to the B2 compartment but as an anergic cell.[32]

Conventional (B2) B cells arise from bone marrow precursors and lack expression of the CD5 molecule. They can develop into either marginal zone B cells, which are present in the spleen but not in the lymph nodes, and which participate in T-cell-independent antibody responses,[33] or follicular B cells, which participate in T-cell-dependent antibody responses. The factors that determine whether a B cell develops as a marginal zone or follicular B cell are not well understood, but are dependent on the microenvironment within the spleen. Recent data suggest that overexpression of BAFF leads to an expansion of marginal zone B cells.[12] Deletion of pyk2,[34] a kinase involved in chemokine receptor signaling in B cells, leads to a loss of marginal zone B cells. In addition, Aiolos-deficient,[35] lymphotoxin alpha-deficient[36] and lyn-deficient mice[37] do not have marginal zone B cells, indicating that the strength of signaling after BCR engagement also influences recruitment of cells into this compartment. Marginal zone B cells respond to type 2 T-independent antigens that express repeating epitopes that can crosslink the BCR. These cells also express the unconventional MHC class I molecule CD1, and thus can act as antigen-presenting cells to CD1-restricted T cells.[33] The nature of the antigenic epitopes presented by CD1 is currently under study, but they appear to be lipid or glycolipid antigens.[38] Thus, these B cells may be involved in presentation of bacterial cell wall moieties to CD1-restricted T cells.

Marginal zone B cells have enhanced signaling through their BCR. Recent data from the NZB/W F1 mouse model of systemic lupus erythematosus (SLE) suggest that marginal zone B cells are expanded early in disease and are involved in the IgM autoantibody production that precedes disease onset.[39] This observation is consistent with the overexpression of BAFF in the serum of NZB/W F1 mice.[40] Under physiologic circumstances, activation of marginal zone B cells results in early transition to short-lived plasma cells that secrete predominantly low-affinity IgM antibodies that are presumably involved in the early immune response to pathogens. Whether marginal zone B cells are fixed in this compartment or can undergo transition to the follicular compartment is not currently known, but active disease in the NZB/W F1 mouse is associated with a decrease in the frequency of marginal zone B cells (Davidson and Porcelli, unpublished findings).

Follicular cells are activated by encounter with antigen coupled with a cognate interaction with T-helper cells. Expression of a series of chemokines and chemokine receptors orchestrates movement of B cells into areas where they can encounter antigen and T-cell help.[41] Upon activation, they enter a specialized milieu, the germinal center (Figure 2.3).[42] Formation of the

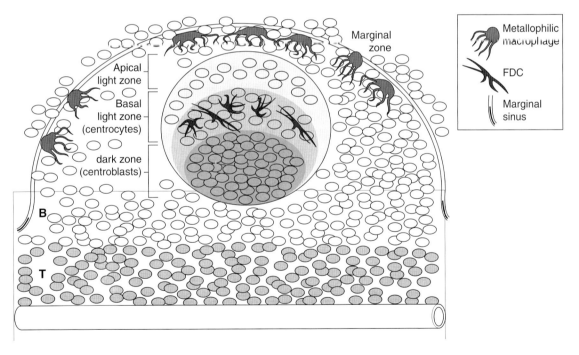

Figure 2.3 Schematic diagram of a B-cell follicle containing a germinal center: B cells enter through the marginal sinus and traffic either to the marginal zone located outside a ring of metallophilic macrophages or to the B-cell area of the follicle. After exposure to antigen, the B cells enter germinal centers, where they come into contact with follicular dendritic cells bearing antigen in the basal light zone and T cells that will facilitate class switching and somatic mutation in the apical light zone. B cells exit the germinal center either as memory cells or as antibody-secreting plasma cells.

germinal center is critically dependent on a number of factors, including costimulatory molecules such as CD40 and possibly BAFF,[43] and cytokines, including TNF-α, lymphotoxin-α and lymphotoxin-$\alpha_1\beta_2$. Within the germinal center environment, B cells undergo both heavy chain class switching to IgG, IgA and IgE and somatic hypermutation. Little is known about the regulation of these events; however, it is clear that CD40–CD40L interactions are essential for this process to occur.[42,44,45] CD40 is a member of the TNF receptor family; its engagement on B cells by T cells expressing CD40L results in rescue of naive B cells from apoptotic cell death and is required for both class switching and somatic mutation to occur.[46] BAFF also may play some role in follicular cell maturation, as mice with BAFF overexpression have increased numbers of germinal centers.[12,47]

Somatic hypermutation is characterized by a series of point mutations occurring within the variable region of an antibody molecule and results in the selective expansion of a B-cell population with higher affinity for the inciting antigen.[48] An increased number of replacement mutations (mutations that alter the amino acid) in complementarity-determining regions, which comprise the antigen-binding site, and an increased number of silent mutations (mutations that do not lead to a change in amino acid) in framework or scaffolding regions of the molecule, are indicative of antigen selection. The role of several DNA polymerases in the process of somatic mutation has been recently described.[49–53] In addition, recent studies of the RNA-editing enzyme AID indicate a crucial role for this enzyme in the class switch and somatic mutation process.[54,55]

While somatic mutation is responsible for affinity maturation of an antibody response, it may also generate novel antibody specificities, including autospecificities. Data from many studies have shown that the autoreactive B cells that are present in patients with rheumatologic disease have accumulated somatic mutations.[56] While there are some rare instances where somatic mutation can occur outside germinal centers,[36] most data suggest that pathogenic autoreactive B cells derive from follicular B cells that have been through a germinal center environment. Furthermore, the mutations are often suggestive of antigen selection, with a high ratio of replacement to silent mutations in complementarity-determining regions.[57]

Germinal center B cells differentiate into either plasma cells, which continue to release antibodies, or memory B cells, which do not secrete immunoglobulin. Memory cells express B7 and surface immunoglobulin.[58] They can differentiate into plasma cells under the influence of T-cell help if there is a second encounter with antigen, but they do not appear to require continued antigen exposure for survival.[59] CD40 ligation favors a memory cell phenotype,[58] and CD27–CD70 interactions may favor plasma cell differentiation,[60] but other factors that determine whether a germinal center B cell becomes a memory or a plasma cell are largely unknown. Plasma cells downregulate CCR7 and express CXCR4, which directs them to areas expressing CXCL12, such as the red pulp of the spleen and the bone marrow.[61] The factors that regulate the differentiation and fate of plasma cells derived from follicular cells have recently been extensively reviewed elsewhere.[61] Plasma cells downregulate a variety of cell surface molecules, including the BCR, but continue to secrete immunoglobulin, some for long periods of time, in an antigen- and costimulation-independent manner.[62,63]

One feature of many autoimmune diseases is the process of lymphoid neogenesis or generation of lymph node- and germinal center-like structures in inflamed target organs. These structures have been described particularly in the diabetic pancreas[64] and the rheumatoid synovium,[65] and are also seen in many murine models of autoimmunity. The factors that contribute to formation of these lymphoid structures are similar to those found in secondary lymphoid organs, with local inflammation inducing upregulation of critical cytokines and chemokines.[66] In the rheumatoid joint, B cells can act to perpetuate the inflammatory response by secretion of rheumatoid factors that form pathogenic immune complexes and by their function as antigen-presenting cells. Dissolution of these germinal center structures using antagonists of crucial trafficking may be a new approach to protect target organs in established autoimmunity.[64]

MECHANISMS THAT REGULATE AUTOREACTIVITY

Data from many laboratories that have described immunoglobulin V region polymorphisms and the process of V(D)J rearrangement suggest that the naive repertoire prior to negative selection does not appreciably differ between healthy individuals and individuals with autoimmune disease. Furthermore, the few studies that have been performed to date do not suggest a major defect in the process of somatic mutation after antigen activation in autoimmune disease.[67] Rather, B-cell autoreactivity appears to result from either a defect in negative selection or from excessive activation of autoreactive cells.[57,68] Defects in negative selection may lead to autoreactivity in the naive B-cell repertoire and/or to autoreactivity in the antigen-activated B-cell repertoire. Knowing whether naive or memory cells play a major role in disease activity and in relapse is critical, as different approaches may be necessary to eliminate, inactivate or alter the function of naive and memory cells. In murine models, there are data demonstrating altered selection of both naive and antigen-activated B cells in autoimmune hosts.[69] In patients with rheumatic disease, there appears to be both abnormal activation of follicular B cells and abnormal negative selection of cells that have undergone germinal center differentiation.[57] It is probable there are also defects in the naive B-cell repertoire.

Given that autospecificities arise twice in the course of B-cell development, first as the naive repertoire is generated, and again following somatic mutation of activated B cells, there need to be mechanisms for screening the B-cell repertoire and eliminating autoreactivity. Mechanisms to maintain self-tolerance in the immature B-cell population have been identified through the analysis of mice expressing transgene-encoded

autoantibodies. Mechanisms that maintain self-tolerance among antigen-activated B cells are less well understood.

There are four potential outcomes for an autoreactive naive or immature B cell: indifference, receptor editing, anergy or deletion.[2,4,70] If limited antigen is available to the B cell or if the affinity of BCR for antigen is low, little BCR ligation occurs, there is insufficient signal transmitted, and the B cell remains a resting B cell. This cell is said to be indifferent or ignorant. It has the potential, however, to become activated upon exposure to a high concentration of antigen and thus to become a pathogenic B cell. For example, if tissue injury exposes sequestered antigen to the immune system, ignorant autoreactive B cells may be activated to secrete antibody and to function as antigen-presenting cells to activate autoreactive T cells. Thus, these autoreactive B cells have the potential to trigger an autoimmune response.

If the naive autoreactive B cell encounters a critical concentration of antigen, signaling through the BCR occurs. The naive B cell will, for a period of time, maintain expression of the RAG genes responsible for V(D)J rearrangement, and therefore the cell has an opportunity to rearrange a second BCR through a process called receptor editing.[71] Because of the nature of the genomic structure of the heavy and light chains, receptor editing occurs much more frequently in light chains than in heavy chains. An upstream Vκ region can undergo a secondary rearrangement to a downstream Jκ, generating a new light chain on the chromosome that has already experienced a VJ rearrangement. Alternatively, rearrangement on the second κ chain locus or on a λ light chain locus can occur. Thus, the B cell can generate a new heavy and light chain combination that may no longer be autoreactive.[72,73] The teleological explanation that has been given for receptor editing is that the difficulty of creating a productively rearranged heavy chain requires that the heavy chain not be squandered, but be given a second opportunity to associate with light chain and form an antibody that may function in immune protection. In addition, it has been suggested that some degree of BCR engagement is needed for B-cell survival and maturation. If the B cell has no affinity for any antigen, receptor editing may occur to generate a cell with a useful BCR.[71] Hallmarks of receptor editing are an increased percentage of light chains utilizing upstream Vκ genes and downstream Jκ genes and an increased number of B cells with λ light chains. Current data would suggest that receptor editing occurs in autoimmune individuals.[74,75]

If receptor editing does not occur, or if the process does not successfully generate a non-autoreactive BCR, anergy or deletion will ensue. Anergy is a state of functional paralysis in which the B cell can no longer be activated through the BCR. The anergic B cell is unable to enter a B-cell follicle, a state termed follicular exclusion, and will die unless rescued by activation through a mitogenic stimulus.[70] Deletion is the elimination of the B cell through programmed cell death. It is currently thought that anergy occurs with less BCR crosslinking and deletion with more BCR crosslinking, although thresholds for each are not entirely understood.

While negative selection mediated through these mechanisms has been extensively studied in the naive B-cell repertoire, mainly through the availability of mice transgenic for an autoantibody, less is known about elimination of B cells that acquire autospecificity after antigen activation as a result of somatic mutation. It is clear that deletion occurs in germinal center B cells, because when B cells are made to overexpress anti-apoptotic genes, it is possible to identify large numbers of autoreactive B cells emerging from antigen-activated responses.[76,77] In these cells, it has been possible to show that high-affinity autoreactivity arises as a consequence of somatic mutation. Currently, there is controversy regarding receptor editing in this population.

The various thresholds for tolerance induction in autoreactive B cells are not static, but can be dynamically altered by immune modulators such as cytokines, hormones or costimulatory molecules, generating a highly flexible system for elimination of autoreactive B cells. In addition to BCR-mediated regulation, there are regulatory cells that cause the death of activated B cells. These include CD4 cells and CD8 cells and appear to function through Fas-dependent and Fas-independent mechanisms.[78–80]

Finally, it is well documented in humans that autoantibodies are present in the circulation in individuals with ongoing infectious processes.[81–83] In most normal individuals, however, these autoreactive responses are not sustained by self-antigens.[83] They diminish over time following the eradication of the infection, suggesting an ongoing process of regulation. The nature of this regulation is currently not well understood, although it may simply reflect the disappearance of T-cell help.

B-CELL COSTIMULATION PATHWAYS

Activation of mature follicular B cells requires both exposure to specific antigen, which binds to the BCR, and additional signals provided by costimulatory pathways (Figure 2.4).[2] Costimulation, in general, is afforded by T-cell help, in the form of interactions between cell surface receptors on the B cell and cell surface molecules from the T cell, such as BAFF–BAFF-R and CD40–CD40L interactions, or by soluble molecules such as cytokines. In general, if antigen exposure occurs in the absence of costimulation as described above, tolerance mechanisms prevail. This is presumably the case for immature naive B cells and for B cells emerging from a germinal center response and entering the memory cell compartment. Since autoreactive T cells are tightly regulated and few survive negative selection to be activated in the periphery, autoreactive B cells will, ordinarily, lack T-cell help.[84] Thus, activation of autoreactive B cells is, in general, unlikely to occur. However, alterations in levels of cell surface signaling molecules can affect thresholds for B-cell activation. If high levels of costimulatory molecules are present, the requirement for a cognate interaction between the B-cell class II complex and the T-cell antigen receptor (TCR) or for antigen ligation of the BCR is likely to be diminished. Thus, regulation of the level of

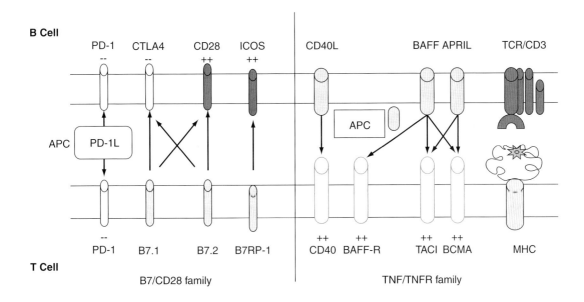

Figure 2.4 Interactions of costimulatory molecules on T cells and B cells: no shading indicates a negative signaling molecule; dark shading indicates a positive signaling molecule. New members of the CD28/B7 family are shown on the left side. A new B7 interacting molecule has been described but not yet identified. In addition, another B7-like molecule B7h3 has been described but its ligand is not yet identified. There are two known ligands for PD-1. Some members of the TNF/TNFR family are shown on the right side. BAFF-R interacts with BAFF, but not with the closely related molecule APRIL (a proliferation-inducing ligand). Many other members of this family, not shown here, are involved in T–B interactions and may be targets for therapy.

costimulatory molecules is critical to an appropriate regulation of autoreactivity.

New data suggest that B-cell costimulation may be provided not just through T-cell help, but also through engagement of other cell surface molecules such as Toll-like receptors (TLRs) (Figure 2.5). These receptors, part of the innate immune response, display pattern recognition of pathogen-associated molecules, which are common to many microbes. Toll-like receptors expressed by B cells include TLR-4, which is part of the cell surface complex that recognizes LPS, a major cell wall component of Gram-negative bacteria,[85] TLR-2, which recognizes lipoproteins in bacterial cell walls,[86] and TLR-9, which recognizes CpG motifs in bacterial DNA.[87,88] Cells deficient in BAFF-R, for example, cannot be activated by BCR signaling but are easily activated by LPS.[13] Recently, it has been demonstrated that cross linking of the BCR

and of TLR-9 can activate B cells. Not all substances that can activate TLRs are microbial derived, as some can be released from damaged tissue in the absence of infection. Nucleosomal fragments from apoptotic cells, for example, will bind TLR-9.[87,89] Thus, apoptotic particles may crosslink TLR-9 and antichromatin BCR, leading to a lupus-like serum response. It is important to note that activation through TLRs is insufficient to activate a high-affinity class-switched and mutated Ig response. Nonetheless, abnormalities of proteins involved in the innate immune response, such as the recently discovered NOD2, which activates NFkB in response to LPS stimulation, can contribute to the genetic susceptibility to the development of autoimmune disease.[90]

The activation of B cells leads not only to antibody secretion, but also to cytokine production. How different pathways of B-cell activation

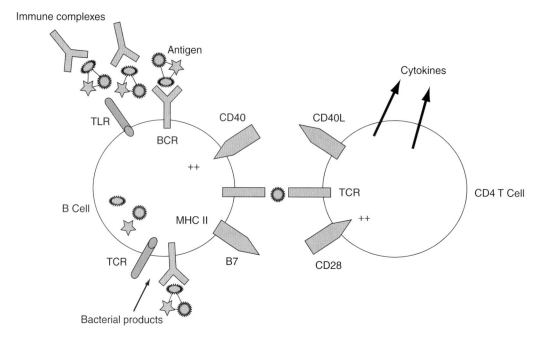

Figure 2.5 B-cell–T-cell interactions: B cells can be activated through interaction of their BCR with antigen, by stimulation of Toll-like receptors by bacterial products, by coligation of the BCR with complement receptors, or by coligation of the BCR with Toll-like receptors by immune complexes containing bacterial DNA or apoptotic particles. B cells present antigen to T cells and receive additional signals through costimulation by CD40L or from secreted cytokines. Memory cells upregulate B7 and can activate T cells to amplify the B-cell response.

affect the pattern of cytokine secretion is an area that needs to be explored.

GENETIC DETERMINANTS OF AUTOREACTIVITY

Recent studies of genetically engineered mice have shown that either deletion or overexpression of a large number of different single genes can give rise to autoantibody production, specifically to the autoantibodies seen in SLE (Table 2.1). These genetic abnormalities affect four aspects of B-cell function: B-cell apoptosis; strength of BCR signaling; strength of B-cell costimulation; and availability of autoantigen, specifically, products of damaged tissues, immune complexes or apoptotic particles (review: Davidson and Diamond[68]).[91–93] These alterations in B-cell function lead to an inability to delete autoreactive cells, to increased B-cell activation through

engagement of the BCR or conventional or nonconventional costimulatory pathways, and to an increased exposure to autoantigen (Table 2.1). It is critical to note that all single genetic alterations that lead to a disease phenotype do so only on particular genetic backgrounds. The clear implication is that multiple genetic pathways must be affected to lead to disease. In addition, resistance genes may modulate disease course.[94] Thus, the likelihood of developing an autoimmune disease depends on the host's genetic load of susceptibility genes and resistance genes, on exposure to environmental triggers, and on the local factors affecting the threshold for signaling through the BCR and through costimulatory pathways (review: Davidson and Diamond[68]). This understanding of the delicate balance of B-cell negative selection and activation suggests that it may be time to re-examine therapeutic strategies in diseases that are mediated by B-cell activation.

Table 2.1   Mutations leading to autoantibody production and SLE-like disease.

Increased B-cell activation
 Increased presence of immune complexes or apoptotic particles
  Dnase I −/−   Nuclease
  SAP −/−   Coats apoptotic particles
  C1q −/−   Clear immune complexes
  C4 −/−   and apoptotic particles
  Tyro 3, Axl, Mer −/−   Tyrosine kinases[92]
 Lack of negative regulation of BCR signals
  CD22 −/−
  lyn −/−   Phosphorylates CD22/recruits SHP-1
  SHP-1 −/−   Tyrosine phosphatase
  FcRIIB −/−   Recruits SHIP[a]
  CD19 tg
  Osteopontin tg   Soluble B-cell activator
 Increased costimulation/T-cell help
  BLyS tg   Costimulates B-cell maturation
  PD-1 −/−   Negative regulator of T cells
  p21 −/−   Cell cycle regulator
  LIGHT tg   Costimulates T cells[93]
Prevention of apoptosis
  Fas −/−   Death signal
  Fas ligand −/−
  Bcl-2 tg   Anti-apoptotic
  Bim −/−   Pro-apoptotic
Inappropriate cytokine expression
  TNF-α −/− (NZB)   TNF-α inhibits T-cell proliferation
  TNF-αR1 −/− (MRL)
  IFN-γ tg (skin promoter)
  TGF-β RII Dom. neg. CD4 specific
Target organ damage
  nrf2 deficiency[91]

*SHIP, SH2-containing inositol 5 phosphatase.
See Davidson and Diamond[68] for a complete list of citations.

NOVEL THERAPEUTIC STRATEGIES

The insight that autoantibodies arise from altered B-cell regulation, i.e. defects in anergy and deletion, and not from alterations in immunoglobulin V gene repertoire or from abnormalities in V(D)J rearrangement, suggests a need for new therapeutic paradigms for B-cell-mediated diseases. While some new therapeutic interventions have been brought to clinical trial, for the most part they have not taken into consideration either the multigenic origin of autoimmune rheumatic diseases or the difference between prevention of an abnormal immune response and attenuation of a fully activated response. For example, established plasma cells that are antigen and costimulation independent can continue to produce autoantibodies for long periods of time once they traffic to the bone marrow,[62,63] and may be resistant to therapies targeting costimulation or BCR signaling.

Pharmacologic agents

Cytotoxic drugs continue to play a major part in the therapy of systemic rheumatic disease. In addition to cyclophosphamide, azathioprine and methotrexate, mycofenolic acid and leflunomide have recently been shown to be effective in the treatment of lupus and rheumatoid arthritis,[95,96] respectively. Fludarabine has been tested in patients with severe lupus, but appears to have an unacceptable toxicity in this population.[97] Whether there is a role for rapamycin in the treatment of rheumatic disease also needs to be explored. While cytotoxic drugs are clearly efficacious in many rheumatic diseases, their specific impact on B-cell survival and function has not been extensively studied.

Biological agents

In recent years, there have been a number of new biological agents successfully brought to the clinic to treat patients with disease (Table 2.2). These include: agents that mediate cytokine blockade or enhancement, such as TNF blockade, which has had great success in the treatment of rheumatoid arthritis[98] and inflammatory bowel disease,[99] or interleukin-1 (IL-1) blockade in rheumatoid arthritis,[98] interferon-beta (IFN-β) administration for multiple sclerosis, or anti-IL-10 administration in SLE;[100] agents that mediate costimulatory blockade, such as the CD28 blocker CTLA4Ig in psoriasis and rheumatoid arthritis[101] and anti-CD40L in SLE;[102,103] agents that mediate depletion of T or B cells or their subsets;[104] and agents that block the migration of immune cells (review: Davidson and

Table 2.2 B-cell-directed biological therapies.

Current
  Cytokine blockade
  Costimulatory blockade (T cell, other)
  Toleragens
  Ablative therapies (with or without reconstitution)
Potential
  Interference with B-cell trafficking
  Blockade of intracellular signaling pathways
    BCR
    Toll-like receptors
    Cytokine receptors
    Costimulatory molecules
    Chemokine receptors

Diamond[68]). In general, these strategies are based on animal models showing that these therapies can either prevent disease onset or decrease disease severity if given early in the disease process. There has been little consideration of the degree of immunosuppression caused by these therapies in murine models. It is clear, however, that TNF blockade causes significant immunosuppression in humans and is associated with a high incidence of mycobacterial infection.[105,106] It is likely that other biological therapies will prove to be similarly immunosuppressive. Furthermore, when these therapies are brought to the clinic, a decrease in end-organ damage has been the measurement of therapeutic efficacy. Thus, there has been little attempt to study in humans how these interventions alter immune regulation. TNF blockade, for example, has unexpectedly led to induction of antinuclear antibodies and, rarely, to SLE[107] and to demyelinating disease in patients who have received this therapy for treatment of rheumatoid arthritis.[108] Why TNF blockade leads to autoantibody production is not clear, but NZB/W lupus-prone mice are characterized by low titers of TNF-α and show a decrease in disease severity when given TNF.[109]

Costimulatory blockade to limit interactions of antigen-presenting cells, T cells and B cells is a promising new approach to the treatment of SLE. Currently, a phase I trial of an antibody that impedes BAFF interactions with its three receptors, TACI, BCMA and BAFF-R, is underway. Antibody to CD40L, a costimulatory molecule that is required for B-cell maturation and germinal center formation, has been used in two separate clinical trials, one in which efficacy was not demonstrated[103] and one in which toxicity precluded completion of the trial.[102] One of these trials was accompanied by studies of peripheral blood B-cell phenotype and of the frequency of B cells spontaneously secreting anti-DNA antibody.[110,111] While these studies were necessarily abbreviated because the trial was discontinued, they demonstrated a marked change in B-cell biology in treated individuals, with a decrease in the frequency of autoantibody-secreting cells and plasma cells in peripheral blood and a decrease in anti-DNA titer. In animal models, it is clear that costimulatory blockade with anti-CD40L or with CTLA-4Ig leads to short-term remission.[112–114] Interestingly, long-term remissions can be achieved with the simultaneous use of two agents, either cyclophosphamide and CTLA-4Ig or anti-CD40L and CTLA-4Ig.[112,115,116] It is likely that combinations of therapeutic agents, each targeting a different pathway or cell population, will improve outcomes in human disease also.

Ablative therapies continue to be central to the treatment of rheumatic disease, despite the obvious fact that they cause global immunosuppression, at least in a transient fashion. B cells are being targeted with monoclonal antibody to the B-cell-specific membrane molecule CD20 in both SLE and rheumatoid arthritis. In a small uncontrolled study of patients with rheumatoid arthritis, long-term remissions were observed in some patients when high-dose cyclophosphamide was used in combination with anti-CD20 antibody.[117] When this combination was used to treat patients with SLE, no decrease in anti-DNA antibody titers was seen early after the onset of therapy.[104] This lack of a serologic response may reflect the fact that plasma cells

express little CD20 and would not be expected to be targeted by this therapy. This therapy, if used long term, is guaranteed to cause significant complications from immunosuppression.

B-cell tolerogens have also been explored in SLE. A multimeric configuration of oligonucleotides has been administered to patients to cause anergy or deletion of anti-DNA-secreting B cells. While the initial trial failed to demonstrate clinical efficacy,[118] a second trial is underway, targeted at those patients with high-affinity anti-DNA antibodies. It is possible that tolerogen-based therapy will be more effective when combined with costimulatory blockade.

The therapeutics described above are most effective at decreasing the induction of autoreactivity. Other strategies focus more on effector functions of activated cells and on decreasing organ damage from inflammation. Approaches that focus exclusively on the effector mechanisms include the use of Cox-2 inhibitors, inhibitors of nitric oxide, inhibitors of complement, inhibitors of cell adhesion or migration and metalloprotease inhibitors. There is some evidence that costimulatory blockade can also affect inflammatory cascades.[119–121] These approaches have not yet shown adequate efficacy in severe disease in humans, but they may have the advantage of causing less global immunosuppression.

OPPORTUNITIES FOR NEW THERAPEUTIC STRATEGIES

Studies of murine models of SLE and rheumatoid arthritis have shown that small perturbations in immune response can cause a non-spontaneously autoimmune animal to develop a disease phenotype. Such perturbations include a 20% increase in expression of Bcl-2, a similarly small increase in expression of CD19 in B cells,[122] or a 30% decrease in the function of the inhibitory costimulatory molecule cytotoxic T-lymphocyte antigen 4 (CTLA-4) which is expressed on T cells and serves to inhibit T-cell activation.[123] Each of these small alterations in gene expression leads to a lupus-like disease only in mice of particular genetic backgrounds. In other mouse strains, these genetic alterations do not cause the development of clinically apparent disease. Similarly, rheumatoid arthritis can be caused in non-spontaneously autoimmune mice by a single exposure to antibody[124] or by immunization with collagen and adjuvant.[125] Again, disease develops only in particular strains of mice.[126] Such studies lead to two significant conclusions. First, it is clear that small changes in cellular function or in microenvironments within the immune system have a major impact on immunologic phenotype. Second, small changes only have a large impact in the context of a particular constellation of disease susceptibility and resistance genes. Simply stated, multiple disease-associated alleles of genes that affect immune cell survival and activation can result in a host who is susceptible to induction of an autoimmune disease.

These insights into the multigenic basis of disease suggest some implications for effective preventive therapy. Since small modulations in multiple pathways of negative selection or lymphocyte activation cause disease, it can be hypothesized that small modulations in multiple pathways will prevent disease. Perhaps small modulations can even reverse established disease and render a host resistant to renewed disease induction. It is highly likely, however, that interventions that modulate pathways of deletion and activation need to be initiated early in the disease progression. Continued activation of the immune system may render the immune system resistant to modulation, because epitope spreading will increase the number of autoreactive cells and cells of multiple autoantigenic specificities. Furthermore, the establishment of a proinflammatory milieu, and the emergence of large numbers of memory and long-lived cells that are resistant to therapies that block the activation of naive cells and the release of multiple previously sequestered autoantigens, may make control of autoreactivity more difficult.[119,120] These concerns suggest that it may be useful to consider immune modulation to help maintain self-tolerance after induction of remission by more aggressive or ablative treatment protocols, or after stem cell transplantation.

One current limitation on designing optimal therapies that target multiple pathways of immune regulation is that we are currently unable to adequately phenotype the immunologic defects in our patients. A second problem is that we cannot use standard pharmacologic approaches to choose the right dose and dosing schedule of a biological reagent. Finally, we measure outcome not by alterations in immune response, but only by reversal or cessation of end-organ destruction. If we were able to analyze such features as B-cell repertoire, the subsets that are involved in disease pathogenesis or resistance, or the extent of somatic mutation and heavy chain class switching, or to measure activation using B- or T-cell membrane markers and to detect susceptibility to apoptotic or activation stimuli, we might be able to identify potentially therapeutic biological reagents. Furthermore, we might obtain information regarding synergy between two or more agents.

In SLE, B-cell activation is a primary cause of disease pathology. BCR signaling, costimulation and accessibility of apoptotic particles might all be targets for therapy. It is reasonable to anticipate efficacy of B-cell-specific kinase inhibitors that will decrease the strength of BCR signaling. There are already multiple reagents to block or activate both positive and negative T- and B-cell costimulation pathways, and there are many more cell surface molecules that could be targeted by antibodies or soluble receptors. Inhibitors of Toll-like receptors might be used to block the activation of B cells through T-cell-independent pathways, and nullify the increased availability of apoptotic particles. If such therapies fail to reverse established disease, they might be used to maintain tolerance following induction of remission with conventional or ablative therapies.

CONCLUSIONS

From this overview, it should be clear that autoreactive B cells arise routinely. With no apparent defect in immune regulation, autoreactive B cells may be activated under certain circumstances, such as during the response to infections. When B cells recognize foreign antigens that are molecular mimics of self-antigens, they may receive costimulation from T cells that are activated by foreign antigen and produce cross-reactive anti-foreign, anti-self antibodies. In general, however, it appears that molecular mimicry accounts for only transient autoreactivity and autoreactive cells fail to enter the memory compartment. For sustained autoreactivity, there needs to be a genetic predisposition that favors activation over tolerance.

The challenge of the coming decade is to develop methods to phenotype patients, to define pathways of immunologic dysfunction that lead to disease, and to target the relevant pathways in defined subsets of patients. While the ultimate test of a therapy will always be disease cessation, it will be necessary to identify small, even subtle, changes in B-cell function mediated by different therapeutic reagents, each of which alone is insufficient to prevent disease progression, but which together may treat disease successfully.[112,127,128] Furthermore, new approaches to therapy need to include recognition that the interventions that work early in disease may differ from those that are effective later in the progression of the disease. Therapy will need to be targeted to particular immunologic phenotypes (or genotypes) and to disease stage. An approach that considers patient phenotype and disease stage, and aims at immunomodulation, rather than more vigorous ablative therapies, would seem to have greater promise in the treatment of disease, and in the prevention of disease flares, while causing limited suppression of protective immune responses. While promising improved therapeutic strategies, this approach requires, above all, new clinical trial methodologies that link classic measures of disease severity with new measures of immunologic status.

ACKNOWLEDGMENT

This work was supported by Grants AI47291 and AI31229 from the National Institutes of Health.

REFERENCES

1. Lipsky PE. Systemic lupus erythematosus: an autoimmune disease of B-cell hyperactivity. *Nat Immunol* 2001; **2**: 764–6.
2. Meffre E, Casellas R, Nussenzweig MC. Antibody regulation of B-cell development. *Nat Immunol* 2000; **1**: 379–85.
3. Hardy RR, Hayakawa K. B-cell development pathways. *Annu Rev Immunol* 2001; **19**: 595–621.
4. Nemazee D. Receptor selection in B and T lymphocytes. *Annu Rev Immunol* 2000; **18**: 19–51.
5. Tonegawa S. The Nobel Lectures in Immunology. The Nobel Prize for Physiology or Medicine, 1987. Somatic generation of immune diversity. *Scand J Immunol* 1993; **38**: 303–19.
6. Loder F, Mutschler B, Ray RJ et al. B-cell development in the spleen takes place in discrete steps and is determined by the quality of B-cell receptor-derived signals. *J Exp Med* 1999; **190**: 75–89.
7. Flaishon L, Hershkoviz R, Lantner F et al. Autocrine secretion of interferon gamma negatively regulates homing of immature B cells. *J Exp Med* 2000; **192**: 1381–8.
8. Cyster JG, Goodnow CC. Antigen-induced exclusion from follicles and anergy are separate and complementary processes that influence peripheral B-cell fate. *Immunity* 1995; **3**: 691–701.
9. MacLennan I, Chan E. The dynamic relationship between B-cell populations in adults. *Immunol Today* 1993; **14**: 29–34.
10. Hasler P, Zouali M. B-cell receptor signaling and autoimmunity. *FASEB J* 2001; **15**: 2085–98.
11. Rolink AG, Schaniel C, Andersson J, Melchers F. Selection events operating at various stages in B-cell development. *Curr Opin Immunol* 2001; **13**: 202–7.
12. Batten M, Groom J, Cachero TG et al. BAFF mediates survival of peripheral immature B lymphocytes. *J Exp Med* 2000; **192**: 1453–66.
13. Rolink AG, Melchers F. BAFFled B cells survive and thrive: roles of BAFF in B-cell development. *Curr Opin Immunol* 2002; **14**: 266–75.

14. Thompson JS, Bixler SA, Qian F et al. BAFF-R, a newly identified TNF receptor that specifically interacts with BAFF. *Science* 2001; **293**: 2108–11.

15. Chung JB, Sater RA, Fields ML, Erikson J, Monroe JG. CD23 defines two distinct subsets of immature B cells which differ in their responses to T-cell help signals. *Int Immunol* 2002; **14**: 157–66.

16. Garside P, Ingulli E, Merica RR, Johnson JG, Noelle RJ, Jenkins MK. Visualization of specific B and T lymphocyte interactions in the lymph node. *Science* 1998; **281**: 96–9.

17. MacLennan IC, Gulbranson-Judge A, Toellner KM et al. The changing preference of T and B cells for partners as T-dependent antibody responses develop. *Immunol Rev* 1997; **156**: 53–66.

18. Reth M. Antigen receptors on B lymphocytes. *Annu Rev Immunol* 1992; **10**: 97–121.

19. Reth M. Antigen receptor tail clue. *Nature* 1989; **338**: 383–4.

20. Gold MR, Matsuuchi L, Kelly RB, DeFranco AL. Tyrosine phosphorylation of components of the B-cell antigen receptors following receptor crosslinking. *Proc Natl Acad Sci USA* 1991; **88**: 3436–40.

21. Jugloff LS, Jongstra-Bilen J. Cross-linking of the IgM receptor induces rapid translocation of IgM-associated Ig alpha, Lyn, and Syk tyrosine kinases to the membrane skeleton. *J Immunol* 1997; **159**: 1096–106.

22. Rowley RB, Burkhardt AL, Chao HG, Matsueda GR, Bolen JB. Syk protein-tyrosine kinase is regulated by tyrosine-phosphorylated Ig alpha/Ig beta immunoreceptor tyrosine activation motif binding and autophosphorylation. *J Biol Chem* 1995; **270**: 11590–4.

23. Maas A, Hendriks RW. Role of Bruton's tyrosine kinase in B-cell development. *Dev Immunol* 2001; **8**: 171–81.

24. Smith KG, Fearon DT. Receptor modulators of B-cell receptor signalling – CD19/CD22. *Curr Top Microbiol Immunol* 2000; **245**: 195–212.

25. Smith KG, Tarlinton DM, Doody GM, Hibbs ML, Fearon DT. Inhibition of the B-cell by CD22: a requirement for Lyn. *J Exp Med* 1998; **187**: 807–11.

26. Doody GM, Justement LB, Delibrias CC et al. A role in B-cell activation for CD22 and the protein tyrosine phosphatase SHP. *Science* 1995; **269**: 242–4.

27. Ansel KM, Harris RB, Cyster JG. CXCL13 is required for B1 cell homing, natural antibody production, and body cavity immunity. *Immunity* 2002; **16**: 67–76.

28. Watanabe N, Ikuta K, Fagarasan S, Yazumi S, Chiba T, Honjo T. Migration and differentiation of autoreactive B-1 cells induced by activated gamma/delta T cells in antierythrocyte immunoglobulin transgenic mice. *J Exp Med* 2000; **192**: 1577–86.

29. Martin F, Kearney JF. B1 cells: similarities and differences with other B-cell subsets. *Curr Opin Immunol* 2001; **13**: 195–201.

30. Poe JC, Hasegawa M, Tedder TF. CD19, CD21, and CD22: multifaceted response regulators of B lymphocyte signal transduction. *Int Rev Immunol* 2001; **20**: 739–62.

31. Qian Y, Santiago C, Borrero M, Tedder TF, Clarke SH. Lupus-specific antiribonucleoprotein B-cell tolerance in nonautoimmune mice is maintained by differentiation to B-1 and governed by B-cell receptor signaling thresholds. *J Immunol* 2001; **166**: 2412–19.

32. Borrero M, Clarke SH. Low-affinity anti-Smith antigen B cells are regulated by anergy as opposed to developmental arrest or differentiation to B-1. *J Immunol* 2002; **168**: 13–21.

33. Martin F, Kearney JF. B-cell subsets and the mature preimmune repertoire. Marginal zone and B1 B cells as part of a 'natural immune memory'. *Immunol Rev* 2000; **175**: 70–9.

34. Guinamard R, Okigaki M, Schlessinger J, Ravetch JV. Absence of marginal zone B cells in Pyk-2-deficient mice defines their role in the humoral response. *Nat Immunol* 2000; **1**: 31–6.

35. Cariappa A, Tang M, Parng C et al. The follicular versus marginal zone B lymphocyte cell fate decision is regulated by Aiolos, Btk, and CD21. *Immunity* 2001; **14**: 603–15.

36. Matsumoto M, Fu YX, Molina H, Chaplin DD. Lymphotoxin-alpha-deficient and TNF receptor-I-deficient mice define developmental and functional characteristics of germinal centers. *Immunol Rev* 1997; **156**: 137–44.

37. Seo S, Buckler J, Erikson J. Novel roles for Lyn in B-cell migration and lipopolysaccharide responsiveness revealed using anti-double-stranded DNA Ig transgenic mice. *J Immunol* 2001; **166**: 3710–16.

38. Benlagha K, Weiss A, Beavis A, Teyton L, Bendelac A. In vivo identification of glycolipid antigen-specific T cells using fluorescent CD1d tetramers. *J Exp Med* 2000; **191**: 1895–903.

39. Zeng D, Lee MK, Tung J, Brendolan A, Strober S. Cutting edge: a role for CD1 in the pathogenesis of lupus in NZB/NZW mice. *J Immunol* 2000; **164**: 5000–4.

40. Gross JA, Johnston J, Mudri S et al. TACI and BCMA are receptors for a TNF homologue implicated in B-cell autoimmune disease. *Nature* 2000; **404**: 995–9.

41. Reif K, Ekland EH, Ohl L et al. Balanced responsiveness to chemoattractants from adjacent zones determines B-cell position. *Nature* 2002; **416**: 94–9.

42. Tarlinton D. Germinal centers: form and function. *Curr Opin Immunol* 1998; **10**: 245–51.

43. Schneider P, MacKay F, Steiner V et al. BAFF, a novel ligand of the tumor necrosis factor family, stimulates B-cell growth. *J Exp Med* 1999; **189**: 1747–56.

44. Han S, Hathcock K, Zheng B, Kepler TB, Hodes R, Kelsoe G. Cellular interaction in germinal centers. Roles of CD40 ligand and B7–2 in established germinal centers. *J Immunol* 1995; **155**: 556–67.

45. Foy TM, Laman JD, Ledbetter JA, Aruffo A, Claassen E, Noelle RJ. gp39–CD40 interactions are essential for germinal center formation and the development of B-cell memory. *J Exp Med* 1994; **180**: 157–63.

46. Grewal IS, Flavell RA. CD40 and CD154 in cell-mediated immunity. *Annu Rev Immunol* 1998; **16**: 111–35.

47. Mackay F, Woodcock SA, Lawton P et al. Mice transgenic for BAFF develop lymphocytic disorders along with autoimmune manifestations. *J Exp Med* 1999; **190**: 1697–710.

48. Wiesendanger M, Scharff MD, Edelmann W. Somatic hypermutation, transcription, and DNA mismatch repair. *Cell* 1998; **94**: 415–18.

49. Poltoratsky V, Woo CJ, Tippin B, Martin A, Goodman MF, Scharff MD. Expression of error-prone polymerases in BL2 cells activated for Ig somatic hypermutation. *Proc Natl Acad Sci USA* 2001; **98**: 7976–81.

50. Diaz M, Verkoczy LK, Flajnik MF, Klinman NR. Decreased frequency of somatic hypermutation and impaired affinity maturation but intact germinal center formation in mice expressing antisense RNA to DNA polymerase zeta. *J Immunol* 2001; **167**: 327–35.

51. Zeng X, Winter DB, Kasmer C, Kraemer KH, Lehmann AR, Gearhart PJ. DNA polymerase eta is an A–T mutator in somatic hypermutation of immunoglobulin variable genes. *Nat Immunol* 2001; **2**: 537–41.

52. Zan H, Komori A, Li Z et al. The translesion DNA polymerase zeta plays a major role in Ig and bcl-6 somatic hypermutation. *Immunity* 2001; **14**: 643–53.

53. Winter DB, Gearhart PJ. Altered spectra of hypermutation in DNA repair-deficient mice. *Philos Trans R Soc Lond B Biol Sci* 2001; **356**: 5–11.

54. Muramatsu M, Kinoshita K, Fagarasan S, Yamada S, Shinkai Y, Honjo T. Class switch recombination and hypermutation require activation-induced cytidine deaminase (AID), a potential RNA editing enzyme. *Cell* 2000; **102**: 553–63.

55. Revy P, Muto T, Levy Y et al. Activation-induced cytidine deaminase (AID) deficiency causes the autosomal recessive form of the Hyper-IgM syndrome (HIGM2). *Cell* 2000; **102**: 565–75.

56. Diamond B, Katz JB, Paul E, Aranow C, Lustgarten D, Scharff MD. The role of somatic mutation in the pathogenic anti-DNA response. *Annu Rev Immunol* 1992; **10**: 731–57.

57. Peeva E, Diamond B, Putterman C. The structure and derivation of antibodies and autoantibodies. In: Wallace D, Hahn B, eds. *Dubois' Lupus Erythematosus.* (Philadelphia: Lippincott, Williams and Wilkins, 2002) 391–413.

58. Arpin C, Banchereau J, Liu YJ. Memory B cells are biased towards terminal differentiation: a strategy that may prevent repertoire freezing. *J Exp Med* 1997; **186**: 931–40.

59. Maruyama M, Lam KP, Rajewsky K. Memory B-cell persistence is independent of persisting immunizing antigen. *Nature* 2000; **407**: 636–42.

60. Jacquot S. CD27/CD70 interactions regulate T dependent B-cell differentiation. *Immunol Res* 2000; **21**: 23–30.

61. Calame KL. Plasma cells: finding new light at the end of B-cell development. *Nat Immunol* 2001; **2**: 1103–8.

62. Manz RA, Radbruch A. Plasma cells for a lifetime? *Eur J Immunol* 2002; **32**: 923–7.

63. Slifka MK, Ahmed R. Long-lived plasma cells: a mechanism for maintaining persistent antibody production. *Curr Opin Immunol* 1998; **10**: 252–8.

64. Wu Q, Salomon B, Chen M et al. Reversal of spontaneous autoimmune insulitis in nonobese diabetic mice by soluble lymphotoxin receptor. *J Exp Med* 2001; **193**: 1327–32.

65. Weyand CM, Goronzy JJ, Takemura S, Kurtin PJ. Cell–cell interactions in synovitis. Interactions between T cells and B cells in rheumatoid arthritis. *Arthritis Res* 2000; **2**: 457–63.

66. Hjelmstrom P. Lymphoid neogenesis: de novo formation of lymphoid tissue in chronic inflammation through expression of homing chemokines. *J Leukoc Biol* 2001; **69**: 331–9.

67. Hahn B, Tsao B. Antibodies to DNA. In: Wallace D, Hahn B, eds. *Dubois' Lupus Erythematosus.* (Philadelphia: Lippincott, Williams and Wilkins, 2002) 425–45.

68. Davidson A, Diamond B. Autoimmune diseases. *N Engl J Med* 2001; **345**: 340–51.

69. Reininger L, Winkler TH, Kalberer CP, Jourdan M, Melchers F, Rolink AG. Intrinsic B-cell defects in NZB and NZW mice contribute to systemic lupus erythematosus in (NZB × NZW)F1 mice. *J Exp Med* 1996; **184**: 853–61.

70. Goodnow CC, Cyster JG, Hartley SB et al. Self-tolerance checkpoints in B lymphocyte development. *Adv Immunol* 1995; **59**: 279–68.

71. Nemazee D. Receptor editing in B cells. *Adv Immunol* 2000; **74**: 89–126.

72. Nussenzweig MC. Immune receptor editing: revise and select. *Cell* 1998; **95**: 875–8.

73. Li H, Jiang Y, Prak EL, Radic M, Weigert M. Editors and editing of anti-DNA receptors. *Immunity* 2001; **15**: 947–57.

74. Itoh K, Meffre E, Albesiano E et al. Immunoglobulin heavy chain variable region gene replacement as a mechanism for receptor revision in rheumatoid arthritis synovial tissue B lymphocytes. *J Exp Med* 2000; **192**: 1151–64.

75. Dorner T, Foster SJ, Farner NL, Lipsky PE. Immunoglobulin kappa chain receptor editing in systemic lupus erythematosus. *J Clin Invest* 1998; **102**: 688–94.

76. Hande S, Notidis E, Manser T. Bcl-2 obstructs negative selection of autoreactive, hypermutated antibody V regions during memory B-cell development. *Immunity* 1998; **8**: 189–98.

77. Smith KG, Light A, O'Reilly LA, Ang SM, Strasser A, Tarlinton D. bcl-2 transgene expression inhibits apoptosis in the germinal center and reveals differences in the selection of memory B cells and bone marrow antibody-forming cells. *J Exp Med* 2000; **191**: 475–84.

78. Singh R, Ebling F, Kumar V, Hahn B. Involvement of regulatory T cells in limiting induction of anti-DNA antibodies in non-autoimmune mice. *Arthritis Rheum* 1999; **42**: S362 (abstract).

79. Singh RR. The potential use of peptides and vaccination to treat systemic lupus erythematosus. *Curr Opin Rheumatol* 2000; **12**: 399–406.

80. Hirose S, Yan K, Abe M et al. Precursor B cells for autoantibody production in genomically Fas-intact autoimmune disease are not subject to Fas-mediated immune elimination. *Proc Natl Acad Sci USA* 1997; **94**: 9291–15.

81. Consigny PH, Cauquelin B, Agnamey P et al. High prevalence of co-factor independent anticardiolipin antibodies in malaria exposed individuals. *Clin Exp Immunol* 2002; **127**: 158–64.

82. Wong RC, Wilson R, Silcock R, Kratzing LM, Looke D. Unusual combination of positive IgG autoantibodies in acute Q-fever infection. *Intern Med J* 2001; **31**: 432–5.

83. Josephson C, Nuss R, Jacobson L et al. The varicella-autoantibody syndrome. *Pediatr Res* 2001; **50**: 345–52.

84. Mandik-Nayak L, Bui A, Noorchashm H, Eaton A, Erikson J. Regulation of anti-double-stranded DNA B cells in nonautoimmune mice: localization to the T–B interface of the splenic follicle. *J Exp Med* 1997; **186**: 1257–67.

85. Hoshino K, Takeuchi O, Kawai T et al. Cutting edge: Toll-like receptor 4 (TLR4)-deficient mice are hyporesponsive to lipopolysaccharide: evidence for TLR4 as the Lps gene product. *J Immunol* 1999; **162**: 3749–52.

86. Takeuchi O, Hoshino K, Kawai T et al. Differential roles of TLR2 and TLR4 in recognition of gram-negative and gram-positive bacterial cell wall components. *Immunity* 1999; **11**: 443–51.

87. Krieg AM. CpG motifs in bacterial DNA and their immune effects. *Annu Rev Immunol* 2002; **20**: 709–60.

88. Carroll M. Innate immunity in the etiopathology of autoimmunity. *Nat Immunol* 2001; **2**: 1089–90.

89. Leadbetter E, Rifkin IR, Hohlbaum AM, Beaudette BC, Shlomchik MJ, Marshak-Rothstein. A. Chromatin–IgG complexes activate B cells by dual engagement of IgM and Toll-like receptors. *Nature* 2002; **416**: 603–7.

90. Beutler B. Autoimmunity and apoptosis: the Crohn's connection. *Immunity* 2001; **15**: 5–14.

91. Yoh K, Itoh K, Enomoto A et al. Nrf2-deficient female mice develop lupus-like autoimmune nephritis. *Kidney Int* 2001; **60**: 1343–53.

92. Lu Q, Lemke G. Homeostatic regulation of the immune system by receptor tyrosine kinases of the Tyro 3 family. *Science* 2001; **293**: 306–11.

93. Wang J, Lo JC, Foster A et al. The regulation of T-cell homeostasis and autoimmunity by T cell-derived LIGHT. *J Clin Invest* 2001; **108**: 1771–80.

94. Wakeland EK, Liu K, Graham RR, Behrens TW. Delineating the genetic basis of systemic lupus erythematosus. *Immunity* 2001; **15**: 397–408.

95. O'Dell JR. Treating rheumatoid arthritis early: a window of opportunity? *Arthritis Rheum* 2002; **46**: 283–5.

96. Wallace D. Current and emerging lupus treatments. *Am J Manag Care* 2001; **7**: 490–5.

97. Kuo GM, Boumpas DT, Illei GG, Yarboro C, Pucino F, Burstein AH. Fludarabine pharmacokinetics after subcutaneous and intravenous administration in patients with lupus nephritis. *Pharmacotherapy* 2001; **21**: 528–33.

98. Feldmann M, Maini RN, Bondeson J, Taylor P, Foxwell BM, Brennan FM. Cytokine blockade in rheumatoid arthritis. *Adv Exp Med Biol* 2001; **490**: 119–27.

99. van Deventer SJ. Transmembrane TNF-alpha, induction of apoptosis, and the efficacy of TNF targeting therapies in Crohn's disease. *Gastroenterology* 2001; **121**: 1242–6.

100. Llorente L, Richaud-Patin Y, Garcia-Padilla C et al. Clinical and biologic effects of anti-interleukin-10 monoclonal antibody administration in systemic lupus erythematosus. *Arthritis Rheum* 2000; **43**: 1790–800.

101. Abrams JR, Lebwohl MG, Guzzo CA et al. CTLA4Ig-mediated blockade of T-cell costimulation in patients with psoriasis vulgaris. *J Clin Invest* 1999; **103**: 1243–52.

102. Boumpas DT, Furie RA, Manzi S, Illei GG, Balw JE, Vaisnaw A. A short course of BG9588 (anti-CD40L antibody) improves serologic activity and decreases hematuria in patients with proliferative glomerulonephritis. *Arthritis Rheum* 2001; **44**: S387 (abstract).

103. Davis JC Jr, Totoritis MC, Rosenberg J, Sklenar TA, Wofsy D. Phase I clinical trial of a monoclonal antibody against CD40-ligand (IDEC-131) in patients with systemic lupus erythematosus. *J Rheumatol* 2001; **28**: 95–101.

104. Anolik J, Campbell D, Ritchlin C et al. B lymphocyte depletion as a novel treatment for systemic lupus erythematosus (SLE): phase I/II trial of Rituximab (Rituxan) in SLE. *Arthritis Rheum* 2001; **44**: S387 (abstract).

105. Keane J, Gershon S, Wise RP et al. Tuberculosis associated with infliximab, a tumor necrosis factor alpha-neutralizing agent. *N Engl J Med* 2001; **345**: 1098–104.

106. Van Den Bosch F, Kruithof E, Baeten D et al. Randomized double-blind comparison of chimeric monoclonal antibody to tumor necrosis factor alpha (infliximab) versus placebo in active spondylarthropathy. *Arthritis Rheum* 2002; **46**: 755–65.

107. Charles PJ, Smeenk RJ, De Jong J, Feldmann M, Maini RN. Assessment of antibodies to double-stranded DNA induced in rheumatoid arthritis patients following treatment with infliximab, a monoclonal antibody to tumor necrosis factor alpha: findings in open-label and randomized placebo-controlled trials. *Arthritis Rheum* 2000; **43**: 2383–90.

108. Mohan N, Edwards ET, Cupps TR et al. Demyelination occurring during anti-tumor necrosis factor alpha therapy for inflammatory arthritides. *Arthritis Rheum* 2001; **44**: 2862–9.

109. Gordon C, Ranges GE, Greenspan JS, Wofsy D. Chronic therapy with recombinant tumor necrosis factor-alpha in autoimmune NZB/NZW F1 mice. *Clin Immunol Immunopathol* 1989; **52**: 421–34.

110. Huang W, Sinha J, Newman J et al. The effect of anti-CD40 ligand antibody on B cells in human SLE. *Arthritis Rheum* 2002; **46**: 1554–62.

111. Grammer AC, Shinohara S, Vazquez E, Gur H, Illei G, Lipsky PE. Normalization of peripheral B cells following treatment of active SLE patients with humanized anti-CD154 MAb (5c8, BG9588). *Arthritis Rheum* 2001; **44**: S282 (abstract).

112. Daikh DI, Finck BK, Linsley PS, Hollenbaugh D, Wofsy D. Long-term inhibition of murine lupus by brief simultaneous blockade of the B7/CD28 and CD40/gp39 costimulation pathways. *J Immunol* 1997; **159**: 3104–8.

113. Mihara M, Tan I, Chuzhin Y et al. CTLA4Ig inhibits T cell-dependent B-cell maturation in murine systemic lupus erythematosus. *J Clin Invest* 2000; **106**: 91–101.

114. Kalled SL, Cutler AH, Datta SK, Thomas DW. Anti-CD40 ligand antibody treatment of SNF1 mice with established nephritis: preservation of kidney function. *J Immunol* 1998; **160**: 2158–65.

115. Daikh DI, Wofsy D. Cutting edge: reversal of murine lupus nephritis with CTLA4Ig and cyclophosphamide. *J Immunol* 2001; **166**: 2913–16.

116. Wang X, Huang W, Mihara M, Sinha J, Davidson A. Mechanism of action of combined short term CTLA4Ig and anti-CD40L in murine SLE. *J Immunol* 2002; **168**: 2046–53.

117. Edwards JC, Cambridge G. Sustained improvement in rheumatoid arthritis following a protocol designed to deplete B lymphocytes. *Rheumatology (Oxford)* 2001; **40**: 205–11.

118. Wallace DJ. Clinical and pharmacological experience with LJP-394. *Expert Opin Investig Drugs* 2001; **10**: 111–17.

119. Burns C, Quesada S, Noelle R, Schned A. CD40–CD154 interactions in the pathogenesis of

murine lupus: the beneficial effects of early and late anti-CD154 antibody treatment appear to be mediated through different mechanisms. *Arthritis Rheum* 2001; **44**: S397.

120. Sinha J, Wang X, Huang W, Schiffer L, Davidson A. Short term costimulatory blockade combined with cyclophosphamide does not abrogate glomerular deposition of antibodies but attenuates the kidney inflammatory response. *Arthritis Rheum* 2001; **44**: S397 (abstract).

121. Becher B, Durell BG, Miga AV, Hickey WF, Noelle RJ. The clinical course of experimental autoimmune encephalomyelitis and inflammation is controlled by the expression of CD40 within the central nervous system. *J Exp Med* 2001; **193**: 967–74.

122. Sato S, Hasegawa M, Fujimoto M, Tedder TF, Takehara K. Quantitative genetic variation in CD19 expression correlates with autoimmunity. *J Immunol* 2000; **165**: 6635–43.

123. Kouki T, Sawai Y, Gardine CA, Fisfalen ME, Alegre ML, DeGroot LJ. CTLA-4 gene polymorphism at position 49 in exon 1 reduces the inhibitory function of CTLA-4 and contributes to the pathogenesis of Graves' disease. *J Immunol* 2000; **165**: 6606–11.

124. Matsumoto I, Maccioni M, Lee DM et al. How antibodies to a ubiquitous cytoplasmic enzyme may provoke joint-specific autoimmune disease. *Nat Immunol* 2002; **3**: 360–5.

125. Luross JA, Williams NA. The genetic and immunopathological processes underlying collagen-induced arthritis. *Immunology* 2001; **103**: 407–16.

126. Wilder RL, Remmers EF, Kawahito Y, Gulko PS, Cannon GW, Griffiths MM. Genetic factors regulating experimental arthritis in mice and rats. *Curr Dir Autoimmun* 1999; **1**: 121–65.

127. Ozkaynak E, Gao W, Shemmeri N et al. Importance of ICOS-B7RP-1 costimulation in acute and chronic allograft rejection. *Nat Immunol* 2001; **2**: 591–6.

128. Trambley J, Bingaman AW, Lin A et al. Asialo GM1(+) CD8(+) T cells play a critical role in costimulation blockade-resistant allograft rejection. *J Clin Invest* 1999; **104**: 1715–22.

3

Macrophages

Peter LEM van Lent and Wim B van den Berg

Introduction • Resident intima macrophages in rheumatoid arthritis • Differentiation and function of macrophages in RA synovium • Activation of synovial macrophages • Macrophages and joint destruction • Depletion of type A intima cells inhibits onset of arthritis • Final remarks • References

INTRODUCTION

Rheumatoid arthritis (RA) is characterized by chronic inflammation in multiple joints and concomitant destruction of cartilage and bone. Macrophages play a crucial role in both the inflammatory process and tissue destruction.[1–3] Macrophages become activated by the RA process in the synovial tissue, either directly through stimulation with bacterial or viral triggers, or indirectly through T- and B-cell-mediated events. The latter responses can be directed to joint-specific autoantigens, but may also include reactions to persistent viral and bacterial elements. Although RA has been considered as an autoimmune process, a crucial autoantigen has not been defined and it seems more likely that we are dealing with multiple candidate triggers. This argues for general therapeutic approaches at a downstream level, making activated macrophages an obvious target.

RA is a systemic disease, with its main expression in body compartments which are surrounded by a synovial lining layer, containing large amounts of macrophages. Such compartments include diarthrodial joints, and

precipitation of the RA process in such areas underlines the crucial role of tissue macrophages in disease onset. During active arthritis, monocytes infiltrate from the blood into the synovium, differentiate into mature macrophages and form the dominant cell type in the inflamed synovium. However, synovial lining macrophages remain a crucial source of inflammatory mediators and contribute significantly to local cytokine and chemokine production. It is of great interest that RA synovial macrophages appear to express deranged levels of Fcγ receptors, and proof is accumulating that an aberrant reaction of macrophages to immune complexes (ICs), leading to prolonged activation, contributes to increased and prolonged release of proinflammatory and cartilage-destructive cytokines. Therapeutic approaches targeting the macrophage itself or its dominant proinflammatory mediators have already been shown to be efficient in the treatment of RA. Inhibition of the macrophage-derived master cytokines tumor necrosis factor alpha (TNF-α) and interleukin-1 (IL-1) created a major breakthrough in the treatment of this crippling disease. Insights into mechanisms of macrophage activation and mediators involved in that process may provide novel targets for further optimization of therapy.

RESIDENT INTIMA MACROPHAGES IN RHEUMATOID ARTHRITIS

The inside of the diarthrodial joint, the preferential site for development of RA, is lined by a layer of cells, usually one to three cells in thickness, called the intima. This layer contains two types of cells, the fibroblast-like type B cell and the macrophage-like type A cell, which interdigitate using cytoplasmic processes.[4] These cells are enclosed within a matrix, probably produced by the lining cell itself, containing collagen type IV, forming a covalently stabilized polygonal framework, and a second interlocking polymer network of laminin. Immunohistologic investigations have shown that three of the four constituents forming a basement membrane (collagen type IV, heparan sulfate proteoglycan and laminin) are present, but that entactin, a sulfated glycoprotein that connects laminin and type IV collagen, is absent. The intima lining sits on compact loose connective tissue bearing a vascular plexus which provides a close contact with the blood vessels. The origin of the type A cell is probably a monocyte, as shown in elegant studies using mice with the Chediak Higashi syndrome. Monocytes of these mice containing crystals were transferred to control mice, and kinetic studies showed accumulation of crystal-containing type A cells in the lining layer.[5] These cells are constantly replaced via the circulation, although the turnover is slow. After selective removal of type A cells in the intima of mice, it takes more than 30 days before the lining cell layer returns to normal levels.[6]

As a first sign of onset of arthritis, intima cells become activated. Intima cells form a strategic barrier within the joint. Substances leaking from the joint, bacterial infections or immune complexes formed within the synovial fluid first meet this layer, and the abundance of receptors expressed by type A cells leads to phagocytosis and activation of these cells. Moreover, this layer lies just above the vascular plexus in the synovium, which makes these cells also very accessible to substances arriving from the bloodstream. Immunolocalization studies have shown that phagocytic intima cells express many proinflammatory factors, like cytokines IL-1α, TNF-α, IL-6 and IL-15 and chemokines like IL-8 or MCP-1, but also growth factors like granulocyte–macrophage colony-stimulating factor (GM-CSF) and transforming growth factor beta (TGF-β).[7] As type A cells produce various chemokines, these cells are involved in attraction of inflammatory cells during the onset of arthritis and probably also in the arrest of inflammatory cells within the synovium during the chronic phase.

DIFFERENTIATION AND FUNCTION OF MACROPHAGES IN RA SYNOVIUM

Activation of the lining layer directs the influx of inflammatory cells, such as polymorphonuclear leucocyte (PMN), lymphocytes (T and B cells) and large amounts of monocytes (Figure 3.1). During RA, a number of alterations in the synovial membrane are observed. Synovial lining cells increase many fold. Type A macrophages still form the predominant population in the hypertrophied intima, approaching 50–70% of cells.[4] Superimposed on this is a highly vascular subintima filled with mononuclear cells, including T and B cells and large numbers of macrophages, often forming aggregates around the blood vessels. Most of the macrophages are thought to stem from monocytes which have infiltrated into the joint, where they differentiate into macrophages.[8] A small proportion may be derived from locally dividing mononuclear phagocytes. Chemokine receptor expression is different on RA monocytes in peripheral blood and synovial fluid (significantly higher CCR3, CCR4 and CCR5 levels in synovial fluid[9]). CCR1 and CCR2 seem to be crucial for monocyte recruitment. CCR3 and CCR5 may play a role in monocyte–macrophage tissue migration or retention. In vivo, generation of monocytes is controlled by various growth factors, including IL-3, GM-CSF and M-CSF. These factors are abundantly present in the RA joint, and are potent stimulators of CD34+ stem cells, which have been found to infiltrate the joints. As such,

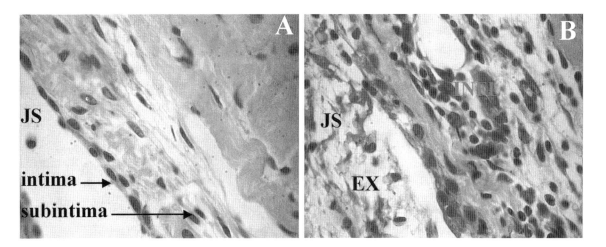

Figure 3.1 Synovial lining layer in knee joints of normal (A) and arthritic (B) mice. JS, joint space; EX, exudate; INFL, infiltrate. Original magnification ×400. Hematoxylin/eosin staining.

local production and maturation may contribute to the total macrophage cell mass.

Monocyte differentiation into macrophages in the RA synovium is highly versatile. Many differentiation stadia are found, reflecting various subpopulations of cells which are probably involved in different aspects of immune and effector mechanisms. Some of the maturation stages are now identified by CD markers, as listed in Tables 3.1 and 3.2. It is a recent finding that an unexpectedly large subpopulation of CD68[+] macrophages express DC-SIGN, a receptor which is normally expressed only on dendritic cells.[10,11] DC-SIGN is a crucial receptor involved in the initial interaction with intercellular adhesion molecule-3 (ICAM-3) expressing naive T cells, which are abundantly present in RA synovia, and blockade of DC-SIGN prevents binding and subsequent antigen presentation. This suggests that these DC-SIGN-positive macrophages contribute to local immune activation, apart from the scant numbers of fully matured dendritic cells.

Expression of different surface markers probably has consequences for macrophage effector function, ranging from more pro- to anti-inflammatory activity. Such a mixture of cell types was found earlier in the chronically

Table 3.1 CD markers on human tissue macrophages.

Functional aspects	CD markers
Adhesion and migration	CD33, CD169, CCR2, CCR5
Cytokine receptors	CD25, CD119, CDw121b, EMR-1
Fcγ and complement receptor (CR)	CD16, CD32, CD64, CD23
Microbial pattern recognition receptors	CD11b, CD204, CD68, CD14, CD206
T-cell activation	MHC class II

Table 3.2 Differences between type 1 and type 2 cytokine polarized macrophages.

Functional aspects	Type 1	Type 2
Adhesion/migration	CCR-5	CCR-2
Microbial pattern recognition receptor	CD206	CD206[++]

inflamed lung, where proinflammatory and suppressor macrophage populations were identified.[12] This diversity is in line with observations in RA tissue, which indicate that many, but certainly not all, CD68+ cells express MRP14, a marker for macrophage activation.[13] Furthermore, it is a consistent finding that only a limited number of cells produce TNF and IL-1, whereas other subpopulations produce no or anti-inflammatory cytokines like IL-6, IL-10 and TGF-β. Further research into the identification of cell surface markers akin to various subgroups of macrophages is warranted, as it may provide targets for more selective anti-inflammatory therapy.

Normal tissue macrophages and young monocytes, recently immigrated into normal tissues, are quiescent. In an activated state, as found in the synovium of RA patients, macrophages acquire multiple functions. First, they elaborate chemokines involved in PMN, monocyte and T-cell migration. Integrins and vascular cell adhesion molecules are upregulated under the influence of IL-1, TNF-α and interferon gamma (IFN-γ) release. Moreover, reactive oxygen and nitrogen intermediates are produced, eliciting local tissue damage. Cytokines like platelet-derived growth factor (PDGF), fibroblast growth factor (FGF) and TNF-α enhance the growth and proliferation of lining macrophages through paracrine interaction with the fibroblast-like lining cells. Activated macrophages also release angiogenesis-promoting factors like TGF-β, angiotropin and vascular endothelial growth factor (VEGF), responsible for neovascularization and further increase of the subintimal layer.

Apart from a role in synovial activation and growth, matured macrophages may function as antigen-presenting cells, initiating local age-specific T- and B-cell responses, and thereby amplifying immune-mediated macrophage activation. Moreover, macrophages producing TNF, IL-1 and destructive enzymes will contribute to cartilage erosion. The ultimate fate of macrophages in the RA synovium is not known, but a large proportion of the CD68+ lining cells show signs of apoptosis.[4] A minority may traffic to other sites, such as remote secondary lymphoid organs.

ACTIVATION OF SYNOVIAL MACROPHAGES

The pathogenic mechanisms involved in synovial macrophage activation are as yet unknown. Theoretically, there is either direct activation by phlogistic stimuli such as bacteria or viruses, or the system is turned on indirectly, as an effector mechanism of immune-mediated events. In principle, the latter can be caused by T- and B-cell-mediated recognition of exogenous antigens reaching the joints, including bacteria and viruses, or by immune responses to joint-specific autoantigens (Figure 3.2). Chronicity of the process of macrophage activation may be due to persistence of stimuli, which is obvious in the case of autoantigens, and/or deranged responsiveness of the cells, which acquire tumor-like properties. In particular, viral stimuli have been suggested to be involved in the latter process, although a viral contribution to chronicity of RA is still to be proven.

Endogenous bacterial fragments enter the joint as a continuous process and, when poorly degraded by the macrophages, do form an obvious, persistent stimulus for macrophage activation. Recently, it was found that bacterial DNA fragments bearing a CpG motif are also powerful stimulants of macrophages.[14,15] In addition to this, when T-cell tolerance against

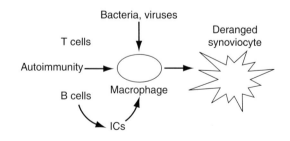

Figure 3.2 Stimuli involved in synovial macrophage activation.

bacterial fragments is lost, T cells are turned on locally and their products activate the macrophage. As a further element of local immune events, antibodies can be generated, forming ICs at the site and stimulating macrophages through their Fc receptors.

In principle, any protein antigen reaching the joint in sufficient quantities and retained in avascular joint structures, due to charge-mediated binding or antibody-mediated trapping, may function as a persistent trigger. As such, the difference between autoantigens of joint structures or endogenous and exogenous proteins sticking to joint structures is mainly semantic, although it may be argued that regulation of tolerance is different.

Animal model studies have identified a number of potential autoantigens, including cartilage-derived collagen type II, proteoglycan and GP-39, citrullinated proteins, and even the ubiquitously expressed enzyme glucose phosphate isomerase (GPI), showing cartilage-adhering potential.[16–19] There is reason to believe that the antigen causing RA might be associated with cartilage, since removal of cartilage at joint replacement is sufficient to silence such a joint, without the need for synovectomy. Nevertheless, it seems unlikely that one particular autoantigen is at the base of RA pathology, and a multiple trigger concept is more obvious. This leaves us with therapeutic options involving interference with general elements of immune functions, such as suppressive T-cell cytokines. Attempts to use joint-specific antigens to induce tolerance and to generate bystander suppression of non-related T-cell responses were successful in animal models, but convincing effects and therapeutic applicability in RA patients have yet to be shown.

Efforts to treat RA by depleting T cells, using monoclonal antibodies or immunotoxins, have been disappointing.[20] No correlation was found between elimination of lymphocytes and clinical responses. One potential explanation may be insufficient depletion of synovial T cells to a level below the minimum threshold needed to sustain joint inflammation. However, during acquired immunodeficiency syndrome, in which profound CD4+ T-cell lymphopenia is evident, RA is not necessarily suppressed.[21]

T-cell macrophage activation and regulating cytokines

The belief in T-cell activation of macrophages was shaken by the difficulty in finding significant amounts of IL-2 or IFN-γ in inflamed RA synovia. However, the recent identification of IL-17 as a Th1-derived cytokine and its clear presence in many RA patients has led to renewed interest.[22,23] This revival of interest is strengthened by the old finding of the virtual absence of the counteracting cytokine IL-4. IL-17 stimulated the production of IL-1 and TNF-α by human macrophages and amplified the effects of IL-1 and TNF-α on synoviocytes. Furthermore, animal model data support the arthritogenic potential of this cytokine. When IL-17 was overexpressed in the joints of mice with experimental collagen type II arthritis (CIA), it strongly aggravated joint inflammation and cartilage destruction, independent of IL-1.[24] In addition, blockade of IL-17 in classic CIA significantly ameliorated the disease.

A further argument for IL-17 and T-cell involvement is the abundance of IL-15 in RA synovia. This cytokine is produced by macrophages and is a major stimulus of T-cell activation. Such IL-15-exposed T cells become TNF-producing cells and are potent activators of macrophage TNF production, in an IL-17- and cell–cell contact-dependent fashion.[25,26]

Additional cytokines involved in boosting T-cell responses are IL-12 and IL-18.[27,28] IL-12 and IL-18, in particular, are found in significant quantities in RA synovia and are products of activated macrophages. Although IL-18 alone is not a potent maturation factor, it markedly synergizes with IL-12 in Th1 maturation. Both mediators are induced in macrophages by bacterial activation, and this provides the intriguing possibility that bacteria are not only phlogistic triggers but also amplify autoimmune responses in the joint through release of IL-12 and IL-18 (Figure 3.3). It may fit with the often suggested relationship between bacterial infections and

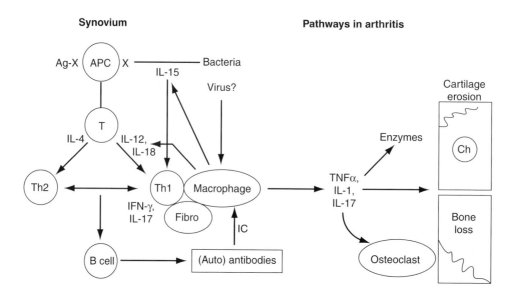

Figure 3.3 Cytokines in synovial activation and tissue destruction. APC, antigen-presenting cell.

arthritis. Apart from septic arthritis, arthritis occurs in patients with Lyme disease and infections of the throat and the gastrointestinal tract. In animal models IL-12 promoted transition from an acute, non-destructive joint inflammation to a chronic, destructive process. Neutralization of IL-12 as well as IL-18 markedly reduced autoimmune CIA, and also non-immune zymosan arthritis, underlining the fact that these cytokines are both immune potentiating as well as directly proinflammatory.[29,30,31]

Apart from promotion of antigen-specific responses through the above-mentioned cytokines, T cells may contribute to macrophage activation in a non-specific way. A vast majority of T cells present in RA synovia are of the naive CD45RA or memory CD45RO type. The abundant presence of the cytokine IL-6, involved in differentiation of the Th2 pathway, may be responsible for inhibiting excessive development of the Th1 subpopulation, with the result that most of the migrated T cells remain in their primary state. The latter cells may, however, still be involved in pathology. Synovial macrophages express large amounts of the receptor DC-SIGN, which can bind with

high affinity to ICAM-3, expressed on naive T cells. We have suggestive evidence that such binding of ICAM-3 to DC-SIGN leads to macrophage activation and TNF production. Earlier in vitro work already identified that fixed T cells, stimulated in an ag-independent manner, induced monocyte production of TNF-α but not IL-10,[26] although the underlying mechanism and contribution of various cell–cell surface ligands remains obscure.

Macrophage activation induced by immune complexes

One of the characteristic features of RA is the presence of high titers of autoantibodies. Impaired B-cell responses have been found within RA synovium and may be caused by impaired antigen presentation or clonal deletion. Autoantibodies are released in large amounts and target many antigens, forming ICs residing in the inflamed joint which contribute to macrophage activation. ICs are found in abundance in the synovial fluid, synovial layer and even the superficial layer of the cartilage. Many potential autoantigens have been defined, including citrullin and IgG. In the latter case, ICs include IgG isotype antibodies directed against the constant part of the IgG isotype. These often large ICs are recognized by Fcγ receptors (FcγR) expressed on the membrane of macrophages.

In the mouse, three FcγR classes have been described. FcγRI is a high-affinity receptor, whereas FcγRII and FcγRIII are low-affinity receptors. FcγRI and FcγRIII are activating receptors. Upon binding, intracellular signaling is mediated by an ITAM motif present in the intracytoplasmic part of the receptor leading to production of syk kinases, resulting in selective activation of genes. In contrast, FcγRII is an inhibiting receptor. Coligation of FcγRII with either FcγRI or FcγRIII leads to inactivation mediated by the ITIM motif present in the intracytoplasmic receptor.[32] All three FcγR classes are expressed on macrophages, and a balance between activating and inhibiting receptors determines the net reaction of the cell if exposed to ICs.

During RA, all three classes of FcγR receptor are elevated on synovial macrophages (Figure 3.4). In humans, two types of FcγRII have been identified, with FcγRIIa being an activating receptor, whereas FcγRIIb is probably the equivalent of the mouse type II inhibitory receptor. To identify which activating FcγRs are important in the onset and prolongation of arthritis, experimental models were studied in various FcγR-knockout mice. When experimental arthritis was passively induced by ICs, FcγRIII appeared to be the dominant FcγR in joint inflammation. Induction of IC arthritis in knee joints of FcγRIII−/− mice completely prevented the onset of arthritis, whereas in FcγRI−/− mice, joint inflammation continued and was not different from controls.[33] In contrast, using a mixture of T-cell and IC-mediated arthritis (antigen-induced arthritis model), we found that not FcγRIII, but FcγRI, was crucial.[34,35] Antigen-induced arthritis (AIA) was not reduced in FcγRIII-knockout mice, but was somewhat suppressed in FcγRI-deficient mice. As CIA is also FcγRIII dependent,[36] this may suggest that the onset of this model is more driven by anti-collagen type II antibodies than by anti-CII T cells.

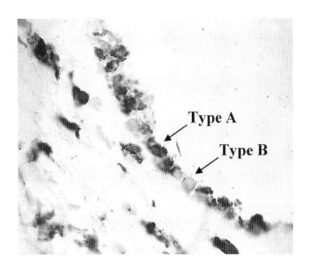

Figure 3.4 FcγRIII expression by macrophage-like type A but not by fibroblast-like type B cells in the intima of knee joints of normal mice.

The contribution of FcγRI and FcγRIII with respect to inflammation and cartilage pathology may differ, and suggestive evidence is accumulating that FcγRI is crucial in destruction, even in FcγRIII-dependent IC arthritis. Cytokines released during arthritis may influence the expression of activatory FcγR. IFN-γ, a cytokine produced mainly by activated Th1 cells but also in smaller amounts by activated macrophages, upregulates FcγRI and may explain why FcγRI becomes the dominant FcγR in the T-cell-mediated arthritis model. Other cytokines found in RA patients may also contribute to skewing of FcγR expression patterns.[37] IL-4 and IL-13 downregulate activating FcR. IL-10 upregulates FcγRI, whereas TGF-β upregulates FcγRIII (Figure 3.5).

Apart from the type of FcγR, the degree of FcγR expression and the relative balance between activatory and inhibitory receptor may be of utmost importance in regulating inflammation. Certain mouse strains appear to be hyperreactive to ICs. IC-mediated arthritis passively induced within knee joints of DBA/1 mice caused a severe phenotype, which became chronic, whereas the same amount of ICs placed

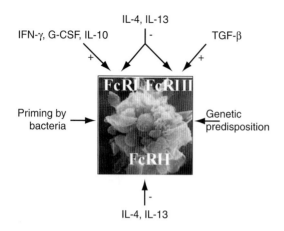

IL-4, IL-13

IFN-γ, G-CSF, IL-10   -   TGF-β

+   +

FcRI FcRII

Priming by bacteria →   ← Genetic predisposition

FcRIII

↑ -

IL-4, IL-13

Figure 3.5   FcγR regulation by cytokines.

into the knee joints of C57BL6 mice only induced a mild arthritis which disappeared after 3 days.[38] As synovial macrophages are crucial for the development of arthritis in both strains, peritoneal macrophages were screened for FcR expression. It appeared that normal macrophages from DBA/1 mice expressed higher FcγRIII and lower FcγRI levels if compared to peritoneal macrophages derived from C57BL6 mice. Upon activation by ICs, a prolonged rise in FcγRI and FcγRIII expression was found, whereas in C57BL6 mice, the rise in FcγR was normalized within 1 day.[39] Upregulation of activatory FcγR had physiologic consequences, since a high prolonged release of IL-1 was found in IC-activated DBA/1 macrophages, whereas release of IL-1 was much lower and only short-lasting in IC-activated BL/6 macrophages. This suggests that genetic differences in macrophages may be responsible for a different regulation of FcγR expression, resulting in prolonged higher expression of activatory receptors and lower expression of the inhibiting FcγRII receptor, leading to an aberrant response upon contact with ICs. A significant correlation was found between genes on the chromosome also containing FcγR and the propensity of mice to develop arthritis.[40,41] In line with this, mice which are not prone to

develop arthritis become highly vulnerable after deletion of the FcγRII gene.[42] Moreover, the ameliorating effect of intravenous IgG treatment is probably mediated by binding to the inhibiting FcγRII, leading to abrogation of intracellular signaling caused by ICs and regulated by the activatory FcR.[43]

MACROPHAGES AND JOINT DESTRUCTION

Destruction of bone and cartilage is a characteristic feature of RA. The number of lining layer macrophages has been found to correlate both with clinical disease activity and radiographic progression in chronic RA.[44] Macrophages may be involved in cartilage destruction by direct release of enzymes, by activation of fibroblasts, and indirectly by activation of catabolic pathways in chondrocytes.

The production of proteolytic enzymes by the inflamed synovium may contribute to the pathogenesis of articular damage,[45] in particular at sites of pannus overgrowth, where there is direct access of activated synovial cells to the cartilage matrix and more limited inhibition by enzyme inhibitors, abundantly present in the synovial fluid. Four families of proteases (metallo, aspartic, cysteine and serine) have been implicated and probably act synergistically to destroy the connective tissue components of the joint. Metalloproteinases (MMPs) are probably the most important group. Several MMPs (MMP-1, 2, 3, 7, 8, 9, 13) have been found to cleave aggrecan, the largest proteoglycan in the cartilage. Amino acid sequence analysis of proteoglycan breakdown products in RA synovial fluid has defined a major site of proteolytic cleavage in aggrecan found within the first interglobular domain of the aggrecan core protein.[46] Cleavage of this site results in the neoepitope VDIPEN, which remains in the cartilage, whereas the other part ending on FFGVG is found within the synovial fluid. Among the many MMP members, collagenase is thought to be of particular importance, since it represents the rate-limiting step in collagen breakdown and eventually leads to cartilage erosions. MMP-1 is strongly elevated in synovial fluid but also in the synovial membrane of patients with RA. More recently, MMP-13 has been identified and implicated in cartilage pathology.[47,48]

Neoepitopes identifying collagenase-mediated collagen breakdown in RA cartilage are abundant, and present also in deep cartilage layers, which may also suggest involvement of bone marrow-derived mediators in the destructive process. Proteolytic enzymes are upregulated in the synovial layer at a very early stage in the course of inflammatory arthritis.[49] The number of MMP 1 and MMP 13 mRNA positive cells in the synovial lining layer was significantly correlated with the development of new joint erosions. Apart from macrophage-derived proteolytic enzymes, fibroblasts stimulated by macrophage interaction are a major source of proteases and believed to contribute to direct matrix attack at the pannus invasive front.[50]

In addition to direct enzyme release, macrophages contribute to cartilage destruction by the production of TNF-α and IL-1. Both IL-1 and TNF-α stimulate surrounding macrophages or fibroblasts to produce MMPs, but these cytokines also modulate the metabolism of chondrocytes. IL-1 is the dominant cytokine involved in inhibition of cartilage proteoglycan and collagen synthesis (Figure 3.6). Moreover, IL-1 stimulates chondrocytes to produce MMPs. MMPs are released in a latent form, are stored in the cartilage matrix, and additionally are activated by as yet unknown factors. Members of other enzyme groups might be involved in this activation step. Cysteine proteases (e.g. cathepsins) or serine proteases (e.g. elastases) can activate pro-MMPs.[51] These enzymes may derive from granulocytes or connective tissue cells but also from the macrophages. In animal models, a crucial role of MMP-3 (stromelysin) is evident in activating pro-MMP-1 inside the cartilage.[52,53] ICs are potent inducers of MMP-3 and crucial in activation of pro-MMPs. Comparing various experimental arthritis models, MMP-mediated cartilage erosion was only found in those models in which ICs were present. Furthermore, in the absence of functional activating FcγR, IC-mediated arthritis did not show cartilage erosion, although latent

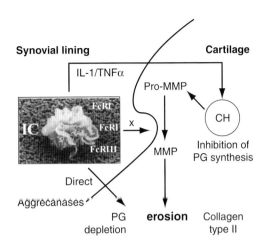

Figure 3.6 Mechanisms involved in cartilage destruction during arthritis. PG, proteoglycan; CH, chondrocyte.

pro-MMPs were present in the cartilage in large amounts. FcγRI appeared to be the dominant activating FcγR in cartilage destruction.[34]

Osteoclasts are the principal effector cells involved in bone resorption. Both maturation of precursor cells and activation of mature cells are highly stimulated by the macrophage-derived cytokines TNF and IL-1, whereas an amplifying role is attributed to T-cell-derived IL-17. Recent studies identified RANKL (receptor activator of nuclear factor kappaB ligand) as a crucial stimulus of osteoclast activation, and the interplay between RANKL, its receptor RANK and OPG (osteoprotegerin), which is the natural inhibitor of RANKL, determines the erosive nature of an arthritic process.

Interestingly, cartilage damage and bone erosion run through different pathways and may occur uncoupled. Bone erosion is completely blocked in arthritis in RANKL-deficient mice, whereas progression of cartilage destruction is evident.[54,55]

DEPLETION OF TYPE A INTIMA CELLS INHIBITS ONSET OF ARTHRITIS

The above studies have identified macrophages as crucial cells in inflammation and joint erosion, thereby providing a rationale for therapeutic macrophage targeting. As intima-type A cells become activated prior to arthritis development and are dominant producers of proinflammatory cytokines, these cells seem to be very important in regulating the early onset of arthritis. Transfer studies, using macrophage-like synovial cells from preinflammatory synovia from rats with developing experimental adjuvant arthritis, were able to transfer arthritis to control rats.[56] The ultimate proof that these cells are crucial in regulating arthritis was provided by selective removal of these cells from the intima.

Several methods to eliminate synovial intima cells have been described. Local deposition of osmium tetroxide[57] or radioisotopes[58] in knee joints showed downregulation of the lining function. However, the disadvantages of these methods are that they are non-selective and often cause side-effects affecting other joint tissues. Another more selective approach is the use of liposomes encapsulating the drug clodronate (dichloromethylene bisphosphonate: Cl_2MDP). This drug belongs to a class of synthetic compounds structurally related to pyrophosphate, an endogenous regulator of calcium metabolism. Macrophages preferentially phagocytose relatively large (1 µm) multilamellar liposomes. Once inside the cell, the lipid bilayer is degraded by enzymes, and clodronate is set free and induces cell death by apoptosis. The exact mechanism whereby clodronate induces apoptosis is not known, but most likely it is due to intracellular arrestment of Fe^{2+}.[59,60] A single injection of 6 µl of liposomes containing 75 µg clodronate into murine knee joints resulted in selective depletion of type A cells. Optimal depletion was found within 6–11 days after liposome injection, but even after 30 days no full recovery of the lining was found. No side-effects were found on cartilage metabolism.[61] The free drug, ^{14}C-labeled clodronate, is not taken up by cells and had no effect on macrophages.

The role of type A intima cells in onset of arthritis was demonstrated in murine experimental arthritis models. Selective depletion of type A intima cells, starting 7 days prior to arthrtis induction, prevented cell influx completely.[61–63] Washouts of the joints showed significantly reduced chemotactic activity and reduced levels of IL-1. The most important reduction was noted in complement factor C5a and IL-1-induced chemokines such as MCP-1.[62] In addition, it was found that elimination of type A lining cells also suppressed the onset of autoimmune collagen arthritis, thus showing that processes initiated by antibodies directed against cartilage epitopes are also dependent on lining cells. Moreover, it markedly reduced joint damage.[63]

As type A cells and macrophages can remain in an activated state in RA for prolonged periods, selective removal might be very beneficial for bringing the inflamed synovium to rest. A serious caveat of targeting lining macrophages selectively during active arthritis is that many PMN and monocytes are then present in the synovial fluid. The abundance of these cells largely prevents proper access of the locally injected liposomes to the intima, and many are destroyed by lipases produced by, for example, PMN. In line with this, injection of an adenoviral vector expressing the reporter gene luciferase only identified infection of exudate cells of the inflamed joint, and the virus failed to reach the synovium. Moreover, injection of an adenoviral IL-1ra vector, which largely prevents the onset of arthritis when given before onset, did not have any effect on arthritis when given during the acute phase.[64] To make it more applicable to the human situation, either synovial fluid aspiration has to be performed before liposome injection, or the joint has to be pretreated with a potent anti-inflammatory drug, e.g. steroid.

It is reassuring to note that clodronate-containing liposomes, injected locally into chronically inflamed murine knee joints, in which only a few exudate cells are present, easily targeted the lining cells. Fluorescent liposomes accumulated in the superficial intima layer when injected into joints of mice with antigen-induced arthritis induced 2 weeks before. The sustained inflammation in the

AIA day 21

AIA day 21: liop treatment

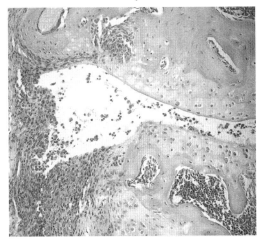
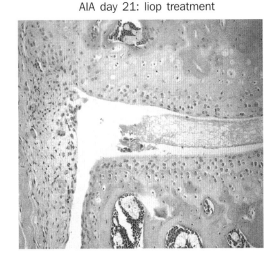

Figure 3.7 Intra-articular injection of clodronate liposomes in mouse arthritic knee joints ameliorates synovitis. Original magnification ×250. Hematoxylin/eosin staining.

synovium was largely resolved 1 week later (Figure 3.7). It is of great interest that exacerbation of the inflammation by oral or intra-articular rechallenge with antigen was largely prevented in these lining-depleted joints, suggesting that, apart from sustaining chronic arthritis, these cells are also crucial players in the flare-up reaction.

Promising results were recently obtained when clodronate liposomes were injected locally into the human RA joint. Seven days after injection, the intima layer was eliminated, whereas the inflammation in the subintima was significantly reduced. The treatment was well tolerated, and no side-effects were found.[65] Optimization of protocols to reduce inflammation are in progress.

Other macrophage-targeted therapies

Apart from liposome targeting of macrophages, more recent approaches are those using gene therapy. Local injection of adenoviral vectors harboring the herpes simplex virus thymidine kinase gene into the knees of rhesus monkeys with developing CIA followed by treatment with gangciclovir for 14 days resulted in increased apoptotic cell death in the synovium. Although the procedure was not associated with any toxic side-effects, the Tk gene therapy approach is not selective for macrophages.[66] Direct intra-articular injection of adenoviral vectors harboring FASL resulted in extensive apoptosis in the synovium without affecting chondrocyte viability.[67] As both type A and type B cells express FAS, this approach might also be not selective for type A cells. Another option for targeting particular cell types more specifically is to use modified viruses or liposomes, e.g. carrying RGD motifs and preferentially touching cells which heavily express adhesion molecules.[68] It is expected that those cells are primarily the ones actively involved in inflammatory mediator release.

Another promising approach to eliminate macrophages is the use of FcγRI as a targeting element. As FcγRs and FcγRI, in particular, are present on macrophages and play an important role in joint inflammation and severe cartilage destruction, this receptor may be used to deplete these cells from the synovium. Since FcγRI is a high-affinity IgG receptor, and is saturated with serum IgG in vivo, conventional antibodies are ineffective in targeting FcγRI. Anti-FcγRI antibodies directed against non-antigen-binding epitopes of the receptor and to which the toxic compound ricin was coupled were found to be very efficient in producing apoptosis of macrophages in vivo in the skin,[69] and studies are ongoing to demonstrate its usefulness for selectively removing FcγRI-expressing macrophages from arthritic joints.

In addition to complete removal of intima macrophages, impairing the function may be sufficient to obtain beneficial consequences for joint inflammation and cartilage destruction. Low-dose non-toxic liposomal clodronate appeared to reduce cartilage proteoglycan loss in experimental arthritis. Low doses of bisphosphonates modulated macrophage-mediated production of proinflammatory cytokines[70] and inhibited MMPs both directly and at the messenger RNA level.[71] Intra-articular injection of glucocorticoids such as methylprednisolone acetate lowered macrophage infiltration and also MMP-1 and MMP-3 and tissue inhibitors of metalloproteinases (TIMPs).[72] Corticoids commonly used in the treatment of RA block transcription by binding to nuclear receptors, inhibiting the transcription of many proinflammatory genes by binding directly to DNA or by binding to transcription factors.[73] Moreover, the classic treatment with gold compounds and probably also the current treatment with methotrexate mainly silence macrophage activity.

Therapeutic scavengers of macrophage mediators

Among the most successful therapeutic approaches to combat RA is blockade of macrophage mediators, such as enzymes and cytokines. As RA is such a versatile disease, it is important to emphasize that therapies directed at one target mediator may be only partially effective.

The most obvious way to block severe cartilage destruction is blockade of MMPs. Using naturally occuring inhibitors has apparent disadvantages. Broad-spectrum inhibitors such as α_2-macroglobulin are too large to penetrate the cartilage matrix. Other inhibitors such as TIMPs, which bind tightly to the active sites of all MMPs, are produced in low amounts, making additional therapy with these, in particular using local gene therapy, an attractive way to combat elevated levels of active MMPs. Experimental data look promising,[74,75] but clinical trials have yet to start. Synthetic MMP inhibitors were developed, but have so far failed to show proper efficacy, or have displayed too many side-effects, such as enhanced tumor spreading or ligament stiffening. It is still unclear whether selective targeting of MMP-13 is beneficial and may eliminate most side-effects. This argues that we do not know enough of the homeostatic functions of most MMPs.

The most successful treatment of RA to date is blocking the macrophage cytokine TNF-α. Given the vast abundance of a whole range of inflammatory mediators in RA synovial tissue, it is encouraging to note that there seems to be a definite hierarchy. TNF-α and IL-1, mainly produced by macrophages, are probably master cytokines regulating inflammation and cartilage destruction. Using culture studies of RA synovial membranes it was claimed that TNF-α drives most of the IL-1 production.[76] Furthermore, it was found that IL-1, rather than TNF-α, regulated cartilage destruction in experimental arthritis. Neutralization of IL-1 activity prevented TNF-induced arthritis, and erosions were absent in a range of arthritis models in IL-1-deficient mice, but not in TNF-deficient mice.[77,78] Moreover, IL-1Ra-deficient mice develop spontaneous arthritis.[79] The dogma that TNF blocking will eliminate most of the IL-1 effect is probably not true in all RA patients, and this suggests the need for additional, IL-1-directed therapy. Recent IL-1Ra trials have shown benefit in RA, including reduction of erosions.[80] Elements of TNF and IL-1 blocking are discussed in more detail in other chapters.

FINAL REMARKS

RA is probably a macrophage-driven disease. Resident synovial macrophages present in the intima become activated, which may be a consequence of aberrant responses to various triggers such as bacterial products or ICs released within the joint. Inflammation starting in the intimal layer attracts blood monocytes, which differentiate into mature macrophages, potentially with deranged function. Genetic preponderance or inadequate feedback mechanisms may be the cause of the aberrant responses to triggers which

are normally cleared without many side-effects. Activated macrophages produce a myriad of mediators, many of which are involved in inflammation and cartilage destruction. As therapies directed at only one target mediator may not be fully effective, selective removal of activated synovial macrophages or treatments leading to inactivation of these cells remain of interest as therapy in this crippling disease.

REFERENCES

1. Kinne RW, Brauer R, Stuhlmuller B, Palombo-Kinne E, Burmester GR. Macrophages in rheumatoid arthritis. *Arthritis Res* 2000; **2**: 189–202.

2. van den Berg WB, van Lent PL. The role of macrophages in chronic arthritis. *Immunobiology* 1996; **195**: 614–23.

3. Burmester GR, Stuhlmuller B, Rittig M. The monocyte/macrophage system in arthritis – leopard tank or Trojan horse? *Scand J Rheumatol Suppl* 1995; **101**: 77–82.

4. Zvaifler NJ. Macrophages and the synovial lining. *Scand J Rheumatol Suppl* 1995; **101**: 67–75.

5. Dreher R. Origin of synovial type A cells during inflammation. An experimental approach. *Immunobiology* 1982; **161**: 232–45.

6. van Lent PL, van den Bersselaar L, van den Hoek AE et al. Reversible depletion of synovial lining cells after intra-articular treatment with liposome-encapsulated dichloromethylene diphosphonate. *Rheumatol Int* 1993; **13**: 21–30.

7. Smolen JS, Tohidast-Akrad M, Gal A et al. The role of T-lymphocytes and cytokines in rheumatoid arthritis. *Scand J Rheumatol* 1996; **25**: 1–4.

8. Gordon S. Macrophage-restricted molecules: role in differentiation and activation. *Immunol Lett* 1999; **65**: 5–8.

9. Katschke KJ Jr, Rottman JB, Ruth JH et al. Differential expression of chemokine receptors on peripheral blood, synovial fluid, and synovial tissue monocytes/macrophages in rheumatoid arthritis. *Arthritis Rheum* 2001; **44**: 1022–32.

10. Geijtenbeek TB, Torensma R, van Vliet SJ et al. Identification of DC-SIGN, a novel dendritic cell-specific ICAM-3 receptor that supports primary immune responses. *Cell* 2000; **100**: 575–85.

11. Steinman RM. DC-SIGN: a guide to some mysteries of dendritic cells. *Cell* 2000; **100**: 491–4.

12. Zeibecoglou K, Ying S, Meng Q, Poulter LW, Robinson DS, Kay AB. Macrophage subpopulations and macrophage-derived cytokines in sputum of atopic and nonatopic asthmatic subjects and atopic and normal control subjects. *J Allergy Clin Immunol* 2000; **106**: 697–704.

13. Youssef P, Roth J, Frosch M et al. Expression of myeloid related proteins (MRP) 8 and 14 and the MRP8/14 heterodimer in rheumatoid arthritis synovial membrane. *J Rheumatol* 1999; **26**: 2523–8.

14. Sester DP, Stacey KJ, Sweet MJ, Beasley SJ, Cronau SL, Hume DA. The actions of bacterial DNA on murine macrophages. *J Leukoc Biol* 1999; **66**: 542–8.

15. Deng GM, Tarkowski A. The role of bacterial DNA in septic arthritis. *Int J Mol Med* 2000; **6**: 29–33.

16. Kraetsch HG, Unger C, Wernhoff P et al. Cartilage-specific autoimmunity in rheumatoid arthritis: characterization of a triple helical B-cell epitope in the integrin-binding-domain of collagen type II. *Eur J Immunol* 2001; **31**: 1666–73.

17. Li NL, Zhang DQ, Zhou KY et al. Isolation and characteristics of autoreactive T cells specific to aggrecan G1 domain from rheumatoid arthritis patients. *Cell Res* 2000; **10**: 39–49.

18. Maccioni M, Zeder-Lutz G, Huang H et al. Arthritogenic monoclonal antibodies from K/BxN mice. *J Exp Med* 2002; **195**: 1071–7.

19. Ji H, Ohmura K, Mahmood U et al. Arthritis critically dependent on innate immune system players. *Immunity* 2002; **16**: 157–68.

20. Weinblatt ME, Maddison PJ, Bulpitt KJ et al. CAMPATH-1H, a humanized monoclonal antibody, in refractory rheumatoid arthritis. An intravenous dose-escalation study. *Arthritis Rheum* 1995; **38**: 1589–94.

21. Choy EH, Pitzalis C, Cauli A et al. Percentage of anti-CD4 monoclonal antibody-coated lymphocytes in the rheumatoid joint is associated with clinical improvement. Implications for the development of immunotherapeutic dosing regimens. *Arthritis Rheum* 1996; **39**: 52–6.

22. Miossec P, van den Berg WB. Th1/Th2 cytokine balance in arthritis. *Arthritis Rheum* 1997; **40**: 2105–15.

23. Chabaud M, Durand JM, Buchs N et al. Human IL-17: a T-cell derived proinflammatory cytokine produced by the RA synovium. *Arthritis Rheum* 1999; **42**: 962–71.

24. Lubberts E, Joosten LA, Oppers B et al. IL-1-independent role of IL-17 in synovial inflammation and joint destruction during collagen-induced arthritis. *J Immunol* 2001; **167**: 1004–13.

25. McInnes IB, Liew FY. IL-15: a proinflammatory role in rheumatoid arthritis synovitis. *Immunol Today* 1998; **19**: 75–9.

26. Dayer JM, Burger D. Cytokines and direct cell contact in synovitis; relevance to therapeutic intervention. *Arthritis Res* 1999; **1**: 17–20.

27. Dinarello CA. Interleukin-18, a proinflammatory cytokine. *Eur Cytokine Netw* 2000; **11**: 483–6.

28. Gracie JA, Forsey RJ, Chan WL et al. A proinflammatory role for IL-18 in rheumatoid arthritis. *J Clin Invest* 1999; **104**: 1393–401.

29. Joosten LA, Lubberts E, Helsen MM, van den Berg WB. Dual role of IL-12 in early and late stages of murine collagen type II arthritis. *J Immunol* 1997; **159**: 4094–102.

30. Joosten LAB, van de Loo FAJ, Lubberts E et al. An IFN-gamma-independent proinflammatory role of IL-18 in murine streptococcal cell wall arthritis. *J Immunol* 2000; **165**: 6553–8.

31. Plater Zyberk C, Joosten LAB, Helsen MMA et al. Therapeutic effect of neutralizing endogenous IL-18 activity in the collagen-induced model of arthritis. *J Clin Invest* 2001; **108**: 1825–32.

32. Ravetch JV, Bolland S. IgG Fc receptors. *Annu Rev Immunol* 2001; **19**: 275–90.

33. Ioan-Facsinay A, de Kimpe SJ, Hellwig SM et al. FcgammaRI (CD64) contributes substantially to severity of arthritis, hypersensitivity responses, and protection from bacterial infection. *Immunity* 2002; **16**: 391–402.

34. van Lent PL, Nabbe K, Blom AB et al. Role of activatory Fc gamma RI and Fc gamma RI and inhibitory Fc gamma RI in inflammation and cartilage destruction during experimental antigen-induced arthritis. *Am J Pathol* 2001; **159**: 2309–20.

35. van Lent PL, van Vuuren AJ, Blom AB et al. Role of Fc receptor gamma chain in inflammation and cartilage damage during experimental antigen-induced arthritis. *Arthritis Rheum* 2000; **43**: 740–52.

36. Kleinau S, Martinsson P, Heyman B. Induction and suppression of collagen-induced arthritis is dependent on distinct fcgamma receptors. *J Exp Med* 2000; **191**: 1611–16.

37. Gerber JS, Mosser DM. Stimulatory and inhibitory signals originating from the macrophage Fcgamma receptors. *Microbes Infect* 2001; **3**: 131–9.

38. Blom AB, van Lent PL, Holthuysen AE, van den Berg WB. Immune complexes, but not streptococcal cell walls or zymosan, cause chronic arthritis in mouse strains susceptible for collagen type II auto-immune arthritis. *Cytokine* 1999; **11**: 1046–56.

39. Blom AB, van Lent PL, van Vuuren H et al. Fc gamma R expression on macrophages is related to severity and chronicity of synovial inflammation and cartilage destruction during experimental immune-complex-mediated arthritis (ICA). *Arthritis Res* 2000; **2**: 489–503.

40. Johansson ACM, Hansson AS, Nandakumar KS, Backlund J, Holmdahl R. IL-10-deficient B10.Q mice develop more severe collagen-induced arthritis, but are protected from arthritis induced with anti-type II collagen antibodies. *J Immunol* 2001; **167**: 3505–12.

41. Ortmann RA, Shevach EM. Susceptibility to collagen-induced arthritis: cytokine-mediated regulation. *Clin Immunol* 2001; **98**: 109–18.

42. Yuasa T, Kubo S, Yoshino T et al. Deletion of fcgamma receptor IIB renders H-2(b) mice susceptible to collagen-induced arthritis. *J Exp Med* 1999; **189**: 187–94.

43. Samuelsson A, Towers TL, Ravetch JV. Anti-inflammatory activity of IVIG mediated through the inhibitory Fc receptor. *Science* 2001; **291**: 484–6.

44. Mulherin D, Fitzgerald O, Bresnihan B. Synovial tissue macrophage populations and articular damage in rheumatoid arthritis. *Arthritis Rheum* 1996; **39**: 115–24.

45. Cawston T. Matrix metalloproteinases and TIMPs: properties and implications for the rheumatic diseases. *Mol Med Today* 1998; **4**: 130–7.

46. Fosang AJ, Last K, Maciewicz RA. Aggrecan is degraded by matrix mtalloproteinases in human arthritis. Evidence that matrix metalloproteinase and aggrecanase activities can be independent. *J Clin Invest* 1996; **98**: 2292–9.

47. Ishiguro N, Ito T, Oguchi T et al. Relationships of matrix metalloproteinases and their inhibitors to cartilage proteoglycan and collagen turnover and inflammation as revealed by analyses of synovial

fluids from patients with RA. *Arthritis Rheum* 2001; **44**: 2503–11.

48. Shingleton WD, Ellis AJ, Rowan AD, Cawston TE. Retinoic acid combines with interleukin-1 to promote the degradation of collagen from bovine nasal cartilage: matrix metalloproteinases-1 and -13 are involved in cartilage collagen breakdown. *J Cell Biochem* 2000; **79**: 519–31.

49. Cunnane G, Fitzgerald O, Beeton C, Cawston TE, Bresnihan B. Early joint erosions and serum levels of matrix metalloproteinase 1, matrix metalloproteinase 3, and tissue inhibitor of metalloproteinases 1 in rheumatoid arthritis. *Arthritis Rheum* 2001; **44**: 2263–74.

50. Pap T, Muller-Ladner U, Gay RE, Gay S. Fibroblast biology. Role of synovial fibroblasts in the pathogenesis of RA. *Arthritis Res* 2000; **2**: 361–7.

51. Okada Y, Nakanishi I. Activation of matrix metalloproteinase 3 (stromelysin) and matrix metalloproteinase 2 ('gelatinase') by human neutrophil elastase and cathepsin G. *FEBS Lett* 1989; **249**: 353–6.

52. van Meurs J, van Lent P, Stoop R et al. Cleavage of aggrecan at the Asn341–Phe342 site coincides with the initiation of collagen damage in murine antigen-induced arthritis: a pivotal role for stromelysin 1 in matrix metalloproteinase activity. *Arthritis Rheum* 1999; **42**: 2074–84.

53. Van Meurs J, van Lent P, Holthuysen A et al. Active matrix metalloproteinases are present in cartilage during immune complex-mediated arthritis: a pivotal role for stromelysin-1 in cartilage destruction. *J Immunol* 1999; **163**: 5633–9.

54. Gravallese EM, Galson DL, Goldring SR, Auron PE. The role of TNF-receptor family members and other TRAF-dependent receptors in bone resorption. *Arthritis Res* 2001; **3**: 6–12.

55. Pettit AR, Ji H, von Stechow D, Muller R et al. TRANCE/RANKL knockout mice are protected from bone erosion in a serum transfer model of arthritis. *Am J Pathol* 2001; **159**: 1689–99.

56. Ramos-Ruiz R, Bernabeu C, Ariza A, Fernandez JM, Larraga V, Lopez-Bote JP. Arthritis transferred by cells derived from pre-inflammatory rat synovium. *J Autoimmun* 1992; **5**: 93–106.

57. Okada Y, Nakanishi I, Kajikawa K. Repair of the mouse synovial membrane after chemical synovectomy with osmium tetroxide. *Acta Pathol Jpn* 1984; **34**: 705–14.

58. Boerbooms AM, Buijs WC, Danen M, van de Putte LB, Vandenbroucke JP. Radio-synovectomy in chronic synovitis of the knee joint in

patients with rheumatoid arthritis. *Eur J Nucl Med* 1985; **10**: 446–9.

59. van Rooijen N, Sanders A. Elimination, blocking, and activation of macrophages: three of a kind? *J Leukoc Biol* 1997; **62**: 702–9.

60. van Rooijen N, Bakker J, Sanders A. Transient suppression of macrophage functions by liposome-encapsulated drugs. *Trends Biotechnol* 1997; **15**: 178–85.

61. Van Lent PL, Van den Hoek AE, Van den Bersselaar LA et al. In vivo role of phagocytic synovial lining cells in onset of experimental arthritis. *Am J Pathol* 1993; **143**: 1226–37.

62. van Lent PL, Holthuysen AE, van den Bersselaar L, van Rooijen N, van de Putte LB, van den Berg WB. Role of macrophage-like synovial lining cells in localization and expression of experimental arthritis. *Scand J Rheumatol Suppl* 1995; **101**: 83–9.

63. van Lent PL, Holthuysen AE, van den Bersselaar LA et al. Phagocytic lining cells determine local expression of inflammation in type II collagen-induced arthritis. *Arthritis Rheum* 1996; **39**: 1545–55.

64. van de Loo FA, van den Berg WB. Gene therapy for rheumatoid arthritis. Lessons from animal models, including studies on interleukin-4, interleukin-10, and interleukin-1 receptor antagonist as potential disease modulators. *Rheum Dis Clin North Am* 2002; **28**: 127–49.

65. Barrera P, Blom A, van Lent PL et al. Synovial macrophage depletion with clodronate-containing liposomes in rheumatoid arthritis. *Arthritis Rheum* 2000; **43**: 1951–9.

66. Goossens PH, Schouten GJ, 't Hart BA et al. Feasibility of adenovirus-mediated nonsurgical synovectomy in collagen-induced arthritis-affected rhesus monkeys. *Hum Gene Ther* 1999; **10**: 1139–49.

67. Yao Q, Glorioso JC, Evans CH et al. Adenoviral mediated delivery of FAS ligand to arthritic joints causes extensive apoptosis in the synovial lining. *J Gene Med* 2000; **2**: 210–19.

68. Bakker AC, Van de Loo FA, Joosten LA et al. A tropism-modified adenoviral vector increased the effectiveness of gene therapy for arthritis. *Gene Ther* 2001; **8**: 1785–93.

69. Thepen T, van Vuuren AJ, Kiekens RC, Damen CA, Vooijs WC, van De Winkel JG. Resolution of cutaneous inflammation after local elimination of macrophages. *Nat Biotechnol* 2000; **18**: 48–51.

70. Makkonen N, Salminen A, Rogers MJ et al. Contrasting effects of alendronate and clodronate on RAW 264 macrophages: the role of a bisphosphonate metabolite. *Eur J Pharm Sci* 1999; **8**: 109–18.

71. Teronen O, Heikkila P, Konttinen YT et al. MMP inhibition and downregulation by bisphosphonates. *Ann NY Acad Sci* 1999; **878**: 453–65.

72. Young L, Katrib A, Cuello C et al. Effects of intraarticular glucocorticoids on macrophage infiltration and mediators of joint damage in osteoarthritis synovial membranes: findings in a double-blind, placebo-controlled study. *Arthritis Rheum* 2001; **44**: 343–50.

73. Firestein GS, Manning AM. Signal transduction and transcription factors in rheumatic disease. *Arthritis Rheum* 1999; **42**: 609–21.

74. Brown PD. Ongoing trials with matrix metalloproteinase inhibitors. *Expert Opin Investig Drugs* 2000; **9**: 2167–77.

75. Brown PD. Clinical studies with matrix metalloproteinase inhibitors. *APMIS* 1999; **107**: 174–80.

76. Feldmann M, Brennan FM, Foxwell BM, Maini RN. The role of TNFα and IL-1 in RA. *Curr Dir Autoimmun* 2001; **3**: 188–99.

77. van den Berg WB. Arguments for interleukin 1 as a target in chronic arthritis. *Ann Rheum Dis* 2000; **59** (suppl 1): 81–4

78. Van den Berg WB, Joosten LAB, van de Loo FAJ. TNFα and IL-1β are separate targets in chronic arthritis. *Clin Exp Rheumatol* 1999; **17** (suppl 18): S105–14.

79. Horai R, Saijo S, Tanioka H et al. Development of chronic inflammatory arthropathy resembling rheumatoid arthritis in interleukin 1 receptor antagonist-deficient mice. *J Exp Med* 2000; **191**: 313–20.

80. Dayer JM, Bresnihan B. Targeting interleukin-1 in the treatment of rheumatoid arthritis. *Arthritis Rheum* 2002; **46**: 574–8.

4

Dendritic cells

Ranjeny Thomas, Angus Thompson, Ela Martin and Brendan O'Sullivan

Introduction • Mechanisms of peripheral tolerance • Regulatory T cells • Mechanisms of regulation • Dendritic cell priming and induction of regulatory T cells in vivo • Common themes that highlight key regulatory pathways • Implications for treatment of autoimmune rheumatic disease • Blockade of dendritic cell function in rheumatic disease • Conclusion • References

INTRODUCTION

Autoimmune rheumatic diseases result from a process involving three distinct but related components – a break in self-tolerance, development of chronic inflammation in one or several organs, and, if ongoing, tissue destruction and its resultant detrimental effects. It has been proposed that dendritic cells (DCs) are the critical decision-making cells in the immune system.[1] Through their role in the generation of central and peripheral tolerance as well as in priming immune responses and stimulation of memory and effector T cells, DCs are likely to play essential roles in both the initiation and perpetuation of autoimmunity and autoimmune diseases. An understanding of the means by which DCs contribute to peripheral tolerance has opened the exciting possibility of harnessing them for antigen-specific immunotherapy of autoimmune diseases and transplantation. This chapter will consider the use of dendritic cells as biological therapy for the induction of tolerance in rheumatic autoimmune diseases. After consideration of the known mechanisms of peripheral tolerance, we will focus on the various means by which effector function is

regulated in the periphery, and distil emerging common themes as the key pathways of regulation. Means and pathways by which DCs have induced peripheral tolerance in autoimmune and transplant models will be discussed, followed by consideration of the potential and relative merits of this approach for future therapy of autoimmune rheumatic diseases. Finally, other strategies for the blockade of DC function will be briefly examined.

MECHANISMS OF PERIPHERAL TOLERANCE

Loss of tolerance to self-antigens is a critical component in the pathogenesis of autoimmunity. Immunologic tolerance is a functional state in which there is either no apparent immune response to self-antigens derived from somatic cells, such as synoviocyte or chondrocyte proteins, or in which an anti-self-immune response exists but does not lead to tissue damage. An anti-nuclear antibody in a healthy individual is an example frequently assessed by rheumatologists. In the fetal and neonatal period, 'central' tolerance is actively maintained in the thymus.[2] Here, T cells reactive to self-antigen presented by medullary DCs are deleted by negative selection above a threshold of affinity for the antigen.[3] Since an affinity threshold applies for central deletion of self-reactive T cells, circulation of low-affinity self-reactive T cells in the periphery is inevitable. Although self-reactive T cells might theoretically escape deletion due to lack of presentation of relevant self-peptide ligands by thymic antigen presenting cells (APCs), this possibility seems small, based on transgenic models in which neo-self-antigens are expressed at ectopic peripheral sites. There is increasing evidence that thymic low-level expression of self-antigens normally expressed by peripheral somatic cells is very common in both normal and transgenic animals.[4]

'Peripheral' tolerance mechanisms exist for the control of self-reactivity outside the thymus. In the periphery, tolerance may be passive, due to 'ignorance' of self-antigens because of presentation below threshold levels of T-cell receptor (TCR) affinity.[5–7] Such antigens may remain sequestered from presentation by DCs, such that potentially autoreactive T cells are not actively regulated – so-called immunologic ignorance.[8] Recently, it has also been proposed that some cases of ignorance may result from presentation of different epitopes or splice variants of the same self-antigen by DCs in the thymus, and by non-APCs in the periphery.[9] Active mechanisms of peripheral tolerance also exist, in which self-reactive cells are either deleted or survive long-term after antigen recognition, but the animal remains tolerant. Deletion of self-reactive cells may occur in lymph nodes draining noninflamed peripheral organs and tissues.[10,11] In other circumstances, TCR signaling may lead to functional unresponsiveness or anergy.[12] However, the regulation of self-reactive effector responses by specialized populations of regulatory T cells constitutes a major mechanism whereby the tolerant state is maintained and autoimmune disease is avoided long term. Several T-cell populations that are able to inhibit the response of other (effector) T cells have been described. Several populations demonstrate a characteristically low proliferative capacity in vitro, including CD4+CD25+ cells, Tr1 cells and Th3 cells. Understanding and harnessing this mechanism using DCs has great potential for therapy of autoimmune disease.

REGULATORY T CELLS

CD4+CD25+ 'natural' regulatory T cells

Mice thymectomized on day 3 after birth develop a syndrome of organ-specific autoimmune disease, including oophoritis, gastritis and/or thyroiditis. The mice can be rescued from illness by transfer of CD4+CD25+ T cells from a syngeneic adult spleen, and depletion of this population from non-thymectomized mice leads to a similar spectrum of autoimmune disease.[13–16] Transfer of CD4+CD25- T cells into syngeneic nude recipients leads to similar autoimmune disease, as well as a wasting syndrome and immune complex-mediated glomerulonephritis in some animals. Transfer of tolerance to thermocytes was first described in the 1960s and 1970s and one cell population responsible for transferable tolerance has been characterized as a sub-population of CD4+CD25+ T-cell. Such cells have the capacity to reduce non-specifically the strength of effector responses.[17,18] By this means, the T cells downregulate immune responses to self-antigens and foreign antigens, and prevent autoimmune disease. Furthermore, their depletion enhances the response to tumor-specific immunotherapeutic maneuvers.[19,20] They constitute 8–12% of murine and human spleen or blood CD4+ T cells. They proliferate poorly in response to mitogen or APCs in vitro, and inhibit CD4+CD25- T-cell proliferative responses in a generally suppressive, antigen-non-specific manner after TCR ligation.[21] Since they are found in umbilical cord blood and neonatal thymus and spleen, they are thought to represent a population of regulatory T cells that arises during fetal life.[17] This population appears to be analogous to the CD4+CD45RB[dim] subset in rat spleen, which can prevent colitis and wasting induced by the CD4+CD45RB[bright] cells transferred into athymic hosts.[22]

Other CD4⁺ regulatory T cells

Tr1 cells

This population of T cells emerges after several rounds of stimulation of human blood T cells by allogeneic monocytes in the presence of IL-10. The clones themselves secrete high levels of IL-10 and moderate levels of transforming growth factor beta (TGF-β) but little inter-leukin-4 (IL-4) or interferon gamma (IFN-γ).[23] Similar populations were induced by stimulation of TCR-transgenic CD4⁺ T cells with cognate peptide and IL-10. More recently, similar T-cell lines emerged after repetitive stimulation of human cord blood T cells with allogeneic immature DCs in vitro.[24] Influenza-specific CD8⁺ T cells with similar cytokine production were also induced in vivo in response to immunization with human immature DCs pulsed with an HLA-A2.1-restricted influenza CTL epitope.[25]

Th3 cells

The so-called Th3 regulatory subpopulation refers to a specific subset induced following antigen delivery via the oral (or other mucosal) route. They produce predominantly TGF-β, and only low levels of IL-10, IL-4 or IFN-γ, and provide specific help for IgA production.[26] They are able to suppress both Th1- and Th2-type effector T cells.

Th2 cells

This subpopulation produces high levels of IL-4, IL-5 and IL-10 but low levels of IFN-γ and TGF-β. Th2 cells are generated in response to a relative abundance of IL-4 and lack of IL-12 in the environment at the time of presentation of their cognate peptide ligands.[27] T-cell signaling by CD86 may also be important for generation of Th2 cells.[28,29] The importance of Th2 cells as a regulatory subset is unclear, but it is likely that the suppressive effects result from deviation away from a Th1-type immune response.

CD8⁺ regulatory T cells

A distinct CD8⁺CD28⁻ regulatory or 'suppressor' subset of T cells can be induced by repetitive

antigenic stimulation in vitro. These cells are also found in vivo in patients with chronic inflammation, transplantation, or tumors such as melanoma.[30–33] They are MHC class I restricted, and suppress CD4⁺ T-cell responses. A related CD4⁺CD28⁻ subset is found in patients with rheumatoid arthritis (RA), particularly in patients with vascular complications. Like CD8⁺CD28⁻ T cells, this subset expresses killer cell immunoglobulin-like receptors (KIRs), including the stimulatory KIR2DS2, which is potentially involved in endothelial damage.[34] However, as yet, no suppressor activity has been reported for the CD4⁺CD28⁻ population.

Natural killer (NK) T cells

This interesting T-cell population, which expresss the NK cell marker CD161, and whose TCR is Vα24JαQ in humans and Vα14Jα281 in mice, is activated specifically by the non-polymorphic CD1d molecule through presentation of a glycolipid antigen.[35] The cells have been shown to be immunoregulatory in a number of experimental systems. They are reduced in number in several autoimmune models before disease onset, and can reduce the incidence of disease upon passive transfer to non-obese diabetic (NOD) mice. Administration of the glycolipid α-galactosyl ceramide (α-gal cer), presented by CD1d, also results in accumulation of NK T cells and amelioration of diabetes in these mice.[36]

γδ T cells

γδ T cells have been implicated in the downregulation of immune responses in various inflammatory diseases and in the suppression of inflammation associated with induction of mucosal tolerance. The tolerance induced by mucosal antigen was transferable to untreated recipient mice by small numbers of γδ T cells.[37,38] Moreover, mucosal tolerance induction was blocked by the administration of the GL3 antibody that blocks γδ T-cell function.[39] However, γδ T cells with a contrasuppressive effect have also been described.[40]

MECHANISMS OF REGULATION

CD4+CD25+ T cells

Both rodent and human CD4+CD25+ T cells have been closely studied, but the mechanism by which they suppress anti-self-responses is still poorly understood – in part because of divergent findings in vitro and in vivo. Much of the analysis of the immunosuppressive mechanism has been done in vitro. Once activated through the TCR, they are capable of suppression of CD4+CD25- T cells in a contact-dependent, non-antigen-specific manner. This does not appear to require direct participation of the APCs, as suppression still occurs in vitro in the presence of fixed or third-party APCs.[18] However, CD4+CD25+ T cells are able to down-regulate the expression of CD80 and CD86 by APC, through cell contact mechanisms.[41] CD4+CD25+ T cells produce low levels of IL-10 and TGF-β, but suppression in vitro cannot usually be overcome by blocking these cytokines or IL-4. In a recent publication, however, they were shown to express high levels of membrane TGF-β, which mediated suppression of CD4+CD25- T-cell effector function.[42] Cytotoxic T-lymphocyte antigen 4 (CTLA-4) is present intra-cellularly in resting CD4+CD25+ T cells and is rapidly translocated to the cell membrane after activation. However, while CTLA-4 is an inhibitory receptor that restricts IL-2 production and cell cycle entry of T cells, blockade of CTLA-4 does not block the suppressive effects of CD4+CD25+ T cells in vitro.[18] Although the functional relevance is as yet uncertain, mRNA for several members of the Notch family of receptors is increased specifically in CD4+CD25+ T cells.[43]

In vivo studies show strikingly different outcomes. CTLA-4 has been shown to play an essential role in the regulation of gut inflammation by CD4+CD25+ T cells in mice.[44] Both IL-4 and TGF-β were essential for the control of thyroiditis in post-thymectomy models in rats,[45] and IL-10 was essential for the control of colitis by CD4+CD45RB^dim regulatory T cells in mice.[46] Furthermore, anti-IL-10R, anti-TGF-β or anti-CTLA-4 monoclonal antibodies (mAbs) prevented disease control. In contrast, neither IL-10 nor TGF-β appears to be involved in the

control of autoimmune gastritis by CD4+CD25+ T cells.[47] CTLA-4 ligation may be required for induction of TGF-β or IL-10 by CD4+CD25+ T cells, or these may be separate coincidental events. IL-2 is likely to be an essential growth factor for CD4+CD25+ T cells, as it reverses the lack of proliferation of these cells in vitro. Furthermore, this population is absent in IL-2- and IL-2Rα-deficient animals.[48–50] Taken together, the data suggest that multiple mechanisms may be involved in the suppression conferred by CD4+CD25+ regulatory T cells, involving inhibitory cytokines and cell–cell interactions, including IL-10, IL-4, TGF-β, and CTLA-4, and potentially affecting T cells as well as APCs. Presumably, the relative importance of these factors differs according to the experimental conditions and tissues involved in vivo.

While CD4+CD25+ T cells clearly suppress the activation of CD4+CD25- effector cells such that purified CD4+CD25- cells can induce autoimmunity upon transfer into nude recipients, this regulatory population may also have regulatory effects – direct or indirect – on other cells. For example, in vitro incubation of CD4+CD25+ T-cell-depleted spleen cells led to the spontaneous generation of activated CD4-CD8- NK cells capable of killing a broad spectrum of tumors in vitro. The NK cells were spontaneously activated by the large amounts of IL-2 secreted by CD25- T cells in the absence of the regulatory T cells.[20] Such NK cells may also be capable of producing significant damage to somatic cells – especially those with low-level MHC class I expression – in autoimmune disease.

Other CD4+ regulatory T cells

Tr1 cells

Tr1 cells stimulated by monocytes in which maturation is suppressed by IL-10 secrete high levels of IL-10 and IL-5, moderate levels of TGF-β and IFN-γ, and low levels of IL-4 and IL-2.[23] The proliferative responses of such clones are suppressed, and TGF-β and IL-10 are partially responsible for the regulation of Th1 cell proliferation in vitro. Transfer of OVA-specific Tr1 clones into *scid* mice reconstituted with

CD4+CD45RB^hi T cells inhibits the development of colitis only in mice that are also fed OVA.[23] Therefore, Tr1 cells, generated in vitro in response to APCs prevented from maturing by IL-10, suppress the generation of colitis in vivo following antigen-specific stimulation – presumably by a gut APC. It is worth noting here that Tr1 clones suppress disease in the same model of colitis that has been shown to be suppressed, in an antigen non-specific way, by CD4+CD45RB^lo or CD4+CD25+ T cells.[44] Thus, it is clear that more than one suppressive pathway exists. Subsequently, Tr1 cells have been shown to inhibit Th2-specific allergic responses to OVA in vivo, again through an IL-10-dependent mechanism.[51] In contrast, regulatory T cells induced from cord blood in vitro by allogeneic adult immature DCs also produce high levels of IL-10 and regulate the proliferation of Th1 clones. However, reminiscent of CD4+CD25+ T cells, this suppression is antigen non-specific, requires cell contact, and can be inhibited by exogenous IL-2.[24]

In vivo, human immature DCs pulsed with influenza matrix peptide induced suppression of previously primed matrix peptide IFN-γ responses. T-cell IL-10 production in response to matrix peptide was increased in vitro.[25] In mice, a single study has been published demonstrating the capacity of TNF-α- and myelin basic protein-pulsed BM-derived DCs to prevent development of experimental allergic encephalomyelitis (EAE). Three doses of 2–2.5 × 10^6 DCs were administered intravenously second daily up to 3 days before induction of disease. The DCs produced little IL-12 and some TGF-β mRNA. CD4+ T cells derived from spleens of treated mice produced IL-10 upon restimulation with antigen, and blockade of IL-10 could partially restore disease development.[52] The mechanism by which this regulation was induced remains obscure.

Th2 cells
IL-4 plays a dominant role in the differentiation of naive T cells towards a Th2-type phenotype, through direct inhibition of IFN-γ produced by Th1 cells.[53] In addition, IL-4 can reduce production of IL-1 and TNF-α by activated macrophages.[54] Administration of IL-4 ameliorates the clinical expression of EAE.[53] Similarly, after adoptive transfer of Th2-type MBP-specific T-cell lines, rats became resistant to the induction of EAE in the context of an accelerated anti-MBP antibody response.[55] Furthermore, Th2-type bystander immune deviation may be sufficient for this effect, as exogenous antigens that can induce Th2 responses can also modify the cytokine environment sufficiently to provide significant protection against EAE.[56]

Th3 cells
In the gut, epithelial cells may preferentially trigger regulatory T-cell function. Although the exact cell type has not been identified, adoptively transferred lamina propria cells induced tolerance in recipient animals. They induce secretion of high levels of IFN-γ (presumably by γβ T cells) and TGF-β (by Th3-type T cells).[57] The intestinal mucosa is rich in IL-4, IL-10 and TGF-β, and their expression is upregulated shortly after administration of oral antigen.[58] This cytokine microenvironment may be important for the stimulation of Th2- and Th3-type T cells in the gut. Inhibition of CD80 and of CTLA-4 signaling can inhibit the induction of oral tolerance under certain circumstances. TGF-β has been shown to reduce the induction of CD40 expression and IL-12 production by cultured macrophages, leading to reduced IFN-γ secretion by antigen-specific T cells in vitro.[59]

CD8+ regulatory T cells

CD8+CD28– regulatory cells inhibit the capacity of CD4+ effector cells to produce IL-2 and to upregulate CD40L expression. The suppression of effector function requires direct interactions between priming APCs and the CD8+CD28– cells. Ig-like inhibitory receptors ILT3 and ILT4, related to NK cell killer inhibitory receptors (KIR), are upregulated by the APCs as a result of this interaction. These receptors negatively signal monocytes and DCs through immunoreceptor tyrosine-based inhibitory motifs (ITIMs).[60–62] CD4+ T-cell-induced NFκB activation of APCs is reduced in the presence of CD8+CD28– T cells, potentially through this signaling pathway.[30] Therefore, two potential mechanisms of tolerance induction by CD8+CD28- T cells through the APCs have been described: reduction of CD40L expression by CD4+ effectors, and reduction of NFκB activation of the APC in the presence of CD4+ effector T cells.

NK T cells

In the context of CD1d and glycolipid ligands, NK T cells rapidly secrete large amounts of Th1- and Th2-type cytokines. The balance of signals processed by the NK T cells can determine the cytokines produced and therefore the immunomodulatory function of NK T cells through stimulatory and inhibitory receptors, including KIR. Treatment of NOD mice with α-gal cer induces recruitment of NK T cells to islets and pancreatic LN. It is of interest that CD8α−CD1d[bright] DCs also accumulate in pancreatic lymph nodes following the treatment.[36] This DC population has been shown to produce less IL-12 than CD8α+ DCs, and may drive production of relatively more IL4, IL-5 and IL-13 by the NK T cells.

γδ T cells

γδ T cells secrete both Th1- and Th2-type cytokines. Aerosol-induced tolerance to OVA was associated with increased IFN-γ production by CD8+ γβ T cells.[37] IL-10-containing γδ T cells have been detected in pancreatic lymph nodes of diabetic mice following treatment with aerosol insulin.[63] Therefore, several mechanisms may exist for suppression of immune responses through γδ T cells after administration of mucosal antigen (see below).

DENDRITIC CELL PRIMING AND INDUCTION OF REGULATORY T CELLS IN VIVO

DC priming

For the priming of immune responses, it is clear that DCs must be functionally differentiated. Proinflammatory signals stimulate differentiation and migration of peripheral DCs via afferent lymphatics to draining lymph nodes, with associated upregulation of molecules required for efficient antigen presentation. Cytokines, including granulocyte–macrophage colony-stimulating factor (GM-CSF), TNF-α and IL-1, pattern-recognition molecules and receptor-mediated phagocytosis may provide differentiating signals to immature DCs, and, in some cases, to peripheral monocytes.[64–67] Upregulated molecules include MHC molecules, costimulatory molecules, adhesion molecules and CCR7, which are important for the interaction of DCs with T cells. Furthermore, upregulation of CCR7 directs the appropriate migration of DCs to the T-cell area of the lymph node for the generation of antigen-specific T cells.[68] In addition to their role in T-cell priming, DCs have been shown to regulate B-cell growth, differentiation and immunoglobulin class switching, in a role that is separate to that played by follicular DC.[69,70]

Induction of CD4+CD25+ regulatory T cells

Despite the overwhelming evidence for the importance of CD4+CD25+ regulatory T cells in the constitutive peripheral suppression of autoreactivity and autoimmune disease, few studies have been able to demonstrate induction of this T-cell subset by vaccination. However, two groups have demonstrated induction of CD4+CD25+ T regulatory cells, by feeding and by intravenous injection of soluble OVA.[71,72] It is of interest that no protocol using injected DCs for induction of peripheral tolerance has yet demonstrated induction of CD4+CD25+ regulatory T cells. CD4+CD25+ cells are generated in the thymus during neonatal life, and thus neonatal thymectomy is associated with autoimmune disease. It is still debatable whether this T-cell subset can be produced outside the thymus – e.g. in the peripheral lymphoid organs – although a recent paper suggests peripheral homeostasis of this subset, potentially mediated by B cells.[73]

Induction of Tr1 CD4+ T cells

There is now a large body of literature demonstrating the induction of regulatory T cells by modified or immature DCs in vivo. The ability of

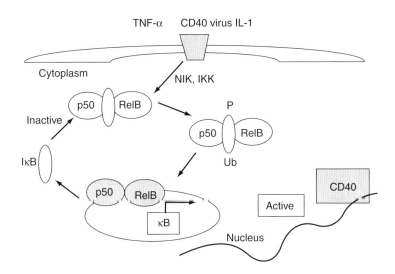

TNF-α CD40 virus IL-1

Cytoplasm

NIK, IKK

p50 RelB

Inactive

IκB

p50 RelB P

Ub

p50 RelB

κB

Active

CD40

Nucleus

Figure 4.1 Control of CD40 expression by RelB. Signals received at the membrane APC induce phosphorylation of IκB, allowing nuclear translocation of p50–RelB heterodimers, and subsequent promotion of transcription of key immunoreceptors, including CD40.

myeloid DCs to induce immunity or tolerance is linked to their maturation state.[24,25,74–76] Immature DCs generated from murine BM induce T-cell unresponsiveness in vitro and can lead to prolongation of cardiac allograft survival in a preventive model.[76] Human immature monocyte-derived myeloid DCs induce CD4+ Tr1-like cells in vitro and CD8+ T regulatory cells in vivo, which each produce high levels of IL-10 and low levels of IFN-γ, but no IL-4.[24,25] Various drugs and cytokines, including IL-10, TGF-β, 1α,25-dihydroxyvitamin D3, cyclosporin A, mycophenolate mofetil, aspirin, glucocorticoids, and inhibitors of NFκB, have been shown to inhibit myeloid DC maturation.[75,77–82] DCs generated in the presence of these agents alter T-cell function in vitro and in vivo, including the promotion of allograft survival.[78,83] Despite this, suppression of previously primed CD4+ T-cell responses by DCs in vivo has been difficult to demonstrate. This is important for therapy of pre-existing autoimmune disease, as CD4+ effector T cells mediate the perpetuation of tissue damage in autoimmune disease through their interactions with monocytes, B cells and local DCs.[84–87]

NFκB activity leads to transcription of a number of genes involved in the immune response.[88,89] RelB activity is required for myeloid DC differentiation.[90–92] We have shown that RelB regulates B-cell APC function through regulation of CD40 and MHC molecule expression.[93,94] Therefore, we investigated whether deficiency of RelB activity in DCs would be sufficient for suppression of immune responses by myeloid DCs. We showed that antigen-exposed myeloid DCs, in which RelB function is inhibited, lack cell surface CD40 expression, prevent priming of immunity, and suppress a previously primed immune response. DCs in which RelB nuclear translocation is inhibited through prevention of IκB phosphorylation, DCs generated from RelB-deficient mice and DCs generated from CD40-deficient mice similarly conferred suppression. Thus CD40, regulated by RelB activity, determines the consequences of presentation of antigen by myeloid DCs (Figure 4.1). Induction of suppression was specific for the antigen to which DC had been exposed. Moreover, this suppression results from induction of antigen-specific regulatory T cells resembling Tr1 cells, as DC immunization increased the proportion of CD4+ IL-10hi T cells in draining lymph nodes. CD4+ splenic T cells from tolerant animals transferred antigen-specific tolerance to primed recipients.

Therefore, the DCs induced an active 'infectious' process of antigen-specific regulation.[95,95a] These observations have significance for immuno-therapeutic suppression of conditions in which ongoing antigen presentation is associated with chronic inflammation, including autoimmune rheumatic disease.

Induction of Th2 CD4[+] T cells or Th2-like effects

In contrast to the control by RelB of myeloid DCs for induction of regulatory T cells, induction of Th2-type T cells by myeloid DCs is most strongly related to reduction of IL-12 p70 production. There are many agents described with this capacity, and many examples in which DCs incubated with pharmacologic or microbial agents have been functionally modified, so that T-cell cytokine production is predominantly skewed towards Th2-type cytokines. One of the most interesting groups of pharmacologic agents to do this signals cAMP in the DCs. Thus, modification of myeloid DC function with prostaglandin E_2, vasointestinal peptide (VIP), cholera toxin and histamine, all of which signal cAMP, leads to the induction of Th2-type T cells in vitro.[96–101] In some cases, these agents have been shown to have immunomodulatory effects in vivo, through induction of Th2-type T cells and cytokine effects. For example, the cAMP analog pentoxifylline stimulates Th2-associated T-cell function in vitro, and oral administration suppresses induction of EAE in rats through this mechanism.[102] Treatment with VIP reduced the incidence and severity of collagen-induced arthritis, associated with selective preservation of Th2-type T-cell function.[103] Previously, DCs derived from CD4[+]CD123[+]CD11c[-] plasmacytoid cells (labeled 'pDC2') were also found to induce Th2-type T-cell differentiation.[104] However, other investigators have demonstrated induction of a predominantly Tr1-type T-cell phenotype in vitro in response to these DCs, and recent in vivo evidence in ovarian cancer supports the idea that plasmacytoid DCs may also induce regulatory T-cell development in the absence of a strong proinflammatory signal.[105,106]

Induction of regulatory cells by the CD8α[+] murine DC subpopulation

Production of indoleamine-2,3-dioxygenase (IDO) by macrophages inhibits T-cell proliferation through depletion of the essential amino acid tryptophan.[107] Monocyte-derived DCs also produce functional IDO after stimulation with exogenous or T-cell-derived IFN-γ.[108] In the mouse, splenic DCs that express the CD8α marker were originally described as a regulatory population, and were found to induce deletion of CD4[+] T cells and to induce lower levels of cytokine production by CD8[+] T cells in vitro than CD8α[-] splenic DCs.[109,110] However, a large amount of evidence subsequently showed CD8α[+] DCs to be the major IL-12-producing murine DC subset. Moreover, it has become clear that certain CD8α[-] DCs express CD8α after activation.[111–113] Recently, however, IFN-γ was found to enhance the regulatory activity of CD8α[+] DCs through enhanced functional activity of IDO and tryptophan degradation, leading to apoptosis of T cells in vitro.[114,115] Since IL-12 can induce IFN-γ secretion by CD8α[+] DCs, it seems possible that this might represent a mechanism for autoregulation of T-cell activity following induction of some Th1-type immune responses.[116] This seems to be the likely mechanism behind the observation made in 1992 that NOD mice were protected from diabetes after receiving DCs derived from pancreatic but not other lymph nodes.[117] Subsequent experiments demonstrated the requirement for IFN-γ treatment of the DCs for the regulatory effect.[118] Taken together, these data suggest that transferred CD8α[+] IDO[+] DCs might regulate diabetes expression, either through the induction of regulatory cells, or through deletion of autoreactive effector CD8[+] T cells. It is of interest that CD40 ligation and IL-6 are able to inhibit the tolerogenic function of CD8α[+] DCs, in part through downregulation of IFN-γR expression. These represent important mediators of the chronic immune inflammatory response in autoimmune arthritis.[86,119] Indeed, mice transgenic for CD40L, driven by the keratin 14 promoter, demonstrate severe skin and systemic autoimmune disease, associated with marked Langerhans cell (LC) activation and lymph node migration.[120]

Genetic engineering of DCs

Several genetic approaches have been taken, largely based on the principles discussed above, for the production of DCs with the capacity for tolerance induction. Peripheral deletional tolerance of antigen-specific T cells has been induced by administration of APCs that express Fas ligand (FasL), and transfusion of FasL-transduced DCs prolongs the survival of MHC-mismatched cardiac allografts.[121,122] DC maturation has been retarded by transduction with either IL-10 or TGF-β, thus leading to induction of regulatory T cells and prolonged renal allograft survival.[123] Blockade of CD80/CD86–CD28 interactions using a DC-like cell line transduced with CTLA-4Ig also improved pancreatic islet allograft survival.[124] Transfection of DCs with NFκB decoy oligo-dinucleotides also prolonged cardiac allograft survival.[83] Finally, deviation of the immune response to production of more IL-4 by splenic T cells was achieved by transduction of DCs with IL-4. Administration of these DCs before disease onset reduced the severity of collagen-induced arthritis through deviation of the T-cell response to a predominant Th2 type.[125]

COMMON THEMES THAT HIGHLIGHT KEY REGULATORY PATHWAYS

Suppression of APCs

The descriptive term 'infectious tolerance' describes a phenomenon of active regulation. After induction of regulatory T cells in vivo by peripheral tolerance mechanisms, CD4+ T cells from tolerant animals can transfer antigen-specific tolerance to naive T cells – either by transfer of naive T cells into the original host, or by transfer of tolerant T cells to naive recipients, potentially over several generations of recipients.[126] What is the basis of the 'infectious' phenomenon? The capacity of both DCs to induce antigen-specific regulatory T cells, and for T cells to transfer tolerance in an antigen-specific way, as well as the requirement for a

continuous antigen supply for regulatory function, strongly suggests both that APCs regulate T cells and that T cells recognize and regulate specific antigen-bearing APCs, for the perpetuation of infectious tolerance. A theme common to the mechanism of regulatory T cells is that of production of molecules, including IL-10 and TGF-β, that can suppress APCs, including DCs. A number of regulatory T cells and NK T cells have the capacity to downregulate NFκB activation and CD40 expression of APCs, including monocytes and DCs. This may also be the case for B cells. Moreover, B cells lacking CD40 or in which CD40 signaling is blocked can induce antigen-specific tolerance in recipient animals.[127,128] Since suppression of RelB activity in myeloid DCs directly suppresses CD40 expression, and the lack of CD40 expression by myeloid DCs is sufficient for induction of regulatory T cells, the NFκB–CD40 pathway represents a key mechanism behind many described models of tolerance induction. Of particular importance, expression of CD40 in response to RelB and induction of RelB by CD40 ligation depicts a positive feedback loop in myeloid DC and B cells[93,94,129] (Figure 4.2). Therefore, blocking either CD40 or NFκB will have similar consequences for the induction of tolerance. Thus, reduction of CD40L expression by T cells, or blockade of CD40–CD40L interactions using mAb, also effectively induces tolerance through this basic mechanism. Several publications have demonstrated the role of regulatory T cells capable of transferring infectious tolerance as a result of blockade of the CD40 pathway.[130,131] Clinical trials of CD40L mAbs in systemic lupus erythematosus (SLE) are ongoing, to determine the effectiveness of this approach in a human autoimmune disease. Suppression of NFκB may also occur through ligation of inhibitory molecules such as KIR.[30]

Suppression of effector T cells and B cells

On the other side of the coin is the requirement of regulatory T cells to downregulate effector T-cell function. This can be mediated by IL-10, CTLA-4 ligation, depletion of tryptophan by IDO – leading to apoptosis – or by IL-4. It is of interest that the

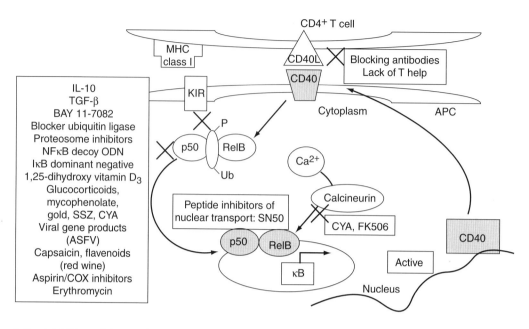

Figure 4.2 Inhibition of the positive feedback loop between CD40 and RelB/p50 in DCs can evoke tolerance. Various described mechanisms of inhibition of the NFκB and CD40 signaling pathway are indicated.[162–165] Some, such as anti-CD40L and DCs treated with various pharmacologic inhibitors of NFκB, have been demonstrated to induce tolerance in vivo. ASFV, African swine fever virus; COX, cyclo-oxygenase.

induction of IDO in DCs appears to be IFN-γ-dependent, and that IFN-γ is produced by Th1 and Tr1 CD4$^+$ T cells, γδ T cells, as well as by IL-12-stimulated DCs themselves.[132] Thus, although multiple types of regulatory cells have been described, and several key APCs have been shown to induce these cells, there appear to be only a limited number of key regulatory mechanisms controlling the decision between tolerance and immunity made by a T cell in contact with an APC. These include the NFκB–CD40 and IFN-γ–IDO pathways in the APC, and IL-10, TGF-β, NFκB and CTLA-4 in the T cells (Figure 4.3). Furthermore, evidence is emerging that one pathway might induce a second pathway, through a type of domino effect, especially as major tolerance pathways in APCs and T cells are regulated by NFκB, and NFκB can be regulated in APCs and T cells by similar upstream molecules, such as IL-10 and TGF-β. Furthermore, ligation of T-cell CTLA-4 leads to profound inhibition of NFκB and AP1 transcription factors.[133] It is of importance that

transgenic mice expressing a transdominant inhibitor of NFκB in T cells, demonstrate that tolerance is induced in transgenic recipients of cardiac allografts and that such a transgene can partially rescue the *gld* (FasL-deficient) autoimmune phenotype.[134,135] Thus, inhibition of NFκB is likely to be a key regulatory pathway mediating tolerance in both APCs and T cells.

Interaction between NK T cells, DCs and T cells

The third major emerging pathway is mediated by NK T cells and the potential functional role of NK receptors, including KIR, CD49b, and others. Not only can CD8$^+$CD28$^-$ T cells induce KIR expression by APCs, but regulatory NK cells, NK T cells and T cells can express these receptors. Currently, most of the evidence identifies these cells by use of NK receptors as markers – for example, suppression of type I diabetes in a murine model requires both CD49b$^+$ and CD49b$^-$

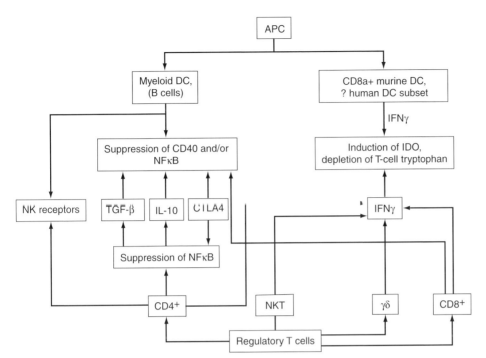

Figure 4.3 Two major mechanisms for tolerance induction by different APC types. The major mechanisms of tolerance described for regulatory T-cell populations and APC (excluding Th2 cells and immune deviation) and the interactions between them are depicted.

CD4[+] T cells.[136] More recently, after administration of antibodies to CD40L, which also suppress type I diabetes, CD49b[+]CD11c[+] DCs from spleens were able to transfer protection.[137] Intriguingly, a few studies have demonstrated induction of KIR expression by CD8[+] T cells following TCR ligation, which could be enhanced in the presence of TGF-β.[138–140] Future studies that define the functional role of these and other NK receptors are anticipated.

As well as the immunotherapeutic possibilities, our studies also suggest a mechanism by which peripheral tolerance might be constitutively maintained by myeloid DCs in which RelB and CD40 are either suppressed or not induced. We have previously demonstrated that, in contrast to inflamed or lymphoid tissues, nuclear RelB[+] cells are absent in non-inflamed, non-lymphoid peripheral tissues.[89,141,142] Therefore, at sites of antigen uptake, myeloid immature DCs lack RelB. Furthermore, a proportion of unmanipulated DCs in both the periphery and lymph nodes has been shown to express little if any CD40 constitutively, and to

rely upon infectious signals for CD40 induction and concomitant IL-12 production.[143] Since DCs containing apoptotic bodies can constitutively migrate from peripheral sites to draining lymph nodes, myeloid DCs may reach lymph nodes lacking RelB activity and cell surface CD40.[144] Cross-presentation of processed self-antigen derived from somatic cells could thereby constitutively induce self-antigen-specific regulatory T cells in lymph nodes draining peripheral tissues (Figure 4.4). Thus, upstream signaling of DCs by infectious antigen through TLR and other pattern-recognition receptors that leads to RelB translocation and CD40 induction provides a key pathway for discrimination by the immune system of antigens loaded and presented or transferred by myeloid peripheral tissue DCs.

IMPLICATIONS FOR TREATMENT OF AUTOIMMUNE RHEUMATIC DISEASE

Why does research in tolerance induction for therapy of autoimmune rheumatic disease lag

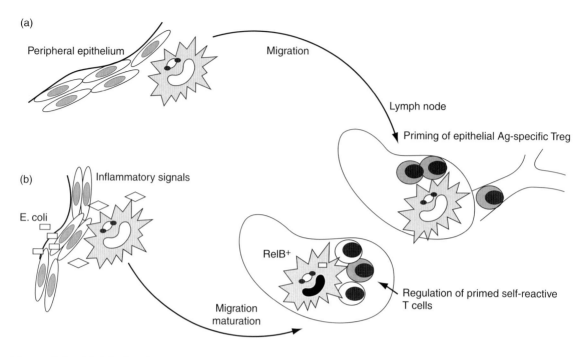

Figure 4.4 Model of peripheral tolerance to endogenously processed somatic self-antigen. (a) Tolerance specific for self-antigen, derived from apoptotic bodies. (b) Prevention of induction of anti-self-responses in response to incidental inflammatory signals by previously primed regulatory T cells.

behind therapy for transplantation or even for type I diabetes? The spectacular early success of non-antigen-specific, anti-cytokine and other anti-inflammatory and anti-destructive therapies, the lack of clear definition of a human pathogenic self-antigen in RA, and the dismal lack of proof-of-principle for disease suppression by tolerance restoration, have led to caution in basic research and biotechnology. These restraints remain in spite of the fact that RA is one of the two most common autoimmune diseases. In contrast, examples exist of suppression of type I diabetes in mice by tolerance to insulin or GAD autoantigens, even after disease onset.[145,146] The development of the exquisite K/B × N mouse model of RA, which is driven by an autoimmune response to the ubiquitous self-antigen glucose-6-phosphate isomerase, provides insight into the difficulties faced in treating autoimmune arthritis with tolerance restoration.[147] This model demonstrates that, following arthritis initiation, subsequent perpet-

uation of disease is antigen and MHC independent – driven by antigen-specific auto- antibodies, immune complexes and complement, which lead to unrestrained proinflammatory and destructive cytokine production.[148,149] Furthermore, an immune response to the same self-antigen is made in a proportion of patients with RA.[150] The pathogenetic concepts illustrated by this model suggest that irreversible suppression of autoimmune arthritis may indeed require both restoration of antigen-specific tolerance and inhibition of key tissue destructive signals – driven especially by immune complexes, and by complement.[151,152]

Using DCs in which RelB activity was suppressed by a soluble inhibitor of NFκB, we treated mice with antigen-induced arthritis, 2–10 days after arthritis induction. The model is driven by immune response to the antigen methylated bovine serum albumin (mBSA). Despite suppression of mBSA responses in all mice when mBSA-pulsed RelB⁻ DCs were

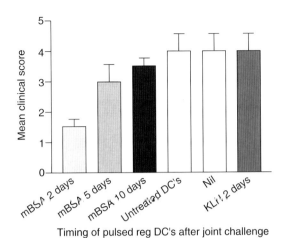

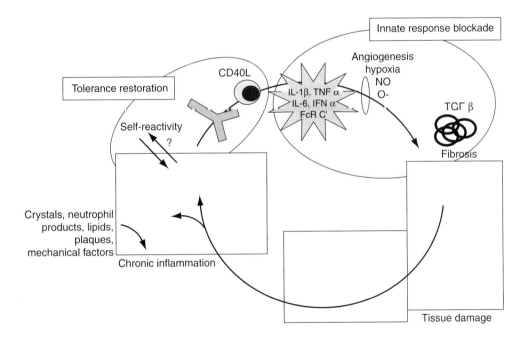

Figure 4.5 Suppression of antigen-induced arthritis (AIA) following induction of disease. C57Bl/6 mice were primed to mBSA, and 8 days later one knee joint was injected with mBSA. Antigen-pulsed BAY-treated DCs were injected subcutaneously between 2 and 10 days later. The clinical score was measured 15 days after arthritis induction.

Figure 4.6 Relationship between inflammation and damage, and implications for immunotherapy.

administered, clinical suppression was effective only when DCs were administered early after induction of disease (Figure 4.5). These data suggest that the window period for arthritis suppression by antigen-specific tolerance is short, and that this therapy is likely to require combination with appropriate anti-destructive therapy to be effective (Figure 4.6).

Finally, an exciting emerging area is the definition of pathogenic autoantibodies in diseases such as Sjogren's syndrome and scleroderma. Thus, anti-muscarinic receptor autoantibodies with the capacity to block function are associated with gut and bladder dysfunction in rheumatic diseases.[153] The possibility exists, once the autoantigens are known, to administer

DCs pulsed with relevant autoantigens or their epitopes, for suppression of such autoantibodies. While this might not cure the disease itself, it may be sufficient to alleviate many disease-associated symptoms.

BLOCKADE OF DENDRITIC CELL FUNCTION IN RHEUMATIC DISEASE

Patients with SLE were recently shown to display major alterations in DC homeostasis, in that plasmacytoid DCs were reduced in blood, and IFN-α-activated monocytes were effective APCs in vitro in these patients.[154] It was speculated that monocyte-derived DCs might efficiently capture apoptotic cells and nucleosomes, present in SLE patients' blood and tissues.[155] In view of the high levels of IFN-α in serum, and its potential detrimental effects in SLE, it has been proposed that IFN-α might represent a potential target for therapeutic intervention in SLE.[156] IFN-α activates not only myeloid cells, including monocytes and myeloid DCs, but also plasmacytoid DCs themselves, which are enriched in the inflammatory site in SLE skin lesions.[157] Other investigators have suggested the blockade of chemokines or chemokine receptors for inhibition of the ectopic lymphoid development characteristic of the chronic inflammatory response in RA and other autoimmune rheumatic diseases. Thus, DCs in perivascular, T-cell enriched areas of synovial tissue are associated with CCL19 and 21 expression and are characterized by CCR7 expression, and immature DCs in the lining and sublining layers are characterized by CCR6 expression and are associated with CCL20 expression.[158] It remains to be seen whether such treatments might be effective in animal models. However, ectopic expression of CCL19 is sufficient for formation of lymphoid tissue.[159] Similarly, BCA-1/CXCL13 is found, predominantly in follicular DCs, in germinal centers in RA synovium. B cells aggregate in these regions, probably attracted by the FDC.[160] The data suggest that blockade of these chemokines would have a marked – but potentially toxic – effect on the process of lymphoid tissue development in synovial tissue.

CONCLUSION

Restoration of tolerance to self-antigens is currently an exciting field. After many years in the doldrums, progress in our understanding of how T-cell regulation occurs and how to control the APCs for generation of regulation has recently surged ahead. There are two major challenges. First, it remains to be seen whether insufficient knowledge of the appropriate self-antigens will hamper progress, or whether creative strategies can be applied by harvesting relevant tissues, as we have learned from clinical trials and animal models of cancer immunotherapy. Second, although TNF-α and IL-1β do drive many pathogenic processes in RA, their blockade is much more effective when combined with other strategies, such as methotrexate.[161] Thus, it remains to be determined whether the upstream drivers of disease can be effectively blocked, sufficient to ablate the antigen-non-specific perpetuation of disease. Only then, we predict, when combined with tolerance restoration, will more permanent therapeutic solutions to autoimmune rheumatic diseases become possible.

REFERENCES

1. Fazekas de St Groth B. The evolution of self-tolerance: a new cell arises to meet the challenge of self-reactivity. *Immunol Today* 1998; **19**: 448–54.
2. Ardavin C. Thymic dendritic cells. *Immunol Today* 1997; **18**: 350–61.
3. Kappler JW, Roehm N, Marrack P. T-cell tolerance by clonal elimination in the thymus. *Cell* 1987; **49**: 273–80.
4. Pugliese A, Brown D, Garza D et al. Self-antigen-presenting cells expressing diabetes-associated autoantigens exist in both thymus and peripheral lymphoid organs. *J Clin Invest* 2001; **107**: 555–64.

5. Hogquist KA, Jameson SC, Heath WR et al. T-cell receptor antagonist peptides induce positive selection. *Cell* 1994; **76**: 17–27.

6. Heath VL, Moore NC, Parnell SM, Mason DW. Intrathymic expression of genes involved in organ specific autoimmune disease. *J Autoimmun* 1998; **11**: 309–18.

7. Anderson AC, Nicholson LB, Legge KL et al. High frequency of autoreactive myelin proteolipid protein-specific T cells in the periphery of naive mice: mechanisms of selection of the self-reactive repertoire. *J Exp Med* 2000; **191**: 761–70.

8. Barker CF, Billingham RE. Immunologically privileged sites. *Adv Immunol* 1977; **25**: 1–54.

9. Diez J, Park Y, Zeller M et al. Differential splicing of the IA-2 mRNA in pancreas and lymphoid organs as a permissive genetic mechanism for autoimmunity against the IA-2 type 1 diabetes autoantigen. *Diabetes* 2001; **50**: 895–900.

10. Kurts C, Kosaka H, Carbone FR et al. Class I-restricted cross presentation of exogenous self antigens leads to deletion of autoreactive CD8+ T cells. *J Exp Med* 1997; **186**: 239–45.

11. Lo D, Freedman J, Hesse S et al. Peripheral tolerance in transgenic mice: tolerance to class II MHC and non-MHC transgene antigens. *Immunol Rev* 1991; **122**: 87–102.

12. Rocha B, Tanchot C, Von Boehmer H. Clonal anergy blocks in vivo growth of mature T cells and can be reversed in the absence of antigen. *J Exp Med* 1993; **177**: 1517–21.

13. Nishizuka Y, Sakakura T. Thymus and reproduction: sex-linked dysgenesia of the gonad after neonatal thymectomy in mice. *Science* 1969; **166**: 753–5.

14. Kojima A, Tanaka-Kojima Y, Sakakura T, Nishizuka Y. Prevention of postthymectomy autoimmune thyroiditis in mice. *Lab Invest* 1976; **34**: 601–5.

15. Itoh M, Takahashi T, Sakaguchi N et al. Thymus and autoimmunity: production of CD25+CD4+ naturally anergic and suppressive T cells as a key function of the thymus in maintaining immunologic self-tolerance. *J Immunol* 1999; **162**: 5317–26.

16. Sakaguchi S, Sakaguchi N, Shimizu J et al. Immunologic tolerance maintained by CD25+ CD4+ regulatory T cells: their common role in controlling autoimmunity, tumor immunity, and transplantation tolerance. *Immunol Rev* 2001; **182**: 18–32.

17. Sakaguchi S, Takahashi T, Yamazaki S et al. Immunologic self tolerance maintained by T-cell-mediated control of self-reactive T cells: implica-tions for autoimmunity and tumor immunity. *Microbes Infect* 2001; **3**: 911–18.

18. McHugh RS, Shevach EM, Thornton AM. Control of organ-specific autoimmunity by immunoregulatory CD4(+)CD25(+) T cells. *Microbes Infect* 2001; **3**: 919–27.

19. Sutmuller RP, van Duivenvoorde LM, van Elsas A et al. Synergism of cytotoxic T lymphocyte-associated antigen 4 blockade and depletion of CD25(+) regulatory T cells in antitumor therapy reveals alternative pathways for suppression of autoreactive cytotoxic T lymphocyte responses. *J Exp Med* 2001; **194**: 823–32.

20. Shimizu J, Yamazaki S, Sakaguchi S. Induction of tumor immunity by removing CD25+CD4+ T cells: a common basis between tumor immunity and autoimmunity. *J Immunol* 1999; **163**: 5211–18.

21. Thornton AM, Shevach EM. Suppressor effector function of CD4+CD25+ immunoregulatory T cells is antigen nonspecific. *J Immunol* 2000; **164**: 183–90.

22. Powrie F, Mason D. OX-22high CD4+ T cells induce wasting disease with multiple organ pathology: prevention by the OX-22low subset. *J Exp Med* 1990; **172**: 1701–8.

23. Groux H, O'Garra A, Bigler M et al. A CD4+ T-cell subset inhibits antigen-specific T-cell responses and prevents colitis. *Nature* 1997; **389**: 737–42.

24. Jonuleit H, Schmitt E, Schuler G et al. Induction of interleukin 10-producing, non-proliferating CD4+ T cells with regulatory properties by repetitive stimulation with allogeneic immature human dendritic cells. *J Exp Med* 2000; **192**: 1213–22.

25. Dhodapkar MV, Steinman RM, Krasovsky J et al. Antigen-specific inhibition of effector T-cell function in humans after injection of immature dendritic cells. *J Exp Med* 2001; **193**: 233–8.

26. Weiner HL. Oral tolerance: immune mechanisms and the generation of Th3-type TGF- beta-secreting regulatory cells. *Microbes Infect* 2001; **3**: 947–54.

27. O'Garra A, Arai N. The molecular basis of T helper 1 and T helper 2 cell differentiation. *Trends Cell Biol* 2000; **10**: 542–50.

28. Lenschow DJ, Herold KC, Rhee L et al. CD28/B7 regulation of Th1 and Th2 subsets in the development of autoimmune diabetes. *Immunity* 1996; **5**: 285–93.

29. Xu H, Heeger PS, Fairchild RL. Distinct roles for B7–1 and B7–2 determinants during priming of effector CD8+ Tc1 and regulatory CD4+ Th2 cells for contact hypersensitivity. *J Immunol* 1997; **159**: 4217–26.

30. Chang CC, Ciubotariu R, Manavalan JS et al. Tolerization of dendritic cells by T(S) cells: the crucial role of inhibitory receptors ILT3 and ILT4. *Nat Immunol* 2002; **3**: 237–43.

31. Becker JC, Vetter CS, Schrama D et al. Differential expression of CD28 and CD94/NKG2 on T cells with identical TCR beta variable regions in primary melanoma and sentinel lymph node. *Eur J Immunol* 2000; **30**: 3699–706.

32. Speiser DE, Valmori D, Rimoldi D et al. CD28–negative cytolytic effector T cells frequently express NK receptors and are present at variable proportions in circulating lymphocytes from healthy donors and melanoma patients. *Eur J Immunol* 1999; **29**: 1990–9.

33. Vallejo AN, Brandes JC, Weyand CM, Goronzy JJ. Modulation of CD28 expression: distinct regulatory pathways during activation and replicative senescence. *J Immunol* 1999; **162**: 6572–9.

34. Yen JH, Moore BE, Nakajima T et al. Major histocompatibility complex class I-recognizing receptors are disease risk genes in rheumatoid arthritis. *J Exp Med* 2001; **193**: 1159–67.

35. Kawano T, Cui J, Koezuka Y et al. CD1d-restricted and TCR-mediated activation of valpha14 NKT cells by glycosylceramides. *Science* 1997; **278**: 1626–9.

36. Naumov YN, Bahjat KS, Gausling R et al. Activation of CD1d-restricted T cells protects NOD mice from developing diabetes by regulating dendritic cell subsets. *Proc Natl Acad Sci USA* 2001; **98**: 13838–43.

37. McMenamin C, McKersey M, Kuhnlein P et al. Gamma delta T cells down-regulate primary IgE responses in rats to inhaled soluble protein antigens. *J Immunol* 1995; **154**: 4390–4.

38. McMenamin C, Pimm C, McKersey M, Holt PG. Regulation of IgE responses to inhaled antigen in mice by antigen-specific gamma delta T cells. *Science* 1994; **265**: 1869–71.

39. Ke Y, Pearce K, Lake JP et al. Gamma delta T lymphocytes regulate the induction and maintenance of oral tolerance. *J Immunol* 1997; **158**: 3610–18.

40. Fujihashi K, Taguchi T, Aicher WK et al. Immunoregulatory functions for murine intraepithelial lymphocytes: gamma/delta T-cell receptor-positive (TCR+) T cells abrogate oral tolerance, while alpha/beta TCR+ T cells provide B-cell help. *J Exp Med* 1992; **175**: 695–707.

41. Cederbom L, Hall H, Ivars F. CD4+CD25+ regulatory T cells down-regulate co-stimulatory molecules on antigen-presenting cells. *Eur J Immunol* 2000; **30**: 1538–43.

42. Nakamura K, Kitani A, Strober W. Cell contact-dependent immunosuppression by CD4(+)CD25(+) regulatory T cells is mediated by cell surface-bound transforming growth factor beta. *J Exp Med* 2001; **194**: 629–44.

43. Ng WF, Duggan PJ, Ponchel F et al. Human CD4(+)CD25(+) cells: a naturally occurring population of regulatory T cells. *Blood* 2001; **98**: 2736–44.

44. Read S, Malmstrom V, Powrie F. Cytotoxic T lymphocyte-associated antigen 4 plays an essential role in the function of CD25(+)CD4(+) regulatory cells that control intestinal inflammation. *J Exp Med* 2000; **192**: 295–302.

45. Seddon B, Mason D. Regulatory T cells in the control of autoimmunity: the essential role of transforming growth factor beta and interleukin 4 in the prevention of autoimmune thyroiditis in rats by peripheral CD4(+)CD45RC– cells and CD4(+)CD8(–) thymocytes. *J Exp Med* 1999; **189**: 279–88.

46. Asseman C, Fowler S, Powrie F. Control of experimental inflammatory bowel disease by regulatory T cells. *Am J Respir Crit Care Med* 2000; **162**: S185–9.

47. Suri-Payer E, Cantor H. Differential cytokine requirements for regulation of autoimmune gastritis and colitis by CD4(+)CD25(+) T cells. *J Autoimmun* 2001; **16**: 115–23.

48. Wolf M, Schimpl A, Hunig T. Control of T-cell hyperactivation in IL-2–deficient mice by CD4(+)CD25(–) and CD4(+)CD25(+) T cells: evidence for two distinct regulatory mechanisms. *Eur J Immunol* 2001; **31**: 1637–45.

49. Sharfe N, Dadi HK, Shahar M, Roifman CM. Human immune disorder arising from mutation of the alpha chain of the interleukin-2 receptor. *Proc Natl Acad Sci USA* 1997; **94**: 3168–71.

50. Singh B, Read S, Asseman C et al. Control of intestinal inflammation by regulatory T cells. *Immunol Rev* 2001; **182**: 190–200.

51. Cottrez F, Hurst SD, Coffman RL, Groux H. T regulatory cells 1 inhibit a Th2-specific response in vivo. *J Immunol* 2000; **165**: 4848–53.

52. Menges M, Rossner S, Voigtlander C et al. Repetitive injections of dendritic cells matured with tumor necrosis factor alpha induce antigen-specific protection of mice from autoimmunity. *J Exp Med* 2002; **195**: 15–21.

53. Racke MK, Bonomo A, Scott DE et al. Cytokine-induced immune deviation as a therapy for

inflammatory autoimmune disease. *J Exp Med* 1994; **180**: 1961–6.

54. Bonder CS, Dickensheets HL, Finlay-Jones JJ et al. Involvement of the IL-2 receptor gamma-chain (gammac) in the control by IL-4 of human monocyte and macrophage proinflammatory mediator production. *J Immunol* 1998; **160**: 4048–56.

55. Ramirez F, Mason D. Induction of resistance to active experimental allergic encephalomyelitis by myelin basic protein-specific Th2 cell lines generated in the presence of glucocorticoids and IL-4. *Eur J Immunol* 2000; **30**: 747–58.

56. Falcone M, Bloom BR. A T helper cell 2 (Th2) immune response against non-self antigens modifies the cytokine profile of autoimmune T cells and protects against experimental allergic encephalomyelitis. *J Exp Med* 1997; **185**: 901–7.

57. Harper HM, Cochrane L, Williams NA. The role of small intestinal antigen-presenting cells in the induction of T-cell reactivity to soluble protein antigens: association between aberrant presentation in the lamina propria and oral tolerance. *Immunology* 1996; **89**: 449–56.

58. Gonnella PA, Chen Y, Inobe J et al. In situ immune response in gut-associated lymphoid tissue (GALT) following oral antigen in TCR-transgenic mice. *J Immunol* 1998; **160**: 4708–18.

59. Takeuchi M, Alard P, Streilein JW. TGF-beta promotes immune deviation by altering accessory signals of antigen-presenting cells. *J Immunol* 1998; **160**: 1589–97.

60. Colonna M, Nakajima H, Cella M. A family of inhibitory and activating Ig-like receptors that modulate function of lymphoid and myeloid cells. *Semin Immunol* 2000; **12**: 121–7.

61. Colonna M, Navarro F, Bellon T et al. A common inhibitory receptor for major histocompatibility complex class I molecules on human lymphoid and myelomonocytic cells. *J Exp Med* 1997; **186**: 1809–18.

62. Colonna M, Samaridis J, Cella M et al. Human myelomonocytic cells express an inhibitory receptor for classical and nonclassical MHC class I molecules. *J Immunol* 1998; **160**: 3096–100.

63. Harrison LC, Dempsey-Collier M, Kramer DR, Takahashi K. Aerosol insulin induces regulatory CD8 gamma delta T cells that prevent murine insulin-dependent diabetes. *J Exp Med* 1996; **184**: 2167–74.

64. Thomas R, Lipsky PE. Dendritic cells: origin and differentiation. *Stem Cells* 1996; **14**: 196–206.

65. Medzhitov R, Janeway CA Jr. Innate immunity: the virtues of a nonclonal system of recognition. *Cell* 1997; **91**: 295–8.

66. Corinti S, Medaglini D, Cavani A et al. Human dendritic cells very efficiently present a heterologous antigen expressed on the surface of recombinant gram-positive bacteria to CD4+ T lymphocytes. *J Immunol* 1999; **163**: 3029–36.

67. Randolph GJ, Beaulieu S, Lebecque S et al. Differentiation of monocytes into dendritic cells in a model of transendothelial trafficking. *Science* 1998; **282**: 480–3.

68. Cyster JG. Chemokines and the homing of dendritic cells to the T-cell areas of lymphoid organs. *J Exp Med* 1999; **189**: 447–50.

69. Dubois B, Vanbervliet B, Fayette J et al. Dendritic cells enhance growth and differentiation of CD40-activated B lymphocytes. *J Exp Med* 1997; **185**: 941–51.

70. Banchereau J, Briere F, Caux C et al. Immunobiology of dendritic cells. *Annu Rev Immunol* 2000; **18**: 767–811.

71. Zhang X, Izikson L, Liu L, Weiner HL. Activation of CD25(+)CD4(+) regulatory T cells by oral antigen administration. *J Immunol* 2001; **167**: 4245–53.

72. Thorstenson KM, Khoruts A. Generation of anergic and potentially immunoregulatory CD25+CD4 T cells in vivo after induction of peripheral tolerance with intravenous or oral antigen. *J Immunol* 2001; **167**: 188–95.

73. Suto A, Nakajima H, Ikeda K et al. CD4(+)CD25(+) T-cell development is regulated by at least 2 distinct mechanisms. *Blood* 2002; **99**: 555–60.

74. Roncarolo M-G, Levings MK, Traversari C. Differentiation of T regulatory cells by immature dendritic cells. *J Exp Med* 2001; **193**: F5–9.

75. Mehling A, Grabbe S, Voskort M et al. Mycophenolate mofetil impairs the maturation and function of murine dendritic cells. *J Immunol* 2000; **165**: 2374–81.

76. Lutz MB, Suri RM, Niimi M et al. Immature dendritic cells generated with low doses of GM-CSF in the absence of IL-4 are maturation resistant and prolong allograft survival in vivo. *Eur J Immunol* 2000; **30**: 1813–22.

77. Steinbrink K, Wolfl M, Jonuleit H et al. Induction of tolerance by IL-10-treated dendritic cells. *J Immunol* 1997; **159**: 4772–80.

78. Griffin MD, Lutz W, Phan VA et al. Dendritic cell modulation by 1alpha,25 dihydroxyvitamin D3 and its analogs: a vitamin D receptor-dependent

pathway that promotes a persistent state of immaturity in vitro and in vivo. *Proc Natl Acad Sci USA* 2001; **98**: 6800–5.

79. Hackstein H, Morelli AE, Larregina AT et al. Aspirin inhibits in vitro maturation and in vivo immunostimulatory function of murine myeloid dendritic cells. *J Immunol* 2001; **166**: 7053–62.

80. Lee JI, Ganster RW, Geller DA et al. Cyclosporine A inhibits the expression of costimulatory molecules on in vitro-generated dendritic cells: association with reduced nuclear translocation of nuclear factor kappa B. *Transplantation* 1999; **68**: 1255–63.

81. de Jong EC, Vieira PL, Kalinski P, Kapsenberg ML. Corticosteroids inhibit the production of inflammatory mediators in immature monocyte-derived DC and induce the development of tolerogenic DC3. *J Leukoc Biol* 1999; **66**: 201–4.

82. Yoshimura S, Bondeson J, Foxwell BM et al. Effective antigen presentation by dendritic cells in NF-kappaB dependent coordinate regulation of MHC, costimulatory molecules and cytokines. *Int Immunol* 2001; **13**: 675–83.

83. Giannoukakis N, Bonham CA, Qian S et al. Prolongation of cardiac allograft survival using dendritic cells treated with NF-κB decoy oligodeoxyribonucleotides. *Mol Ther* 2000; **1**: 430–7.

84. Dayer JM, Burger D. Cytokines and direct cell contact in synovitis: relevance to therapeutic intervention. *Arthritis Res* 1999; **1**: 17–20.

85. Feldmann M. Pathogenesis of arthritis: recent research progress. *Nat Immunol* 2001; **2**: 771–3.

86. MacDonald KPA, Nishioka N, Lipsky PE, Thomas R. Functional CD40-ligand is expressed by T cells in rheumatoid arthritis. *J Clin Invest* 1997; **100**: 2404–14.

87. Sakata A, Sakata K, Ping H et al. Successful induction of severe destructive arthritis by the transfer of in vitro-activated synovial fluid T cells from patients with rheumatoid arthritis (RA) in severe combined immunodeficient (SCID) mice. *Clin Exp Immunol* 1996; **104**: 247–54.

88. Neumann M, Fries H, Scheicher C et al. Differential expression of Rel/NF-kappaB and octamer factors is a hallmark of the generation and maturation of dendritic cells. *Blood* 2000; **95**: 277–85.

89. Pettit AR, Quinn C, MacDonald KP et al. Nuclear localization of RelB is associated with effective antigen-presenting cell function. *J Immunol* 1997; **159**: 3681–91.

90. Burkly L, Hession C, Ogata L et al. Expression of relB is required for the development of thymic medulla and dendritic cells. *Nature* 1995; **373**: 531–6.

91. Weih F, Carrasco D, Durham SK et al. Multiorgan inflammation and hematopoietic abnormalities in mice with a targeted disruption of RelB, a member of the NF-kappaB/Rel family. *Cell* 1995; **80**: 331–40.

92. Wu L, A DA, Winkel KD et al. RelB is essential for the development of myeloid-related CD8alpha-dendritic cells but not of lymphoid-related CD8-alpha+ dendritic cells. *Immunity* 1998; **9**: 839–47.

93. O'Sullivan BJ, MacDonald KP, Pettit AR, Thomas R. RelB nuclear translocation regulates B-cell MHC molecule, CD40 expression, and antigen-presenting cell function. *Proc Natl Acad Sci USA* 2000; **97**: 11421–6.

94. Pai S, O'Sullivan BJ, Cooper L et al. RelB nuclear translocation mediated by C-terminal activator regions of Epstein–Barr virus-encoded latent membrane protein 1 and its effect on antigen-presenting function in B cells. *J Virol* 2002; **76**: 1914–21.

95. Cobbold S, Waldmann H. Infectious tolerance. *Curr Opin Immunol* 1998; **10**: 518–24.

95a. Martin E, O'Sullivan BJ, Low P, Thomas R. Antigen-specific suppression of a primed immune response by dendritic cells mediated by regulatory T cells secreting interleukin-10. *Immunology* 2002 (in press).

96. de Jong EC, Vieira PL, Kalinski P et al. Microbial compounds selectively induce Th1 cell-promoting or Th2 cell-promoting dendritic cells in vitro with diverse th cell-polarizing signals. *J Immunol* 2002; **168**: 1704–9.

97. Kalinski P, Hilkens CM, Snijders A et al. IL-12-deficient dendritic cells, generated in the presence of prostaglandin E2, promote type 2 cytokine production in maturing human naive T helper cells. *J Immunol* 1997; **159**: 28–35.

98. Kalinski P, Schuitemaker JHN, Hilkens CMU, Kapsenberg ML. Prostaglandin E2 induces the final maturation of IL-12-deficient CD1a+CD83+ dendritic cells: the levels of IL-12 are determined during the final dendritic cell maturation and are resistant to further modulation. *J Immunol* 1998; **161**: 2804–9.

99. Kalinski P, Hilkens CM, Wierenga EA, Kapsenberg ML. T-cell priming by type-1 and type-2 polarized dendritic cells: the concept of a third signal. *Immunol Today* 1999; **20**: 561–7.

100. Mazzoni A, Young HA, Spitzer JH et al. Histamine regulates cytokine production in maturing dendritic cells, resulting in altered T-cell polarization. *J Clin Invest* 2001; **108**: 1865–73.

101. Caron G, Delneste Y, Roelandts E et al. Histamine polarizes human dendritic cells into Th2 cell-promoting effector dendritic cells. *J Immunol* 2001; **167**: 3682–6.

102. Rott O, Cash E, Fleischer B. Phosphodiesterase inhibitor pentoxifylline, a selective suppressor of T helper type 1- but not type 2-associated lymphokine production, prevents induction of experimental autoimmune encephalomyelitis in Lewis rats. *Eur J Immunol* 1993; **23**: 1745–51.

103. Delgado M, Abad C, Martinez C et al. Vasoactive intestinal peptide prevents experimental arthritis by downregulating both autoimmune and inflammatory components of the disease. *Nat Med* 2001; **7**: 563–8.

104. Rissoan MC, Soumelis V, Kadowaki N et al. Reciprocal control of T helper cell and dendritic cell differentiation. *Science* 1999; **283**: 1183–6.

105. Zou W, Machelon V, Coulomb-L'Hermin A et al. Stromal-derived factor-1 in human tumors recruits and alters the function of plasmacytoid precursor dendritic cells. *Nat Med* 2001; **7**: 1339–46.

106. Kuwana M, Kaburaki J, Wright TM et al. Induction of antigen-specific human CD4(+) T-cell anergy by peripheral blood DC2 precursors. *Eur J Immunol* 2001; **31**: 2547–57.

107. Munn DH, Shafizadeh E, Attwood JT et al. Inhibition of T-cell proliferation by macrophage tryptophan catabolism. *J Exp Med* 1999; **189**: 1363–72.

108. Hwu P, Du MX, Lapointe R et al. Indoleamine 2,3-dioxygenase production by human dendritic cells results in the inhibition of T-cell proliferation. *J Immunol* 2000; **164**: 3596–9.

109. Kronin V, Winkel K, Suss G et al. A subclass of dendritic cells regulates the response of naive CD8 T cells by limiting their IL-2 production. *J Immunol* 1996; **157**: 3819–27.

110. Suss G, Shortman K. A subclass of dendritic cells kills CD4 T cells via Fas/Fas-ligand-induced apoptosis. *J Exp Med* 1996; **183**: 1789–96.

111. Martinez del Hoyo G, Martin P, Arias CF et al. CD8alpha+ dendritic cells originate from the CD8alpha– dendritic cell subset by a maturation process involving CD8alpha, DEC-205, and CD24 up-regulation. *Blood* 2002; **99**: 999–1004.

112. Merad M, Fong L, Bogenberger J, Engleman EG. Differentiation of myeloid dendritic cells into CD8alpha-positive dendritic cells in vivo. *Blood* 2000; **96**: 1865–72.

113. Maldonaldo-Lopez R, De Smedt T, Michel P et al. CD8α⁺ and CD8α⁻ subclasses of dendritic cells direct the development of distinct T helper cells in vivo. *J Exp Med* 1999; **189**: 587–92.

114. Fallarino F, Vacca C, Orabona C et al. Functional expression of indoleamine 2,3-dioxygenase by murine CD8alpha(+) dendritic cells. *Int Immunol* 2002; **14**: 65–8.

115. Grohmann U, Fallarino F, Silla S et al. CD40 ligation ablates the tolerogenic potential of lymphoid dendritic cells. *J Immunol* 2001; **166**: 277–83.

116. Ohteki T, Fukao T, Suzue K et al. Interleukin 12-dependent interferon gamma production by CD8alpha+ lymphoid dendritic cells. *J Exp Med* 1999; **189**: 1981–6.

117. Clare-Salzler MJ, Brooks J, Chai A et al. Prevention of diabetes in nonobese diabetic mice by dendritic cell transfer. *J Clin Invest* 1992; **90**: 741–8.

118. Shinomiya M, Fazle Akbar SM, Shinomiya H, Onji M. Transfer of dendritic cells (DC) ex vivo stimulated with interferon-gamma (IFN-gamma) down-modulates autoimmune diabetes in non-obese diabetic (NOD) mice. *Clin Exp Immunol* 1999; **117**: 38–43.

119. Ohshima S, Saeki Y, Mima T et al. Interleukin 6 plays a key role in the development of antigen-induced arthritis. *Proc Natl Acad Sci USA* 1998; **95**: 8222–6.

120. Mehling A, Loser K, Varga G et al. Over-expression of CD40 ligand in murine epidermis results in chronic skin inflammation and systemic autoimmunity. *J Exp Med* 2001; **194**: 615–28.

121. Zhang H-G, Su X, Liu D et al. Induction of specific T-cell tolerance by Fas ligand-expressing antigen-presenting cells. *J Immunol* 1999; **162**: 1423–30.

122. Min WP, Gorczynski R, Huang XY et al. Dendritic cells genetically engineered to express Fas ligand induce donor-specific hyporesponsiveness and prolong allograft survival. *J Immunol* 2000; **164**: 161–7.

123. Gorczynski RM, Yu K, Clark D. Receptor engagement on cells expressing a ligand for the tolerance-inducing molecule OX2 induces an immunoregulatory population that inhibits alloreactivity in vitro and in vivo. *J Immunol* 2000; **165**: 4854–60.

124. O'Rourke RW, Kang SM, Lower JA et al. A dendritic cell line genetically modified to express CTLA4–IG as a means to prolong islet allograft survival. *Transplantation* 2000; **69**: 1440–6.

125. Morita Y, Yang J, Gupta R et al. Dendritic cells genetically engineered to express IL-4 inhibit murine collagen-induced arthritis. *J Clin Invest* 2001; **107**: 1275–84.

126. Waldmann H, Cobbold S. Regulating the immune response to transplants. A role for CD4+ regulatory cells? *Immunity* 2001; **14**: 399–406.

127. Buhlmann JE, Foy TM, Aruffo A et al. In the absence of a CD40 signal, B cells are tolerogenic. *Immunity* 1995; **2**: 645–53.

128. Hollander GA, Castigli E, Kulbacki R et al. Induction of alloantigen-specific tolerance by B cells from CD40-deficient mice. *Proc Natl Acad Sci USA* 1996; **93**: 4994–8.

129. O'Sullivan BJ, Thomas R. CD40 ligation conditions dendritic cell antigen presenting function through sustained activation of NFkB. *J Immunol* 2002; **168**: 5491–8.

130. Graca L, Honey K, Adams E et al. Cutting edge: anti-CD154 therapeutic antibodies induce infectious transplantation tolerance. *J Immunol* 2000; **165**: 4783–6.

131. Taylor PA, Noelle RJ, Blazar BR. CD4(+)CD25(+) immune regulatory cells are required for induction of tolerance to alloantigen via costimulatory blockade. *J Exp Med* 2001; **193**: 1311–18.

132. Stober D, Schirmbeck R, Reimann J. IL-12/IL-18-dependent IFN-gamma release by murine dendritic cells. *J Immunol* 2001; **167**: 957–65.

133. Fraser JH, Rincon M, McCoy KD, Le Gros G. CTLA4 ligation attenuates AP-1, NFAT and NF-kappaB activity in activated T cells. *Eur J Immunol* 1999; **29**: 838–44.

134. Vallabhapurapu S, Ryseck RP, Malewicz M et al. Inhibition of NF-kappaB in T cells blocks lymphoproliferation and partially rescues autoimmune disease in gld/gld mice. *Eur J Immunol* 2001; **31**: 2612–22.

135. Finn PW, Stone JR, Boothby MR, Perkins DL. Inhibition of NF-kappaB-dependent T-cell activation abrogates acute allograft rejection. *J Immunol* 2001; **167**: 5994–6001.

136. Gonzalez A, Andre-Schmutz I, Carnaud C et al. Damage control, rather than unresponsiveness, effected by protective DX5+ T cells in autoimmune diabetes. *Nat Immunol* 2001; **2**: 1117–25.

137. Homann D, Jahreis A, Wolfe T et al. CD40L blockade prevents autoimmune diabetes by induction of bitypic NK/DC regulatory cells. *Immunity* 2002; **16**: 403–15.

138. Huard B, Karlsson L. A subpopulation of CD8+ T cells specific for melanocyte differentiation antigens expresses killer inhibitory receptors (KIR) in healthy donors: evidence for a role of KIR in the control of peripheral tolerance. *Eur J Immunol* 2000; **30**: 1665–75.

139. Huard B, Karlsson L. KIR expression on self-reactive CD8+ T cells is controlled by T-cell receptor engagement. *Nature* 2000; **403**: 325–8.

140. Bertone S, Schiavetti F, Bellomo R et al. Transforming growth factor-beta-induced expression of CD94/NKG2A inhibitory receptors in human T lymphocytes. *Eur J Immunol* 1999; **29**: 23–9.

141. Pettit AR, MacDonald KPA, O'Sullivan B, Thomas R. Differentiated dendritic cells expressing nuclear RelB are predominantly located in rheumatoid synovial tissue perivascular mononuclear cell aggregates. *Arthritis Rheum* 2000; **43**: 791–800.

142. Thompson AG, Pettit AR, Padmanabha J et al. Nuclear RelB+ cells are found in normal lymphoid organs and in peripheral tissue in the context of inflammation, but not under normal resting conditions. *Immunol Cell Biol* 2002; **80**: 164–9.

143. Schulz O, Edwards DA, Schito M et al. CD40 triggering of heterodimeric IL-12 p70 production by dendritic cells in vivo requires a microbial priming signal. *Immunity* 2000; **13**: 453–62.

144. Huang FP, Platt N, Wykes M et al. A discrete subpopulation of dendritic cells transports apoptotic intestinal epithelial cells to T-cell areas of mesenteric lymph nodes. *J Exp Med* 2000; **191**: 435–44.

145. Chatenoud L, Thervet E, Primo J, Bach JF. Anti-CD3 antibody induces long-term remission of overt autoimmunity in nonobese diabetic mice. *Proc Natl Acad Sci USA* 1994; **91**: 123–7.

146. Chatenoud L, Primo J, Bach JF. CD3 antibody-induced dominant self tolerance in overtly diabetic NOD mice. *J Immunol* 1997; **158**: 2947–54.

147. Kouskoff V, Korganow AS, Duchatelle V et al. Organ-specific disease provoked by systemic autoimmunity. *Cell* 1996; **87**: 811–22.

148. Matsumoto I, Staub A, Benoist C, Mathis D. Arthritis provoked by linked T and B-cell recognition of a glycolytic enzyme. *Science* 1999; **286**: 1732–5.

149. Korganow AS, Ji H, Mangialaio S et al. From

systemic T-cell self-reactivity to organ-specific autoimmune disease via immunoglobulins. *Immunity* 1999; **10**: 451–61.

150. Schaller M, Burton DR, Ditzel HJ. Autoantibodies to GPI in rheumatoid arthritis: linkage between an animal model and human disease. *Nat Immunol* 2001; **2**: 746–53.

151. Matsumoto I, Maccioni M, Lee DM et al. How antibodies to a ubiquitous cytoplasmic enzyme may provoke joint-specific autoimmune disease. *Nat Immunol* 2002; **18**: 18.

152. Ji H, Ohmura K, Mahmood U et al. Arthritis critically dependent on innate immune system players. *Immunity* 2002; **16**: 157–68.

153. Waterman SA, Gordon TP, Rischmueller M. Inhibitory effects of muscarinic receptor autoantibodies on parasympathetic neurotransmission in Sjogren's syndrome. *Arthritis Rheum* 2000; **43**: 1647–54.

154. Blanco P, Palucka AK, Gill M et al. Induction of dendritic cell differentiation by IFN-alpha in systemic lupus erythematosus. *Science* 2001; **294**: 1540–3.

155. Amoura Z, Piette JC, Chabre H et al. Circulating plasma levels of nucleosomes in patients with systemic lupus erythematosus: correlation with serum antinucleosome antibody titers and absence of clear association with disease activity. *Arthritis Rheum* 1997; **40**: 2217–25.

156. Vallin H, Blomberg S, Alm GV et al. Patients with systemic lupus erythematosus (SLE) have a circulating inducer of interferon-alpha (IFN-alpha) production acting on leucocytes resembling immature dendritic cells. *Clin Exp Immunol* 1999; **115**: 196–202.

157. Farkas L, Beiske K, Lund-Johansen F et al. Plasmacytoid dendritic cells (natural interferon-alpha/beta-producing cells) accumulate in cutaneous lupus erythematosus lesions. *Am J Pathol* 2001; **159**: 237–43.

158. Page G, Lebecque S, Miossec P. Anatomic localization of immature and mature dendritic cells in an ectopic lymphoid organ: correlation with selective chemokine expression in rheumatoid synovium. *J Immunol* 2002; **168**: 5333–41.

159. Fan L, Reilly CR, Luo Y et al. Cutting edge: ectopic expression of the chemokine TCA4/SLC is sufficient to trigger lymphoid neogenesis. *J Immunol* 2000; **164**: 3955–9.

160. Shi K, Hayashida K, Kaneko M et al. Lymphoid chemokine B cell-attracting chemokine-1 (CXCL13) is expressed in germinal center of ectopic lymphoid follicles within the synovium of chronic arthritis patients. *J Immunol* 2001; **166**: 650–5.

161. Lipsky PE, van der Heijde DM, St Clair EW et al. Infliximab and methotrexate in the treatment of rheumatoid arthritis. Anti-Tumor Necrosis Factor Trial in Rheumatoid Arthritis with Concomitant Therapy Study Group. *N Engl J Med* 2000; **343**: 1594–602.

162. Yamamoto Y, Gaynor RB. Therapeutic potential of inhibition of the NF-kB pathway in the treatment of inflammation and cancer. *J Clin Invest* 2001; **107**: 135–42.

163. Koski GK, Lyakh LA, Cohen PA, Rice NR. CD14+ monocytes as dendritic cell precursors: diverse maturation-inducing pathways lead to common activation of NF-kappab/RelB. *Crit Rev Immunol* 2001; **21**: 179–89.

164. Palanki MS. Inhibitors of AP-1 and NF-kappa B mediated transcriptional activation: therapeutic potential in autoimmune diseases and structural diversity. *Curr Med Chem* 2002; **9**: 219–27.

165. Powell PP, Dixon LK, Parkhouse RM. An IkappaB homolog encoded by African swine fever virus provides a novel mechanism for downregulation of proinflammatory cytokine responses in host macrophages. *J Virol* 1996; **70**: 8527–33.

5

Mast cells

Peter Valent and Hans-Peter Kiener

Introduction • Origin of mast cells and regulation of growth • Distribution in normal and pathologic tissues • Activation-linked antigens and phenotypic heterogeneity • Proinflammatory mediators and control of secretion • Interactions with anti-inflammatory drugs • Emerging pathogenetic concepts • References

INTRODUCTION

Mast cells (MCs) are multifunctional effector cells of the immune system.[1–3] They produce an array of proinflammatory and vasoactive compounds, including histamine, prostaglandin-D_2, and tumor necrosis factor-alpha (TNF-α).[1–6] MCs also express a number of biologically active cell surface membrane receptors, such as the high-affinity receptor for IgE (FcϵRI).[7–10] In response to activating stimuli, MCs release their chemical mediators in the tissues, thereby contributing to inflammatory reactions and respective clinical symptoms.[1–10] Likewise, the MC plays a crucial role as effector cell in IgE-dependent allergies. In addition, MCs have been implicated in chronic inflammatory processes, host defense, (neo)angiogenesis, fibrosis, wound healing, atherosclerosis, and vascular thrombosis.[11–15] Respective molecular mechanisms involve a complex network of cytokines, mediators, matrix molecules, and specific target receptors.[11–15] This chapter provides a survey of our knowledge on MCs, with special reference to their role in rheumatoid disorders and respective pathogenetic and pharmacologic concepts.

ORIGIN OF MAST CELLS AND REGULATION OF GROWTH

Origin from hemopoietic progenitors

The MC was originally described as a tissue-fixed metachromatic cell by Paul Ehrlich,[16] who also described the metachromatic leukocyte in the blood (blood basophil). Based on their morphology and staining properties, Paul Ehrlich proposed a relationship between MCs and basophils. For a long time, however, the exact origin of MCs remained an enigma. Today, it is generally appreciated that MCs are of hemopoietic origin. This concept is based on the notion that transplanted hemopoietic progenitors give rise to MCs in mice[17] and humans.[18] In addition, human and murine MCs grow in mixed colonies derived from multipotent CD34+ precursor cells.[19–21] These progenitors are detectable in the bone marrow as well as in the peripheral blood. However, MCs are not derived from blood monocytes or blood basophils.[21] Rather, MCs are replenished from MC-committed precursor cells which, in turn, derive from precommitted (CD34+/FcϵRI–) stem cells.[19–24] MC differentiation takes a significant time (weeks to months), with an extremely long life-span (up to years)[3,18] compared to the lifespan of basophils (few days or weeks). Confirming their hemopoietic origin, MCs and their progenitors express the pan leukocyte antigen CD45.[10]

Mast cells are myeloid cells and form a separate myeloid lineage

Based on expression of lineage-restricted antigens and CD phenotype, MCs are myeloid cells.[10,25,26] In fact, MCs express myeloid CD antigens, but do not express 'lymphoid' determinants (Table 5.1).[10,25,26] Interestingly, MCs share a number of functionally important cell surface membrane antigens with blood monocytes and blood basophils.[10] Notably, MCs and basophils as well as monocytes in atopic individuals display FcεRI. However, despite coexpression of distinct surface structures, MCs differ from basophils and monocytes when comparing the overall profile of surface CD

Table 5.1 Expression of lineage-associated and other CD antigens on mast cells and their progenitors: comparison with other hemopoietic cells.

		Expression on						
CD	Antigen	MC progenitor	MC	BA	EO	MO	B cell	T cell
02	LFA 2	–	–	–	–	–	–	+/–
03	TcR	–	–	–	–	–	–	+
04	T4	+/–	–	–	–	+/–	–	+
09	MRP-1	+	+	+	+	+	+	+
13	AP-N	+	–	+	+	+	–	–
14	LPSR	NK	–	–	–	+	–	–
15	3FAL	+/–	–	–	+	+	–	–
17	LCM	NK	–	+	–	+/–	–	–
19	B4	–	–	–	–	–	+	–
20	B1	NK	–	–	–	–	+	–
21	CR1	–	–	–	–	–	+	–
25	IL-2Rα	+/–	–	+	+/–	+/–	+	+
33	Siglec-3	+	+	+	+	+	–	–
35	CR1	+/–	–	+	+	+	+/–	+/–
45	LCA	+	+	+	+	+	+	+
116	GM-CSFRα	+/–	–	+	+	+	–	–
117	KIT	+	+	–	–	–	–	–
121b	IL-1RII	NK	–	+	+	+	+	+
123	IL-3Rα	+/–	–	+	+	+	+/–	–

MC, mast cell; BA, blood basophil; EO, eosinophil granulocyte; MO, monocyte. Data refer to published antibody-staining results obtained with the respective cell types.[10,26,106–109,117,134,135,145,203,204] +, majority of cells reactive; +/–, only a subset of cells reactive; –, no significant reactivity found; NK, not known; LFA, leukocyte function-associated antigen; IL, interleukin; GM-CSF, granulocyte–macrophage colony-stimulating factor.

antigens (Table 5.1).[10,25,26] Thus, based on their origin and CD antigen phenotype, MCs constitute a separate myeloid lineage within the hemopoietic cell system. The term 'tissue basophil' should not be used to denominate MCs.

Growth factors

Various cytokines are involved in the regulation of differentiation and maturation of MCs. In the murine system, interleukin-3 (IL-3), IL-4, stem cell factor (SCF), IL-9, IL-10 and nerve growth factor (NGF) promote the development of MCs from their progenitors (Table 5.2).[27–31] Under physiologic conditions, SCF appears to be the most important cytokine. Thus, mice with a functionally inactive *SCF* gene (Sl/Sl[d]) are virtually MC deficient.[32] Moreover, SCF is a major and specific differentiation and survival factor for human MCs.[33–36] Correspondingly, injection of SCF into patients[37] (or in experimental animals[31]) is associated with MC differentiation and MC hyperplasia. The effects of SCF on MCs and their progenitors are exerted through a transmembrane tyrosine kinase receptor (SCF receptor = KIT = CD117) encoded by the *c-kit* proto-oncogene.[38–40] The SCF receptor is expressed on CD34[+] (precommitted) progenitors, on MC-committed progenitors, as well as on mature MCs.[10,40] Functional defects in the *c-kit* gene (W/W[v]) are associated with profound MC deficiency.[41] All in all, the SCF receptor KIT, and its ligand, SCF (KIT ligand), appear to be essential for MC differentiation and growth as well as MC survival. The MC growth factor SCF is produced by microenvironmental cells such as (activated) fibroblasts or vascular endothelial cells.[42,43] In line with this notion, MC development often occurs in association with blood vessels or stromal cells in vivo.[3]

IL-3 was originally described as a major differentiation factor for murine MCs.[3,27] In fact, IL-3 promotes the differentiation and growth of immature MC-lineage cells in mouse bone marrow culture.[27] However, late-stage MC progenitors can develop independently of IL-3,[44] and additional factors (cytokines) seem to be required for further MC differentiation and maturation.[28–31] Also, under physiologic conditions, IL-3 is not required for MC development in the mouse – in fact, IL-3-knockout mice

---

Table 5.2   Effects of growth factors on differentiation and maturation of mast cells.

Growth factor	Human mast cells		Murine mast cells	
	Induces differentiation	Promotes maturation	Induces differentiation	Promotes maturation
SCF	+	+	+	+
IL-3	–	–	+	+
IL-4	–	+	+/–	+
IL-5	–	–	–	+/–
IL-6	–	+/–	–	+
IL-7	–	–	–	–
IL-9	–	–	+	+
IL-10	–	–	+	+
NGF	–	+/–	+	+

SCF, stem cell factor; NGF, nerve growth factor.

exhibit almost normal numbers of MCs in the tissues.[45] However, when infected with a nematode, the resulting increase in mouse tissue (gastrointestinal) MCs and blood basophils appears to be IL-3 dependent.[45] In the human system, IL-3 is a major differentiation factor for basophils, but not for human MCs (Table 5.2).[46–48] In line with this notion, human basophils express high-affinity IL-3-binding sites,[49] whereas human MCs usually do not express IL-3 receptors (Table 5.1).[26,48] However, these cells may acquire IL-3 receptor under certain circumstances, i.e. after activation by distinct cytokines (unpublished).

In contrast to other hemopoietic cells, MCs complete their differentiation and maturation in extramedullary organs.[3,40] The process of terminal maturation is associated with expression of distinct granular (cytoplasmic) molecules and distinct profiles of cell surface antigens.[1–3,10] Likewise, depending on their maturation stage and other factors, human MC subsets differ from each other in their content of the MC-specific enzyme chymase.[50,51] Recent data suggest that terminal maturation of MCs is regulated by interleukins. In the murine system, IL-4, IL-9 and IL-10 have been implicated in the generation of MC subsets defined by expression of distinct protease profiles, distinct functions, and various staining properties.[28,52–55] In the human system, IL-4 appears to be a critical factor. Thus, IL-4 promotes the expression of chymase as well as expression of important surface molecules, including FcεRI, in developing (SCF-dependent) human MCs.[51,56] The effects of IL-4 on MCs and their progenitors are mediated through a specific receptor (IL-4 receptor).[56]

DISTRIBUTION IN NORMAL AND PATHOLOGIC TISSUES

Physiologic distribution

Under physiologic conditions, MCs are detectable in almost all organ systems.[3,57] The number of MCs varies, however, depending on the tissue examined. The lung, skin, and gastrointestinal tract are rich in MCs (Figure 5.1). Other organs,

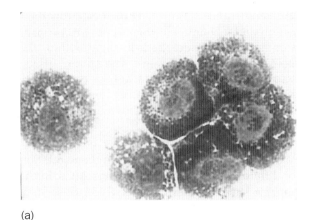

(a)

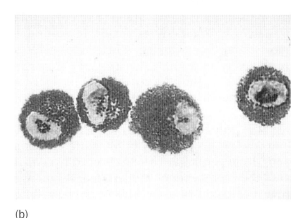

(b)

Figure 5.1 MCs enriched from human lung tissue. Isolated MCs were stained with Wright–Giemsa (a) and an antibody against MC tryptase (b).

like the brain, contain only a few MCs. Remarkably, the physiologic number of MCs detectable in primary hemopoietic tissues (bone marrow, spleen) is rather low.[58] Also, in contrast to other hemopoietic cells and MC progenitors, mature MCs are not detectable in the blood.[3,57] In local tissues, MCs exhibit a certain affinity for distinct cells and cell-based structures. Notably, MCs are often found in close apposition to small blood vessels, capillaries, and postcapillary venules.[2,3,57] Also, MCs are frequently detectable in association with nerves or foci of fibrohistio-cytic cells.[3,59,60] Some of these associations may be due to direct cell–cell interactions.[3,57] Others may be due to an affinity of MCs for cell-derived matrix molecules, cell-derived chemotactic factors, or cell-derived growth factors.[3,15,57] Thus, the MC growth factor SCF is produced by various (activated) stromal cells including vascular endothelial cells.[42,43] Interestingly, SCF is expressed in these cells in membrane-bound or soluble form, and thus can act as either a chemoattracting cytokine (soluble) or an adhesion receptor (membrane-bound form) for MCs and their progenitors.[42,43,61] Based on histologic aspects, the baseline numbers of MCs in the tissues may be regarded as low.[58] However, the calculated volume of a hypothetical organ that would contain all MCs in a given individual (man) at one site would reach the size of the spleen.

Mast cell accumulation in inflamed tissues

Depending on the condition and pathogen, the baseline levels of tissue MCs can change in inflammatory reactions. During acute inflammation (especially anaphylactic reactions), the numbers of detectable MCs may decrease, due to massive degranulation with loss of metachromasia.[62,63] However, these 'phantom mast cells' have the capacity to recover and to regranulate.[64,65] The so-called 'late-phase reaction' following an anaphylactic response is frequently accompanied by an increase in metachromatic cells.[66] Some of these cells may be MCs – most of them, however, are basophils.[66]

During chronic inflammation, the number of MCs often increases (Figure 5.2).[67–85] Such an increase in MCs is observed in chronic arthritides,[67,68,80,81,83] Crohn's disease,[69] inflammatory hepatobiliary diseases,[71,72] (glomerulo)nephritides,[73–75] dermatitides,[78,79] or worm infections.[76] In most conditions, the MC hyperplasia is a local phenomenon restricted to the affected organ site(s). The mechanisms underlying MC accumulation in chronic inflammation are not well understood. Based on several observations, the increase is most likely due to both an accumulation (chemotaxis) of mature MCs and influx and local differentiation of MC progenitors. In fact, MCs detectable at sites of ongoing inflammation often represent a mixture of mature and

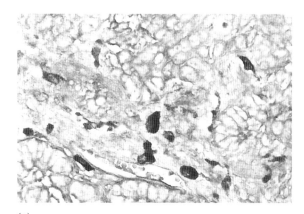

(a)

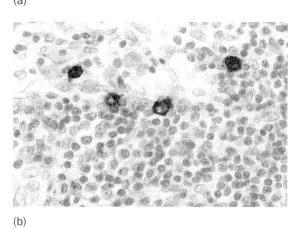

(b)

Figure 5.2 Increase in MCs in chronic inflammation. (a) Wright–Giemsa-stained tissue section obtained from a patient with chronic gastrointestinal inflammation. (b) A tissue section obtained from a patient with rheumatoid arthritis – this tissue section was stained with an antibody against MC tryptase.

immature cells. So far, little is known, however, about factors regulating the transmigration and homing of MC progenitors, their differentiation, and MC chemotaxis in inflamed tissues. One critical factor may be SCF. In fact, this 'MC-targeting' cytokine is produced by activated stromal cells[42,43] and is upregulated in chronically inflamed tissues.[81–85] However, apart from SCF, other cytokines (ILs, others), chemokines, complement factors and adhesion molecules may also be involved in MC accumulation.[3,15,57]

Mast cells in fibrosis, vascular thrombosis, and (neo)angiogenesis

Apart from inflammation, a number of other pathologic conditions may also lead to an increase and accumulation of MCs. Most of these conditions are characterized by activation of local fibroblasts or vascular endothelial cells. Since inflammation is also characterized by activation of stromal cells, the molecular mechanisms underlying MC accumulation in diverse pathologies may be quite similar, and most of them may involve SCF. MC accumulation is specifically found in wound healing,[86–88] fibrosis,[89–91] angiogenesis,[92–94] atherosclerosis,[95,96] thrombosis,[14,15,97] and growth of certain tumors.[92–94,98,99] In several of these conditions, MCs may not only accumulate, but may also play an active pathogenetic role. Likewise, MCs are capable of producing and secreting fibrogenic and angiogenic cytokines (fibroblast growth factor (FGF), vascular endothelial growth factor (VEGF) and others).[100–103] In addition, MCs produce and release repair molecules such as anti-thrombotic heparin or profibrinolytic tissue-type plasminogen activator (tPA).[15,104,105] Thus, MCs may also participate actively in various pathologic conditions associated with activation or/and growth of stromal cells, fibrin deposition, and tissue repair.[15] With regard to angiogenesis and fibroblast proliferation, it is difficult to define for each pathology whether the increase in MCs is a cause or result of the stroma cell accumulation.[91] In most of the disease models examined, however, it turned out that MCs increased in response to a primary accumulation (and activation) of stromal cells.[91,97] Based on the notion that MCs express repair molecules (heparin, tPA and others) and increase in local affected areas, it is tempting to speculate that these cells can act as important repair cells in vivo.[15]

Expression of adhesion molecules and homing receptors

The distribution and spread of various leukocytes in the tissues is regulated in part by expression of adhesion receptors. MCs and their progenitors express a number of cell–cell- and cell–matrix-type adhesion antigens on their surface.[10,56,106–111] The immature (circulating) MC progenitor is supposedly capable of rolling on selectins and transmigrating through the endothelial cell layer.[40] In line with this concept, MC progenitors express selectin ligands and β_2 integrins known to bind to endothelial cell surface antigens (Table 5.3).[110,111] Tissue-specific homing of MC progenitors may be facilitated by distinct adhesion receptors.[111] After migration and differentiation, MCs adhere to various cell-based and matrix-based structures. Thus, mature (tissue) MCs can bind to laminin, vitronectin, fibrinogen and fibronectin, and express respective receptors, including β_1 and β_3 integrins.[10,106–116] They also express a number of intercellular adhesion molecules, including ICAM-1 (CD54), on their surface (Table 5.3).[10,56,106–109] Remarkably, the ICAM-3 antigen (CD50) is detectable on lung MCs, whereas skin MCs express only low or undetectable amounts of ICAM-3.[117] In contrast to blood basophils (and other leukocytes), mature tissue MCs do not express substantial amounts of β_2 integrins as resting cells.[10,56,106–109] Expression of multiple adhesion receptors may explain why MCs are primarily tissue-fixed cells after maturation. However, expression of adhesion receptors on MCs may change in response to cell activation (by cytokines or other stimuli).[10,56,118] Moreover, MCs reportedly have the capacity to relocate and even to transmigrate from one organ site to another.[119]

Response to chemotactic stimuli

A number of observations suggest that MCs can migrate within tissues and accumulate in response to chemotactic factors.[3,119] Thus, chemotaxis may contribute to the MC accumulation observed in inflammatory or other tissue reactions. A number of MC-chemotactic factors have been identified in the past. Murine MCs chemotax against several compounds, including cytokines, chemokines, and even matrix-derived molecules (laminin).[3,120,121] Human tissue MCs show a chemotactic response to SCF, certain

Table 5.3   Adhesion receptor expression on human mast cells (MCs): comparison to basophils (BA).

Structure	CD	Major ligand(s)	Lung MCs	Skin MCs	BA
β_1 integrin β-chain	29	Matrix molecules, CAMs	+	+	+
VLA-1α	49a	Collagen, laminin-1	–	–	+
VLA-2α	49b	Collagen, laminin	–	–	–
VLA-3α	49c	Laminin-5, Fn, collagen	+	+	–
VLA-4α	49d	CD106, MAdCAM	+	+	+
VLA-6α	49f	Laminins, invasin, CD104	–	–	–
β_2 integrin β-chain	18	CAMs, matrix molecules	–	–	+
LFA-1α	11a	ICAM-1, -2, -3	–	–	+
C3biRα	11b	C3bi, Fgen, ICAM-1	–	–	+
CR4α	11c	C3bi, ICAM-1	–	–	+
β_3 integrin β-chain	61	Vitronectin, Fgen, vWF	+	+	–
VNRα	51	Vitronectin, Fgen, vWF	+	+	–
GPIIb/αIIb-integrin	41	Fgen, Fn, vWF	–	–	–
β_4 integrin	104	Laminins, CD49f	–	–	–
HML-1α	103	E-cadherin, β_7 integrin	–	–	–
LFA-2	02	LFA-3/CD58, CD48	–	–	–
PECAM-1	31	CD38	–	–	+
ICAM-1	54	CD11/LFA-1/Mac-1	+	+	+
ICAM-2	102	LFA-1	+/–	+/–	+
ICAM-3	50	LFA-1	+	+/–	+
LFA-3	58	LFA-2/CD2	+	+	+
VCAM-1	106	$\alpha_4\beta_1$ integrin	–	–	–
MRP-1, DRAP-1	09	CD81, CD82, CD63	+	+	+
3-FAL	15	Selectins, CD62	–	–	–
sLe^x	15s	P, E-selectins	–	–	+
HPCA-1	34	L-selectin/CD62L	–	–	–
PSGL-1	162	P, E-selectins	–	–	+
Leukosialin	43	Hyaluronan	+	+	+
Pgp-1	44	Hyaluronan, Fn	+	+	+
IAP	47	SIRPα/CD172a	+	+	+
L-selectin	62L	MAdCAM, CD34	–	–	+
LIMP	63	VLAs, CD81	+	+	+
PETA-3	151	β_1 integrins	+	+	+
BST-1	157	Unknown	+	+	+
ALCAM	166	CD6	–	–	–
SIRPα	172a	CD47	+	+	+/–

Data refer to published antibody-staining results obtained with the respective cell types.[10,26,106–109,117,128–130] +, majority of cells reactive; +/–, only a subset of cells reactive; –, no significant reactivity found.

chemokines, urokinase, and C5a.[43,122–126] The effects of the chemotaxins on MCs are mediated through specific receptors.[121–126] Whereas SCF appears to induce chemotaxis in all types of MCs (MCs almost invariably express SCF receptors), C5a and the chemokines only induce chemotaxis in distinct subsets of MCs, i.e. those expressing specific receptors.[125–130] With regard to chemokines, immature and activated MCs may express significant numbers of target receptors on their cell surface.[126,127] The chemotactic C5a receptor (CD88) is variably expressed on human MCs, depending on the condition and type of disease.[125,128–130]

ACTIVATION-LINKED ANTIGENS AND PHENOTYPIC HETEROGENEITY

A number of different observations in mice and humans support the concept of MC heterogeneity. In fact, depending on the environment and other factors, MCs differ in their staining properties, expression of mediators, and response to certain stimuli.[131–134] MCs also are heterogeneous cells in terms of their cell surface antigen phenotype.[10,128–130] Some of these differences may be due to an organ-specific heterogeneity of MCs. Other differences may be due to cell activation or different stages of maturation.[134] Likewise, a number of observations made with cultured immature MCs (in humans or mice) could not be reconfirmed when normal mature tissue MCs (in the same species) were examined. When comparing results in the literature, it is also of importance to take into account that MCs from different species do not behave in the same way in all respects and may express different patterns of cytoplasmic and cell surface antigens.

Cytokine receptors

MCs and their progenitors express a number of cytokine receptors on their surface. Uncommitted and precommitted MC progenitors express multiple sites, including receptors for SCF, IL-3, IL-4, IL-6, granulocyte–macrophage colony-stimulating factor (GM-CSF), and many

more.[10,24,26,135] In contrast to other myeloid lineages, MCs exhibit the SCF receptor (KIT) throughout development.[10,40,135] Receptors for IL-4 may also be expressed throughout mastopoiesis. Other cytokine receptors, however, decrease in expression or are lost during MC differentiation, at least in the human system.[10,26,135] Thus, mature human MCs lack many cytokine receptors (GM-CSF receptor, G-CSF receptor, IL receptors) otherwise detectable on granulocytic or monocytic cells.[10,26,48] With regard to the IL-3 receptor, major differences between human and murine MCs have been reported.[26,48] In fact, IL-3 receptors are detectable on murine MCs, but usually not on human MCs.[26,48] However, more recent data suggest that human MCs may express IL-3 receptors when exposed to distinct cytokines, i.e. SCF plus IL-4 (unpublished). Interestingly, exposure of MCs to IL-4 is also followed by a decrease in expression of KIT.[38] Thus, expression of growth factor receptors on human MCs may be regulated by the cytokine network. Another interesting phenomenon is that the KIT ligand SCF itself is capable of downmodulating its own specific receptor at both the mRNA and protein levels.[61,136] All in all, multiple mechanisms and factors appear to be responsible for differential expression of cytokine receptors on MCs and their progenitors.[134]

Complement receptors

MCs in various organs express surface receptors for distinct components of complement.[10,26,117,129,130,137,138] Human MCs constitutively express membrane cofactor protein, MCP (CD46),[130,137] decay accelerating factor, DAF (CD55),[130,137] and membrane attack complex inhibitory factor, MACIF (CD59)[130,137] on their surface (Table 5.4). Other complement receptors, such as the C3bi receptor (CD11b) or CR1 (CD35), are only expressed on MCs under certain conditions (activated MCs, mastocytosis).[118,139] The lymphocyte C3d receptor CR2 (CD21) is not detectable on human MCs.[10] Human MCs (derived from lung or skin) also lack significant amounts of the phagocytic C1q receptor CD93.[117]

Table 5.4 Complement receptors expressed on mast cells (MCs): comparison to basophils.

Complement receptor	CD	Ligand(s)	Lung MCs	Synovial MCs (RA)	Synovial MCs (OA)	Basophils
C1qR	93	C1(2)	–	NK	NK	–
CR1	35	C3b	–	–	–	+
CR2	21	C3d	–	–	–	–
CR3α/C3biRα	11b	C3bi	–	–	–	+
CR4α	11c	C3bi, C3d,g	–	–	–	+
CR3/4 β-chain	18	C3	–	–	–	+
MCP	46	C3b, C4b	+	+	+	+
DAF	55	C4b/2a, C3b/Bb	+	+	+	+
MACIF	59	C5b-8, C5b-9	+	+	+	+
C5aR	88	C5a	–	+	–	+

RA, rheumatoid arthritis; OA, osteoarthritis; NK, not known. Data refer to published antibody-staining results obtained with respective cells.[10,26,106–109,117,128–130]

Under physiologic conditions, the C5a receptor (CD88) is expressed on foreskin MCs,[117] and a small subset of cardiac MCs,[140] but is usually not detectable on lung MCs, synovial MCs, or MCs in other organ systems.[117,129,130,134] Remarkably, in rheumatoid arthritis, synovial MCs express substantial amounts of C5a receptor (CD88), whereas MCs in osteoarthritis display only low levels of CD88 (Table 5.4).[129] Thus, the C5a receptor apparently represents an activation-linked cell surface membrane antigen expressed on MCs in inflamed tissues. The factor(s) that contribute(s) to expression of C5a receptor on (synovial) MCs in chronic (rheumatoid) inflammation have not been identified yet.

The high-affinity receptor for IgE

MCs in various organs express the high-affinity receptor for IgE (FcεRI).[1–10] Expression of FcεRI on MCs is dependent on several factors. During differentiation from their progenitors and consecutive maturation, MCs acquire FcεRI in a cytokine-dependent manner.[3,10] In the murine system, several cytokines (IL-3, IL-4, SCF) may be involved. In the human system, IL-4 is considered to be a critical cytokine promoting expression of FcεRI during SCF-dependent differentiation of MC progenitors.[51] Mature MCs express FcεRI in a constitutive manner.[7–9] However, the levels of expressed FcεRI vary depending on the environment and presence of IgE. Thus, when occupied with IgE, FcεRI on MCs and basophils exhibits a longer half-life and a reduced rate of internalization compared to the unoccupied receptor.[141,142] In line with this concept, the serum levels of IgE in atopic individuals correspond well with the levels of FcεRI detectable on the surface of blood basophils.[143] Thus, IgE itself appears to be involved in the regulation of expression of high-affinity IgE-binding sites on mature MCs and basophils.

Apart from FcεRI, MCs also express other Fc receptors. In particular, it has been shown that distinct subsets of MCs, especially cutaneous MCs, constitutively express the low-affinity FcγRI (CD32).[117] This observation points to organ-specific expression of Fcγ receptors on MCs. Other observations suggest, however, that expression of Fcγ receptors on MCs is regulated by distinct cytokines. Likewise, the high-affinity IgG receptor FcγRI is expressed in considerable amounts on human MCs after exposure to interferon gamma (IFN-γ).[144] Expression of IgG receptors on MCs may explain why not all antigen-triggered, MC-dependent reactions are mediated through IgE. The low-affinity FcεRI (CD23) is not expressed by human MCs.[10,25,26]

Receptors for microbial antigens

Human MCs express a number of CD determinants known to bind viral or bacterial antigen. Respective CDs detectable on human tissue MCs include the herpesvirus-8 (HHV-8) receptor CD29/CD49c,[109] the major rhinovirus receptor CD54 (ICAM-1),[56,106] the measles virus receptor CD46 (identical with MCP),[117,130,137] the Coxsackie B/echovirus receptor CD55 (identical with DAF),[117,130,137] the African swine virus receptor CD59,[117,130,137] and the hepatitis C virus receptor CD81 (Table 5.5).[117] Human tissue MCs do not express the echovirus-1 binding site CD49b, the lymphocyte Epstein–Barr virus (EBV) receptor (CD21), the herpes simplex (HS) virus receptors CD111 and CD112, or poliovirus receptor (PVR = CD155) (Table 5.5).[10,109,128,130,137] Some of the virus receptors appear to be expressed on immature MC progenitors rather than on mature MCs. Likewise, the Corona virus/cytomegalovirus (CMV) receptor CD13 and the HIV coreceptors CXCR4 (CD184) and CCR3 are expressed on immature cultured MCs.[126,127,145–147] Also, these progenitors may express low levels of HIV receptor CD4.[147] By contrast, mature tissue MCs do not express substantial amounts of CD4, CD13 or CXCR4.[10,117,128]

Bacterial antigens may also bind to MCs via distinct CD molecules. Notably, MCs express CD48, a GPI-linked receptor that has been implicated in the binding to FimH-expressing *Escherichia coli*.[26,117,148] MCs also express CD55, which binds to *E. coli* antigen in a specific manner. Moreover, MCs can be activated by *E. coli* derived antigen.[148,149] Other bacterial receptors, including lipopolysaccharide (LPS) receptors CD14 and CD180 as well as Shiga toxin 1 receptor (CD77), are not detectable on human MCs[10,26,117] (Table 5.5). Also, MCs fail to express receptors for *Plasmodium falciparum* (CD36, CD236).[10,26,117]

Apart from binding to CD antigens, all types of bacteria and viruses can bind to MCs through specific IgE and the high-affinity IgE receptor (FcεRI).

Activation-linked antigens

Activation of MCs or basophils is often associated with (followed by) an increased expression of distinct (surface) molecules. During the past decade, a number of such activation-linked antigens have been identified. In response to crosslinking of the FcεRI, murine and human MCs, as well as basophils, express increased amounts of CD63 on their surface.[150,151] This increase is probably due to a translocation of CD63 from intracellular (granule-associated) stores. The CD63 test is widely used to measure IgE-dependent (specific) responses to an allergen.[151,152] Another activation-linked antigen appears to be CD203c. This antigen has recently been identified as ectonucleotide pyrophosphatase/phosphodiesterase 3 (E-NPP3).[153,154] E-NPP3 is expressed on basophils and MCs as well as on MC- and basophil-progenitor cells.[153] In response to IgE receptor crosslinking, the levels of CD203c increase significantly.[153]

PROINFLAMMATORY MEDIATORS AND CONTROL OF SECRETION

Spectrum of mediators

MCs produce an array of vasoactive and proinflammatory mediator substances, including histamine, cytokines, and prostaglandin-D_2.[1–6] In addition, MCs produce various repair molecules such as heparin, tPA, or biologically active proteases, including tryptase and chymase.[1–6,50,100–105] In general, the MC-derived mediators can be divided into several groups based on production requirement(s). Some mediators (histamine, β-tryptase, TNF-α) are

Table 5.5   Expression of binding sites for viral and bacterial antigens.

CD	Antigen	Ligand	Expression on human		
			MC precursor	Tissue MC	Basophil
04	T4	HIV	+/−	−	−
13	AP-N	Coronavirus, CMV	+	−	+
21	CR2	EBV	NK	−	−
46	MCP	Measles virus	+	+	+
49b	VLA-2α	Echo virus-1	NK	−	−
49c	VLA-3	Herpes virus-8/KSHV	NK	+	−
54	ICAM-1	Rhino virus	NK	+	+
55	DAF	Coxsackie-B/echo virus-70	NK	+	+
59	MACIF	African swine virus	NK	+	+
81	HCVR	HCV	NK	+	+/−
111	PRR1	Env gD of HSV	NK	−	−
112	PRR2	Env gD of HSV	NK	−	−
155	PVR	Polio virus	NK	−	−
184	CXCR4	HIV (coreceptor)	+	−	+/−
195	CCR5	HIV (coreceptor)	NK	−	−
14	LPS-R	LPS	NK	−	−
35	CR1	Mycobacterial antigen	+/−	−	+
48	Blast-1	FimH of *Escherichia coli*	NK	+	+
66	NCA	Opa of *Neisseria* m/g	NK	−	−
77	Gb3	Shiga toxin-1	NK	−	−
90	Thy-1	*A.h.* aerolysin	NK	−	−
180	RP105	LPS	NK	−	−
36	ThrSpR	*Plasmodium falciparum*	NK	−	−
236	GlycphC	*Plasmodium falciparum*	NK	−	−

HIV, human immunodeficiency virus; HCV, hepatitis C virus; CMV, cytomegaly virus; EBV, Epstein–Barr virus; HSV, herpes simplex virus; LPS, lipopolysaccharide; NK not known. Data refer to published antibody-staining results obtained with respective cells.[10,26,106–109,117,128–130]

primarily produced during MC differentiation or during the recovery phase after degranulation. In mature resting MCs, these mediators are stored within secretory granules, and are released from MCs during cell activation. A second group of mediators (prostaglandin D_2, interleukins) are produced (and consecutively released) during activation of MCs, but not in resting cells.[1,3–6,155,156] A third group of mediators (α-protryptase, tPA) seem to be constitutively produced and released in resting tissue MCs. These mediators can be measured in biological fluids (especially serum samples) in health and disease. Likewise, the levels of α-protryptase are considered to reflect the total burden of MCs in healthy subjects (normal serum α-protryptase levels average about 5 ng/ml) as well as in those suffering from (systemic) mastocytosis.[157] Table 5.6 provides a short summary of mediators expressed in MCs.

Cytokine-dependent secretion of mediators

In the murine system, several different cytokines have been reported to induce or promote secretion of mediators in MCs. In the human system, SCF upregulates IgE-dependent secretion of histamine (and of other mediators and

Table 5.6	Mediators of human mast cells: major functions and biological effects.
Mediator	**Biological effects and resulting clinical findings**
Histamine	Capillary leak/edema formation, vascular instability, induces selectin expression on endothelial cells, and thereby margination (rolling) of activated leukocytes
Heparin	Anti-thrombotic effect (AT-III cofactor activity), cofactor for tryptase, tPA (fibrinolytic), and FGF (angiogenic), anti-inflammatory effects, tissue repair
Tryptases	Fibrinogenolytic, matrix degradation, activate pro-uPA, induce fibroblast proliferation and mediate angiogenesis
Chymases	Matrix degradation, activation of several prohormones, inactivates thrombin (anti-thrombotic effect)
tPA	Induces plasminogen activation and fibrinolysis (thrombolysis)
Prostaglandin D_2	Induces smooth muscle cell contraction and mediates vascular instability, inhibits platelet aggregation
TNF-α	Induces endothelial cell activation and CAM expression, mediates leukocyte transmigration and invasion in local tissue sites, mediator of constitutional symptoms, fever, cachexia, shock as well as of chronic inflammation
VEGF	Activates endothelial cells, induces capillary leak and edema formation, induces (neo)angiogenesis
bFGF	Induces fibrosis, wound healing, and angiogenesis
TGF-β	Induces tissue fibrosis and wound healing
ILs, CSFs	Mediate granulopoiesis and recruitment of proinflammatory effector cells into local tissue sites
Chemokines (MCP-1, IL-8, others)	Induce chemotaxis of various leukocytes and their accumulation in local tissue sites, induce leukocyte activation and mediator release from phagocytes

tPA, tissue-type plasminogen activator; VEGF, vascular endothelial growth factor; bFGF, basic fibroblast growth factor; TGF-β, transforming growth factor beta; ILs, interleukins; CSFs, colony-stimulating factors.

cytokines) in various organs.[117,137,138,140,158–163] Moreover, after long exposure (> 90 min), SCF induces mediator secretion in MCs in the absence of other stimuli.[159,163] However, in contrast to IgE-dependent (anaphylactic) degranulation, the SCF-induced release of mediators from MCs is not associated with a rapid and complete loss of their granular content. Rather, SCF induces a slow release of mediators into the extracellular space. The effects of SCF on mediator secretion in MCs are mediated through the SCF receptor, KIT [158–163] The process of activation is initiated by dimerization of KIT by its dimeric ligand, SCF.

IgE-dependent mediator release

Crosslinking of the IgE receptor on MCs by an exogenous allergen or an autoantigen (autoallergen) is mediated through specific (receptor-bound) IgE, and is followed by (rapid) secretion of multiple mediators.[7–9] After antigen challenge, specific IgE is produced by B cells and is provided to MCs in the tissues. Once bound to FcεRI on MCs, IgE exhibits a very long half-life.[7] Exposure to a specific allergen can result in massive (anaphylactic) degranulation of MCs.[7–10] Mechanistically, crosslinkage of FcεRI on MCs leads to Ca^{2+} influx, cytoskeletal changes, surface membrane ruffling, and granule exocytosis (degranulation).[7–9] Severe systemic IgE-dependent reactions involving MCs can be life-threatening.[1,4,5] In other cases, the release reaction is less pronounced or is a chronic process. This may particularly hold true for patients who display autoantigens as a basis of chronic inflammation (severe atopy, autoimmune disorders). In fact, in these patients several different phenomena, including desensitization, cytokine interactions, and also drug effects, may contribute to the actual responsiveness of IgE-bearing effector cells (MCs).

Mast cell activation by anaphylatoxins

The anaphylatoxins C3a and C5a can also induce mediator secretion in human MCs under certain conditions. In fact, these compounds induce histamine release in MCs expressing a specific receptor. Notably, human foreskin MCs and MCs in rheumatoid arthritis express C5a receptor (CD88) and release histamine when exposed to C5a.[129,130] The notion that CD88 is only expressed on synovial MCs in rheumatoid arthritis but not in other synovial disorders suggests that the C5a receptor is an activation-linked antigen with specificity for distinct pathologies.[129] Human basophils invariably express C5aR and release histamine in response to C5a.[130]

Signal transduction events

Depending on the type of stimuli and other factors, MC activation is associated with a number of signal transduction events. In general, KIT- and FcεRI-dependent activation appear to use overlapping and in part identical pathways of signaling. In murine MCs, signaling events following IgE receptor crosslinking include activation of the tyrosine kinases Lyn and Syk, activation of phospholipase C (PLC) with subsequent generation of inositol polyphosphate- and diacylglycerol-type second messengers, activation of protein kinase C (PKC), activation of PI-3 kinase, mobilization of intracellular Ca^{2+}, and activation of the calmodulin–calcineurin–NFAT pathway.[164–168] Also, FcεRI crosslinking is followed by activation of the Ras–Raf–MEK–ERK pathway.[169] However, unlike KIT, FcεRI lacks endogenous signaling capacity. Rather, signaling through FcεRI is initiated by phosphorylation and recruitment of receptor-independent effector molecules. Apart from tyrosine kinases and other 'prosecretory' antigens, several counteracting molecules may also play a role in FcεRI activation. Of importance may be inhibitory surface molecules (which may directly interact with the IgE receptor) and distinct tyrosine phosphatases like SHP-1 or SHIP.[170–172] SHIP, especially, has been described as a gatekeeper of FcεRI-dependent mediator secretion in MCs.[172] With regard to SCF/KIT-dependent MC activation, distinct members of the signal inhibitory receptor protein (SIRP) family (CD172) and SHP-1 may play an important role. All in all, FcεRI-dependent and KIT-dependent signaling in MCs involves a number of pathways and factors, and the final reaction defining what and how much mediator is released from MCs (releasability) may be a product of multiple biochemical processes. This may also explain why MCs react quite differently to certain stimuli, depending on the overall status of the cell, the environment, and the type of disease.[3,133,134]

INTERACTIONS WITH ANTI-INFLAMMATORY DRUGS

Most of the anti-inflammatory drugs used in clinical medicine, such as the non-steroidal anti-inflammatory drugs (NSAIDs), corticosteroids, or cyclosporin A (CSA), exhibit profound inhibitory effects on MCs. These drugs interfere with signal transduction events contributing to mediator production and/or secretion. Some anti-inflammatory drugs also interfere with MC differentiation or expression of critical surface molecules such as FcεRI. In fact, most drugs exhibit multiple effects on MCs and MC progenitors. However, the anti-inflammatory drugs also interact with other immune cells such as T cells, B cells, basophils, eosinophils, and macrophages. Therefore, it is difficult to specify whether (and to which extent) a given clinical response to a drug is due to interaction with MCs or due to interaction with additional proinflammatory cells.

Glucocorticosteroids

Glucocorticosteroids are potent immunosuppressive drugs and exhibit profound inhibitory effects on growth and function of MCs.[173–178] These effects are based on multiple actions on signal transduction events. Corticosteroids reportedly inhibit IgE-dependent mediator secretion in murine MCs as well as their capacity to produce cytokines.[173–177] A remarkable effect of the steroids is their inhibitory action on TNF-α production in MCs.[176,177] Another important aspect of the glucocorticoid-type drugs is that they are capable of inhibiting surface expression of FcεRI on MCs.[178] Moreover, glucocorticoids inhibit the development of MCs in vitro as well

as in vivo.[68,179] This interesting steroid effect appears to be due to inhibition of expression of MC growth factor SCF in local cells in the tissues rather than to a direct inhibitory effect on MCs or MC progenitors.[179] Corticosteroids are widely used to treat inflammatory reactions associated with MC activation and mediator release. In addition, these drugs are used to treat patients with the aggressive form of MC proliferative disorders.

Cyclosporin A (CSA) and FK506

Both CSA and FK506 exhibit potent inhibitory effects on MCs in mice and humans.[180–186] Most significantly, these drugs block the capacity of MCs to produce cytokines in response to IgE receptor crosslinking.[184,185] Moreover, both CSA and FK506 downmodulate IgE-dependent and SCF-mediated secretion of histamine in human MCs.[180–183] The effects of CSA and FK506 on MCs are mediated through specific acceptor-molecules (cyclophilins, FKBPs) and at least in part through disruption of the calmodulin–calcineurin–NFAT pathway.[180,184–186] Both drugs are widely used for the treatment of T-cell-mediated autoimmune reactions. However, some of the beneficial effects of CSA and FK506 seen in autoimmune diseases may primarily be due to deactivation of MCs and basophils. Neither CSA nor FK506 inhibit SCF-induced in vitro differentiation of human MCs.[183]

NSAIDs and other drugs

NSAIDs and various anti-rheumatic drugs exhibit some striking effects on MCs.[187–190] Likewise, the cyclo-oxygenase inhibitors (indomethacin, salicylic acid, and others) suppress the production of prostaglandin D_2 in MCs.[187–190] Interestingly, in contrast to other NSAIDs, nimesulide also inhibits IgE-dependent release of preformed mediators in (synovial) MCs.[190] Of the many effects of other drugs on MCs to be mentioned is the inhibitory action of pentoxyfylline on TNF-α production.[177] In contrast to glucocorticoids, pentoxyfylline inhibits TNF synthesis in murine MCs at the transcriptional level.[177]

EMERGING PATHOGENETIC CONCEPTS

Apart from their well-known role as effector cells of allergic reactions, MCs have been implicated in the pathogenesis of autoimmune diseases, chronic inflammatory (rheumatic) processes, cardiovascular diseases, bacterial and viral infections, and local tissue repair (Table 5.7). These novel concepts are based on recently discovered MC mediators and MC receptors, and interactions between these receptors and their specific ligands. Notably, MCs have

recently been identified as a direct target of several viruses, bacteria, and endogenous autoantigens. Novel MC-derived mediators include tPA and several cytokines and chemokines known to be critically involved in the pathogenesis of inflammatory reactions. A major emerging concept is that MCs are critical regulators in rheumatic inflammation processes.

Mast cells as effector cells of inflammation in rheumatic diseases

A number of observations suggest that MCs can interact with autoantigens through specific IgE and thereby contribute to autoimmune

Table 5.7 Pathogenetic concepts: role of mast cells and mast cell-derived mediators.

Disease	Important MC-derived mediators	Target cell(s)	Pathologic finding(s)
Type I allergy	Vasoactive mediators, (histamine, VEGF)	Vascular endothelium	Edema formation Allergic shock
Autoimmune disorders and resulting chronic inflammation	Multiple cytokines and chemokines, proteases as well as vasoactive mediators and repair molecules	Stromal cells Fibroblasts Endothelium Macrophages Lymphocytes	Chronic edema Leukocyte infiltrate Tissue destruction Tissue repair Fibrosis
Bacterial or viral infection	Cytokines (TNF-α, ILs), chemokines (MCP-1), vasoactive mediators	Phagocytes Lymphocytes Capillaries	Leukocyte infiltrate Pus formation Edema
Helminth infection	Cytokines, chemokines proteases	Leukocytes Endothelium	Leukocyte infiltrate
Tumor invasion	Angiogenic molecules (VEGF, bFGF, tryptase)	Endothelial progenitors	Neovascularization Tumor angiogenesis
Atherosclerosis	Cytokines, proteases, heparin, tPA, TNF-α	Vascular cells Macrophages	Foam cell formation Plaque alteration
Thromboembolic diseases	Heparin, tPA Cytokines, TNF-α Proteases	Endothelial and other vascular cells	Thrombolysis Neovascularization Tissue repair

reactions.[80,191] Some of the antigen-triggered symptoms may even be MC dependent. In addition, MCs can bind various types of immune complexes through diverse Fc receptors. Also, MCs accumulate and participate in chronic inflammatory reactions through interactions with stroma cell-derived factors and cytokines.[67–80] Thus, MCs accumulate at sites of inflammation and show signs of degranulation in chronically inflamed tissues (Figure 5.2).[67–80] A widely accepted hypothesis is that MCs actively participate in chronic inflammatory processes by providing proinflammatory mediators and multifunctional cytokines in response to antigen-induced activation or in response to other, less specific stimuli (SCF, complement components and others).[3–6,67–80,192]

Of particular importance may be MC-derived TNF-α, which is upregulated in various autoimmune diseases and considered as a 'key player' and important therapeutic target in rheumatoid arthritis.[193,194] Especially in an early phase of disease or acute disease progression, MC-derived TNF may play a crucial role. Notably, TNF-α is selectively stored in MCs in the tissues and, after release, induces rapid endothelial cell activation, with consecutive influx of leukocytes from the peripheral blood into local tissue sites.[3,195,196] Other important MC-derived mediators are histamine, prostaglandin D_2, leukotrienes, chemokines, ILs, and VEGF.[4–6,101–103,155,156,160,197] All these mediators and cytokines appear to cooperate in preparing and

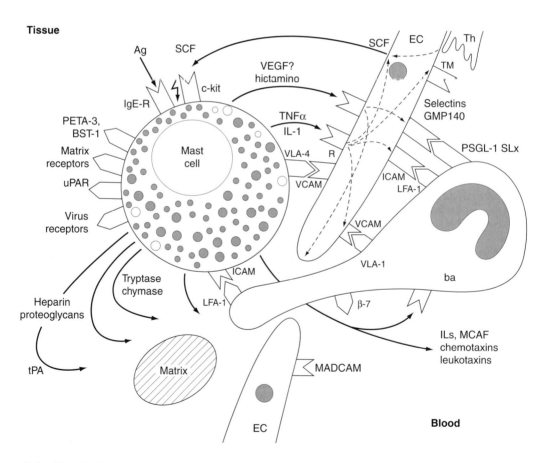

Figure 5.3 Hypothetical scheme of the role of the MC in acute and chronic inflammatory reactions and related repair processes. EC, endothelial cell; ILs, interleukins.

mediating the influx of white blood cells. In fact, histamine induces expression of selectins on endothelial cells with consecutive margination and rolling of leukocytes. In a next step, the leukocytes firmly bind to vascular endothelial cells via cytoadhesive molecules (ICAMs, VCAMs, and others). These CAMs reportedly increase in response to MC-derived TNF-α.[198,199] Histamine and VEGF promote the permeability of the capillary wall and thereby facilitate transmigration of leukocytes into the tissues. MC-derived chemokines and ILs then induce chemotaxis of invading leukocytes, resulting in their accumulation at the sites of ongoing disease.[160] MC-derived proteases (tryptases, chymases, tPA) together with heparin may facilitate leukocyte locomotion in the tissues by matrix degradation and inhibition of fibrin deposition. All in all, the MC appears to be a major regulator of leukocyte invasion during inflammatory reactions (Figure 5.3; Tables 5.6 and 5.7).

Indeed, rheumatoid lesions (synovitis) as well as other rheumatic processes are often characterized by a significant (local) infiltration of blood-derived leukocytes. A special aspect of rheumatoid synovitis (arthritis) is the resulting mesenchymal reaction leading to the formation of a hyperplastic synovium that encroaches over and invades the cartilage (then often referred to as synovial pannus). Since MCs also produce important (matrix-degrading) enzymes and interact with fibroblasts and other stromal cells by producing TNF-α and other compounds, these cells may also be involved in the destruction of local tissue elements seen in rheumatoid arthritis.

So far, little is known about cytokines and other factors leading to the accumulation and activation of MCs in rheumatoid arthritis. SCF may be one critical factor.[83] Another potential factor may be C5a. In particular, MCs in rheumatoid arthritis, but not in osteoarthritis, express C5aR and are responsive against C5a.[129] In this regard, it is noteworthy that C5a is not only upregulated in patients with rheumatoid arthritis but has also been identified as a most critical pathogenetic factor in autoimmune-type experimental arthritis.[200] Thus, it is tempting to speculate that MCs and the C5a–C5aR system play a crucial role in the pathogenesis of rheumatoid arthritis.

Possible role of mast cells in bacterial and viral infection

MCs can bind bacterial or viral antigen through specific IgE. In addition, various microbial antigens may directly bind to distinct CD antigens expressed on the surface of MCs. It therefore has been hypothesized that MCs are involved in respective infectious diseases. In bacterial infections, MCs have been implicated as major regulators of the rapid influx of phagocytes (neutrophils, monocytes) into inflamed areas.[11,12] The mechanisms appear to be similar to those of the MC-dependent influx of leukocytes in other antigen-triggered inflammatory processes (Figure 5.3). Again, MC-derived TNF-α is considered to play a key role, together with other MC-derived mediators and cytokines.[11,12] Whether MCs have the capacity to take up and kill bacteria is still under discussion. The biological significance of such phenomena may be questionable, since patients with severe neutropenia after high-dose chemotherapy have normal numbers of tissue MCs but cannot defend against bacterial invasion.

Similarly, little is known about the role of MCs in viral infections. Several observations have led to the assumption that MCs may be involved in HIV infection.[146,147,201] First, in these patients, the levels of IgE often increase, and viral antigen may induce IgE-dependent or indepedent mediator release. In addition, it has been shown that MC progenitors express CD4 and HIV coreceptors, and can be infected with HIV in vitro.[147] Moreover, distinct populations of MCs (subset of gastrointestinal MCs which may be IL dependent) in these patients may decrease in number during infection.[202] All these data suggest that the MC lineage may be involved in HIV infection. Whether, indeed, MCs play a role in the pathogenesis or progression of HIV infection, however, remains, at present, unknown.

Another important aspect is that MCs express receptors for diverse types of other viruses, including CMV receptor (CD13), hepatitis C virus receptor (CD81), and many more (Table 5.5).

Mast cells and cardiovascular disorders

Several previous and more recent studies suggest that MCs play a role in the pathogenesis and progression of cardiovascular disorders, including atherosclerosis, ischemic heart diseases, and vascular thrombosis.[14,15,95–97] In most of these conditions, MCs accumulate at the sites of ongoing disease. However, it still remains unclear whether MCs are contributing to the pathologic process as a trigger of the disease or as important repair cells. Likewise, the different mediators produced by MCs can either promote or counteract atherogenesis. Mediators that possibly may be pro-atherogenic in vivo include TNF-α (activates endothelial cells and macrophages), ILs (leukocyte activation), and histamine (induces platelet aggregation) (Tables 5.6 and 5.7). MC-derived mediators that may counteract atherosclerosis in vivo include heparin (anti-thrombotic), tPA (fibrinolytic), and other proteases (proteolysis, degradation of matrix molecules) (Tables 5.6 and 5.7). Thus, MCs and their products may be pro- or anti-atherogenic, depending on the overall situation, type of disease, and many other

factors. Likewise, the degrading effects of MC proteases, which may otherwise counteract atherosclerosis, may be fatal in case of a progressive plaque with high risk of local rupture.[96]

Mast cells as repair cells

MCs express a number of important repair molecules, including heparin, tryptases, tPA, bFGF and VEGF (Table 5.6).[100–105] Based on this notion, it has been proposed that MCs play a role in diverse repair processes, including wound healing, angiogenesis, local (physiologic) fibrosis, or endogenous fibrinolysis (Tables 5.6 and 5.7). In all these processes, MCs accumulate in local areas. After complete reconstitution and healing, the levels of MCs may decrease back to normal levels. An interesting concept has recently been proposed with regard to MC-dependent fibrinolysis. In particular, it was found that thrombin activates endothelial cells to produce soluble SCF, which in turn leads to an accumulation of MCs.[14,15,43] The accumulated MCs then provide heparin and tPA, thereby inducing fibrinolysis and counteracting further fibrin generation.[15] Thus, MC-derived heparin and tPA may play a role in chronic inflammation associated with fibrin deposition. Notably, the numbers of MCs are inversely related to the amount of fibrin deposits in the synovial tissue in rheumatoid arthritis.[68]

REFERENCES

1. Schwartz LB. The mast cell. In: Kaplan AP, ed. *Allergy*, 1st edn. (Churchill Livingstone: New York, Edinburgh, London, and Melbourne, 1985) 53–92.
2. Parwaresch MR, Horny HP, Lennert K. Tissue mast cells in health and disease. *Path Res Pract* 1985; **179**: 439–61.
3. Galli SJ. Biology of disease: new insights into 'the riddle of the mast cells': microenvironmental regulation of mast cell development and phenotypic heterogeneity. *Lab Invest* 1990; **62**: 5–33.
4. Lewis RA, Austen KF. Mediation of homeostasis and inflammation by leukotrienes and other mast cell dependent compounds. *Nature* 1981; **293**: 103–8.
5. Serafin WE, Austen KF. Mediators of immediate hypersensitivity reactions. *N Engl J Med* 1987; **317**: 30–4.
6. Gordon JR, Burd PR, Galli SJ. Mast cells as a source of multifunctional cytokines. *Immunol Today* 1990; **11**: 458–64.
7. Ishizaka T, Ishizaka K. Activation of mast cells for mediator release through IgE receptors. *Prog Allergy* 1984; **34**: 188–235.
8. Metzger H, Alcaraz G, Hohman R et al. The receptor with high affinity for immunoglobulin E. *Annu Rev Immunol* 1986; **4**: 419–70.
9. Kinet JP. The high affinity IgE receptor (FcεRI): from physiology to pathology. *Ann Rev Immunol* 1999; **17**: 931–72.

10. Valent P, Bettelheim P. Cell surface structures on human basophils and mast cells: Biochemical and functional characterization. *Adv Immunol* 1992; **52**: 333–421.

11. Zhang Y, Ramos BF, Jakschik BA. Neutrophil recruitment by tumor necrosis factor from mast cells in immune complex peritonitis. *Science* 1992; **258**: 1957–9.

12. Malaviya R, Ikeda T, Ross E, Abraham SN. Mast cell modulation of neutrophil influx and bacterial clearance at sites of infection through TNFα. *Nature* 1996; **381**: 77–80.

13. Blair RJ, Meng H, Marchese MJ et al. Human mast cells stimulate vascular tube formation. Tryptase is a novel, potent angiogenic factor. *J Clin Invest* 1997; **99**: 2691–700.

14. Bankl HC, Radaszkiewicz Th, Klappacher GW et al. Increase and redistribution of mast cells in auricular thrombosis: possible role of kit ligand. *Circulation* 1995; **91**: 275–83.

15. Valent P, Sillaber C, Baghestanian M et al. What have mast cells to do with edema formation, the consecutive repair, and fibrinolysis? *Int Arch Allergy Immunol* 1998; **115**: 2–8.

16. Ehrlich P. Beiträge zur Kenntnis der granulierten Bindegewebszellen und der eosinophilen Leukozyten. *Arch Anat Physiol* 1879; **3**: 166–9.

17. Kitamura Y, Shimada M, Hatanaka K, Miyano Y. Development of mast cells from grafted bone marrow cells in irradiated mice. *Nature* 1977; **268**: 442–3.

18. Födinger M, Fritsch G, Winkler K et al. Origin of human mast cells: development from transplanted hemopoietic stem cells after allogeneic bone marrow transplantation. *Blood* 1994; **84**: 2954–9.

19. Kitamura Y, Yokoyama M, Matsuda H, Ohno T, Mori KJ. Spleen colony forming cell as common precursor for tissue mast cells and granulocytes. *Nature* 1981; **291**: 159–60.

20. Kirshenbaum AS, Goff JP, Kessler SW et al. Effects of IL-3 and stem cell factor on the appearance of human basophils and mast cells from CD34+ pluripotent progenitor cells. *J Immunol* 1992; **148**: 772–7.

21. Agis H, Willheim M, Wilfing A et al. Monocytes do not make mast cells when cultured in the presence of SCF. Characterization of the circulating mast cell progenitor as a c-kit+, CD34+, Ly–, CD14–, CD17–, colony forming cell. *J Immunol* 1993; **151**: 4221–7.

22. Rodewald HR, Dessing M, Dvorak AM, Galli SJ. Identification of a committed precursor for the mast cell lineage. *Science* 1986; **271**: 818–22.

23. Rottem M, Okada T, Goff JP, Metcalfe DD. Mast cells cultured from peripheral blood of normal donors and patients with mastocytosis originate from a CD34+/FcεRI− cell population. *Blood* 1994; **84**: 2489–96.

24. Kempuraj D, Saito H, Kaneko A et al. Characterization of mast cell-committed progenitors present in human umbilical cord blood. *Blood* 1999; **93**: 3338–46.

25. Valent P, Ashman LK, Hinterberger W et al. Mast cell typing: demonstration of a distinct hemopoietic cell type and evidence for immunophenotypic relationship to mononuclear phagocytes. *Blood* 1989; **73**: 1778–85.

26. Agis H, Füreder W, Bankl HC et al. Comparative phenotypic analysis of human mast cells, blood monocytes and blood basophils: dissection of three distinct myeloid cell lineages. *Immunology* 1996; **87**: 535–43.

27. Ihle JN, Keller J, Oroszlan S et al. Biologic properties of homogeneous interleukin-3. I. Demonstration of WEHI-3 growth factor activity, mast cell growth factor activity, P cell-stimulating factor activity, colony-stimulating factor activity, and histamine-producing cell-stimulating factor activity. *J Immunol* 1983; **131**: 282–7.

28. Hamaguchi Y, Kanakura Y, Fujita J et al. Interleukin-4 is an essential factor for in vitro clonal growth of murine connective tissue-type mast cells. *J Exp Med* 1987; **165**: 268–73.

29. Hültner L, Druez C, Moeller J et al. Mast cell growth-enhancing activity (MEA) is structurally related and functionally identical to the novel mouse T-cell growth factor P40/TCGFIII (interleukin 9). *Eur J Immunol* 1990; **20**: 1413–16.

30. Thompson-Snipes L, Dhar V, Bond MW et al. Interleukin-10: a novel stimulatory factor for mast cells and their progenitors. *J Exp Med* 1991; **173**: 507–10.

31. Tsai M, Shih LS, Newlands GF et al. The rat c-kit ligand, stem cell factor, induces the development of connective tissue-type and mucosal mast cells in vivo. Analysis by anatomical distribution, histochemistry, and protease phenotype. *J Exp Med* 1991; **174**: 125–31.

32. Kitamura Y, Go S. Decreased production of mast cells in Sl/Sl^d mice. *Blood* 1979; **53**: 492–7.

33. Mitsui H, Furitsu T, Dvorak AM et al. Development of human mast cells from umbilical cord blood cells by recombinant human and murine c-kit ligand. *Proc Natl Acad Sci USA* 1993; **90**: 735–9.

34. Valent P, Spanblöchl E, Sperr WR et al. Induction of differentiation of human mast cells from bone marrow and peripheral blood mononuclear cells by recombinant human stem cell factor (SCF)/kit ligand (KL) in long term culture. *Blood* 1992; **80**: 2237–45.

35. Irani AM, Nilsson G, Miettinen U et al. Recombinant human stem cell factor stimulates differentiation of human mast cells from dispersed fetal liver cells. *Blood* 1992; **80**: 3009–16.

36. Saito H, Ebisawa M, Tachimoto H et al. Selective growth of human mast cells induced by steel factor, IL-6, and prostaglandin E2 from cord blood mononuclear cells. *J Immunol* 1996; **157**: 343–50.

37. Costa JJ, Demetri GD, Harrist TJ et al. Recombinant human stem cell factor (kit ligand) promotes human mast cell and melanocyte hyperplasia and functional activation in vivo. *J Exp Med* 1996; **183**: 2681–6.

38. Sillaber C, Bevec D, Ashman LK et al. IL-4 regulates c-kit gene product expression in human myeloid- and mast cell progenitors. *J Immunol* 1991; **147**: 4224–8.

39. Galli SJ, Tsai M, Wershil BK. The c-kit receptor, stem cell factor, and mast cells. What each is teaching us about the others. *Am J Pathol* 1993; **142**: 965–74.

40. Valent P. The riddle of the mast cell: kit(CD117)-ligand as the missing link? *Immunol Today* 1994; **15**: 111–14.

41. Kitamura Y, Go S, Hatanaka K. Decrease of mast cells in W/Wᵛ mice and their increase by bone marrow transplantation. *Blood* 1978; **52**: 447–52.

42. Flanagan JG, Chan DC, Leder P. Transmembrane form of kit ligand growth factor is determined by alternative splicing and is missing in the Sld mutant. *Cell* 1991; **64**: 1025–35.

43. Baghestanian M, Hofbauer R, Kress HG et al. Thrombin augments vascular cell-dependent migration of human mast cells: role of MGF. *Thromb Haemostas* 1997; **77**: 577–84.

44. Jarboe DL, Marshall JS, Randolph TR, Kukolja A, Huff TF. The mast cell-committed progenitor. I. Description of a cell capable of IL-3-independent proliferation and differentiation without contact with fibroblasts. *J Immunol* 1989; **142**: 2405–17.

45. Lantz CS, Boesiger J, Song CH et al. Role for inter-leukin-3 in mast-cell and basophil development and in immunity to parasites. *Nature* 1998; **392**: 90–3.

46. Valent P, Schmidt G, Besemer J et al. Interleukin-3 is a differentiation factor for human basophils. *Blood* 1989; **73**: 1763–9.

47. Sillaber C, Sperr WR, Agis H et al. Inhibition of stem cell factor dependent formation of human mast cells by interleukin-3 and interleukin-4. *Int Arch Allergy Immunol* 1994; **105**: 264–8.

48. Valent P, Besemer J, Sillaber C et al. Failure to detect interleukin-3 binding sites on human mast cells. *J Immunol* 1990; **145**: 3432–7.

49. Valent P, Besemer J, Muhm M et al. Interleukin-3 activates human blood basophils via high affinity binding sites. *Proc Natl Acad Sci USA* 1989; **86**: 5542–6.

50. Irani AA, Schechter NM, Craig SS, DeBlois G, Schwartz LB. Two types of human mast cells that have distinct neutral protease compositions. *Proc Natl Acad Sci USA* 1986; **83**: 4464–8.

51. Xia HZ, Du Z, Craig S et al. Effects of recombinant human IL-4 on tryptase, chymase, and Fc epsilon receptor type I expression in recombinant human stem cell factor-dependent fetal liver-derived human mast cells. *J Immunol* 1997; **159**: 2911–21.

52. Gurish MF, Ghildyal N, McNeil HP et al. Differential expression of secretory granule proteases in mouse mast cells exposed to inter-leukin-3 and c-kit ligand. *J Exp Med* 1992; **175**: 1003–12.

53. Ghildyal N, McNeil HP, Stechschulte S et al. IL-10 induces transcription of the gene for mouse mast cell protease-1, a serine protease preferentially expressed in mucosal mast cells of Trichinella spiralis-infected mice. *J Immunol* 1992; **149**: 2123–9.

54. Ghildyal N, McNeil HP, Gurish MF, Austen KF, Stevens RL. Transcriptional regulation of the mucosal mast cell-specific protease gene, MMCP-2, by interleukin-10 and interleukin-3. *J Biol Chem* 1992; **267**: 8473–7.

55. Eklund KK, Ghildyal N, Austen KF, Stevens RL. Induction by IL-9 and suppression by IL-3 and IL-4 of the levels of chromosome 14-derived transcripts that encode late-expressed mouse mast cell proteases. *J Immunol* 1993; **151**: 4266–73.

56. Valent P, Bevec D, Maurer D et al. Interleukin-4 promotes expression of mast cell ICAM-1 antigen. *Proc Natl Acad Sci USA* 1991; **88**: 3339–42.

57. Valent P, Sillaber C, Bettelheim P. The growth and differentiation of human mast cells. *Prog Growth Factor Res* 1991; **3**: 27–41.

58. Horny H-P, Valent P. Diagnosis of mastocytosis: general histopathological aspects, morphological criteria, and immunohistochemical findings. *Leuk Res* 2001; **25**: 543–51.

59. Bienenstock J, Perdue M, Blennerhassett M et al. Inflammatory cells and the epithelium. Mast cell/nerve interactions in the lung in vitro and in vivo. *Am Rev Resp Dis* 1988; **138**: S31–4.

60. Botchkarev VA, Eichelmuller S, Peters EM et al. A simple immunofluorescence technique for simultaneous visualization of mast cells and nerve fibers reveals selectivity and hair cycle-dependent changes in mast cell–nerve fibre contacts in murine skin. *Arch Dermatol Res* 1997; **289**: 292–302.

61. Adachi S, Tsujimura T, Jippo T et al. Inhibition of attachment between cultured mast cells and fibroblasts by phorbol 12-myristate 13-acetate and stem cell factor. *Exp Hematol* 1995; **23**: 58–65.

62. Dvorak AM, Massey W, Warner J et al. IgE-mediated anaphylactic degranulation of isolated human skin mast cells. *Blood* 1991; **77**: 569–78.

63. Claman HN, Choi KL, Sujansky W, Vatter AE. Mast cell 'disappearance' in chronic murine graft-vs-host disease (GVHD) – ultrastructural demonstration of 'phantom mast cells'. *J Immunol* 1986; **137**: 2009–13.

64. Dvorak AM, Kissel S. Granule changes of human skin mast cells characteristic of piecemeal degranulation and associated with recovery during wound healing in situ. *J Leukoc Biol* 1991; **49**: 197–210.

65. Dvorak AM, Morgan ES, Schleimer RP, Lichtenstein LM. Diamine oxidase–gold ultrastructural localization of histamine in isolated human lung mast cells stimulated to undergo anaphylactic degranulation and recovery in vitro. *J Leukoc Biol* 1996; **59**: 824–34.

66. Bascom R, Wachs M, Naclerio RM et al. Basophil influx occurs after nasal antigen challenge: effects of topical corticosteroid pretreatment. *J Allergy Clin Immunol* 1988; **81**: 580–9.

67. Malone DG, Irani AM, Schwartz LB, Barrett KE, Metcalfe DD. Mast cell numbers and histamine levels in synovial fluids from patients with diverse arthritides. *Arthritis Rheum* 1986; **29**: 956–63.

68. Malone DG, Wilder RI, Saavedra-Delgado AM, Metcalfe DD. Mast cell numbers in rheumatoid synovial tissues. Correlations with quantitative measures of lymphocytic infiltration and modulation by antiinflammatory therapy. *Arthritis Rheum* 1987; **30**: 130–7.

69. Dvorak AM, Monahan RA, Osage JE, Dickersin GR. Crohn's disease: transmission electron microscopic studies. II. Immunologic inflammatory response. Alterations of mast cells, basophils, eosinophils, and the microvasculature. *Hum Pathol* 1980; **11**: 606–19.

70. Feltis JT, Perez-Marrero R, Emerson LE. Increased mast cells of the bladder in suspected cases of interstitial cystitis: a possible disease marker. *J Urol* 1987; **138**: 42–3.

71. Matsunaga Y, Tereda T. Mast cell subpopulations in chronic inflammatory hepatobiliary diseases. *Liver* 2000; **20**: 152–6.

72. Nakamura A, Yamazaki K, Suzuki K, Sato S. Increased portal tract infiltration of mast cells and eosinophils in primary biliary cirrhosis. *Am J Gastroenterol* 1997; **92**: 2245–9.

73. Toth T, Toth-Jakatics R, Jimi S, Takebayashi S. Increased density of interstitial mast cells in amyloid A renal amyloidosis. *Mod Pathol* 2000; **13**: 1020–8.

74. Hiromura K, Kurosawa M, Yano S, Naruse T. Tubulointerstitial mast cell infiltration in glomerulonephritis. *Am J Kidney Dis* 1998; **32**: 593–9.

75. Colvin RB, Dvorak AM, Dvorak HF. Mast cells in the cortical tubular epithelium and interstitium in human renal disease. *Hum Pathol* 1974; **5**: 315–26.

76. Gustowska L, Ruitenberg EJ, Elgersma A, Kociecka W. Increase of mucosal mast cells in the jejunum of patients infected with Trichinella spiralis. *Int Arch Allergy Appl Immunol* 1983; **71**: 304–8.

77. Turlington BS, Edwards WD. Quantitation of mast cells in 100 normal and 92 diseased human hearts. Implications for interpretation of endomyocardial biopsy specimens. *Am J Cardiovasc Pathol* 1988; **2**: 151–7.

78. Hawkins RA, Claman HN, Clark RA, Steigerwald JC. Increased dermal mast cell populations in progressive systemic sclerosis: a link in chronic fibrosis? *Ann Intern Med* 1985; **102**: 182–6.

79. Toyry S, Fraki J, Tammi R. Mast cell density in psoriatic skin. The effect of PUVA and corticosteroid therapy. *Arch Dermatol Res* 1988; **280**: 282–5.

80. Gruber BL. Immunoglobulin E, mast cells, endogenous antigens, and arthritis. *Rheum Dis Clin North Am* 1991; **17**: 333–42.

81. Ceponis A, Konttinen YT, Takagi M et al. Expression of stem cell factor (SCF) and SCF receptor in synovial membrane in arthritis: correlation with synovial mast cell hyperplasia and inflammation. *J Rheumatol* 1998; **25**: 2304–14.

82. Esposito I, Friess H, Kappeler A et al. Mast cell distribution and activation in chronic pancreatitis. *Hum Pathol* 2001; **32**: 1174–83.

83. Kiener HP, Hofbauer R, Tohidast-Akrad M et al. TNFα promotes the expression of stem cell factor in synovial fibroblasts and their capacity to induce mast cell migration. *Arthritis Rheum* 2000; **43**: 164–74.

84. Tsunemyama K, Kono N, Yamashiro M et al. Abberrant expression of stem cell factor on biliary epithelial cells and peribiliary infiltration of c-kit-expressing mast cells in hepatolithiasis and primary sclerosing cholangitis: a possible contribution to bile duct fibrosis. *J Pathol* 1999; **189**: 609–14.

85. El-Koraie AF, Baddour NM, Adam AG et al. Role of stem cell factor and mast cells in the progression of chronic glomerulonephritides. *Kidney Int* 2001; **60**: 167–72.

86. Matsuda H, Kitamura Y. Migration of stromal cells supporting mast-cell differentiation into open wound produced in the skin of mice. *Exp Hematol* 1981; **9**: 38–43.

87. Kischer CW, Bunce H, Shetlah MR. Mast cell analysis in hypertrophic scars, hypertrophic scars treated with pressure and mature scars. *J Invest Dermatol* 1978; **70**: 355–7.

88. Trabucchi E, Radaellie E, Marazzi M et al. The role of mast cells in wound healing. *Int J Tissue React* 1988; **10**: 367–72.

89. Choi KL, Claman HN. Mast cells, fibroblasts, and fibrosis. New clues to the riddle of mast cells. *Immunol Res* 1987; **6**: 145–52.

90. Li QY, Raza-Ahmed A, MacAulay MA et al. The relationship of mast cells and their secreted products to the volume of fibrosis in posttransplant hearts. *Transplantation* 1992; **53**: 1047–51.

91. Okazaki T, Hirota S, Xu ZD et al. Increase of mast cells in the liver and lung may be associated with but not a cause of fibrosis: demonstration using mast cell-deficient Ws/Ws rats. *Lab Invest* 1998; **78**: 1431–8.

92. Ribatti D, Vacca A, Nico B et al. The role of mast cells in tumor angiogenesis. *Br J Haematol* 2001; **115**: 514–21.

93. Takanami I, Takeuchi K, Naruke M. Mast cell density is associated with angiogenesis and poor outcome in pulmonary adenocarcinoma. *Cancer* 2000; **88**: 2686–92.

94. Meininger CJ, Zetter BR. Mast cells and angiogenesis. *Semin Cancer Biol* 1992; **3**: 73–9.

95. Kovanen PT. Role of mast cells in atherosclerosis. *Chem Immunol* 1995; **62**: 70.

96. Kovanen PT, Kaartinen M, Paavonen T. Infiltrates of activated mast cells at the site of coronary atheromatous erosion or rupture in myocardial infarction. *Circulation* 1995; **92**: 1084–8.

97. Bankl HC, Großsschmidt K, Pikula B, Bankl H, Lechner K, Valent P. Mast cells are augmented in deep vein thrombosis and express a pro-fibrinolytic phenotype. *Hum Pathol* 1999; **30**: 188–94.

98. Yamamoto T, Katayama I, Nishioka K. Expression of stem cell factor in basal cell carcinoma. *Br J Dermatol* 1997; **137**: 709–13.

99. Ribatti D, Vacca A, Marzullo A et al. Angiogenesis and mast cell density with tryptase activity increase simultaneously with pathologic progression of B-cell non-Hodgkin's lymphomas. *Int J Cancer* 2000; **85**: 171–5.

100. Qu Z, Liebler JM, Powers MR et al. Mast cells are a major source of basic fibroblast growth factor in chronic inflammation and cutaneous hemangioma. *Am J Pathol* 1995; **147**: 564–73.

101. Reed JA, Albino AP, McNutt NS. Human cutaneous mast cells express basic fibroblast growth factor. *Lab Invest* 1995; **72**: 215–22.

102. Boesiger J, Tsai M, Maurer M et al. Mast cells can secrete vacular permeability factor/vascular endothelial cell growth factor and exhibit enhanced release after immunoglobulin E-dependent upregulation of Fc epsilon receptor I expression. *J Exp Med* 1998; **188**: 1135–45.

103. Grutzkau A, Kruger-Krasagakes S, Baumeister H et al. Synthesis, storage, and release of vascular endothelial growth factor/vascular permeability factor (VEGF/VPF) by human mast cells: implications for the biological significance of VEGF. *Mol Biol Cell* 1998; **9**: 875–84.

104. Yurt RW, Leid RW, Austen KF, Silbert JE. Native heparin from rat peritoneal mast cells. *J Biol Chem* 1977; **252**: 518–21.

105. Sillaber C, Baghestanian M, Bevec D et al. The mast cell as site of tissue type plasminogen activator production and fibrinolysis. *J Immunol* 1999; **162**: 1032–41.

106. Valent P, Majdic O, Maurer D et al. Further characterization of surface membrane structures expressed on human basophils and mast cells. *Int Arch Allergy Appl Immunol* 1990; **91**: 198–203.

107. Sperr WR, Agis H, Cerwenka K et al. Differential expression of cell surface integrins on human mast cells and basophils. *Ann Hematol* 1992; **65**: 10–16.

108. Guo CB, Kagey-Sobotka A, Lichtenstein LM, Bochner BS. Immunophenotypic and functional analysis of purified human uterine mast cells. *Blood* 1992; **79**: 708–12.

109. Wimazal F, Ghannadan M, Müller MR et al. Expression of homing receptors and related molecules on human mast cells and basophils: a comparative analysis using multi-color flow cytometry and toluidine blue/immunofluorescence staining technique. *Tissue Antigens* 1999; **54**: 499–507.

110. Tachimoto H, Hudson SA, Bochner BS. Acquisition and alteration of adhesion molecules during cultured human mast cell differentiation. *J Allergy Clin Immunol* 2001; **107**: 302–9.

111. Gurish MF, Tao H, Abonia JP et al. Intestinal mast cell progenitors require CD49dbeta7 (alpha4beta7 integrin) for tissue-specific homing. *J Exp Med* 2001; **194**: 1243–52.

112. Dastych J, Costa JJ, Thompson HL, Metcalfe DD. Mast cell adhesion to fibronectin. *Immunology* 1991; **73**: 478–84.

113. Thompson HL, Burbelo PD, Segui-Real, Yamada Y, Metcalfe DD. Laminin promotes mast cell attachment. *J Immunol* 1989; **143**: 2323–7.

114. Bianchine PJ, Burd PR, Metcalfe DD. IL-3-dependent mast cells attach to plate-bound vitronectin. Demonstration of augmented proliferation in response to signals transduced via cell surface vitronectin receptors. *J Immunol* 1992; **149**: 3665–71.

115. Columbo M, Bochner BS. Human skin mast cells adhere to vitronectin via the alphavbeta3 integrin receptor (CD51/CD61). *J Allergy Clin Immunol* 2001; **107**: 554.

116. Shimizu Y, Irani AM, Brown EJ, Ashman LK, Schwartz LB. Human mast cells derived from fetal liver cells cultured with stem cell factor express a functional CD51/CD61 (alpha v beta 3) integrin. *Blood* 1995; **86**: 930–9.

117. Ghannadan M, Baghestanian M, Wimazal F et al. Phenotypic characterization of human skin mast cells by combined staining for toluidine blue and CD antibodies. *J Invest Dermatol* 1998; **111**: 689–95.

118. Toru H, Kinishi T, Ra C et al. Interleukin-4 induces homotypic aggregation of human mast cells by promoting LFA-1/ICAM-1 adhesion molecules. *Blood* 1997; **89**: 3296–302.

119. Friend DS, Gurish MF, Austen KF, Hunt J, Stevens RL. Senescent jejunal mast cells and eosinophils in the mouse preferentially translocate to the spleen and draining lymph node, respectively, during the recovery phase of helminth infection. *J Immunol* 2000; **165**: 244–52.

120. Meininger CJ, Yano H, Rottapel R et al. The c-kit receptor ligand functions as a mast cell chemoattractant. *Blood* 1992; **79**: 958–63.

121. Thompson HL, Burbelo PD, Yamada Y, Kleinman HK, Metcalfe DD. Mast cell chemotax to laminin with enhancement after IgE-mediated activation. *J Immunol* 1989; **143**: 4188–92.

122. Nillson G, Butterfield JH, Nilsson K, Siegbahn A. Stem cell factor is a chemotactic factor from human mast cells. *J Immunol* 1994; **153**: 3717–23.

123. Sillaber Ch, Baghestanian M, Hofbauer R et al. Molecular and functional characterization of the urokinase receptor on human mast cells. *J Biol Chem* 1997; **272**: 7824–32.

124. Hartmann K, Henz BM, Kruger-Krasagakes S et al. C3a and C5a stimulate chemotaxis of human mast cells. *Blood* 1997; **89**: 2863–70.

125. Nilsson G, Johnell M, Hammer CH et al. C3a and C5a are chemotactic for human mast cells and act through distinct receptors via pertussis toxin-sensitive signal transduction pathways. *J Immunol* 1996; **157**: 1693–8.

126. Nilsson G, Mikovits JA, Metcalfe DD, Taub DD. Mast cell migratory response to interleukin-8 is mediated through interaction with chemokine receptor CXCR2/interleukin-8RB. *Blood* 1999; **93**: 2791–7.

127. Juremalm M, Hjertson M, Olsson N et al. The chemokine receptor CXCR4 is expressed within the mast cell lineage and its ligand stromal cell-derived factor-1 alpha acts as a mast cell chemotaxin. *Eur J Immunol* 2000; **30**: 3614–22.

128. Ghannadan M, Hauswirth A, Schernthaner G-H et al. Detection of novel CD antigens on the surface of human mast cells and basophils. *Int Arch Allergy Immunol* 2002; **127**: 299–307.

129. Kiener H, Baghestanian M, Dominkus M et al. Expression of C5a-receptor (CD88) on synovial mast cells in rheumatoid arthritis. *Arthritis Rheum* 1998; **41**: 233–45.

130. Füreder W, Agis H, Willheim M et al. Differential expression of complement receptors on human mast cells and basophils: evidence for mast cell heterogeneity and C5aR/CD88 expression on skin mast cells. *J Immunol* 1995; **155**: 3152–60.

131. Bienenstock J, Befus D, Denburg J et al. Comparative aspects of mast cell heterogeneity in different species and sites. *Int Arch Allergy Appl Immunol* 1985; **77**: 126–9.

132. Befus D, Goodacre R, Dyck N, Bienenstock J. Mast cell heterogeneity in man. I. Histologic studies of the intestine. *Int Arch Allergy Appl Immunol* 1985; **76**: 232–6.

133. Kitamura Y. Heterogeneity of mast cells and phenotypic change between subpopulations. *Annu Rev Immunol* 1989; **7**: 59–76.

134. Valent P, Scherntrhaner GH, Sperr WR et al. Variable expression of activation-linked surface antigens on human mast cells in health and disease. *Immunol Rev* 2001; **179**: 74–81.

135. Ochi H, Hirani WM, Yuan Q et al. T helper cell type 2 cytokine-mediated comitogenic response and CCR3 expression during differentiation of human mast cells in vitro. *J Exp Med* 1999; **190**: 267–80.

136. Baghestanian M, Agis H, Bevec D et al. Stem cell factor-induced downregulation of c-kit in human lung mast cells and HMC-1 cells. *Exp Hematol* 1996; **24**: 1377–86.

137. Füreder W, Bankl HC, Toth J et al. Immunophenotypic and functional characterization of human tonsillar mast cells. *J Leukocyte Biol* 1997; **61**: 592–9.

138. Beil WJ, Füreder W, Wiener H et al. Phenotypic and functional characterization of mast cells derived from renal tumor tissues. *Exp Hematol* 1998; **26**: 158–69.

139. Escribano L, Díaz-Agustín B, Bellas C et al. Utility of flow cytometric analysis of mast cells in the diagnosis and classification of adult mastocytosis. *Leuk Res* 2001; **25**: 563–70.

140. Sperr WR, Bankl HC, Mundigler G et al. The human cardiac mast cell: Localization, isolation, phenotype and functional characterization. *Blood* 1994; **84**: 3876–84.

141. Furuichi K, Rivera J, Isersky C. The receptor for immunoglobulin E on rat basophilic leukemia cells: effects of ligand binding on receptor expression. *Proc Natl Acad Sci USA* 1985; **82**: 1522–5.

142. Yamaguchi M, Lantz CS, Oettgen HC et al. IgE enhances mouse mast cell Fc(epsilon)RI expression in vitro and in vivo: evidence for a novel amplification mechanism in IgE-dependent reactions. *J Exp Med* 1997; **185**: 663–72.

143. Malveaux FJ, Conroy MC, Adkinson NF, Lichtenstein LM. IgE receptors on human basophils: relationship to serum IgE concentrations. *J Clin Invest* 1978; **62**: 176–81.

144. Okayama Y, Kirshenbaum AS, Metcalfe D. Expression of a functional high-affinity IgG receptor, Fc gamma RI, on human mast cells: up-regulation by IFN-gamma. *J Immunol* 2000; **164**: 4332–9.

145. Kirshenbaum AS, Goff JP, Semere T et al. Demonstration that human mast cells arise from a progenitor cell population that is CD34+, c-kit+, and expresses aminopeptidase N (CD13). *Blood* 1999; **94**: 2333–42.

146. Marone G, Florio G, Petraroli A, Triggiani M, de Paulis A. Human mast cells and basophils in HIV-1 infection. *Trends Immunol* 2001; **22**: 229–32.

147. Bannert N, Farzan M, Friend DS et al. Human mast cell progenitors can be infected by macrophagetropic human immunodeficiency virus type 1 and retain virus with maturation in vitro. *J Virol* 2001; **75**: 10808–14.

148. Malaviya R, Gao Z, Thankavel K, van der Merwe PA, Abraham SN. The mast cell tumor necrosis factor alpha response to FimH-expressing Escherichia coli is mediated by the glycosylphosphatidylinositol-anchored molecule CD48. *Proc Natl Acad Sci USA* 1999; **96**: 8110–15.

149. Malaviya R, Abraham SN. Mast cell modulation of immune responses to bacteria. *Immunol Rev* 2001; **179**: 16–24.

150. Furuno T, Teshima R, Kitani S, Sawada J, Nakanishi M. Surface expression of CD63 antigen (AD1 antigen) in P815 mastocytoma cells by transfected IgE receptors. *Biochem Biophys Res Commun* 1996; **219**: 740–4.

151. Knol EF, Mul FP, Jansen H, Calafat J, Roos D. Monitoring basophil activation via CD63 monoclonal antibody 435. *J Allergy Clin Immunol* 1991; **88**: 328–38.

152. Pâris-Köhler A, Demoly P, Persi L et al. In vitro diagnosis of cypress pollen allergy by using cytofluorimetric analysis of basophils (Basotest). *J Allergy Clin Immunol* 2000; **105**: 339–45.

153. Bühring HJ, Simmons PJ, Pudney M et al. The monoclonal antibody 97A6 defines a novel surface antigen expressed on human basophils and their multi- and unipotent progenitors. *Blood* 1999; **94**: 2343–56.

154. Bühring HJ, Seiffert M, Giesert C et al. The basophil activation marker defined by antibody 97A6 is identical with the ecto-nucleotide pyrophosphatase/phosphodiesterase 3 (E-NPP3). *Blood* 2001; **97**: 3303–5.

155. Wodnar-Filipowicz A, Heusser CH, Moroni C. Production of the haemopoietic growth factors GM-CSF and interleukin-3 by mast cells in response to IgE receptor-mediated activation. *Nature* 1989; **339**: 150–2.

156. Plaut M, Pierce JH, Watson CJ et al. Mast cell lines produce lymphokines in response to cross-linking of Fc epsilon RI or to calcium ionophores. *Nature* 1989; **339**: 64–7.

157. Schwartz LB, Sakai K, Bradford TR et al. The alpha form of human tryptase is the predominant type present at baseline in normal subjects and is elevated in those with systemic mastocytosis. *J Clin Invest* 1995; **96**: 2702–10.

158. Bischoff SC, Dahinden CA. c-kit ligand: a unique potentiator of mediator secretion by human lung mast cells. *J Exp Med* 1992; **175**: 237–44.

159. Columbo M, Horowitz EM, Botana LM et al. The human recombinant c-kit receptor ligand, rhSCF, induces mediator release from human cutaneous mast cells and enhances IgE-dependent mediator release from both skin mast cells and peripheral blood basophils. *J Immunol* 1992; **149**: 599–608.

160. Baghestanian M, Hofbauer R, Kiener H et al. The c-kit ligand stem cell factor and anti-IgE promote expression of monocyte chemoattractant protein 1 (MCP-1) in human lung mast cells. *Blood* 1997; **90**: 4438–49.

161. Bischoff SC, Schwengberg S, Wordelmann K et al. Effects of c-kit ligand, stem cell factor, on mediator release by human intestinal mast cells isolated from patients with inflammatory bowel disease and controls. *Gut* 1996; **28**: 104–14.

162. de Paulis A, Marino I, Ciccarelli A et al. Human synovial mast cells. I. Ultrastructural in situ and in vitro immunologic characterization. *Arthritis Rheum* 1996; **39**: 1222–33.

163. Sperr WR, Czerwenka K, Mundigler C et al. Specific activation of human mast cells by the ligand of c-kit: comparison between lung-, uterus- and heart mast cells. *Int Arch Allergy Appl Immunol* 1993; **102**: 170–5.

164. Eiseman E, Bolen JB. Engagement of the high affinity IgE receptor activates src protein-related tyrosine kinases. *Nature* 1992; **355**: 78–80.

165. White HR, Pluznik DH, Ishizaka K, Ishizaka T. Antigen-induced increase in protein kinase C activity in plasma membrane of mast cells. *Proc Natl Acad Sci USA* 1985; **82**: 8193–7.

166. Kihara H, Siraganian RP. Src homology 2 domains Syk and Lyn bind to tyrosine-phosphorylated subunits of the high affinity IgE receptor. *J Biol Chem* 1994; **269**: 22427–32.

167. Turner H, Kinet JP. Signalling through the high-affinity IgE receptor FcεRI. *Nature* 1999; **402**: B24–30.

168. Nadler MJ, Matthews SA, Turner H, Kinet JP. Signal transduction by the high-affinity immunoglobulin E receptor Fc epsilon RI. *Adv Immunol* 2000; **76**: 325–55.

169. Graham TE, Pfeiffer JR, Lee RJ. MEK and ERK activation in ras-disabled RBL-2H3 mast cells and novel roles for geranylgeranylated and farnesylated proteins in Fc epsilonRI-mediated signaling. *J Immunol* 1998; **161**: 6733–44.

170. Fleming TJ, Donnadieu E, Song CH et al. Negative regulation of FcεRI-mediated degranulation by CD81. *J Exp Med* 1997; **186**: 1307–14.

171. Kimura T, Sakamoto H, Appella E, Siraganian RP. The negative signaling molecule SH2 domain-containing inositol-polyphosphate 5-phosphatase (SHIP) binds to the tyrosine-phosphorylated β subunit of the high affinity IgE receptor. *J Biol Chem* 1997; **272**: 13991–6.

172. Huber M, Helgason CD, Damen JE et al. The src homology 2-containing inositol phosphatase (SHIP) is the gatekeeper of mast cell degranulation. *Proc Natl Acad Sci USA* 1998; **95**: 11330–5.

173. Robin JL, Seldin DC, Austen KF, Lewis RA. Regulation of mediator release from mouse bone marrow-derived mast cells by glucocorticoids. *J Immunol* 1985; **135**: 2719–26.

174. Daeron M, Sterk AR, Hirata F, Ishizaka T. Biochemical analysis of glucocorticoid-induced inhibition of IgE-mediated histamine release from mouse mast cells. *J Immunol* 1982; **129**: 1212–18.

175. Wershil BK, Furuta GT, Lavigne JA et al. Dexamethasone or cyclosporin A suppress mast cell–leukocyte cytokine cascades. Multiple mechanisms of inhibition of IgE- and mast cell-dependent cutaneous inflammation in the mouse. *J Immunol* 1995; **154**: 1391–8.

176. Eklund KK, Humphries DE, Xia Z et al. Glucocorticoids inhibit the cytokine-induced proliferation of mast cells, the high-affinity IgE receptor-mediated expression of TNF-α, and the IL-10-induced expression of chymase. *J Immunol* 1997; **158**: 4373–80.

177. Schmidt-Choudhury A, Furuta GT, Lavigne JA, Galli SJ, Wershil BK. The regulation of tumor necrosis factor-alpha production in murine mast cells: pentoxifylline or dexamethasone inhibits IgE-dependent production of TNF-alpha by distinct mechanisms. *Cell Immunol* 1996; **171**: 140–6.

178. Yamaguchi M, Hirai K, Komiya A et al. Regulation of mouse mast cell surface FcεRI

expression by dexamethasone. *Int Immunol* 2001; **13**: 843–51.

179. Finotto S, Mekori YA, Metcalfe DD. Glucocorticoids decrease tissue mast cell number by reducing the production of the *c-kit* ligand, stem cell factor, by resident cells: *in vitro* and *in vivo* evidence in murine systems. *J Clin Invest* 1987; **99**: 1721–8.

180. Cirillo R, de Paulis A, Ciccarelli A, Triggiani M, Marone G. Ciclosporin A inhibits mediator release from human Fc epsilon RI+ cells by interacting with cyclophilin. *Int Arch Allergy Appl Immunol* 1991; **94**: 76–7.

181. de Paulis A, Cirillo R, Ciccarelli A, Condorelli M, Marone G. FK-506, a potent novel inhibitor of the release of proinflammatory mediators from human Fc epsilon RI+ cells. *J Immunol* 1991; **146**: 2374–81.

182. Stellato C, de Paulis A, Ciccarelli A et al. Anti-inflammatory effects of cyclosporin A on human skin mast cells. *J Invest Dermatol* 1992; **98**: 800–4.

183. Sperr WR, Agis H, Czerwenka K et al. Effects of cyclosporin A and FK-506 on c-kit ligand/SCF dependent activation and growth of human mast cells. *J Allergy Clin Immunol* 1996; **98**: 389–99.

184. Kaye RE, Fruman DA, Bierer BE et al. Effects of cyclosporin A and FK506 on Fc epsilon receptor type I-initiated increases in cytokine mRNA in mouse bone marrow-derived progenitor mast cells: resistance to FK506 is associated with a deficiency in FK506–binding protein FKBP12. *Proc Natl Acad Sci USA* 1992; **89**: 8542–6.

185. Fruman DA, Bierer BE, Benes JE et al. The complex of FK506–binding protein 12 and FK506 inhibits calcineurin phosphatase activity and IgE activation-induced cytokine transcripts, but not exocytosis, in mouse mast cells. *J Immunol* 1995; **154**: 1846–51.

186. Hultsch T, Brand P, Lohmann S et al. Direct evidence that FK506 inhibition of FcepsilonRI-mediated exocytosis from RBL mast cells involves calcineurin. *Arch Dermatol Res* 1998; **290**: 258–63.

187. Peters SP, MacGlashan DW, Schleimer RP et al. The pharmacologic modulation of the release of arachidonic acid metabolites from purified human lung mast cells. *Am Rev Respr Dis* 1985; **132**: 367–73.

188. Obata T, Nagakura T, Kanbe M et al. IgE-anti-IgE-induced prostaglandin D2 release from cultured human mast cells. *Biochem Biophys Res Commun* 1996; **225**: 1015–20.

189. Gomes JC, Pearce FL. Comparative studies on the effects of non-steroidal anti-inflammatory drugs (NSAID) on histamine release from mast cells of the rat and guinea pig. *Agents Actions* 1988; **24**: 266–71.

190. de Paulis A, Ciccarelli A, Marino I, de Crescenzo G, Marino D, Marone G. Human synovial mast cells. II. Heterogeneity of the pharmacologic effects of antiinflammatory and immunosuppressive drugs. *Arthritis Rheum* 1997; **40**: 469–78.

191. Valenta R, Duchenne M, Pettenburger K et al. Identification of profilin as a novel pollen allergen: IgE autoreactivity in sensitized individuals. *Science* 1991; **253**: 557–60.

192. Woolley DE, Tetlow LC. Mast cell activation and its relationship to proinflammatory cytokines in the rheumatoid lesion. *Arthritis Res* 2000; **2**: 65–74.

193. Brennan FM, Maini RN, Feldmann M. TNF alpha – a pivotal role in rheumatoid arthritis? *Br J Rheumatol* 1992; **31**: 293–8.

194. Feldmann M, Brennan FM, Elliott MJ, Williams RO, Maini RN. TNF alpha is an effective therapeutic target for rheumatoid arthritis. *Ann NY Acad Sci* 1995; **766**: 272–8.

195. Yano H, Wershil BK, Arizono N, Galli SJ. Substance P-induced augmentation of cutaneous vascular permeability and granulocyte infiltration in mice is mast cell dependent. *J Clin Invest* 1989; **84**: 1276–86.

196. Nishida M, Uchikawa R, Tegoshi T et al. Migration of neutrophils is dependent on mast cells in nonspecific pleurisy in rats. *APMS* 1999; **107**: 929–36.

197. Malaviya R, Abraham SN. Role of mast cell leukotrienes in neutrophil recruitment and bacterial clearance in infectious peritonitis. *J Leukocyte Biol* 2000; **67**: 841–6.

198. Walsh LJ, Trinchieri G, Waldorf HA, Whitaker D, Murphy GF. Human dermal mast cells contain and release tumor necrosis factor α, which induces endothelial leucocyte adhesion molecule 1. *Proc Natl Acad Sci USA* 1991; **88**: 4220–4.

199. Klein LM, Lavker RM, Matis WL, Murphy GF. Degranulation of human mast cells induces an endothelial cell antigen central to leukocyte adhesion. *Proc Natl Acad Sci USA* 1989; **86**: 8972–6.

200. Hong J, Ohmura K, Mahmood U et al. Arthritis critically dependent on innate immune system players. *Immunity* 2002; **16**: 157–68.

201. Marone G, de Paulis A, Florio G et al. Are mast cells MASTers in HIV-1 infection? *Int Arch Allergy Immunol* 2001; **125**: 89–95.

202. Irani AM, Craig SS, DeBlois G et al. Deficiency of the tryptase-positive, chymase-negative mast cell type in gastrointestinal mucosa of patients with defective T lymphocyte function. *J Immunol* 1987; **138**: 4381–6.

203. Schlossman SF, Boumsell L, Gilks W et al (eds). *Leucocyte Typing V*. (Oxford University Press: Oxford, New York, Tokyo, 1995).

204. Kishimoto T, Kikutani H, von dem Borne AEG et al (eds). *Leucocyte Typing VI*. (Garland Publishing: New York, 1998).

6

Angiogenesis

Judah Folkman

Introduction • What is the evidence for neovascularization in the arthritic joint? • How does normal cartilage resist vascular invasion? • How is angiogenesis mediated in arthritis? • What therapeutic angiogenesis inhibitors are useful or may become useful in rheumatoid arthritis? • Acknowledgment • Summary • References

INTRODUCTION

A useful operational distinction between acute and chronic inflammation is that the latter is angiogenesis dependent.[1] The hallmarks of acute inflammation are vasodilation and increased permeability of pre-existing microvessels. In contrast, new microvessels are recruited into a site of chronic inflammation. These new vessels provide conduits for continuous delivery of inflammatory cells into the site.[2]

The field of angiogenesis research began with a hypothesis that tumor growth is angiogenesis dependent.[3] This concept is now supported by a wide variety of experiments and has been proved genetically.[4-8] Lessons from the study of tumor angiogenesis are being extended to other angiogenesis-dependent diseases, of which arthritis is one.

Correlations between tumor angiogenesis and angiogenesis in rheumatoid arthritis were described in 1980.[9] A vascular hypothesis for the pathogenesis of arthritis was proposed in 1982.[10] In 1983 a partially purified angiogenesis factor was isolated from synovial fluid in various joint diseases.[11] Since then, numerous reports have appeared that demonstrate a critical role for angiogenesis in the progression of arthritis – rheumatoid arthritis more so than osteoarthritis. For recent reviews see Refs 12–19.

A prevailing view in rheumatology has been that an inflammatory cellular infiltrate emerges in the synovium and in synovial fluid and must be present for some time before the angiogenesis can be induced, i.e. that angiogenesis is a relatively late event in the pathogenesis of rheumatoid arthritis. This thinking is based in part on the fact that there are fewer synovial biopsies in the very early stages of disease, and in part on patterns of inflammation due to infection, where acute inflammation (cellular infiltrate and edema) commonly precedes chronic inflammation (neovascularization – 'granulation tissue'). An example of acute inflammation preceding chronic inflammation would be pneumococcal pneumonia followed by empyema.

However, angiogenesis may be among the earliest triggering factors in rheumatoid arthritis. Synovial tissues from a patient with monoarthritis who was subsequently found to have rheumatoid arthritis showed vascular endothelial cell proliferation without a detectable inflammatory infiltrate[20] (reviewed in Ref. 21). Although this hypothesis may be difficult to confirm in humans because of the paucity of synovial biopsies at a very early stage in the disease, it does fit with our current knowledge of the cell biology of the onset of angiogenesis. In angiogenesis driven by an immune reaction (i.e. antigen on the surface of endothelial cells), lymphocytes adhere to endothelium of post-capillary venules, and this adhesion and subsequent lymphocyte transmigration can activate angiogenesis.[22] In fact, lymphocytes can cleave E-selectin and vascular adhesion molecule-1 (VCAM-1) from the endothelial cell surface. The resulting chemoattractant effect on endothelial cells in the neighborhood of these molecules may potentiate angiogenesis. In the case of angiogenesis driven by tumor hypoxia, the release of vascular endothelial growth factor (VEGF) from tumor cells also causes mononuclear cells to adhere to microvessels in the tumor bed.[23] Furthermore, in collagen-induced arthritis in mice, overexpression of VEGF in affected joints appeared early and tracked with the severity of disease.[24]

WHAT IS THE EVIDENCE FOR NEOVASCULARIZATION IN THE ARTHRITIC JOINT?

In rheumatoid arthritis, the synovium becomes hyperplastic. Mononuclear cells infiltrate the synovial sublining. This process is followed by neovascularization in a vascular pannus which invades cartilage. The vascular pannus contains intense capillary growth with endothelial proliferation.[16,25,26] A variety of experimental studies also demonstrate the presence of angiogenesis in arthritis. Endothelial cells from this pannus have been grown in vitro.[27] The vascular pannus from human synovium has been grafted into SCID mice and revascularizes.[28] Synovitis induced by carrageenan in the rat is accompanied by vascular endothelial cell proliferation.[29]

HOW DOES NORMAL CARTILAGE RESIST VASCULAR INVASION?

In the mid-1970s Eisenstein and Kuettner were the first to show that normal cartilage was resistant to invasion by vascular endothelial cells in vitro[30] and to invasion by vascular mesenchyme in vivo.[31] In our laboratory, normal cartilage implanted in a rabbit cornea[32] inhibited neovascularization induced by an implanted tumor.[33,34]

An angiogenesis inhibitor was isolated from cartilage.[35] The partially purified protein inhibited tumor angiogenesis (and tumor growth) when infused into a rabbit.[36] From these in vivo studies, two angiogenesis inhibitors were subsequently purified to completion from cartilage in our laboratory: (i) a tissue inhibitor of metalloproteinase,[37] and (ii) tropinin I,[189] a 22 kD subunit of the troponin complex (troponin-C and troponin-T being the other two members). Tropinin I is a specific inhibitor of angiogenesis. The thrombospondins, which inhibit angiogenesis, have also been identified in cartilage.[6,38–40] The cellular source of thrombospondin-1 in normal cartilage is mainly from mid-zone chondrocytes. These cells also express CD36, one of the receptors for thrombospondin-1.[41] It remains to be seen whether other inhibitors will be identified in cartilage. Nevertheless, these three angiogenesis inhibitors help to explain how normal cartilage can resist angiogenesis and why osteoarthritis cartilage loses its ability to remain avascular.[42] Furthermore, it is well known that osteogenic sarcoma rarely invades the growth plate. A recently proposed mechanism of resistance of normal cartilage to such an aggressive tumor is that growth plate chondrocytes inhibit angiogenesis.[43]

HOW IS ANGIOGENESIS MEDIATED IN ARTHRITIS?

For a neovascular pannus to develop, the endogenous inhibitors that normally guard cartilage against invasion by endothelial cells must be counter-balanced by pro-angiogenic factors, mainly proteins, which are produced at the local site, or which are brought to the site by macrophages or other inflammatory cells.

Pro-angiogenic factors

Vascular endothelial growth factor (VEGF)
A significant portion of the synovial fluid angiogenic activity in rheumatoid arthritis is due to

VEGF.[44] VEGF was first reported in 1983 as vascular permeability factor (VPF) by Dvorak and co-workers[45] and its amino acid sequence was reported in 1989 by Ferrara and Henzel.[46] There are currently six isoforms of VEGF, but VEGF-165 appears to be the most widely distributed and most extensively studied. (For reviews of VEGF see Refs 45, 47, 48). Of all the pro-angiogenic proteins, VEGF is the most specific mitogen for vascular endothelial cells and also stimulates endothelial cell migration. It is one of the most potent inducers of increased permeability of the microvasculature – more potent than histamine and equivalent to platelet activating factor (Shea Soker, personal communication). VEGF activity is transmitted by three major tyrosine kinase receptors: Flt-1 (VEGF-R1), Flk-1/KDR (VEGF-R2) and Flt-4, (VEGF-R3).[47,49] The ligands for VEGF-R3 are VEGF-C and VEGF-D which mediate lymphangiogenesis. We have recently shown that in the mouse cornea low-dose basic fibroblast growth factor (bFGF) stimulates lymphangiogenesis completely through VEGF-D and angiogenesis through VEGF-A (VEGF-A includes VEGF-165, VEGF-121 and VEGF-145) (Arja Kaipainen et al, personal communication). Furthermore, the effects of VEGF-A and VEGF-D do not overlap in vivo, and lymphangiogenesis is not dependent on angiogenesis. Although little is known about lympangiogenesis in rheumatoid arthritis, it is now possible to study angiogenesis and lymphangiogenesis separately under experimental conditions.

Neuropilin-1 binds VEGF and acts as a co-receptor for VEGF.[50,51] The source of VEGF in rheumatoid arthritis appears to be synovial lining cells, as well as macrophages. In fact, circulating mononuclear cells in patients with rheumatoid arthritis overexpress VEGF.[52]

In rheumatoid arthritis synovial tissue supernatents, more than 25% of the mitogenic activity for endothelial cells was inhibited by incubation of the supernatents with anti-VEGF.[44] Synoviocytes in rheumatoid arthritis secrete VEGF,[14] and synovial fluid in these patients contains abnormally high levels of VEGF (higher than in osteoarthritis) as reported by several groups.[12,14,40] VEGF found in human synovial fluid targets endothelium in rheumatoid arthritis.[44] Of interest is that VEGF is highly expressed in osteoarthritis cartilage (from the tibial plateau) (approximately 240 pg/100 mg tissue), but not in normal cartilage.[53] In one study, the isoform VEGF-121 was constituitively expressed in the synovial tissues (as determined by RT-PCR analysis) in all rheumatoid arthritis patients (17/17) and in all osteoarthritis patients (8/8). In contrast, the isoform VEGF-165 was observed in 41% of rheumatoid arthritis synovia (7/17), but in no osteoarthritis patients (0/8).[54]

A variety of stimuli increase VEGF expression. Tumor necrosis factor alpha (TNF-alpha) appears to be a major inducer of VEGF from blood monocytes.[52,14] Platelet-derived growth factor (PDGF), bFGF, transforming growth factor beta (TGF-beta) and interleukin 1-beta also induce VEGF expression in epithelial cells and smooth muscle cells.[14] However, VEGF expression is most sensitive to hypoxia,[55,48] a response mediated by upregulation of hypoxia-inducible factor-1 (HIF-1 alpha).[55] Synovial fluid appears to be hypoxic as a possible result of increased oxygen demands by inflammatory cells in the joint.[12]

Ets1 transcription factor is expressed in vascular endothelial cells during angiogenesis of different types, including inflammatory angiogenesis and tumor angiogenesis.[56] VEGF induces expression of the *Ets1* transcription factor in endothelial cells. There is a significant upregulation of *Ets1* transcript in rheumatoid compared to osteoarthritic synovial membranes.[57] Osteoarthritis has significantly less neovascularization than rheumatoid arthritis. Both *Ets1* RNA and *Ets1* protein were co-localized to capillary endothelial cells of newly formed blood vessels (by in situ hybridization and immunohistochemistry). Mature vessels were negative for *Ets1* in both rheumatoid arthritis and osteoarthritis. During angiogenesis, *Ets1* up-regulates, among other genes, collagenase 1 and the urokinase-type plasminogen activator. Both enzymes participate in the matrix degradation necessary for formation of capillary sprouts.[58] *Ets1* can also cooperate with the activator protein 1 (Fos/Jun) transcription factor complex during transactivation.[57] Like *Ets1*, activator protein 1 transactivates several genes that encode matrix-degrading proteases. These are some examples of the molecular mechanisms by which a neovascular pannus can destroy cartilage. These phenomena suggest a hypothesis that cartilage destruction in rheumatoid arthritis may be angiogenesis dependent.

TNF-alpha

TNF-alpha, a 17 kD protein,[59,60] is secreted by activated macrophages[59,61] and by T-cells and is also found in synovial fluid. It is pro-angiogenic in vivo. TNF-alpha also induces *Ets1* in endothelial cells in vitro and in angiogenic endothelium.[56,58] Treatment of rheumatoid arthritis patients with an approved antibody against TNF-alpha (infliximab) decreased VEGF in the serum, and reduced vascularity in the synovium accompanied by reduced markers for endothelium (i.e. von Willebrand factor, CD31) and reduced expression of the integrin $alpha_v beta_3$ in the neovasculature.[62]

TNF-alpha has many other activities in arthritis besides its pro-angiogenic activity. TNF-alpha also induces changes of expression in a variety of cytokines in rheumatoid arthritis. These include pro-inflammatory factors such as interleukin-1 (IL-1), IL-6, IL-8, granulocyte macrophage colony stimulating factor (GNM-CSF) and others, and anti-inflammatory factors (counter-regulatory factors) IL-10, IL1ra and soluble TNF-receptor (solTNFR).[63] It should be emphasized that several cytokines and mitogens induced by TNF-alpha are also expressed by proliferating endothelial cells (in a tumor bed). These include, among others, bFGF, PDGF, heparin-binding growth factor (HB-EGF), IGF-1, G-CSF and IL-6.[64–66] Therefore, it remains to be demonstrated whether any of the pro- or anti-inflammatory cytokines induced by TNF-alpha are in fact mediated by endothelium or are endothelium dependent.

IL-8

IL-8 (40 kD) is a member of the C-X-C family of chemokines in which the first two cysteines are separated by a nonconserved amino acid residue.[67] The motif Glu-Leu-Arg (ELR motif) in the NH_2 terminus confers angiogenic activity on C-X-C chemokines (as well as the ability to recruit polymorphonuclear neutrophils).[68] Synovial tissue homogenates from rheumatoid arthritis joints overproduce IL-8, as well as another C-X-C chemokine, ENA-78 (epithelial neutrophil activating peptide). These angiogenic proteins were also found to be overexpressed by macrophages which were often in direct proximity to synovial vessels in the rheumatoid arthritis joints. Furthermore, both of the proteins were chemotactic to endothelial cells.[68]

Fractalkine

This chemokine, named for its fractal geometry, is the only member of the CX_3C family which contains three amino acids between the two terminal cysteines. Recently fractalkine has been found to stimulate endothelial cell migration in vitro in the pmol/l range and its receptor has been identified on endothelial cells (CX_3CR1).[69] It stimulates angiogenesis in vivo in Matrigel plugs implanted into mice. Immunodepletion of fractalkine from rheumatoid arthritis synovial tissue homogenates significantly inhibited their angiogenic activity in the in vivo Matrigel assay. Soluble fractalkine also functions as a chemoattractant for natural killer cells, lymphocytes and monocytes.

Hepatocyte growth factor

Hepatocyte growth factor (HGF) is a motogen and a mitogen for endothelial cells and other cells including hepatocytes. It has structural homology to plasminogen, but has no coagulation functions. It is synthesized in an inactive pro-HGF form and becomes active in the presence of a proteolytic enzyme HGF activator (HGFA). It induces angiogenesis when it binds to its receptor c-Met on endothelial cells (hepatocytes and other cells also have the c-Met receptor).[70] HGF, HGFA and c-Met are strongly expressed in macrophages, endothelial cells and synovial lining cells (and fibroblasts), in rheumatoid arthritis and in osteoarthritis. HGF itself is only faintly expressed in macrophages and fibroblasts, and not at all by endothelial cells. However, its activation by HGFA induces angiogenesis in rheumatoid arthritis and osteoarthritis. Other pro-angiogenic proteins which may play a role in rheumatoid arthritis are PDGF, angiopoietins-1 and -2, angiogenin, pleiotrophin and placental growth factor.[12]

Fibroblast growth factors

Basic fibroblast growth factor (bFGF), the bioactivity of which was originally described by Gospodarowicz and co-workers,[71] was first isolated and purified in our laboratory from a chrondrosarcoma in 1984 and shown to have a high affinity for heparin.[72] The amino acid sequence was subsequently reported by Guillemin and co-workers.[73] Acidic FGF (aFGF or FGF-1 (16.4 kD)) was discovered by Maciag et al (for reviews see Refs 74–76), and there is now an extensive literature on the FGFs and their receptors.[77] Acidic and basic FGFs stimulate endothelial cell mitosis and migration in vitro and are among the most potent angiogenic proteins in vivo. They have high affinity for heparin and heparan sulfate, are stored in extracellular matrix,[78] but lack a signal sequence for secretion. bFGF is present in normal cartilage. Proteinases or heparanases can mediate release of FGF from extracellular matrix.[78,79] Furthermore, macrophages[80] can be activated to secrete bFGF.[81] Mast cells found in synovial fluid have a high heparin content and could sequester bFGF.[81] However, while bFGF has been localized to the rheumatoid arthritis joint by immunohistochemistry, it has not been found in synovial fluid. Therefore its role, in the pathogenesis of arthritis angiogenesis has not been defined.[82]

Angiopoietins

Only endothelial cells express the Tie-2 receptor, a tyrosine kinase. Its ligands are members of the angiopoietin family discovered by Yancopoulos and colleagues (for a review see Ref. 83). Angiopoietin-1 is a 70 kD ligand for Tie-2, which induces endothelial cells to recruit pericytes and smooth muscle cells which become incorporated in the vessel wall. Pericyte and smooth muscle

recruitment are mediated by endothelial production of PDGF-BB (and probably other factors) when Tie-2 is activated by angiopoietin-1. In mice that overexpress angiopoietin-1 in their skin, vascularization is significantly increased.[84] The dermal vessels are significantly larger than normal and the skin is reddened. The vessels do not leak and there is no skin edema, in contrast to dermal vessels of mice overexpressing VEGF. In double transgenic mice expressing both angiopoietin-1 and VEGF in the skin, dermal angiogenesis is increased in an additive manner, but the vessels do not leak.[85]

Angiopoietin-2 blocks the Tie-2 receptor and acts to oppose the recruitment of pericytes and smooth muscle. In a tumor bed, angiopoietin-2 is produced by vascular endothelium. High angiopoietin-2 production causes new microvessels to be unstable, i.e. they will grow in the presence of VEGF, but regress when it is withdrawn. In contrast, high angiopoietin-1 production (by mesenchymal cells) stabilizes microvessels, making them less responsive to VEGF or to other growth factors, and less likely to undergo regression.

In rheumatoid synovial tissues angiopoietin-1, angiopoietin-2 and Tie-2 were elevated compared to osteoarthritis or to normal synovium.[86] In the early stages of rheumatoid arthritis, where vigorous angiogenesis was underway, angiopoietin-2 expression by synovial tissue was very high (70–120-fold increase). However, in the late stages of rheumatoid arthritis, angiopoietin-1 predominated in synovial tissues.[87] These findings suggest that increased synovial fluid in a rheumatoid joint may in part be the result of very high angiopoetin-2 expression by synovial tissues (mainly vascular endothelium) during the early stages of the disease.

Other mediators of angiogenesis in arthritis

Endoglin

Endoglin is a glycoprotein which is a receptor for TGF-beta on endothelial cells. Alisa Koch's laboratory has shown that endoglin is upregulated in rheumatoid arthritis synovial cells, compared to normal synovial tissue endothelial cells.[88]

Matrix metalloproteinases (MMPs)

MMP-1, MMP-2 and MMP-13 are produced at increased levels in the rheumatoid arthritis synovium. In these patients there was also a small increased production of tissue inhibitor of metalloproteinases 1 (TIMP 1), although this was exceeded by activity of the three enzymes.[89] After endothelial cells are activated by a given mitogen (e.g. VEGF), they increase their expression of metalloproteinases. This facilitates invasion through type IV collagen in the vascular basement membrane, and also permits penetration of endothelial cells and capillary loops through the extracellular matrix. However, some of these metalloproteinases also cleave plasminogen to angiostatin (Figure 6.1). In the current model of angiostatin formation,[90] urokinase plasminogen activator (from tumor or other sources) cleaves plasminogen to plasmin. Phosphoglycerate kinase from hypoxic tissue converts plasmin to reduced plasmin from which kringle 1-4.5 is generated by the action of either a serine protease (from tumor) or plasmin. MMP-3, -7, -9 and 12 can cleave kringle 1-4.5 to kringle 1-4. MMP-2 and -12 can generate kringle 1-3 from kringle 1-4.5. It is not yet understood for rheumatoid angiogenesis to what extent the production of angiostatin by proliferating invading endothelium is counter-regulatory to the angiogenic process in the joint. Nor is it clear whether angiostatin production in one joint can inhibit angiogenesis in a remote joint because of circulating angiostatin, similar to the mechanism by which a primary tumor can inhibit angiogenesis in a remote tumor.[91,92] Nevertheless, this is a key point for clinicians, because the therapeutic use of metalloproteinase inhibitors in some forms of arthritis may be problematic unless blood or urine can be tested for angiostatin concentration.

WHAT THERAPEUTIC ANGIOGENESIS INHIBITORS ARE USEFUL OR MAY BECOME USEFUL IN RHEUMATOID ARTHRITIS?

Anti-arthritis agents that were found to inhibit angiogenesis after they were already in general use for arthritis

Gold thiomalate

Gold compounds have been used empirically in rheumatoid arthritis. Gold sodium thiomalate has been shown to inhibit DNA synthesis in endothelial cells in vitro at concentrations as low as 1 µg/ml. Auranofin inhibited endothelial cells at 0.1 µg/ml. Both levels are attainable in blood and synovium of patients.[93] In a subsequent experiment, corneal neovascularization was potently inhibited in rabbits injected intravenously every other day with gold sodium thiomalate at 3 mg/kg or auranofin at

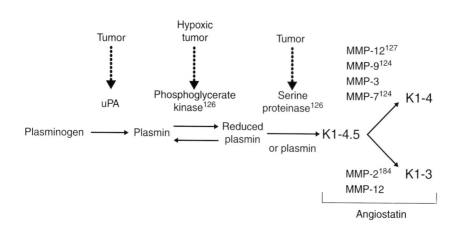

Figure 6.1 Current model of angiostatin formation. (Adapted from Lay et al. *Nature* 2000; **408**: 469–73.[90])

1 mg/kg.[94] These doses maintained serum gold levels at 2–5 µg/ml and less than 2 µg/ml for these two drugs, respectively. No inhibition of corneal neovascularization was observed when non-steroidal anti-inflammatory drugs were injected intravenously on a daily basis, e.g. acetylsalicylic acid at 20 mg/kg/day, ibuprofen at 10 mg/kg/day or indomethacin at 10 mg/kg/day. However, others have reported antiangiogenic activity in vivo with indomethacin.[95,96]

Penicillamine

An antiangiogenic mechanism for D-penicillamine has been proposed based on *in vitro* and in vivo studies.[97] D-penicillamine at concentrations attainable in the serum and tissues of patients suppressed DNA synthesis of endothelial cells in vitro in a dose-dependent manner, but only in the presence of copper sulfate in the tissue culture medium. The inhibition was blocked by catalase or horseradish peroxidase, but not when these enzymes were heat-inactivated by boiling. Neither D-penicillamine nor copper sulfate alone significantly affected endothelial cell DNA synthesis. Corneal neovascularization was also inhibited in rabbits injected intravenously with D-penicillamine daily at the per kilogram dosage administered to rheumatoid patients. A hypothetical mechanism is that D-penicillamine and copper generate local hydrogen peroxide which inhibits endothelial proliferation. Like other angiogenesis inhibitors, quiescent, non-proliferating endothelial cells in the rest of the body are not affected.

Sulfasalazine

Sulfasalazine is a combination of the antibiotic sulfapyridine and 5-aminosalicylic acid. Several potential mechanisms of action have been suggested for the efficacy of sulfasalazine, including inhibition of neutrophil adhesion to endothelial cells, inhibition of fibroblast proliferation and prevention of cartilage destruction. Recent experiments reveal that sulfasalazine or its metabolite sulfapyridine, but not 5-aminosalicylic acid, inhibited basal proliferation of human microvascular endothelial cells and chemotaxis in vitro.[98] Sulfasalazine suppressed

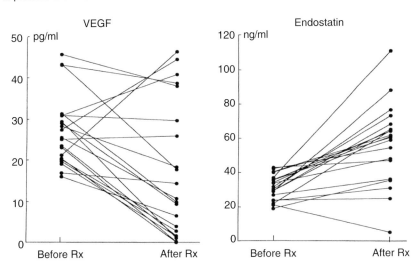

Imbalance in production between vascular endothelial growth factor and endostatin in patients with rheumatoid arthritis

Treatment of patients with prednisolone 5 mg/day plus salazosulfapyridine 1000 mg/day

Figure 6.2 VEGF and endostatin response to salazosulfapyridine and prednisolone treatment of rheumatoid arthritis. In rheumatoid arthritis patients treated for 4 to 5 months with salazosulfapyridine and prednisolone, abnormally elevated levels of VEGF in the peripheral blood and in joint fluids decreased significantly, and endostatin blood levels increased. (Adapted from Nagashima et al. *J Rheumatol* 2000; **27**: 2339–42.[99])

bFGF-induced proliferation of endothelial cells and inhibited tube formation of endothelial cells. Sufapyridine inhibited cytokine-stimulated endothelial cell expression of IL-8 and monocyte chemoattractant protein-1 (MCP-1).

Of interest is the observation that in rheumatoid arthritis patients treated with 'salazosulfapyridine 1000 mg/day and prednisolone 5 mg/day', abnormally elevated levels of VEGF in the peripheral blood decreased signifcantly, and endostatin blood levels increased after 4 or 5 months of treatment[99] (Figure 6.2). There was a similar finding in joint fluids. This result suggests that the efficacy of sulfasalazine (with prednisolone) in rheumatoid arthritis may be mediated by suppression of an endogenous pro-angiogenic protein (VEGF) and stimulated production of an endogenous inhibitor of angiogenesis (endostatin). We can ask whether other treatment regimens for rheumatoid arthritis may be mediated by a similar mechanism. Also, could other endogenous inhibitors of angiogenesis, such as angiostatin, platelet factor 4, interferon alpha or tumstatin (see below), increase as a result of a given conventional therapy for rheumatoid arthritis?

Methotrexate
Methotrexate at doses below the conventional chemotherapeutic dose has been effective in long-term therapy of rheumatoid arthritis. The prevailing view of the mechanism of action has been inhibition of humoral and cellular immune responses. However, it has also been proposed that low-dose methotrexate may inhibit angiogenesis in rheumatoid arthritis.[100] A low concentration of methotrexate (5×10^{-9} M), which is similar to serum concentrations in patients on low-dose methotrexate, inhibited DNA synthesis in human vacular endothelial cells in vitro. Low doses of methotrexate administered intramuscularly in rabbits (0.3 or 0.7 mg/kg), effectively suppressed corneal neovascularization induced by locally implanted endothelial cell growth factors.

Antimalarials
Antimalarials such as chloroquine and hydroxychloroquine sulfate have been used successfully in some patients with rheumatoid arthritis or with lupus erythematosus. However, the mechanism of action has not been clear. Recent studies show that chloroquine inhibits proliferation and induces apoptosis in human endothelial cells in vitro, in a concentration-dependent manner.[101] Indomethacin at concentrations sufficient to inhibit endogenous production of prostacyclin did not interfere with the antiproliferative effect of chloroquine. Fibroblasts, osteoblasts and monocytes did not undergo apoptosis. These results suggest that antimalarial therapy in rheumatoid arthritis may act in part by inhibiting angiogenesis.

Cylooxygenase-2 inhibitors
Cylooxygenase-2 inhibitors, developed mainly for rheumatoid arthritis and then approved for this use by the FDA, were subsequently discovered to inhibit angiogenesis in animal models. Oral administration of a cyclooxygenase-2 inhibitor (celecoxib) inhibited angiogenesis in the cornea and inhibited tumor growth based on its antiangiogenic activity.[102] Currently, celecoxib in combination with other angiogenesis inhibitors or with conventional chemotherapy (often at low dose) is being studied in a variety of clinical trials for patients with advanced metastatic cancer. As oncologists gain experience in determining the most effective and least toxic combinations of cyclooxygenase-2 inhibitors with other types of angiogenesis inhibitors, these therapeutic approaches may also eventually become applicable to rheumatoid arthritis.

Angiogenesis inhibitors currently in clinical trial for cancer

TNP-470
Donald Ingber in our laboratory reported in 1990 that a fungal contaminant (*Aspergillus fumigatus*) of an endothelial cell culture strikingly inhibited motility and proliferation of endothelial cells without killing the cells. The active principle, fumagillin was isolated in collaboration with scientists at Takeda Chemical Industries (Osaka, Japan)[103] (Table 6.1). Takeda

Table 6.1 Angiogenesis inhibitors (1980–1999).

		Reference
1980	Interferon α/β, new activity	159
1982	Platelet factor 4 Protamine	185
1985	Angiostatic steroids	186
1990	TNP-470 a fumagillin analogue (with Takeda)	103
1994	Angiostatin	91
1994	Thalidomide	187
1994	2-Methoxyestradiol	172
1997	Endostatin	142
1999	Cleaved antithrombin III	188

Angiogenesis inhibitors discovered in the author's laboratory from 1980 to 1999 beginning with the finding that interferon α/β inhibits endothelial cell motility in vitro. Seven of the nine angiogenesis inhibitors are currently in clinical trial for cancer.

made a synthetic analogue (angiogenesis modulator-470, AGM-470) which was less toxic and more potent as an endothelial inhibitor than fumagillin. Subsequently, they produced kilogram quantities of this small molecule for clinical use, TNP-470 (Takeda Neoplastic Product-470). TNP-470 is a potent angiogenesis inhibitor with broad spectrum antitumor activity in mice (human and murine tumors), rats and rabbits.[104] TNP-470 is currently in phase II clinical trials for cancer. Its wide use is limited because it diffuses into the cerebrospinal fluid and causes neurotoxicity in some patients at higher doses. However, this problem may soon be solved based on a polymeric conjugate with TNP-470 (by Ronit Satchi-Fainaro in our laboratory, unpublished data), which prevents access to the cerebrospinal fluid and increases antitumor efficacy.

Brahn et al first used TNP-470 in an animal model of collagen-induced arthritis and demonstrated effective suppression of angiogenesis and prevention of cartilage destruction.[105,106] Others have also observed reductions in cartilage and bone destruction. In one report, the protective effect persisted up to 80 days after injections of TNP-470 were discontinued in KRN/NOD mice which spontaneously develop arthritis.[107]

Angiostatin
Angiostatin is a 38 kD internal fragment of plasminogen that was purified from serum and urine of mice bearing a subcutaneous Lewis lung carcinoma that suppressed growth of its lung metastases by inhibiting their angiogenesis.[91] For a review see Ref. 108.

Angiostatin is not secreted by tumor cells, but is generated through proteolytic cleavage of circulating plasminogen by a series of enzymes released from the tumor cells (Figure 6.1). Other types of tumors have since been reported to generate angiostatin, e.g. human prostate cancer.[110]

Angiostatin and its isoforms induce cell arrest and apoptosis of endothelial cells;[109–115] inhibit endothelial migration;[116,117] inhibit angiogenesis in vitro;[118] inhibit angiogenesis in the quail chorioallantoic membrane, which provides a quantitative bioassay;[119] can be generated by different enzymes and by other cell types;[92,110,120–127] can inhibit other tumor types;[128–133] decrease activity of the mitogen-activated protein kinase ERK-1 and ERK-2 in endothelial cells;[134] upregulate E-selectin in proliferating endothelial cells;[135] can be delivered in vivo by gene therapy;[127,136] bind specifically to ATP synthase, a transmembrane protein expressed by vascular endothelial cells;[137] bind to a fragment of vitronectin;[138] and potentiate radiation therapy of experimental tumors.[139,140]

A provocative recent finding is that angiostatin inhibits proliferation of circulating precursor endothelial cells at a significantly lower concentration than it inhibits endothelial cells isolated from tissues.[141] Because precursor endothelial cells from bone marrow can home to angiogenic sites and participate in new vessel formation in a tumor (see above), it has been speculated that at least one mechanism of angiostatin is to inhibit this subpopulation of endothelium, and that these cells may be employed as a sensitive bioassay for the identification of novel antiangiogenic molecules.

Angiostatin is currently in phase II clinical trials for patients with advanced cancer that has failed all conventional therapy.

Endostatin

Endostatin[142,143] is a 20–22 kDa internal fragment of collagen XVIII.[144,145] (Table 6.1). For a review see Ref. 108 briefly summarized here. Endostatin was isolated and sequenced from conditioned medium of murine hemangioendothelioma[146] based on the same strategy employed for the discovery of angiostatin, i.e. hemangioendothelioma suppressed secondary tumors. It is a specific inhibitor of endothelial cell proliferation and migration like angiostatin. The crystal structures for mouse endostatin[147] and for human endostatin[148] have been elucidated. One of the enzymes produced from medium conditioned by hemangioendothelioma cells has been identified as an elastase.[149] Endostatin is present in basement membranes and vessel walls and is especially rich in elastic fibers of the aorta and sparse elastic fibers of veins.[150] Some, but not all capillaries or arterioles show weak labeling for endostatin. Within the elastic fibers, endostatin is colocalized with fibulin-2, fibulin-1 and nidogen-2 and binds to these components of the elastic fibers. Systemic administration of endostatin to APO-E-deficient mice inhibits angiogenesis in atherosclerotic plaques and inhibits plaque growth.[151]

Endostatin has no effect on wound healing in mice (Jennifer Marler and J. Folkman, unpublished data), nor on pregnancy. Pregnant mice bearing tumors and treated with endostatin have their tumors inhibited, but deliver normal babies. Furthermore, the babies grow normally (Robert D'Amato, unpublished data).

When human recombinant endostatin was injected into the joints of SCID mice carrying a graft of human rheumatoid arthritis tissue, synovial volume was significantly reduced, the number of inflammatory cells was significantly reduced in a dose-dependent manner and microvesssel density was decreased. Apoptotic cells were increased in the synovium.[152]

When mice with arthritis received endostatin gene therapy directly into their joints (endostatin-expressing lentiviral vector), angiogenesis and pannus formation was significantly inhibited.[153] In fact, systemic gene therapy with endostatin has recently been successful in inhibiting tumor growth in mice.[154–156]

Patients with Down's syndrome have abnormally elevated levels of endostatin because of three copies of the collagen XVIII gene.[157] When 17,897 Americans with Down's syndrome were studied recently, they were found to have less than 10% of the expected incidence of all solid tumors in comparison to the rest of the US population,[158] even though they lived to middle age. This raises the interesting question of whether Down's patients have a different pattern of rheumatoid arthritis because of constantly elevated levels of circulating endostatin throughout their life. Normal serum levels of endostatin are approximately 20–30 ng/ml.

Recombinant human endostatin produced in yeast entered phase I clinical trial in October 1999, for patients with advanced cancer. It is currently in phase I/II. Serum endostatin levels of 250 ng/ml or higher correlate with stable disease or tumor regression. There have been virtually no drug related side-effects since these clinical trials began.

Interferon alpha

Interferon alpha therapy at low dose (3 million units/m²/day subcutaneously) has been found to inhibit angiogenesis, based on in vitro data and animal studies in the 1980s[159–161] and on its use to treat children with life-threatening hemangiomas.[162–165] Proliferating cutaneous hemangiomas were also found to be deficient in interferon beta. During spontaneous regression of hemangiomas, interferon beta increased to normal levels.[166] This inverse relationship between angiogenesis and endogenous interferon beta[167] raised the speculation that if interferon beta could be considered as an endogenous inhibitor of angiogenesis, then administration of interferon alpha could be a form of replacement therapy.[168]

It was recently reported that mice genetically deficient in interferon beta exhibit severe loss of bone mass. Conversely, under physiologic conditions interferon alpha/beta contributes to maintenance of normal bone mass by down-regulating osteoclast bone resorption.[169] Furthermore, local administration of interferon beta into a site of experimental endotoxin-induced bone destruction in mice results in marked inhibition of osteoclast formation and inhibition of bone resorption. Interferon alpha also downregulates tumor cell production of at least one angiogenic factor, bFGF (both mRNA and protein are markedly decreased).

From these results it remains to be determined whether osteoclast function is endothelial cell dependent. In patients whose multiple myeloma was being held in a stable phase by interferon alpha therapy, addition of bisphosphonates inhibited osteoclastic activity, and induced bone formation.[170] It may be fruitful to ask whether combinations of very low-dose interferon alpha and bisphosphonates could be employed in severe cases of rheumatoid arthritis refractory to other therapies.

2-Methoxyestradiol and angiostatic steroids

2-Methoxyestradiol is a mammalian metabolite of estradiol, but it is extremely weak in binding to cytosol estrogen receptors. It was found to inhibit endothelial cell proliferation in vitro[171] and angiogenesis in vivo.[172] It binds to the colchicine site of tubulin and, depending on reaction conditions, either inhibits assembly or seems to be incorporated into a polymer with altered stability properties.[172] 2-Methoxyestradiol inhibits proliferation and induces apoptosis of endothelial cells (and some tumor cells) independently of estrogen receptors alpha and beta.[173]

2-Methoxyestradiol is currently in phase II clinical trials (called Panzem) as an oral preparation for patients with metastatic prostate cancer and breast cancer.[174] It has not been used in rheumatoid arthritis, but it is a potential candidate as an angiogenesis inhibitor for arthritis.

Avastin

Avastin (Bevacizumab)[175] is a neutralizing antibody to VEGF. It is in phase II/III clinical trials for patients with advanced cancer. In the future, this antibody or other inhibitors of VEGF could possibly be injected into the synovial cavity in the earliest stages of rheumatoid arthritis. The rationale for this speculation is: (i) abnormally elevated VEGF in the synovial cavity is a

common early feature of rheumatoid arthritis; (ii) bFGF induction of angiogenesis may be VEGF dependent (Arja Kaipainen et al, unpublished data); and (iii) the VEGF-producing cells in rheumatoid arthritis are genetically stable, in contrast to cancer cells, so that 'drug resistance' to a VEGF antibody is less likely to develop in the treatment of non-neoplastic diseases.

Antiangiogenic chemotherapy

It was recently reported that the antiangiogenic activity of a cytotoxic chemotherapeutic agent (e.g. cyclophosphamide) could be improved by administering the drug at low, frequent doses instead of at the conventional maximum tolerated dose.[176] Drug resistance was avoided and antitumor efficacy was significantly increased by the *antiangiogenic chemotherapy* schedule in comparison to the *conventional chemotherapy* schedule. Antiangiogenic activity can also be increased in other cytotoxic chemotherapeutic agents by this change in dose and schedule to maximize cytotoxic activity against proliferating endothelial cells in the tumor bed.[177,178] When antiangiogenic chemotherapy was administered with a pure angiogenesis inhibitor (e.g. TNP-470), tumors that were resistant to cyclophosphamide and were inhibited by 60% by TNP-470 alone underwent complete regression when the two agents were administered together.[176] This principle is being tested in a clinical trial for cancer pateints who receive three orally administred agents daily: low-dose cyclophosphamide (interchanged with etoposide every 21 days) in combination with thalidomide and celecoxib (Mark Kieran, personal communication).

Orally available angiogenesis inhibitors in clinical trial for ocular angiogenesis

Currently, five angiogenesis inhibitors are in clinical trials to treat macular degeneration which has failed conventional therapy (Table 6.2). The growth of new blood vessels from the choroid can cause blindness from microhemorrhages. This neovascularization can be suppressed, and in some cases regressed, by angiogenesis inhibitors administered either

Table 6.2   Eye disease: angiogenesis inhibitors in clinical trials. Updated February 2002.

Drug	Sponsor	Mechanism	Phase	Location
Anecortave acetate (local)	Alcon	Angiostatic steroid	Phase II macular degeneration	USA
LY33531 (oral)	Lilly	Protein kinase C β inhibitor (anti-VEGF)	Phase III diabetic retinopathy	USA
rhuFab (local)	Genentech	Anti-VEGF F(ab)$_2$	Phase I macular degeneration	USA
AG3340 (oral)	Agouron	Inhibitor of MMP 2 and 9	Phase II macular degeneration	USA
EYE001 (local)	EyeTECH	Anti-VEGF aptamer	Phase III macular degeneration	USA, Europe, Australia, Japan
EYE001 (local)	EyeTECH	Anti-VEGF aptamer	Phase II diabetic retinopathy	USA

systemically or locally. Three of the inhibitors are administered orally: anecortave acetate, an angiostatic steroid; Ly33531, a protein kinase C inhibitor which blocks VEGF production; and AG3340, an inhibitor of metalloproteinases 2 and 9. An interesting analogy between ocular angiogenesis and rheumatoid angiogenesis is that because they are both non-neoplastic diseases which may require long-term or life-long management, the clinical experience of using angiogenesis inhibitors for non-neoplastic diseases may be shared between ophthalmologists and rheumatologists.

Candidates for surrogate markers of efficacy of angiogenesis inhibitors

As new angiogenesis inhibitors have been introduced into clinical trials for cancer, there has been an increasing need for surrogate markers of efficacy that do not depend solely on tumor imaging. For example, can a decrease of circulating progenitor endothelial cells from the bone marrow predict whether an angiogenesis inhibitor will be effective, or whether a given dose is optimal, before there is a tumor response? This hypothesis is being studied in animals and in clinical trials.

If angiogenesis inhibitors are employed in rheumatoid arthritis there may be a similar need for surrogate markers of efficacy of antiangiogenic activity per se. Two possible candidates may be considered. CD146 (MUC18) is a marker of tumor progression and metastasis formation in human melanoma. CD146 is expressed almost exclusively by vascular endothelium.[179] It is significantly elevated in synovial fluid of patients with rheumatoid arthritis, psoriatic arthritis and osteoarthritis, but not in patients with traumatic joint injury. Patients with early rheumatoid arthritis (< 1 year after diagnosis) revealed the highest levels. In rheumatoid arthritis, CD146 correlated significantly with morning stiffness, the number of tender joints, and the number of swollen joints, but not with the erythrocyte sedimentation rate. Tetranectin is a tetrameric protein that specificly binds to kringle 4 of plasminogen and enhances plasminogen activation by tissue-type plasminogen activator (t-PA).[180] Tetranectin blood levels were significantly lower in rheumatoid arthritis patients. Tetranectin decrease was correlated with increased severity of disease.

SUMMARY

The variety of different drugs that were successfully employed for rheumatoid arthritis before they were found to inhibit angiogensis (gold thiomalate, sulfasalazine, antimalarials, etc.) suggests that the microvascular endothelial cell is central to the pathogenesis of rheumatoid arthritis and that rheumatoid arthritis may be angiogenesis dependent.

New insights into mechanisms of angiogenesis in rheumatoid arthritis may be gained by asking if any lessons learned from studying tumor angiogenesis could be applied to rheumatoid angiogenesis. For example, the new proliferating endothelial cells in a tumor bed originate partly from the local neighborhood and partly from circulating progenitor bone marrow-derived endothelial cells.[7,8] Do any endothelial cells in the vascular pannus of a rheumatoid joint originate from the bone marrow? Can endothelium in a vascular pannus be targeted as tumor endothelium has been, by taking advantage of the increased expression of alpha$_v$beta$_3$ integrins on activated or proliferating endothelial cells?[181,182] If angiostatin or endostatin are produced in one joint during the angiogenic process, could they circulate and suppress angiogenesis in remote joints analogous to some tumors?[183] This mechanism operates in some tumors because the half-life of VEGF is short (cleared from the circulation in approximately 3 minutes), compared to a half-life of hours for angiostatin or endostatin. Within a primary tumor, VEGF exceeds the inhibitor, but in the circulation the inhibitor gradually accumulates and is in excess of circulatng VEGF. This phenomenon of a primary tumor suppressing a remote metastasis was called 'concomitant immunity' in the 1950s and 1960s, but is now understood in terms of angiogenic mechanisms.[184]

Peripheral blood mononuclear cells from patients with rheumatoid arthritis spontaneously secrete VEGF. TNF-alpha specifically upregulates this secretion in synovial fluid.[52] Do these cells infiltrate other tissues (e.g. skin, eye) to establish remote angiogenic sites?

In treating tumor angiogenesis there is a great need for reliable surrogate markers of efficacy of antiangiogenic therapy. Many laboratories are working on this problem. Preliminary data suggest that VEGF-secreting tumors induce increased circulating endothelial cells.

Even if these endothelial cells do not traffic to a tumor, counting them may indicate the presence of an angiogenic site. Furthermore, if it becomes feasible to distinguish in a blood sample between apoptotic mature endothelial cells exiting a tumor and young progenitor endothelial cells coming out of the bone marrow, this may provide further quantification of therapeutic efficacy. By analogy, do any of these questions apply to a rheumatoid joint that is secreting VEGF into the circulation, or generating VEGF-producing cells that circulate?

As newer angiogenesis inhibitors become more widely available after they have become approved drugs, will any of them be candidates for treating arthritis? An analogy is macular degeneration. There are currently five different angiogenesis inhibitors in clinical trial to treat macular degeneration (Table 6.2). Two of them are already in phase III. They all originated from angiogenesis inhibitors developed for cancer and they work by the same mechanism as angiogenesis inhibitors employed to treat cancer.

A long-term goal of antiangiogenic therapy in cancer is to reduce the harsh side-effects of conventional cytotoxic chemotherapy, to reduce the risk of drug resistance and to try to convert cancer to a chronic manageable disease. Because most of these objectives are already being achieved in rheumatoid arthritis, it can be considered a model for the next step in cancer therapy.

ACKNOWLEDGMENT

This study was supported by the National Institutes of Health grants 5P01 CA45548 and 5R01 CA37395 and a grant to Children's Hospital from EntreMed, Inc., Rockville, MD. J.F. would like to thank Alison Clapp, Wendy Foss and Sarah Schmidt for administrative support and help with the references.

REFERENCES

1. Folkman J. Angiogenesis in cancer, vascular, rheumatoid and other disease. *Nature Med* 1995; **1**: 27–31.
2. Folkman J, Brem H. Angiogenesis and inflammation. In: Gallin JI, Goldstein IM, Snyderman R, eds. *Inflammation: Basic Principles and Clinical Correlates* (Raven Press: New York, 1992) 821–39.
3. Folkman J. Tumor angiogenesis: therapeutic implications. *N Engl J Med* 1971; **285**: 1182–6.
4. Folkman J. Angiogenesis. In: Braunwald E, Fauci AS, Kasper DL et al, eds. *Harrison's Textbook of Internal Medicine*, 15th edn (McGraw-Hill: New York, 2001) 517–30.
5. Carmeliet P, Jain RK. Angiogenesis in cancer and other diseases. *Nature* 2000; **407**: 249–57.
6. Streit M, Riccardi L, Velasco P et al. Thrombospondin-2: a potent endogenous inhibitor of tumor growth and angiogenesis. *Proc Natl Acad Sci USA* 1999; **96**: 14888–93.
7. Lyden D, Young AZ, Zagzag D et al. Id1 and Id3 are required for neurogenesis, angiogenesis and vascularization of tumour xenografts. *Nature* 1999; **401**: 670–7.
8. Lyden D, Hattori K, Dias S et al. Impaired recruitment of bone marrow-derived endothelial and hematopoietic precursor cells blocks tumor angiogenesis and growth. *Nature Med* 2001; **7**: 1194–201.
9. Folkman J, Ausprunk D, Langer R. Connective tissue: small blood vessels and capillaries. In: Kelley WN, Harris ED, Ruddy S, Sledge CB, eds. *Textbook of Rheumatology* (W.B. Saunders: Philadelphia, 1980) 210–20.
10. Rothschild BM, Masi AT. Pathogenesis of rheumatoid arthritis: a vascular hypothesis. *Semin Arthritis Rheum* 1982; **12**: 11–31.
11. Brown RA, Tomlinson IW, Hill CR et al. Relationship of angiogenesis factor in synovial fluid to various joint diseases. *Ann Rheum Dis* 1983; **42**: 301–7.
12. Paleolog EM. Angiogenesis in rheumatoid arthritis. *Arthritis Res* 2002; **4**: S81–90.
13. Walsh DA, Haywood L. Angiogenesis: a therapeutic target in arthritis. *Curr Opin Investig Drugs* 2001; **2**: 1054–63.
14. Brenchley PE. Antagonising angiogenesis in rheumatoid arthritis. *Ann Rheum Dis* 2001; **60**: iii71–iii74.
15. Walsh DA, Pearson CI. Angiogenesis in the pathogenesis of inflammatory joint and lung diseases. *Arthritis Res* 2001; **3**: 147–53.
16. Koch AE. The role of angiogenesis in rheumatoid arthritis: recent developments. *Ann Rheum Dis* 2000; **59**: i65–i71.
17. Griffioen AW, Molema G. Angiogenesis: potentials for pharmacologic intervention in the treatment of cancer, cardiovascular diseases, and chronic inflammation. *Pharmacol Rev* 2000; **52**: 237–68.
18. Brown RA, Weiss JB, Tomlinson IW et al. Angiogenic factor from synovial fluid resembling that from tumors. *Lancet* 1980; **1**: 682–5.
19. Walsh DA. Angiogenesis and arthritis. *Rheumatology* 1999; **38**: 103–12.
20. Hirohata S, Sakakibara JK. Angiogenesis as a possible elusive triggering factor in rheumatoid arthritis. *Lancet* 1999; **353**: 1331.
21. Weber AJ, De Bandt M. Angiogenesis: general mechanisms and implications for rheumatoid arthritis. *Joint Bone Spine* 2000; **67**: 366–83.
22. Koch AM, Halloran MM, Haskell CJ et al. Angiogenesis mediated by soluble forms of E-selectins and vascular adhesion molecule-1. *Nature* 1995; **376**: 517–19.
23. Griffioen AW, Tromp SC, Hillen HF. Angiogenesis modulates the tumour immune response. *Int J Exp Pathol* 1998; **76**: 363–8.
24. Lu J, Kasama T, Kobayashi K et al. Vascular endothelial growth factor expression and regulation of murine collagen-induced arthritis. *J Immunol* 2000; **164**: 5922–7.
25. Paleolog EM. Angiogenesis: a critical process in the pathogenesis of RA – a role for VEGF? *Br J Rheumatol* 1996; **35**: 917–19.
26. Kimball ES, Gross JL. Angiogenesis in pannus formation. *Agents Actions* 1991; **34**: 329–31.
27. Jackson CJ, Garbett PK, Marks RM et al. Isolation and propagation of endothelial cells derived from rheumatoid synovial microvasculature. *Ann Rheum Dis* 1989; **48**: 733–6.
28. Scola MP, Imagawa T, Boivin GP et al. Expression of angiogenic factors in juvenile rheumatoid arthritis: correlation revascularization of human synovium engrafted into SCID mice. *Arthritis Rheum* 2001; **44**: 794–801.
29. Walsh DA, Rodway HA, Claxson A. Vascular turnover during carrageenan synovitis in the rat. *Lab Invest* 1998; **78**: 1513–21.
30. Eisenstein R, Kuettner KE, Neapolitan C et al. The resistance of certain tissues to invasion. III. Cartilage extracts inhibit the growth of fibroblasts

and endothelial cells in culture. *Am J Pathol* 1975; **81**: 337–47.

31. Sorgente N, Kuettner KE, Soble LW et al. The resistance of certain tissues to invasion. II. Evidence for extractable factors in cartilage which inhibit invasion by vascularized mesenchyme. *Lab Invest* 1975; **32**: 217–22.

32. Gimbrone MA Jr, Cotran RS, Leapman SB, Folkman J. Tumor growth and neovascularization: an experimental model using rabbit cornea. *J Natl Cancer Inst* 1974; **52**: 413–27.

33. Brem H, Folkman J. Inhibition of tumor angiogenesis mediated by cartilage. *J Exp Med* 1975; **141**: 427–39.

34. Brem H, Arensman R, Folkman J. Inhibition of tumor angiogenesis by a diffusible factor from cartilage. In: Slavkin HC, Greulich RC, eds. *Extracellular Matrix Influences on Gene Expression* (Academic Press: New York, 1975) 767–72.

35. Langer R, Brem H, Falterman K et al. Isolation of a cartilage factor which inhibits tumor neovascularization. *Science* 1976; **193**: 70–2.

36. Langer R, Conn H, Vacant J et al. Control of tumor growth in animals by infusion of an angiogenesis inhibitor. *Proc Natl Acad Sci USA* 1980; **77**: 4331–5.

37. Moses MA, Sudhalter J, Langer R. Identification of an inhibitor of neovascularization from cartilage. *Science* 1990; **248**: 1408–10.

38. Good DJ, Polverini PJ, Rastinejad F et al. A tumor suppressor-dependent inhibitor of angiogenesis is immunologically and functionally indistinguishable from a fragment of thrombospondin. *Proc Natl Acad Sci USA* 1990; **87**: 6624–8.

39. Miller RR, McDevitt CA. Thrombospondin is present in articular cartilage and is synthesized by articular chondrocytes. *Biochem Biophys Res Commun* 1988; **153**: 708–14.

40. Koch AE, Szekanecz Z, Friedman J et al. Effects of thrombospondin-1 on disease course and angiogenesis in rat adjuvant-induced arthritis. *Clin Immunol Immunopathol* 1998; **86**: 199–208.

41. Iruela-Arispe ML, Liska DJ, Sage EH, Bornstein P. Differential expression of thrombospondin 1, 2, and 3 during murine development. *Dev Dyn* 1993; **197**: 40–56.

42. Fenwick SA, Gregg PJ, Rooney P. Osteoarthritis cartilage loses its ability to remain avascular. *Osteoarthritis Cartilage* 1999; **7**: 441–52.

43. Cheung WH, Lee KM, Fung KP, Leung KS. Growth plate chondrocytes inhibit neo-angiogenesis: a possible mechanism for tumor control. *Cancer Lett* 2001; **163**: 25–32.

44. Koch AE, Harlow LA, Haines GK et al. Vascular endothelial growth factor: a cytokine modulating endothelial function in rheumatoid arthritis. *J Immunol* 1994; **152**: 4149–56.

45. Senger DR, Galli SJ, Dvorak AM et al. Tumor cells secrete a vascular permeability factor that promotes accumulation of ascites fluid. *Science* 1983; **219**: 983–5.

46. Ferrara N, Henzel WJ. Pituitary follicular cells secrete a novel heparin-binding growth factor specific for vascular endothelial cells. *Biochem Biophys Res Commun* 1989; **161**: 851–5.

47. Ferrara N. Role of vascular endothelial growth factor in regulation of physiological angiogenesis. *Am J Cell Physiol* 2001; **280**: C1358–66.

48. Shima DT, Adamis AP, Yeo K-T et al. Hypoxic induction of endothelial cell growth factors in retinal cells: identification and characterization of vascular endothelial growth factor (VEGF) as the mitogen. *Mol Med* 1995; **1**: 182–93.

49. Neufeld G, Cohen T, Gengrinovitch S, Poltorak Z. Vascular endothelial growth factor (VEGF) and its receptors. *FASEB J* 1999; **13**: 9–22.

50. Gagnon ML, Bielenberg DR, Gechtman Z et al. Identification of a natural soluble neuropilin-1 that binds vascular endothelial growth factor: in vivo expression and anti-tumor activity. *Proc Natl Acad Sci USA* 2000; **97**: 2573–8.

51. Miao H-Q, Klagsbrun M. Neuropilin is a mediator of angiogenesis. *Cancer Metastasis Rev* 2000; **29**: 29–37.

52. Bottomley MJ, Webb NJ, Watson CJ et al. Peripheral blood mononuclear cells from patients with rheumatoid arthritis spontaneously secrete vascular endothelial growth factor (VEGF): specific up-regulation by tumour necrosis factor-alpha (TNF-alpha) in synovial fluid. *Clin Exp Immunol* 1999; **117**: 171–6.

53. Pufe T, Petersen W, Tillmann B, Mentlein R. The splice variants VEGF121 and VEGF189 of the angiogenic peptide vascular endothelial growth factor are expressed in osteoarthritic cartilage. *Arthritis Rheum* 2001; **44**: 1082–8.

54. Ikeda M, Hosoda Y, Hirose S et al. Expression of vascular endothelial growth factor isoforms and their receptors Flt-1, KDR, and Neuropilin-1 in synovial tissues of rheumatoid arthritis. *J Pathol* 2000; **191**: 426–33.

55. Shweiki D, Itin A, Soffer D, Keshet E. Vascular endothelial growth factor induced by hypoxia may mediate hypoxia-initiated angiogenesis. *Nature* 1992; **359**: 843–5.

56. Wernert N, Raes MB, Lassalle P et al. C-ets1 proto-oncogene is a transcription factor expressed in endothelial cells during tumor vascularization and other forms of angiogenesis in humans. *Am J Pathol* 1992; **140**: 119–27.

57. Wernert N, Justen HP, Rothe M et al. The Ets 1 transcription factor is upregulated during inflammatory angiogenesis rheumatoid arthritis. *J Mol Med* 2002; **80**: 258–66.

58. Iwasaka C, Tanaka K, Abe M, Sato Y. Ets-1 regulates angiogenesis by inducing the expression of urokinase-type plasminogen activator and matrix metalloproteinase-1 and the migration of vascular endothelial cells. *J Cell Physiol* 1996; **169**: 522–31.

59. Fràter-Schröder M, Risau W, Hallmann R et al. Tumor necrosis factor type alpha, a potent inhibitor of endothelial cell growth in vitro, is angiogenic in vivo. *Proc Natl Acad Sci USA* 1987; **84**: 5277–81.

60. Leibovich SJ, Polverini PJ, Shepard HM et al. Macrophage-induced angiogenesis is mediated by tumour necrosis factor-alpha. *Nature* 1987; **329**: 630–2.

61. Stavrl GT, Zachary IC, Baskerville PA et al. Basic fibroblast growth factor upregulates the expression of vascular endothelial growth factor in vascular smooth muscle cells. Synergistic interaction with hypoxia. *Circulation* 1995; **92**: 11–14.

62. Maini RN, Taylor PC, Paleolog E et al. Anti-tumor necrosis factor specific antibody (infliximab) treatment provides insights into the pathophysiology of rheumatoid arthritis. *Ann Rheum Dis* 1999; **58**(suppl 1): 156–60.

63. Feldmann M, Maini RN. Anti-TNF alpha therapy of rheumatoid arthritis: what have we learned? *Annu Rev Immunol* 2001; **19**: 163–96.

64. Nicosia RF, Tchao R, Leighton J. Angiogenesis-dependent tumor spread in reinforced fibrin clot culture. *Cancer Res* 1983; **43**: 2159–66.

65. Hamada J, Cavanaugh PG, Lotan O, Nicolson GL. Separable growth and migration factors for large-cell lymphoma cells secreted by microvascular endothelial cells derived from target organs for metastasis. *Br J Cancer* 1992; **66**: 349–54.

66. Rak JW, St Croix BD, Kerbel RS. Consequences of angiogenesis for tumor progression, metastasis and cancer therapy. *Anti-cancer Drugs* 1995; **6**: 3–18.

67. Belperio JA, Keane MP, Arenberg DA et al. CXC chemokines in angiogenesis. *J Leukoc Biol* 2000; **68**: 1–8.

68. Koch AE, Volin MV, Woods JM et al. Regulation of angiogenesis by the C-X-C chemokines interleukin-8 and epithelial neutrophil activating peptide 78 in the rheumatoid joint. *Arthritis Rheum* 2001; **44**: 31–40.

69. Volin MV, Woods JM, Amin MA et al. Fractalkine: a novel angiogenic chemokine in rheumatoid arthritis. *Am J Pathol* 2001; **150**: 1521–30.

70. Nagashima M, Hasegawa J, Kato K et al. Hepatocyte growth factor (HGF), HGF activator, and c-Met in synovial tissues in rheumatoid arthritis and osteoarthritis. *J Rheumatol* 2001; **28**: 1772–8.

71. Gospodarowicz D, Zetter BR. The use of fibroblast and epidermal growth factors to lower the serum requirement for growth of normal diploid cells in early passage: a new method for cloning. *Dev Biol Stand* 1976; **37**: 109–30.

72. Shing Y, Folkman J, Sullivan R et al. Heparin affinity: purification of a tumor-derived capillary endothelial cell growth factor. *Science* 1984; **223**: 1296–8.

73. Ueno N, Baird A, Esch F et al. Purification and partial characterization of a mitogenic factor from bovine liver; structural homology with basic fibroblast growth factor. *Regul Pept* 1986; **16**: 135–45.

74. Christofori G. The role of fibroblast growth factors in tumour progression and angiogenesis. In: Bicknell R, Lewis CE, Ferrara N, eds. *Tumour Angiogenesis* (Oxford University Press: Oxford, 1996) 201–37.

75. Friesel RE, Maciag T. Molecular mechanisms of angiogoenesis: fibroblast growthfactor signal. *FASEB J* 1995; **9**: 919–25.

76. Folkman J, Shing Y. Angiogenesis. *J Biol Chem* 1992; **267**: 10931–4.

77. Griffioen AW, Molema G. Angiogenesis: potentials for pharmacologic intervention in the treatment of cancer, cardiovascular diseases and chronic inflammation. *Pharmacol Rev* 2000; **52**: 237–68.

78. Folkman J, Klagsbrun M, Sasse J et al. A heparin-binding angiogenic protein – basic fibroblast growth factor – is stored within basement membrane. *Am J Pathol* 1988; **130**: 393–400.

79. Vlodavsky I, Bashkin PK, Korner G et al. Extracellular matrix-resident growth factors and enzymes: relevance to angiogenesis and metastasis. *Proc Annu Meet Am Assoc Cancer Res* 1990; **31**: 491–3.

80. Polverini P, Leibovich S. Induction of neovascularization in vivo and endothelial proliferation in vitro by tumor-associated macrophages. *Lab Invest* 1984; **51**: 635–42.

81. Norrby K. Mast cells and de novo angiogenesis: angiogenic capability of individual mast-cell mediators such as histamine, TNF, IL-8 and bFGF. *Inflamm Res* 1997; **46**: S7–S8.

82. Qu Z, Huang XN, Ahmadi P et al. Expression of basic fibroblast growth factor in synovial tissue from patients with rheumatoid arthritis and degenerative joint disease. *Lab Invest* 1995; **73**: 339–46.

83. Davis S, Aldrich TH, Jones PF et al. Isolation of angiopoietin-1, a ligand for the TIE2 receptor, by secretion-trap expression cloning. *Cell* 1996; **87**: 1161–9.

84. Suri C, McClain J, Thurston G et al. Increased vascularization in mice overexpressing angiopoietin-1. *Science* 1998; **282**: 468–71.

85. Thurston G, Suri C, Smith K et al. Leakage-resistant blood vessels in mice transgenically overexpressing angiopoietin-1. *Science* 1999; **286**: 2511–14.

86. Shahrara S, Volin MV, Connors MA et al. Differential expression of the angiogenic Tie receptor family in arthritis and normal synovial tissue. *Arthritis Res* 2002; **4**: 201–8.

87. Scott BB, Zaratin PF, Colombo A et al. Constitutive expression of the angiopoietin-1 and -2 and modulation of their expression by inflammatory cytokines in rheumatoid arthritis synovial fibroblasts. *J Rheumatol* 2002; **29**: 230–9.

88. Szekanecz Z, Haines GK, Harlow LA et al. Increased synovial expression of TGF-beta receptor endoglin and TGF-beta1 in rheumatoid arthritis. *Clin Immunol Immunopathol* 1995; **76**: 187–94.

89. Jain A, Nanchahal J, Troeberg L et al. Production of cytokines, vascular endothelial growth factor, matrix metalloproteinases, and tissue inhibitor of metalloproteinases 1 by tenosynovium demonstrates its potential for tendon destruction in rheumatoid arthritis. *Arthritis Rheum* 2001; **44**: 1754–60.

90. Lay AJ, Jiang X-M, Kisker O et al. Phosphoglycerate kinase acts in tumour angiogenesis as a disulphide reductase. *Nature* 2000; **408**: 869–73.

91. O'Reilly MS, Holmgren L, Shing Y et al. Angiostatin: a novel angiogenesis inhibitor that mediates the suppression of metastases by a Lewis lung carcinoma. *Cell* 1994; **79**: 315–28.

92. Cornelius LA, Nehring LC, Harding E et al. Matrix metalloproteinases generate angiostatin: effects on neovascularization. *J Immunol* 1998; **161**: 6845–52.

93. Matsubara T, Ziff M. Inhibition of human endothelial cell proliferation by gold compounds. *J Clin Invest* 1987; **79**: 1440–6.

94. Saura R, Matsubara T, Mizuno K. Inhibition of neovascularization in vivo by gold compounds. *Rheumatol Int* 1994; **14**: 1–7.

95. Silverman KJ, Lund DP, Zetter BR et al. Angiogenic activity of adipose tissue. *Biochem Biophys Res Commun* 1988; **154**: 205–12.

96. Haynes WL, Proia AD, Klintworth GK. Effect of inhibitors of arachidonic acid metabolism on corneal neovascularization in the rat. *Invest Ophthalmol Vis Sci* 1989; **30**: 1588–93.

97. Matsubara T, Saura R, Hirohata K, Ziff M. Inhibition of human endothelial cell proliferation in vitro and neovascularization in vivo by D-penicillamine. *J Clin Invest* 1989; **83**: 158–67.

98. Volin MV, Harlow LA, Woods JM et al. Treatment with sulfasalazine or sulfapyridine, but not 5-aminosalicylic acid inhibits basic fibroblast growth factor-induced endothelial cell chemotaxis. *Arthritis Rheum* 1999; **42**: 1927–35.

99. Nagashima M, Asano G, Yoshino S. Imbalance in production between vascular endothelial growth factor and endostatin in patients with rheumatoid arthritis. *J Rheumatol* 2000; **27**: 2339–42.

100. Hirata S, Matsubara T, Saura R et al. Inhibition of in vitro vascular endothelial cell proliferation and in vivo neovascularization by low-dose methotrexate. *Arthritis Rheum* 1989; **32**: 1065–73.

101. Potvin F, Petitclerc E, Marceu F, Poubelle P. Mechanisms of action of antimalarials in inflammation. Induction of apoptosis in human endothelial cells. *J Immunol* 1997; **158**: 1872–9.

102. Masferrer JL, Leahy KM, Koki AT et al. Antiangiogenic and antitumor activities of cyclooxygenase-2 inhibitors. *Cancer Res* 2000; **60**: 1306–11.

103. Ingber D, Fujita T, Kishimoto S et al. Synthetic analogues of fumagillin that inhibit angiogenesis and suppress tumour growth. *Nature* 1990; **348**: 555–7.

104. Folkman J. Tumor angiogenesis. In: Wells SA, Jr, Sharp PA, eds. *Accomplishments in Cancer Research* (Lippincott Williams & Wilkins: Philadelphia, 1998) 32–44.

105. Peacock DJ, Banquerigo ML, Brahn E. Angiogenesis inhibition suppresses collagen arthritis. *J Exp Med* 1992; **175**: 1135–8.

106. Oliver SJ, Brahn E. Combination therapy in rheumatoid arthritis: the animal model perspective. *J Rheumatol* 1996; **44**: 56–60.

107. de Bandt M, Grossin M, Weber AJ et al. Suppression of arthritis and protection from bone destruction by treatment with TNP-470/AGM-1470 in a transgenic mouse model of rheumatoid arthritis. *Arthritis Rheum* 2000; **43**: 2056–63.

108. Folkman J. Tumor angiogenesis. In: Holland JF, Frei E III, Bast RC Jr et al, eds. *Cancer Medicine*, 5th edn (B. C. Decker: Ontario, 2000) 132–52.

109. Lu H, Dhanabal M, Volk R et al. Kringle 5 causes cell cycle arrest and apoptosis of endothelial cells. *Biochem Biophys Res Commun* 1999; **258**: 668–73.

110. Gately S, Twardowski P, Stack MS et al. Human prostate carcinoma cells express enzymatic activity that converts human plasminogen to the angiogenesis inhibitor, angiostatin. *Cancer Res* 1996; **56**: 4887–90.

111. Lucas R, Holmgren L, Garcia I et al. Multiple forms of angiostatin induce apoptosis in endothelial cells. *Blood* 1998; **92**: 4730–41.

112. Griscelli F, Li H, Bennaceur-Griscelli A et al. Angiostatin gene transfer: inhibition of tumor growth in vivo by blockage of endothelial cell proliferation associated with a mitosis arrest. *Proc Natl Acad Sci USA* 1998; **95**: 6367–72.

113. Claesson-Welsh L, Welsh M, Ito N et al. Angiostatin induces endothelial cell apoptosis and activation of focal adhesion kinase independently of the integrin-binding motif RGD. *Proc Natl Acad Sci USA* 1998; **95**: 5579–83.

114. Wu Z, O'Reilly MS, Folkman J, Shing Y. Suppression of tumor growth with recombinant murine angiostatin. *Biochem Biophys Res Commun* 1997; **236**: 651–4.

115. Cao Y, Chen A, An SSA et al. Kringle 5 of plasminogen is a novel inhibitor of endothelial cell growth. *J Biol Chem* 1997; **272**: 22924–8.

116. Ji WR, Castellino FJ, Chang Y et al. Characterization of kringle domains of angiostatin as antagonists of endothelial cell migration, an important process in angiogenesis. *FASEB J* 1998; **12**: 1731–8.

117. Ji WR, Barrientos LG, Llinas M et al. Selective inhibition by kringle 5 of human plasminogen on endothelial cell migration, an important process in angiogenesis. *Biochem Biophys Res Commun* 1998; **247**: 414–19.

118. Barendsz-Janson AF, Griffioen AW, Muller AD et al. In vitro tumor angiogenesis assays: plasminogen lysine binding site 1 inhibits in vitro tumor-induced angiogenesis. *J Vasc Res* 1998; **35**: 109–14.

119. Parsons-Wingerter P, Lwai B, Yang MC et al. A novel assay of angiogenesis in the quail chorioallantoic membrane: stimulation by bFGF and inhibition by angiostatin according to fractal dimension and grid intersection. *Microvasc Res* 1998; **55**: 201–14.

120. Falcone DJ, Khan KM, Layne T, Fernandes L. Macrophage formation of angiostatin during inflammation. A byproduct of the activation of plasminogen. *J Biol Chem* 1998; **273**: 31480–5.

121. O'Mahony CA, Albo D, Tuszynski GP, Berger DH. Transforming growth factor-beta 1 inhibits generation of angiostatin by human pancreatic cancer cells. *Surgery* 1998; **24**: 388–93.

122. O'Mahony CA, Seidel A, Albo D et al. Angiostatin generation by human pancreatic cancer. *J Surg Res* 1998; **77**: 55–8.

123. Lijnen HR, Ugwu F, Bini A, Collen D. Generation of an angiostatin-like fragment from plasminogen by stromelysin-1 (MMP-3). *Biochem* 1998; **37**: 4699–702.

124. Patterson BC, Sang QA. Angiostatin-converting enzyme activities of human matrilysin (MMP-7) and gelatinase B/type IV collagenase (MMP-9). *J Biol Chem* 1997; **272**: 28823–5.

125. Gately S, Twardowski P, Stack MS et al. The mechanism of cancer-mediated conversion of plasminogen to the angiogenesis inhibitor angiostatin. *Proc Natl Acad Sci USA* 1997; **94**: 10868–72.

126. Stathakis P, Fitzgerald M, Matthias LJ et al. Generation of angiostatin by reduction and proteolysis of plasmin. Catalysis by a plasmin reductase secreted by cultured cells. *J Biol Chem* 1997; **272**: 20641–5.

127. Dong Z, Kumar R, Yang X, Fidler IJ. Macrophage-derived metalloelastase is responsible for the generation of angiostatin in Lewis lung carcinoma. *Cell* 1997; **88**: 801–10.

128. Cao R, Wu HL, Veitonmaki N et al. Suppression of angiogenesis and tumor growth by the inhibitor K1-5 generated by plasmin-mediated proteolysis. *Proc Natl Acad Sci USA* 1999; **96**: 5728–33.

129. Stack S, Gately S, Bafetti LM et al. Angiostatin inhibits endothelial and melanoma cellular invasion by blocking matrix-enhanced plasminogen activation. *Biochem J* 1999; **340**: 77–84.

130. Kirsch M, Strasser J, Allende R et al. Angiostatin suppresses malignant glioma growth in vivo. *Cancer Res* 1998; **58**: 4654–9.

131. Sim BK, O'Reilly MS, Liang H et al. A recombinant human angiostatin protein inhibits experimental primary and metastatic cancer. *Cancer Res* 1997; **57**: 1329–34.

132. Lannutti BJ, Gately ST, Quevedo ME et al. Human angiostatin inhibits murine hemangioendothelioma tumor growth in vivo. *Cancer Res* 1997; **57**: 5277–80.

133. Joe YA, Hong YK, Chung DS et al. Inhibition of human malignant glioma growth in vivo by human recombinant plasminogen kringles 1-3. *Int J Cancer* 1999; **82**: 694–9.

134. Redlitz A, Daum G, Sage EH. Angiostatin diminishes activation of the mitogen-activated protein kinases ERK-1 and ERK-2 in human dermal microvascular endothelial cells. *J Vasc Res* 1999; **36**: 28–34.

135. Luo J, Lin J, Paranya G, Bischoff J. Angiostatin upregulates E-selectin in proliferating endothelial cells. *Biochem Biophys Res Commun* 1998; **245**: 906–11.

136. Tanaka T, Cao Y, Folkman J, Fine HA. Viral vector-targeted anti-angiogenic gene therapy utilizing an angiostatin complementary DNA. *Cancer Res* 1998; **58**: 3362–9.

137. Moser TL, Stack MS, Asplin I et al. Angiostatin binds ATP synthase on the surface of human endothelial cells. *Proc Natl Acad Sci USA* 1999; **96**: 2811–16.

138. Kost C, Benner K, Stockmann A et al. Limited plasmin proteolysis of vitronectin. Characterization of the adhesion protein as morpho-regulatory and angiostatin-binding factor. *Eur J Biochem* 1996; **236**: 682–8.

139. Gorski DH, Mauceri HJ, Salloum RM et al. Potentiation of the antitumor effect of ionizing radiation by brief concomitant exposures to angiostatin. *Cancer Res* 1998; **58**: 5686–9.

140. Mauceri HJ, Hanna NN, Beckett MA et al. Combined effects of angiostatin and ionizing radiation in antitumour therapy. *Nature* 1998; **394**: 287–91.

141. Ito H, Rovira II, Bloom ML et al. Endothelial progenitor cells as putative targets for angiostatin. *Cancer Res* 1999; **59**: 5875–7.

142. O'Reilly MS, Boehm T, Shing Y et al. Endostatin: An endogenous inhibitor of angiogenesis and tumor growth. *Cell* 1997; **88**: 277–85.

143. Boehm T, Folkman J, Browder T, O'Reilly MS. Antiangiogenic therapy of experimental cancer does not induce acquired drug resistance. *Nature* 1997; **390**: 404–7.

144. Oh SP, Kamagata Y, Muragaki Y et al. Isolation and sequencing of cDNAs for proteins with multiple domains of Gly-Xaa-Yaa repeats identify a distinct family of collagenous proteins. *Proc Natl Acad Sci USA* 1994; **91**: 4229–33.

145. Rehn M, Pihlajaniemi T. a1(XVIII), a collagen chain with frequent interruptions in the collagenous sequence, a distinct tissue distribution, and homology with type XV collagen. *Proc Natl Acad Sci USA* 1994; **91**: 4234–8.

146. Obeso J, Weber J, Auerbach R. A hemangioendothelioma-derived cell line: its use as a model for the study of endothelial cell biology. *Lab Invest* 1990; **63**: 259–69.

147. Hohenester E, Sasaki T, Olsen BR, Timpl R. Crystal structure of the angiogenesis inhibitor endostatin at 1.5 Å resolution. *EMBO J* 1998; **17**: 1656–64.

148. Ding Y-H, Javaherian K, Lo K-M et al. Zinc-dependent dimers observed in crystals of human endostatin. *Proc Natl Acad Sci USA* 1998; **95**: 10443–8.

149. Wen W, Moses MA, Wiederschain D et al. The generation of endostatin is mediated by elastase. *Cancer Res* 1999; **59**: 6052–6.

150. Miosge N, Sasaki T, Timpl R. Angiogenesis inhibitor endostatin is a distinct component of elastic fibers in vessel walls. *FASEB J* 1999; **13**: 1743–50.

151. Moulton KS, Heller E, Konerding MA et al. Angiogenesis inhibitors endostatin and TNP-470 reduce intimal neovascularization and plaque growth in apolipoprotein E-deficient mice. *Circulation* 1999; **99**: 1726–32.

152. Matsuno H, Yudoh K, Uzuki M et al. Treatment with the angiogenesis inhibitor endostatin: a novel therapy in rheumatoid arthritis. *J Rheumatol* 2002; **29**: 890–5.

153. Yin G, Liu W, An P et al. Endostatin gene transfer inhibits joint angiogenesis and pannus formation in inflammatory arthritis. *Mol Ther* 2002; **5**: 547–54.

154. Indraccolo S, Gola E, Rosato A et al. Differential effects of angiostatin, endostatin and interferon-alpha1 gene transfer on in vivo growth of human breast cancer cells. *Gene Ther* 2002; **9**: 867–78.

155. Calvo A, Feldman AL, Libutti SK, Green JE. Adenovirus-mediated endostatin delivery results in inhibition of mammary gland tumor growth in C3 (1)/SV40 T-antigen transgenic mice. *Cancer Res* 2002; **62**: 3934–8.

156. Shi W, Teschendorf C, Muzyczka N, Siemann DW. Adeno-associated virus-mediated gene transfer of endostatin inhibits angiogenesis and tumor growth in vivo. *Cancer Gene Ther* 2002; **9**: 513–21.

157. Zorick TS, Mustacchi Z, Bando SY et al. High serum endostatin levels in Down syndrome: implications for improved treatment and prevention of solid tumors. *Eur J Hum Genet* 2001; **9**: 811–14.

158. Yang Q, Rasmussen SA, Friedman JM. Mortality associated with Down's syndrome in the USA from 1983–1997: a population-based study. *Lancet* 2002; **359**: 1019–25.

159. Brouty-Boye D, Zetter B. Inhibition of cell motility by interferon. *Science* 1980; **208**: 516–18.

160. Dvorak HF, Gresser I. Microvascular injury in the pathogenesis of intereron induced necrosis of subcutaneous tumors in mice. *J Natl Cancer Inst* 1989; **81**: 497–502.

161. Sidky YA, Borden EC. Inhibition of angiogenesis by interferons: effects on tumor- and lympho-cyte-induced vascular diseases. *Cancer Res* 1987; **47**: 5155–61.

162. White CW, Sondheimer IIM, Crouch EC et al. Treatment of pulmonary hemangiomatosis with recombinant intereron alpha-2a. *N Engl J Med* 1989; **320**: 1197–200.

163. Folkman J. Successful treatment of an angiogenic disease. *N Engl J Med* 1989; **320**: 1211–12.

164. Ezekowitz RAB, Mulliken JB, Folkman J. Interferon alpha-2a therapy for life-threatening hemangiomas of infancy. *N Engl J Med* 1992; **326**: 1456–63. [Erratum *N Eng J Med* 1994; **330**: 300; *N Eng J Med* 1995; **333**: 595.]

165. Mulliken JB, Boon LM, Takahashi K et al. Pharmacologic therapy for endangering hemangiomas. *Curr Opin Derm* 1995; **2**: 109–13.

166. Bielenberg DR, Bucana CD, Sanchez R et al. Progressive growth of infantile cutaneous hemangiomas is directly correlated with hyperplasia and angiogenesis of adjacent epidermis and inversely correlated with expression of the endogenous angiogenesis inhibitor, IFN-beta. *Int J Oncol* 1999; **14**: 401–8.

167. Singh RK, Fidler IJ. Systemic administration of interferons for inhibition of cancer metastasis. In: Stuart-Harris R, Penny R, eds. *Clinical Applications of the Interferons* (Chapman & Hall: London, 1997) 391–404.

168. Folkman J, Mulliken JB, Ezekowitz RAB. Antiangiogenic therapy of hemangiomas with interferon alpha. In: Stuart-Harris R, Penny R, eds. *Clinical Applications of the Interferons* (Chapman & Hall: London, 1997) 255–65.

169. Takayanagi H, Kim S, Matsuo K et al. RANKL maintains bone homeostasis through c-Fos-dependent induction of interferon-β. *Nature* 2002; **416**: 744–9.

170. Terpos E, Palermos J, Viniou N et al. Pamidronate increses markers of bone formation in patients with multiple myeloma in plateau phase under interferon-alpha treatment. *Calcif Tissue Int* 2001; **68**: 285–90.

171. Fotsis T, Zhang Y, Pepper MS et al. 2-Methoxy-estradiol, an endogenous estrogen metabolite, inhibits angiogenesis and suppresses tumor growth. *Nature* 1994; **368**: 237–9.

172. D'Amato RJ, Lin CM, Flynn E et al. 2-Methoxy-estradiol, an endogenous mammalian metabolite, inhibits tubulin polymerization by interacting at the colchicine site. *Proc Natl Acad Sci USA* 1994; **91**: 3964–8.

173. LaVallee TM, Zhan XH, Herbstritt CJ et al. 2-Methoxyestradiol inhibits proliferation and induces apoptosis independently of estrogen receptors alpha and beta. *Cancer Res* 2002; **62**: 3691–7.

174. Figg WD, Kruger EA, Price DK et al. Inhibition of angiogenesis: treatment options for patients with metastatic prostate cancer. *Invest New Drugs* 2002; **20**: 183–94.

175. Rosen LS. Clinical experience with angiogenesis signaling inhibitors: focus on vascular endothelial growth factor (VEGF) blockers. *Cancer Control* 2002; **9**: 36–44.

176. Browder T, Butterfield CE, Kräling BM et al. Antiangiogenic scheduling of chemotherapy improves efficacy against experimental drug-resistant cancer. *Cancer Res* 2000; **60**: 1878–86.

177. Klement G, Barucel S, Rak J et al. Continuous low-dose therapy with vinblastine and VEGF receptor-2 antibody induces sustained tumor regression without overt toxicity. *J Clin Invest* 2000; **105**: R15–24.

178. Man S, Bocci G, Francia G et al. Antitumor effects in mice of low-dose (metronomic) cyclophosphamide administered continuously through the drinking water. *Cancer Res* 2002; **62**: 2731–5.

179. Neidhart M, Wehrli R, Bruhlmann P et al. Synovial fluid CD146 (MUC18), a marker for synovial membrane angiogenesis in rheumatoid arthritis. *Arthritis Rheum* 1999; **42**: 622–30.

180. Kamper EF, Kopeikina LT, Koutsoukos V et al.

Plasma tetranectin levels and disease activity in patients with rheumatoid arthritis. *J Rheumatol* 1997; **24**: 262–8.

181. Hood JD, Bednarshi M, Frausto R et al. Tumor regression by targeted gene delivery to the neovasculature. *Science* 2002; **296**: 2404–7.

182. Gerlag DM, Borger E, Tak PP et al. Suppression of murine collagen-induced arthritis by targeted apoptosis of synovial neovasculature. *Arthritis Res* 2001; **3**: 357–61.

183. Holmgren L, O'Reilly MS, Folkman J. Dormany of micrometastases: balanced proliferation and apoptosis in the presence of angiogenesis suppression. *Nature Med* 1995; **1**: 149–53.

184. O'Reilly MA, Wiederschain D, Stetler-Stevenson WG et al. Regulation of angiostatin production by matrix metalloproteinase-2 in a model of concomitant resistance. *J Biol Chem* 1999; **274**: 29568–71.

185. Taylor S, Folkman J. Protamine is an inhibitor of angiogenesis. *Nature* 1982; **297**: 107–12.

186. Crum R, Szabo S, Folkman J. A new class of steroids inhibit angiogenesis in the presence of heparin and heparin fragment. *Science* 1985; **230**: 1375–8.

187. D'Amato RJ, Loughnan MS, Flynn E, Folkman J. Thalidomide is an inhibitor of angiogenesis. *Proc Natl Acad Sci USA* 1994; **91**: 4082–5.

188. O'Reilly M, Pirie-Shepherd S, Lane WS, Folkman J. Antiangiogenic activity of the cleaved conformation of the serpin antithrombin *Science* 1999; **295**: 1296–8.

189. Moses M, Wiederschain D, Wu I et al. Troponin I is present in human cartilage and inhibits angiogenesis. *Proc Natl Acad Sci USA* 1999; **96**: 2645–50.

7

Fibroblasts

Sang-Heon Lee and Gary S Firestein

Introduction • Fibroblast heterogeneity • Fibroblast biology • Biological relevance to rheumatic disease • Conclusion • References

INTRODUCTION

Fibroblasts are mesenchymal-derived cells that play an integral role in tissue structure, injury and repair. Although once considered relatively passive participants that created the structural framework of tissues, it is now clear that these cells play a crucial and very active role in immune responses and extracellular matrix regulation. Fibroblasts certainly do synthesize matrix proteins such as collagen, fibronectin and proteoglycans under the influence of local growth factors. However, they also produce an array of cytokines and small molecule mediators that can recruit inflammatory cells and alter the function of other cells in the vicinity. The extent of extracellular matrix production is usually determined by the fibroblast environment, with local injury resulting in wound repair and normal fibrosis or unknown stimuli contributing to pathogenic processes such as scleroderma.[1] The mesenchymal-derived cells can also release a variety of matrix-degrading enzymes, such as the metalloproteinase involved in tissue remodeling, or, in extreme cases, tissue destruction.[2] Finally, fibroblasts can actively participate in immune responses through the elaboration of soluble products and by interacting with other immune cells through adhesion molecules.

Fibroblasts are readily identified after in vitro cultivation based on their ability to adhere to various surfaces (plastic, glass, etc.) as well as their characteristic elongated shape and oval nuclei (Figure 7.1). They usually require an adherent surface to survive in culture, and

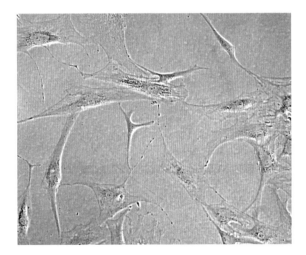

Figure 7.1 Cultured fibroblast-like synoviocytes using phase-contrast microscopy. The cells generally form monolayers in culture and exhibit spindle-shaped morphology with oval nuclei.

growth subsequently arrests once confluence is attained ('contact inhibition'). Fibroblasts are generally derived from mesenchymal precursors. These primitive cells express specific patterns of bone morphogenic protein (BMP) receptors and endoglin, lack CD34, and are present in both tissues and in blood.[3] Under the influence of local factors, pluripotential cells differentiate into tissue-specific fibroblasts with certain unique characteristics depending on the location. For instance, synovial lining fibroblasts (type B synoviocytes) express distinctive surface markers like CD55 and VCAM-1, and possess the machinery for prodigious proteoglycan synthesis. Similarly, fibroblasts in other locations such as the lung or skin have their own specific properties.

FIBROBLAST HETEROGENEITY

Fibroblasts do not form a single homogeneous population, but are composed of discrete subpopulations with unique phenotypes and functions. Furthermore, aberrant function of these subsets are associated with unique clinical syndromes (Table 7.1). For instance, activation of pulmonary fibroblasts with excessive production of extracellular matrix (ECM) can result in pulmonary fibrosis, while dermal fibroblast abnormalities can contribute to scleroderma. In contrast, dysfunctional fibroblasts in rheumatoid arthritis lead to destruction of the articular structures rather than fibrosis. Early studies support the concept of 'tissue-specific fibroblasts', where unique characteristics can be observed for each type of tissue. Fibroblasts from skin differ from those from lung in terms of morphology, proliferation rates, and synthesis of cytokines and ECM components.[4] Fibroblasts are also heterogeneous in their proliferation rate and biosynthetic activity within the same anatomic site.[5,6] The synovium is an example of this phenomenon, and fibroblasts in the intimal lining (type B fibroblast-like synoviocytes) are distinct from the sublining fibroblasts that reside in the interstitium (see below).

The study of fibroblast heterogeneity is technically difficult, although several methods

Table 7.1 Fibroblast phenotype in human diseases.

Rheumatoid arthritis
   Anchorage-independent growth ↑
   Contact inhibition ↓
   Oncogene expression ↑
   Cartilage invasion in SCID mice ↑
   Tumor suppressor gene function ↓
   Anti-apoptotic molecules ↑
Scleroderma
   Collagen production (type I, III, VI) ↑
   TGF-β receptors ↑
   IL-6 ↑
   IL-1 receptor ↑
   ICAM-1 ↑
Pulmonary fibrosis
   Thy1$^+$ population ↑
   Myofibroblast phenotype ↑

TGF, transforming growth factor; IL, interleukin.

have been used to distinguish subsets. In some cases, organ-specific diseases provide the opportunity to identify and characterize previously unrecognized phenotypes or determine specific functional abnormalities in fibroblasts isolated from the site of disease. Among the techniques that have been utilized, clonal expansion after limiting dilution, evaluation of cellular morphology, immunocytochemistry, determination of synthetic activity and responsiveness of prostaglandin E_2 (PGE$_2$), collagen synthesis, and fluorescence-activated cell sorting (FACS) have identified specific fibroblast subpopulations.[6] FACS has been especially valuable and has permitted the establishment of phenotypically stable subtypes even when cultured for many passages.[5,7]

The function and heterogeneity of lung fibroblasts has been extensively studied using many of these techniques. Fibroblasts isolated from lungs of patients with pulmonary fibrosis have a more aggressive growth rate than those from normal lung tissue.[8] A unique subset of pulmonary fibroblasts that expresses the surface marker Thy-1, a 25-kDa glycoprotein expressed on murine T lymphocytes, has been characterized.[7] The Thy-1[+] lung fibroblasts produce 2–3-fold more collagen than the Thy-1[-] subset; this difference is potentiated by interleukin-4 (IL-4) and suppressed by interferon gamma (IFN-γ).[9] The Thy-1[+] cells also synthesize greater amounts of fibronectin.[10] In addition, Thy-1 distinguishes lung fibroblasts based on their responses to cytokines. Upon stimulation of TNF-α, IL-1 protein is only detected in the supernatant of the Thy-1[-] subset, whereas IL-6 is produced by both subpopulations.[6] IFN-γ only induces class II MHC antigens in the Thy-1[-] subset.[7] In idiopathic pulmonary fibrosis, alveolar fibroblasts reveal myofibroblast phenotype characterized by smooth muscle actin immunofluorescence labeling.[11]

Dermal fibroblasts have also been divided into distinct subsets. Based on morphology, seven fibroblast subtypes can be defined that probably reflect stages of differentiation. F I, F II and F III are mitotic fibroblasts. F I are spindle shaped and rapidly proliferate, while the smaller F III exhibit a rounded phenotype with decreased proliferation. F IV F V, and F VI are more mature postmitotic subtypes that have a large rounded appearance and can ultimately differentiate into degenerating cells known as F VII.[12] These fibroblast subtypes have distinct protein synthesis patterns, and terminally differentiated F VI cells synthesize the greatest number of proteins. Further studies on skin fibroblast clones have shown a fivefold difference in proliferation rate among clones, which is related to the growth-suppressing effect of PGE$_2$ synthesis.[13] Clonal fibroblast populations vary significantly in collagen synthesis, which correlates with morphology. Mitototic phenotypes (F I, II, III) usually produce low levels of collagen, whereas the highest collagen production is observed in postmitotic types (F IV, F V, F VI).[14] Although the molecular basis for differences between clones of fibroblasts is not clear, clones may differ in intracellular signaling following

exposure to a given stimulus. Heterogeneity in responses involving cell surface receptors for parathyroid hormones or PGE$_2$ also exist in substrains from human neonatal dermal fibroblasts, demonstrated by different cAMP responses.[15] Other evidence of heterogeneity is found in C1q binding affinity (high affinity showing faster growth and more protein synthesis) and PGE$_2$ synthesis (inverse correlation with collagenase production).[16]

The synovium also shows clear evidence of fibroblast heterogeneity. In normal human synovium, fibroblasts display two main phenotypes based on their location within the tissue.[17] Intimal lining and subintimal fibroblasts are difficult to distinguish in tissue culture, so the definition of fibroblast populations has relied upon histochemical studies on intact tissue. There is no reliable sublining fibroblast marker, although the presence of non-vascular cells in synovium lacking CD45 identifies most sublining fibroblasts. Intimal fibroblasts express a specialized range of gene products, including uridine diphosphoglucose dehydrogenase (UDPGD), VCAM-1 and complement decay accelerating factor (DAF; CD55). Perhaps the defining feature of intimal fibroblasts is their high level of production of hyaluronan, reflected by the high activity of the enzyme UDPGD.[18] Normal intimal fibroblasts also generally do not express matrix metalloproteinases (MMPs) in situ. However, intimal lining fibroblasts in diseased tissue secrete massive amounts of MMPs.

The synovial intimal fibroblasts share the ability to express DAF with coelomic linings such as the pericardium and pleura. DAF expression in the intima is associated with local macrophage expression of FcγRIIIa, a molecule involved in immune complex clearance. DAF is also a ligand for the macrophage surface protein CD97, which is expressed by neighboring macrophage-like synoviocytes in the lining. Similarities between synovial and bone marrow fibroblasts have been observed. These include production of bone marrow stromal factor 1, stromal cell-derived factor 1 and bone morphogenic protein 2.[19,20] Contiguity between synovium and bone marrow probably does allow mixing of populations, and some fibroblasts or precursor cells can migrate through pores that connect the two compartments. Mesenchymal stem cells in the synovium can be derived either directly through these channels or from the circulating blood.[21]

FIBROBLAST BIOLOGY

Extracellular matrix regulation

Tissue fibroblasts are normally quiescent, with little cell proliferation and a low level of matrix production required to replace and maintain the stroma. In response to injury, fibroblasts rapidly proliferate, migrate to the sites of damage, and exhibit a marked increase in metabolic activity. The signals responsible for sensing damage are not fully elucidated but can involve release of growth factors by platelets (such as platelet-derived growth factor; PDGF) as well as mediators produced by damaged endothelium and pattern recognition mechanisms known as innate immunity (Figure 7.2). The cells then synthesize or degrade molecules in the ECM that are most appropriate for the specific injured tissue, including various forms of collagen, fibronectin, proteoglycan and glycoproteins. Type I and type III collagen are the main types synthesized by skin and interstitial fibroblasts, but types V, VI and VII are also produced as key proteins involved in collagen fibril organization.[22]

Transcriptional regulation of the genes encoding the α_1 (COL1A1) and α_2 (COL1A2) subunits of type I collagen help define the ECM produced by fibroblasts. The most widely studied cytokine involved in collagen deposition is transforming growth factor beta (TGF-β). This growth factor increases collagen synthesis when the cognate nuclear protein complex (TbRC) binds to upstream promoter element at −378/−108 bp (TbRE) of COL1A2. Sp1, one of the TbRC components, is required for the immediate early response of COL1A2 to TGF-β.[23] Oncostatin M (OSM), a member of the hematopoietic cytokine family produced by activated T cells and monocytes, shares many biological effects of TGF-β and may play important roles in ECM accumulation. OSM stimulates COL1A2 gene transcription through a constitutive-positive cis-response element in the collagen promoter, which interacts with two members of the Sp family of transcription factor (Sp1 and Sp3).[24]

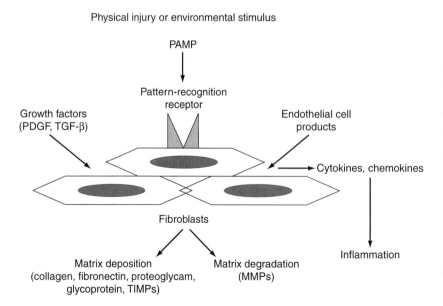

Figure 7.2 The environmental signals that influence fibroblast activation and metabolism. In response to physical injury or stimulus, fibroblasts can sense the damage through growth factors, endothelial products and pathogen-associated molecular pattern (PAMP), followed by expression of matrix proteins, cytokines and MMPs. Depending on the signals and the type of responding fibroblasts, either matrix deposition or degradation occurs. MMP, matrix metalloproteinase; TIMP, tissue inhibitor of metalloproteinase.

IFN-γ is the most potent inhibitor of collagen production by human mesenchymal cells.[25] IFN-α and IFN-β exert strong inhibitory effects on fibroblast collagen production, although less than than IFN-γ.[26] IFN-γ also abrogates the stimulatory effects of TGF-β on collagen production through both transcriptional and post-transcriptional mechanisms. IL-1 has variable effects on collagen synthesis in adult dermal fibroblasts depending on cell type and the local milieu.[27] The signal transduction pathways activated by IL-1 that result in modulation of collagen gene expression involve protein kinase C as well as feedback mechanisms utilizing endogenous prostaglandin production. Administration of the natural IL-1 antagonist IL-1Ra prevents lung fibrosis induced by bleomycin in mice, suggesting that IL-1 might play a profibrotic role in some circumstances.[28]

In addition to elaborating matrix proteins, fibroblasts are also primary sources of the tissue inhibitors of metalloproteinases (TIMPs) that protect the ECM from the proteolytic action of metalloproteinases. TGF-β is an especially potent inducer of TIMP.[29] Thus, TGF-β has an overall matrix-promoting effect, augmenting production of collagen and MMP inhibitors while suppressing collagenase production (see below). TIMP expression in fibroblasts can also be induced by IL-6 and IL-11,[30–32] while the effect of IL-1 is variable.

Cytokines released from neighboring cells affect fibroblast activation and are key determinants of their destructive or reparative potential. In contrast to TGF-β, which appears to direct fibroblasts towards fibrosis and repair, proinflammatory cytokines such as IL-1 and TNF-α released by endothelial cells and resident macrophages direct the cells along a more aggressive path. While these cytokines can stimulate proliferation, the effects are relatively modest compared with TGF-β or PDGF.[33] Degradation of the ECM is largely mediated by the production of MMPs by fibroblasts under the influence of proinflammatory cytokines. Members of this large family of enzymes, which include collagenases, stromelysins and gelatinases, have well-defined substrate specificities

and are, as a group, able to degrade most of the proteins present in normal tissues. They are secreted as latent proenzymes and subsequently activated in the extracellular space (Chapter 28). Native collagens require collagenases such as MMP-1 and MMP-13 to initiate the process (an exception is cathepsin K, which can also digest native collagen). Once cleaved, the denatured collagen can be further degraded by constitutively produced gelatinases, such as MMP-2 (72-kDa gelatinase), or induced proteases, such as MMP-9, stromelysin and pump-1 (uterine MMP). In addition to collagen, other ECM proteins, like proteoglycan, fibronectin, laminin and cartilage link protein, can be degraded by broad-spectrum MMPs such as the stromelysins.[31] Hence, the stroma and all of its constituents can be digested by the MMPs and ultimately replaced or remodeled as directed by the cytokine profile (Table 7.2).

Table 7.2   Regulation of extracellular matrix balance by cytokines.

	Induction	Suppression
Matrix protein	TGF-β	IFN-γ
	OSM	
MMPs	IL-1	TGF-β
	TNF-α	OSM
	IL-17	IL-4
	LIF	IL-10
		IL-13
		IFN-γ
TIMP	TGF-β	
	IL-6	
	IL-11	

TGF-β, transforming growth factor beta; IFN-γ, interferon gamma; OSM, oncostatin M; MMP, matrix metalloproteinases; LIF, leukemia inhibitory factor; TIMP, tissue inhibitor of metalloproteinase.

IL-1 is the most potent of the matrix-degrading cytokines. Very low concentrations markedly induce MMP gene expression and protein production. While TNF-α can also increase MMP expression, the concentrations required are often several orders of magnitude higher. The relatively greater impact of IL-1 on MMP expression might contribute to the observation that IL-1 is more intimately implicated in joint destruction, while TNF-α plays a prominent role in the inflammation.[34] In contrast, IFN-γ inhibits both collagen synthesis and synthesis of collagenase and stromelysin.[35,36] TGF-β, a potent stimulator of collagen synthesis, also suppresses production of collagenase and stromelysin,[37] whereas IL-4 can inhibit IL-1-mediated induction of MMPs.[38] Many other cytokines can alter MMP production by fibroblasts, including IL-17 and leukemia inhibitory factor (LIF) (which induce MMPs) and IL-10 and IL-13 (which suppress MMPs). Therefore, the cytokine profile plays a critical role in the balance between matrix production and release of the enzymes responsible for its destruction.

The mechanisms of MMP induction by IL-1 in fibroblasts have been carefully studied and involve the MAP kinase signal transduction pathways. This group of kinases includes three main families: c-Jun N-terminal kinase (JNK), p38 and extracellular regulated kinase (ERK). JNK, in particular, appears to play a crucial role in collagenase gene expression in fibroblasts by virtue of its ability to phosphorylate c-Jun, a key component of the AP-1 transcription factor complex.[39] AP-1-binding sites are present in virtually all of the MMP promoters and play a major role as initiators of mRNA transcription. ERK also contributes to the transcriptional regulation of MMPs, while the role of p38 is highly variable and depends on the individual cell lineage. The proinflammatory transcription factor NF-κB also regulates MMP expression in fibroblasts and, when activated, can enhance MMP production.[40,41] This pathway is regulated by IκB kinase-2 (IKK-2), an enzyme that can phosphorylate the endogenous NF-κB inhibitor IκB. Activation of IKK-2 alone is sufficient to induce MMP and cytokine expression (e.g. IL-6

and IL-8), and IKK-2 inhibition using dominant negative constructs blocks these same functions.[42] While MMP transcription plays a primary role in fibroblast MMP production, post-transcriptional events are also crucial. In addition to the requirement for post-translational modification, IL-1 can also stabilize MMP-1 mRNA and thereby increase steady-state levels.[43,44] This process can be suppressed (along with decreased MMP production) by engagement of A2b adenosine receptors.

Role of fibroblasts in cytokine networks

Cytokines are protein mediators that can either be released into the extracellular milieu or displayed on the surface of cells. These factors modulate cellular functions by binding to specific membrane receptors on the originating cell (autocrine), a neighboring cell (paracrine) or a distant cell (endocrine). As noted above, many cytokines can activate or modulate fibroblast function. Similarly, fibroblasts can serve as a rich source of cytokines that contribute to the inflammatory or reparative environment. For instance, cultured fibroblasts constitutively produce factors like TGF-β, fibroblast growth factor (FGF), stromal-derived factor-1 (SDF-1) and IL-6. Stimulation of fibroblasts by proinflammatory cytokines also leads to expression of other cytokines that can either enhance or suppress the process. In addition to induction of IL-1 and TNF-α, colony-stimulating factors like GM-CSF are rapidly produced, enhancing macrophage HLA-DR display and antigen presentation.[22,45] IL-1 and TNF-α synergistically stimulate fibroblast IL-6 production, which serves to stimulate the acute-phase response and activate plasma cells.[46] IL-17, a cytokine derived from stimulated T cells, can synergize with TNF-α or IL-1 and is able to induce inflammatory cytokines, including IL-6, IL-1 and IL-8.[47]

Fibroblasts also release chemokines and angiogenic factors into the microenvironment to recruit leukocytes to sites of inflammation. Following cytokine stimulation and/or engagement of CD40, synovial fibroblasts release chemoattractant molecules such as MCP-1 (monocytes), IL-8 (neutrophil), RANTES (monocytes), and IL-16 (CD4 T cells), which attract leukocytes into the synovium.[48] Another characteristic feature of inflamed tissue is new blood vessel formation. Hypoxia-driven expression of the angiogenesis factor vascular endothelial growth factor (VEGF) by fibroblasts is augmented by IL-1, but not by TNF-α.[49] Other cytokines and proteins released by mesenchymal cells can stimulate blood vessel growth, including TGF-β, PDGF, IL-8, soluble VCAM-1 and GM-CSF.[50]

Anti-inflammatory factors can be produced by fibroblasts and serve to terminate or downregulate an inflammatory reaction. For instance, IL-1Ra is constitutively produced by cultured fibroblasts. In addition to the secreted form of IL-1Ra, synovial fibroblasts also contain substantial amounts of an alternatively spliced intracellular form (icIL-1Ra).[51] Fibroblasts express and release soluble cytokine receptors that can inhibit the function of TNF-α or IL-1. IL-10, a potent anti-inflammatory cytokine, is produced by synovial fibroblasts, although the amount is insufficient to suppress production of inflammatory cytokines in synovitis.[52] Other suppressive cytokines, including TGF-β which can block T-cell activation, are also in the fibroblast armamentarium and can prevent antigen-specific responses.[53]

Small molecular mediator production

Fibroblasts can synthesize small molecular mediators such as prostaglandin and leukotrienes, which modulate turnover, vascular permeability and inflammatory cell recruitment. For instance, IL-1 and TNF-α stimulate fibroblast PGE_2 synthesis.[54] The prostanoid can inhibit the function or production of certain cytokines, such as IFN-γ. PGE_2 also suppresses fibroblast proliferation and collagen production. Regulation of prostaglandin production by cytokines in fibroblasts is primarily mediated through the expression of the inducible form of cyclo-oxygenase (COX2).[55] While COX1 is constitutively expressed, the marked increase in arachidonic acid mediators requires transcrip-

tional activation of the COX2 gene along with activation of cytosolic phospholipase A_2.[56] COX2 induction is blocked by corticosteroids and NF-κB inhibitors.

Leukotrienes, which are arachidonic acid metabolites produced through the lipoxygenase pathway, also exert a wide spectrum of biological activities. Among several types of leukotriene, leukotriene B_4 (LTB_4) plays a critical role in inflammation through its action as a chemotactic factor for leukocytes. In addition to leukocyte chemotaxis, LTB_4 promotes differentiation and chemotaxis of fibroblasts. Overexpression of 5-lipoxygenase (LOX), a key enzyme for the production of LTB_4, in fibroblasts is a critical pathway for leukotriene production in scleroderma.[57] Constitutive production of LTB_4 in several types of human fibroblasts has been reported,[58,59] and calcium ionophores can increase the release of LTB_4.[57] The production of leukotrienes in fibroblasts requires translocation of 5-LOX to the nuclear membrane, as well as binding to an integral membrane protein designated '5-LOX activating protein' (FLAP).[60] FLAP is expressed in cells that express 5-LOX is expressed and is regulated by activator protein 2.[61]

Cell–cell contact

Communication between cells is often mediated by soluble factors such as cytokines, although it has become increasingly clear that direct cell–cell contact is critically important for cell survival, trafficking and function. The interaction of immune cells with fibroblasts in tissues requires three steps (Figure 7.3): (1) leukocyte adherence to microvascular endothelium under the influence of chemotactic factors; (2) emigration from the vasculature into the extravascular space; and (3) adherence to fibroblasts or the ECM through specific ligand–receptor interactions.[22] As described above, fibroblasts can indirectly contribute to the first two phases through the elaboration of potent chemokines as well as cytokines that can induce the expression of cell adhesion molecules on endothelium. The subsequent anchoring of cells to the ECM produced by fibroblasts requires the expression

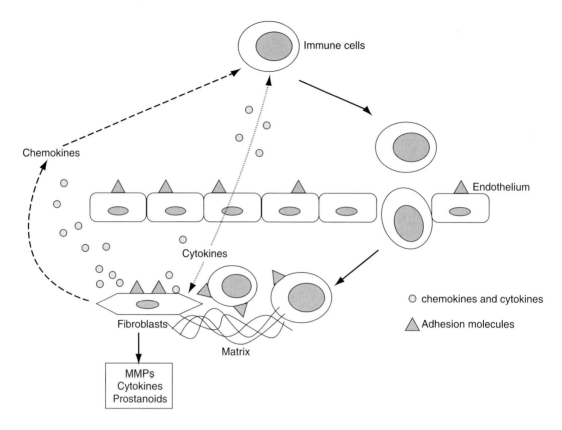

Figure 7.3 Interaction of immune cells with fibroblasts in tissues. The localization of immune cells in tissue requires cellular activation (by chemokines and/or cytokines), emigration from the vasculature, and binding to cellular and matrix component. These contact interactions are mediated through adhesion receptors, and are followed by activation of fibroblasts marked by production of MMPs (matrix metalloproteinases), cytokines and prostanoids.

of several additional adhesion molecules, including the hyaluronate receptor CD44 and integrins that bind to matrix proteins.[62] The β_1 family, including α_5/β_1, play especially important functions in this process.[63] Fibroblasts express many of these same receptors and utilize them to maintain their position within the tissue and prevent egress into the blood or lymphatics.

Leukocytes can also bind to and interact directly with fibroblasts. T cells and macrophages express α_4/β_1 integrin, which binds to VCAM-1 and an alternatively spliced form of fibronectin called CS-1 displayed on the synovial fibroblasts.[64] Engagement of the α_4/β_1 integrins on synoviocytes by fibronectin can

markedly enhance MMP gene expression, accounting for up to 5% of protein produced.[65] IL-1, TNF-α, IFN-γ and IL-4 induce the expression of other integrin counter-receptors on fibroblasts.[64] One of these, ICAM-1, is constitutively expressed by fibroblasts and can be markedly induced within hours after cytokine stimulation. ICAM-1 serves as a ligand for β_2 integrins on neutrophils and mononuclear cells. It can help retain inflammatory cells in the tissue and provide integrin-mediated signals that activate immune cells.

The interactions between the fibroblasts and T cells can also serve as survival signals. Normally, T cells undergo apoptosis, or programmed cell death, when cultured in vitro. In the presence of fibroblasts, however, this process is significantly delayed. The mechanism involves direct cell–cell contact and integrins, including those that bind to the RGD motif of several matrix proteins.[66] Mesenchymal cells also produce a variety of trophic factors that can support the survival of lymphocytes. Finally, fibroblasts that have been activated by IFN-γ (and express class II MHC antigens) are able to present antigens directly to T cells.[67] Therefore, interstitial fibroblasts have a complex task within the tissues that involves attraction and retention of immune cells as well as prolonging cell survival and contributing to their activation state under appropriate conditions.

The signaling between fibroblasts and other cells is bidirectional. Contact between T cells and fibroblasts can enhance cytokine, metalloproteinase and prostanoid production.[68] This interaction does not require viable T cells, since purified cell membranes or non-viable cells can perform the same function. Such activities involve surface proteins, including membrane-bound cytokines such as TNF-α and adhesion molecules such as leukocyte function-associated antigen-1 (LFA-1).[68] Therefore, T cells can orchestrate an inflammatory response through an antigen-independent mechanism.

BIOLOGICAL RELEVANCE TO RHEUMATIC DISEASE

Rheumatoid arthritis

There is growing evidence that activated fibroblast-like synoviocytes (FLS) play an important role in the pathogenesis of RA. Recently, significant progress has been made in elucidating the specific characteristics of these specialized fibroblasts. Along with neighboring macrophage-like cells, FLS form a productive paracrine–autocrine unit that is responsible for most of the inflammatory and destructive mediators produced in the rheumatoid joint.[69] In addition to serving as the primary source of MMPs, prostaglandins and complement, FLS

also produce cytokines that can stimulate adjacent cells or serve as autocrine factors.[70]

What is not clear is whether this process is entirely autonomous or whether the RA FLS must be continuously stimulated to achieve this level of activation. Are RA fibroblasts permanently imprinted by their environment, or are they passively responding to an inflammatory milieu? There is some evidence supporting both hypotheses,[69] although the former is especially intriguing in light of the marked expansion and invasive properties of RA synovium (Table 7.1) RA FLS exhibit anchorage-independent growth in vitro, especially in the presence of PDGF or high concentrations of serum.[71] Certain genes associated with cell transformation, including early growth response gene-1 (*egr-1*), c-*fos*, c-*jun* and c-*myc*, are expressed by RA synovial fibroblasts.[72] Inhibition of c-*myc* expression using antisense oligodeoxynucleotides suppresses proliferation and induces apoptosis of RA FLS.[73] Other distinctive features of RA FLS include increased IL-6 production[74] and monoclonal or oligoclonal expansion at the invasive front of synovium.[75]

The invasive properties of synoviocytes are maintained even after they have been cultured for many months. Elegant studies by Müller-Ladner and colleagues demonstrated that RA FLS, but not osteoarthritis or normal FLS, invade cartilage explants in severe combined immunodeficient (SCID) mice.[76] A similar phenotype can be induced in normal synoviocytes by inactivation of the p53 tumor suppressor gene. Other proteins involved in cell cycle regulation and cell death are also abnormal in RA fibroblasts. For instance, expression of *PTEN*, which is a tumor suppressor protein, is low in RA synovial fibroblasts.[77] The anti-apoptotic protein sentrin is found predominantly in the intimal layer of RA synovium, whereas normal synoviocytes express very little.[78] Taken together, these data suggest that FLS might be altered in RA and results in a cell phenotype that is invasive and resistant to apoptosis.

Because several lines of evidence suggest permanent alterations in RA FLS, the possibility of somatic mutations has been extensively explored. Most of the data focus on the role of the p53 tumor suppressor gene in RA and FLS. Several studies have demonstrated that p53 protein is overexpressed in RA synovial tissues or FLS compared with samples of osteoarthritis and other inflammatory joint diseases such as reactive arthritis.[79,80] p53 mutations in RA synovial tissue and FLS have been reported, although there is some variability in the number of mutations identified. Loss of p53 function in FLS enhances proliferation, cartilage invasion and anchorage-independent growth while suppressing apoptosis, thereby recapitulating the rheumatoid phenotype. The notion that p53 is a key homeostatic protein in inflammation and fibroblast function was confirmed in p53-knockout mice.[81] Collagen-induced arthritis is more destructive in p53-knockout mice than in wild-type animals. Enhanced synovitis is marked by higher cytokine (IL-1 and IL-6) and MMP expression in the mice lacking p53.

Scleroderma

Scleroderma is a systemic disease marked by excessive deposition of matrix proteins in skin and other organs. While the pathogenesis of the disease remains controversial, one possibility is that dermal fibroblasts develop a distinct phenotype that causes the production of an abnormal ECM. Cultured fibroblasts from patients with scleroderma are characterized by the overproduction of matrix components, especially type I, III and VI collagen. These cells produce 2–3-fold more collagen relative to normal fibroblasts (Table 7.1).[82] The persistence of the biosynthetically activated phenotype in scleroderma fibroblasts in vitro in the absence of exogenous activating signals suggests fundamental alterations regulating ECM gene expression.

Although it is not clear which stimuli contribute to fibroblast activation in scleroderma, certain cytokines and growth factors have been implicated. Cultured scleroderma fibroblasts express increased amounts of TGF-β receptors,

suggesting that sensitivity to this growth factor might contribute to the exaggerated TGF-β responses in scleroderma.[83] TGF-β induces expression of the type I and type III collagen genes (COL1A1, COL3A1) in scleroderma fibroblasts through the action of protein kinase C-δ which binds to a 129-bp promoter region encompassing nucleotides −804 to −675.[84]

Other abnormalities noted in scleroderma fibroblasts include higher production of IL-6,[85] increased responsiveness to IL-1,[86] increased expression of IL-1 receptors,[87] and increased expression of ICAM-1.[6] It is not certain whether this represents clonal expansion of a unique subset, a growth advantage resulting in polyclonal expansion of a particular subset, or the cells responding passively to their environment. The last of these seems less likely, since the scleroderma fibroblasts maintain their phenotype long after they are removed from the patient. Although there is no definite evidence of clonality, the increased proportion of high-collagen-producing cells in scleroderma compared with normal cells suggests the possibility of either clonal selection or selective activation.[88]

CONCLUSION

Previous views suggesting that fibroblasts form a homogeneous population of cells that passively respond to stress are untenable. These cells represent a dynamic force that constantly creates and re-creates its environment and interacts with immune cells to regulate inflammatory responses. Certain diseases are marked by a predominance of effector molecules produced by fibroblasts, suggesting that this cell lineage represents a reasonable target for therapeutic intervention. While it is very likely that fibroblast-targeted treatments can modify a pathogenic process, it is not clear whether 'irreversible' damage due to alterations in the ECM can be remodeled in the appropriate cytokine milieu.

REFERENCES

1. Agelli M, Wahl SM. Cytokines and fibrosis. *Clin Exp Rheumatol* 1986; **4**: 379–88.

2. Westhoff CS, Freudiger D, Petrow P et al. Characterization of collagenase 3 (matrix metalloproteinase 13) messenger RNA expression in the synovial membrane and synovial fibroblasts of patients with rheumatoid arthritis. *Arthritis Rheum* 1999; **42**: 1517–27.

3. Jorgensen C, Noel D, Gross G. Could inflammatory arthritis be triggered by progenitor cells in the joints? *Ann Rheum Dis* 2002; **61**: 6–9,

4. Ko SD, Page RC, Narayanan AS. Fibroblast heterogeneity and prostaglandin regulation of subpopulations. *Proc Natl Acad Sci USA* 1977; **74**: 3429–32.

5. Bordin S, Page RC, Narayanan AS. Heterogeneity of normal human diploid fibroblasts: isolation and characterization of one phenotype. *Science* 1984; **223**: 171–3.

6. Fries KM, Blieden T, Looney RJ et al. Evidence of fibroblast heterogeneity and the role of fibroblast subpopulations in fibrosis. *Clin Immunol Immunopathol* 1994; **72**: 283–92.

7. Phipps RP, Penney DP, Keng P et al. Characterization of two major populations of lung fibroblasts: distinguishing morphology and discordant display of Thy 1 and class II MHC. *Am J Respir Cell Mol Biol* 1989; **1**: 65–74.

8. Jordana M, Schulman J, McSharry C et al. Heterogeneous proliferative characteristics of human adult lung fibroblast lines and clonally derived fibroblasts from control and fibrotic tissue. *Am Rev Respir Dis* 1988; **137**: 579–84.

9. Sempowski GD, Derdak S, Phipps RP. Interleukin-4 and interferon-gamma discordantly regulate collagen biosynthesis by functionally distinct lung fibroblast subsets. *J Cell Physiol* 1996; **167**: 290–6.

10. Derdak S, Penney DP, Keng P et al. Differential collagen and fibronectin production by Thy 1+ and Thy 1– lung fibroblast subpopulations. *Am J Physiol* 1992; **263**: L283–90.

11. Fireman E, Shahar I, Shoval S et al. Morphological and biochemical properties of alveolar fibroblasts in interstitial lung diseases. *Lung* 2001; **179**: 105–17.

12. Bayreuther K, Rodemann HP, Hommel R et al. Human skin fibroblasts in vitro differentiate along a terminal cell lineage. *Proc Natl Acad Sci USA* 1988; **85**: 5112–16.

13. Korn JH, Torres D, Downie E. Clonal heterogeneity in the fibroblast response to mononuclear cell derived mediators. *Arthritis Rheum* 1984; **27**: 174–9.

14. Jelaska A, Strehlow D, Korn JH. Fibroblast heterogeneity in physiological conditions and fibrotic disease. *Springer Semin Immunopathol* 1999; **21**: 385–95.

15. Goldring SR, Stephenson ML, Downie E et al. Heterogeneity in hormone responses and patterns of collagen synthesis in cloned dermal fibroblasts. *J Clin Invest* 1990; **85**: 798–803.

16. Maxwell DB, Grotendorst CA, Grotendorst GR, LeRoy EC. Fibroblast heterogeneity in scleroderma: Clq studies. *J Rheumatol* 1987; **14**: 756–9.

17. Edwards JC. Fibroblast biology. Development and differentiation of synovial fibroblasts in arthritis. *Arthritis Res* 2000; **2**: 344–7.

18. Wilkinson LS, Pitsillides AA, Worrall JG, Edwards JC. Light microscopic characterization of the fibroblast-like synovial intimal cell (synoviocyte). *Arthritis Rheum* 1992; **35**: 1179–84.

19. Shimaoka Y, Attrep JF, Hirano T et al. Nurse-like cells from bone marrow and synovium of patients with rheumatoid arthritis promote survival and enhance function of human B cells. *J Clin Invest* 1998; **102**: 606–18.

20. Fowler MJ Jr, Neff MS, Borghaei RC et al. Induction of bone morphogenetic protein-2 by interleukin-1 in human fibroblasts. *Biochem Biophys Res Commun* 1998; **248**: 450–3.

21. Corr M, Zvaifler NJ. Mesenchymal precursor cells. *Ann Rheum Dis* 2002; **61**: 3–5.

22. Korn JH, Lafyatis R. Fibroblast function and fibrosis. In: Ruddy S, Harris ED, Sledge CB, eds. *Kelley's Textbook of Rheumatology*, 6th edn. (WB Saunders: Philadelphia, 2001) 263–74.

23. Greenwel P, Inagaki Y, Hu W et al. Sp1 is required for the early response of alpha2(I) collagen to transforming growth factor-beta1. *J Biol Chem* 1997; **272**: 19738–45.

24. Ihn H, LeRoy EC, Trojanowska M. Oncostatin M stimulates transcription of the human alpha2(I) collagen gene via the Sp1/Sp3–binding site. *J Biol Chem* 1997; **272**: 24666–72.

25. Granstein RD, Murphy GF, Margolis RJ et al. Gamma-interferon inhibits collagen synthesis in vivo in the mouse. *J Clin Invest* 1987; **79**: 1254–8.

26. Jimenez SA, Freundlich B, Rosenbloom J. Selective inhibition of human diploid fibroblast

collagen synthesis by interferons. *J Clin Invest* 1984; **74**: 1112–16.

27. Mauviel A, Heino J, Kahari VM et al. Comparative effects of interleukin-1 and tumor necrosis factor-alpha on collagen production and corresponding procollagen mRNA levels in human dermal fibroblasts. *J Invest Dermatol* 1991; **96**: 243–9.

28. Piguet PF, Vesin C, Grau GE, Thompson RC. Interleukin 1 receptor antagonist (IL-1ra) prevents or cures pulmonary fibrosis elicited in mice by bleomycin or silica. *Cytokine* 1993; **5**: 57–61.

29. Gunther M, Haubeck HD, van de Leur E et al. Transforming growth factor beta 1 regulates tissue inhibitor of metalloproteinases-1 expression in differentiated human articular chondrocytes. *Arthritis Rheum* 1994; **37**: 395–405.

30. DiBattista JA, Pelletier JP, Zafarullah M et al. Interleukin-1 beta induction of tissue inhibitor of metalloproteinase (TIMP-1) is functionally antagonized by prostaglandin E2 in human synovial fibroblasts. *J Cell Biochem* 1995; **57**: 619–29.

31. Sato T, Ito A, Mori Y. Interleukin 6 enhances the production of tissue inhibitor of metalloproteinases (TIMP) but not that of matrix metallo proteinases by human fibroblasts. *Biochem Biophys Res Commun* 1990; **170**: 824–9.

32. Maier R, Ganu V, Lotz M. Interleukin-11, an inducible cytokine in human articular chondrocytes and synoviocytes, stimulates the production of the tissue inhibitor of metalloproteinases. *J Biol Chem* 1993; **268**: 21527–32.

33. Schmidt JA, Mizel SB, Cohen D, Green I. Interleukin 1, a potential regulator of fibroblast proliferation. *J Immunol* 1982; **128**: 2177–82.

34. Kuiper S, Joosten LA, Bendele AM et al. Different roles of tumour necrosis factor alpha and interleukin 1 in murine streptococcal cell wall arthritis. *Cytokine* 1998; **10**: 690–702.

35. Varga J, Yufit T, Brown RR. Inhibition of collagenase and stromelysin gene expression by interferon-gamma in human dermal fibroblasts is mediated in part via induction of tryptophan degradation. *J Clin Invest* 1995; **96**: 475–81.

36. Alvaro-Gracia JM, Zvaifler NJ, Firestein GS. Cytokines in chronic inflammatory arthritis. V. Mutual antagonism between interferon-gamma and tumor necrosis factor-alpha on HLA-DR expression, proliferation, collagenase production, and granulocyte macrophage colony-stimulating factor production by rheumatoid arthritis synoviocytes. *J Clin Invest* 1990; **86**: 1790–8.

37. Overall CM, Wrana JL, Sodek J. Independent regulation of collagenase, 72-kDa progelatinase, and metalloendoproteinase inhibitor expression in human fibroblasts by transforming growth factor-beta. *J Biol Chem* 1989; **264**: 1860–9.

38. Borghaei RC, Rawlings PL Jr, Mochan E. Interleukin-4 suppression of interleukin-1-induced transcription of collagenase (MMP-1) and stromelysin 1 (MMP-3) in human synovial fibroblasts. *Arthritis Rheum* 1998; **41**: 1398–406.

39. Han Z, Boyle DL, Chang L et al. c-Jun N-terminal kinase is required for metalloproteinase expression and joint destruction in inflammatory arthritis. *J Clin Invest* 2001; **108**: 73–81.

40. Han Z, Boyle DL, Manning AM, Firestein GS. AP-1 and NF-kappaB regulation in rheumatoid arthritis and murine collagen-induced arthritis. *Autoimmunity* 1998; **28**: 197–208.

41. Vincenti MP, Coon CI, Brinckerhoff CE. Nuclear factor kappaB/p50 activates an element in the distal matrix metalloproteinase 1 promoter in interleukin-1beta-stimulated synovial fibroblasts. *Arthritis Rheum* 1998; **41**: 1987–94.

42. Aupperle K, Bennett B, Han Z et al. NF-kappa B regulation by I kappa B kinase-2 in rheumatoid arthritis synoviocytes. *J Immunol* 2001; **166**: 2705–11.

43. Rutter JL, Benbow U, Coon CI, Brinckerhoff CE. Cell-type specific regulation of human interstitial collagenase-1 gene expression by interleukin-1 beta (IL-1 beta) in human fibroblasts and BC-8701 breast cancer cells. *J Cell Biochem* 1997; **66**: 322–36.

44. Boyle DL, Han Z, Rutter JL et al. Posttranscriptional regulation of collagenase-1 gene expression in synoviocytes by adenosine receptor stimulation. *Arthritis Rheum* 1997; **40**: 1772–9.

45. Lorenzo JA, Jastrzebski SL, Kalinowski JF et al. Tumor necrosis factor alpha stimulates production of leukemia inhibitory factor in human dermal fibroblast cultures. *Clin Immunol Immunopathol* 1994; **70**: 260–5.

46. Elias JA, Lentz V. IL-1 and tumor necrosis factor synergistically stimulate fibroblast IL-6 production and stabilize IL-6 messenger RNA. *J Immunol* 1990; **145**: 161–6.

47. Katz Y, Nadiv O, Beer Y. Interleukin-17 enhances tumor necrosis factor alpha-induced synthesis of interleukins 1, 6, and 8 in skin and synovial fibroblasts: a possible role as a 'fine-tuning cytokine' in inflammation processes. *Arthritis Rheum* 2001; **44**: 2176–84.

48. Smith RS, Smith TJ, Blieden TM, Phipps RP. Fibroblasts as sentinel cells. Synthesis of chemokines and regulation of inflammation. *Am J Pathol* 1997; **151**: 317–22.

49. Jackson JR, Minton JA, Ho ML et al. Expression of vascular endothelial growth factor in synovial fibroblasts is induced by hypoxia and interleukin 1beta. *J Rheumatol* 1997; **24**: 1253–9.

50. Ritchlin C. Fibroblast biology. Effector signals released by the synovial fibroblast in arthritis. *Arthritis Res* 2000; **2**: 356–60.

51. Firestein GS, Boyle DL, Yu C et al. Synovial inter-leukin-1 receptor antagonist and interleukin-1 balance in rheumatoid arthritis. *Arthritis Rheum* 1994; **37**: 644–52.

52. Ritchlin C, Haas-Smith SA. Expression of inter-leukin 10 mRNA and protein by synovial fibrob-lastoid cells. *J Rheumatol* 2001; **28**: 698–705.

53. Chu CQ, Field M, Abney E et al. Transforming growth factor-beta 1 in rheumatoid synovial membrane and cartilage/pannus junction. *Clin Exp Immunol* 1991; **86**: 380–6.

54. Elias JA, Gustilo K, Baeder W, Freundlich B. Synergistic stimulation of fibroblast prostaglandin production by recombinant inter-leukin 1 and tumor necrosis factor. *J Immunol* 1987; **138**: 3812–16.

55. Crofford LJ, Wilder RL, Ristimaki AP et al. Cyclooxygenase-1 and -2 expression in rheuma-toid synovial tissues. Effects of interleukin-1 beta, phorbol ester, and corticosteroids. *J Clin Invest* 1994; **93**: 1095–101.

56. Mehindate K, al-Daccak R, Dayer JM et al. Superantigen-induced collagenase gene expres-sion in human IFN-gamma-treated fibroblast-like synoviocytes involves prostaglandin E2. Evidence for a role of cyclooxygenase-2 and cytosolic phospholipase A2. *J Immunol* 1995; **155**: 3570–7.

57. Kowal-Bielecka O, Distler O, Neidhart M et al. Evidence of 5-lipoxygenase overexpression in the skin of patients with systemic sclerosis: a newly identified pathway to skin inflammation in systemic sclerosis. *Arthritis Rheum* 2001; **44**: 1865–75.

58. Koyama S, Sato E, Masubuchi T et al. Human lung fibroblasts release chemokinetic activity for monocytes constitutively. *Am J Physiol* 1998; **275**: L223–30.

59. Bonnet C, Bertin P, Cook-Moreau J et al. Lipoxygenase products and expression of 5-lipoxygenase and 5-lipoxygenase-activating

protein in human cultured synovial cells. *Prostaglandins* 1995; **50**: 127–35.

60. Dixon RA, Diehl RE, Opas E et al. Requirement of a 5-lipoxygenase-activating protein for leuko-triene synthesis. *Nature* 1990; **343**: 282–4.

61. Kennedy BP, Diehl RE, Boie Y et al. Gene charac-terization and promoter analysis of the human 5-lipoxygenase-activating protein (FLAP). *J Biol Chem* 1991; **266**: 8511–16.

62. Murakami S, Okada H. Lymphocyte–fibroblast interactions. *Crit Rev Oral Biol Med* 1997; **8**: 40–50.

63. Sarkissian M, Lafyatis R. Transforming growth factor-beta and platelet derived growth factor regulation of fibrillar fibronectin matrix forma-tion by synovial fibroblasts. *J Rheumatol* 1998; **25**: 613–22.

64. Morales-Ducret J, Wayner E, Elices MJ et al. Alpha 4/beta 1 integrin (VLA-4) ligands in arthritis. Vascular cell adhesion molecule-1 expression in synovium and on fibroblast-like synoviocytes. *J Immunol* 1992; **149**: 1424–31.

65. Huhtala P, Humphries MJ, McCarthy JB et al. Cooperative signaling by alpha 5 beta 1 and alpha 4 beta 1 integrins regulates metallopro-teinase gene expression in fibroblasts adhering to fibronectin. *J Cell Biol* 1995; **129**: 867–79.

66. Salmon M, Scheel-Toellner D, Huissoon AP et al. Inhibition of T-cell apoptosis in the rheumatoid synovium. *J Clin Invest* 1997; **99**: 439–46.

67. Boots AM, Wimmers-Bertens AJ, Rijnders AW. Antigen-presenting capacity of rheumatoid synovial fibroblasts. *Immunology* 1994; **82**: 268–74.

68. Burger D, Rezzonico R, Li JM et al. Imbalance between interstitial collagenase and tissue inhibitor of metalloproteinases 1 in synoviocytes and fibroblasts upon direct contact with stimu-lated T lymphocytes: involvement of membrane-associated cytokines. *Arthritis Rheum* 1998; **41**: 1748–59.

69. Firestein GS. Invasive fibroblast-like synovio-cytes in rheumatoid arthritis. Passive responders or transformed aggressors? *Arthritis Rheum* 1996; **39**: 1781–90.

70. Firestein GS, Zvaifler NJ. How important are T cells in chronic rheumatoid synovitis? *Arthritis Rheum* 1990; **33**: 768–73.

71. Lafyatis R, Remmers EF, Roberts AB et al. Anchorage-independent growth of synoviocytes from arthritic and normal joints. Stimulation by exogenous platelet-derived growth factor and inhibition by transforming growth factor-beta and retinoids. *J Clin Invest* 1989; **83**: 1267–76.

72. Müller-Ladner U, Kriegsmann J, Gay RE, Gay S. Oncogenes in rheumatoid arthritis. *Rheum Dis Clin North Am* 1995; **21**: 675–90.

73. Hashiramoto A, Sano H, Maekawa T et al. C-myc antisense oligodeoxynucleotides can induce apoptosis and down-regulate Fas expression in rheumatoid synoviocytes. *Arthritis Rheum* 1999; **42**: 954–62.

74. Baumann H, Kushner I. Production of interleukin-6 by synovial fibroblasts in rheumatoid arthritis. *Am J Pathol* 1998; **152**: 641–4.

75. Imamura F, Aono H, Hasunuma T et al. Monoclonal expansion of synoviocytes in rheumatoid arthritis. *Arthritis Rheum* 1998; **41**: 1979–86.

76. Müller-Ladner U, Kriegsmann J, Franklin BN et al. Synovial fibroblasts of patients with rheumatoid arthritis attach to and invade normal human cartilage when engrafted into SCID mice. *Am J Pathol* 1996; **149**: 1607–15.

77. Pap T, Franz JK, Hummel KM et al. Activation of synovial fibroblasts in rheumatoid arthritis: lack of expression of the tumour suppressor PTEN at sites of invasive growth and destruction. *Arthritis Res* 2000; **2**: 59–64.

78. Franz JK, Pap T, Hummel KM et al. Expression of sentrin, a novel antiapoptotic molecule, at sites of synovial invasion in rheumatoid arthritis. *Arthritis Rheum* 2000; **43**: 599–607.

79. Firestein GS, Nguyen K, Aupperle KR et al. Apoptosis in rheumatoid arthritis: p53 overexpression in rheumatoid arthritis synovium. *Am J Pathol* 1996; **149**: 2143–51.

80. Tak PP, Smeets TJ, Boyle DL et al. p53 overexpression in synovial tissue from patients with early and longstanding rheumatoid arthritis compared with patients with reactive arthritis and osteoarthritis. *Arthritis Rheum* 1999; **42**: 948–53.

81. Yamanishi Y, Boyle DL, Pinkoski MJ et al. Regulation of joint destruction and inflammation by p53 in collagen-induced arthritis. *Am J Pathol* 2002; **160**: 123–30.

82. LeRoy EC. Increased collagen synthesis by scleroderma skin fibroblasts in vitro: a possible defect in the regulation or activation of the scleroderma fibroblast. *J Clin Invest* 1974; **54**: 880–9.

83. Kawakami T, Ihn H, Xu W et al. Increased expression of TGF-beta receptors by scleroderma fibroblasts: evidence for contribution of autocrine TGF-beta signaling to scleroderma phenotype. *J Invest Dermatol* 1998; **110**: 47–51.

84. Jimenez SA, Gaidarova S, Saitta B et al. Role of protein kinase C-delta in the regulation of collagen gene expression in scleroderma fibroblasts. *J Clin Invest* 2001; **108**: 1395–403.

85. Feghali CA, Bost KL, Boulware DW, Levy LS. Mechanisms of pathogenesis in scleroderma. I. Overproduction of interleukin 6 by fibroblasts cultured from affected skin sites of patients with scleroderma. *J Rheumatol* 1992; **19**: 1207–11.

86. Denton CP, Xu S, Black CM, Pearson JD. Scleroderma fibroblasts show increased responsiveness to endothelial cell-derived IL-1 and bFGF. *J Invest Dermatol* 1997; **108**: 269–74.

87. Kawaguchi Y, Harigai M, Hara M et al. Increased interleukin 1 receptor, type I, at messenger RNA and protein level in skin fibroblasts from patients with systemic sclerosis. *Biochem Biophys Res Commun* 1992; **184**: 1504–10.

88. Jelaska A, Arakawa M, Broketa G, Korn JH. Heterogeneity of collagen synthesis in normal and systemic sclerosis skin fibroblasts. Increased proportion of high collagen-producing cells in systemic sclerosis fibroblasts. *Arthritis Rheum* 1996; **39**: 1338–46.

8

Origin of the invasive rheumatoid arthritis synovial fibroblasts

John D Mountz, Hui-Chen Hsu and Huang-Ge Zhang

Introduction • Chronic inflammatory disease and autoimmune disease in *lpr* and *gld* mice • Post-*Mycoplasma pulmonis* inflammation and arthritis • Antigen-presenting cell (APC)–FasL cell gene therapy to treat *M. pulmonis*-induced arthritis • APC–FasL treatment in a collagen II (CII) arthritis model • CII pulse is required for elimination of CII response T cells using APC–AdFasLp35Tet treatment • Molecular defects associated with rheumatoid arthritis synovial fibroblasts • Regulation of apoptosis in RASFs, defects in NFκB and ubiquitin proteosome degradation • Increased proliferation of RASF-intrinsic defect in phosphorylated Akt • Summary • Acknowledgment • References

INTRODUCTION

There is now a substantial body of evidence to indicate that both genetic factors and environmental agents are involved in the initiation and perpetuation of rheumatoid arthritis (RA). The most likely environmental factors include those that can trigger an inflammatory response, and may have some tropism towards inducing joint inflammation. The inflammatory response is unique in RA and involves neovascularization and infiltration of macrophages, T cells and B cells. The second phase of developmental RA involves hyperplasia of synovial lining cells and development of synovial fibroblasts which exhibit the property of increased proliferation and growth as well as expression of collagenase and stromelysin that can lead to erosion of cartilage and bone. Once initiated, the process is difficult to arrest, due either to ongoing episodes of synovial inflammation, or diminished regulatory capacity of the rheumatoid arthritis synovial fibroblasts (RASFs). In this chapter, we will outline animal models that lead to initiation of a chronic erosive arthritis that follow these two sequences of events. Second, we will describe genetic changes that occur in human RASFs that lead to either increased hyperplasia and invasive potential or decreased susceptibility to regulation by apoptosis.

CHRONIC INFLAMMATORY DISEASE AND AUTOIMMUNE DISEASE IN *lpr* AND *gld* MICE

Ten years have passed since the identification of *fas* and *fas* ligand (*fasL*) genes in the murine model of autoimmune disease in *lpr* (lympho-proliferation) and *gld* (generalized lymphopro-liferative disease) mice, respectively.[1-3] Autoimmune disease in *lpr* and *gld* mice consists primarily of nephritis and pneumonitis, but, on some genetic backgrounds, the mice also develop arthritis and a Sjögren's-like syndrome inflammation of the salivary gland.[4-6] In addition, these mice develop myositis, cerebritis and vasculitis, and are also predisposed to ocular inflammatory diseases after infection.[7,8] Therefore, these mice exhibit a generalized defect in elimination of inflammatory, autoreactive T cells.

We previously observed that a Fas apoptosis defect of T cells and other inflammatory cells can lead to an inability to downmodulate systemic infection initiated by a murine cytomegalovirus (MCMV) viral inflammatory response in the lung, liver, salivary gland and kidney, resulting in the development of a chronic inflammation.[9,10] This chronic inflammation was not seen in resistant B6 wild-type mice, but only in Fas apoptosis-deficient B6-*lpr/lpr* and B6-*gld/gld* mice.[9,10] Furthermore, this inflammation was not related to defective clearance of MCMV from these tissues, and clearance of the virus was nearly equivalent in these mice.[10] We therefore proposed that progressing factor leading to a chronic inflammation after an acute inflammatory response to an infectious agent is associated with a defect in the Fas/FasL apoptosis pathway, leading to a failure to downmodulate the inflammatory response. The rapid clearance of the inciting infectious agent despite persistent inflammation may explain the difficulty in isolating infectious agents in mid- to late-stage chronic inflammatory disease.

POST-*MYCOPLASMA PULMONIS* INFLAMMATION AND ARTHRITIS

It also has been difficult to identify an infectious etiology of RA. This may be due to clearance of the organism after initiation of arthritis but failure to downmodulate the arthritis process. Post-infectious arthritis resulting from Gram-negative infection has been extensively studied

in humans.[11-14] Most of these studies indicate that, although knowledge of a trigger for reactive arthritis is important, arthritis is an uncommon outcome of these infections, and the development of chronic arthritis, as distinct from brief arthritis, is very rare and the predisposing factors leading to development of chronic arthritis are unknown. Similarly, recent studies by Schumacher et al[15] and Gerard et al[16] have provided evidence that chronic arthritis can have an infectious etiology and, in a small percentage of cases, the etiologic agent could be identified. However, in the majority of patients, no evidence of any viable infectious agent can be identified. One problem is that, in most cases, only late-stage arthritis has been evaluated, and it is possible that an infectious agent may trigger the arthritis and then be cleared. In this case, it is not clear what the genetic or susceptibility factors are that lead to persistence of arthritis after an initial triggering event by a proposed infectious agent.

Mycoplasma, like *Chlamydia* and *Yersinia*, is an intracellular pathogen that has been reported to be associated with reactive arthritis (ReA) in humans and animals.[17-19] Henry et al[20] and Keystone et al[21] previously reported the recovery of *Mycoplasma* from the joints of patients with ReA. However, most animal studies show this correlation only during the acute phase, and not in the chronic phase, and, in some studies, only few or no viable *Mycoplasma* organisms could be isolated from the joints of infected animals during the chronic phase.[22,23] This suggests that, in addition to persistent infection, there are other cellular factors that are important for the development of post-*Mycoplasma* infectious arthritis. The molecular mechanisms that predispose animals to post-*Mycoplasma* infectious arthritis are not clear. High immune responder strains of mice have been reported to exhibit higher resistance to *Mycoplasma*-induced arthritis compared to low responder mice.[24] This suggests that systemic activation of lymphocytes is an important factor either for the elimination of *Mycoplasma* or prevention of arthritis.

Modulation of apoptosis appears to play an important role in the pathogenesis of inflammatory arthritis. The occurrence of apoptosis in

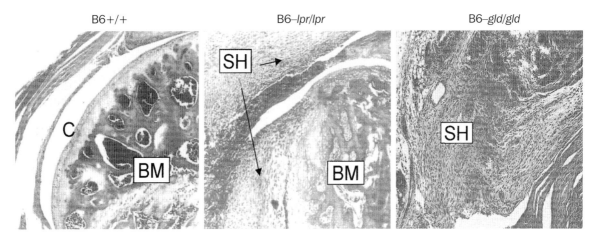

Figure 8.1 Arthritis in *M. pulmonis*-infected B6-*lpr/lpr* and B6-*gld/gld* mice, but not B6+/+ mice. Mice were sacrificed 4 weeks after infection with a moderate dose of *M. pulmonis* (1×10^7 CFU). Sagittal sections through the knee joint of infected B6+/+, B6-*lpr/lpr* and B6-*gld/gld* mice were prepared and stained with hematoxylin and eosin (H&E). C, cartilage; SH, synovial hyperplasia; BM, bone marrow cavity. Magnification $\times$ 800. (Reproduced with permission from Hsu et al, *Arthritis Rheum* 2001; **44**(9): 2146–59.[27])

rheumatoid synovial tissue and the ability of RA synovial cells to undergo anti-Fas-induced apoptosis have been demonstrated in several recent studies.[25,26] Defective apoptosis can lead to tolerance loss in both T and B cells, thus enhancing the inflammatory response. These observations suggest that Fas-mediated apoptosis may be a natural protective strategy to prevent progression of an inflammatory response to arthritis, and that activation of Fas-mediated apoptosis may be an effective strategy for prevention and treatment of patients with inflammatory arthritis. To explore this possibility, we infected wild-type B6+/+ mice, Fas-deficient B6-*lpr/lpr* or Fas ligand-deficient B6-*gld/gld* mice with a moderate dose of *M. pulmonis* and subsequently evaluated the development of both acute joint damage and chronic post-infectious arthritis in these mice. Our study shows that infection of B6-*lpr/lpr* and B6-*gld/gld* mice with *M. pulmonis* resulted in an acute-phase inflammation of the synovium that later developed into a chronic erosive arthritis. Similar infection of B6+/+ mice resulted only in an acute joint inflammatory response that resolved (Figure 8.1).[27] Chronic arthritis in B6-*gld/gld* mice was not due to persistent infection,

since there was no difference in the clearance rate of *Mycoplasma* from the joints of B6-*gld/gld* or B6-*lpr/lpr* mice compared to B6+/+ mice. This finding therefore presents an infectious chronic arthritis model, which is highly associated with the genetic component regulating the apoptosis pathway mediated by Fas and FasL of the host.

ANTIGEN-PRESENTING CELL (APC)–FasL CELL GENE THERAPY TO TREAT *M. PULMONIS*-INDUCED ARTHRITIS

The *Mycoplasma* infection-induced arthritis in *gld* mice could be due to the ongoing inflammatory response or could be due to an apoptosis defect in synovial lining cells or synovial fibroblasts that lead to chronic inflammation. To support the hypothesis that defective apoptosis is an important mechanism associated with post-*Mycoplasma* infection-induced arthritis and to identify the major cell type that is associated with the development of arthritis in this model, we used a cell–gene therapy strategy to deliver expression of high levels of functional cell surface FasL in lymphoid organs of B6-*gld/gld* mice.[27] To achieve very high levels of FasL expression in almost 100%

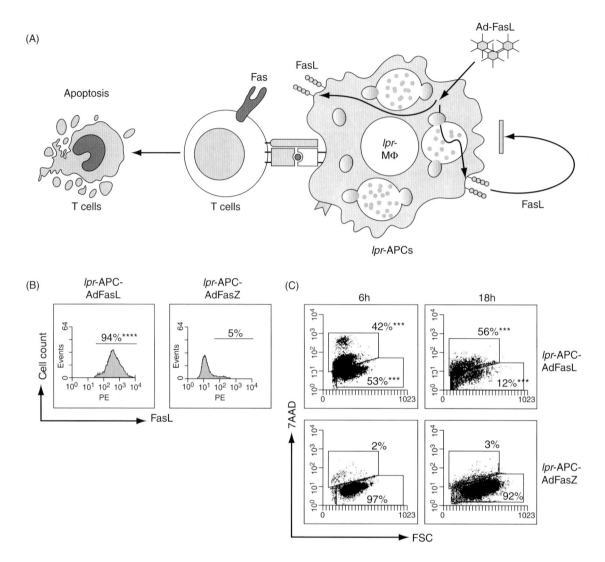

Figure 8.2 Induction of T-cell apoptosis using the *lpr*-APC–AdFasL strategy. (A) The *lpr*-APC–AdFasL gene therapy was made possible by the development of an adenovirus that could express FasL and easily transfect it into macrophages derived from *lpr* mice, which lacked expression of Fas and therefore would not undergo autocrine apoptosis. (B) Transfection of AdFasL into macrophages from B6-*lpr/lpr* mice resulted in high levels of FasL expression. Macrophages from *lpr* mice were transfected with either AdCMVLoxpFasL+ AdCANCre (*lpr*-APC–AdFasL) or AdCMVLoxpFasL+ AdCANLacZ (*lpr*-APC–AdLacZ) at 5 PFU/cell of each virus for 1 h at 37°C, and the transfected cells were further incubated at 37°C for 18 h. Fluorescine-activated cell sorting (FACS) analysis indicated that more than 90% of the AdFasL-transfected *lpr*-APC expressed FasL ($p < 0.0001$ versus *lpr*-APC–AdLacZ group). The results presented here are representative of three independent experiments. (C) The function of the transfected AdFasL was determined by the induction of apoptosis upon co-culture with the Fas-apoptosis-sensitive Jurkat T cells. Apoptosis of Jurkat T cells 6 h and 18 h after co-culturing with *lpr*-APC–AdFasL or *lpr*-APC–AdLacZ was determined by flow cytometry using 7-amino-actinomycin D staining. Co-culture of Jurkat cells with *lpr*-APC–AdFasL resulted in a significant increase in the percentage of Jurkat T cells undergoing apoptosis compared to that in the *lpr*-APC–AdLacZ group ($p < 0.001$). The results presented here are representative of three independent experiments.

of infected APCs, we have utilized APCs transfected with AdLoxpFasL plus AxCANCre (APC–AdFasL[28–30]) (Figure 8.2). The high efficiency of FasL expression accomplished by this technique is due, in part, to the ability to produce very high titers of both viruses in the 293 cells resulting from the lack of FasL expression by AdLoxpFasL, which requires co-infection with an AxCANCre virus.[30] In addition, this two-virus system was used to infect an APC cell line derived from B6-lpr/lpr mice; consequently, these lpr APCs can express high levels of FasL (lpr-APC–AdFasL) without undergoing autocrine suicide. We previously showed that administration of lpr-APC–AdFasL (1 × 10[6] cells/mouse) through the intravenous route did not cause any liver toxicity to B6+/+ mice. This is explained by the migration pattern of APCs, whereby intravenous injection of lpr-APCs leads to the homing of lpr-APCs to spleen, but not to liver.[31,32] We have previously used this strategy and demonstrated that administration of lpr-APC–AdFasL (1 × 10[6] cells/mouse for five doses) can induce tolerance of adenovirus-specific T cells and also MCMV-induced chronic inflammatory disease.[31,32]

Our study demonstrated that intraperitoneal injection of lpr-APC–AdFasL inhibited the development of chronic arthritis (Figure 8.3).[27] This therapy also induced a potent apoptosis effect in vivo in lymph node T cells of Mycoplasma-infected B6-gld/gld mice. There was a dramatic reduction of both T and B cells in the peripheral blood of B6-gld/gld mice as early as 24 h after administration of the lpr-APC–AdFasL. In addition, there was a significant decrease in the percentage of the autoreactive B220[+] T cells in the lymph nodes of B6-gld/gld mice after administration of five doses of lpr-APC–AdFasL.[27] We propose that this correlates with the migration of lpr-APCs into the lymph nodes of the injected mice. There was, however, no enhancement of apoptosis of synovial cells in lpr-APC–AdFasL-treated mice compared to lpr-APC–AdLacZ-treated mice. Taken together, these results indicate that defective deletion of activated T cells triggered by M.

pulmonis infection is an important pathogenic mechanism for the induction of M. pulmonis-induced murine arthritis in Fas/FasL apoptosis. These results are also consistent with our previous results showing that administration of lpr-APC–AdFasL to normal B6+/+ mice resulted in the homing of lpr-APC–AdFasL to the lymphoid organs,[32] and suggest that elimination of T cells in the lymphoid organ before their emigration to the target organs can be effective in preventing acute and chronic arthritis triggered by infectious pathogens. Together, these results indicate that the on going inflammatory response, even in the absence of microorganisms, is necessary to sustain the synovial cell hyperplasia.

APC–FasL TREATMENT IN A COLLAGEN II (CII) ARTHRITIS MODEL

In addition to proinflammatory cytokine production by T cells,[33–35] autoantibodies such as rheumatoid factor are produced in patients with RA.[36,37] To determine the relative role of T cells, or autoantibodies, APC–FasL therapy or an adenovirus expressing soluble transmembrane activator and calcium modulator and cyclophilin ligand interactor (AdsTACI) therapy, which blocks B-cell activation, was used to treat a CII arthritis model.[38]

CII-induced arthritis in DBA/1j mice is mediated by both CII-reactive T cells and anti-CII antibody-producing B cells.[39–43] To determine the relative roles of these processes in the development of arthritis, we specifically eliminated CII-reactive T cells by treating the mice with CII-pulsed syngeneic macrophages that had been transfected with a binary adenovirus system.[29–32,44] To develop a generally applicable strategy in which autocrine apoptosis of APCs is inhibited and FasL is inducibly expressed, an improved binary adenovirus system was constructed (Figure 8.4A).[38] One of the adenoviruses contains the fas ligand gene under the regulation of the tetracycline response element (TRE)[45–47] and the apoptosis inhibitory p35 gene[48,49] under the regulation of the cytomegalovirus (CMV) promoter (Figure 8.4A). The other adenovirus contains the

(A)

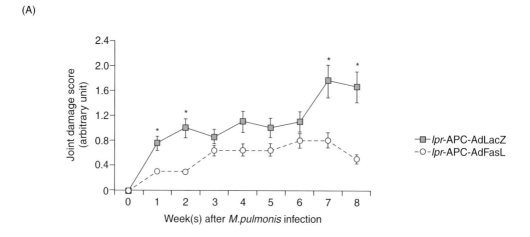

(B)

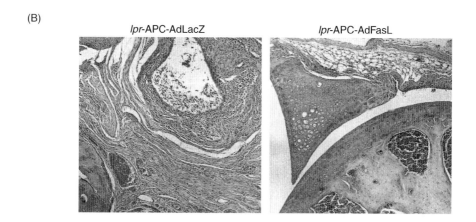

Figure 8.3 Reduced arthritis in the joint of *lpr*-APC–AdFasL-treated B6-*gld/gld* mice. (A) Reduction of the severity of joint damage in response to *M. pulmonis* infection in *lpr*-APC–AdFasL-treated *gld* mice. The foot pads and paws of all the infected mice were evaluated blindly on a weekly basis for severity of arthritis triggered by *M. pulmonis*. The severity of arthritis was evaluated according to the following scale: 0, no swelling and redness; 1, mild swelling and redness; 2, severe swelling and redness; and 3, ankylosis and deformity of joint. At least 10 mice were evaluated per time point per group. There was a significantly reduced joint-swelling response in the FasL group versus the LacZ group at weeks 1, 2, 7 and 8 (*$p < 0.05$). (B) Mice were sacrificed 8 weeks after the infection with *M. pulmonis* and after treatment with either *lpr*-APC–AdFasL or *lpr*-APC–AdLacZ. Knee joint sections were prepared and stained with H&E. Representative histologic analysis is shown for *lpr*-APC–AdLacZ-treated (left panel) or *lpr*-APC–AdFasL-treated (right panel) B6-*gld/gld* mice. Magnification ×80. (Reproduced with permission from Hsu et al, *Arthritis Rheum* 2001; **44**(9): 2146–59.[27])

reverse tetracycline transactivator (rtTA) under the regulation of the CMV promoter, leading to high expression of rtTA.[50] This binary adenovirus system will be referred to as AdFasLp35Tet. Macrophages transfected with AdFasLp35Tet will be referred to as APC–AdFasL. In combination, these adenoviruses enable doxycycline-inducible expression of FasL with concomitant expression of the *p35* anti-apoptosis gene product to prevent autocrine apoptosis of the transfected macrophages.

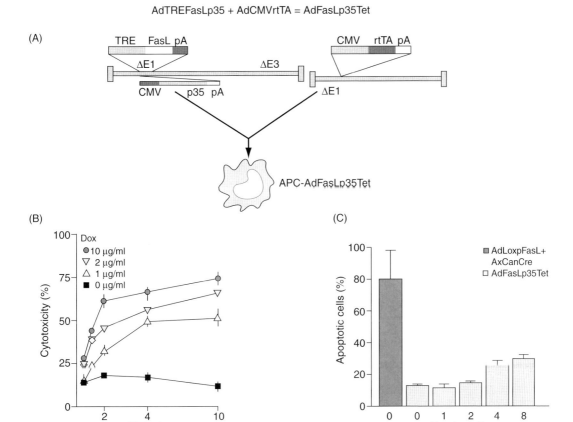

Figure 8.4 Inducible expression of murine Fas ligand (mFasL) on macrophages without induction of autocrine suicide. (A) Antigen-specific T cells were eliminated by using CII-pulsed DBA/1j macrophages that had been transfected with a tetracycline-inducible FasL construct that also expresses the p35 anti-apoptosis gene (CII–APC–AdFasLp35Tet). This enables a high level of production of FasL on CII-pulsed DBA/1j macrophages and, thus, specific elimination of T cells that interact with CII that is processed and presented on these DBA/1j antigen-presenting cells. (B) To confirm that the expressed mFasL is functional, ^{51}Cr-labeled A20 target cells (1×10^5) were mixed with AdTREFasLp35 plus AdCMVrtTA (AdFasLp35Tet)-transfected DBA/1j macrophages at different target/effector cell (E/T) ratios and at different concentrations of doxycycline (Dox) and co-cultured for 8 h. The target cell cytotoxicity was determined by measuring the radioactivity in the cell culture supernatants (cytotoxicity = (c.p.m.^{exp} − c.p.m.^{spon})/(c.p.m.^{max} − c.p.m.^{spon}) × 100). Results are representative of three experiments. (C) The effectiveness of p35 in preventing autocrine suicide of the transfected macrophages at different concentrations of doxycycline was confirmed using the ATP-Lite assay. Results are representative of three experiments. (Adapted with permission from Zhang et al, *J Immunol* 2002; **168**(8): 4164–72.[38])

To confirm the inducibility of biologically active FasL in this system, peritoneal macrophages (1×10^6) from DBA/1j mice were transfected with 50 PFU/cell of AdFasLp35Tet and then incubated with various concentrations of doxycycline for 18 h. The expression of functional FasL on the surface of the transfected cells was then evaluated by co-culture at different effector cells to target cells (E/T) ratios with chromium-51-labeled A20 target cells. Only low levels of cytotoxicity of the A20 target cells were observed on incubation with the transfected macrophages in the absence of doxycycline (Figure 8.4B). The addition of doxycycline resulted in a doxycycline dose-dependent increase in the death of the A20 target cells at 18 h, which was evident at doses of doxycycline that ranged from 1 µg/ml to 10 µg/ml.[38]

To test whether the AdFasLp35Tet construct effectively prevents autocrine apoptosis, the viability of the DBA/1j macrophages transfected with AdFasLp35Tet was evaluated after incubation with 0.0–8.0 µg/ml of doxycycline for 18 h, as determined in an ATP-Lite assay. As a control, DBA/1j macrophages were transfected with the AdLoxpFasL plus AxCANCre, which results in expression of FasL independently of doxycycline induction and in the absence of the anti-apoptosis gene *p35*. As anticipated, the control macrophages transfected with AdLoxPFasL plus AxCANCre underwent 80% of apoptosis (Figure 8.4C). In contrast, the macrophages transfected with AdFasLp35Tet

exhibited only low levels of apoptosis even in the presence of high levels of doxycycline (Figure 8.4C).[38]

To find whether treatment of CII–APC–AdFasLp35Tet can prevent CII-induced arthritis, the macrophages were pulsed with bovine collagen II and then transfected with AdFasLp35Tet.[38] These macrophages were then used to treat DBA/1j mice, commencing 2 weeks after the mice had been immunized with CII in complete Freund's adjuvant at 9 weeks of age. Mice received a total of four doses of macrophages (10[6] cells/dose) over a 2-week time period. At the same time, the mice (10 mice/group) received 1.5 mg/ml of doxycycline administered in the drinking water with 4% sucrose or 0.3% ethanol in water with 4% sucrose as a control. The mice were next immunized with CII in incomplete Freund's adjuvant 4 weeks after the first immunization at 11 weeks of age, and the development of arthri-

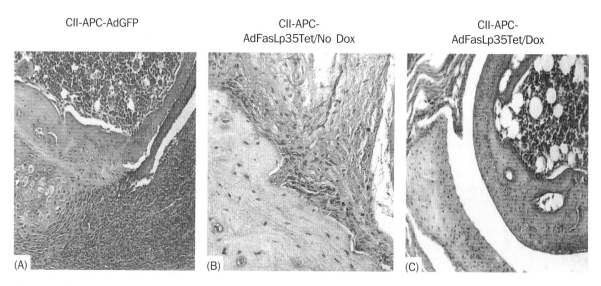

Figure 8.5 CII–APC–AdFasLp35Tet prevents CII arthritis. DBA/1j mice were immunized with bovine CII or ovalbumin (OVA) plus Complete Freund's Adjuvant (CFA) at 7 weeks of age and boosted with CII or ovalbumin (OVA) plus IFA 4 weeks later. Four doses of control (A) CII–APC–AdGFP (1 × 10[6] APCs/dose), or CII–APC–AdFasLp35Tet were administered between weeks 9 and 11 with drinking water containing either (B) 0.3% ethanol as a control or (C) doxycycline (1.5 mg/ml). The mice were analyzed at different time points and then sacrificed at 20 weeks of age. DBA/1j mice immunized with CII and treated with either CII–APC–AdGFP (A) or CII–APC–AdFasLp35Tet without doxycycline (B) or with doxycycline (C) were sacrificed at 20 weeks of age, sectioned and stained with H&E. Magnification ×100. (Adapted with permission from Zhang et al, *J Immunol* 2002; **168**(8): 4164–72.[38])

tis was assessed weekly up to 20 weeks of age. The administration of doxycycline alone in the range of 1.0–8.0 mg/ml confirmed that the administration of doxycycline alone had no effect on the development of arthritis. As anticipated, the control groups of mice treated with either CII–APC or CII–APC–AdGFP developed severe arthritis 9 weeks after the second immunization with CII in incomplete Freund's adjuvant (Figure 8.5A). Histologic examination of the joints of the mice sacrificed at 9 weeks after CII–APC–AdFasLp35Tet or control treatment confirmed that the control groups of mice that were treated with either CII–APC–AdGFP or CII–APC–AdFasLp35Tet/no doxycycline exhibited histologic changes indicative of severe arthritis, with nearly all the joints showing pronounced synovial hyperplasia, cartilage erosion, and ankylosis (Figure 8.5B). These histologic features were significantly less apparent in the group of mice treated with CII–APC–AdFasLp35Tet plus doxycycline (Figure 8.5C). The severity of arthritis in the groups of mice treated with CII–APC–AdFasLp35Tet plus doxycycline was significantly lower than in the control groups. Interestingly, mice that were treated with CII–APC–AdFasLp35Tet without doxycycline inducer also showed less severe arthritis at the first 3 weeks after the treatment but not afterwards indicating that low-level expression of FasL may occur in the absence of doxycycline and is sufficient to decrease the initial severity of CII-induced arthritis.

CII PULSE IS REQUIRED FOR ELIMINATION OF CII RESPONSE T CELLS USING APC–AdFasLp35Tet TREATMENT

To test if loading of APC–AdFasLp35Tet with CII is necessary for inhibition of arthritis and deletion of CII-specific T cells, APC–AdFasLp35Tet treatment with or without CII was carried out. CD3 T-cell staining showed that there was extensive T-cell infiltration of the joints of the group of mice treated with APC–AdFasLp35Tet without CII (Figure 8.6A).[38] T-cell infiltration and arthritis were greatly reduced in mice treated with CII-pulsed APC–AdFasLp35Tet (Figure 8.6B). B220-positive B-cell infiltration of the joints was minimal regardless of the treatments at 9 weeks after the CII boost. The requirement of CII-pulsed APC–AdFasLp35Tet treatment was further demonstrated by an in vitro T-cell proliferation assay and interleukin-2 (IL-2) induction. T-cell proliferation was determined at different times after stimulation by pulsing with

APC-AdFasLp35Tet

CII-APC-AdFasLp35Tet

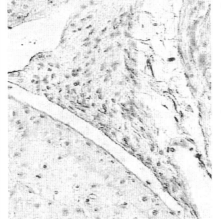

(A)

(B)

Figure 8.6 Deletion of CII-specific T cells in the joint by CII-pulsed APC–AdFasLp35Tet. DBA/1j mice were immunized with CII or OVA and treated as described in Figure 8.5. The mice were sacrificed at 20 weeks of age. Anti-CD3 antibody staining of the joints of mice treated with APC–AdFasLp35Tet pulsed (A) without CII or (B) with CII. The photographs were taken using a DigiSpot camera system. Original magnification ×20. (Adapted with permission from Zhang et al, *J Immunol* 2002; **168**(8): 4164–72.[38])

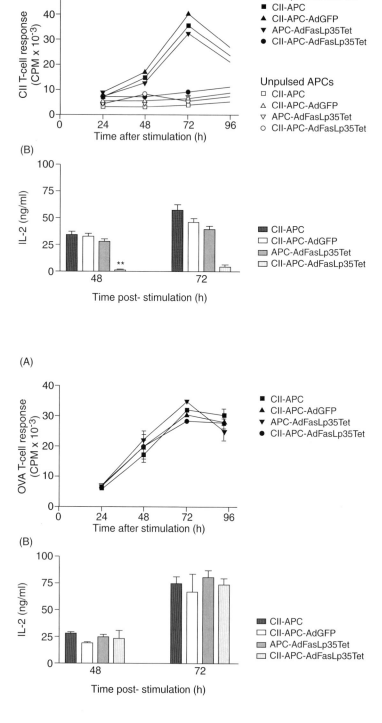

Figure 8.7 CII-pulsed APC–AdFasLp35Tet is required for induction of CII-specific deletion of T cells. (A) Draining lymph node T cells were isolated from mice at the time of sacrifice (20 weeks of age) and were stimulated with irradiated APCs from DBA/1j mice that were either pulsed with CII or unpulsed (stimulator/responder ratio = 1:10). The proliferation of the T cells from mice treated with CII–APC, CII–APC–AdGFP or APC–AdFasLp35Tet pulsed with or without CII was determined at different times after an 18-h pulse of [³H]thymidine. The counts were determined using a scintillation counter. (B) IL-2 was determined in the supernatant at 48 and 72 h after culture. The results represent the mean ± standard error of the mean (SEM) of duplicate cultures of five mice per group analyzed separately. **P < 0.01; *P < 0.05. (Adapted with permission from Zhang et al, *J Immunol* 2002; **168**(8): 4164–72.[38])

Figure 8.8 CII-pulsed APC–AdFasLp35Tet does not induce deletion of OVA-specific T cells. (A) Draining lymph node T-cell proliferation and (B) IL-2 induction after OVA stimulation in vitro were carried out as described in Figure 8.7. The results represent the mean ± SEM of duplicate cultures of five mice per group analyzed separately. (Adapted with permission from Zhang et al, *J Immunol* 2002; **168**(8): 4164–72.[38])

[³H]thymidine 18 h prior to harvest of the supernatants at 48 and 72 h after stimulation (Figure 8.7A). There was a significant decrease in T-cell proliferation, as indicated by decreased [³H]thymidine uptake and a significant decrease in IL-2 production at 48 and 72 h in the group of mice treated with CII–APC–AdFasLp35Tet compared to APC–AdFasLp35Tet-treated mice (Figure 8.7B). There was no T-cell proliferation or IL-2 induction when the stimulator APCs were not pulsed with CII, indicating that CII was required (Figure 8.7). Thus, the results indicated that CII-loaded APC–AdFasLp35Tet treatment is necessary to achieve higher specificity, since both [³H]thymidine uptake and IL-2 induction

were much higher in the group of mice treated with APC–AdFasLp35Tet.

To determine whether treatment of CII–APC–AdFasLp35Tet impairs an irrelevant T-cell-dependent antigen response, DBA/1j mice were immunized with both CII and OVA at 7 and 11 weeks of age and treated with CII–APC–AdFasLp35Tet plus doxycycline from 9 to 11 weeks of age, as above. Draining lymph node T cells isolated from these mice were co-cultured with OVA-pulsed APCs. Neither T-cell proliferation nor induction of IL-2 in response to OVA was impaired after treatment with CII–APC–AdFasLp35Tet plus doxycycline, indicating that the decreased IL-2 response for CII is specific for CII (Figure 8.8).

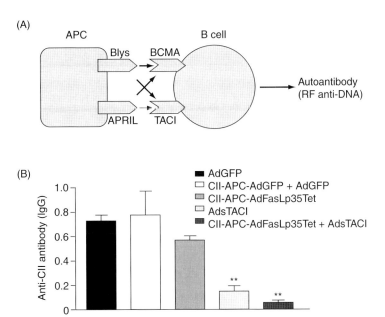

Figure 8.9 Blocking the production of anti-CII antibody using CII–APC–AdFasL + AdCMVsTACI. (A) The interaction of APCs, including macrophages, with B cells is mediated by the expression by the APCs of Blys, APRIL and BAFF, which interact with the transmembrane activator and calcium modulator and cyclophilin ligand (CAML) interactor (TACI), B-cell maturation antigen (BCMA) and B-cell activating factor belonging to the TNF family (BAFF) receptor on the B cells. Interaction of these molecules on APCs and B cells has been postulated to be a mechanism leading to the production of autoantibodies, including rheumatoid factor (RF) and anti-DNA antibodies in arthritis. (B) DBA/1j mice were immunized with CII and underwent treatment with AdCMVsTACI, CII–APC–AdFasLp35Tet or combined treatment with CII–APC–AdFasLp35Tet + AdCMVsTACI. Control DBA/1j mice were immunized with CII and treated with AdGFP or CII–APC–AdGFP + AdGFP. Sera were collected at the time of sacrifice (20 weeks of age) and analyzed for anti-CII antibody by an ELISA assay using an IgG. The results represent the mean ± SEM of two individual determinations on five mice per group determined separately. (Adapted with permission from Zhang et al, *J Immunol* 2002; **168**(8): 4164–72.[38])

Stimulation of B cells by the transmembrane activator and calcium modulator and cyclophilic ligand interactor (TACI)–B-lymphocyte stimulator (Blys), and B-cell maturation antigen (BCMA)–proliferation-inducing ligand (APRIL) leads to autoantibody production (Figure 8.9A).[51–55] Treatment with CII–APC–AdFasLp35Tet alone or in combination with a single dose of AdCMVsTACI prevented the development of CII-induced arthritis and T-cell infiltration in the joint. The elimination of T cells was specific, in that a normal T-cell response was observed on stimulation with ovalbumin (OVA) after treatment with CII–APC–AdFasLp35Tet. Treatment with AdCMVsTACI alone prevented production of detectable levels of circulating anti-CII autoantibodies and reduced the severity of arthritis but did not prevent its development (Figure 8.9B). These results indicate that the CII-reactive T cells play a crucial role in the development of CII-induced arthritis, and that the anti-CII antibodies act to enhance the development of CII induced arthritis.

These results agree with results obtained in the *M. pulmonis* model, where the chronic T-cell inflammatory response is primarily necessary to maintain an arthritis triggered by CII injection in the tail of the mouse. This model is different from the infection-induced model, and may constitute a second method of induction of arthritis in humans. However, in either case, the APC–FasL gene therapy elimination of the chronic inflammatory T cells was sufficient to reverse the arthritis.

MOLECULAR DEFECTS ASSOCIATED WITH RHEUMATOID ARTHRITIS SYNOVIAL FIBROBLASTS

Thus far, this chapter has dealt with the role of T cells in initiation and perpetuation of chronic inflammatory arthritis. Relatively low migration of T cells appears to be sufficient to sustain the immune response, either after clearance of a microorganism or after injection of CII, and leads to the development of synovial fibroblasts that exhibit unusual features such as increased prolif-

eration and invasion of cartilage and bone. In both of the models described above, the synovial fibroblast development of arthritis may be abnormal. This is especially true in the DBA/1j CII arthritis model. RASFs were therefore isolated from human patients, and unique molecular and cellular abnormalities were determined relative to osteoarthritis fibroblasts (OASFs). Using affymetrix gene chip analysis, we analyzed different genes in RASFs and OASFs. We analyzed gene expression in three separate samples of RNA isolated from RASFs treated with either a control AdTet or an Ad inhibitor of NFκB (IκB) dominant negative (DN) followed by treatment with tumour necrosis factor alpha (TNF-α) for 3 h. The U95Av2 gene chip can analyze 12 500 genes. RASFs expressed approximately 4500 genes that can be compared under conditions of high and low apoptosis susceptibility. Significant gene expression changes were considered only if the altered expression was comparable in all three RNA samples from controls and all three samples from treated RASFs. This has led to identification of groups of genes that are significantly downregulated if TNF-α-mediated NF-κB release from IκB is inhibited. These genes fall into different groups including anti-apoptosis genes, including inhibitor of apoptosis protein (IAP), genes encoding adhesion molecules, including ICAM-1 and VCAM-1 and cytokine genes. These genes have the common feature of being regulated by NFκB, or may be closely linked genes on chromosomal segments that are regulated by NFκB. These results indicate that NFκB orchestrates high production of families of anti-apoptosis and proinflammatory genes, and dysfunctional signaling in RASFs plays an important role in the pathogenesis of RA.

REGULATION OF APOPTOSIS IN RASFS, DEFECTS IN NFκB AND UBIQUITIN PROTEOSOME DEGRADATION

TNF-α signaling provides potent growth and inflammatory signals for RASFs.[56] TNF-α signals TNFR-1 and TNFR-2. Soluble TNF receptor is an efficacious treatment for RA, indicating the importance of TNF-α in promoting RA lesions.[57,58]

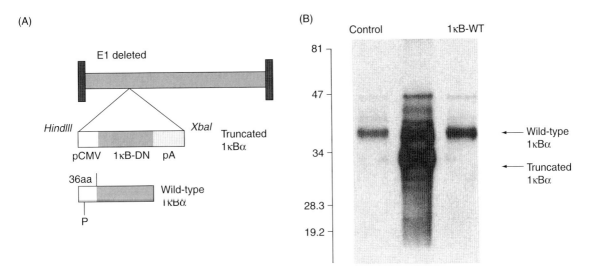

Figure 8.10   Construction of AdCMVIκBα-DN (dominant negative). (A) AdCMVIκBα-DN was constructed by recombination of the mutated inhibitor of NFκB (IκB) plasmid, pF-IκBα, into the E1 site of pCA13 to produce pCA13IκBα. The pCA13IκBα was then recombined with pJM17 in 293 cells to produce the recombinant adenovirus-expressing mutant IκB, denoted AdCMVIκBα-DN. (B) Western blot IκBα-DN expression by AdCMVIκBα-DN. An RA synovial fibroblast cell line was transfected, and cell lysate was analyzed for expression of IκBα by Western blot analysis. Control = control RASF; IκBα-DN = AdCMVIκBα-DN-transfected RASF at 10 PFU/cell; IκB-WT = pcDNA3-expressing wild-type IκB. (Reproduced with permission from Zhang et al, *Arthritis Rheum* 2000; **43**(5): 1094–105.[64])

We analyzed TNF receptor signaling in RASFs and looked at both the pro-apoptosis and the anti-apoptosis pathways.[59] These studies indicate that the anti-apoptosis pathway of signaling through RASFs is mediated by Akt and NFκB.

To study signals through NFκB, RASFs were treated with an AdIκB-DN.[59] This resulted in high susceptibility to TNF-α-induced apoptosis. TNF-α increased the survival and proliferation of human RA cell lines.[60–62] These experiments were designed to determine if inhibition of NFκB nuclear translocation leads to increased apoptosis of TNF-α-treated human RA cell lines. We constructed an IκB dominant negative (AdCMVIκB-DN) (Figure 8.10) and an X-linked inhibitor of apoptosis protein (XIAP) antisense (AdCMV XIAP-AS) adenovirus. Primary RASFs were transfected in vitro and SV40-transformed RA synovial cell lines in SCID mice were transfected in vivo.[63] Cells were treated with TNF-α and analyzed for apoptosis. There was no apoptosis of primary RASFs transfected in vitro with AdCMVIκB-DN alone. In contrast, there was

apoptosis of more than 85% of cells treated with both AdCMVIκB-DN and TNF-α (Figure 8.11). SV40-transformed RASFs in SCID mice also exhibited high levels of apoptosis after in vivo transfection with AdCMVIκB-DN followed by treatment with TNF-α. There was no apoptosis after treatment with AdCMVIκB-DN in the absence of TNF-α. XIAP is an inhibitor of apoptosis, which was upregulated by TNF-α, and this upregulation was inhibited by AdCMVIκB-DN + TNF-α. Transfection of an AdCMV XIAP antisense by gene therapy resulted in increased TNF-α-induced apoptosis (Figure 8.12). These results indicate that AdCMVIκB-DN gene therapy greatly enhances apoptosis due to inhibition of an NFκB-mediated anti-apoptosis signaling pathway, and that XIAP is a TNF-α-inducible specific inhibitor of apoptosis in RASF lines. This and other modulators of TNF receptor or the Fas apoptosis pathway may be therapeutically beneficial to facilitate apoptosis of synovial tissue in patients with RA. These results are consistent

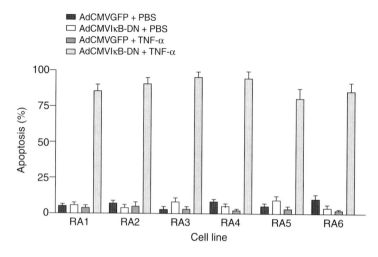

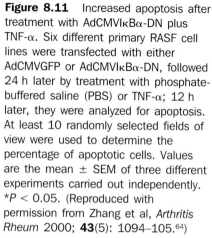

Figure 8.11 Increased apoptosis after treatment with AdCMVIκBα-DN plus TNF-α. Six different primary RASF cell lines were transfected with either AdCMVGFP or AdCMVIκBα-DN, followed 24 h later by treatment with phosphate-buffered saline (PBS) or TNF-α; 12 h later, they were analyzed for apoptosis. At least 10 randomly selected fields of view were used to determine the percentage of apoptotic cells. Values are the mean ± SEM of three different experiments carried out independently. *P < 0.05. (Reproduced with permission from Zhang et al, *Arthritis Rheum* 2000; **43**(5): 1094–105.[64])

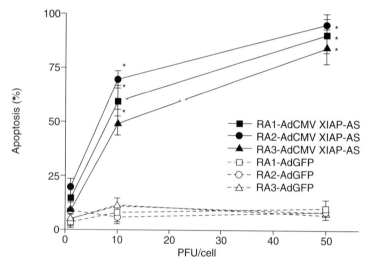

Figure 8.12 Increased TNF-α-induced apoptosis of RASFs after treatment with AdCMVXIAP-AS (antisense). Three different primary RASF cell lines were transfected with either AdCMVGFP or AdCMXIAP-AS at different concentrations, followed 24 h later by treatment with TNF-α; 12 h later they were analyzed for apoptosis. The percentage of apoptotic cells was determined as the number of apoptotic cells divided by the total number of cells in each field of view. At least 10 randomly selected fields of view were used to determine the percentage of apoptotic cells. Values are the mean ± SEM of three different experiments carried out independently. *P < 0.05 versus AdCMVGFP-transfected cells. (Reproduced with permission from Zhang et al, *Arthritis Rheum* 2000; **43**(5): 1094–105.[64])

with the gene chip analysis data, which indicate that NFκB-mediated anti-apoptosis signaling plays an important role in perpetuation of the survival of the RASF.

INCREASED PROLIFERATION OF RASF-INTRINSIC DEFECT IN PHOSPHORYLATED Akt

We propose that gene therapy can be used to dissect important pathways and mechanisms of

human RA. These results include the growth of human RASFs and OASFs. In addition, these RASFs and OASFs were transfected with different gene therapy agents to analyze the apoptosis-resistant state and induce apoptosis.[64] We first utilized AdNFκB-DN, which resulted in reversal of the apoptosis-resistant state of RASFs after exposure to TNF-α. To further understand the origin of NFκB and anti-apoptosis signaling in RASFs, we analyzed the Akt pathway. Akt is phosphorylated through the phosphatidylinositol (PI) 3–kinase pathway and has numerous downstream targets, including NFκB but also inhibitors of apoptosis and cell cycle regulation.[65–67] We observed that there was increased

phosphorylated Akt and primary cell lines produced from RASFs compared to OASFs.[59]

To analyze the role of Akt and the induction of apoptosis in RASFs, we constructed an Ad-Akt-DN. RASFs produced higher levels of Akt,

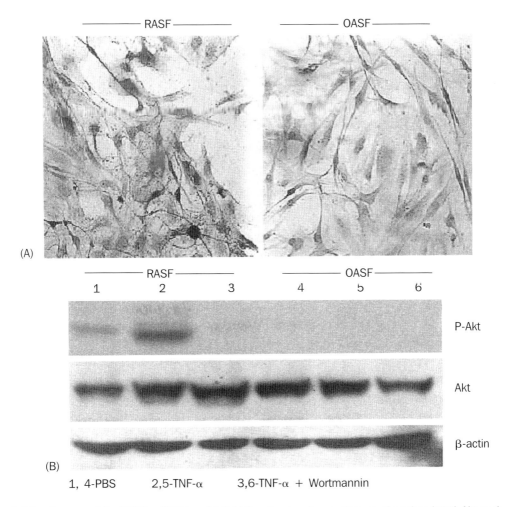

1, 4-PBS   2,5-TNF-α   3,6-TNF-α + Wortmannin

Figure 8.13 Compared to OASFs, RASFs exhibit higher levels of endogenous phosphorylated Akt and increased phosphorylation of Akt in response to TNF-α treatment that can be inhibited by wortmannin. (A) Primary RASFs (left panel) and OASFs (right panel) were grown to confluence and stimulated with TNF-α (10 ng/ml). After 6 h, the cells were washed and stained with an anti-phosphorylated Akt (Thr308) antibody and revealed by DAB substrate. Cells were photographed at ×40. The photograph illustrates a representative field of view. (B) Cellular extracts were prepared from RASFs and OASFs treated with PBS, TNF-α, or TNF-α plus wortmannin as described above. The levels of phosphorylated Akt were determined by Western blot analysis of lysates from RASF and OASF cell lines. Identical blots were probed with an antibody for: upper panel, phosphorylated Akt (P-Akt); middle panel, total Akt protein; and lower panel, anti-β-actin. Lane 1, RASFs treated with PBS; lane 2, RASFs treated with TNF-α (10 ng/ml); lane 3, RASFs treated with TNF-α (10 ng/ml) + wortmannin (50 nM); lane 4, OASFs treated with PBS; lane 5, OASFs treated with TNF-α (10 ng/ml); lane 6, OASFs treated with TNF-α (10 ng/ml) + wortmannin (50 nM). (Reproduced with permission from Zhang et al, *Arthritis Rheum* 2001; **44**(7); 1555–67.[59])

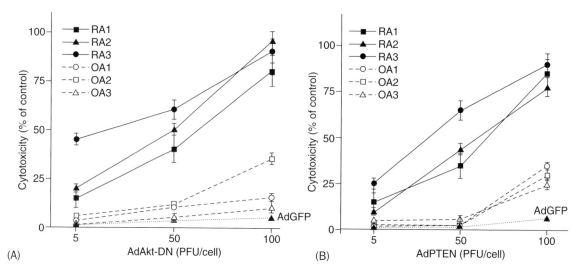

Figure 8.14 Increased cytotoxicity of RASFs transfected by AdAkt-DN and adenovirus expressing phosphatase and tensin homolog deleted on chromosome ten (AdPTEN) in the presence of TNF-α. (A) Cytotoxicity of three different RASF and OASF cell lines was determined at different amounts of PFU/cell of AdAkt-DN. Cytotoxicity was quantitated using the ATP-Lite assay. There was no significant cytotoxicity of either RASFs or OASFs 18 h after transfection with AdGFP in the presence of TNF-α (10 ng/ml) (dashed line). The results represent the mean ± SEM of at least two experiments using each cell line. (B) Apoptosis of three different RASF and OASF cell lines was determined at different amounts of PFU/cell of AdPTEN. Cytotoxicity was quantitated using the ATP-Lite assay. There was no significant cytotoxicity of either RASFs or OASFs 18 h after transfection with AdGFP followed by incubation with TNF-α (dashed line). The results represent the mean ± SEM of at least two experiments using each cell line. (Reproduced with permission from Zhang et al, *Arthritis Rheum* 2001; **44**(7); 1555–67.[59])

which could be suppressed by an AdAkt-DN or an adenovirus expressing phosphatase and tensin homolog deleted on chromosome ten (AdPTEN), which is the natural inhibitor of Akt. This resulted in downmodulation of the phosphorylated Akt protein and increased susceptibility of apoptosis of RASFs to TNF-α.[68] To determine if TNF-α-driven proliferation of rheumatoid synovial fibroblasts is associated with upregulation of the serine/threonine kinase B (PKB)/Akt activity and RASF survival, staining of phosphorylated Akt in TNF-α-treated RASFs was done using antiphosphorylated Thr308-Akt antibody. Phosphorylated Akt was analyzed by immunohistochemical staining and Western blot, and Akt activity was analyzed using a kinase assay. The levels of phosphorylated Akt are higher in RASFs than in OASFs, as demonstrated by immunohistochemical staining, immunoblot analysis and an Akt kinase

assay (Figure 8.13A). The levels of phosphorylated Akt and Akt kinase activity were increased by stimulation of primary RASFs with TNF-α (10 ng/ml) (Figure 8.13B). The cytotoxicity of TNF-α treatment or TNF-α plus Akt activity inhibitor wortmannin, TNF-α plus AdAkt-DN or AdPTEN was analyzed by TUNEL staining. Treatment of RASFs with the PI 3-kinase inhibitor wortmannin (50 nM) plus TNF-α resulted in apoptosis of 75% ± 8% of RASFs within 24 h. This pro-apoptosis effect was specific for Akt, as equivalent levels of apoptosis were observed upon TNF-α treatment of RASFs transfected with AdAkt-DN and with an AdPTEN, which opposes the action of Akt (Figure 8.14). These results indicate that phosphorylated Akt acts as a survival signal in RASFs and contributes to the stimulatory effect of TNF-α on these cells by inhibiting the apoptosis response. This effect was not observed in

OASFs, and may reflect the pathophysiologic changes associated with the proliferating synovium in RA.

SUMMARY

These results indicate that RA is caused by an inflammatory trigger. This inflammatory trigger can be an infectious agent such as *M. pulmonis* or an antigen such as CII. In the appropriate background, these immunologic stimuli can lead to a chronic erosive arthritis. In addition to the triggering agent, there are specific properties of the RASFs, including increased proliferation and decreased susceptibility to apoptosis. Some of the molecules involved include cell cycle proteins as determined by gene chip analysis. Other pathways include anti-apoptosis pathways mediated by NFκB and phosphory-lated Akt. This chapter clearly indicates that specific elimination of T-cell responses, and, potentially, other inflammatory cells, can prevent and greatly limit the development of synovial cell hyperplasia and the development of synovial fibroblasts that have properties of invasion of cartilage and bone. Once the second phase of developmental RASF hyperplasia has been initiated, a potential therapeutic option will be direct induction of apoptosis to RASFs.

ACKNOWLEDGMENT

We thank Ms Linda Flurry for excellent secretarial work. This work was supported by NIH grants R01 AG 11653 and N01 AR 6-2224, and a Birmingham VAMC Merit Review Grant. H.-G. Zhang is a recipient of an Arthritis Foundation Investigator Award.

REFERENCES

1. Watanabe-Fukunaga R, Brannan CI, Copeland NG et al. Lymphoproliferation disorder in mice explained by defects in Fas antigen that mediates apoptosis. *Nature* 1992; **356**(6367): 314–17.
2. Takahashi T, Tanaka M, Brannan CI et al. Generalized lymphoproliferative disease in mice, caused by a point mutation in the Fas ligand. *Cell* 1994; **76**(6): 969–76.
3. Wu J, Zhou T, He J et al. Autoimmune disease in mice due to integration of an endogenous retrovirus in an apoptosis gene. *J Exp Med* 1993; **178**(2): 461–8.
4. Steinberg AD, Raveche ES, Laskin CA et al. NIH conference. Systemic lupus erythematosus: insights from animal models. *Ann Intern Med* 1984; **100**(5): 714–27.
5. Matsumura R, Umemiya K, Kagami M et al. Glandular and extraglandular expression of the Fas–Fas ligand and apoptosis in patients with Sjogren's syndrome. *Clin Exp Rheumatol* 1998; **16**(5): 561–8.
6. Cohen PL, Eisenberg RA. The lpr and gld genes in systemic autoimmunity: life and death in the Fas lane. *Immunol Today* 1992; **13**(11): 427–8.
7. Bamberger AM, Schulte HM, Thuneke I et al. Expression of the apoptosis-inducing Fas ligand (FasL) in human first and third trimester placenta and choriocarcinoma cells. *J Clin Endocrinol Metab* 1997; **82**(9): 3173–5.
8. Wahlsten JL, Gitchell HL, Chan CC et al. Fas and Fas ligand expressed on cells of the immune system, not on the target tissue, control induction of experimental autoimmune uveitis. *J Immunol* 2000; **165**(10): 5480–6.
9. Fleck M, Kern ER, Zhou T et al. Murine cytomegalovirus induces a Sjogren's syndrome-like disease in C57Bl/6–lpr/lpr mice. *Arthritis Rheum* 1998; **41**(12): 2175–84.
10. Fleck M, Kern ER, Zhou T et al. Apoptosis mediated by Fas but not tumor necrosis factor receptor 1 prevents chronic disease in mice infected with murine cytomegalovirus. *J Clin Invest* 1998; **102**(7): 1431–43.
11. Marker-Hermann E, Hohler T. Pathogenesis of human leukocyte antigen B27-positive arthritis. Information from clinical materials. *Rheum Dis Clin North Am* 1998; **24**(4): 865–81, xi.
12. Burmester GR, Daser A, Kamradt T et al. Immunology of reactive arthritides. *Annu Rev Immunol* 1995; **13**: 229–50.
13. Leirisalo-Repo M, Helenius P, Hannu T et al. Long-term prognosis of reactive salmonella arthritis. *Ann Rheum Dis* 1997; **56**(9): 516–20.
14. Yli-Kerttula T, Tertti R, Toivanen A. Ten-year follow up study of patients from a Yersinia pseudotuberculosis III outbreak. *Clin Exp Rheumatol* 1995; **13**(3): 333–7.

15. Schumacher HR Jr, Gerard HC, Arayssi TK et al. Lower prevalence of Chlamydia pneumoniae DNA compared with Chlamydia trachomatis DNA in synovial tissue of arthritis patients. *Arthritis Rheum* 1999; **42**(9): 1889–93.

16. Gerard HC, Schumacher HR, El-Gabalawy H et al. Chlamydia pneumoniae present in the human synovium are viable and metabolically active. *Microb Pathog* 2000; **29**(1): 17–24.

17. Horowitz S, Evinson B, Borer A et al. Mycoplasma fermentans in rheumatoid arthritis and other inflammatory arthritides. *J Rheumatol* 2000; **27**(12): 2747–53.

18. Johnson S, Sidebottom D, Bruckner F et al. Identification of Mycoplasma fermentans in synovial fluid samples from arthritis patients with inflammatory disease. *J Clin Microbiol* 2000; **38**(1): 90–3.

19. Haier J, Nasralla M, Franco AR et al. Detection of mycoplasmal infections in blood of patients with rheumatoid arthritis. *Rheumatology* (Oxford) 1999; **38**(6): 504–9.

20. Henry CH, Hughes CV, Gerard HC et al. Reactive arthritis: preliminary microbiologic analysis of the human temporomandibular joint. *J Oral Maxillofac Surg* 2000; **58**(10): 1137–42; discussion 1143–4.

21. Keystone EC, Taylor-Robinson D, Osborn MF et al. Effect of T-cell deficiency on the chronicity of arthritis induced in mice by Mycoplasma pulmonis. *Infect Immun* 1980; **27**(1): 192–6.

22. Schutze E, Laber G, Walzl H. Clinical and histopathological findings in mycoplasmal polyarthritis of rats. III. Course of infection during the weeks 7–30 and 54–61. *Zentralbl Bakteriol* 1976; **234**(1): 91–104.

23. Keystone EC, Taylor-Robinson D, Metcalfe A et al. Role of viable mycoplasmas in the pathogenesis of arthritis induced by M. pulmonis. *Br J Exp Pathol* 1981; **62**(4): 350–6.

24. Evengard B, Sandstedt K, Bolske G et al. Intranasal inoculation of Mycoplasma pulmonis in mice with severe combined immunodeficiency (SCID) causes a wasting disease with grave arthritis. *Clin Exp Immunol* 1994; **98**(3): 388–94.

25. Kobayashi T, Okamoto K, Kobata T et al. Tumor necrosis factor alpha regulation of the FAS-mediated apoptosis-signaling pathway in synovial cells. *Arthritis Rheum* 1999; **42**(3): 519–26.

26. Kobayashi T, Okamoto K, Kobata T et al. Differential regulation of Fas-mediated apoptosis of rheumatoid synoviocytes by tumor necrosis

factor alpha and basic fibroblast growth factor is associated with the expression of apoptosis-related molecules. *Arthritis Rheum* 2000; **43**(5): 1106–14.

27. Hsu HC, Zhang HG, Song GG et al. Defective Fas ligand-mediated apoptosis predisposes to development of a chronic erosive arthritis subsequent to Mycoplasma pulmonis infection. *Arthritis Rheum* 2001; **44**(9): 2146–59.

28. Zhang HG, Bilbao G, Zhou T et al. Application of a Fas ligand encoding a recombinant adenovirus vector for prolongation of transgene expression. *J Virol* 1998; **72**(3): 2483–90.

29. Zhang HG, Liu D, Heike Y et al. Induction of specific T-cell tolerance by adenovirus-transfected, Fas ligand-producing antigen presenting cells. *Nat Biotechnol* 1998; **16**(11): 1045–9.

30. Zhang HG, Su X, Liu D et al. Induction of specific T-cell tolerance by Fas ligand-expressing antigen-presenting cells. *J Immunol* 1999; **162**(3): 1423–30.

31. Zhang HG, Fleck M, Kern ER et al. Antigen presenting cells expressing Fas ligand down-modulate chronic inflammatory disease in Fas ligand-deficient mice. *J Clin Invest* 2000; **105**(6): 813–21.

32. Fleck M, Zhang HG, Kern ER et al. Treatment of chronic sialadenitis in a murine model of Sjogren's syndrome by local fasL gene transfer. *Arthritis Rheum* 2001; **44**(4): 964–73.

33. Arend WP. Physiology of cytokine pathways in rheumatoid arthritis. *Arthritis Rheum* 2001; **45**(1): 101–6.

34. Feldmann M, Brennan FM, Maini RN. Role of cytokines in rheumatoid arthritis. *Annu Rev Immunol* 1996; **14**: 397–440.

35. Yamamura Y, Gupta R, Morita Y et al. Effector function of resting T cells: activation of synovial fibroblasts. *J Immunol* 2001; **166**(4): 2270–5.

36. Mustila A, Paimela L, Leirisalo-Repo M et al. Antineutrophil cytoplasmic antibodies in patients with early rheumatoid arthritis: an early marker of progressive erosive disease. *Arthritis Rheum* 2000; **43**(6): 1371–7.

37. Goronzy JJ, Weyand CM. T and B cell-dependent pathways in rheumatoid arthritis. *Curr Opin Rheumatol* 1995; **7**(3): 214–21.

38. Zhang H-G, Yang P, Xie X et al. Depletion of collagen II-reactive T cells and blocking of B-cell activation prevents collagen II- induced arthritis in DBA/1j mice. *J Immunol* 2002; **168**: 4164–72.

39. Stuart JM, Townes AS, Kang AH. Nature and specificity of the immune response to collagen in

type II collagen-induced arthritis in mice. *J Clin Invest* 1982; **69**(3): 673–83.

40. Terato K, Hasty KA, Reife RA et al. Induction of arthritis with monoclonal antibodies to collagen. *J Immunol* 1992; **148**(7): 2103–8.

41. Holmdahl R, Bailey C, Enander I et al. Origin of the autoreactive anti-type II collagen response. II. Specificities, antibody isotypes and usage of V gene families of anti-type II collagen B cells. *J Immunol* 1989; **142**(6): 1881–6.

42. Burkhardt H, Holmdahl R, Deutzmann R et al. Identification of a major antigenic epitope on CNBr-fragment 11 of type II collagen recognized by murine autoreactive B cells. *Eur J Immunol* 1991; **21**(1): 49–54.

43. Hom JT, Stuart JM, Chiller JM. Murine T cells reactive to type II collagen. I. Isolation of lines and clones and characterization of their antigen-induced proliferative responses. *J Immunol* 1986; **136**(3): 769–75.

44. Mountz JD, Hsu H, Matsuki Y et al. Apoptosis and rheumatoid arthritis: past, present, and future directions. *Curr Rheumatol Rep* 2001; **3**(1): 70–8.

45. Gossen M, Bujard H. Tight control of gene expression in mammalian cells by tetracycline-responsive promoters. *Proc Natl Acad Sci USA* 1992; **89**(12): 5547–51.

46. Gossen M, Freundlieb S, Bender G et al. Transcriptional activation by tetracyclines in mammalian cells. *Science* 1995; **268**(5218): 1766–9.

47. Baron U, Bujard H. Tet repressor-based system for regulated gene expression in eukaryotic cells: principles and advances. *Methods Enzymol* 2000; **327**: 401–21.

48. Beidler DR, Tewari M, Friesen PD et al. The baculovirus p35 protein inhibits Fas- and tumor necrosis factor-induced apoptosis. *J Biol Chem* 1995; **270**(28): 16526–8.

49. Seshagiri S, Vucic D, Lee J et al. Baculovirus-based genetic screen for antiapoptotic genes identifies a novel IAP. *J Biol Chem* 1999; **274**(51): 36769–73.

50. Bohl D, Salvetti A, Moullier P et al. Control of erythropoietin delivery by doxycycline in mice after intramuscular injection of adeno-associated vector. *Blood* 1998; **92**(5): 1512–17.

51. Yu G, Boone T, Delaney J et al. APRIL and TALL-I and receptors BCMA and TACI: system for regulating humoral immunity. *Nat Immunol* 2000; **1**(3): 252–6.

52. Thompson JS, Bixler SA, Qian F et al. BAFF-R, a newly identified TNF receptor that specifically interacts with BAFF. *Science* 2001; **293**(5537): 2108–11.

53. Wang H, Marsters SA, Baker T et al. TACI-ligand interactions are required for T-cell activation and collagen-induced arthritis in mice. *Nat Immunol* 2001; **2**(7): 632–7.

54. Moore PA, Belvedere O, Orr A et al. BLyS: member of the tumor necrosis factor family and B lymphocyte stimulator. *Science* 1999; **285**(5425): 260–3.

55. Marsters SA, Yan M, Pitti RM et al. Interaction of the TNF homologues BLyS and APRIL with the TNF receptor homologues BCMA and TACI. *Curr Biol* 2000; **10**(13): 785–8.

56. Firestein GS. Invasive fibroblast-like synoviocytes in rheumatoid arthritis. Passive responders or transformed aggressors? *Arthritis Rheum* 1996; **39**(11): 1781–90.

57. Feldman M, Taylor P, Paleolog E et al. Anti-TNF alpha therapy is useful in rheumatoid arthritis and Crohn's disease: analysis of the mechanism of action predicts utility in other diseases. *Transplant Proc* 1998; **30**(8): 4126–7.

58. Moreland LW, Baumgartner SW, Schiff MH et al. Treatment of rheumatoid arthritis with a recombinant human tumor necrosis factor receptor (p75)-Fc fusion protein. *N Engl J Med* 1997; **337**(3): 141–7.

59. Zhang HG, Wang Y, Xie JF et al. Regulation of tumor necrosis factor alpha-mediated apoptosis of rheumatoid arthritis synovial fibroblasts by the protein kinase Akt. *Arthritis Rheum* 2001; **44**(7): 1555–67.

60. Sioud M, Mellbye O, Forre O. Analysis of the NF-kappa B p65 subunit, Fas antigen, Fas ligand and Bcl-2-related proteins in the synovium of RA and polyarticular JRA. *Clin Exp Rheumatol* 1998; **16**(2): 125–34.

61. Han Z, Boyle DL, Manning AM et al. AP-1 and NF-kappaB regulation in rheumatoid arthritis and murine collagen-induced arthritis. *Autoimmunity* 1998; **28**(4): 197–208.

62. Chu ZL, McKinsey TA, Liu L et al. Suppression of tumor necrosis factor-induced cell death by inhibitor of apoptosis c-IAP2 is under NF-kappaB control. *Proc Natl Acad Sci USA* 1997; **94**(19): 10057–62.

63. Zhang HG, Blackburn WD Jr, Minghetti PP. Characterization of a SV40-transformed rheumatoid synovial fibroblast cell line which retains genotypic expression patterns: a model for evaluation of anti-arthritic agents. *In Vitro Cell Dev Biol Anim* 1997; **33**(1): 37–41.

64. Zhang HG, Huang N, Liu D et al. Gene therapy that inhibits nuclear translocation of nuclear factor kappaB results in tumor necrosis factor alpha-induced apoptosis of human synovial fibroblasts. *Arthritis Rheum* 2000; **43**(5): 1094–105.

65. Li J, Yen C, Liaw D et al. PTEN, a putative protein tyrosine phosphatase gene mutated in human brain, breast, and prostate cancer. *Science* 1997; **275**(5308): 1943–7.

66. Franke TF, Kaplan DR, Cantley LC. PI3K: downstream AKTion blocks apoptosis. *Cell* 1997; **88**(4): 435–7.

67. Hemmings BA. Akt signaling: linking membrane events to life and death decisions. *Science* 1997; **275**(5300): 628–30.

68. Olschwang S, Serova-Sinilnikova OM, Lenoir GM et al. PTEN germ-line mutations in juvenile polyposis coli. *Nat Genet* 1998; **18**(1): 12–14.

9

Complement receptors

V Michael Holers

Introduction • Background • Review of complement receptors • Complement receptor targeting strategies and associated therapeutic opportunities • Summary • References

INTRODUCTION

This review serves as a companion to Chapter 26. As compared to that chapter, though, in which blockade of serum complement proteins is discussed, herein are reviewed the therapeutic options afforded by targeting the receptors for complement activation fragments.

BACKGROUND

The classical, alternative and lectin pathways of the complement system are activated by several

mechanisms relevant to the immunopathogenesis of rheumatoid arthritis, systemic lupus erythematosus and other rheumatic diseases.

The complement system can be activated by each of three distinct pathways: the classical, alternative and lectin pathways (Figure 9.1). Although the classical pathway is typically thought of as activated only by pathogens or immune complexes that contain antigen and IgM or complement-fixing isotypes of IgG, many situations have been described in which this complement pathway is initiated (Table

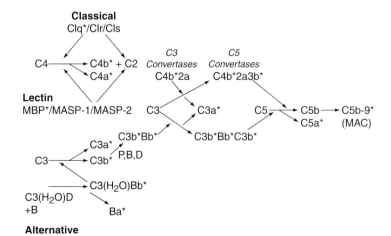

Figure 9.1 Schematic of the complement activation pathways. *indicates complement activation fragments for which known or proposed receptors have been described as outlined in this chapter. MASP, mannose-binding lectin-associated serum protease; MAC, membrane attack complex; MBP, mannose binding protein.

Table 9.1   Biologically relevant complement pathway activators.

Classical	Alternative	Lectin
Immune complexes (natural IgM, IgG)	'Tickover'	Repeating simple sugars
C-reactive protein (CRP)	Polysaccharides	
Serum amyloid P protein	Endotoxin	
β-amyloid fibrils/tau protein	IgA immune complexes	
Apoptotic bodies	Cobra venom factor (CVF)	
	Amplification pathway	

9.1). For example, the classical pathway is activated in the complete absence of antibody directly through the actions of C-reactive protein (CRP) and serum amyloid P (SAP) protein, members of the pentraxin family.[1] Classical pathway activation occurs when either of these proteins binds microbial pathogens or nuclear constituents such as chromatin released from necrotic or dying cells, which then allows C1 to be directly bound and the pathway activated. SAP also serves to block chromatin and DNA degradation.[2] The classical pathway may also be activated when apoptotic bodies derived from cells directly bind C1q,[3] or when β-amyloid fibrils or the tau protein bind C1q.[4,5] C1q is part of the C1 molecule and is found in serum physically associated in a calcium-dependent complex with two other components, C1r and C1s, with a stoichiometry of $C1q_1C1r_2C1s_2$ (review: Sim and Reid[6]). C1q itself is a 460-kDa molecule that includes six strands, each strand formed by unique ~23-kDa A, B and C chains. Each C1q strand has two primary domains, globular 'heads' and collagen-like 'tails', that interact with unique receptors. Complement is activated by C1q when it binds IgM- and IgG-containing immune complexes via the head regions, or when the tails interact with molecules such as CRP or SAP protein. This is followed by conformational changes and sequential activation of the C1r and C1s proteases.

The alternative pathway is activated on surfaces of pathogens that have neutral or positive charge characteristics and do not express or contain complement inhibitors. This is due to a process termed 'tickover' of C3 that occurs spontaneously, involves the interaction of conformationally altered C3 with factor B, and results in the fixation of active C3b on pathogens or other surfaces (review: Muller–Eberhard[7]). The alternative pathway can, however, also be initiated by IgA isotype antibody-containing immune complexes. The alternative pathway is also activated by a mechanism called the 'amplification loop', when C3b that is deposited onto targets via the classical or lectin pathways then serves to bind factor B and also propagate activation of the pathway by this pathway. Certain autoantibodies, termed C3 nephritic factors, also greatly enhance activation of the alternative pathway because they act by stabilizing the C3 convertase C3bBbP and do not allow it to spontaneously decay at a normal rate. Because of the ability of the alternative pathway to auto-activate, the continuous presence of complement regulatory proteins, both in the soluble phase and on cell membranes, is crucial to normal homeostasis.

The lectin pathway is initiated by the binding of mannose-binding lectin (MBL) to repeating carbohydrate moieties found primarily on the surface of microbial pathogens (review: Reid and Turner[8]). MBL is physically associated with proteases called mannose-binding lectin-associated serum protease (MASP)-1, MASP-2 and MASP-3, which act like C1r and C1s of the classical pathway.[9] Once MBL is bound to its target, MASP-1 and MASP-2 are activated, resulting in the cleavage of C4 and C2, which is then followed by the assembly of the remainder of the complement pathway. In addition to this mechanism involving C4 and C2, direct activation of C3 has been reported.

Using these recognition and activation mechanisms, the complement pathway is one of the major means by which the body recognizes foreign antigens and pathogens as well as tissue injury, ischemia, apoptosis and necrosis.[10] This capacity places the complement system at the center of many clinically relevant responses to foreign pathogens and, relevant to this chapter, to rheumatic diseases such as systemic lupus erythematosus (SLE) and rheumatoid arthritis, which are characterized by tissue injury mediated by humoral immune mechanisms (see Chapter 32 for lists of diseases for which complement inhibition may be relevant).

Convergence of the three activation pathways on the C3 protein results in a common pathway of effector functions

C3 is the first point at which each of the three pathways converges. Therefore, without activating C3, the pathway is not efficiently propagated to C5b-9. Because of this, inhibition of C3 activation has a particularly profound biological effect. Although direct C5a activation by non-complement proteases has been previously proposed,[11] and bypass pathways in the early classical pathway have also been proposed that would allow C3 activation to proceed even in a complete deficiency state,[12] the biological relevance of these additional complement activation and propagation mechanisms is uncertain.

Activation of C3 by any of the three pathways leads to cleavage of C3, with generation of the fragments C3a and C3b. C3a is a small anaphylatoxin that binds to receptors on leukocytes and other cells, resulting in activation and release of soluble inflammatory mediators (review: Hugli[13]). C3b and its further sequential cleavage fragments, iC3b and C3d, are ligands for complement receptors 1 and 2 (CR1 and CR2) and the β_2 integrins, CD11b/CD18 (CR3) and CD11c/CD18 (CR4), which are present on a variety of phagocytic and immune accessory cells (reviews: Brown[14] and Holers[15]).

C3b attaches covalently to targets, and this is followed by assembly of the classical and alternative pathway C5 convertases, with subsequent cleavage of C5 to C5a and C5b. C5a is a potent soluble inflammatory anaphylatoxic and chemotactic peptide that promotes the recruitment and activation of neutrophils, monocytes and other cells (review: Wetsel[16]). Binding of C5b to the target initiates the assembly of the C5b-9 membrane attack complex (MAC). Insertion of the C5b-9 MAC can result in cell lysis or, on nucleated cells, activation of specific signaling pathways through the recruitment of heterotrimeric G proteins.[17] Cell activation by the MAC may be the most important event in some disease states, such as glomerulonephritis and renal ischemia–reperfusion injury.[18,19]

REVIEW OF COMPLEMENT RECEPTORS

C1q receptors

C1q has been reported to demonstrate many biological effects manifested through at least four receptors (Table 9.2; Figure 9.2), though other reports have suggested that there may be additional C1q receptors or receptor complexes that interact with collagen-like tails[20] and globular heads.[21,22] C1q receptors play an important role by enhancing Fc receptor- and CR1-mediated phagocytosis. In addition, C1q receptors are expressed on endothelial cells and appear to mediate the upregulation of adhesion molecules on these cells after interacting with C1q-containing immune complexes.[23]

The 33-kDa C1q receptor (designated in some reports as gC1qR for its interaction with globular heads) is found on most leukocytes, platelets and endothelial cells. A second receptor, which interacts with C1q collagen-like tails, designated

Table 9.2   Complement receptors.

Protein		Ligand(s)	Size (kDa)	Family	Distribution
C1q receptors	gC1qR	C1q heads	33	–	Platelets, leukocytes, vascular endothelium
	C1qR$_P$	C1q tails	126	–	Myeloid (mono, macro) vascular endothelium
	cC1qR	C1q tails SP-A MBL SP-D	60	–	Leukocytes, platelets, vascular endothelium, fibroblasts, epithelium, alveolar type II, smooth muscle, mesangial
CR1 (CD35)		C3b > iC3b C4b C1q MBL	190 220	RCA	E, B and T cells, thymocyte, mono, macro, neutrophils, FDC, podocytes, Kuppfer
CR2 (CD21)		C3d = iC3b EBV CD23 IFN-α	145	RCA	B cells, T cells, FDC, basophils, keratinocytes, epithelial
CR3 (CD11b/CD18)		iC3b > C3b >> C3d ICAM-1 Factor X Fibrinogen Other	165, 95	Integrin	Mono, macro, lymphocyte subset, FDC
CR4 (CD11c/CD18)		iC3b > C3b	150, 95	Integrin	Mono, macro
C5aR (CD88)		C5a	50	Rhodopsin	Eosinophils, neutrophils, mono, macro, platelets, mast, hepatocytes, vascular smooth muscle, bronchial/alveolar epithelial, vascular endothelium, astrocytes, mast
C3aR		C3a	65	Rhodopsin	Eosinophils, neutrophils, mono, macro, platelets, mast, adipocytes

MBL, mannose-binding lectin; EBV, Epstein–Barr virus; IFN, interferon; FDC, follicular dendritic cell.

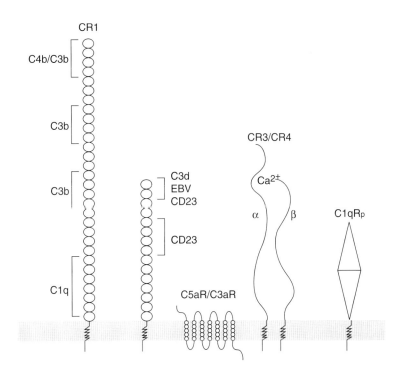

Figure 9.2 Schematic representation of complement receptors whose structures are known at the molecular level. EBV, Epstein–Barr virus.

C1qR$_P$, has been described as a 126-kDa molecule whose expression is limited to myeloid cells (neutrophils and monocytes/macrophages) and endothelial cells.[24–26] A third C1q receptor, designated cC1qR, to reflect its interaction with collagen-like tails, is a 60-kDa molecule that is very widely distributed.[6,27,28] This receptor has been identified on all types of leukocytes, platelets, endothelial cells, fibroblasts, epithelial cells, alveolar type II cells, smooth muscle cells and glomerular mesangial cells. Interestingly, this receptor has also been shown to interact with a family of proteins designated the collectins.[6] This family is characterized by lectin-binding activity through a specific domain and the presence in each of an additional collagen-like region.[29] Members of the collectin family include MBL, conglutinin, and surfactant proteins A (SP-A) and D (SP-D).

In addition, complement receptor type 1 (CR1) has also been shown to interact with C1q[30] in a unique domain outside of its interaction site with C4b and C3b.[31] In addition to C1q, MBL has also been found to bind CR1, resulting in enhanced phagocytosis of IgG-opsonized bacteria by macrophages.[32]

CRP and SAP receptor

CRP, along with its related pentraxin family member SAP, has been shown to interact with Fcγ receptors.[33,34] The interaction of CRP- and SAP-bound particles with Fc receptors results in enhanced phagocytosis by leukocytes. The biological outcomes of such interactions can vary, resulting in either enhanced injury of target organs such as the ischemic myocardium,[35] or conversely, protection from the development of humoral autoimmunity.[2]

Complement receptor type 1 (CR1, C3b/C4b receptor, CD35)

CR1 is a relatively widely distributed complement receptor that binds, in addition to C1q and MBL, the C3b form of C3 as well as the C4b form of C4 (Table 9.2) (reviews: Ahearn and Fearon,[36] Carroll[37] and Ross[38]). CR1 has a lower affinity for the more proteolytically cleaved iC3b form of C3. The structure of CR1 consists of a linear series of structurally related modules, designated short consensus repeats (SCRs), followed by a transmembrane and short intracytoplasmic domain. CR1 is expressed on erythrocytes, B cells, a subset of peripheral T cells (~15%), thymocytes (~25%), monocytes, macrophages, neutrophils, follicular dendritic cells (FDCs), eosinophils, glomerular podocytes, and Kuppfer cells.

CR1 has a number of biological roles. Erythrocyte CR1 binds large circulating immune complexes that have fixed complement, and transports them to the liver and spleen for further processing.[39] CR1 on monocytes, macrophages and neutrophils promotes the phagocytosis of C3-bound targets.[14] CR1 on FDCs is believed to play a role in the trapping of immune complexes within germinal centers in lymphoid organs, and CR1 on B cells promotes B-cell activation in addition to facilitating antigen binding and presentation to T cells (review: Carroll[37]). A potentially interesting observation has been that CR1 on T cells and thymocytes interacts with complement-opsonized HIV, resulting in CD4-independent infection of these cells.[40,41]

Complement receptor type 2 (C3d receptor, CD21)

Human CR2 is a receptor for the C3d/C3d,g and iC3b forms of C3 as well as the Epstein–Barr virus (EBV) (Table 9.2).[36,37] CR2 mediates EBV infection and immortalization of B cells through its interactions with the EBV surface protein gp350/220. Studies have also shown that CR2 is a receptor for soluble or membrane-bound CD23.[42] Like CR1, CR2 is composed of a series of repeating SCRs and is a member of the RCA family.[43] CR2 is expressed on mature B lymphocytes, FDCs, a small subset of peripheral T cells, early thymocytes, basophils, keratinocytes, and many types of epithelial cells (nasopharyngeal, oropharyngeal, cervical, lacrimal, and ocular surface).[15]

CR2 has a number of biological roles. On B cells, CR2 interacts with C3d/iC3b-bound antigens and promotes B-cell activation and differentiation through associations with CD19 and TAPA-1 (CD81).[44,45] The major role of this CR2–CD19–CD81 complex is to lower thresholds of B-cell activation to foreign[46–48] and likely self-antigens.[49,50] In addition, by binding CD23, CR2 may enhance B-cell class switching to IgE and antigen presentation by CR2-expressing B cells to CD23-positive T cells.[51]

Complement receptor type 3 (CR3, CD11b/CD18) and type 4 (CR4, CD11c/CD18)

CR3 and CR4 are members of the integrin family and share common β-chains of the β_2 form.[52] The CR3 α-chain is 87% identical with the CR4 α-chain. CR3 and CR4 are expressed on neutrophils, monocytes, macrophages, FDCs, a subset of lymphocytes, and eosinophils. CR3 is the primary receptor for iC3b and interacts less well with C3b and C3d, while CR4 is a receptor for iC3b and C3b (Table 9.2).[14] CR3, in particular, has many non-complement-dependent functions in cellular adhesion and also interacts with a variety of ligands, including ICAM-1, factor X, and fibrinogen.[14] CR3 also mediates adherence to plastic and many types of clinically used biomaterials, and mediates inside-out signaling in phagocytes. In addition, CR3 mediates a portion of the adhesive interactions of neutrophils with endothelium in both a C3 ligand-dependent and C3—independent manner. An additional important interaction of CR3 may be with CD23.[53]

C5a receptor (C5aR/CD88)

C5a is a potent 74 amino acid fragment of C5 that is released upon activation by either the classical or alternative pathway C5 convertases (Figure 9.1) (review: Wetsel[16]). The biological effects of C5a and other anaphylatoxins such as C3a include leukocyte chemotaxis, cell activation and synthesis of acute-phase reactants. The C5a receptor is a ~50-kDa protein expressed on a variety of cell types (Table 9.2). C5a utilizes a receptor (C5aR, CD88) that is a G-protein-linked member of the heptahelical seven transmembrane spanning protein family.[54] Expression of the C5aR, although initially thought to be limited to neutrophils, monocytes and eosinophils, has been shown to be quite widespread (review: Wetsel[16]). Cells now known to express C5aR include liver parenchymal cells, in which C5aR binding mediates increased acute-phase gene expression, vascular smooth muscle cells, renal mesangial cells, bronchial and alveolar cells in the lung, and astrocytes.

C3a receptor (C3aR)

The C3aR, like the C5aR, is a G-protein-coupled member of the tetraspan family.[55–57] The C3aR is 65 kDa in size and is expressed on platelets, eosinophils, mast cells, neutrophils, macrophages, adipocytes, brain and many other tissues. Biological roles of the C3aR include chemotaxis of eosinophils, macrophages and mast cells as well as stimulation of the respiratory burst. In whole-organ systems, C3a causes cardiac dysfunction[58] and the induction of bronchospasm.[59]

COMPLEMENT RECEPTOR TARGETING STRATEGIES AND ASSOCIATED THERAPEUTIC OPPORTUNITIES

Chapter 32 reviews therapeutic opportunities by targeting the activation of complement proteins using soluble CR1 (sCR1), anti-C5 monoclonal antibody and other means such as peptides and recombinant soluble C3 and C5 convertase inhibitors. Clearly, a major beneficial effect of those targeting strategies is to decrease interactions of downstream complement activation fragments such as C5a with their receptors. In contrast, herein I will focus on therapeutic strategies that target a specific complement receptor. There are relative advantages and disadvantages to targeting either the soluble proteins in the pathway or individual receptors. The major advantage of targeting activation pathways is that several downstream receptor–ligand interactions are usually diminished. For example, by blocking C3 activation, C3a, C3b, C5a and MAC interactions are all diminished. Therefore, there may be a more profound immunomodulatory and suppressive effect. The disadvantage of this strategy is that, in addition to blocking the deleterious effects of complement, one may also affect the protective aspects of complement without gaining any additional therapeutic benefit. By targeting a specific ligand–receptor interaction that plays a key role in disease in the target organ(s), one might gain therapeutic benefit without the expense of potential complications. Indeed, one of the major directions of study in the complement area is to define the specific and unique contributions of individual complement components and receptor–ligand interactions to each disease process.

C1q receptors

Except for one monoclonal antibody that blocks the function of a C1q receptor-related molecule,[25] there are no currently available therapeutics that specifically target C1q receptors. There are two major reasons for this. The first is that there are many apparent C1q receptors, and the biological roles and consequences of inhibition are incompletely understood. The second is that a major effect of C1q receptor interactions appears to be protective, either by recognition of foreign pathogens such as bacteria and viruses, or by recognizing and clearing immune complexes or self-antigens containing chromatin and DNA. Therefore, rather than blocking C1q receptor interactions, perhaps increasing the expression or binding capacity of C1q receptors in order to enhance the clearance of C1q-containing self-antigens may be a more rational therapeutic strategy to improve autoimmune diseases. The use of such a strategy, though, requires further characterization of these complement receptors at a molecular level and increased understanding of which of these postulated receptors are relevant to unique C1q effects.

There is one emerging area, though, in which inhibition of C1q activities, or C1q receptors, may be beneficial. Studies have shown that C1q–/– (C1q-deficient) mice are relatively protected from the peripheral inoculation of prions in experimental models of disease.[60] The mechanism may be due to decreasing the targeting to and retention of prions by FDCs in peripheral immune tissue, an event that appears to be key to the pathogenesis of this condition. Whatever the mechanism, though, better understanding of the role of C1q and other complement components and receptors in the central nervous and peripheral immune system handling of infectious prion particles[60] is an important undertaking with substantial therapeutic potential.

CRP and SAP receptor

There are no current strategies that specifically target CRP and SAP receptors, for many of the same reasons as outlined above for C1q receptors. There is a potential benefit of blocking CRP activities in ischemia–reperfusion injury of the heart.[35] In addition, as for C1q, improving the expression levels of CRP may be beneficial in autoimmune[2] or infectious diseases.[61] However, with regard to their receptors, despite the in vitro data that support a relevant interaction, it is not clear what is the contribution of specific receptors, Fc or others, as compared to direct complement activation to the specific disease or immune phenotypes reported by manipulating CRP and/or SAP levels.

CR1/CD35

As outlined in Chapter 32, CR1 is primarily being used therapeutically as a soluble recombinant protein that blocks complement C3 and C5 activation. In addition, similar to C1q, because of the relative deficiencies of CR1 in autoimmune diseases such as SLE, increasing binding of immune complexes to CR1 using strategies such as heteropolymers of anti-CR1 and DNA may be one means to improve the clearance of pathogenic autoantibodies and immune complexes.[62] This strategy may also be used to facilitate the clearance of microbial pathogens from the blood.

There are certain circumstances, though, in which one might be able to block CR1 activities in a therapeutically beneficial manner. The first involves the role of erythrocyte CR1 as a mediator of the rosetting that is associated with severe malaria.[63] Here, CR1 mediates erythrocyte agglutination, which may contribute to central nervous system and other tissue injury. The second is in HIV-1 infection, where, as outlined below, there may be an unanticipated important role in pathogenesis, related to either the infection of cells using CR1 as the receptor for C3-bound HIV-1, or to the retention of infectious HIV-1 for prolonged periods of time on FDCs in vivo. One complicating feature of the inhibition of CR1 using monoclonal antibodies (mAbs) is the presence of spatially separated repeating domains, several of which appear to bind C3 fragments.[64]

CR2/CD21

Therapeutic targeting of this receptor is possible in several situations. First, because the CR2–CD19–CD81 complex is essential to the development of humoral immunity for foreign antigens, blocking unwanted humoral immune responses to antigens may be possible by interfering with CR2. Second, certain autoimmune diseases in which responses to foreign antigens trigger autoimmunity by either epitope spreading or molecular mimicry may also benefit from such a strategy. The experimental model that has been used to test this idea is murine myocarditis that is initiated by immunization with cardiac myosin or infection with cardiotropic virus.[65] In this model, myocarditis was greatly diminished in association with profound changes in T-cell autoimmunity, the development of antibodies cross-reactive with myosin, and the elaboration of pathogenic inflammatory cytokines.

A third use of CR2 inhibitors may be in the amelioration of EBV infection, either during the primary clinical phase of mononucleosis, or by decreasing the likelihood of developing EBV-related lymphoproliferative diseases in immunocompromised individuals, including those who are HIV-1 infected. In these settings, the relative role of new viral infection versus reactivation of already EBV-infected cells requires better definition. In addition, the relative benefits of receptor blockade versus enhancement of cytotoxic T lymphocyte (CTL) function need to be evaluated. A fourth potential role of CR2 inhibition involves blocking the B-cell effects of CD23 that are related to class switching to IgE, or form part of the process of antigen presentation to CD23-positive T cells. In addition, as noted above, both CR1 and CR2 on T cells and thymocytes can interact with complement-opsonized HIV, resulting in CD4-independent infection of these cells. This may represent an important alternative infection mechanism. Finally, as outlined above, complement C3 and CR2 have also been shown to be essential for HIV binding to FDCs in germinal centers or circulating B cells. CR2 appears to play a particularly important role in the binding of infectious HIV-1-containing immune complexes to FDCs and B cells.[66,67]

With regard to SLE, it may be possible to improve the levels of B-cell tolerance to self-antigens by targeting these antigens more effectively to CR2, or potentially CR1. This conclusion is based on the findings that the absence of CR2/CR1,[50] or the presence of a dysfunctional CR2/CR1 allele,[49] results in loss of self-tolerance. Finally, targeting of C3d-bound antigens to CR2 greatly increases the immunogenicity of foreign proteins,[68] and this is being pursued in various vaccine development strategies.

Strategies for blocking CR2 function include inhibitory monoclonal antibodies,[69,70] soluble proteins containing the C3d ligand-binding domain,[71] and, potentially, small molecule inhibitors based on the recently solved CR2–C3d structure.[72]

CR3/CR4

Targeting of CR3 and CR4 as a therapeutic strategy has been attempted using several means, including antibodies, small molecules and activators of CR3 function such as β-glucan.[73]

CR3 plays a major role in the adhesive interactions of neutrophils with activated endothelium, and, consistent with this effect, blocking receptor function with a mAb resulted in decreased inflammation in a model of colitis.[74] β-Glucan has been used to activate cytotoxic function in cells expressing CR3 that interact with targets such as tumor cells.[73] In addition, blocking the CD23–CR3 interaction on macrophages would probaby decrease the synthesis of proinflammatory cytokines.[53]

C5aR/CD88

By using inhibitory antibodies, single-chain reagents and mice in which expression of the C5aR has been eliminated,[75] C5a has been shown to play a central role in the reverse passive Arthus reaction,[76,77] contact sensitivity,[78] pulmonary inflammation,[79] thrombotic glomerulonephritis[80] and inflammatory arthritis.[81] Recently, an orally active cyclic peptide inhibitor of C5a has been described.[82] This reagent blocks murine models of disease, including the reverse passive Arthus reaction and endotoxic shock. Interestingly, in mice, and perhaps humans, the effects of C5a appear to have a relative tissue specificity, with inflammation in kidney, lung and joints being the most dependent upon C5aR.

C3aR

C3a analogs with altered cell-binding and biological effects have been created, and the structure of the C3a anaphylatoxin itself is well understood.[13] Recently, by using *C3aR–/–* mice, the C3aR has been shown to play an unexpectedly important role in experimental models of asthma.[83] By using a non-peptide antagonist of the C3aR, a role in lipopolysaccharide (LPS)-induced airway neutrophilia and adjuvant-induced arthritis has been identified.[84] In contrast to the therapeutic potential of blocking C3aR function, though, this receptor has been shown to play an important role in protection from the lethal effects of LPS, as shown by the increased lethality in *C3aR–/–* mice.[85]

Inhibition of MAC activities

Incorporation of the C5b-9 MAC into cell membranes has pronounced effects on cell function. MAC binding activates several signal transduction pathways, resulting in increases in arachidonic acid mobilization, generation of diacyl glyceride and ceramide, and activation of protein kinase C, mitogen-activated protein kinase (MAPK) and Ras.[17,18] Proinflammatory and tissue-damaging phenotypic outcomes following these signaling events include proliferation as well as the release of reactive oxygen intermediates, leukotrienes, thromboxane, basic fibroblast growth factor (bFGF), platelet-derived growth factor (PDGF), von Willebrand factor and GMP-140. Because of these potentially deleterious effects, inhibitors of MAC activation have been pursued. A major strategy has involved inhibition of C5, and thus subsequent C5b-9 activation using anti-C5 mAb. However, blocking activation of the MAC without the C5aR is possible, either by using soluble targeted forms of the C8/C9 inhibitor CD59,[86] or potentially by blocking components such as C6 from being incorporated into the MAC. In addition, because MAC incorporation into cell membranes involves a series of increasingly hydrophobic interactions as the complex is assembled, interference with membrane binding is also theoretically possible.

Other potential receptor targets

Finally, there are other potential ligand–receptor interactions in the complement system that may serve as good targets. Currently, there is little understanding of the molecular structure of the receptor(s) that might be involved; however, if these receptors are truly present in humans, inhibition of their activities could have very important and beneficial effects. One example is factor B receptors that may interact with the Bb and Ba activation fragments, which have been described by function only. These receptors may be important because factor B-deficient mice are resistant to both the development of renal injury in the MRL/*lpr* model of SLE[87] and to arthritis in a passive transfer model of rheumatoid arthritis.[81] Although the effects of factor B deficiency may be due only to direct activation of the alternative pathway by pathogenic immunoglobulin, or to amplification of the classical pathway, one compelling idea is that factor B receptors may mediate the biological effects. Another example is the C4a receptor, which has only been described by functional effects but is likely to be distinct from C5aR C3aR.[88] In this circumstance, given the great importance of the C5a and C3a anaphylatoxins, it is likely that the structurally homologous C4a protein will interact with a similar receptor and mediate clinically important effects.

SUMMARY

Reviewed herein and in Chapter 32 have been several lines of evidence that support the likelihood that complement inhibition should have benefit in several clinical diseases. Whether targeting soluble proteins or complement receptors is the most effective strategy remains to be determined. It is likely that, similar to the situation with cytokine antagonists, strategies that are relatively unique to each disease process will ultimately have to be pursued. In addition, it is likely that other complement components such as factor D and properdin play currently underappreciated roles in certain diseases. Blockade of these proteins may provide additional therapeutic opportunities.

REFERENCES

1. Gewurz H, Zhang X-H, Lint TF. Structure and function of the pentraxins. *Curr Opin Immunol* 1996; **7**: 54–64.

2. Bickerstaff MC, Botto M, Hutchinson WL et al. Serum amyloid P component controls chromatin degradation and prevents antinuclear autoimmunity. *Nature Med* 1999; **5**: 694–7.

3. Navratil JS, Watkins SC, Wisnieski JJ, Ahearn JM. The globular heads of C1q specifically recognize surface blebs of apoptotic vascular endothelial cells. *J Immunol* 2001; **166**: 3231–9.

4. Bradt BM, Kolb WP, Cooper NR. Complement-dependent proinflammatory properties of the Alzheimer's disease beta-peptide. *J Exp Med* 1998; **188**: 431–8.

5. Shen Y, Lue L, Yang L et al. Complement activation by neurofibrillary tangles in Alzheimer's disease. *Neurosci Lett* 2001; **305**: 165–8.

6. Sim RB, Reid KBM. C1: molecular interactions with activating systems. *Immunol Today* 1991; **12**: 307–11.

7. Muller-Eberhard HJ. Molecular organization and function of the complement system. *Annu Rev Biochem* 1988; **57**: 321–47.

8. Reid KBM, Turner MW. Mammalian lectins in activation and clearance mechanisms involving the complement system. *Springer Semin Immunopathol* 1994; **15**: 307–25.

9. Matsushita M, Fujita T. Activation of the classical complement pathway by mannose-binding protein in association with a novel C1s-like serine protease. *J Exp Med* 1992; **176**: 1497–502.

10. Fearon DT, Locksley RM. The instructive role of innate immunity in the acquired immune response. *Science* 1996; **272**: 50–4.

11. Wetsel RA, Kolb WP. Expression of C5a-like biological activities by the fifth component of human complement (C5) upon limited digestion with noncomplement enzymes without release of polypeptide fragments. *J Exp Med* 1983; **157**: 2029–48.

12. Fries LF, O'Shea JJ, Frank MM. Inherited deficiencies of complement and complement related proteins. *Clin Immunol Immunopathol* 1986; **40**: 37–49.

13. Hugli TE. Structure and function of C3a anaphylatoxin. *Curr Top Microbiol Immunol* 1989; **153**: 181–208.

14. Brown EJ. Complement receptors and phagocytosis. *Curr Opin Immunol* 1991; **3**: 76–82.

15. Holers VM. Complement. In: Rich R, ed. *Principles and Practices of Clinical Immunology* (Mosby: St Louis, MO, 2001) 21.1–21.8.

16. Wetsel RA. Structure, function and cellular expression of complement anaphylatoxin receptors. *Curr Opin Immunol* 1995; **7**: 48–53.

17. Shin ML, Rus HG, Nicolescu FI. Membrane attack by complement: assembly and biology of terminal complement complexes. *Biomembranes* 1996; **4**: 123–49.

18. Morgan BP. Effects of the membrane attack complex of complement on nucleated cells. *Curr Topics Microbiol Immunol* 1992; **178**: 115–40.

19. Zhou W, Farrar CA, Abe K et al. Predominant role for C5b-9 in renal ischemia/reperfusion injury. *J Clin Invest* 2000; **105**: 1363–71.

20. Siegel RC, Schumaker VN. Measurement of the association constants of the complexes formed between intact C1q or pepsin-treated C1q stalks and the unactivated or activated C1r2C1s2 tetramers. *Mol Immunol* 1983; **20**: 53–66.

21. Ghebrehiwet B, Lim BL, Peerschke EIB, Willis AC, Reid KBM. Isolation, cDNA cloning, and overexpression of a 33-kD cell surface glycoprotein that binds to the globular 'heads' of C1q. *J Exp Med* 1994; **179**: 1809–21.

22. Reid KB, Kishore U. C1q: structure, function, and receptors. *Immunopharmacology* 2000; **49**: 159–70.

23. Lozada C, Levin RI, Huie M et al. Identification of C1q as the heat-labile serum cofactor required for immune complexes to stimulate endothelial expression of the adhesion molecules E-selectin and intercellular and vascular cell adhesion molecules. *Proc Natl Acad Sci USA* 1995; **92**: 8378–82.

24. Guan E, Robinson SL, Goodman EB, Tenner AJ. Cell-surface protein identified on phagocytic cells modulates the C1q-mediated enhancement of phagocytosis. *J Immunol* 1994; **152**: 4005–16.

25. Nepomuceno RR, Henschen-Edman AH, Burgess WH, Tenner AJ. cDNA cloning and primary structure analysis of C1qR(P), the human C1q/MBL/SPA receptor that mediates enhanced phagocytosis in vitro. *Immunity* 1997; **6**: 119–29.

26. Nepomuceno RR, Tenner AJ. C1qRP, the C1q receptor that enhances phagocytosis, is detected specifically in human cells of myeloid lineage, endothelial cells and platelets. *J Immunol* 1998; **160**: 1929–35.

27. Chen A, Gaddipati S, Hong Y, Volkman DJ,

Peerschke EIB, Ghebrehiwet B. Human T cells express specific binding sites for C1q. Role in T-cell activation and proliferation. *J Immunol* 1994; **153**: 1430–40.

28. Ghebrehiwet B, Kew RR, Gruber BL, Marchese MJ, Peerschke EIB, Reid KBM. Murine mast cells express two types of C1q receptors that are involved in the induction of chemotaxis and chemokinesis. *J Immunol* 1995; **155**: 2614–19.

29. Holmskov U, Malhotra R, Sim RB, Jensenius JC. Collectins: collagenous C-type lectins of the innate immune defense system. *Immunol Today* 1994; **15**: 67–74.

30. Klickstein LB, Barbashov SF, Nicholson-Weller A, Liu T, Jack RM. Complement receptor type 1 (CR1, CD35) is a receptor for C1q. *Immunity* 1997; **7**: 345–55.

31. Tas SW, Klickstein LB, Barbashov SF, Nicholson-Weller A. C1q and C4b bind simultaneously to CR1 and additively support erythrocyte adhesion. *J Immunol* 1999; **163**: 5056–63.

32. Ghiran I, Barbashov SF, Klickstein LB, Tas SWJJC, Nicholson-Weller A. Complement receptor 1/CD35 is a receptor for mannan-binding lectin. *J Exp Med* 2000; **192**: 1797–808.

33. Bharadwaj D, Stein M-P, Volzer M, Mold C, Du Clos TW. The major receptor for C-reactive protein on leukocytes is Fc receptor II. *J Exp Med* 1999; **150**: 585–90.

34. Bharadwaj D., Mold C, Markham E, Du Clos TW. Serum amyloid P component binds to Fc gamma receptors and opsonizes particles for phagocytosis. *J Immunol* 2001; **166**: 6735–41.

35. Griselli M, Herbert J, Hutchinson WL et al. C-reactive protein and complement are important mediators of tissue damage in acute myocardial infarction. *J Exp Med* 1999; **190**: 1733–40.

36. Ahearn JM, Fearon DT. Structure and function of the complement receptors, CR1 (CD35) and CR2 (CD21). *Adv Immunol* 1989; **46**: 183–219.

37. Carroll MC. CD21/CD35 in B-cell activation. *Semin Immunol* 1998; **10**: 279–86.

38. Ross GD. Complement receptor type 1. *Curr Top Microbiol Immunol* 1992; **178**: 31–44.

39. Hebert LA, Cosio FG, Birmingham DJ, Mahan JD. Biologic significance of the erythrocyte complement receptor: a primate perquisite. *J Lab Clin Med* 1991; **118**: 301–8.

40. Stoiber H, Kacani L, Speth C, Wurzner R, Dierich MP. The supportive role of complement in HIV pathogenesis. *Immunol Rev* 2001; **180**: 168–76.

41. Delibrias CC, Kazatchkine MD, Fischer E. Evidence for the role of CR1 (CD35), in addition to CR2 (CD21), in facilitating infection of human T cells with opsonized HIV. *Scand J Immunol* 1993; **38**: 183–9.

42. Aubry J-P, Pochon S, Gauchat J-F et al. CD23 interacts with a new functional extracytoplasmic domain involving *N*-linked oligosaccharides on CD21. *J Immunol* 1994; **152**: 5806–13.

43. Hourcade D, Holers VM, Atkinson JP. The regulators of complement activation (RCA) gene cluster. *Adv Immunol* 1989; **45**: 381–416.

44. Fearon DT, Carter RH. The CD19/CR2/TAPA-1 complex of B lymphocytes: linking natural to acquired immunity. *Annu Rev Immunol* 1995; **13**: 127–49.

45. Tedder TF, Zhou L-J, Engel P. The CD19/CD21 signal transduction complex of B lymphocytes. *Immunol Today* 1994; **15**(9): 437–42.

46. Carter RH, Fearon DT. CD19: lowering the threshold for antigen receptor stimulation of B lymphocytes. *Science* 1992; **256**: 105–7.

47. Ahearn JM, Fischer MB, Croix DA et al. Disruption of the *Cr2* locus results in a reduction in B-1a cells and in an impaired B-cell response to T-dependent antigen. *Immunity* 1996; **4**: 251–62.

48. Molina H, Holers VM, Li B et al. Markedly impaired humoral immune response in mice deficient in complement receptors 1 and 2. *Proc Natl Acad Sci USA* 1996; **93**: 3357–61.

49. Boackle SA, Holers VM, Chen X et al. *Cr2*, a candidate gene in the murine Sle1c lupus susceptibility locus, encodes a dysfunctional protein. *Immunity* 2001; **15**: 775–85.

50. Prodeus A, Goerg S, Shen L-M et al. A critical role for complement in maintenance of self-tolerance. *Immunity* 1998; **9**: 721–31.

51. Aubry JP, Pochon S, Graber P, Jansen KU, Bonnefoy JY. CD21 is a ligand for CD23 and regulates IgE production. *Nature* 1992; **358**: 505–7.

52. Kishimoto TK, O'Connor K, Lee A, Roberts TM, Springer TA. Cloning of the β subunit of the leukocyte adhesion proteins: homology to an extracellular matrix receptor defines a novel supergene family. *Cell* 1987; **48**: 681–90.

53. Rezonnico R, Chicheportiche R, Imbert V, Dayer JM. Engagement of CD11b and CD11c beta2 integrin by antibodies or soluble CD23 induces IL-1beta production on primary human monocytes through mitogen-activated protein kinase-dependent pathways. *Blood* 2000; **95**: 3868–77.

54. Gerard NP, Gerard C. The chemotactic receptor

for human C5a anaphylatoxin. *Nature* 1991; **349**: 614–17.

55. Roglic A, Prossnitz ER, Cavanagh SL, Pan Z, Zou A, Ye RD. cDNA cloning of a novel G protein-coupled receptor with a large extracellular loop structure. *Biochim Biophys Acta* 1996; **1305**: 39–43.

56. Crass T, Raffetseder U, Martin U et al. Expression cloning of the human C3a anaphylatoxin receptor (C3aR) from differentiated U-937 cells. *Eur J Immunol* 1996; **26**: 1944–50.

57. Ames RS, Li Y, Sarau HM et al. Molecular cloning and characterization of the human anaphylotoxin C3a receptor. *J Biol Chem* 1996; **271**: 20231–4.

58. del Balzo U, Sakuma I, Levi R. Cardiac dysfunction caused by recombinant human C5a anaphylatoxin: mediation by histamine, adenosine and cyclooxygenase arachidonate metabolites. *J Pharmacol Exp Ther* 1990; **2253**: 171–9.

59. Watson JW, Drazen JM, Stimler-Gerard NP. Synergism between inflammatory mediators in vivo. Induction of airway hyperresponsiveness to C3a in the guinea pig. *Am Rev Respir Dis* 1988; **137**: 636–40.

60. Klein MA, Kaeser PS, Schwarz P et al. Complement facilitates early prion pathogenesis. *Nature Med* 2001; **7**: 488–92.

61. Szalai AJ, Briles DE, Volanakis JE. Human C-reactive protein is protective against fatal Streptococcus pneumoniae infection in transgenic mice. *J Immunol* 1995; **155**: 2557–63.

62. Lindorfer MA, Schuman TA, Craig ML, Martin EN, Taylor RP. A bispecific dsDNA × monoclonal antibody construct for clearance of anti-dsDNA IgG in systemic lupus erythematosus. *J Immunol Methods* 2001; **248**(125): 138.

63. Rowe JA, Moulds JM, Newbold CI, Miller LH. P. falciparum rosetting mediated by a parasite-variant erythrocyte membrane protein and complement-receptor 1. *Nature* 1997; **388**: 292–5.

64. Krych M, Hauhart R, Atkinson JP. Structure–function analysis of the active sites of complement receptor type 1. *J Biol Chem* 1998; **273**: 8623–9.

65. Kaya Z, Afanasyeva M, Wang Y et al. Contribution of the innate immune system to autoimmune myocarditis: a role for complement. *Nature Immunol* 2001; **2**: 739–45.

66. Kacani L, Prodinger WM, Sprinzl GM et al. Detachment of human immunodeficiency virus type 1 from germinal centers by blocking complement receptor type 2. *J Virol* 2000; **74**: 7997–8002.

67. Moir S, Malaspina A, Li Y et al. B cells of HIV-1-infected patients bind virions through CD21-complement interactions and transmit infectious virus to activated T cells. *J Exp Med* 2000; **192**: 637–46.

68. Dempsey P, Allison M, Akkaraju S, Goodnow C, Fearon D. C3d of complement as a molecular adjuvant: bridging innate and acquired immunity. *Science* 1996; **271**: 348–50.

69. Guthridge JM, Young K, Gipson MG et al. Epitope mapping using the x-ray crystallographic structure of complement receptor type 2 (CR2/CD21): identification of a highly inhibitory monoclonal antibody that directly recognizes the CR2–C3d interface. *J Immunol* 2001; **167**: 5758–66.

70. Prodinger WM, Schwendinger MG, Schoch J, Kochle M, Larcher C, Dierich MP. Characterization of C3d,g binding to a recess formed between SCR 1 and SCR 2 of complement receptor type 2. *J Immunol* 1998; **161**(9): 4604–10.

71. Hebell T, Ahearn JM, Fearon DT. Suppression of the immune response by a soluble complement receptor of B lymphocytes. *Science* 1991; **254**: 102–5.

72. Szakonyi G, Guthridge JM, Li D, Young K, Holers VM, Chen XS. Structure of complement receptor 2 in complex with its C3d ligand. *Science* 2001; **292**: 1725–8.

73. Yan J, Vetvicka V, Xia Y et al. Beta-glucan, a 'specific' biologic response modifier that uses antibodies to target tumors for cytotoxic recognition by leukocyte complement receptor type 3 (CD11b/CD18). *J Immunol* 1999; **163**: 3045–52.

74. Palmen MJ, Dijkstra CD, van der Ende MB, Pena AS, van Rees EP. Anti-CD11b/CD18 antibodies reduce inflammation in acute colitis in rats. *Clin Exp Immunol* 1995; **101**: 351–6.

75. Hopken UE, Lu B, Gerard NP, Gerard C. The C5a chemoattractant receptor mediates mucosal defence to infection. *Nature* 1996; **383**: 86–8.

76. Hopken UE, Lu B, Gerard NP, Gerard C. Impaired inflammatory responses in the reverse arthus reaction through genetic deletion of the C5a receptor. *J Exp Med* 1997; **185**: 749–56.

77. Heller T, Hennecke M, Baumann U et al. Selection of a C5a receptor antagonis from phage libraries attenuating the inflammatory response in immune complex disease and ischemia/reperfusion injury. *J Immunol* 1999; **163**: 985–94.

78. Tsuji RF, Kikuchi M, Askenase PW. Possible involvement of C5/C5a in the efferent and elicitation phases of contact sensitivity. *J Immunol* 1996; **156**: 4644–50.

79. Mulligan MS, Schmid E, Beck-Schimmer B et al. Requirement and role of C5a in acute lung

inflammatory injury in rats. *J Clin Invest* 1996; **98**: 503–12.

80. Kondo C, Mizuno M, Nishikawa K, Yuzawa Y, Hotta N, Matsuo S. The role of C5a in the development of thrombotic glomerulonephritis in rats. *Clin Exp Immunol* 2001; **124**: 323–9.

81. Ji H, Ohmura J, Mahmood U et al. Arthritis critically dependent on innate immune system players. *Immunity* 2002; **16**: 157–68.

82. Strachan AJ, Woodruff TM, Haaima G, Fairlie DP, Taylor SM. A new small molecule C5a receptor antagonist inhibits the reverse-passive Arthus reaction and endotoxic shock in rats. *J Immunol* 2000; **164**: 6560–5.

83. Humbles AA, Lu B, Nilsson CA et al. A role for the C3a anaphylatoxin receptor in the effector phase of asthma. *Nature* 2000; **406**: 998–1001.

84. Ames RS, Lee D, Foley JJ et al. Identification of a selective nonpeptide antagonist of the anaphylatoxin C3a receptor that demonstrates

antiinflammatory activity in animal models. *J Immunol* 2001; **166**: 6341–8.

85. Kildsgaard J, Hollman TJ, Matthews KW, Bian K, Murad F, Wetsel RA. Targeted disruption of the C3a receptor gene demonstrates a novel protective anti-inflammatory role for C3a in endotoxin-shock. *J Immunol* 2000; **165**: 5406–9.

86. Zhang H-F, Yu J, Bajwa E, Morrison SL, Tomlinson S. Targeting of functional antibody–CD59 fusion proteins to a cell surface. *J Clin Invest* 1999; **103**: 55–61.

87. Watanabe H, Garnier G, Circolo A et al. Modulation of renal disease in MRL/lpr mice genetically deficient in the alternative complement pathway factor B. *J Immunol* 2000; **164**: 786–94.

88. Ames RS, Tornetta MA, Foley JJ, Hugli TE, Sarau HM. Evidence that the receptor for C4a is distinct from the C3a receptor. *Immunopharmacology* 1997; **38**: 87–92.

10

Fc receptors

Jane Salmon

Introduction • FcγR structure and expression • FcγR signaling • FcγR in efferent and afferent responses: lessons from FcγR-deficient mice • Regulation of human FcγR expression and function • FcγR as targets for treatment of autoimmune disease • Summary • References

INTRODUCTION

Receptors for IgG constitute the link between humoral and cellular aspects of the immune cascade and play an integral part in afferent and efferent immune response. These cell-based binding sites for antibodies, termed Fcγ receptors (FcγR), interact with the constant region (Fc portion) of the IgG heavy chain, irrespective of its antigen specificity. Antibodies are adaptors that bind antigens to non-committed inflammatory cells and direct their destructive effector responses. Accessory cells that lack intrinsic specificity, such as neutrophils, macrophages, and mast cells, are recruited to participate in inflammatory responses through the interaction of their FcγR with antigen-specific antibodies. FcγR provide the means by which opsonized material, both foreign and endogenous, is identified and destroyed. One would expect that interfering with this interaction would limit immune complex-mediated tissue damage. Similarly, therapies directed at the afferent limb of the immune response, specifically targeting FcγR on B cells and antigen-presenting cells, can modulate humoral immune responses and peripheral tolerance. Recent progress in elucidating the physiology of FcγR has underscored

their importance in rheumatic diseases, such as systemic lupus erythematosus (SLE) and rheumatoid arthritis (RA).[1–3] Although specific receptors exist for each antibody class, this chapter will focus on human receptors for IgG: FcγR.

FcγR form a diverse group of receptors, expressed as hematopoetic cell surface molecules. Our current understanding of FcγR has been greatly enhanced by the cloning of human genes, the recent description of the crystal structure of receptor and ligand complexes, and studies in mice deficient in FcγR.[4–7] Two general classes of FcγR are recognized, stimulatory and inhibitory; they are often coexpressed on effector cells and act in concert.[8] Triggering stimulatory FcγR initiates phagocytosis, antibody-dependent cell-mediated cytotoxicity (ADCC), and phagocyte release of inflammatory mediators such as cytokines, reactive oxidants, and proteases. Through these mechanisms, stimulatory FcγR play an essential role in initiating type II and III hypersensitivity reactions.

Inhibitory FcγR, which modulate thresholds for activation and terminate stimulatory signals, form a key element in the regulation of effector function.[9–11] Because stimulatory and inhibitory FcγR bind IgG with similar affinity, coengagement of both signaling pathways occurs. When co-aggregated with stimulatory receptors on the cell surface, inhibitory FcγR can abolish cellular signaling, whereas when self-aggregated, they do not trigger effector functions. Inhibitory FcγR play a central role in afferent and efferent immune responses as negative regulators of both antibody production and immune complex-triggered activation.

Experiments in mice deficient in either receptor have established the importance of balanced function of stimulatory and inhibitory receptors. In vivo murine studies have demonstrated that stimulatory FcγR are both necessary and sufficient to trigger the Arthus reaction, autoimmune glomerulonephritis, cytopenia, and antigen-induced arthritis.[9] In contrast, mice deficient in inhibitory FcγR demonstrate enhanced antibody responses, a proclivity to autoimmunity, and increased inflammation in all three types of antibody-mediated hypersensitivity reactions.[9–12] Given that inhibitory and stimulatory FcγR are often coexpressed, the effector response to a specific stimulus in a particular cell represents the balance between stimulatory and inhibitory signals. Therapeutic interventions to alter this balance may minimize FcγR-mediated tissue damage, maintain tolerance, and influence antibody repertoire.

FcγR STRUCTURE AND EXPRESSION

FcγR are encoded by members of the immunoglobulin superfamily of genes. In humans, eight genes for FcγR are clustered on the long arm of chromosome 1 (1221–23). Extensive structural diversity among FcγR family members leads to differences in ligand-binding capacity, distinct signal transduction pathways, and cell-type-specific expression patterns.[1–3,8] Such diversity allows IgG complexes to activate a broad program of cell functions relevant to autoimmunity, inflammation, and host defense against microbes and cancer. In addition, allelic variation within genes provides an inherited basis for a predisposition to inflammatory diseases.

The three families of FcγR – FcγRI, FcγRII and FcγRIII (Figure 10.1) – are encoded by distinct

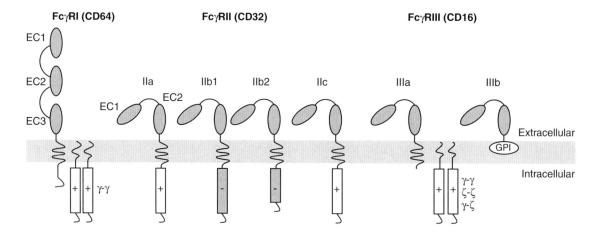

Figure 10.1 Schematic representation of the human FcγR receptor family members. FcγR α-chains contain two or three disulfide-linked immunoglobulin-like extracellular domains (ellipses) which mediate binding to IgG. The cytoplasmic domains of FcγR or their associated subunits are responsible for signal transduction. FcγRIIIb is the only FcγR that lacks a cytoplasmic tail. FcγRI and FcγRIIIa are multichain receptors that associate with immunoreceptor tyrosine-based activation motif (ITAM)-bearing γ- or ζ-chain dimers (white rectangles) to mediate positive signaling. FcγRIIa and FcγRIIc are single-chain stimulatory receptors containing ITAM motifs in their cytoplasmic tails. FcγRIIb1 and FcγRIIb2 are single-chain inhibitory receptors containing immunoreceptor tyrosine-based inhibitory motif (ITIM) motifs in their cytoplasmic tail (grey rectangles).

genes on human chromosome 1. As members of the immunoglobulin supergene family, these families share the common structural motif of two or three immunoglobulin-like disulfide-linked domains in the extracellular portion of the receptor. While these receptors share similar (though not identical) extracellular domains, their transmembrane and cytoplasmic tails are very different (Figure 10.1). Such diversity is responsible for the variety of functions that these receptors can elicit.

Stimulatory FcγR

Stimulatory FcγR trigger cellular activation. They possess intracellular activation motifs, termed immunoreceptor tyrosine-based activation motifs (ITAMs), similar to those of B-cell receptors (BCRs) and T-cell receptors (TCRs).[13,14] Stimulatory FcγR, expressed predominantly on myeloid cells, are typically multichain receptors composed of a ligand-binding α-subunit, which confers ligand specificity and affinity, and associated signaling subunits with ITAMs in the cytoplasmic domain (Figure 10.1). The α-

subunits, encoded by seven genes, are transmembrane molecules that share the structural motif of two or three extracellular immunoglobulin-like domains, but vary in their affinity for IgG and in their preference for binding different IgG subclasses (IgG$_1$, IgG$_2$, IgG$_3$ and IgG$_4$). Allelic variations in the ligand-binding region of specific FcγR that influence their ability to bind certain IgG subclasses and dramatically alter the effector responses of phagocytes to IgG-opsonized antigens have been described (Figure 10.2).[15-18] The transmembrane domains of the α subunits contain a basic residue that mediates the interaction with associated signaling chains required for efficient expression and signal transduction.

The two multichain FcγR isoforms are termed FcγRI, a high-affinity receptor for IgG that binds monomeric IgG, and FcγRIIIa, an intermediate-affinity receptor that binds only multivalent IgG. Homodimeric γ-chains are transducing modules for FcγRI and FcγRIIIa on mononuclear phagocytes (Figure 10.1). Heterodimers of γ–ζ chains or ζ–ζ-chain homodimers can also transduce signals through FcγRIIIa in human natural killer (NK)

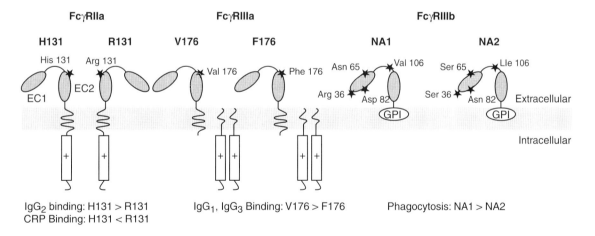

Figure 10.2 Allelic variants of human FcγR. The FcγRIIa polymorphism is a consequence of an arginine (R131) to histidine (H131) substitution at amino acid position 131 in the extracellular domain which causes differences in binding affinity for human IgG$_2$ and C-reactive protein (CRP). The FcγRIIIa polymorphism is the consequence of a valine (V176) to phenylalanine (F176) substitution at position 176 leading to changes in binding affinity for human IgG$_1$ and IgG$_3$. The NA1 and NA2 polymorphism of FcγRIIIb reflects four amino acid substitutions with consequent differences in N-linked glycosylation sites and quantitative differences in phagocytic function.

cells. FcγRI, expressed on monocytes, macrophages and interferon gamma (IFN-γ)-stimulated polymorphonuclear leukocytes, is distinguished by three extracellular, immunoglobulin-like domains and high affinity for IgG. It is the only FcγR that binds monomeric IgG, and it is also a receptor for C-reactive protein (CRP).[19] FcγRI triggers phagocyte activation and may play a role in antigen processing on monocytes, macrophages, and dendritic cells. FcγRIIIa, found on NK cells and mononuclear phagocytes (including mesangial cells), is an intermediate-affinity receptor. FcγRIIIa displays codominantly expressed biallelic variants, F176 and V176, which differ in one amino acid at position 176 in the extracellular domain (phenylalanine or valine, respectively), leading to differences in IgG$_1$ and IgG$_3$ binding: V176 homozygotes bind IgG$_1$ and IgG$_3$ more avidly than F176 (Figure 10.2).[18,20] This variability in IgG binding has implications for antibody-mediated immune surveillance, ADCC, antibody-mediated host defense against pathogens, and autoimmune disease. The low-binding FcγRIIIa–F176 allele has been associated with SLE, the prototypic immune complex disease, and this gene may constitute an inherited susceptibility factor in some populations.[18,21,22]

It is thought that immune complexes present within the joints of patients with RA activate macrophages to promote articular damage. In murine models of RA, FcγRIIIa is required for cartilage damage.[23–25] A study of the distribution of FcγRIIIa variants in patients with RA showed an increased frequency of genotypes homozygous for FcγRIIIa–F176.[26] The mechanism by which the low-binding FcγR allele expressed on macrophages and NK cells influences disease pathogenesis is unclear.

In addition to multichain receptors, there are three other types of activating FcγR, all unique to humans: FcγRIIa, FcγRIIc, and FcγRIIIb. FcγRIIa and FcγRIIc are highly homologous, single-chain, low-affinity receptors that include an extracellular ligand-binding domain and ITAM in the cytoplasmic domain (Figure 10.1). FcγRIIa is widely expressed, and is present on neutrophils (PMN), monocytes, macrophages, eosinophils, mast cells, dendritic cells and platelets. It interacts most effectively with multivalent IgG immune complexes and IgG-opsonized particles. There are two codominantly expressed allelic forms of FcγRIIa (H131 and R131), which differ at amino acid position 131 in the extracellular domain (histidine or arginine, respectively), a region that strongly influences ligand binding (Figure 10.2). These allelic variants differ substantially in their ability to bind human IgG$_2$.[15,17] H131 is the high-binding allele, R131 is low binding, while heterozygotes have intermediate function. Because IgG$_2$ is a poor activator of the classical complement pathway, FcγRIIa–H131 is essential for handling IgG$_2$-opsonized antigens. FcγRIIa has considerable clinical importance for host defense against infection, with encapsulated bacteria known to elicit IgG$_2$ responses and for removal of immune complexes of self-antigens and IgG$_2$-containing autoantibodies.[1,27] Low-binding FcγRIIIa–R131 alleles are enriched in certain groups of SLE patients, particularly in patients with IgG$_2$ anti-C1q antibodies.[28–31] That FcγRIIa is the main receptor for CRP, taken together with the recent report of a reciprocal relationship between the binding affinities of IgG$_2$ and CRP for FcγRIIa alleles, raises the possibility that handling of nucleosomes bound to CRP may also be influenced by allelic polymorphisms[32,33] (Figure 10.2).

FcγRIIIb provides the most dramatic example of structural divergence within the FcγR family. It has neither an ITAM nor a transmembrane domain, but is retained in the plasma membrane outer leaflet by a glycosyl phosphatidylinositol anchor (Figure 10.1). FcγRIIIb, expressed exclusively on PMN, is a low-affinity receptor that, like FcγRII, binds immune complexes. There are two alleles of FcγRIIIb (termed NA1 and NA2, reflecting their initial description as neutrophil-associated antigens). They differ by five nucleotides, which results in a substitution of four amino acids in the membrane-distant first extracellular domain.[34] Neutrophils from NA1-homozygous individuals have more robust FγR-mediated phagocytic responses and a greater capacity for PMN priming, despite comparable expression and equivalent ligand binding by NA1 and NA2.[16,35,36] As in the polymorphisms of FcγRIIA and FcγRIIIA, FcγRIIIb, alleles are expressed in a codominant fashion (Figure 10.2).

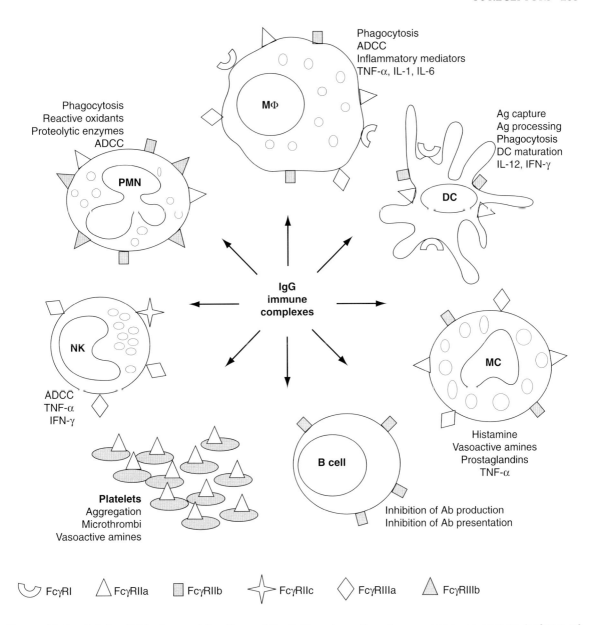

Figure 10.3 Cellular distribution and functions of FcγR. Hematopoetic cells expressing one or more isoforms of FcγR: monocytes and macrophages (Mφ), dendritic cells (DC), mast cells (MC), B lymphocytes (B), platelets, natural killer cells (NK) and polymorphonuclear leukocytes (PMN). The effects of FcγR engagement by immune complexes are cell specific. TNF, tumor necrosis factor; IFN, interferon; IL, interleukin; Ab, antibody; Ag, antigen.

Biological responses triggered by stimulatory FcγR appear to depend more on the cells that express the receptor than on the receptor itself (Figure 10.3). For example, macrophages, the most efficient professional phagocytes, express FcγRIa, FcγRIIa, and FcγRIIIa, each of which initiates the same responses in these cells: internalization, respiratory burst, release of proteases and lipid mediators, and production of inflammatory cytokines. On PMN, both FcγRIIa and FcγRIIIb work in concert to activate the neutrophil to generate reactive oxidants, release granular contents, and internalize opsonized antigens. In Wegener's granulomatosis, antineutrophil cytoplasmic antibodies engage both FcγRIIa and FcγRIIIb on neutrophils to trigger cell activation.[37] Conversely, when expressed on different cells, a particular receptor isoform triggers cell-type-specific functions. Thus, while FcγRIIa trigger respiratory burst and internalization by neutrophils, on platelets they trigger aggregation and degranulation. Activating FcγR on mast cells triggers the secretion of tumor necrosis factor alpha (TNF-α), which contributes to the pathogenesis of autoantibody-mediated vasculitis.[38] On dendritic cells, ITAM-bearing FcγR mediate endocytic transport of antigen–antibody complexes and induce efficient processing and presentation of antigen[39] (Figure 10.3). Murine studies have shown that targeting different FcγR results in the selection of different epitopes for presentation.[39,40] Internalization of immune complexes via activating FcγR appears to influence the epitopes that are presented by antigen-presenting cells, and thus alter the T-cell response, particularly when otherwise cryptic epitopes are revealed. Such targeting of antigens at specific FcγR might prove an effective strategy to enhance the response to vaccination.

Soluble FcγR

Normal sera contain soluble FcγRII and FcγRIII, derived either from alternative splicing of mRNA (FcγRIIa) or from proteolytic release from circulating cells (FcγRIII).[41,42] It has been proposed that one biological function of plasma FcγR is to suppress IgG production on B cells. A striking property of soluble FcγRII is its ability to completely suppress immune complex-induced inflammation in the reverse passive Arthus reaction.[43] Soluble FcγRIIIb may also modulate PMN function through interactions between the lectin-like domain of PMN complement receptor 3 (CR3) and the carbohydrates on

soluble receptors. However, the physiologic significance of these circulating IgG-binding proteins in IgG production and immune complex handling is not yet clear. Soluble FcγR binding to immune complexes might affect their clearance by changing the size of complexes, altering their solubility, or modifying their ability to activate complement and capture C3b and, in consequence, altering their capacity to interact with surface FcγR and complement receptors. Soluble FcγR, chosen for specific binding properties (such FcγRIIa–H131, which recognizes IgG₂), could be a useful treatment for diseases induced by autoantibodies.

Inhibitory FcγR

Inhibitory FcγR, FcγRIIb, are single-chain low-affinity receptors characterized by extracellular domains highly homologous to their activating counterparts and cytoplasmic domains containing an immunoreceptor tyrosine-based inhibitory motif (ITIM) (Figure 10.1). They are encoded by a single gene on chromosome 1q23–24. Alternative splicing generates two isoforms, FcγRIIb1 and FcγRIIb2, which differ in their intracytoplasmic regions, their cellular expression, and their functional capacities.[44] FcγRIIb1 contains an insertion of 19 amino acids. FcγRIIb2 participates in endocytosis of multivalent ligands by phagocytes and antigen-presenting cells, while the intracytoplasmic insertion of FcγRIIb1 inhibits internalization.[45] Neither isoform can trigger cell activation. Instead, both isoforms of FcγRIIb are negative regulators of activation. In order to inhibit cell activation, a multivalent ligand must co-aggregate FcγRIIb with the activation-inducing ITAM-expressing receptors.[2,8] FcγRIIb can modulate cell activation by stimulatory FcγR as well as responses triggered by BCRs and Fc receptors for IgE.[46,47]

FcγRIIb1 is present only on B cells and it is the only FcγR expressed on B lymphocytes. FcγRIIb1 influences the state of B-cell activation and B-cell survival. Coligation of FcγRIIb1 with BCRs by antibody–antigen complexes inhibits B-cell proliferation and antibody production.[48,49] Because follicular dendritic cells retain antigen in the form of immune complexes, antigen can interact with B cells either through BCRs and FcγRIIb1 (when there is high-affinity cognate antigen binding) or through FcγRIIb1 alone (low-affinity cognate antigen binding). In the germinal center, coligation of BCR and FcγRIIb1 promotes B-cell survival, whereas homo-aggregation of FcγRIIb is a proapoptotic signal.[49] FcγRIIb1 can therefore provide a mechanism to discriminate between the rare, somatically mutated germinal center B cells and the predominant population of B cells, with low affinity antigen binding and potentially cross-reactive specificities. Thus FcγRIIb1 can contribute to affinity maturation of B cells and maintenance of peripheral tolerance by promoting deletion of low-affinity self-reactive lymphocytes.

FcγRIIb2, expressed on most myeloid cells, regulates the threshold and magnitude of immune complex-initiated inflammatory responses (Figure 10.3). For example, co-aggregation of FcγRIIb2 with FcγRIIa by IgG-opsonized particles blocks phagocytosis and generation of reactive oxygen intermediates.[50] FcγRIIb-mediated negative regulation of ITAM-dependent cell activation endows IgG-containing immune complexes with the capacity to regulate B cells and inflammatory cells.[48] As yet, deficiency of inhibitory FcγRIIb function in antibody-mediated human disease has not been reported. Since the balance between stimulatory and inhibitory input determines cellular response, altering this balance represents a strategy for treating rheumatic disease.

FcRn

FcRn, initially identified as the neonatal gut IgG transport receptor, is now recognized as an integral part of the mechanism that prevents catabolism of IgG.[51–53] It is a heterodimer of β_2-microglobulin and an α-chain closely related to MHC class I, that binds IgG most efficiently in the acidic milieu of the endosome. FcRn is expressed ubiquitously in adult tissues, with particularly high levels on endothelial cells, considered by some investigators to be the site of IgG homeostasis.

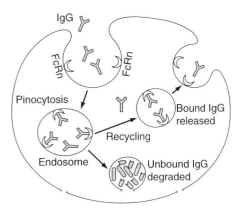

Figure 10.4 FcRn as an IgG homeostat. Endothelial cells, on which FcRn is highly expressed, internalize IgG through pinocytosis. In the acidic environment of the endosome, IgG molecules bind FcRn. Bound IgG is recycled in its transport vesicle and released at the neutral pH of the cell surface, which is not permissive of the IgG–FcRn interaction. Unbound IgG is transferred to lysosomes for degradation.

A model for how FcRn might function as an IgG homeostat is shown in Figure 10.4. IgG is taken up from plasma by endothelial cells through non-specific pinocytosis and then enters acidic endosomes. The IgG that binds to FcRn in the endocytic vesicles is salvaged from lysosomal degradation and subsequently returned intact to the circulation. In the absence of such a protective mechanism, IgG that entered the lysosome would be degraded. This model describes how FcRn acts as a finely tuned homeostat to regulate serum IgG levels.[51,52] As IgG levels increase, more FcRn becomes saturated and an increased proportion of pinocytosed IgG is degraded. Thus, individual IgG molecules are eliminated from the circulation in direct proportion to their concentration in plasma.

Saturation of FcRn in hypergammaglobulinemia accelerates catabolism of IgG and may explain the temporary benefit from intravenous gammaglobulin in autoimmune diseases characterized by type II and type II hypersensitivity reactions.[54] The discovery that FcRn regulates plasma IgG levels has provided a new target for depleting pathogenic IgG in antibody-mediated autoimmune disease.

FcγR SIGNALING

Stimulatory FcγR

Effector cell activation is initiated when FcγR are clustered at the cell surface by multivalent antigen–antibody complexes. The requirement for crosslinking of at least two receptors on the cell surface in order to trigger intracellular signaling prevents circulating IgG from stimulating cells in the absence of antigen. Although stimulatory FcγR have no intrinsic enzymatic activity, they are associated with membrane-anchored Src family kinases. The cytoplasmic domain of FcγR, or their associated signaling subunits, contains the ITAM, common to numerous immunologically important receptors, including TCRs and BCRs. The ITAM is characterized by a tyrosine–X–X–leucine repeat (where X is any amino acid) separated by seven variable residues (or 12 in the case of FcγRIIa and FcγRIIc).[1-3] Crosslinking of the ligand-binding extracellular domains leads to phosphorylation of the ITAM by members of the Src family of tyrosine kinases, but the specific kinases involved vary with different cell types. For example, FcγRIIIa aggregation activates Lck in NK cells, while FcγRIIa or FcγRIIIa activate Lyn and Hck in monocytes and mast cells.[55,56]

Phosphorylated tyrosine–X–X–leucine forms a docking site for other signaling intermediates which contain a Src-homology domain type 2 (SH2), most notably Syk family of tyrosine kinases. That each ITAM-containing molecule differs in the flanking amino acids provides specificity in the recruitment of additional signaling intermediates and in subsequent downstream signaling events. For instance, Syk is activated in mast cells and macrophages, whereas the related kinase ZAP70 is activated in NK cells.[56,57] Subsequent signaling pathways associated with cellular activation by FcγR are similar to those described for other ITAM-containing receptors, including BCRs and TCRs.

Tyrosine kinases phosphorylate many intracellular substrates, including phospholipid kinases, phospholipases, adaptor molecules, and cytoskeletal proteins. Activation of phosphatase C and phosphatidylinositol-3 kinase (P13K) by Syk leads to the production of phosphoinositol messengers and a sustained increase in cytoplasmic Ca^{2+} [59] (Figure 10.5a). Recruitment of the adaptor protein Shc allows signals triggered by FcγR to reach the nucleus via the ras pathway, leading to phosphorylation of MAP kinase, activation of transcription factors, and induction of gene expression.[60] These critical signaling molecules are potential targets for pharmacologic inhibition of immune complex-initiated inflammation, and such a therapeutic approach could be narrowly focused, based on distinctive signaling elements that characterize the various cell types.

The mechanism by which the glycosyl-phosphatidylinositol-linked FcγRIIIb engages intracellular signaling molecules is still unknown. Possibilities include interaction with another transmembrane protein, direct association with an Src-family kinase residing in membrane lipid domains, or an extracellular carbohydrate–lectin interaction with CR3.

Figure 10.5 Signaling pathways triggered by co-aggregation of positive- and negative-signaling FcγR. (a) Crosslinking of stimulatory FcγR leads to (1) phosphorylation (P) of the tyrosines in the ITAM motif by Src kinases, (2) recruitment of the SH2-domain tyrosine kinase Syk, and (3) activation of PI3 kinase (PI3K). This leads to a series of downstream events that result in an influx of calcium from intracellular and extracellular sources, cytoskeletal changes, release of inflammatory mediators, and activation of transcription factors. (b) Co-aggregation of inhibitory FcγRIIb with ITAM-bearing FcγR leads to (1) phosphorylation of tyrosine in the ITIM, (2) recruitment of the SH2-domain inositol phosphatase SHIP, and (3) hydrolysis of phosphatidylinositol-3,4,5-triphosphate (PIP_3) into phosphatidylinositol-4,5-biphosphate (PIP_2). The latter results in abrogation of Ca^{2+} influx and inhibition of the downstream events of activation cascade.

Since most cells express more than one FcγR isoform, it is likely that antigen–antibody complexes co-aggregate more than one type of receptor. Co-clustering of stimulatory FcγR represents a mechanism whereby different FcγR cooperate to amplify signals and produce more efficient activation of effector cells. FcγR that act synergistically transphosphorylate each other,

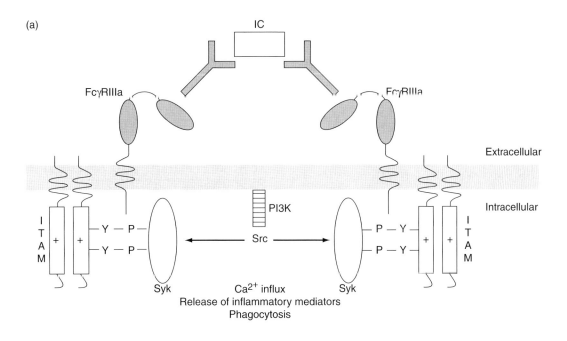

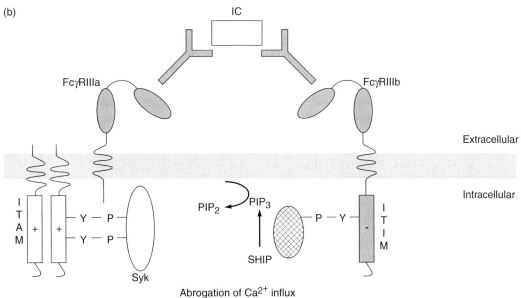

leading to activation of tyrosine kinases and downstream substrates and initiation of $[Ca^{2+}]_i$ transients, with subsequent cytoskeletal changes and transcriptional activation (Figure 10.5a).

Inhibitory FcγR

FcγRIIb isoforms are important negative regulators of ITAM-dependent activation and establish the threshold for effector cell activation. Inert when self-aggregated, inhibitory FcγRIIb abolish cellular signals when coligated with stimulatory receptors (Figure 10.5b). The ITIM motif (V/IxYxxL: valine/isoleucine–X–tyrosine–X–X–leucine), contained in a 13 amino acid sequence present in the intracytoplasmic domain of both FcγRIIb1 and FcγRIIb2, is essential for the negative regulatory properties of FcγRIIb and other inhibitory receptors.[61–63] Like ITAMs, ITIMs, once phosphorylated by protein tyrosine kinases, recruit SH2-containing cytoplasmic molecules. By providing activated protein tyrosine kinases to phosphorylate the ITIM of FcγRIIb, stimulatory FcγR play a role in their own inhibition. Thus, inhibitory function requires the recruitment of phosphatases to the phosphorylated ITIM. Although the protein tyrosine phosphatases SHP-1 and SHP-2 bind to FcγRIIb-phosphorylated ITIMs, the inositol phosphorylate-5′-phosphatase SHIP has been shown to be preferentially recruited to FcγRIIb and appears to play the predominant role in FcγRIIb-mediated inhibition by preventing Ca^{2+} influx[64–66] (Figure 10.5b). The importance of SHIP in the transduction of inhibitory signaling by FcγRIIb isoforms has been most carefully studied in B cells and mast cells, but, given that SHIP is expressed in phagocytes, it is also likely to mediate inhibition by FcγRIIb2 in monocytes and PMN. By altering the local composition of the phosphoinositide pools, SHIP regulates membrane targeting of kinases required to open Ca^{2+} channels and allow the influx of extracellular calcium.[67] Blockade of calcium influx inhibits calcium-dependent processes, such as degranulation, phagocytosis, ADCC, and cytokine release. In cells that express both stimulatory and inhibitory receptors for IgG, the relative levels of these two receptor types determine the state of cell activation in response to immune complexes.

Arrest of B-cell proliferation induced by co-crosslinking BCRs with FcγRIIb1 is mediated by a distinct ITIM-dependent pathway that leads to MAP kinase inactivation.[61] A third inhibitory activity of FcγRIIb1, generated by homo-aggregation of FcγRIIb1, produces apoptotic signals in B cells. This mechanism is B-cell specific and ITIM independent. That the proapoptotic signal is blocked by SHIP recruitment (induced when FcγRIIb1 is co-clustered with BCR) suggests a means for maintaining peripheral tolerance of B cells that have undergone hypermutation.[49]

FcγR IN EFFERENT AND AFFERENT RESPONSES: LESSONS FROM FcγR-DEFICIENT MICE

Studies in mice deficient in activating or inhibiting FcγR have revealed the crucial role these receptors play in immune complex-triggered inflammation. Mice with targeted deletion of the γ-subunit of (FcRγ–/–) do not express activating FcγR, FcγRI and FcγRIII. Their macrophages are incapable of FcγR-mediated phagocytosis and, consequently, they manifest reduced autoantibody-dependent experimental hemolytic anemia and thrombocytopenia, antigen–antibody immune complex Arthus reactions, and ADCC against tumor cells.[68–70] Notably, FcRγ–/– mice are protected from fatal glomerulonephritis induced by passive transfer of antiglomerular basement membrane antibodies and severe cartilage destruction in experimental antigen-induced arthritis[23,71] and arthritigenic (anti-glucose-6-phosphate isomerase) antibody-induced disease.[25] In disease models with endogenously generated autoantibodies, such as NZB/NZW, FcRγ–/– mice also have attenuated disease despite the presence of autoantibodies, circulating immune complexes, and glomerular deposition of IgG.[72] These murine models emphasize the importance of FcγR activation in initiating tissue injury at sites of immune complex deposition and identify this class of receptors as targets for interventions to prevent IgG-mediated damage.

Disruption of FcγRIIb by gene targeting has the opposite effect: it is proinflammatory.

FcγRIIb–/– mice have augmented type II and type III hypersensitivity responses, manifested in experimental models by enhanced immune complex-mediated alveolitis and accelerated antibody-induced glomerulonephritis.[10,11,71] Mice deficient in FcγRIIb also show alterations in afferent immune responses. They exhibit elevated IgG levels in response to thymus-dependent and thymus-independent antigens as well as a proclivity towards autoimmunity.[10] For example, mice with MHC class II genes associated with resistance to collagen-induced arthritis are rendered susceptible to autoimmune arthritis when FcγRIIb is deleted.[73] Furthermore, on specific genetic backgrounds, FcγRIIb–/– mice develop autoantibodies and autoimmune glomerulonephritis.[12] This autoimmune phenotype has been shown to be associated with B cells, suggesting that deficiency of FcγRIIb-mediated inhibitory signals in B cells leads to spontaneous autoimmune disease in a strain-dependent fashion. These observations suggest that FcγRIIb plays a role in maintaining immune tolerance and preventing autoimmune disease.

Recent work has revealed that deletions are present in the promoter region of FcγRIIb in all major autoimmune-prone mice strains, underscoring the concept that the balance between stimulatory and inhibitory FcγR is a determinant of susceptibility to and severity of immune complex-induced inflammatory disease. FcγRIIb promoter deletions are associated with a reduction in the expression and function of FcγRIIb on macrophages and activated B cells, defects that would be expected to promote autoimmunity.[74,75] Further studies have shown that FcγRIIb promoter and intronic polymorphisms identified in mice prone to autoimmunity correlate with downregulation of FcγRIIb1 expression on germinal center B cells on stimulation with antigen and upregulation of IgG antibody responses.[76]

REGULATION OF HUMAN FcγR EXPRESSION AND FUNCTION

The total absence of specific FcγR isoforms is extremely rare in humans. Indeed, as a consequence of the redundancy of function among FcγR, individuals identified as lacking certain stimulatory receptors (FcγRI or FcγRIIIb) are generally healthy.[77,78] However, it is possible that differences in the relative expression of ITAM- and ITIM-containing FcγR impact on the susceptibility to and severity of autoimmune disease in a particular individual.

Cytokines elaborated during an immune response have been shown to alter FcγR expression and functional capacity. For example, IFN-γ and granulocyte colony-stimulating factor (G-CSF) upregulate FcγRI on monocytes and induce its expression on PMN, whereas interleukin-4 (IL-4) inhibits the expression of all ITAM-bearing FcγR.[79,80] GM-CSF specifically increases FcγRIIa, and transforming growth factor beta (TGF-β) increases FcγRIIIa.[81] In contrast to their effects on stimulatory receptors, IFN-γ decreases and IL-4 increases the expression of the inhibitory receptor, FcγRIIb2, on circulating human monocytes.[82] That IFN-γ (a prototypic Th1 cytokine) and IL-4 (a prototypic Th2 cytokine) differentially regulate the expression of FcγR isoforms with opposite functions provides a mechanism for regulation of activating and inhibitory signals delivered by FcγR on phagocytes. Hence, cytokines released within the inflammatory milieu act in an autocrine and paracrine manner to modulate effector cell function.

In contrast to cytokine-induced changes in receptor expression, which occur over hours or days, reactive oxidants and proteases modulate FcγR function more rapidly, probably over a time frame of minutes. Reactive oxygen intermediates, such as H_2O_2, augment phagocytosis mediated by FcγRI and FcγRIIa without altering receptor density.[35,83] Serine proteases rapidly activate FcγRIIa-binding capacity and thereby augment effector function, such as TNF-α release.[84] In an inflammatory environment, reactive oxidants and serine proteases secreted by PMN and monocytes rapidly stimulate quiescent cells to increase effector functions. For antimicrobial host defense, oxidant- and protease-initiated increases in phagocytosis are protective. In contrast, at sites of immune complex deposition, such as the kidney in SLE and the joint in RA, augmentation of FcγRI- and FcγRIIa-triggered release of inflammatory mediators is likely to directly promote injury. The definition of oxidants and serine proteases as amplifiers of FcγR function provides distinct new targets for prevention of immune complex-mediated organ damage.

FcγR AS TARGETS FOR TREATMENT OF AUTOIMMUNE DISEASE

The structural heterogeneity and complex nature of FcγR isoforms and their variant alleles reflect the diverse functions mediated by these receptors. Recognition of the role of FcγR in the pathogenesis of immune-mediated disease suggests multiple avenues for potential therapeutic intervention (Table 10.1). That allelic variants of FcγR are considered susceptibility factors or disease accelerants in SLE, RA and

---

Table 10.1   Targeting FcγR to modulate immune responses.

Decrease inflammatory responses triggered by stimulatory FcγR

    Interference with FcγR–ligand interactions

        Soluble FcγR

        Fc domain binding peptides

    Blockade of FcγR

        Monoclonal anti-FcγR antibodies

        Peptide antagonists of FcγR

    Inhibition FcγR signaling

        Selective inhibition of protein tyrosine kinases

        SHIP agonists to block ITAM signaling

        Inhibition of reactive oxidants and serine proteases

Increase anti-inflammatory responses

    Increase in expression of inhibitory FcγR

        Th2 cytokines (IL-4)

        Intravenous gammaglobulin

    Tether activating and inhibiting FcγR with bispecific antibodies

---

Wegener's granulomatosis underscores their importance in the pathogenesis and progression of these diseases.

Interfering with FcγR–IgG interaction can prevent triggering of stimulatory FcγR by immune complexes that initiate tissue injury in SLE and RA. Thus, soluble FcγR may prove to be novel anti-inflammatory agents. In animal models, infusion of soluble FcγR inhibits immune complex-mediated activation of phagocytes by blocking access to FcγR on effector cells. With the development of soluble TNF receptors and soluble complement receptors as therapeutic modalities, one can envision the use of soluble FcγR to block antibody-mediated tissue injury. Indeed, circulating forms of FcγRII and FcγRIII are present in normal individuals.[85,86] The unique properties of different FcγR, such as their affinity and IgG subclass preferences, could be exploited to target specific pathogenic antibodies with specific soluble FcγR variants. One could develop a panel of soluble FcγR with diverse properties, e.g. the H131 allele of FcγRIIa that binds IgG_2 or the F158 allele of FcγRIIIa that binds IgG_1 and IgG_3 with higher affinity, to block FcγR–ligand interactions of specific disease-associated autoantibodies. The striking observation that soluble FcγR block active inflammatory reactions implies that soluble receptors have considerable potential as therapeutic agents. Alternatively, peptides that bind the Fc domain of pathogenic antibodies could be engineered. Such compounds have been shown to prevent disease in MRL/lpr mice[87] and may prove effective in humans.

Infusion of monoclonal antibodies that block the ligand-binding domain of stimulatory FcγR is another approach to inhibit the initiation of effector cell responses to immune complexes. There are reports that anti-FcγRIII and anti-FcγRI antibodies have been used with benefit in small idiopathic thrombocytopenia purpura (ITP).[88] Blockade of FcγR–ligand interactions to prevent phagocytosis of opsonized platelets by splenic and hepatic macrophages has also been achieved in patients with ITP with intravenous gammaglobulin or infusions with anti-D (in Rh-positive individuals).[89] Synthetic peptide ligands that bind FcγR with higher affinity than immune complexes could also be developed for this purpose. Evidence that FcγRIIIa plays a dominant role in murine models of type II and type III hypersensitivity reactions and in murine models of RA argues that receptor-blocking interventions should be directed at FcγRIIIa in these diseases.[8,24] The contribution of FcγRIIa cannot be examined in these models because this receptor is not expressed in mice.

An alternative approach to modulating immune complex triggered inflammation is to alter the balance of stimulatory and inhibitory FcγR expressed on phagocytes with cytokines or pharmacologic agents. The administration of cytokines that increase the ratio of expression of inhibitory FcγR relative to stimulatory FcγR, such as IL-4 and other Th2 cytokines, represents a new approach for the treatment of autoimmune disease.[82] Indeed, a recently described effect of intravenous gammaglobulin, required for successful treatment of ITP in a murine model, is the induction of increased expression of FcγRIIb relative to ITAM-bearing FcγR on monocytes.[90] Because immune complexes can either enhance or suppress the humoral immune response, depending on the FcγR type engaged and the cell type involved (B cells or antigen-presenting cells), alterations in the balance of FcγR expression can also influence afferent responses.

Downregulation of FcγR γ-chain and FcγRIIa downstream signaling pathways or upregulation of the FcγRIIb inhibitory pathway would also limit antibody-mediated damage. Targeted pharmacologic inhibition of protein tyrosine kinases or phosphatases could block ITAM signaling. The fact that different Src family tyrosine kinases characterize cells provides focused targets for signaling blockade. The development of therapeutics specifically for FcγRIIb or its effector SHIP may also lead to effective treatments for immune complex-mediated inflammation. These could include biologics, such as bispecific antibodies that constitutively tether activating and inhibiting receptors such that normally activating stimuli trigger the inhibitory loop, and

small molecule agonists of SHIP, to inhibit all signaling responses initiated by ITAM-bearing receptors.

An alternative approach to limit FcγR–immune complex interactions is to decrease the levels of autoantibodies by targeting FcRn. Intravenous gammaglobulin has been shown to accelerate catabolism of IgG, presumably by saturating FcRn and permitting degradation of IgG to occur in proportion to its total concentration in the plasma, leading to preferential removal of high titer autoantibodies[54] (Figure 10.4). Novel strategies for the depletion of IgG include neutralizing monoclonal antibodies designed to modify FcRn covalently, synthetic peptide ligands with a higher affinity than IgG for FcRn to saturate FcRn, and antisense nucleotides to downregulate the expression of FcRn.

Recent advances in understanding the interactions between FcγR and IgG based on the crystal structures of FcγR family members may make it possible to design Fc regions of chimeric proteins to discriminate among FcγR isoforms and alleles or even block FcγR-binding sites.[6,7] For example, to minimize cell depletion as a consequence of treatment with Fc-containing proteins, such as T-cell-targeted antibodies, the Fc portion might be modified to prevent its binding to cell surface FcγR. Alternatively, to optimize in vivo cytotoxicity against specific cell populations, the Fc portion of an antibody or chimeric protein could be fashioned to bind preferentially to activating FcγR and minimally to inhibitory FcγR.[70] In addition, altering the interaction of a therapeutic IgG with FcRn could increase its survival in the serum. Ultimately, the specificity of biological agents administered therapeutically will vary with the receptor to be targeted and the FcγR genotypes of the host. The opportunities for therapeutic intervention are abundant and wide-ranging.

SUMMARY

The structural diversity of FcγR provides a mechanism by which IgG can elicit a broad range of cell responses. FcγR vary in their affinity for IgG, their preference for IgG subclasses, the cell types where they are expressed, and the intracellular signals which they elicit – stimulatory or inhibitory. Rapid expansion in our knowledge of their structure–function relationships has identified FcγR as valuable targets for therapeutic modulation of the immune system.

REFERENCES

1. Salmon JE, Pricop L. Human receptors for immunoglobulin G. Key elements in the pathogenesis of rhematic disease. *Arthritis Rheum* 2000; **44**: 739–50.

2. Daeron M. Fc receptor biology. *Annu Rev Immunol* 1997; **15**: 203–34.

3. Hulett MD, Hogarth PM. Molecular basis of Fc receptor function. *Adv Immunol* 1994; **57**: 1–127.

4. Brooks DG, Qiu WQ, Luster AD et al. Structure and expression of human IgG FcRII(CD32). Functional heterogeneity is encoded by the alternatively spliced products of multiple genes. *J Exp Med* 1989; **170**: 1369–85.

5. Hibbs ML, Bonandonna L, Scott BM et al. Molecular cloning of a human immunoglobulin G Fc receptor. *Proc Natl Acad Sci USA* 1988; **85**: 2240–4.

6. Sondermann P, Huber R, Jacob U. Crystal structure of the soluble form of the human FcγRIIb: a new member of the immunoglobulin superfamily at 1.7 A resolution. *EMBO J* 1999; **18**: 1095–103.

7. Maxwell KF, Powell MS, Hulett MD et al. Crystal structure of the human leukocyte Fc receptor, FcγRIIa. *Nat Struct Biol* 1999; **6**: 437–42.

8. Ravetch JV, Bolland S. IgG Fc receptors. *Annu Rev Immunol* 2001; **19**: 275–90.

9. Ravetch JV, Clynes RA. Divergent roles for Fc receptors and complement in vivo. *Annu Rev Immunol* 1998; **16**: 421–32.

10. Takai T, Ono M, Hikida M, Ohmori H, Ravetch JV. Augmented humoral and anaphylactic responses in Fc gamma RII-deficient mice. *Nature* 1996; **379**: 346–9.

11. Glynes R, Maizes JS, Guinamard R, Ono M, Takai T, Ravetch JV. Modulation of immune complex-induced inflammation in vivo by the coordinate expression of activation and inhibitory Fc receptors. *J Exp Med* 1999; **189**: 179–86.

12. Bolland S, Ravetch JV. Spontaneous autoimmune disease in Fc(gamma)RIIB-deficient mice results from strain-specific epistasis. *Immunity* 2000; **13**: 277–85.

13. Van den Herik-Oudijk IE, Capel PJ, van der Bruggen T, Van de Winkel JG. Identification of signaling motifs within human Fc gamma RIIa and Fc gamma RIIb isoforms. *Blood* 1995; **85**: 2202–11.

14. Gambier JC. Antigen and Fc receptor signaling. The awesome power of the immunoreceptor tyrosine-based activation motif (ITAM). *J Immunol* 1995; **155**: 3281–5.

15. Warmerdam PA, van de Winkel JG, Vlug A et al. A single amino acid in the second Ig-like domain of the human Fc gamma receptor II is critical for human IgG2 binding. *J Immunol* 1991; **147**: 1338–43.

16. Salmon JE, Edberg JC, Brogle NL, Kimberly RP. Allelic polymorphisms of human Fc gamma receptor IIA and Fc gamma receptor IIIB. Independent mechanisms for differences in human phagocyte function. *J Clin Invest* 1992; **89**: 1274–81.

17. Salmon JE, Millard S, Schachter LA et al. Fc gamma RIIa alleles are heritable risk factors for lupus nephritis in African Americans. *J Clin Invest* 1996; **97**: 1348–54.

18. Wu J, Edberg JC, Redecha PB et al. A novel polymorphism of FcgammaRIIIa (CD16) alters receptor function and predisposes to autoimmune disease. *J Clin Invest* 1997; **100**: 1059–70.

19. Marnell LL, Mold C, Volzer MA et al. C-reactive protein binds to Fc gamma RI in transfected COS cells. *J Immunol* 1995; **155**: 2185–93.

20. Koene HR, Kleijer M, Algra J et al. Fc gammaRIIIa–158V/F polymorphism influences the binding of IgG by natural killer cell Fc gammaRIIIa, independently of the Fc GammaRIIIa–48L/R/H phenotype. *Blood* 1997; **90**: 1109–14.

21. Koene HR, Kleijer M, Swaak AJ et al. The Fc gammaRIIIA–158F allele is a risk factor for systemic lupus erythematosus. *Arthritis Rheum* 1998; **41**: 1813–18.

22. Lehrnbecher T, Foster CB, Zhu S et al. Variant genotypes of the low-affinity Fcgamma receptors in two control populations and a review of low-affinity Fcgamma receptor polymorphisms in control and disease populations. *Blood* 1999; **94**: 4220–32.

23. Van Lent PL, Van Vuuren AJ, Blom AB et al. Role of Fc receptor gamma chain in inflammation and cartilage damage during experimental antigen-induced arthritis. *Arthritis Rheum* 2000; **43**: 740–52.

24. Kleinau S, Martinsson P, Heyman B. Induction and suppression of collagen-induced arthritis is dependent on distinct Fcγ receptors. *J Exp Med* 2000; **191**: 1611–16.

25. Ji H, Ohmura K, Mahmood U et al. Arthritis critically dependent on innate immune system players. *Immunity* 2002; **16**: 157–68.

26. Nieto A, Caliz R, Pascual M et al. Involvement of Fc gamma receptor IIIA genotypes in susceptibility to rheumatoid arthritis. *Arthritis Rheum* 2000; **43**: 735–9.

27. Yee AM, Ng SC, Sobel RE, Salmon JE. Fc gammaRIIA polymorphism as a risk factor for invasive pneumococcal infections in systemic lupus erythematosus. *Arthritis Rheum* 1997; **40**: 1180–2.

28. Haseley LA, Wisnieski JJ, Denburg MR et al. Antibodies to C1q in systemic lupus erythematosus: characteristics and relation to Fc gamma RIIA alleles. *Kidney Int* 1997; **52**: 4075–82.

29. Norsworthy P, Theodoridis E, Botto M et al. Over-representation of the Fcgamma receptor type IIa R131/R131 genotype in caucasoid systemic lupus erythematosus patients with autoantibodies to C1q and glomerulonephritis. *Arthritis Rheum* 1999; **42**: 1828–32.

30. Manger K, Repp R, Spriewald BM et al. Fcgamma receptor IIa polymorphism in Caucasian patients with systemic lupus erythematosus: association with clinical symptoms. *Arthritis Rheum* 1998; **41**: 1181–9.

31. Song YW, Han CW, Kang SW et al. Abnormal distribution of Fc gamma receptor type IIa polymorphisms in Korean patients with systemic lupus erythematosus. *Arthritis Rheum* 1998; **41**: 421–6.

32. Stein MP, Edberg JC, Kimberly RP et al. C-reactive protein binding to FcgammaRIIa on human monocytes and neutrophils is allele-specific. *J Clin Invest* 2000; **105**: 369–76.

33. Bharadwaj D, Stein MP, Volzer M, Mold C, Du Clos TW. The major receptor for C-reactive protein on leukocytes is Fcgamma receptor II. *J Exp Med* 1999; **190**: 585–90.

34. Ory PA, Goldstein IM, Kwoh EE, Clarkson SB. Characterization of polymorphic forms of Fc receptor III on human neutrophils. *J Clin Invest* 1989; **83**: 1676–81.

35. Salmon JE, Edberg JC, Kimberly RP. Fc gamma receptor III on human neutrophils. Allelic variants have functionally distinct capacities. *J Clin Invest* 1990; **85**: 1287–95.

36. Salmon JE, Millard SS, Brogle NL, Kimberly RP. Fc gamma receptor IIIb enhances Fc gamma receptor IIa function in an oxidant-dependent and allele-sensitive manner. *J Clin Invest* 1995; **95**: 2877.

37. Kocher M, Edberg JC, Fleit HB, Kimberly RP. Antineutrophil cytoplasmic antibodies preferentially engage Fc gamma RIIIB on human neutrophils. *J Immunol* 1998; **161**: 6909–14.

38. Watanabe N, Akikusa B, Park SY et al. Mast cells induce autoantibody-mediated vasculitis syndrome through tumor necrosis factor production upon triggering Fcgamma receptors. *Blood* 1999; **94**: 3855–63.

39. Amigorena S, Bonnerot C. Fc receptor signaling and trafficking: a connection for antigen processing. *Immunol Rev* 1999; **172**: 279–84.

40. Regnault A, Lankar D, Lacabanne V et al. Fcγ receptor-mediated induction of dendritic cell maturation and major histocompatibility complex class I-restricted antigen presentation after immune-complex internalization. *J Exp Med* 1999; **189**: 371–80.

41. Huizinga TW, de Haas M, Kleijer M et al. Soluble Fc gamma receptor III in human plasma originates from release by neutrophils. *J Clin Invest* 1990; **86**: 416–23.

42. Galon J, Paulet P, Galinha A et al. Soluble Fc gamma receptors: interaction with ligands and biological consequences. *Int Rev Immunol* 1997; **16**: 87–111.

43. Ierino FL, Powell MS, McKenzie IF, Hogarth PM. Recombinant soluble human Fc gamma RII: production, characterization, and inhibition of the Arthus reaction. *J Exp Med* 1993; **178**: 1617–28.

44. Brooks DG, Qiu WQ, Luster AD, Ravetch JV. Structure and expression of human IgG FcRII(CD32). Functional heterogeneity is encoded by the alternatively spliced products of multiple genes. *J Exp Med* 1989; **170**: 1369–85.

45. Van Den Herik-Oudijk IE, Westerdaal NA, Henriquez NV et al. Functional analysis of human Fc gamma RII (CD32). *J Immunol* 1994; **152**: 574–85.

46. Daeron M, Malbec O, Latour S et al. Regulation of high-affinity IgE receptor-mediated mast cell activation by murine low-affinity IgG receptors. *J Clin Invest* 1995; **95**: 577–85.

47. Daeron M, Latour S, Malbec O et al. The same tyrosine-based inhibition motif, in the intracytoplasmic domain of Fc RIIB, regulates negatively BCR-, TCR-, and FcR-dependent cell activation. *Immunity* 1995; **3**: 635–46.
48. Phillips NE, Parker DC. Cross-linking of B lymphocyte Fc gamma receptors and membrane immunoglobulin inhibits anti-immunoglobulin-induced blastogenesis. *J Immunol* 1984; **132**: 627–32.
49. Pearse RN, Kawabe T, Bolland S et al. SHIP recruitment attenuates FcγRIIB-induced B cell apoptosis. *Immunity* 1999; **10**: 753–60.
50. Hunters S, Indik ZK, Kim MK et al. Inhibition of Fcgamma receptor-mediated phagocytosis by a nonphagocytic Fcgamma receptor. *Blood* 1998; **91**: 1762–8.
51. Ghetie V, Ward ES. Multiple roles for the major histocompatibility complex class I-related receptor FcRn. *Annu Rev Immunol* 2000; **18**: 739–66.
52. Sell S, Fahey JL. Relationship between γ-globulin metabolism and low serum γ-globulin in germ-free mice. *J Immunol* 1964; **93**: 81–7.
53. Junghan RP, Anderson CL. The protection receptor for IgG catabolism is the β2-microglobulin containing neonatal interstinal transport receptor. *Proc Natl Acad Sci USA* 1996; **93**: 5512–16.
54. Yu Z, Lennon VA. Mechanism of intravenous immune globulin therapy in antibody-mediated autoimmune diseases. *N Engl J Med* 1999; **340**: 227–8.
55. Ghazizadeh S, Bolen JB, Fleit HB. Physical and functional association of Src-related protein tyrosine kinases with FcγRII in monocytic THP-1 cells. *J Biol Chem* 1994; **269**: 8878–84.
56. Salcedo TW, Kurosaki T, Kanakara J et al. Physical and functional association of p56lck with FcγRIIIA (CD16) in natuiral killer cells. *J Exp Med* 1993; **177**: 1475–80.
57. Agarwal A, Salem P, Robbins KC. Involveent of p72syk, a protein kinase, in Fcγ receptor signaling. *J Biol Chem* 1999; **268**: 15900–5.
58. Cone JC, Lu Y, Trevillyan JM et al. Association of the p56lck protein tyrosine kinase with the FcγRIIIa/CD16 complex in human natural killer cells. *Eur J Immunol* 1993; **23**: 2488–97.
59. Lowry MB, Duchemin AM, Coggeshall KM et al. Chimeric receptors composed of phosphoinositide 3-linase domains and Fcγ receptor ligand-binding domains mediate phagocytosis in COS fibroblasts. *J Biol Chem* 1998; **273**: 24513–20.
60. Karimi K, Lennartz MR. Mitogen-activated protein kinase is activated during IgG-mediated phagocytosis, but is not required for target ingestion. *Inflammation* 1998; **22**: 67–82.
61. Bolland S, Ravtech JV. Inhibitory pathways triggered by ITIM-containing receptors. *Adv Immunol* 1999; **72**: 149–77.
62. Malbec O, Fridman WH, Daeron M. Negative regulation of hematopoietic cell activation and proliferation by Fc gamma RIIB. *Curr Top Microbiol Immunol* 1994; **244**: 13–27.
63. Coggeshall KM. Negative signaling in health and disease. *Immunol Res* 1999; **19**: 47–64.
64. Ono M, Bollard S, Tempst P, Ravetch JV. Role of the inositol phosphatase SHIP in negative regulation of the immune system by the receptor FcγRIIB. *Nature* 1996; **383**: 263–6.
65. Bolland S, Pearse RN, Kurosaki T, Ravetch JV. SHIP modulates immune receptor responses by regulating membrane association of Btk. *Immunity* 1998; **8**: 509–16.
66. Chacko GW, Tridandapani S, Damen JE et al. Negative signaling in B lymphocytes induces tyrosine phosphorylation of the 145-kDa inositol polyphosphate 5-phosphatase, SHIP. *J Immunol* 1996; **157**: 2234–8.
67. Scharenberg AM, El-Hillal O, Fruman DA et al. Phosphatidylinositol-3,4,5-trisphosphate (PtdIns-3,4,5-P3)/Tec kinase-dependent calcium signaling pathway: a target for SHIP-mediated inhibitory signals. *EMBO J* 1998; **17**: 1961–72.
68. Sylvestre DL, Ravetch JV. Fc receptors initiate the Arhtus reaction: redefining the inflammatory cascade. *Science* 1994; **265**: 1095–8.
69. Clynes R, Ravetch JV. Cytotoxic antibodies trigger inflammation through Fc receptors. *Immunity* 1995; **3**: 21–6.
70. Clynes RA, Towers TL, Presta LG. Inhibitory Fc receptors modulate in vivo cytoxicity against tumor targets. *Nat Med* 2000; **6**: 443–6.
71. Suzuki Y, Shirato I, Okumura K et al. Distinct contribution of Fc receptors and angiotensin II-dependent pathways in anti-GBM glomerulonephritis. *Kidney Int* 1998; **54**: 1166–74.
72. Clynes R, Dumitru C, Ravetch JV. Uncoupling of immune complex formation and kidney damage in autoimmune glomerulonephritis. *Science* 1998; **279**: 1052–4.
73. Yuasa T, Kubo S, Yoshino T et al. Deletion of Fcgamma receptor IIB renders H-2(b) mice susceptible to collagen-induced arthritis. *J Exp Med* 2000; **191**: 303–11.
74. Luan JJ, Monteiro RC, Sautes C et al. Defective Fc gamma RII gene expression in macrophages of

NOD mice: genetic linkage with up-regulation of IgG1 and IgG2b in serum. *J Immunol* 1996; **157**: 4607–16.

75. Pritchard NR, Cutler AJ, Uribe S et al. Autoimmune-prone mice share a promoter haplotype associated with reduced expression and function of the Fc receptor FcgammaRII. *Curr Biol* 2000; **10**: 227–30.

76. Jiang Y, Hirose S, Abe M et al. Polymorphisms in IgG Fc receptor IIB regulatory regions associated with autoimmune susceptibility. *Immunogenetics* 2000; **51**: 429–35.

77. Ceuppens JL, Baroja ML, Van Vaeck F, Anderson CL. Defect in the membrane expression of high affinity 72-Kd Fc gamma receptors on phagocytic cells in four healthy subjects. *J Clin Invest* 1988; **82**: 571–8.

78. De Haas M, Kleijer M, van Zwieten R et al. Neutrophil FcγRIIIb deficiency, nature, and clinical consequences: a study of 21 individuals from 14 families. *Blood* 1995; **86**: 2403–13.

79. Pan LY, Mendel DB, Zurlo J, Guyre PM. Regulation of the steady state level of Fc gamma RI mRNA by IFN-gamma and dexamethasone in human monocytes, neutrophils, and U-937 cells. *J Immunol* 1990; **145**: 267–75.

80. te Velde AA, Huijbens RJ, de Vries JE, Figdor CG. IL-4 decreases Fc gamma R membrane expression and Fc gamma R-mediated cytotoxic activity of human monocytes. *J Immunol* 1990; **144**: 3046–51.

81. Welch GR, Wong HL, Wahl SM. Selective induction of Fc gamma RIII on human monocytes by transforming growth factor-beta. *J Immunol* 1990; **144**: 3444–8.

82. Pricop L, Redecha P, Teillard J-L et al. Differential modulation of stimulatory and inhibitory Fc gamma receptors on human monocytes by TH1 and TH2 cytokines. *J Immunol* 2001; **166**: 531–7.

83. Pricop L, Gokhale J, Redecha P, Ng SC. Reactive oxygen intermediates enhance Fc gamma receptor signaling and amplify phagocytic capacity. *J Immunol* 1999; **162**: 7041–8.

84. Debets JM, Van de Winkel JG, Ceuppens JL et al. Cross-linking of both Fc gamma RI and Fc gamma induces secretion of tumor necrosis factor by human monocytes, requiring high affinity Fc–Fc gamma R interactions. Functional activation of Fc gamma RII by treatment with proteases or neuraminidase. *J Immunol* 1990; **144**: 1304–10.

85. Huizinga TW, de Haas M, Kleijer M et al. Soluble Fc gamma receptor III in human plasma originates from release by neutrophils. *J Clin Invest* 1990; **86**: 416–23.

86. De Haas M, Kleijer M, Minchinton RM et al. Soluble Fc gamma RIIIa is present in plasma and is derived from natural killer cells. *J Immunol* 1994; **152**: 900–7.

87. Marino M, Ruvo M, De Falco S et al. Prevention of systemic lupus erythematosus in MRL/lpr mice by administration of an immunoglobulin-binding peptide. *Nat Biotechnol* 2000; **18**: 735–9.

88. Bussel JB. Fc receptor blockade and immune thrombocytopenia purpura. *Semin Hematol* 2000; **37**: 26.

89. Cines DB, Blanchette VS. Medical progress: immune thrombocytopenic purpura. *N Engl J Med* 2002; **346**: 995–1008.

90. Samuelsson A, Towers TL, Ravtech JV. Anti-inflammatory activity of IVIG mediated through the inhibitory Fc receptor. *Science* 2001; **291**: 445–6.

Section II

Cytokines, chemokines and other effector molecules

11

TNFα

Marc Feldmann and Ravinder N Maini

Introduction • Cytokines and RA • Cytokine expression in rheumatoid synovium • Cytokine gene regulation in synovium • Studies in animal models confirm that TNFα is a good therapeutic target in arthritis • The future: what controls upregulated TNFα production in RA patients? • References

INTRODUCTION

The mechanisms of autoimmune disease are quite diverse. In some diseases, antibodies are of major importance in driving the pathogenesis of the disease; these include myasthenia gravis disease, Graves' disease, Goodpasture's syndrome, and autoimmune haemolytic anaemia.[1,2] In others T cells appear to be more important; these include multiple sclerosis and type I diabetes.[3,4] However, in human diseases the mechanisms are usually complex, and there are usually huge gaps in our knowledge. For diseases where antibodies are important, often there is clear-cut evidence; for example, improvement upon removing the antibody by plasmapheresis (e.g. in Goodpasture's syndrome), or mother-to-foetus transfer of disease due to transfer of pathogenic antibody. In other instances, if antibody-mediated pathology is not clearly defined, it is assumed that T cells are important. However, in human diseases, in contrast to animal models, the data needed to establish this point are usually circumstantial. In animal models transfer of T cells or antibody is possible in order to verify

mechanisms. Collagen-induced arthritis, a model of rheumatoid arthritis (RA), is transferable by both T cells and antibodies.[5] However, other models differ. K/BxN arthritis is transferable by serum or purified antibodies to glucose-6-phosphate isomerase.[6] TNFα transgenic arthritis is transferable in the absence of T or B cells, as it can be backcrossed to T and B cell deficit RAG knockout mice.[7] Hence studies in animal models are inherently incapable of providing definitive answers as to the pathogenesis of complex heterogeneous multigenic diseases, such as RA.

For RA the mechanism of disease has been the subject of many different hypotheses with the role of T cells emphasized by some,[8–10] of antibody and B cells,[11] and of synovial fibroblast-like cells by others.[12,13] These conflicting hypotheses reflect the fact that there is much left to learn about pathogenic processes, let alone how these processes are engaged by the causative 'aetiological' interactions of genes and environment.

The first attempts to evaluate directly the role of T cells in human autoimmune diseases such as RA by using therapeutic monoclonal antibodies to CD4 were not successful, and so failed to confirm their role.[14,15] However, more encouraging results appear to be forthcoming for non-lytic antibodies to CD4,[16] and possibly to CD3,[17] and concepts are emerging that might explain the failure of the early anti-CD4 experiments. These include the removal of CD4[+] regulatory T cells, many of which express CD25.[18] This may also explain the failure of IL-2 toxin to be beneficial.[19] Furthermore, while lytic antibodies to CD4 were very effective in reducing CD4[+] counts in blood, this was not the case in terms of synovial T cells.[20,21]

CYTOKINES AND RA

Our work which led up to defining TNFα as a useful therapeutic target is based on considering concepts of the pathogenesis of autoimmune disease. In 1983 we published a hypothesis based on immunohistological analysis of diseased tissue, overexpressing MHC class II, suggesting that autoimmune disease involved upregulation of antigen presentation.[22] The only molecules known at the time to upregulate MHC class II expression were cytokines such as IFNγ, and thus we postulated that local cytokine production was a critical early step in the pathogenesis of autoimmunity (Figure 11.1). Our concept was based mostly on thyroid disease, but was also compatible with diabetes and RA[23-25] in which upregulation of MHC class I and II has also been noted. This hypothesis attracted a lot of attention, and

Cytokines
Short range protein mediators
Involved in: immunity, inflammation, cell growth, differentiation, repair, fibrosis
Produced in response to 'stress'
About 150 currently defined, probably ~300 in total

Proinflammatory cytokines drive inflammation
(e.g. TNF, IL-1, IL-6, GM-CSF)
Induce activation and accumulation of leukocytes
These produce mediators which cause pain, swelling, stiffness and initiate tissue damage

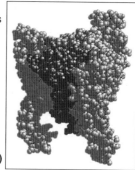

TNFα bound to receptor

Figure 11.1 Cytokines as mediators of inflammation.

experimental support. Thus it was found that transgenic mice[26] expressing IFNγ in the islet of Langerhans under the control of the insulin promoter developed an autoimmune diabetes. In contrast transgenic mice expressing MHC class I antigen in the islet had islet damage,[27] but this was due to an autoimmune response. Subsequently transgenic mice overexpressing IFNγ in many sites were found to develop local inflammatory autoimmune disease in the eye and CNS (Figure 11.2).[28,29]

To explore these hypothetical mechanisms of autoimmunity, and to investigate whether our

Upregulation of HLA-DR in rheumatoid synovium

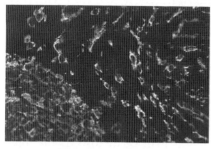 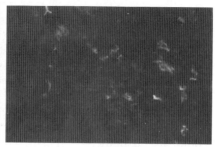

Figure 11.2 Sections of synovial tissue labelled with rabbit anti-HLA-DR antibody and using FITC labelled anti-rabbit as second antibody. (Klareskog L et al. *Proc Natl Acad Sci USA* 1982; **79**: 3632–6.[25])

Rheumatoid arthritis   Osteoarthritis

Expression of HLA-DR on cells usually negative indicates presence of inducers = cytokines

concept was correct, we performed a number of studies in human systems. The first set of experiments was performed using thyroid tissue taken at operation from Graves' disease patients. With this tissue our colleague Marco Londei was able to clone autoreactive T cells from the thyroid tissue that recognized, and were restimulated, by thyroid epithelial cells from diseased patients[30] or normal thyroid epithelial cells induced to express HLA class II. This result was interesting and controversial as it demonstrated that an epithelial cell, once it was induced by cytokines, was able to stimulate already activated T cells. Influenza-specific T cell clones were also able to be stimulated by thyroid epithelial cells,[31] if these were appropriately HLA matched. Proinflammatory cytokine expression in Graves' disease tissue[32] was detectable and cytokine injection induced thyroiditis, and so the outline of this concept of autoimmune induction was established. However, attempts to use this information for patient benefit failed, as there is not much 'unmet medical need' in Graves' disease as judged by the pharmaceutical industry and hence no commercial interest. In RA there was also evidence of a local immune and inflammatory response as judged by the nature of the cell infiltrate, and upregulated MHC expression. In contrast there was a significant unmet medical need, and also the opportunity to study the disease tissue at various stages, including at the height of the local disease process, which is not possible in most human diseases.

CYTOKINE EXPRESSION IN RHEUMATOID SYNOVIUM

Cytokines, short-range protein messenger molecules involved in immunity, inflammation, fibrosis, repair, etc., were first cloned in the early 1980s. With the cloning of cDNA for cytokines, assays specific for these molecules were developed; for example, detection of mRNA by Northern blotting. Detection of the protein was made possible by the generation of specific monoclonal and polyclonal antibodies generated using the cytokine proteins obtained in

pure form by expression from cDNA. Hence the function of cytokines could now be studied in vivo and in vitro, in the absence of contaminating signals. This led to a rapid expansion in cytokine research, which is still ongoing, and to the deeper understanding of multiple biological processes of high relevance to arthritis, including inflammation, immunity, and cell proliferation. Based on this understanding, the use of cytokines and anti-cytokines in medicine has been established. This was initially with the use of haemopoietic factors, such as erythropoetin (EPO)[33] and granulocyte colony-stimulating factor (G-CSF),[34] and the interferons.[35,36]

Synovial joints, which are relatively acellular in health, with a lining layer of fibroblast-like cells and macrophages, are infiltrated by a massive accumulation of blood-borne cells in RA. These cells are chiefly T lymphocytes (20–30%) and macrophages (30–40%), with B lymphocytes, plasma cells, and dendritic cells.[37] To sustain this new tissue mass, angiogenesis is a prominent feature.[38–40] As multiple activated cell types are present in this tissue, it is not surprising that using appropriate technology it is found that there is abundant cytokine expression in the rheumatoid synovium (Table 11.1).

Table 11.1 Many cytokines are produced in rheumatoid synovium.

Proinflammatory
    e.g. IL-1, IL-6, TNFα, IL-12, IL-15, IL-17, IL-18, IFNγ, IL-2, OncoM, GM-CSF

Anti-inflammatory
    e.g. IL-10, IL-1Ra, TGFβ, IL-11, IL-13

Chemokines
    e.g. IL-8, MIP-1α, MCP-1, RANTES, ENA-78, GROα

Growth factors
    e.g. VEGF, PDGF, FGF

Almost all cytokines are present in RA synovium except IL-4

Cytokine analysis in RA engaged a number of research groups, assaying different aspects in various ways. The initial groups studied cytokines in synovial fluid. Interleukin-1 (IL-1) was the first cytokine to be detected in RA, using a bioassay, by Fontana et al.[41] Other groups studied cytokine mRNA expression by in situ hybridization,[42] whereas the approach in our laboratory was to look for local mRNA expression by blotting.[43] The rationale for this was that locally produced cytokines were most likely to be important in the disease process. Having detected a plethora of cytokine mRNAs by in situ hybridization or blotting, it was important to establish that the relevant proteins were, indeed, synthesized in the synovium. Several approaches were useful. Immunostaining of biopsies was successful,[44] as were assays of cytokine protein in synovial fluids.[45–47] We also found that short-term unstimulated cultures of cells dissociated from the whole synovial membrane (a complex cell mixture) yielded cytokine-rich supernatants for assay.[37,43] These studies using multiple approaches verified that a great number of proinflammatory cytokines such as IL-1, TNFα, IL-6, GM-CSF, and IL-8 were locally produced.[43,48–50] This was found in essentially all the rheumatoid synovial membrane samples assayed regardless of the duration of disease or its treatment.

In normal circumstances proinflammatory cytokines are expressed for a short period of time in response to extrinsic stimuli such as lipopolysaccharide (LPS). Thus their consistent presence in biopsies or operative samples suggested that, unlike normal stimulation, cytokine synthesis in rheumatoid synovial tissue may be 'constitutive'. This was also the first clue that cytokines may be important, as their production was disregulated compared to normal cells in culture. However, analysis of the results also revealed that there were a number of proinflammatory cytokines such as TNFα, IL-1, IL-6, and GM-CSF with closely related biological properties in active rheumatoid synovium. This raised the question as to which, if any, might be rate limiting, and hence might be a useful therapeutic target. If the concepts generated thus far

in vitro were correct, then blocking a single cytokine might not be useful, as the proinflammatory activity would still be driven by the remaining proinflammatory cytokines.

We, and others, also studied the expression of anti-inflammatory cytokines such as IL-10, IL-1ra, and TGFβ in rheumatoid synovium.[50–53] This was relevant, as it was possible that the chronic inflammation of RA was due to anti-inflammatory cytokines not being expressed there, and the proinflammatory mediators not being counterbalanced by anti-inflammatory mediators. The production of anti-inflammatory mediators such as IL-10, TGFβ1, soluble TNF receptor, IL-1 receptor antagonist, and IL-11 in rheumatoid synovium was found to be considerably upregulated.[50–53] For example, levels of up to 1 ng/ml of IL-10 were found in rheumatoid synovial cultures. These quantities were found to be biologically significant from neutralizing antibody studies, using anti-IL-10 in synovial cultures, in a mirror image of the anti-TNFα work described below. It was found that anti-IL-10 antibody augmented the amounts of TNFα and IL-1 produced by the synovial cultures 2–3 fold.[50] Thus the IL-10 endogenously produced was partially downregulating the major proinflammatory cytokines. In a converse set of experiments it was shown that adding IL-10 to synovial cultures was anti-inflammatory, suggesting that IL-10 might be a useful therapeutic agent. This was indeed the case in animal models,[54] but in humans the therapeutic effect at tolerable doses was modest.[55]

The amounts of TGFβ1 are high in synovial culture, approximately 10 ng/ml.[56] It appears that this is a plateau level, as adding more has an insignificant effect on production. As the immunoregulatory effects of TGFβ are moderately long-lived in vitro, it is not possible to demonstrate any worsening of cytokine in synovial cultures on its neutralization, and so its role in the pathogenesis of RA is still not understood. In animal models there is convincing evidence that TGFβ has both proinflammatory and anti-inflammatory roles,[57] and regrettably the profibrotic effects of TGFβ1 have halted its use in clinical trials.[58]

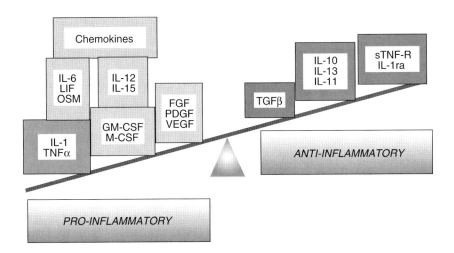

Figure 11.3 Cytokine disequilibrium. Both pro- and anti-inflammatory cytokines are upregulated in rheumatoid synovium but the balance is in favour of proinflammatory cytokines promoting inflammation. (Reproduced with permission from Feldmann M, Brennan FM, Maini RN. Cell 1996; **85**(3): 307–10.)

The production of anti-inflammatory mediators in rheumatoid synovium appears to be partly under the regulation of the proinflammatory mediators, as blocking TNFα partly inhibited production of IL-10, solTNF-R, and IL-1ra.[43,50] This appears to be also true in vivo, as judged by clinical trial data, most dramatically for IL-1ra,[59] somewhat less so for solTNF-R and IL-10. The implications of this are not fully understood, but it may explain why blocking TNFα exerts only a temporary effect in patients due to the concomitant downregulation of the IL-10, IL-1ra, and solTNF-R homeostatic mechanisms in the disequilibrium of cytokines, as shown in Figure 11.3.

Other anti-inflammatory cytokines appear to be poorly expressed. The presence of IL-4 in rheumatoid synovial tissue is occasional, and most studies do not report it.[60] This may be of relevance to the Th1 preponderance that is reported in rheumatoid patients as IL-4 is the most potent cytokine skewing towards the Th2 phenotype and inhibiting Th1 cells. IL-13 is reported to be present in some studies,[61] but not others.[62] The inconsistent results are not understood, but the heterogeneity of RA is well known.

CYTOKINE GENE REGULATION IN SYNOVIUM

To test if the pathology in RA is due to the disregulated and prolonged production of cytokines, dissociated cell cultures of rheumatoid synovium were used to study cytokine regulation in the diseased tissue. The cells were found to reaggregate rapidly, and produced proinflammatory cytokines such as TNFα, IL-1, and IL-6 continuously over the 6- or 7-day period that they were studied before the cell composition changed from its original mixture.[37,43] This culture system generated an in vitro model for studying the proinflammatory gene regulation in synovium and evaluating whether it was indeed abnormal or prolonged.

Faced with a plethora of candidate cytokines, the problem was which cytokine to study first. The properties of TNFα and IL-1 are consistent with many features of RA. Because IL-1 (also described in the 1970s as 'catabolin') had been demonstrated to be involved in damage to the joints in a variety of experimental situations,[63–65] and hence presumably in RA, our colleague Fionula Brennan studied IL-1 regulation by TNFα in these dissociated rheumatoid synovium cell cultures. It was found that adding neutralizing anti-TNFα antibodies (polyclonal at the time)[66] at the beginning of cultures abrogated their IL-1 production, assessed at protein or mRNA level (Figure 11.4). This was not the case for the IL-1 produced by osteoarthritic synovium. These data provided the first clue that TNFα might be of particular importance in the mechanism of inflammation. Subsequent experiments revealed

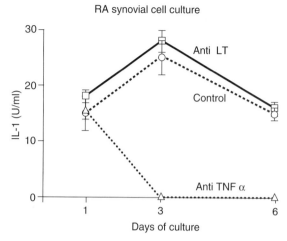

Approach
Operative sample synovium, active RA cells isolated, placed in 'tissue culture'

Observation
Spontaneous production of many mediators of disease – cytokines, enzymes etc.

Experiment
Antibody to TNF inhibits production of other pro-inflammatory cytokines

Figure 11.4 IL-1 synthesis is downregulated in cultures of synovial tissue from patients with RA but not osteoarthritis. (Reproduced with permission from Brennan FM et al. *Lancet* 1989; **2**: 244–7.[66])

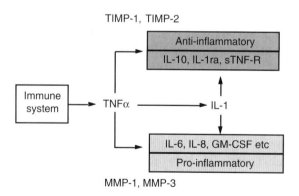

Figure 11.5 Cytokine cascade in RA. Pro- and anti-inflammatory cytokines interact in a 'network' or 'cascade'. (Adapted with permission from Feldmann M, Brennan FM, Maini RN. *Cell* 1996; **85**(3): 307–10.)

the widespread regulatory effects of anti-TNFα antibody in synovial cultures, e.g. downregulating other proinflammatory cytokines, such as IL-6, GM-CSF, and IL-8.[67–69]

The simplest interpretation for the widespread effects of anti-TNF on multiple cytokines is that TNFα is at the apex of a proinflammatory 'cascade'. This concept is illustrated in Figure 11.5. The results raised the possibility that blocking TNFα, just one of the multitude of proinflammatory cytokines, might, by its downstream effect on other cytokines, have a major influence on the complex disease process. Hence these results suggested that blocking TNFα might be therapeutically useful, and this idea was subsequently tested.

It is important to stress that this work involved the use of mixed unpurified synovial cultures, and not cultured rheumatoid synovial fibroblasts. Most studies prior to this time had focused on rheumatoid synovial fibroblasts, but we felt that these cells, undoubtedly important, were not representative of the complexity in the cell mixture synovium, and did not reflect the important contribution of blood borne cells capable of driving inflammation and immunity.

STUDIES IN ANIMAL MODELS CONFIRM THAT TNFα IS A GOOD THERAPEUTIC TARGET IN ARTHRITIS

A number of studies in animal models have yielded consistent data indicating that TNFα is intimately involved in the generation of arthritis. The properties of TNFα are consistent with this concept.[70,71] One set of important studies has come from George Kollias' laboratory.[72] Beutler and Cerami[70] had reported that the 3' untranslated region of TNFα was rich in A and U nucleotides. This AU-rich motif, AUUUA, was found in a great number of cytokines and proto-oncogenes. Shaw and Kamen[73] demonstrated that this motif reduced the half-life of mRNA, and it was shown that it was involved in macrophage expression. Kollias' group made transgenic mice that expressed a human TNFα gene lacking the 3' untranslated region of TNF, replacing it with a β

Model

Genetically susceptible mice (DBA/1)

Injected with collagen type II
(major constituent of cartilage)

About 21 days later arthritis
appears and then spreads

Inflammation damages joints

Results

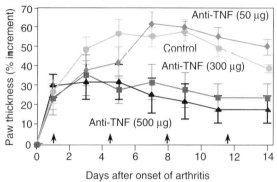

Histology

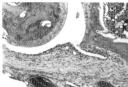

Anti-TNF treated

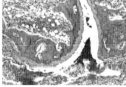

Isotype IgG control

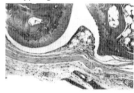

Normal

Figure 11.6 Animal model of collagen-induced arthritis. The graph shows the effects of different doses of anti-TNF on clinical progression of established arthritis. Arrows indicate time of injections of anti-TNF. Paw width was measured using calipers and increase in thickness expressed as a percentage compared with baseline. Histology: paraffin sections of paws were stained with haematoxylin. Bottom: normal joint; middle: severe arthritis; top: mouse treated with anti-TNF. (Reproduced with permission from Williams RO, Feldmann M, Maini RN. *Proc Natl Acad Sci USA* 1992; **89**: 9784–8.[78])

globin 3′ untranslated region. This led to many lines of mice with disregulated and upregulated TNFα production, and the transgenic mice were all found to develop an erosive arthritis, with some lines also having inflammatory bowel disease and skin inflammation.[73,74] This rather local inflammation was a different phenotype from the diffuse inflammation of the TGFβ1[75] knockouts. It is still not clear why the joints in these mice are the major site of inflammation, despite many years of subsequent studies.

A different but complementary set of studies came from neutralizing TNFα after disease onset in mice with a disease resembling RA. Injection of collagen type II into genetically susceptible mouse strains such as DBA/1 yielded an erosive arthritis with histological features resembling human RA.[76] Anti-TNFα antibody injected at adequate doses (but not at low dose) after disease onset was found to ameliorate disease activity. The degree of footpad swelling, a measure of inflammation, the clinical score (production of degree of inflammation by number of affected paws), as well as the histology, all assessments of disease, were improved.

Histologically there was less leucocyte infiltration of the joints, less damage to cartilage, and less erosion of bone (Figure 11.6).

Similar studies in this model were reported within a few months of each other by the late Jeanette Thorbecke's group,[77] Richard Williams of our group,[78] and Pierre Piguet's group.[79] These animal studies were an important part of establishing the rationale for testing anti-TNFα in human RA.

Proinflammatory cytokines, especially TNFα, are very rapidly produced after stimulation, for example by the ubiquitous LPS. Hence it was of importance to verify that the studies performed with human synovial tissue in vitro reflected the situation in vivo. A key experiment was to freeze biopsy tissue from joints within minutes of its extraction. In these few minutes TNFα synthesis could not take place, and hence TNFα expression in vivo could be inferred from these studies with fresh frozen tissue. A representative analysis is shown in Figure 11.7. These studies showed that TNF was expressed before removal from the body,[44] as were TNF receptors.[80] These studies provided a rationale for anti-TNFα

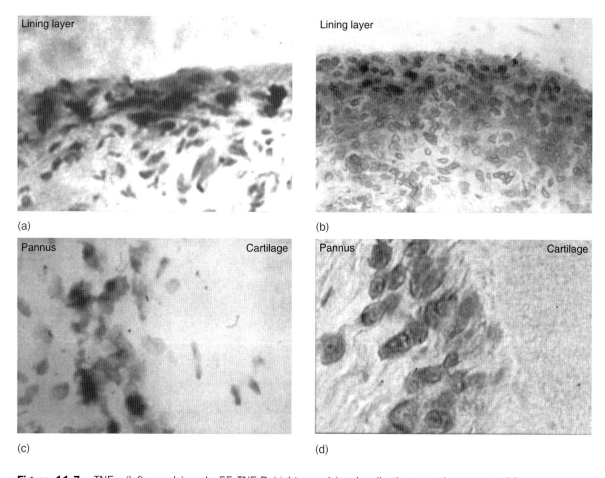

Figure 11.7 TNFα (left panels) and p55 TNF-R (right panels) colocalization was demonstrated by immunohistology in synovial lining layer (a,b) and at the cartilage–pannus junction (c,d). (Adapted with permission from Chu et al. *Arthritis Rheum* 1989; **34**: 1125–32 and Delewan et al. *Arthritis Rheum* 1992; **35**: 1170–78.)

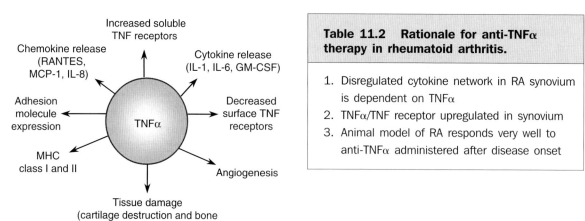

Figure 11.8 TNFα actions relevant to the pathogenesis of rheumatoid arthritis.

Table 11.2 Rationale for anti-TNFα therapy in rheumatoid arthritis.

1. Disregulated cytokine network in RA synovium is dependent on TNFα
2. TNFα/TNF receptor upregulated in synovium
3. Animal model of RA responds very well to anti-TNFα administered after disease onset

therapy in RA (Table 11.2). With hindsight it is evident that the actions of TNFα mimic many processes occurring in RA (Figure 11.8).

THE FUTURE: WHAT CONTROLS UPREGULATED TNFα PRODUCTION IN RA PATIENTS?

An understanding of the control of TNFα production at sites of inflammation is a very interesting question, with considerable impact on therapeutic strategies for the future. This question can be studied at multiple levels. At the cellular level there is agreement that it is macrophages that make most of the TNFα in rheumatoid synovium. But what drives them to do it? This has been studied in cellular terms and it has been recently reported that an atypical subset of T cells, which behave like T cells activated not by antigen but by cytokines, were

important in inducing TNFα in cell–cell contact mechanisms.[81]

In molecular terms, a number of studies have suggested that IL-15[82] and IL-18[83] might be 'upstream' of TNFα. These studies are promising, but are by no means conclusive, as they are difficult to perform in synovial tissue. Nevertheless, these molecules might be therapeutic targets.

In terms of intracellular mechanisms, a number of pathways have been reported to regulate TNFα production. The best studied is the p38 MAP kinase,[84] others include the other MAP kinases p42/44 ERK[85] and JNK[86] stress activated kinase. Other interesting pathways include the NFκB pathway[87,88] and the phosphotidyl inositol 3 kinase pathway.[88] However, in all these cases, these pathways control many biological processes, and so there may be costs in terms of safety in their excessive blockade.

REFERENCES

1. Weetman AP. Graves' disease. *N Engl J Med* 2000; **343**: 1236–48.
2. Salama AD, Levy JB, Lightstone L, Pusey CD. Goodpasture's disease. *Lancet* 2001; **385**: 1374.
3. Steinman L. Multiple sclerosis: a co-ordinated immunological attack against myelin in the central nervous system. *Cell* 1996; **85**: 299–302.
4. Tisch R, McDevitt H. Insulin dependent diabetes mellitus. *Cell* 1996; **85**: 291–7.
5. Muller-Ladner U, Gay RE, Gay S. Activation of synoviocytes. *Curr Opin Rheumatol* 2000; **12**: 186–94.
6. Kouskoff V, Korganow A-S, Duchatelle V et al. Organ-specific disease provoked by systemic autoimmunity. *Cell* 1996; **87**: 811–22.
7. Plows D, Kontogeorgos G, Kollias G. Mice lacking mature T and B lymphocytes develop arthritis lesions after immunization with type II collagen. *J Immunol* 1999; **162**: 1018–23.
8. Coakley G, Iqbal M, Brooks D et al. CD8+, CD57+ T cells from healthy elderly subjects suppress neutrophil development in vitro: implications for the neutropenia of Felty's and large granular lymphocyte syndromes. *Arthritis Rheum* 2000; **43**: 834–43.
9. Seckinger P, Isaaz S, Dayer JM. A human inhibitor of tumor necrosis factor alpha. *J Exp Med* 1988; **167**: 1511–16.
10. Cope AP. Exploring the pathogenesis of rheumatoid arthritis in transgenic and mutant mice. *Curr Dir Autoimmun* 2001; **3**: 64–93.
11. Edwards JC, Cambridge G, Abrahams VM. Do self-perpetuating B lymphocytes drive human autoimmune disease? *Immunology* 1999; **97**: 188–96.
12. Yamanishi Y, Firestein GS. Pathogenesis of rheumatoid arthritis: the role of synoviocytes. *Rheum Dis Clin North Am* 2001; **27**: 355–71.
13. Pap T, Aupperle KR, Gay S et al. Invasiveness of synovial fibroblasts is regulated by p53 in the SCID mouse in vivo model of cartilage invasion. *Arthritis Rheum* 2001; **44**: 676–81.
14. Moreland L, Pratt P, Mayes M. Minimal efficacy of a depleting chimaeric anti-CD4 (cM-T412) in treatment of patients with refractory rheumatoid arthritis (RA) receiving concomitant methotrexate (MTX). *Arthritis Rheum* 1993; **36**: 39.
15. Van de Lubbe PA, Dijkmans BAC, Markusse HM et al. A randomized double-blind, placebo-controlled study of CD4 monoclonal antibody therapy in early rheumatoid arthritis. *Arthritis Rheum* 1995; **38**: 1097–106.
16. Schulze-Koops H, Davis LS, Haverty TP et al. Reduction of Th1 cell activity in the peripheral circulation of patients with rheumatoid arthritis

after treatment with a non-depleting humanized monoclonal antibody to CD4. *J Rheumatol* 1998; **25**: 2065–76.

17. Chatenoud L, Thervet E, Primo J, Bach JF. Anti CD3 antibody induces long-term remission of overt autoimmunity in nonobese diabetic mice. *Proc Natl Acad Sci USA* 1994; **91**: 123–7.

18. Shevach EM, McHugh RS, Piccirillo CA, Thornton AM. Control of T cell activation by CD4+ CD25+ suppressor T cells. *Immunol Rev* 2001; **182**: 58–67.

19. Strom TB, Kelley VR, Murphy JR et al. Interleukin-2 receptor-director therapies: antibody- or cytokine-based targeting molecules. *Ann Rev Med* 1993; **44**: 343–53.

20. Moreland LW, Heck LWJ, Koopman WJ. Biologic agents for treating rheumatoid arthritis. Concepts and progress. *Arthritis Rheum* 1997; **40**: 397–409.

21. Williams RO, Mason LJ, Feldmann M, Maini RN. Synergy between anti-CD4 and anti-tumor necrosis factor in the amelioration of established collagen-induced arthritis. *Proc Natl Acad Sci USA* 1994; **91**: 2762–6.

22. Bottazzo GF, Pujol-Borrell R, Hanafusa T, Feldmann M. Role of aberrant HLA-DR expression and antigen presentation in induction of endocrine autoimmunity. *Lancet* 1983; **2**: 1115–19.

23. Pujol-Borrell R, Todd I, Londei M et al. Inappropriate major histocompatibility complex class II expression by thyroid follicular cells in thyroid autoimmune disease and by pancreatic beta cells in type I diabetes. *Mol Biol Med* 1986; **3**: 159–65.

24. Janossy G, Panayai G, Duke O et al. Rheumatoid arthritis: a disease of T-lymphocyte/macrophage immunoregulation. *Lancet* 1981; **ii**: 839–41.

25. Klareskog L, Forsum U, Scheynius A et al. Evidence in support of a self perpetuating HLA-DR dependent delayed type cell reaction in rheumatoid arthritis. *Proc Natl Acad Sci USA* 1982; **72**: 3632–6.

26. Sarvetnick N, Shizuru J, Liggitt D et al. Loss of pancreatic islet tolerance induced by β-cell expression of interferon-γ. *Nature* 1990; **346**: 844–7.

27. Allison J, Campbell IL, Morahan G et al. Diabetes in transgenic mice resulting from over-expression of class I histocompatibility molecules in pancreatic beta cells. *Nature* 1988; **333**: 529–33.

28. Geiger K, Howes E, Gallina M et al. Transgenic mice expressing IFN-gamma in the retina

29. Antel JP, Owens T. Immune regulation and CNS autoimmune disease. *J Neuroimmunol* 1999; **100**: 181–90.

30. Taylor DJ, Whitehead RJ, Evanson JM et al. Effect of recombinant cytokines on glycolysis and fructose 2,6-bisphosphate in rheumatoid synovial cells in vitro. *Biochem J* 1988; **250**: 111–15.

31. Londei M, Lamb JR, Bottazzo GF, Feldmann M. Epithelial cells expressing aberrant MHC class II determinants can present antigen to cloned human T cells. *Nature* 1984; **312**: 639–41.

32. Grubeck-Loebenstein B, Buchan G, Chantry D et al. Analysis of intrathyroidal cytokine production in thyroid autoimmune disease: thyroid follicular cells produce IL-1 alpha and interleukin-6. *Scand J Rheum* 1989; **77**: 324–30.

33. Cody J. Recombinant human erythropoietin for chronic renal failure anaemia in pre-dialysis patients. *Cochrane Database Sys Rev* 2001; **4**: CD003266.

34. Morstyn G, Foote MA, Walker T, Molineux T. Filgrastim (r-metHuG-CSF) in the 21st century: SD/01. *Acta Haematol* 2001; **105**: 151–5.

35. Herrine SK. Approach to the patient with chronic hepatitis C virus infection. *Ann Intern Med* 2002; **136**: 747–57.

36. Bagnato F, Pozzilli C, Scagnolari C et al. A one year study on the pharmacodynamic profile of interferon-beta 1a in MS. *Neurology* 2002; **59**: 1409–11.

37. Brennan FM, Chantry D, Jackson AM et al. Cytokine production in culture by cells isolated from the synovial membrane. *J Autoimmun* 1989; **2** (suppl): 177–86.

38. Brenchley PEC. Antagonising angiogenesis in rheumatoid arthritis. *Ann Rheum Dis* 2001; **60** (suppl 3): 71–4.

39. Koch AE. The role of angiogenesis in rheumatoid arthritis: recent developments. *Ann Rheum Dis* 2000; **59** (suppl 1): 65–71.

40. Paleolog EM, Young S, Stark AC et al. Modulation of angiogenic vascular endothelial growth factor by tumor necrosis factor alpha and interleukin-1 in rheumatoid arthritis. *Arthritis Rheum* 1998; **41**: 1258–65.

41. Fontana A, Hengartner H, Weber E et al. Interleukin 1 activity in the synovial fluid of patients with rheumatoid arthritis. *Rheumatol Int* 1982; **2**: 49–53.

42. Wood NC, Symons JA, Dickens E, Duff GW. In situ hybridization of IL-6 in rheumatoid arthritis. *Clin Exp Immunol* 1992; **87**: 183–9.

43. Feldmann M, Brennan FM, Maini RN. Role of cytokines in rheumatoid arthritis. [Review] [226 refs]. *Annu Rev Immunol* 1996; **14**: 397–440.

44. Chu CQ, Field M, Feldmann M, Maini RN. Localization of tumor necrosis factor α in synovial tissues and at the cartilage–pannus junction in patients with rheumatoid arthritis. *Arthritis Rheum* 1991; **34**: 1125–32.

45. Hopkins SJ, Humphreys M, Jayson MI. Cytokines in synovial fluid. I. The presence of biologically active and immunoreactive IL-1. *Clin Exp Immunol* 1988; **72**: 422–7.

46. Saxne T, Palladino MA Jr, Heinegard D et al. Detection of tumor necrosis factor α but not tumor necrosis factor β in rheumatoid arthritis synovial fluid and serum. *Arthritis Rheum* 1988; **31**: 1041–5.

47. Arend WP, Dayer JM. Cytokines and cytokine inhibitors or antagonists in rheumatoid arthritis. *Arthritis Rheum* 1990; **33**: 305–15.

48. Koch AE, Kunkel SL, Harlow LA et al. Enhanced production of monocyte chemoattractant protein-1 in rheumatoid arthritis. *J Clin Invest* 1992; **90**: 772–9.

49. Brennan FM, Zachariae CO, Chantry D et al. Detection of interleukin 8 biological activity in synovial fluids from patients with rheumatoid arthritis and production of interleukin 8 mRNA by isolated synovial cells. *Eur J Immunol* 1990; **20**: 2141–4.

50. Katsikis PD, Chu CQ, Brennan FM et al. Immunoregulatory role of interleukin 10 in rheumatoid arthritis. *J Exp Med* 1994; **179**: 1517–27.

51. Wahl SM, Allen JB, Wong HL et al. Antagonistic and agonistic effects of transforming growth factor-β and IL-1 in rheumatoid synovium. *J Immunol* 1990; **145**: 2514–19.

52. Fava R, Olsen N, Keski-Oja J et al. Active and latent forms of transforming growth factor β activity in synovial effusions. *J Exp Med* 1989; **169**: 291–6.

53. Arend WP. Interleukin-1 receptor antagonist. *Adv Immunol* 1993; **54**: 167–227.

54. Walmsley M, Katsikis PD, Abney E et al. Interleukin-10 inhibition of the progression of established collagen-induced arthritis. *Arthritis Rheum* 1996; **39**: 495–503.

55. Maini RN, Paulus H, Breedveld FC et al. rHUIL-10 in subjects with active rheumatoid arthritis (RA): a phase I and cytokine response study. *Arthritis Rheum* 1997; **40** (suppl): S224.

56. Brennan FM, Chantry D, Turner M et al. Transforming growth factor-β in rheumatoid arthritis synovial tissue: lack of effect on spontaneous cytokine production in joint cell cultures. *Clin Exp Immunol* 1990; **81**: 278–85.

57. Allen JB, Manthey CL, Hand AR et al. Rapid onset synovial inflammation and hyperplasia induced by transforming growth factor β. *J Exp Med* 1990; **171**: 231–47.

58. Gambaro G, Weigert C, Ceol M, Schleicher ED. Inhibition of transforming growth factor-beta 1 gene overexpression as a strategy to prevent fibrosis. *Contrib Nephrol* 2001; **131**: 107–13.

59. Charles P, Elliott MJ, Davis D et al. Regulation of cytokines, cytokine inhibitors, and acute-phase proteins following anti-TNF-alpha therapy in rheumatoid arthritis [In Process Citation]. *J Immunol* 1999; **163**: 1521–8.

60. Simon AK, Seipelt E, Sieper J. Divergent T-cell cytokine patterns in inflammatory arthritis. *Proc Natl Acad Sci USA* 1994; **91**: 8562–6.

61. Isomaki P, Luukkainen R, Toivanen P, Punnonen J. The presence of interleukin-13 in rheumatoid synovium and its antiinflammatory effects on synovial fluid macrophages from patients with rheumatoid arthritis. *Arthritis Rheum* 1996; **39**: 1693–702.

62. Woods JM, Haines GK, Shah MR et al. Low level production of interleukin-13 in synovial fluid and tissue from patients with arthritis. *Clin Immunol Immunopathol* 1997; **85**: 210–20.

63. Fell HB, Jubb RW. The effect of synovial tissue on the breakdown of articular cartilage in organ culture. *Arthritis Rheum* 1977; **20**: 1359–71.

64. Dingle JT, Saklatvala J, Hembry R et al. A cartilage catabolic factor from synovium. *Biochem J* 1979; **184**: 177–80.

65. Saklatvala J, Sarsfield SJ, Townsend Y. Purification of two immunologically different leucocyte proteins that cause cartilage resorption lymphocyte activation and fever. *J Exp Med* 1985; **162**: 1208–15.

66. Brennan FM, Chantry D, Jackson A et al. Inhibitory effect of TNF alpha antibodies on synovial cell interleukin-1 production in rheumatoid arthritis. *Lancet* 1989; **2**: 244–7.

67. Butler DM, Maini RN, Feldmann M, Brennan FM. Modulation of proinflammatory cytokine release in rheumatoid synovial membrane cell cultures. Comparison of monoclonal anti-TNFα antibody

with the IL-1 receptor antagonist. *Eur Cytokine Network* 1995; **6**: 225–30.

68. Haworth C, Brennan FM, Chantry D et al. Expression of granulocyte-macrophage colony-stimulating factor in rheumatoid arthritis: regulation by tumor necrosis factor-alpha. *Eur J Immunol* 1991; **21**: 2575–9.

69. Alvaro-Garcia JM, Zvaifler NJ, Brown CB et al. Cytokines in chronic inflammatory arthritis. VI. Analysis of the synovial cells involved in granulocyte-macrophage colony stimulating factor production and gene expression in rheumatoid arthritis and its regulation by IL-1 and TNFα. *J Immunol* 1991; **146**: 3365–71.

70. Beutler B, Cerami A. Cachectin: more than a tumor necrosis factor. *N Engl J Med* 1987; **316**: 379–85.

71. Vassalli P. The pathophysiology of tumor necrosis factors. *Annu Rev Immunol* 1992; **10**: 411.

72. Keffer J, Probert L, Cazlaris H et al. Transgenic mice expressing human tumour necrosis factor: a predictive genetic model of arthritis. *EMBO J* 1991; **10**: 4025–31.

73. Shaw G, Kamen R. A conserved AU sequence from the 3′ untranslated region of GM-CSF mRNA mediates selective mRNA degradation. *Cell* 1986; **46**: 659.

74. Douni E, Akassoglou K, Alexopoulou L et al. Transgenic and knockout analyses of the role of TNF in immune regulation and disease pathogenesis. *J Inflamm* 1995–96; **47**: 27–38.

75. Christ M, McCartney-Francis NL, Kulkarni AB et al. Immune dysregulation in TGF-beta 1-deficient mice. *J Immunol* 1994; **153**: 1936–46.

76. Holmdahl R, Andersson M, Goldschmidt TJ et al. Type II collagen autoimmunity in animals and provocations leading to arthritis. *Immunol Rev* 1990; **118**: 193–232.

77. Thorbecke GJ, Shah R, Leu CH et al. Involvement of endogenous tumor necrosis factor alpha and transforming growth factor beta during induction of collagen type II arthritis in mice. *Proc Natl Acad Sci USA* 1992; **89**: 7375–9.

78. Williams RO, Feldmann M, Maini RN. Anti-tumor necrosis factor ameliorates joint disease in murine collagen-induced arthritis. *Proc Natl Acad Sci USA* 1992; **89**: 9784–8.

79. Piguet PF, Grau GE, Vesin C et al. Evolution of collagen arthritis in mice is arrested by treatment with anti-tumour necrosis factor (TNF) antibody or a recombinant soluble TNF receptor. *Immunology* 1992; **77**: 510–14.

80. Deleuran BW, Chu CQ, Field M et al. Localization of tumor necrosis factor receptors in the synovial tissue and cartilage–pannus junction in patients with rheumatoid arthritis. Implications for local actions of tumor necrosis factor alpha. *Arthritis Rheum* 1992; **35**: 1170–8.

81. Brennan FM, Hayes AL, Ciesielski CJ et al. Evidence that rheumatoid arthritis synovial T cells are similar to cytokine-activated T cells. *Arthritis Rheum* 2002; **46**: 31–41.

82. McInnes IB, Leung BP, Sturrock RD et al. Interleukin-15 mediates T cell-dependent regulation of tumor necrosis factor-alpha production in rheumatoid arthritis. *Nat Med* 1997; **3**: 189–95.

83. Gracie JA, Forsey RJ, Chan WL et al. A proinflammatory role for IL-18 in rheumatoid arthritis. *J Clinical Invest* 1999; **104**: 1393–401.

84. Saklatvala J, Dean J, Finch A. Protein kinase cascades in intracellular signalling by interleukin-I and tumour necrosis factor [In Process Citation]. *Biochem Soc Symp* 1999; **64**: 63–77.

85. Schett G, Tohidast-Akrad M, Smolen JS et al. Activation, differential localization and regulation of the stress-activated protein kinases, extracellular signal-regulated kinase, c-JUN N-terminal kinase, and p38 mitogen-activated protein kinase, in synovial tissue and cells in rheumatoid arthritis. *Arthritis Rheum* 2000; **43**: 2501–12.

86. Derijard B, Hibi M, Wu IH et al. JNK1: a protein kinase stimulated by UV light and Ha-Ras that binds and phosphorylates the c-Jun activation domain. *Cell* 1994; **76**: 1025–37.

87. Foxwell B, Browne K, Bondeson J et al. Efficient adenoviral infection with IkBa reveals that macrophage tumor necrosis factor a production in rheumatoid arthritis is NF-kB dependent. *Proc Natl Acad Sci USA* 1998; **95**: 8211–15.

88. Bondeson J, Foxwell B, Brennan F, Feldmann M. Defining therapeutic targets by using adenovirus: blocking NF-κB inhibits both inflammatory and destructive mechanisms in rheumatoid synovium but spares anti-inflammatory mediators. *Proc Natl Acad Sci USA* 1999; **96**: 5668–73.

12

Interleukin-1

Cem Gabay and William P Arend

Introduction • IL-1 family members and receptors • The balance between IL-1 and IL-1Ra • Summary • References

INTRODUCTION

Interleukin-1 (IL-1) is a key cytokine in host defense that also possesses potent inflammatory properties. There are two agonist forms of IL-1, IL-1α and IL-1β. This family also includes a natural inhibitor, the IL-1 receptor antagonist (IL-1Ra), a structural variant that binds to IL-1 receptors but fails to activate target cells.[1-3] IL-1 is an important mediator of tissue damage in multiple chronic inflammatory diseases, including rheumatoid arthritis (RA) and osteoarthritis (OA) (Figure 12.1). Thus, inhibiting the production or effects of IL-1 represents a significant therapeutic goal.

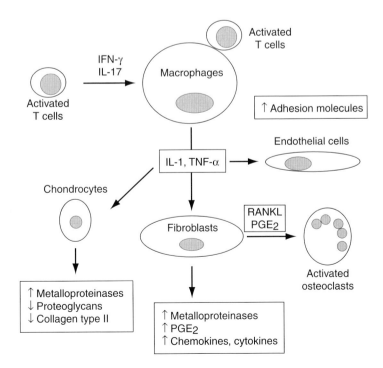

Figure 12.1 Potential role of IL-1 in rheumatoid arthritis. Activated CD4+ T lymphocytes present in the rheumatoid synovium stimulate synovial macrophages either through the release of the lymphokines interferon-γ (IFN-γ) and IL-17 or by direct cell–cell interactions. Stimulated macrophages produce both tumour necrosis factor alpha (TNF-α) and IL-1. These cytokines stimulate production of chemokines and expression of adhesion molecules on endothelial cells, thus leading to the recruitment of inflammatory cells in the joints. In addition, TNF-α and IL-1 exert catabolic effects on articular cartilage. IL-1 also contributes directly and indirectly through the release of prostaglandin E_2 (PGE_2) and receptor activation of nuclear factor kappa B ligand (RANKL) to the development of bone erosions.

This chapter on targeting IL-1 in disease consists of five sections, discussing IL-1 family members and receptors, IL-1 in animal models of inflammatory arthritis and in RA, the balance between IL-1 and IL-1Ra, exogenous IL-1Ra in the treatment of RA, and other approaches to targeting IL-1 or signaling. Each section will briefly review the relevant background information and present in more detail recent findings and areas of current development.

IL-1 FAMILY MEMBERS AND RECEPTORS

IL-1 ligands and receptors

The IL-1 ligands and receptors are summarized in Table 12.1. The three members of the IL-1 family are highly homologous to each other and are tightly conserved across species. The amino acid identities between these human proteins are: IL-1α and IL-1β 22%, IL-1α and IL-1Ra 18%, and IL-1β and IL-1Ra 26%. Moreover, human IL-1α is ~55% identical to the murine and rat forms of this molecule, with IL-1β being ~78% identical and IL-1Ra ~76% identical. The genes for these three members of the IL-1 family are quite similar, indicating an origin by gene duplication. The genes for IL-1α, IL-1β, and IL-1Ra are located close to each other in the human chromosome 2q14 region.[3,4] Further analysis of the protein structures suggests that IL-1Ra separated from a primordial IL-1 molecule ~360 million years ago, whereas the separation between IL-1α and IL-1β is a more recent event, occurring ~285 million years ago.[5]

Table 12.1 IL-1 ligands and receptors.

Ligands
  Agonists: IL-1α and IL-1β
  Antagonists: IL-1Ra, with four described
    structural variants

Receptors
  Type I IL-1R, membrane bound and soluble
  Type II IL-1R, membrane bound and soluble

There are two IL-1 receptors (IL-1R). The 80-kDa type I IL-1R (IL-1RI) has a long cytoplasmic domain of 215 residues and is biologically active,[1] whereas the 60-kDa type II IL-1R (IL-1RII) possesses a short cytoplasmic region of 29 residues and is biologically inert.[1,6] IL-1RII is a natural inhibitor of IL-1, either on the cell surface or in the cell microenvironment as a soluble form after enzymatic cleavage of the extracellular portion.[7] A second receptor subunit, the IL-1 receptor accessory protein (IL-1R AcP), forms a complex with IL-1R after binding of IL-1α or IL-1β and is involved in activation of signal transduction pathways.[8,9] However, binding of IL-1Ra to IL-1RI prevents subsequent interaction of the complex with IL-1R AcP, explaining the mechanism of action of IL-1Ra. IL-1 activates cells through the nuclear factor κB (NFκB), c-Jun N-terminal kinase (JNK)/AP-1 and p38 mitogen-activated protein kinase (MAPK) signal transduction pathways. After formation of the complex between IL-1, IL-1RI and IL-1R AcP at the plasma membrane, two cytosolic proteins, MyD88 and Tollip are recruited to the complex.[10] These molecules recruit IL-1 receptor-associated kinase (IRAK), a serine–threonine kinase, which is then phosphorylated at the receptor complex and dissociates to interact with TNF receptor-associated factor 6 (TRAF6). To activate the NFκB pathway, TRAF6 associates with the MAPKK kinase TAK1, leading to phosphorylation of nuclear factor κB-inducing kinase (NIK) with stimulation of kinase activity. IκB kinase (IKK) in turn phosphorylates IκB, causing dissociation of this inhibitor from NFκB with subsequent movement of this protein complex to the nucleus and activation of transcription of multiple target genes.[11] However, TRAF6 also activates the JNK/AP-1 pathway through a different domain from that involved in the NFκB pathway which does not require TRAF6 phosphorylation.[10]

IL-1 is produced by most nucleated cells, with the more important sources including monocytes, macrophages, neutrophils, microglial cells, astrocytes, endothelial cells, epithelial cells, and dendritic cells.[1] IL-1 production is stimulated by endotoxin, other bacterial cell wall products, viral products, complement fragments, cytokine themselves, and other proteins.[1] Both IL-1α and IL-1β are synthesized as larger precursor proteins in the cytoplasm, but do not contain leader sequences. Most IL-1α is placed on the plasma membrane or traffics to the nucleus, whereas IL-1β is largely secreted from cells through unclear mechanisms. The most characterized functions for IL-1 in normal physiology include host resistance to intracellular organisms (*Mycobacterium tuberculosis*, *Listeria*, etc.), regulation of the sleep–wake cycle in the central nervous system (CNS), the reproductive cycle in the uterus, induction of fever, and stimulation of turnover of matrix components of connective tissue. However, excess or unopposed production of IL-1 may lead to tissue damage in many chronic inflammatory diseases. The major pathophysiologic effects of IL-1 include induction of adhesion molecule expression on endothelial cells, with the subsequent migration of inflammatory and immune cells from the blood into tissues, and induction of the production of enzymes that destroy connective tissue proteins.

IL-1 receptor antagonist

IL-1Ra was originally described as IL-1 inhibitory bioactivities in the supernatant of monocyes cultured on IgG[12] and in the urine of patients with myelomonocytic leukemia.[13] The semi-purified protein from both sources was shown to function as a specific receptor antagonist of IL-1.[14,15] The IL-1Ra protein was purified from the supernatants of monocytes cultured on IgG[16] and from the supernatants from phorbol miristate acetate (PMA)-differentiated U937 cells, a human myelomonocytic cell line.[17] A cDNA was cloned and expressed for a 17-kDa form of IL-1Ra that was secreted as variably glycosylated species of 22–25 kDa.[17,18] Additional isoforms of IL-1Ra have subsequently been described, with the original secreted form now termed sIL-1Ra (Figure 12.2). An 18-kDa intracellular isoform, created by alternative transcriptional splice of an upstream exon, termed icIL-1Ra1, is a major protein in keratinocytes and other epithelial cells,

monocytes, macrophages, fibroblasts, and endothelial cells.[19] An mRNA for icIL-1Ra2, also formed by alternative transcriptional splice from another upstream exon, was cloned from human cells.[20] However, it is unlikely that this mRNA is translated in vivo, as no naturally occurring IL-1Ra protein with the predicted molecular mass of 25 kDa has been described. A third 16-kDa intracellular isoform of IL-1Ra, termed icIL-1Ra3, was found in human monocytes, neutrophils, and hepatocytes.[21,22] This low-molecular-weight species of IL-1Ra may be formed by alternative translational initiation[22] or by an alternative transcriptional splice mechanism.[23] Both sIL-1Ra and icIL-1Ra1 bind avidly to IL-1RI and IL-1RII, whereas icIL-1Ra3 binds very weakly. Some icIL-1Ra1 may be released from keratinocytes under certain conditions and inhibit receptor binding of IL-1, but it is possible that the intracellular isoforms of IL-1Ra carry out additional and unique functions inside cells.

IL-1Ra is produced by most cells that also are sources of IL-1, including monocytes, macrophages, neutrophils, keratinocytes and other epithelial cells. The stimuli for IL-1Ra production vary with the cell and include endotoxin, adherent IgG, direct contact with Th2 cells, and granulocyte–macrophage colony-stimulating factor (GM-CSF) and other cytokines.[24] Some stimuli exhibit reciprocal regulation, with IL-4 inhibiting IL-1 production by monocytes and macrophages while enhancing IL-1Ra production.

Further molecules with sequence similarities to IL-1 or IL-1Ra have been described, but none of the molecules characterized to date possesses IL-1 agonist or receptor antagonist activities. However, the possibility remains that further functional members of the IL-1 family may exist.

IL-1 in animal models of arthritis and in rheumatoid arthritis

Extensive evidence exists to incriminate IL-1 in pathophysiologic events in both animal models of inflammatory arthritis and in RA (reviews: Arend and Dayer[25,26]) (Table 12.2). Early studies demonstrated that pig cartilage released factors

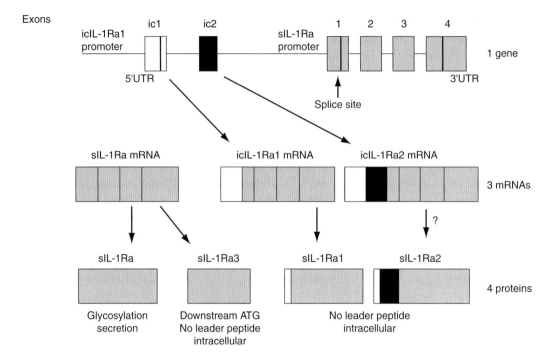

Figure 12.2 IL-1Ra structural variants. The IL-1Ra gene contains six exons and codes for three different mRNAs and four structurally different IL-1Ra proteins. icIL-1Ra1 and sIL-1Ra mRNA transmission start at two different exons: ic1 and 1, respectively. The splice acceptor site for the first exon of icIL-1Ra1 is located in the region coding for the leader peptide. Therefore, icIL-1Ra1 lacks a complete leader peptide and remains intracellular. icIL-1Ra2 mRNA includes the presence of an additional exon of 66 bp, ic2, located between the icIL-1Ra1 and sIL-1Ra first exons. However, endogenous production of icIL-1Ra2 has not been confirmed yet. icIL-1Ra3 is a smaller peptide that is generated by alternative translation initiation, mainly from sIL-1Ra mRNA. After cleavage of the leader peptide, sIL-1Ra is glycosylated and secreted as a 22–25-kDa protein. UTR, untranslated region.

Table 12.2   Evidence for role of IL-1 in RA.

Experimental animal models of RA
   IL-1 found in synovial tissue and fluid
   Intra-articular injection of IL-1 causes
      inflammatory arthritis
   Delivery of IL-1Ra protein or cDNA decreases
      severity of arthritis
   Antibodies to IL-1Ra worsen arthritis

RA in humans
   IL-1 bioactivities and protein present in
      synovial tissue and fluids
   IL-1Ra production by synovial tissue not
      sufficient to effectively inhibit IL-1
   Administration of IL-1Ra protein decreases
      disease activity and tissue damage

that induced the destruction of proteoglycans from articular cartilage by activating chondrocytes.[27] This bioactivity, called catabolin or mononuclear cell factor, was later shown to be IL-1. Subsequently, IL-1 bioactivity was described in the synovial fluids from patients with RA or other forms of inflammatory arthritis.[28,29] IL-1 bioactivities were produced by cultured synovial fluid macrophages,[30] and such activities were released from human rheumatoid synovial tissue during cell isolation[31] or after cell culture.[32] Injection of recombinant human IL-1 into normal rabbit knees led to an influx of polymorphonuclear and mononuclear leukocytes into the joint space and to the loss of proteoglycans from the articular cartilage.[33] The proteoglycan loss from articular cartilage after the intra-articular injection of IL-1 was due to both enhancement of degradation and inhibition of synthesis.[34] Collagen degradation was also induced by culture of bovine articular cartilage with IL-1, with pericellular loss of collagen demonstrated both in these cartilage pieces in vitro and in rheumatoid cartilage in vivo.[35] These studies, published in 1989, proved that IL-1-stimulated chondrocytes were the source of the matrix-degrading enzymes.

Additional experimental results accumulated over the past decade have further characterized the presence and role of IL-1 in inflammatory arthritis. IL-1 immunoreactivity was present in macrophages in the rheumatoid synovium, with localization in the lining layer, particularly at the pannus–cartilage junction, and in perivascular and loose connective tissue areas.[36,37] Intracellular staining for IL-1α and IL-1β was described in macrophages in the rheumatoid synovium, in both the lining and sublining areas, indicating that these cytokines were synthesized in this tissue.[38] Both the quantities and patterns of cytokine presence, as determined by immunohistochemical techniques, were highly heterogeneous in rheumatoid synovia between patients, despite similar macroscopic and histologic features of inflammation.[39] Injection of IL-1β-neutralizing antisera markedly reduced the cellular infiltration, reversed the inhibition of proteoglycan synthesis, and decreased the loss in proteoglycan content in articular cartilage in antigen-induced arthritis in mice.[40–42] Finally, clinical and histologic changes highly similar to those seen in RA were induced in rabbits by intra-articular gene transfer of human IL-1β[43] and in mice transgenic for human IL-1α.[44]

Extensive studies on IL-1Ra have further clarified the importance of IL-1 as a pathophysiologic

mediator in RA (reviews: Dinarello[1] and Arend et al[24]). Abundant IL-1Ra protein and mRNA were localized to macrophages in the lining, sublining and perivascular areas,[38,45–47] as well as to endothelial cells in the rheumatoid synovium.[38] High levels of IL-1Ra protein were present in the synovial fluids of 80% of patients with RA, and less commonly in other forms of inflammatory arthritis.[48] IL-1Ra levels were correlated with the synovial fluid neutrophil concentrations in these studies, and these cells are capable of producing IL-1Ra.[49] Cultured rheumatoid synovial fluid mononuclear cells also produced IL-1Ra in vitro.[50] IL-1Ra inhibited IL-1-induced prostaglandin E_2 (PGE_2) and collagenase production by cultured rheumatoid synovial cells[51] and reversed the inhibition of proteoglycan synthesis.[52] Thus, IL-1Ra is present in significant amounts in the rheumatoid synovial fluid and tissue and can inhibit the pathophysiologic effects of IL-1 on synovial fibroblasts in vitro.

IL-1Ra treatment of animal models of arthritis

Administration of recombinant IL-1Ra has prevented or dramatically ameliorated a variety of experimental animal models of inflammatory arthritis. The chronic phase of streptococcal cell wall (SCW) arthritis in rats was markedly reduced by intraperitoneal injections of IL-1Ra at the time of reactivation of the disease.[53] Although IL-1Ra was found not to reduce inflammation in murine SCW arthritis, continuous intraperitoneal infusion of IL-1Ra led to a marked reversal of the inhibition of proteoglycan synthesis as well as to decreased inflammatory cell influx and proteoglycan depletion in articular cartilage.[54]

The greater effect of IL-1Ra on reducing cartilage and bone destruction rather than on decreasing signs of inflammation, in contrast to the effects of tumour necrosis factor (TNF) inhibition, were described in immune complex-induced arthritis in mice,[55] antigen-induced arthritis in rabbits,[56] and collagen-induced arthritis (CIA) in mice.[57,58] IL-1Ra treatment in CIA in mice, an experimental model with many similar features to RA, led to reduced incidence, delayed onset, and decreased severity.[59] The maintenance of sustained blood levels of IL-1Ra was shown to be important in the successful treatment of established CIA.[60] The combination of IL-1Ra and methotrexate gave more dramatic inhibition of inflammation and bone resorption in adjuvant arthritis in rats than did either therapy alone.[61] Furthermore, combination therapy with IL-1Ra and a soluble TNF-α receptor exhibited synergistic effects in adjuvant arthritis in rats,[62,63] and in CIA in rats.[63] Finally, decreasing endogenous production of IL-1β through the administration of an inhibitor of IL-1β-converting enzyme delayed the onset and decreased the severity of murine CIA.[64]

All of the above studies indicate that inflammatory arthritis in experimental animal models is significantly prevented or ameliorated by blocking IL-1. These successful therapeutic approaches have been complemented by the recent use of gene therapy techniques to deliver IL-1Ra to the joint. Ex vivo gene therapy has been carried out by transfection of the IL-1Ra cDNA into cultured rabbit synovial fibroblasts, and then injection of the cells into the knee. The cells are taken up by the synovial lining, and secrete IL-1Ra into the synovial fluid, preventing IL-1-induced migration of neutrophils[65,66] and proteoglycan degradation in the articular cartilage.[66,67] Ex vivo gene therapy with IL-1Ra also suppressed antigen-induced arthritis in rabbits,[68] bacterial cell wall-induced arthritis in rats,[69] and both ipsilateral and contralateral arthritis in CIA in mice.[70] Gene transfer carried out by injection of viral vectors containing the IL-1Ra cDNA directly into the joint was successful in adjuvant arthritis in rats,[71] antigen-induced arthritis in rabbits,[72] IL-1-induced arthritis in rabbits,[73] and lipopolysaccharide (LPS)-induced arthritis in rats.[74] Finally, systemic gene therapy with soluble IL-1RII decreased clinical and histologic parameters of disease activity in CIA in mice.[75]

Although this chapter has focused on RA, IL-1 has also been incriminated in the cartilage damage in OA, and IL-1 inhibition has been efficacious in animal models of this disease.

Transplantation of IL-1Ra-transduced chondrocytes onto the articular surface of osteoarthritic cartilage organ cultures protected against IL-1-induced proteoglycan degradation.[76] The progression of experimental OA in dogs was prevented by IL-1Ra administered by intra-articular injections of recombinant protein,[77] ex vivo gene therapy,[78] or in vivo gene therapy.[79]

This chapter has reviewed some of the data indicating an important role for IL-1 in mediating inflammation and tissue destruction in inflammatory arthritis in animals, in RA in patients, and in an experimental animal model of OA. Inhibition of IL-1 by blocking IL-1 production, preventing receptor binding of IL-1 with neutralizing antibodies, or competing for receptor binding with IL-1Ra, have all proven efficacious in animal models of RA or OA. Many of these treatments have been, or currently are being, evaluated in patients with these diseases.

THE BALANCE BETWEEN IL-1 AND IL-1RA

The role of endogenous IL-1Ra

The balance between IL-1 and IL-1Ra plays a critical role in the course of a variety of inflammatory diseases. The levels of IL-1 and IL-1Ra were examined in the intestine of patients with inflammatory bowel disease. Freshly homogenized biopsies from involved tissue in patients with inflammatory bowel disease exhibited a lower IL-1β/IL-1Ra ratio than control and uninvolved tissue in inflammatory bowel disease.[80] Using explant cultures, in vitro production of IL-1β was higher in supernatants from inflammatory bowel disease and increased with disease severity, whereas IL-1Ra secretion was not higher in involved samples as compared with controls.[80] The expression of IL-1Ra in comparison to that of IL-1β appeared to be relatively low in the colonic tissue of patients with Crohn's disease as compared to patients with self-limited colitis.[81] IL-1Ra is produced by hepatocytes in response to IL-1β and IL-6 in vitro and in vivo.[82,83] The circulating levels of IL-1Ra were also elevated in patients with liver diseases and correlated with markers of disease activity.[84] High serum levels of IL-1β and IL-1Ra were observed in patients with fulminant hepatic failure and acute hepatitis. Interestingly, IL-1Ra/IL-1β ratios were markedly higher in patients who survived than in those who did not, suggesting that IL-1Ra, probably produced in the liver, influences the outcome of severe liver diseases.[85] Defective production of IL-1Ra is observed in patients with acute liver graft rejection resistant to steroid therapy.[86]

An important anti-inflammatory role for endogenous IL-1Ra in arthritis was also suggested by a study that compared the clinical course of knee arthritis in patients with Lyme disease. Patients with high concentrations of synovial fluid IL-1Ra and low concentrations of IL-1β had rapid resolution of acute attacks of arthritis, whereas patients with the reverse pattern of cytokine concentrations had a more protracted course.[87] In addition, several studies demonstrated that the IL-1Ra/IL-1β ratio was low in RA, thus leading to the perpetuation of articular inflammation and subsequent tissue destruction.[45,88,89] We recently showed that the IL-1β/IL-1Ra ratio was elevated in the synovium of mice with collagen-induced arthritis and that this ratio correlated with the severity of joint score. In contrast, the IL-1β/IL-1Ra ratio decreased at later time points. These changes were associated with a progressive reduction in the levels of inflammatory activity in the joints, thus further emphasizing the role of the balance between IL-1 and IL-1Ra in the modulation of the inflammatory response.[90]

The physiologic function of endogenous IL-1Ra has been further demonstrated in several studies by stimulating production of endogenous IL-1Ra, blocking endogenous IL-1Ra with specific antibodies, or deleting the gene for IL-1Ra. Injection of IL-4 from the time of the initial SCW injection in mice largely suppressed the chronic phase of this disease, primarily through stimulating the endogenous production of IL-1Ra.[91] Exogenous or endogenous IL-10 was found to be an even more potent stimulant of endogenous IL-1Ra than IL-4 in SCW arthritis in mice.[92] Injection of neutralizing F(ab')₂ anti-IL-1Ra antibodies led to enhanced leukocyte infiltration and protein leakage into synovial fluid in LPS-induced arthritis in rabbits.[93] Mice lacking the expression of IL-1Ra were more susceptible to endotoxin-induced lethality.[94] IL-1Ra-knockout mice had a significantly earlier onset of collagen-induced arthritis and more severe synovitis, often accompanied by bony erosions.[95] Most interestingly, the absence of IL-1Ra by gene deletion in BALB/cA mice was associated with the spontaneous development of chronic polyarthritis with the presence of autoantibodies, thus reproducing some of the clinical and biological features of RA.[96] An arterial inflammatory disease resembling polyarteritis nodosa spontaneously developed in IL-1Ra-knockout mice bred on an MFI × 129 background.[97] Taken together, these findings indicate that an imbalance between IL-1 and IL-1Ra may predispose to inflammatory diseases and that endogenous IL-1Ra may serve an important role in preventing or limiting organ damage in IL-1-mediated diseases.

IL-1Ra gene polymorphism and human diseases

A polymorphism is present in intron 2 of the human IL-1Ra gene, due to the presence of variable numbers of 86-bp tandem repeats (VNTR).[98] Five alleles have been described, and this allelic region contains three potential binding sites, suggesting possible functional significance. The two-repeat allele (IL-1RN*2) has been associated with a variety of human diseases (Table 12.3). It is of interest that these diseases are primarily diseases of epithelial cells. Recently, associations between IL-1RN*2 and coronary artery disease[99,100] and polymyalgia rheumatica[101] have also been reported. In addition, an increased risk of gastric cancer in IL-1RN*2 homozygotes has also been described.[102] The mechanism of IL-1RN*2 association with diseases has been investigated. The results of different studies showed that the effect of IL-1RN*2 genotype on IL-1Ra production varies according to the cell type. IL-1RN*2 was associated with increased production of sIL-1Ra

Table 12.3 Association of IL-1RN*2 with diseases.
Ulcerative colitis
Alopecia areata
Lichen sclerosis
Psoriasis
Lupus erythematosus skin lesions
Graves' disease
Diabetic nephropathy
Sjogren's syndrome
Coronary artery disease
Polymyalgia rheumatica
Gastric cancer
Severe Henoch Schönlein purpura

by monocytes in culture,[103] whereas icIL-1Ra1 mRNA levels were not altered in keratinocytes from individuals possessing different intron 2 alleles.[98] In contrast, human endothelial cells homozygous for the IL-1RN*2 allele produced three times less icIL-1Ra1 protein than cells of other genotypes.[104] This finding and the results of recent epidemiologic studies showing an increased risk of coronary events in patients with the IL-1RN*2 allele suggest that deficient production of IL-1Ra by endothelial cells may predispose to the development of atherosclerosis and other inflammatory diseases of blood vessels. Another polymorphism has also been discovered as a single base pair change in exon 2 that does not modify the amino acid sequence. This second polymorphism is invariably linked to the presence of the two-repeat allele.[105]

Administration of IL-1Ra in the treatment of RA

Recombinant human sIL-1Ra, also known as anakinra, is produced by AMGEN (USA). Anakinra has been recently approved for the treatment of RA by the United States Food and Drug Administration and is now commercially available as Kineret®.

IL-1Ra administration by daily subcutaneous injections has been examined in phase I and II clinical trials in patients with RA. An initial randomized, double-blind study was performed in 172 patients with RA.[106] The treatment was well tolerated, with the most frequent adverse effect being injection-site reactions. The patients receiving the daily injections of IL-1Ra appeared to exhibit some clinical improvement and exhibited decreased serum levels of C-reactive protein.

In a subsequent randomized, double-blind, placebo-controlled, multicenter trial, 472 patients with RA received daily subcutaneous injections of placebo or three different doses of IL-1Ra for 24 weeks.[107] The group receiving the largest dose (150 mg/injection) demonstrated ~35% improvement in various clinical parameters in comparison to the placebo group at 24 weeks. Furthermore, patients receiving the highest dose of IL-1Ra demonstrated a reduced frequency and severity of radiologic joint erosions. A 24-week extension of this study was carried out where IL-1Ra was also given to the placebo group. The results of this extension showed that administration of IL-1Ra to the placebo patients resulted in new clinical improvement and that the patients who previously received IL-1Ra maintained the improvement seen in the first 24-week trial.[108]

There has been growing interest over the past few years in the combined use of several anti-rheumatic drugs in the treatment of RA. The treatment of experimental animal models of arthritis with IL-1Ra and methotrexate together, or with IL-1Ra combined with a soluble TNF receptor, is reviewed above. The effect of IL-1Ra in combination with methotrexate has been studied recently in a randomized, double-blind, placebo-controlled, multicenter trial. Four hundred and nineteen patients with active RA despite being treated with methotrexate received either subcutaneous injections of placebo or different doses of IL-1Ra.[109] The results demonstrated that the group of patients receiving 1 mg/kg of IL-1Ra had a better clinical response than the placebo group, indicating that IL-1Ra provides additional clinical improvement to RA patients not responding to methotrexate alone. No additional side-effects were observed in patients receiving the combination therapy.

The results of a confirmatory study were recently presented. Nine hundred and six patients with active RA despite treatment with methotrexate were randomized to receive anakinra 100 mg/day or placebo. After 6 months, a significantly higher percentage of patients treated with the combination of anakinra and methotrexate achieved the ACR20 response as compared with those in the placebo group. These results were confirmed by using more stringent criteria such as the ACR50 and ACR70 responses.

Combination therapy targeting both IL-1 and TNF-α was recently studied in a phase II open trial in 58 RA patients. These patients demonstrated active disease despite treatment with etanercept, a fusion protein containing the extracellular domain of TNF receptor p75 and the Fc region of human IgG class 1, and received anakinra at a dosage of 1 mg/kg per day while continuing etanercept 25 mg subcutaneously twice weekly. After 24 weeks, various clinical and biological parameters of disease activity were ameliorated by the combination of anakinra and etanercept. However, approximately one-third of the patients discontinued this treatment. Eleven of 58 patients demonstrated serious side-effects, including four cases with severe infection.[110] Of note, no cases of tuberculosis or opportunistic infections have been reported to date in patients treated with anakinra alone. An increased frequency of infectious adverse events is a concern with the use of anti-cytokine treatment and has been observed in post-marketing surveillance of the anti-TNF therapies. Studies performed in experimental animal models indicated that combinations of low doses of cytokine inhibitors had a synergistic effect on clinical and histologic signs of arthritis. Thus, the objective of future studies is to define an appropriate dosage of cytokine inhibitors that will be effective in the treatment of RA with a minimal risk of infections.

The therapeutic use of IL-1Ra may be limited by the fact that high amounts of IL-1Ra are necessary to block the effects of IL-1. Thus, different authors have considered the possibility of delivering IL-1Ra by local gene therapy in arthritic joints. The successful application of gene therapy in several experimental animal models of arthritis is reviewed above. The anti-arthritic effects of intra-articular gene transfer were also observed in contralateral untreated joints, indicating that local gene therapy can be used in the treatment of a polyarticular and systemic disease.[70] The results of clinical trials of gene therapy with IL-1Ra in patients with RA demonstrated the successful transfer of ex vivo transduced synoviocytes, resulting in intra-articular expression of IL-1Ra.[111] However, two important issues involving the safety and the transient nature of cDNA expression in transduced cells need to be resolved to enhance the feasibility of gene therapy for the treatment of RA.

Other options for targeting IL-1 and IL-1 signaling

A list of some possible strategies intended to inhibit the production of IL-1, to block IL-1 in the extracellular space, to interfere with the binding of IL-1 to its cell surface receptors, or to block intracellular signaling induced by IL-1 after binding to type I IL-1 receptors, is given in Table 12.4 (Figure 12.3).

Inhibition of IL-1 production and secretion
A variety of currently used therapeutic approaches inhibit the production of IL-1 in vivo and in vitro. Glucocorticoids are known to inhibit the in vitro transcription of several proinflammatory cytokines in monocytes or macrophages, such as IL-1β and TNF-α. In human volunteers treated with glucocorticoids, the circulating levels of IL-1β in response to an intravenous injection of LPS were significantly lower than in untreated controls.[112] In addition, peripheral blood mononuclear cells (PBMC) of rheumatoid patients treated with methotrexate produced less IL-1 in vitro; this decrease was correlated with clinical improvement.[113] Gold sodium thiomalate or auranofin inhibited the production of IL-1 by LPS-stimulated PBMC and increased the production of

Table 12.4   Strategies to block IL-1 in rheumatoid arthritis.

Decrease production of IL-1
  Corticosteroids
  IL-4, IL-10, IL-13
  Block IL-1β-converting enzyme (ICE)
  Methotrexate, gold compounds

Inhibit extracellular IL-1
  Soluble IL-1R type II
  IL-1 TRAP

Interfere with IL-1R binding
  IL-1Ra
  Synthetic peptides with IL-1Ra activity

Block intracellular response to IL-1
  Inhibit JNK and p38 MAPK pathways
  Block NFκB activation or DNA binding

IL-1Ra, thus modifying favorably the balance between IL-1 and IL-1Ra.[114] IL-1 production may be decreased both in vitro and in vivo by other cytokines such as IL-4, IL-10, and IL-13. In contrast, these cytokines enhanced the production of IL-1Ra.[115] The administration of IL-10 was safe; however, whereas a positive response to treatment with IL-10 was observed for psoriasis, psoriatic arthritis did not improve.[116]

Interfere with extracellular IL-1

The two types of IL-1R exist as both membrane-bound and soluble forms. Both receptors belong to the immunoglobulin superfamily and possess some homology in their extracellular domains. Soluble IL-1R type II binds to IL-1Ra with much lower affinity than IL-1β and may supplement the anti-inflammatory effects of IL-1Ra.[117] The administration of soluble IL-1R type II in experimental animal models of arthritis resulted in a marked inhibition of joint swelling and joint damage.[75,118] In addition, recent data indicate

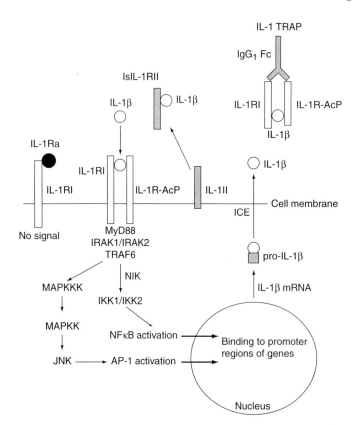

Figure 12.3   Different options to block the biological effects of IL-1. (i) To inhibit production of mature IL-1β at the level of gene expression or by blocking IL-1β-converting enzyme activity. (ii) To block extracellular IL-1β with soluble IL-1R type II (IL-1RI). IL-1RI binds IL-1β with high affinity and prevents its interaction with cell surface IL-1R type I. In addition, IL-1RI binds IL-1β with a higher affinity than IL-1Ra, which may potentially increase the anti-inflammatory effects of IL-1Ra. Another approach to binding extracellular IL-1 is the development of a reagent called the IL-1 TRAP, consisting of a combination of the extracellular portions of the type I IL-1R and the IL-1R AcP bound to the Fc portion of human IgG$_1$. (iii) To inhibit the interaction of IL-1 with membrane-bound receptor type I using IL-1Ra or another synthetic molecule having similar properties. (iv) To block the post-receptor effects of IL-1 by interfering with NFκB or AP-1 activation pathways or the binding of these transcription factors to the promoter regions of target genes.

that soluble IL-1R type II may exert a chondroprotective effect in vitro. Thus, the administration of soluble IL-1R type II may be an interesting approach in the treatment of RA and other IL-1-mediated diseases. In contrast, the administration of soluble IL-1R type I in RA patients exhibited no efficacy.[119]

Another approach to binding extracellular IL-1 is the development of a reagent called the IL-1 TRAP, consisting of a combination of the extracellular portions of the type I IL-1R and the IL-1R AcP bound to the Fc portion of human IgG$_1$. This material exhibits a high affinity for IL-1 and can be administered in a single weekly subcutaneous injection.[120] A phase II clinical trial with the IL-1 TRAP in RA is in progress.

Inhibit IL-1-induced intracellular signaling

IL-1 and TNF-α are able to stimulate some common post-receptor events that play an important role in cell activation. Thus, it is conceivable that strategies aimed at interfering with these intracellular signaling pathways should be beneficial for the treatment of arthritis. NFκB is a well-studied transcription factor that mediates the effects of TNF-α and IL-1 in inflammatory diseases. The spontaneous production of proinflammatory cytokines was decreased in cells expressing high levels of a NFκB inhibitor, whereas production of anti-inflammatory cytokines such as IL-10, IL-11 and IL-1Ra was not influenced by NFκB. In addition, IκBα overexpression inhibited production of matrix metalloproteinases 1 and 3 but had no effect on their tissue inhibitor.[121] The oral use of proteosome inhibitors, which block the degradation of IκB, reduced the severity of peptidoglycan polysaccharide-induced arthritis in female Lewis rats.[122] This treatment attenuated the synovial infiltrate and the formation of pannus as well as bone and cartilage destruction. Recently, the oral administration of IKK2 inhibitors decreased the severity of arthritis in two different experimental animal models of arthritis.[123,124]

IL-1 induces activation of stress-activated protein kinases (SAPKs), c-Jun N-terminal kinases (JNKs) and p38 mitogen-activated protein kinases (MAPKs). These signaling pathways result in activation of transcription factors. JNKs activate different members of the AP-1 transcription factor family (c-Fos and c-Jun). Activation of AP-1 plays an important role in the mechanisms of joint damage. Inhibition of AP-1 binding to its consensus DNA site decreased joint destruction in mice with CIA.[125] p38 MAPK is involved in expression of IL-1 and TNF-α, as well as in downstream members of the cytokine cascade, including IL-6 and IL-8. Accordingly, the administration of p38 MAPK inhibitors decreased the severity of adjuvant-induced arthritis in the rat.[126]

SUMMARY

The IL-1 family consists of two agonists, a receptor antagonist with three structural variants, and three receptors. Extensive evidence both in animal models of inflammatory arthritis and in patients with RA indicates that IL-1 is a key mediator of inflammation and tissue destruction. The delivery of IL-1Ra by either protein injection or gene therapy approaches is efficacious in decreasing inflammation as well as cartilage and bone destruction. In addition, other strategies for targeting IL-1 production and signaling are promising for the treatment of RA.

REFERENCES

1. Dinarello CA. Interleukin-1 and interleukin-1 antagonism. *Blood* 1991; **77**: 1627–52.
2. Arend WA. Interleukin-1 receptor antagonist. *Adv Immunol* 1993; **54**: 167–227.
3. Steinkasserer A, Spurr NK, Cox S et al. The human IL-1 receptor antagonist gene (IL1RN) maps to chromosome 2q14–q21, in the region of the IL-1α and IL-1β loci. *Genomics* 1992; **13**: 654–7.
4. Patterson D, Jones C, Hart I et al. The human interleukin-1 receptor antagonist (IL1RN) gene is located in the chromosome 2q14 region. *Genomics* 1993; **15**: 173–6.

5. Eisenberg SP, Brewer MT, Verderber E et al. Interleukin 1 receptor antagonist is a member of the interleukin 1 gene family: evolution of a cytokine control mechanism. *Proc Natl Acad Sci USA* 1991; **88**: 5232–6.

6. Sims JE, Giri JG, Dower SK. Short analytical review. The two interleukin-1 receptors play different roles in IL-1 actions. *Clin Immunol Immunopathol* 1994; **72**: 9–14.

7. Colotta F, Dower SK, Sims JE, Mantovani A. The type II 'decoy' receptor: a novel regulatory pathway for interleukin 1. *Immunol Today* 1994; **15**: 562–6.

8. Greenfeder SA, Nunes P, Kwee L et al. Molecular cloning and characterization of a second subunit of the interleukin 1 receptor complex. *J Biol Chem* 1995; **270**: 13757–65.

9. Huang J, Gao X, Li S, Cao Z. Recruitment of IRAK to the interleukin 1 receptor complex requires interleukin 1 receptor accessory protein. *Proc Natl Acad Sci USA* 1997; **94**: 12829–32.

10. Li X, Commane M, Jiang Z, Stark GR. IL-1-induced NFκB and c-Jun N-terminal kinase (JNK) activation diverge at IL-1 receptor-associated kinase (IRAK). *Proc Natl Acad Sci USA* 2001; **98**: 4461–5.

11. Ninomiya-Tsuji J, Kishimoto K, Hiyama A et al. The kinase TAK1 can activate the NIκ-1B as well as the MAP kinase cascade in the IL-1 signalling pathway. *Nature* 1999; **398**: 252–6.

12. Arend WP, D'Angelo S, Massoni RJ, Joslin FG. Interleukin 1 production by human monocytes: effects of different stimuli. In: Kluger MJ, Oppenheim JJ, Powanda MC, eds. *The Physiologic, Metabolic, and Immunologic Actions of Interleukin-1.* (Alan R. Liss: New York, 1985) 399–407.

13. Balavoine J-F, de Rochemonteix B, Cruchaud A, Dayer J-M. Collagenase- and PGE$_2$-stimulating activity (interleukin-1-like) and inhibitor in urine from a patient with monocytic leukaemia. In: Kluger MJ, Oppenheim JJ, Powanda MC, eds. *The Physiologic, Metabolic, and Immunologic Actions of Interleukin-1.* (Alan R. Liss: New York, 1985) 429–36.

14. Seckinger P, Lowenthal JW, Williamson K et al. A urine inhibitor of interleukin 1 activity that blocks ligand binding. *J Immunol* 1987; **139**: 1546–9.

15. Arend WP, Joslin FG, Thompson RC, Hannum CH. An IL-1 inhibitor from human monocytes production and characterization of biologic properties. *J Immunol* 1989; **143**: 1851–8.

16. Hannum Ch, Wilcox CJ, Arend WP et al. Interleukin-1 receptor antagonist activity of a human interleukin-1 inhibitor. *Nature* 1990; **343**: 336–40.

17. Carter DB, Deibel MR, Dunn CJ et al. Purification, cloning, expression and biological characterization of an interleukin-1 receptor antagonist protein. *Nature* 1990; **344**: 633–8.

18. Eisenberg SP, Evans RJ, Arend WP et al. Primary structure and functional expression from complementary DNA of a human interleukin-1 receptor antagonist. *Nature* 1990; **343**: 341–6.

19. Haskill S, Martin G, Van Le L et al. cDNA cloning of an intracellular form of the human interleukin 1 receptor antagonist associated with epithelium. *Proc Natl Acad Sci USA* 1991; **88**: 3681–5.

20. Muzio M, Polentarutti N, Sironi M et al. Cloning and characterization of a new isoform of the interleukin 1 receptor antagonist. *J Exp Med* 1995; **182**: 623–8.

21. Malyak M, Guthridge JM, Hance KR et al. Characterization of a low molecular weight isoform of IL-1 receptor antagonist. *J Immunol* 1998; **161**: 1997–2003.

22. Malyak M, Smith MF, Abel AA et al. The differential production of three forms of IL-1 receptor antagonist by human neutrophils and monocytes. *J Immunol* 1998; **161**: 2004–10.

23. Weissbach L, Tran K, Colquhoun SA et al. Detection of an interleukin-1 intracellular receptor antagonist mRNA variant. *Biochem Biophys Res Commun* 1998; **244**: 91–5.

24. Arend WP, Malyak M, Guthridge CJ, Gabay C. Interleukin-1 receptor antagonist: role in biology. *Ann Rev Immunol* 1998; **16**: 27–55.

25. Arend WP, Dayer J-M. Cytokines and cytokine inhibitors or antagonists in rheumatoid arthritis. *Arthritis Rheum* 1990; **33**: 305–15.

26. Arend WP, Dayer J-M. Inhibition of the production and effects of interleukin-1 and tumor necrosis factor α in rheumatoid arthritis. *Arthritis Rheum* 1995; **38**: 151–60.

27. Fell H, Jubb RW. The effect of synovial tissue on the breakdown of articular cartilage in organ culture. *Arthritis Rheum* 1977; **20**: 1359–71.

28. Fontana A, Hengartner H, Weber E. Interleukin 1 activity in the synovial fluid of patients with rheumatoid arthritis. *Rheumatol Int* 1982; **2**: 49–53.

29. Wood DD, Ihrie EJ, Dinarello CA, Cohen PL. Isolation of an interleukin-1-like factor from human joint effusions. *Arthritis Rheum* 1983; **26**: 975–83.

30. Poubelle P, Damon M, Blotman F, Dayer J-M. Production of mononuclear cell factor by mononuclear phagocytes from rheumatoid synovial fluid. *J Rheumatol* 1985; **12**: 412–17.

31. Wood DD, Ihrie EJ, Hamerman D. Release of interleukin-1 from human synovial tissue in vitro. *Arthritis Rheum* 1985; **28**: 853–62.

32. Miyasaka N, Sato K, Goto M et al. Augmented interleukin-1 production and HLA-DR expression in the synovium of rheumatoid arthritis patients. *Arthritis Rheum* 1988; **31**: 480–6.

33. Pettipher ER, Higgs GA, Henderson B. Interleukin 1 induces leukocyte infiltration and cartilage proteoglycan degradation in the synovial joint. *Proc Natl Acad Sci USA* 1986; **83**: 8749–53.

34. van de Loo AAJ, van den Berg WB. Effects of murine recombinant interleukin 1 on synovial joints in mice: measurement of patellar cartilage metabolism and joint inflammation. *Ann Rheum Dis* 1990; **49**: 238–45.

35. Dodge GR, Poole AR. Immunohistochemical detection and immunochemical analysis of type II collagen degradation in human normal, rheumatoid, and osteoarthritic articular cartilages and in explants of bovine articular cartilage cultured with interleukin 1. *J Clin Invest* 1989; **83**: 647–61.

36. Farahat MN, Yanni G, Poston R, Panayi GS. Cytokine expression in synovial membranes of patients with rheumatoid arthritis and osteoarthritis. *Ann Rheum Dis* 1993; **52**: 870–5.

37. Chu CQ, Field M, Allard S et al. Detection of cytokines at the cartilage/pannus junction in patients with rheumatoid arthritis: implications for the role of cytokines in cartilage destruction and repair. *Br J Rheumatol* 1992; **31**: 653–61.

38. Ulfgren A-K, Lindblad S, Klareskog L et al. Detection of cytokine producing cells in the synovial membrane from patients with rheumatoid arthritis. *Ann Rheum Dis* 1995; **54**: 654–61.

39. Ulfgren A-K, Grondal L, Lindblad S et al. Interindividual and intra-articular variation of proinflammatory cytokines in patients with rheumatoid arthritis: potential implications for treatment. *Ann Rheum Dis* 2000; **59**: 439–77.

40. van de Loo FAJ, Arntz OJ, Otterness IG, van den Berg WB. Protection against cartilage proteoglycan synthesis inhibition by antiinterleukin 1 antibodies in experimental arthritis. *J Rheumatol* 1992; **19**: 348–56.

41. van de Loo AAJ, Arntz OJ, Bakker AC et al. Role of interleukin 1 in antigen-induced exacerbation of murine arthritis. *Am J Pathol* 1995; **146**: 239–49.

42. van de Loo FAJ, Joosten LAB, van Lent PLEM et al. Role of interleukin-1, tumor necrosis factor α, and interleukin-6 in cartilage proteoglycan metabolism and destruction. *Arthritis Rheum* 1995; **38**: 164–72.

43. Ghivizzani SC, Kang R, Georgescu HI et al. Constitutive intra-articular expression of human IL-1β following gene transfer to rabbit synovium produces all major pathologies of human rheumatoid arthritis. *J Immunol* 1997; **159**: 3604–12.

44. Niki Y, Yamada H, Seki S et al. Macrophage-and neutrophil dominant arthritis in human IL-1 transgenic mice. *J Clin Invest* 2001; **107**: 1127–35.

45. Deleuran BW, Chu CQ, Field M et al. Localization of interleukin-1, type 1 interleukin-1 receptor and interleukin-1 receptor antagonist in the synovial membrane and cartilage/pannus junction in rheumatoid arthritis. *Br J Rheumatol* 1992; **31**: 801–9.

46. Firestein GS, Berger AE, Tracey DE et al. IL-1 receptor antagonist protein production and gene expression in rheumatoid arthritis and osteoarthritis synovium. *J Immunol* 1992; **149**: 1054–62.

47. Koch AE, Kunkel SL, Chensue SW et al. Expression of interleukin-1 and interleukin-1 receptor antagonist by human rheumatoid synovial tissue macrophages. *Clin Immunol Immunopathol* 1992; **65**: 23–9.

48. Malyak M, Swaney RE, Arend WP. Levels of synovial fluid interleukin-1 receptor antagonist in rheumatoid arthritis and other arthropathies. *Arthritis Rheum* 1993; **36**: 781–9.

49. Beaulieu AD, McColl SR. Differential expression of two major cytokines produced by neutrophils, interleukin-8 and the interleukin-1 receptor antagonist, in neutrophils isolated from the synovial fluid and peripheral blood of patients with rheumatoid arthritis. *Arthritis Rheum* 1994; **37**: 855–9.

50. Roux-Lombard P, Modoux C, Vischer T et al. Inhibitors of interleukin 1 activity in synovial fluids and in cultured synovial fluid mononuclear cells. *J Rheumatol* 1992; **19**: 517–23.

51. Seckinger P, Kaufmann M-T, Dayer J-M. An interleukin 1 inhibitor affects both cell-associated interleukin-1 induced T-cell proliferation and PGE$_2$/collagenase production by human dermal fibroblasts and synovial cells. *Immunobiology* 1990; **180**: 316–27.

52. Seckinger P, Yaron I, Meyer FA et al. Modulation of the effects of interleukin-1 on glycosaminoglycan synthesis by the urine-derived interleukin-1 inhibitor, but not by interleukin-6. *Arthritis Rheum* 1990; **33**: 1807–14.

53. Schwab JH, Anderle SK, Brown RR et al. Pro- and anti-inflammatory roles of interleukin-1 in recurrence of bacterial cell wall-induced arthritis in rats. *Infection Immunity* 1991; **59**: 4436–42.

54. Kuiper S, Joosten LAB, Bendele AM et al. Different roles of tumour necrosis factor α and interleukin 1 in murine streptococcal cell wall arthritis. *Cytokine* 1998; **10**: 690–702.

55. van Lent PLEM, van de Loo FAJ, Holthuysen AEM et al. Major role for interleukin 1 but not for tumor necrosis factor α in early cartilage damage in immune complex arthritis in mice. *J Rheumatol* 1995; **22**: 2250–8.

56. Arner EC, Harris RR, DiMeo TM et al. Interleukin-1 receptor antagonist inhibits proteoglycan breakdown in antigen induced but not polycation induced arthritis in the rabbit. *J Rheumatol* 1995; **22**: 1338–46.

57. Joosten LAB, Helsen MMA, van de Loo FAJ, van den Berg WB. Anticytokine treatment of established type II collagen-induced arthritis in DBA/1 mice. *Arthritis Rheum* 1996; **39**: 797–809.

58. Joosten LAB, Helsen MMA, Saxne T et al. IL-1 blockade prevents cartilage and bone destruction in murine type II collagen-induced arthritis, whereas TNF-blockade only ameliorates joint inflammation. *J Immunol* 1999; **163**: 5049–55.

59. Wooley PH, Whalen JD, Chapman DL et al. The effect of an interleukin-1 receptor antagonist protein on type II collagen-induced arthritis and antigen-induced arthritis in mice. *Arthritis Rheum* 1993; **36**: 1305–14.

60. Bendele A, McAbee T, Sennello G et al. Efficacy of sustained blood levels of interleukin-1 receptor antagonist in animal models of arthritis. *Arthritis Rheum* 1999; **42**: 498–506.

61. Bendele A, Sennello G, McAbee T et al. Effects of interleukin 1 receptor antagonist alone and in combination with methotrexate in adjuvant arthritic rats. *J Rheumatol* 1999; **26**: 1225–9.

62. Feige U, Hu Y-L, Gasser J et al. Anti-interleukin-1 and anti-tumor necrosis factor-α synergistically inhibit adjuvant arthritis in Lewis rats. *Cell Mol Life Sci* 2000; **57**: 1457–70.

63. Bendele AM, Chlipala ES, Scherrer J et al. Combination benefit of treatment with the cytokine inhibitors interleukin-1 receptor antagonist and PEGylated soluble tumor necrosis factor receptor type I in animal models of rheumatoid arthritis. *Arthritis Rheum* 2000; **43**: 2648–59.

64. Ku G, Faust T, Lauffer LL et al. Interleukin-1β converting enzyme inhibition blocks progression of type II collagen-induced arthritis in mice. *Cytokine* 1996; **8**: 377–86.

65. Bandara G, Mueller GM, Galea-Lauri J et al. Intraarticular expression of biologically active interleukin 1-receptor-antagonist protein by *ex vivo* gene transfer. *Proc Natl Acad Sci USA* 1993; **90**: 10764–8.

66. Hung GL, Galea-Lauri J, Mueller GM et al. Suppression of intra-articular responses to interleukin-1 by transfer of the interleukin-1 receptor antagonist gene to synovium. *Gene Ther* 1994; **1**: 64–9.

67. Roessler BJ, Hartman JW, Vallance DK et al. Inhibition of interleukin-1-induced effects in synoviocytes transduced with the human IL-1 receptor antagonist cDNA using an adenoviral vector. *Hum Gene Ther* 1995; **6**: 307–16.

68. Otani K, Nita I, Macaulay W et al. Suppression of antigen-induced arthritis in rabbits by ex vivo gene therapy. *J Immunol* 1996; **156**: 3558–62.

69. Makarov SS, Olsen JC, Johnston WN et al. Suppression of experimental arthritis by gene transfer of interleukin 1 receptor antagonist cDNA. *Proc Natl Acad Sci USA* 1996; **93**: 402–6.

70. Bakker AC, Joosten LAB, Arnta OJ et al. Prevention of murine collagen-induced arthritis in the knee and ipsilateral paw by local expression of human interleukin-1 receptor antagonist protein in the knee. *Arthritis Rheum* 1997; **40**: 893–900.

71. Nguyen KHY, Boyle DL, McCormack JE et al. Direct synovial gene transfer with retroviral vectors in rat adjuvant arthritis. *J Rheumatol* 1998; **25**: 1118–25.

72. Ghivizzani SC, Lechman ER, Kang R et al. Direct adenovirus-mediated gene transfer of interleukin 1 and tumor necrosis factor soluble receptors to rabbit knees with experimental arthritis has local and distal anti-arthritic effects. *Proc Natl Acad Sci USA* 1998; **95**: 4613–18.

73. Oligino T, Ghivizzani SC, Wolfe D et al. Intra-articular delivery of a herpes simplex virus IL-1Ra gene vector reduces inflammation in a rabbit model of arthritis. *Gene Ther* 1996; **6**: 1713–20.

74. Pan RU-YU, Chen S-Li, Xiao X et al. Therapy and prevention of arthritis by recombinant adeno-associated virus vector with delivery of inter-leukin-1 receptor antagonist. *Arthritis Rheum* 2000; **43**: 289–97.

75. Bessis N, GuÈry L, Mantovani A et al. The type II decoy receptor of IL-1 inhibits murine collagen-induced arthritis. *Eur J Immunol* 2000; **30**: 867–75.

76. Baragi VM, Renkiewicz RR, Jordan H et al. Transplantation of transduced chondrocytes protects articular cartilage from interleukin-1-induced extracellular matrix degradation. *J Clin Invest* 1995; **96**: 2454–60.

77. Caron JP, Fernandes JC, Martel-Pelletier J et al. Chondroprotective effect of intraarticular injec-tions of interleukin-1 receptor antagonist in experimental osteoarthritis. *Arthritis Rheum* 1996; **39**: 1535–44.

78. Martel-Pelletier J, Caron JP, Evans C et al. In vivo suppression of early experimental osteoarthritis by IL-1 receptor antagonist using gene therapy. *Arthritis Rheum* 1997; **40**: 1012–19.

79. Fernandes J, Tardif G, Martel-Pelletier J et al. In vivo transfer of interleukin-1 receptor antagonist gene in osteoarthritic rabbit knee joints. Prevention of osteoarthritis progression. *Am J Pathol* 1999; **154**: 1159–69.

80. Dionne S, D'Agata ID, Hiscott J, Vanoudou T, Seidman EG. Colonic explant production of IL-1 and its receptor antagonist is imbalanced in inflammatory bowel disease (IBD). *Clin Exp Immunol* 1998; **112**: 435–42.

81. Casini-Raggi V, Kam L, Chong YJT, Fiocchi C, Pizarro TT, Cominelli F. Mucosal imbalance of IL-1 and IL-1 receptor antagonist in inflamma-tory bowel disease. A novel mechanism of chronic intestinal inflammation. *J Immunol* 1995; **154**: 2434–40.

82. Gabay C, Smith Jr MF, Eidlen D, Arend WP. Interleukin-1 receptor antagonist is an acute-phase protein. *J Clin Invest* 1997; **99**: 2930–40.

83. Gabay C, Gigley JP, Sipe J, Arend WP, Fantuzzi G. Production of interleukin-1 receptor antago-nist by hepatocytes is regulated as an acute-phase protein in vivo. *Eur J Immunol* 2001; **31**: 490–9.

84. Tilg H, Vogel W, Wiedermann CJ et al. Circulating interleukin-1 and tumor necrosis factor antagonists in liver diseases. *Hepatology* 1993; **18**: 1132–8.

85. Sekiyama KD, Yoshiba M, Thompson AW. Circulating proinflammatory cytokines (IL-1β, TNF-α, and IL-6) and IL-1 receptor antagonist (IL-1Ra) in fulminant hepatic failure and acute hepatitis. *Clin Exp Immunol* 1994; **98**: 71–7.

86. Conti F, Breton S, Batteux F et al. Defective interleukin-1 receptor antagonist production is associated with resistance of acute liver graft rejection to steroid therapy. *Am J Pathol* 2000; **157**: 1685–92.

87. Miller LC, Lynch EA, Isa S, Logan JW, Dinarello CA, Steere AC. Balance of synovial fluid IL-1β and IL-1 receptor antagonist and recovery from Lyme arthritis. *Lancet* 1993; **341**: 146–8.

88. Firestein GS, Boyle DL, Yu C et al. Synovial inter-leukin-1 receptor antagonist and interleukin-1 balance in rheumatoid arthritis. *Arthritis Rheum* 1994; **37**: 644–52.

89. Chikanza IC, Roux-Lombard P, Dayer J-M, Panayi G. Dysregulation of the in vivo produc-tion of interleukin-1 receptor antagonist in patients with rheumatoid arthritis. *Arthritis Rheum* 1995; **38**: 642–8.

90. Gabay C, Marinova-Mutafchieva L, Williams RO et al. Increased production of intracellular inter-leukin-1 receptor antagonist type I in the synovium of mice with collagen-induced arthri-tis. A possible role in the resolution of arthritis. *Arthritis Rheum* 2001; **44**: 251–62.

91. Allen JB, Wong HL, Costa GL, Bienkowski MJ, Wahl SM. Suppression of monocyte function and differential regulation of IL-1 and IL-1Ra by IL-4 contribute to resolution of experimental arthritis. *J Immunol* 1993; **151**: 4344–51.

92. Lubberts E, Joosten LAB, Helsen MMA, van den Berg WB. Regulatory role of interleukin 10 in joint inflammation and cartilage destruction in murine streptococcal cell wall (SCW) arthritis. More therapeutic benefit with IL-4/IL-10 combi-nation therapy than with IL-10 treatment alone. *Cytokine* 1998; **10**: 361–9.

93. Fukumoto T, Matsukawa A, Ohkawara S, Takagi K, Yoshinaga M. Administration of neutralizing antibody against rabbit IL-1 receptor antagonist exacerbates lipopolysaccharide-induced arthritis in rabbits. *Inflamm Res* 1996; **45**: 479–85.

94. Hirsch E, Irikura VM, Paul SM, Hirsh D. Functions of interleukin 1 receptor antagonist in gene knockout and overproducing mice. *Proc Natl Acad Sci USA* 1996; **93**: 11008–13.

95. Ma Y, Thornton S, Boivin GP, Hirsh D, Hirsch R, Hirsch E. Altered susceptibility to collagen induced arthritis in transgenic mice with aberrant expression of IL-1 receptor antagonist. *Arthritis Rheum* 1998; **41**: 1798–805.

96. Horai R, Saito S, Tanioka H et al. Development of chronic inflammatory polyarthropathy resembling rheumatoid arthritis in interleukin-1 receptor antagonist-deficient mice. *J Exp Med* 2000; **191**: 313–20.

97. Nicklin MJH, Hughes DE, Barton JL, Ure JM, Duff GW. Arterial inflammation in mice lacking the interleukin 1 receptor antagonist gene. *J Exp Med* 2000; **191**: 303–11.

98. Clay FE, Tarlow JK, Cork MJ, Cox A, Nicklin MJH, Duff GW. Novel interleukin-1 receptor antagonist exon polymorphisms and their use in allele-specific mRNA assessment. *Hum Genet* 1996; **97**: 723–6.

99. Manzoli A, Andreotti F, Varlotta C et al. Allelic polymorphism of the interleukin-1 receptor antagonist gene in patients with acute or stable presentation of ischemic heart disease. *Cardiologia* 1999; **44**: 825–30.

100. Francis SE, Camp NJ, Dewberry RM et al. Interleukin-1 receptor antagonist gene polymorphism and coronary artery disease. *Circulation* 1999; **99**: 861–6.

101. Boiardi L, Salvarani C, Timms JM, Silvestri T, Macchioni PL, Di Giovine FS. Interleukin-1 cluster and tumor necrosis factor-α gene polymorphisms in polymyalgia rheumatica. *Clin Exp Rheumatol* 2000; **18**: 675–81.

102. El-Omar EM, Carrington M, Chow W-H et al. Interleukin-1 polymorphism associated with increased risk of gastric cancer. *Nature* 2000; **404**: 398–402.

103. Danis VA, March LM, Nelson DS, Brooks PM. Interleukin-1 secretion by peripheral blood monocytes and synovial macrophages from patients with rheumatoid arthritis. *J Rheumatol* 1987; **14**: 33–9.

104. Dewberry R, Holden H, Crossman D, Francis S. Interleukin-1 receptor antagonist expression in human endothelial cells and atherosclerosis. *Arterioscler Thromb Vasc Biol* 2000; **20**: 2394–400.

105. Clay FE, Tarlow JK, Cork MJ, Duff GW. Quantification of interleukin-1 receptor antagonist (IL-1ra) gene allele-specific transcripts in keratinocytes. *Cytokine* 1994; **6**: A35.

106. Campion GV, Lebsack ME, Lookabaugh J, Gordon G, Catalano MA. Dose-range and dose-frequency study of recombinant human interleukin-1 receptor antagonist in patients with rheumatoid arthritis. *Arthritis Rheum* 1996; **39**: 1092–101.

107. Bresnihan B, Alvaro-Gracia JM, Cobby M et al. Treatment of rheumatoid arthritis with recombinant human interleukin-1 receptor antagonist. *Arthritis Rheum* 1998; **41**: 2196–204.

108. Bresnihan B, Newmark RD, Robbins S, McCabe D, Genant HK. Anakinra reduces the rate of joint destruction after 1 year of treatment in a randomized controlled cohort of patients with rheumatoid arthritis. *Ann Rheum Dis* 2001; **60**(suppl I): 168.

109. Cohen S, Hurd E, Cush JJ et al. Treatment of interleukin-1 receptor antagonist in combination with methotrexate in rheumatoid arthritis patients. *Arthritis Rheum* 2002; **46**: 614–24.

110. Schiff MH, Bulpitt K, Weaver AA et al. Safety of combination therapy with anakinra and etanercept in patients with rheumatoid arthritis. *Arthritis Rheum* 2001; **44**: S79 (abstract).

111. Ghivizzani SC, Kang R, Muzzonigro T et al. Gene therapy for arthritis – treatment of the first three patients. *Arthritis Rheum* 1997; **40**: S223 (abstract).

112. Rock CS, Coyle SM, Keogh CV et al. Influence of hypercortisolemia on the acute-phase protein response to endotoxin in humans. *Surgery* 1992; **112**: 467.

113. Seitz M, Loetcher P, Dewald B et al. Interleukin 1 (IL-1) receptor antagonist, soluble tumor necrosis factor receptors, IL-1β, and IL-8 markers of remission in rheumatoid arthritis during treatment with methotrexate. *J Rheumatol* 1996; **23**: 1512–16.

114. Shingu M, Fujikawa Y, Wada T, Nonaka S, Nobunaga M. Increased IL-1 receptor antagonist (IL-1ra) production and decreased IL-1β/IL-1ra ratio in mononuclear cells from rheumatoid arthritis patients. *Br J Rheumatol* 1995; **34**: 24–30.

115. Dinarello CA. Biologic basis for interleukin-1 in disease. *Blood* 1996; **87**: 2095–147.

116. McInnes IB, Illei GG, Danning CL et al. IL-10 improves skin disease and modulates endothelial activation and leukocyte effector function in patients with psoriatic arthritis. *J Immunol* 2001; **167**: 4075–82.

117. Burger D, Chicheportiche R, Giri JG, Dayer J-M. The inhibitory activity of human interleukin-1 receptor antagonist is enhanced by type II interleukin-1 soluble receptor and hindered by type I interleukin-1 soluble receptor. *J Clin Invest* 1995; **96**: 38–41.

118. Dawson J, Engelhardt P, Kastelic T, Cheneval D, Mackenzie A, Ramage P. Effects of soluble interleukin-1 type II receptor on rabbit antigen-induced arthritis: clinical, biochemical and histological assessment. *Rheumatology* 1999; **38**: 401–6.

119. Drevlow BE, Lovis R, Haag MA et al. Recombinant human interleukin-1 receptor type I in the treatment of patients with active rheumatoid arthritis. *Arthritis Rheum* 1996; **39**: 257–65.

120. Guler H-P, Caldwell J, Littlejohn III et al. A phase I, single dose escalation study of IL-1 TRAP in patients with rheumatoid arthritis. *Arthritis Rheum* 2001; **44**: S370 (abstract).

121. Bondeson J, Foxwell B, Brennan F, Feldmann M. Defining therapeutic targets by using adenovirus: blocking NF-κB inhibits both inflammatory and destructive mechanisms in rheumatoid synovium but spares anti inflammatory mediators. *Proc Natl Acad Sci USA* 1999; **96**: 5668–73.

122. Conner EM, Fuseler JW, Davis JM et al. Selective proteasome inhibition attenuates experimental polyarthritis via inhibition of nuclear transcription factor κB (NFκB) activation. *Arthritis Rheum* 1997; **40**: S322.

123. Sagot Y, Sattonet-Roche P, Bhagwat SS, Grimshaw CE, Dreano M, Plater-Zyberk C. Two IKK2 inhibitors are orally active small molecules decreasing severity of collagen-induced arthritis in DBA/1 mice. *Arthritis Rheum* 2001; **44**: S368 (abstract).

124. Bhagwat SS, Bennett BL, Satoh Y et al. The small molecule IKK2 inhibitor SPC 839 is efficacious in an animal model of arthritis. *Arthritis Rheum* 2001; **44**: S213 (abstract).

125. Shiozawa S, Shimizu K, Tanaka K, Hino K. Studies on the contribution of c-fos/AP-1 to arthritic joint destruction. *J Clin Invest* 1997; **99**. 1210–16.

126. Badger AM, Griswold DE, Kapadia R et al. Disease-modifying activity of SB 242235, a selective inhibitor of p38 mitogen-activated protein kinase, in rat adjuvant-induced arthritis. *Arthritis Rheum* 2000; **43**: 175–83.

13

Interleukin-6

Norihiro Nishimoto, Kazuyuki Yoshizaki and Tadamitsu Kishimoto

Introduction • Pathological significance of IL-6 in immunological disorders • Clinical studies with anti-IL-6R antibody • Potential problems • Conclusion • References

INTRODUCTION

Over the past 10 years, immunological defects in rheumatoid arthritis (RA) have been clarified considerably. RA is a common autoimmune disease characterized by persistent synovitis with synovial cell proliferation and emergence of rheumatoid factors.[1] The exact causes are unknown, but autoreactive T cells are thought to contribute to the development of RA.[2] Shortcomings in the specific recognition of non-self- and self-antigens by T cells may occur due to incomplete clonal deletion in the thymus or to elimination of the anergy of autoreactive T cells, resulting in the activation of autoreactive T cells.[3,4] Once the autoreactive T cells are activated, various cytokines and/or mediators of inflammation are released, inducing proliferation and differentiation of immunocompetent cells and production of autoreactive antibodies which present autoimmune phenomena. These inflammatory mediators further amplify the autoimmune response. In the affected joints, constitutive production of inflammatory cytokines induces proliferation of vascular endothelial cells, fibroblasts and articular synovial cells to generate pathological features characteristic of RA. They also induce activation of osteoclasts and production of proteases, resulting in irreversible destructive changes in the bone and cartilage of the joints. Furthermore, since such inflammatory cytokines are soluble, they diffuse into the blood and generate systemic inflammatory manifestations such as fever and malaise, in addition to abnormal laboratory findings such as elevation of C-reactive protein (CRP) and erythrocyte sedimentation rate (ESR). They may also cause extra-articular complications such as glomerulonephritis, interstitial pneumonia and secondary amyloidosis.

Identification of antigen epitopes which autoreactive T cells recognize would make it possible to antagonize T-cell recognition prior to autoimmune response. However, such epitopes have not yet been fully identified. On the other hand, interference with inflammatory cytokines, which enhance autoimmune response and inflammation, and consequently generate pathological changes, may constitute a strategy in the treatment of RA. Interleukin-6 (IL-6) is one of the target cytokines whose functions need to be blocked in such treatment.

PATHOLOGICAL SIGNIFICANCE OF IL-6 IN IMMUNOLOGICAL DISORDERS

Multifunction of IL-6

IL-6 was originally identified as a B-cell differentiation factor[5] which induces activated B cells to produce immunoglobulins. The cDNA of IL-6 was cloned in 1986.[6] Since recombinant IL-6 and monoclonal antibodies against IL-6 became available, studies on IL-6 biology have made remarkable progress. IL-6 has been shown to be produced by various types of cells, such as T cells, B cells, monocytes, fibroblasts, endothelial cells, and several kinds of tumor cells, and also has a wide range of biological activities on various target cells.[7] IL-6 is a differentiation factor of T cells through the induction of IL-2 receptor.[8,9] In addition to T and B cells, IL-6 has been shown to induce terminal differentiation of macrophages in murine myeloid leukemia cell line M1 cells.[10,11] It differentiates megakaryocytes to produce platelets[12] and acts on hematopoietic stem cells synergistically with IL-3 to support the formation of multilineage blast cell colonies.[13,14] IL-6 also plays important roles in the acute-phase reaction. It stimulates hepatocytes to produce acute-phase proteins such as CRP, fibrinogen, α_1-antitrypsin, and serum amyloid A (SAA), while it simultaneously suppresses production of albumin.[15–17] It induces leukocytosis and fever when it is administered in vivo[18] and, in the presence of soluble IL-6 receptor (sIL-6R), induces osteoclast precursor cells to become authentic osteoclasts characterized by the presence of tartrate-resistant acid phosphatase (TRAP) activity, calcitonin receptors, and pit formation in dentine slices.[19] In addition, IL-6 acts as a growth factor for mesangial cells,[20] epidermal keratinocytes,[21,22] and various tumor cells such as malignant lymphoma cells,[23] multiple myeloma cells,[24] and renal carcinoma cells.[25] Besides the functions described above, IL-6 has multiple biological actions in both physiological and pathological conditions. The signal for IL-6 to exert these pleiotropic actions is mediated by the IL-6 receptor (IL-6R).

IL-6 receptor system

The IL-6R system consists of two functional membrane proteins: an 80-kDa ligand-binding chain (IL-6R, IL-6R α-chain, CD126)[26] and a 130-kDa non-ligand-binding but signal-transducing

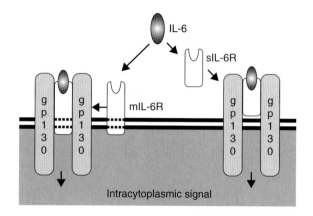

Figure 13.1 Schematic model for IL-6R system. IL-6, when bound to membrane IL-6R (mIL-6R), induces homodimerization of gp130, leading to a high-affinity functional receptor complex of IL-6, IL-6R and gp130. The soluble form of IL-6R (sIL-6R) also induces homodimerization of gp130. IL-6 binding to either mIL-6R or sIL-6R can mediate IL-6 signals into the cells.

chain (gp130, IL-6R β-chain, CD130).[27,28] When bound to cell surface IL-6R, IL-6 induces homodimerization of gp130, and produces a high-affinity functional receptor complex of IL-6, IL-6R, and gp130. The soluble form of IL-6R (sIL-6R), lacking the intracytoplasmic portion of IL-6R, is also capable of signal transduction as a ligand-binding receptor. Since a very short intracytoplasmic portion of IL-6R containing only 82 amino acids is not essential for signal transduction, the complex of IL-6 and sIL-6R also induces homodimerization of gp130.[27,28] Thus, IL-6 binding to either a membrane-anchored or soluble form of IL-6R can mediate IL-6 signals into cells as long as they express gp130 (Figure 13.1). In fact, considerable amounts of sIL-6R are observed both in the serum and in the synovial fluids,[29,30] and they may play a physiological role as well as a pathological role in the autoimmune response.

The receptor system of IL-6 is also useful in understanding the overlapping functions of IL-6 and IL-6-family cytokines such as interleukin-11 (IL-11), leukemia inhibitory factor (LIF), oncostatin M (OSM), ciliary neurotrophic factor (CNTF), and cardiotrophin-1 (CT-1).[31] In a similar manner to IL-6, these cytokines exert multiple biological actions in immunological reactions, inflammation, hematopoiesis, oncogenesis, etc. In fact, gp130 is shared by these cytokines as a common signal transducer. Based on an understanding of this unique receptor system of IL-6, a strategy has been established to inhibit IL-6 functions.

IL-6 in animal models

IL-6 transgenic mice

Since many of IL-6's biological activities have been shown in vitro, it was of interest to discover what kind of manifestations might arise if IL-6 were constitutively produced in vivo. We can find the answer to this question from IL-6 transgenic mice. Transgenic mice were produced by the introduction of the human IL-6 gene into C57BL/6 mice under the transcriptional control of the immunoglobulin μ heavy chain enhancer (Eμ)[32] or histocompatibility class I (H2-Ld) promoter.[33] The IL-6 transgenic mice showed polyclonal hypergamma-globulinemia with massive plasmacytosis in the spleen and lymph nodes, an increase in serum levels of fibrinogen, and a reduction in serum albumin. The mice also showed an elevated number of megakaryocytes in the bone marrow, mesangial proliferative glomerulonephritis in the kidney,[32,34] and lymphocytic interstitial pneumonia in the lung.[35] The data confirmed that IL-6 could function in vivo in the same way as in vitro. Furthermore, it is interesting to note that the abnormal findings observed in IL-6 transgenic mice represent some of the features of human inflammatory diseases such as Castleman's disease and RA, although the mice do not always show arthritis.

Collagen-induced arthritis as a model for rheumatoid arthritis

Animal models for arthritis have been used to study the pathological significance of IL-6 as well as the therapeutic effects of some agents in blocking IL-6 functions. Collagen-induced arthritis (CIA) in DBA/1J mice is an experimental model widely used for human RA. Alonzi et al showed that the IL-6 gene knockout mice were completely resistant to CIA.[36] That is to say, IL-6 is essential in developing CIA. Later on, Sasai et al reported that IL-6 gene knockout delayed the onset of CIA and also reduced its severity.[37] Although the susceptibility of the mice to CIA differed between the two reports, they both indicate that IL-6 plays an important role in CIA. However, inactivation of the IL-6 gene affected the total immune response in mice, and therefore makes it difficult to identify the actual mechanism for decreasing susceptibility to and/or the severity of CIA. Furthermore, it is impossible to predict the therapeutic effect of anti-IL-6 therapy for RA from the IL-6 knockout study.

The effect of anti-IL-6R antibody on arthritis was also examined in CIA models, and this study was more useful in predicting the efficacy of anti-IL-6R therapy for RA. Administration of rat anti-mouse IL-6R monoclonal antibody, MR16-1, to DBA/1J mice suppressed both the incidence and severity of CIA and prevented destruction of the joints.[38] Similarly, the effects of humanized anti-human IL-6R monoclonal antibody, MRA, were examined in CIA in cynomolgus monkeys, as MRA cross-reacts with monkey IL-6R. MRA treatment decreased both the incidence and the severity of CIA in the monkeys and consequently prevented the destructive changes in the joint[39] (Figure 13.2). These data indicate that blocking IL-6 function prevents joint destruction caused by CIA. In the study of mouse CIA, however, the effect was observed only when anti-IL-6R antibody was injected within 3 days after immunization of bovine type II collagen, but not when it was injected 7 days after immunization.[38] Therefore, anti-IL-6R antibody acts mainly by suppressing immunization of bovine type II collagen. If this is the mechanism by which anti-IL-6R antibody treatment prevents arthritis, we need to address the question as to whether or not anti-IL-6R antibody is indeed therapeutically effective in human RA, as the autoimmune response is already established in RA patients before they visit a clinic for treatment.

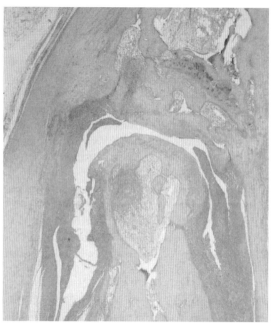
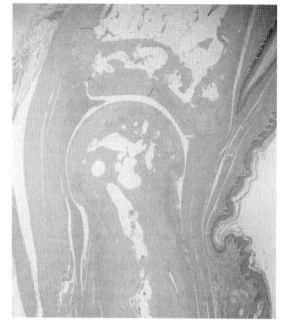

Non-treated   MRA-treated

Figure 13.2 Histological examination of monkey CIA. Cynomolgus monkeys were immunized with bovine type II collagen to induce CIA. Humanized anti-IL-6R antibody, MRA, treatment (10 mg/kg) prevented the destructive changes of the joint in monkey CIA.

Severe combined immunodeficiency mice transplanted with RA joint tissue

Severe combined immunodeficiency (SCID) mice transplanted with joint tissue from human RA pannus can maintain histological features identical to those of human RA in the transplants.[40] Since the transplanted tissue is taken from humans, therapeutic agents such as monoclonal antibodies, which react specifically to human antigens, can be examined for their efficacy in this model. The model was used to examine the therapeutic usefulness of humanized anti-human IL-6R monoclonal antibody, MRA, for RA.[41] Weekly administration of MRA (100 μg/body) for a period of 1 month significantly decreased the number of infiltrating inflammatory cells, matrix metalloproteinase (MMP)-9-positive cells and TRAP-positive cells in the implanted synovium as well as decreasing the volume of implanted tissue. Therefore, IL-6

blockade may be able to eliminate the inflammation of RA synovitis and prevent joint destruction by decreasing MMP production and the number of osteoclasts in RA. Furthermore, the data suggest that MRA is effective in the treatment of RA patients even though their autoimmune response is already established.

IL-6 in human immune inflammatory diseases

Castleman's disease

In order to find out if IL-6 is involved in the pathogenesis of human diseases, we first studied Castleman's disease. Castleman's disease is a benign lymphoproliferative disease characterized by chronic inflammatory manifestations and immunological disorders such as general fatigue, fever, anemia, an increased ESR, elevated levels of CRP and fibrinogen, and

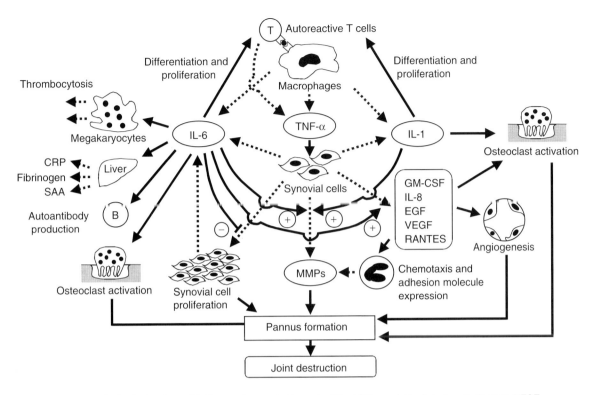

Figure 13.3 Pathological roles of inflammatory cytokines in RA. EGF, endothelial growth factor; VEGF, vascular endothelial growth factor; RANTES, regulated upon activation, normal T cell expressed and secreted.

polyclonal hypergamma-globulinemia, and is frequently associated with autoantibodies to red blood cells and platelets.[42,43] Patients with Castleman's disease often show lymphocytic interstitial pneumonia or mesangial prolifera- tive glomerulonephritis (MPGN) as complica- tions. These findings resemble those seen in the IL-6 transgenic mice as described above. Although the causes of this disease are not known, we found in 1989 that uncontrolled IL-6 hyperproduction from the affected lymph nodes was involved in its pathogenesis.[44] It is of special interest that, if there was a solitary swollen lymph node, resection of the affected lymph node normalized serum IL-6 activity and immediately improved all the inflammatory symptoms and laboratory findings in the patients. The findings indicated that the specific blockade of IL-6 function by utilizing antibody

may constitute a new therapeutic strategy for Castleman's disease and perhaps for inflamma- tory diseases, including RA.

Rheumatoid arthritis
IL-6, as well as other inflammatory cytokines such as tumor necrosis factor alpha (TNF-α) and IL-1, is thought to be profoundly involved in the pathogenesis of RA. The repetition of ameliora- tion and exacerbation observed in RA suggests that the antigen stimulation for autoimmune response continues intermittently in vivo in patients. IL-6 is essential for the initial autoim- mune response as a factor that induces prolifera- tion and differentiation of autoreactive T cells and differentiation of macrophages. IL-6 as a B- cell differentiation factor contributes to the emergence of antibodies which react with autol- ogous tissues, including anti-immunoglobulin

autoantibody, rheumatoid factor. IL-6 is also involved in the infiltration of immunocompetent cells by modulating the expression of cell adhesion molecules.[45] Continuous stimulation of autoimmune reactions results in persistent synovitis in multiple joints, where IL-6 is produced mainly by the synovial cells under the stimulation of TNF-α,[46,47] and extremely large amounts of IL-6 can be found in the synovial fluids.[48–51] This overproduction of IL-6 further amplifies the autoimmune response. In a similar way to IL-1 and TNF-α, IL-6 activates osteoclasts and induces bone absorption, resulting in osteo-porosis and joint destruction in RA. IL-6 may induce angiogenesis and contribute to pannus formation. On the other hand, IL-6 suppresses the proliferation of synovial fibroblastic cells in vitro and competes with TNF-α, a growth inducer of synovial cells. Since IL-6 is produced by synovial cells under the stimulation of TNF-α, IL-6 may act as a negative-feedback regulator of TNF-α-induced synovial cell proliferation.[52] To understand the pathological roles of IL-6, we need to consider the interaction of cytokines with individual functions at the same time.

In extra-articular manifestations, IL-6 causes a subfebrile state and body weight loss. Over-production of IL-6 induces polyclonal hyper-gamma-globulinemia and thrombocytosis as well as an increase in acute-phase proteins such as CRP, fibrinogen and SAA, and a decrease in albumin in the serum. Continuous stimulation of the kidney by IL-6 may cause MPGN in the kidney.

A schematic model of the pathological actions of IL-6 and other mediators in RA is shown in Figure 13.3.

CLINICAL STUDIES WITH ANTI-IL-6R ANTIBODY

Humanized anti-IL-6R monoclonal antibody

The therapeutic value of mouse antibody in human chronic diseases remains limited because chronic diseases require repetitive administra-tion of the antibody, resulting in the emergence of neutralizing human antibodies against mouse

antibody. Such neutralizing antibodies reduce therapeutic efficacy or induce an allergic reaction to the mouse antibody. We therefore attempted to block IL-6 signal transduction by utilizing humanized monoclonal antibody against IL-6R in order to obtain an effective therapeutic agent that can be administered to patients in repeated doses. MRA is a humanized antibody obtained by grafting the complemen-tarity-determining regions from the murine anti-IL-6R monoclonal antibody into human IgG, thereby creating a functioning antigen-binding site in a reshaped human antibody.[41] It inhibited the growth of IL-6-dependent human myeloma cells with an affinity similar to that of the origi-nal mouse antibody and polyclonal anti-IL-6R antibody.[41,53]

Treatment of Castleman's disease

Beck et al showed that the in vivo administration of murine anti-IL-6 monoclonal antibody to a patient with Castleman's disease was therapeu-tically effective, thus confirming the in vivo function of IL-6 in this disease.[54] However, they used murine anti-IL-6 antibody, and therefore it was difficult to continue the treatment.

We treated a number of patients with Castleman's disease utilizing humanized anti-IL-6R antibody, MRA, with the approval of the ethics committee of Osaka University and with the consent of the patients. Treatment with 50–100 mg/body of MRA either once or twice weekly immediately improved systemic symptoms such as fever and malaise. It also normalized the levels of CRP, fibrinogen, albumin, and hemoglobin. After 3 months of treatment, hypergamma-globulinemia and lymphadenopathy were remarkably alleviated.[55] Treatment was well tolerated, with only transient leukopenia. Histopathological exami-nation revealed that MRA treatment reduced follicular hyperplasia and vascularity after treat-ment. Therefore, the pathological significance of IL-6 in Castleman's disease was confirmed, and the blockade of the IL-6 signal by MRA was thought to have potential as a new therapy.

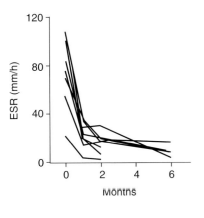

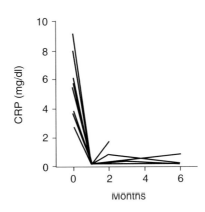

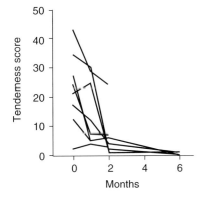

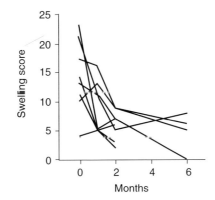

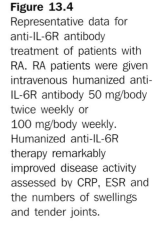

Figure 13.4
Representative data for anti-IL-6R antibody treatment of patients with RA. RA patients were given intravenous humanized anti-IL-6R antibody 50 mg/body twice weekly or 100 mg/body weekly. Humanized anti-IL-6R therapy remarkably improved disease activity assessed by CRP, ESR and the numbers of swellings and tender joints.

Treatment of rheumatoid arthritis

Wendling et al reported that the administration of mouse anti-human IL-6 monoclonal antibody to patients with RA resulted in improvements of the symptoms and laboratory findings of RA.[56] This confirmed that IL-6 plays an important role in this disease, although the effects were transient because mouse antibody was used.

We treated 11 patients with refractory RA compassionately with humanized anti-IL-6R antibody, MRA, after obtaining the permission of the ethical committee of our institute before we started the clinical trial of MRA.[35,57] All the patients had active disease resistant to conventional therapy using various disease-modifying anti-rheumatic drugs (DMARDs), including methotrexate and low-dose corticosteroids. The patients were treated with MRA in the same regimen as used in Castleman's disease. In the eight patients who received MRA treatment for more than 8 weeks, both clinical and laboratory findings improved during treatment. Representative data for the MRA therapy are shown in Figure 13.4. The remarkable improvement in objective markers, CRP and ESR, indicates the high efficacy of MRA in RA. At 2 months, the clinical response was 88% assessed by ACR20 criteria, and 50% by ACR50. A similar response was obtained in four patients who received MRA treatment for 6 months. The therapy was relatively well tolerated. Appearance of anti-idiotypic antibody was observed in one case, who was therefore withdrawn. Two additional patients were withdrawn: one because of the occurrence of an attack of angina, the relationship of which to MRA administration could not be classified, and the other for personal reasons. A transient decrease in neutrophil counts, mostly within the normal range, was observed in most of the cases on the day after MRA administration, similar to patients with Castleman's disease. These results indicate that MRA is relatively safe and useful in the treatment of RA. On the basis of our data, a phase I clinical trial in the UK and a phase I/II study in Japan were performed. In these studies, the safety and efficacy of humanized anti-IL-6R antibody were proven.[58,59] Double-blind randomized placebo-controlled phase II studies for RA both in Europe and in Japan are now in progress.

POTENTIAL PROBLEMS

The first problem is that we have been unable to determine whether or not MRA can prevent joint destruction in patients with RA. It is already known that TNF-α blockade can prevent joint destruction,[60,61] and therefore it is important to determine the difference between the anti-IL-6 and anti-TNF-α therapy. The second problem is the possibility of side-effects. Since IL-6 is essential for host defense, the clinical trials need to examine the incidence of serious infections and malignant diseases. In the phase I/II clinical trial, an increase in total cholesterol was observed.[59] IL-6 may play a critical role in the metabolism of fat. The third problem is that MRA still possesses the mouse sequence in the CDR portion that may be antigenic in human. There is a possibility of the emergence of anti-MRA neutralizing antibody and the occurrence of an allergic reaction. The fourth problem is the extremely high cost of the production of recombinant protein, which is a common problem among recombinant biological therapeutic agents. For MRA to become a standard therapy for RA, these problems need to be resolved in the near future.

CONCLUSION

Success in humanized anti-IL-6R antibody therapy for RA confirmed that IL-6 plays an important role in the development of RA. However, the mechanism of the action by which MRA exerts its therapeutic effect is still not fully understood. We have just started therapy utilizing this new biological agent for RA, a chronic disease that lasts for years. The final decision on whether the therapy is successful or not will be made on the basis on the long-term treatment of the disease. In addition to RA, various kinds of diseases, such as Castleman's disease, Crohn's disease, multiple myeloma, MPGN, psoriasis and Kaposi's sarcoma, are thought to be related to IL-6 overproduction. These could be possible targets for humanized anti-IL-6R antibody in the future.

REFERENCES

1. Harris ED Jr. Rheumatoid arthritis: pathophysiology and implications for therapy. *N Engl J Med* 1990; **322**: 1277–89.
2. Feldmann M, Londei M, Leech Z et al. Analysis of T cell clones in rheumatoid arthritis. *Springer Semin Immunopathol* 1988; **10**: 157–67.
3. Smilek DE, Lock CB, McDevitt HO. Antigen recognition and peptide-mediated immunotherapy in autoimmune disease. *Immunol Rev* 1990; **118**: 37–71.
4. Aichele P, Bachmann MF, Hengartner H, Zinkernagel RM. Immunopathology or organ-specific autoimmunity as a consequence of virus infection. *Immunol Rev* 1996; **152**: 21–45.
5. Yoshizaki K, Nakagawa T, Kaieda T et al. Induction of proliferation and Igs-production in human B leukemic cells by anti-immunoglobulins and T cell factors. *J Immunol* 1982; **128**: 1296–301.
6. Hirano T, Yasukawa K, Harada H et al. Complementary DNA for a novel human interleukin (BSF-2) that induces B lymphocytes to produce immunoglobulin. *Nature* 1986; **324**: 73–6.
7. Akira S, Taga T, Kishimoto T. Interleukin-6 in biology and medicine. *Adv Immunol* 1993; **54**: 1–78.

8. Noma T, Mizuta T, Rosen A et al. Enhancement of the interleukin-2 receptor expression on T cells by multiple B-lymphotropic lymphokines. *Immunol Lett* 1987; **15**: 249–53.

9. Okada M, Kitahara M, Kishimoto S et al. IL-6/BSF-2 functions as killer helper factor in the *in vitro* induction of cytotoxic T cells. *J Immunol* 1988; **141**: 1543–9.

10. Miyaura C, Onozaki K, Akiyama Y et al. Recombinant human interleukin 6 (B-cell stimulatory factor 2) is a potent inducer of differentiation of mouse myeloid leukemia cells (M1). *FEBS Lett* 1988; **234**: 17–21

11. Shabo Y, Lotem J, Rubinstein M et al. The myeloid blood cell differentiation-inducing protein MGI-2A is interleukin-6. *Blood* 1988; **72**: 2070–3.

12. Ishibashi T, Kimura H, Shikama Y et al. Interleukin-6 is a potent thrombopoietic factor in vivo in mice. *Blood* 1989; **74**: 1241–4.

13. Ikebuchi K, Wong GG, Clark SC et al. Interleukin-6 enhancement of interleukin-3-dependent proliferation of multipotential hemopoietic progenitors. *Proc Natl Acad Sci USA* 1987; **84**: 9035–9.

14. Koike K, Nakahata T, Takagi M et al. Synergism of BSF2/interleukin-6 and interleukin-3 on development of multipotential hemopoietic progenitors in serum free culture. *J Exp Med* 1988; **168**: 879–90.

15. Gauldie J, Richards C, Harnish D et al. Interferon-β_2/B cell-stimulatory factor type 2 shares identity with monocyte-derived hepatocyte stimulating factor and regulates the major acute phase protein response in liver cells. *Proc Natl Acad Sci USA* 1987; **84**: 7251–5.

16. Andus T, Geiger T, Hirano T et al. Recombinant human B cell stimulatory factor 2 (BSF-2/INFβ2) regulates β-fibrinogen and albumin mRNA levels in Fao-9 cell. *FEBS Lett* 1987; **221**: 18–22.

17. Castell JV, Gomez-Lechon MJ, David M et al. Recombinant human interleukin-6(IL-6/BSF-2/HSF) regulates the synthesis of acute phase proteins in human hepatocytes. *FEBS Lett* 1988; **232**: 347–50.

18. Ulich TR, del Castillo J, Guo KZ. *In vivo* hematologic effects of recombinant interleukin-6 on hematopoiesis and circulating numbers of RBCs and WBCs. *Blood* 1989; **73**: 108–10.

19. Tamura T, Udagawa N, Takahashi N et al. Soluble interleukin-6 receptor triggers osteoclast formation by interleukin 6. *Proc Natl Acad Sci USA* 1993; **90**: 11924–8.

20. Horii Y, Muraguchi A, Iwano M et al. Involvement of interleukin-6 in mesangial proliferation of glomerulonephritis. *J Immunol* 1989; **143**: 3949–55.

21. Grossman RM, Krueger J, Yourish D et al. Interleukin 6 is expressed in high levels in psoriasis skin and stimulates proliferation of cultured human keratinocytes. *Proc Natl Acad Sci USA* 1989; **86**: 6367–71.

22. Yoshizaki K, Nishimoto N, Matsumoto K et al. Interleukin-6 and expression of its receptor on the epidermal keratinocytes. *Cytokine* 1990; **2**: 381–7

23. Yee C, Biondi A, Wang XH et al. A possible autocrine role for interleukin-6 in two lymphoma cell lines. *Blood* 1989; **74**: 798–804.

24. Kawano M, Hirano T, Matsuda T et al. Autocrine generation and requirement of BSF-2/IL-6 for human multiple myelomas. *Nature* 1988; **332**: 83–5.

25. Miki S, Iwano M, Miki Y et al. Interleukin-6 (IL-6) functions as an in vitro autocrine growth factor in renal cell carcinomas. *FEBS Lett* 1989; **250**: 607–10.

26. Yamasaki K, Taga T, Hirata Y et al. Cloning and expression of the human interleukin-6 (BSF-2/INF b2) receptor. *Science* 1988; **241**: 825–8.

27. Taga T, Hibi M, Hirata Y et al. Interleukin-6 triggers the association of its receptor with a possible signal transducer, gp130. *Cell* 1989; **58**: 573–81.

28. Hibi M, Murakami M, Saito M et al. Molecular cloning and expression of an IL-6 signal transducer, gp130. *Cell* 1990; **63**: 1149–57.

29. Uson J, Balsa A, Pascual-Salcedo D et al. Soluble interleukin 6 (IL-6) receptor and IL-6 levels in serum and synovial fluid of patients with different arthropathies. *J Rheumatol* 1997; **24**: 2069–75.

30. Desgeorges A, Gabay C, Silcci P et al. Concentration and origins of soluble interleukin 6 receptor-a in serum and synovial fluid. *J Rheumatol* 1997; **24**: 1510–16.

31. Kishimoto T, Akira S, Narazaki M, Taga T. Interleukin-6 family of cytokines and gp130. *Blood* 1995; **86**: 1243–54.

32. Suematsu S, Matsuda T, Aozasa K et al. IgG1 plasmacytosis in interleukin-6 transgenic mice. *Proc Natl Acad Sci USA* 1989; **86**: 7547–51.

33. Suematsu S, Matsusaka T, Matsuda T et al. Generation of plasmacytomas with the chromosomal translocation t(12;15) in interleukin-6 transgenic mice. *Proc Natl Acad Sci USA* 1992; **89**: 232–5.

34. Katsume A, Miyai T, Suzuki H et al. Interleukin-6 overexpression cannot generate serious disorders in severe combined immunodefficiency mice. *Clin Immunol Immunopathol* 1997; **82**: 117–24.

35. Nishimoto N, Kishimoto T, Yoshizaki K. Anti-interleukin 6 antibody treatment in rheumatic disease. *Ann Rheum Dis* 2000; **59**: 121–7.

36. Alonzi T, Fattori E, Lazzaro D et al. Interleukin-6 is required for the development of collagen-induced arthritis. *J Exp Med* 1998; **187**: 461–8.

37. Sasai M, Saeki Y, Ohshima S et al. Delayed onset and reduced severity of collagen-induced arthritis in interleukin-6-deficient mice. *Arthritis Rheum* 1999; **42**: 1635–43.

38. Takagi N, Mihara M, Moriya Y et al. Blockage of interleukin-6 receptor ameliorates joint disease in murine collagen-induced arthritis. *Arthritis Rheum* 1998; **41**: 2117–21.

39. Mihara M, Kotoh M, Nishimoto N et al. Humanized antibody to human interleukin-6 receptor inhibits the development of collagen arthritis in cynomolgus monkeys. *Clin Immunol* 2001; **98**: 319–26.

40. Matsuno H, Sawai T, Nezuka T et al. Treatment of rheumatoid synovitis with anti-reshaping human interleukin-6 receptor monoclonal antibody. *Arthritis Rheum* 1998; **41**: 2014–21.

41. Sato K, Tsuchiya M, Saldanha J et al. Reshaping a human antibody to inhibit the interleukin 6-dependent tumor cell growth. *Cancer Res* 1993; **53**: 851–6.

42. Castleman B, Iverson L, Menendez VP. Localized mediastinal lymphnode hyperplasia resembling thymoma. *Cancer* 1956; **9**: 822–30.

43. Keller AR, Hochholzer L, Castleman B. Hyalin-vascular and plasma-cell types of giant lymph node hyperplasia of the mediastinum and other locations. *Cancer* 1972; **29**: 670–83.

44. Yoshizaki K, Matsuda T, Nishimoto N et al. Pathogenic significance of interleukin-6(IL-6/BSF-2) in Castleman's disease. *Blood* 1989; **74**: 1360–7.

45. Yamamoto M, Yoshizaki K, Kishimoto T, Ito H. IL-6 is required for the development of Th1 cell-mediated murine colitis. *J Immunol* 2000; **164**: 4878–82.

46. Guerne P-A, Zuraw BL, Vaughan JH et al. Synovium as a source of interleukin 6 in vitro. Contribution to local and systemic manifestations of arthritis. *J Clin Invest* 1988; **83**: 585–92.

47. Harigai M, Hara M, Kitani A et al. Interleukin 1 and tumor necrosis factor-alpha synergistically increase the production of interleukin 6 in human synovial fibroblast. *J Clin Lab Immunol* 1991; **34**: 107–13.

48. Hirano T, Matsuda T, Turner M et al. Excessive production of interleukin 6/B cell stimulatory factor-2 in rheumatoid arthritis. *Eur J Immunol* 1988; **18**: 1797–801.

49. Houssiau FA, Devogelaer JP, Van Damme J et al. Interleukin-6 in synovial fluid and serum of patients with rheumatoid arthritis and other inflammatory arthritis. *Arthritis Rheum* 1988; **31**: 784–8.

50. Sack U, Kinne R, Marx T et al. Interleukin-6 in synovial fluid is closely associated with chronic synovitis in rheumatoid arthritis. *Rheumatol Int* 1993; **13**: 45–51.

51. Madhok R, Crilly A, Watson J, Capell HA. Serum interleukin 6 levels in rheumatoid arthritis: correlation with clinical and laboratory indices of disease activity. *Ann Rheum Dis* 1993; **52**: 232–4.

52. Nishimoto N, Ito A, Ono M et al. Interleukin-6 inhibits the proliferation of fibroblastic synovial cells from rheumatoid arthritis patients in the presence of soluble interleukin-6 receptor. *Int Immunol* 2000; **12**: 187–93.

53. Nishimoto N, Ogata A, Shima Y et al. Oncostatin M, leukemia inhibitory factor, and interleukin 6 induce the proliferation of human plasmacytoma cells via the common signal transducer, gp130. *J Exp Med* 1994; **179**: 1343–7.

54. Beck JT, Hsu SM, Wijdenes J et al. Brief report: alleviation of systemic manifestations of Castleman's disease by monoclonal anti-interleukin-6 antibody. *N Engl J Med* 1994; **330**: 602–5.

55. Nishimoto N, Sasai M, Shima Y et al. Improvement in Castleman's disease by humanized anti-IL-6 receptor antibody therapy. *Blood* 2000; **95**: 56–61.

56. Wendling D, Racadot E, Wijenes J. Treatment of severe rheumatoid arthritis by anti-interleukin-6 monoclonal antibody. *J Rheumatol* 1993; **20**: 259–62.

57. Yoshizaki K, Nishimoto N, Mihara M, Kishimoto T. Therapy of RA by blocking IL-6 signal transduction with humanized anti-IL-6 receptor antibody. *Springer Semin Immunopathol* 1998; **20**: 247–59.

58. Choy EH, Isenberg DA, Farrow S et al. A double-blind, randomized, placebo-controlled trial of anti-interleukin-6 (IL-6) receptor monoclonal antibody in rheumatoid arthritis (RA). *Arthritis Rheum* 2001; **44**(suppl): S84.

59. Nishimoto N, Maeda K, Kuritani T et al. Safety and efficacy of repetitive treatment with humanized anti-interleukin-6 receptor antibody (MRA) in rheumatoid arthritis (RA). *Arthritis Rheum* 2001; **44**(suppl): S84.

60. Bathon JM, Martin RW, Fleischmann RM et al. A comparison of etanercept and methotrexate in patients with early rheumatoid arthritis. *N Engl J Med* 2000; **343**: 1586–93.

61. Lipsky PE, van der Heijde DM, St Clair EW et al. Infliximab and methotrexate in the treatment of rheumatoid arthritis. Anti-tumor necrosis factor trial in rheumatoid arthritis with concominant therapy study group. *N Engl J Med* 2000; **343**: 1594–602.

14

Interleukin-12, Interleukin-23 and Interleukin-27

Masato Moriguchi, Naresh Chauhan, Alison Finnegan, Warren Strober, David M Frucht, Massimo Gadina and John J O'Shea

Introduction • Structure and regulation of IL-12, IL-23 and IL-27 • Structure and expression of IL-12, IL-23 and IL-27 receptors • Biological effects of IL-12 and IL-23 • Signal transduction • Phenotypes associated with deficiency of IL-12 and related signaling molecules • IL-12 and the pathogenesis of autoimmune disease • Targeting IL-12 • References

INTRODUCTION

It is now well established that cytokines play critical roles in regulating all aspects of immune responses. Processes such as lymphoid development, homeostasis, differentiation, tolerance and memory are all regulated by different cytokines. Interleukin (IL)-12 is especially important in the differentiation of naive CD4[+] T cells to T helper 1 (Th1) cells that produce IFN-γ, which in turn is critical in host defense and promoting cell-mediated immunity. Not surprisingly, IL-12 is important in the pathogenesis of a variety of autoimmune disorders. In this chapter we review the basic biology of IL-12 and the related cytokines IL-23 and IL-27, their receptors, their modes of signaling and their biological activities. We also review what is known about the role of IL-12 in selected autoimmune diseases and conclude by briefly describing therapies that target IL-12.

STRUCTURE AND REGULATION OF IL-12, IL-23 AND IL-27

IL-12 comprises two disulfide-linked subunits designated p40 and p35 (Figure 14.1).[1–6] Interestingly, p40 has homology to cytokine receptors, whereas the p35 subunit has homology to IL-6 and G-CSF. Together, these subunits form the biologically active p70 heterodimer. The genes encoding human p35 and p40 map to distinct chromosomes, 3p12–3p13.2 and 5q31–5q33, respectively. The subunit p35 is expressed ubiquitously, whereas p40 expression is more limited. Consequently, IL-12 production is essentially regulated by the level of p40 transcription.[7–10] The p40 gene is highly inducible and its promoter binds a number of transcription factors including NF-κB, IRF-1 and Ets-family members.[11–14] IRF-9 (ICSBP) is also critical for IL-12 production.[15]

IL-12 is produced by a variety of cells, but most importantly is made by antigen presenting

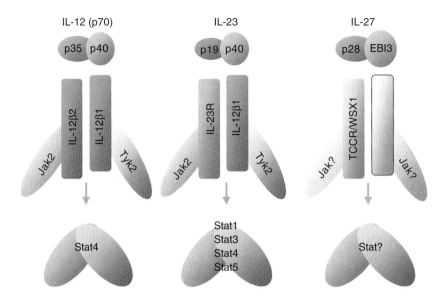

Figure 14.1 Structure of ligands and receptors and signaling molecules. IL-12 is a heterodimeric cytokine composed of IL-12p35 associated with a receptor-like subunit p40 which is also shared with IL-23 (p19 associated with p40). IL-27 is also a heterodimeric cytokine. IL-12 and IL-23 also share the receptor subunit IL-12Rb1 but also have distinct ligand-specific subunits. IL-27 utilizes a subunit designated TCCR/WSX1; whether another subunit is employed is unknown. These receptors associate with the Jaks and Stats shown. Stat4 is especially important for IL-12 signaling; just how important it is for the other cytokines is not known.

cells, particularly dendritic cells (DCs) and macrophages (Figure 14.2). A variety of different pathogenic organisms induce IL-12 production, including gram positive and gram negative organisms, *M. tuberculosis*, *L. monocytogenes*, *T. gondii* and *L. major*. Products of these organisms bind to Toll-like receptors and the mechanisms involved in signaling via these receptors are active areas of research.[16-19] IL-12 production is also induced by crosslinking CD40, CD80 and CD58. Conversely, IL-12 production is inhibited by IL-10, IL-11, IL-13 and type I IFNs. There is some controversy as to whether IL-4 inhibits IL-12 production. In some cases it clearly does,[20-23] whereas in other circumstances pretreatment with IL-4 can enhance IL-12 production.[24-27] G-protein-coupled receptors (GPCRs) including the receptors for monocyte chemoattractant protein 1 (MCP-1), prostaglandin E2, histamine and ligands for phagocytic receptors also inhibit IL-12 production, although some GPCRs such as

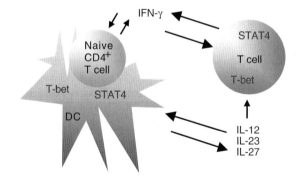

Figure 14.2 Model of interactions between lymphocytes and antigen presenting cells (APCs). IL-12, IL-23 and IL-27 are all produced by antigen presenting cells. These cytokines act both on T cells and on APCs to promote cell-mediated immunity (see text for details).

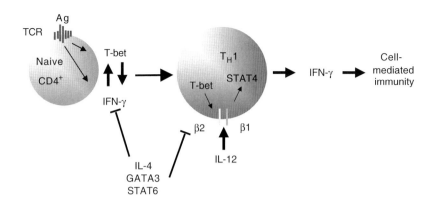

Figure 14.3 Regulation of T helper cell development by cytokines and transcription factors. Activation of naive CD4$^+$ T cells through the T cell antigen receptor induces expression of IL-12Rβ1, IL-12Rβ2, T-bet and Stat4. Antigen stimulation also induces IFN-γ production; T-bet and IFN-γ promote each other's expression. T-bet stabilizes IL-12Rβ2 expression, allowing continued responsiveness to IL-12 and further induction of IFN-γ. In contrast, IL-4 downregulates expression of IL-12Rβ2.

CCR5 positively regulate production.[28] Similarly, cholera toxin and measles infection downregulate IL-12 production.

A new complexity pertaining to IL-12 biology is the existence of a recently identified subunit, p19. Identified by computational searches for IL-6-related cytokines, it is homologous to IL-12p35 and, in fact, p19 associates with p40 to form a cytokine designated IL-23.[29] The human p19 gene is localized to 12q13.13 and, like p35, p19 is produced by macrophages, DCs, T cells and endothelial cells and is inducible by bacterial products (Figure 14.1).

IL-27, the newest member of this family of cytokines, is also a heterodimeric cytokine.[30] It comprises subunits encoded by two genes, designated EBI3 (Epstein–Barr virus-induced gene 3) and p28. EBI3 is related to the IL-12p40-related gene and so has homology to cytokine receptors.[31,32] p28 is homologous to IL-12p35 and, like the related heterodimeric cytokines IL-12 and IL-23, EBI3 coexpression appears to be required for secretion of p28. IL-27 is produced by antigen presenting cells with the highest levels of p28 and EBI3-occurring LPS-activated monocytes and monocyte-derived DCs. Like IL-12, both subunits are required for efficient secretion.

STRUCTURE AND EXPRESSION OF IL-12, IL-23 AND IL-27 RECEPTORS

The IL-12 receptor (IL-12R) consists of at least two receptor subunits, β1 and β2, which have structural features of the type I cytokine receptor superfamily and are homologous to gp130.[33–36] The loci encoding β1 and β2 reside on chromosomes 19p13.1 and 1p31.2, respectively. Coexpression of both β1 and β2 subunits is required for the generation of human high-affinity IL-12 binding sites. The receptor-like subunit, IL-12p40, interacts with the β1 subunit, whereas p35 interacts predominantly with the β2 subunit. The β2 subunit functions as the primary signal transducing component, as it contains three intracellular tyrosine residues that recruit signaling molecules; tyrosine 800 is the site that binds STAT4 (signal transducer and activator of transcription).[37] In contrast, IL-12Rβ1 has no intracellular tyrosine residues. IL-12Rβ1 and IL-12Rβ2 are expressed on T cells, NK cells and DCs.[38]

IL-12R expression is tightly controlled on T cells. Resting T cells do not express β1 or β2 but these subunits are induced upon activation of T cells (Figure 14.3). Additionally, the control of IL-12Rβ2 expression is an important aspect of helper T cell regulation (see below). IFN-γ stimulation upregulates the transcription factor T-bet, which in turn maintains IL-12Rβ2 chain expression.[39,40] In contrast, IL-4 downregulates IL-12Rβ2 expression.[41–43] Thus, the counter-regulation of IL-12 receptor expression by IFN-γ and IL-4 is one important factor that governs Th1/Th2 differentiation. However, it should be noted that transgenic expression of IL-12Rβ2 alone is not sufficient to drive Th1 differentiation, implying that other factors play a role in Th differentiation.[44,45]

IL-23 binds a receptor composed of IL-12Rβ1 and a second subunit designated IL-23R; IL-23 does not utilize IL-12Rβ2 as part of its receptor.[46] The IL-23R gene is on human chromosome 1 within 150 kb of IL-12Rβ2. IL-23R is expressed at rather low levels, but is present on T cells, NK cells, monocytes and DCs. Interestingly, murine CD4+ CD45Blow memory T cells express IL-23R and low levels of IL-12Rβ2 whereas murine CD4+CD45RBhigh cells express IL-12Rβ2 but not IL-23R. IL-23R contains seven intracellular tyrosine residues that could potentially be involved in signaling.

IL-27 has recently been shown to bind the orphan receptor WSX-1/TCCR, another receptor with homology to members of the gp130 family.[30,47,48] Interestingly, mice nullizygous for this receptor had been generated prior to the discovery of the ligand. These mice exhibit impaired Th1 development and IFN-γ production in response to antigen stimulation. Moreover, these mice exhibit increased susceptibility to infection with intracellular pathogens such as *Listeria monocytogenes* and *Leishmania major*.

BIOLOGICAL EFFECTS OF IL-12 AND IL-23

The developmental regulation of naive CD4+ T cells to either Th1 or Th2 cells is critically important for the effective acquired immunity and cytokines play a key role in this process. Th1 cells produce IFN-γ and promote cell-mediated immunity, which is essential for the response against intracellular pathogens and IL-12 is a key cytokine that regulates this differentiation (Figures 14.2 and 14.3). IL-12 has a number of important actions that serve to promote cell-mediated immunity.[49–54]

IL-12 induces production of IFN-γ in NK cells and IFN-γ production in both T and NK cells is enhanced by an unrelated cytokine, IL-18, the combination of these cytokines being highly synergistic. Notably, IL-12 also enhances expression of the IL-18 receptor.[55] IL-12, especially in conjunction with IL-18, can also induce IFN-γ production in macrophages, thereby activating

these cells and promoting Th1 differentiation.[56,57] IL-27 also synergizes with IL-12 to trigger IFN-γ production by T cells.[30] IL-12 and IFN-γ antagonize Th2 differentiation and the production of IL-4, IL-5 and IL-13. Moreover, IL-12 acts on DCs to induce further production of IL-12;[38] IL-23 has similar effects on DCs.[58] IL-12 also promotes the maturation of skin Langerhans cells.

Addititonally, IL-12 enhances the cytolytic activity of NK and T cells and induces T cell proliferation. Like IL-12, IL-27 preferentially acts on naive CD4+ T cells to induce their differentiation and expansion. This differs from IL-23, which exerts its effect preferentially on memory CD4+ T cells, consistent with the expression of its receptor. Finally, IL-12 is an indirect inhibitor of angiogenesis due to production of IP-10.

SIGNAL TRANSDUCTION

Unlike other cytokine receptors in which multiple pathways emanating from the receptor are apparent, rather few IL-12-mediated biochemical events have been identified. Like other cytokine receptors, however, IL-12R lacks intrinsic enzymatic activity. Instead, signaling through IL-12R involves activation of Janus kinases (JAKs) (Figure 14.1).[51] JAK2 associates with IL-12Rβ2, whereas TYK2 interacts with the β1 subunit.[59,60] JAKs phosphorylate the IL-12R on tyrosines located in the intracellular domain. STATs play a central role in cytoplasmic IL-12 signaling cascades. STATs bind the site of phosphorylated tyrosines on IL-12R and are tyrosine phosphorylated by JAKs. The phosphorylated STATs form themselves into hetero- or homodimers, translocate into the nucleus, bind DNA and modulate gene expression. Although STAT1, STAT3 and STAT4 have all been reported to be activated by IL-12, STAT4 appears to be most critical for IL-12 signaling[61,62] (see below).

IL-23 activates JAK2, TYK2, STAT1, STAT3, STAT4 and STAT5. However, STAT4 phosphorylation induced by IL-23 is weak compared to IL-12.[46] IL-23R associates constitutively with JAK2 in a similar manner as IL-12Rβ2.

IL-12 stimulation of cells also activates the Src family protein tyrosine kinase Lck. In addition,

IL-12 activates the MAPK p38.[63–65] One target of p38 appears to be STAT4 itself on S721; mutation of this site disrupts IFN-γ production and Th1 differentiation. In contrast to cytokines like IL-2, IL-12 does not induce phosphorylation of Shc, Gab2 and SHP-2 and apparently does not activate ERK1/2.

PHENOTYPES ASSOCIATED WITH DEFICIENCY OF IL-12 AND RELATED SIGNALING MOLECULES

The phenotypes of the IL-12p35, p40 and IL-12Rβ1 knockout mice are similar in many respects. The mice are viable and display no obvious development abnormalities.[66–69] However, IFN-γ secretion, Th1 development and enhancement of NK lytic activity are greatly impaired, whereas generation of Th2 cells is moderately enhanced. These mice can still produce small amounts of IFN-γ in some circumstances. Knocking out p40 and IL-12Rβ1 would be expected to abrogate both IL-12 and IL-23 signaling. Consequently, the phenotype of p40 knockouts should therefore be more severe than deficiency of IL-12p35 or IL-12Rβ1 and, in fact, several recent studies indicate than p40$^{-/-}$ mice are more immunocompromised than IL-12p35$^{-/-}$ mice.[70–73] Interestingly, some patients with atypical mycobacterial and salmonella infections have been found to have mutations of the genes encoding IL-12p40 (also designated *IL12B*) and IL-12 Rβ1 (*IL12RB1*).[74,75]

STAT4 knockout mice are viable but have defective IL-12 responses, production of IFN-γ and Th1 differentiation.[76,77] These mice also have impaired expression of IL-12R, IL-18R, CCR5, E-selectin and P-selectin ligand.[55,78–81] Even though the basis for the physiological actions of STAT4 is not yet entirely clear, STAT4 appears to bind to the IFN-γ promoter; exactly how it contributes to the regulation of transcription remains to be determined. Recent data demonstrate that co-stimulation with IL-12 and IL-18 results in a nuclear complex of activated STAT4 and AP-1, which serve to upregulate the IFN-γ promoter.[82]

JAK2 is associated with a number of cytokine receptors. Deficiency of JAK2 is embryonically lethal because it is essential for the actions of erythropoietin.[83,84] The phenotype of TYK2 knockout mice is surprisingly benign.[85,86] Thought to be crucial for interferon signaling, this is apparently not the case. TYK2 deficiency is associated with impaired IL-12 signaling.

IL-12 AND THE PATHOGENESIS OF AUTOIMMUNE DISEASE

As is clear from the above, a wealth of evidence supports the role of IL-12 in promoting Th1 differentiation and cell-mediated immunity. Importantly though, there is also a body of information that supports a role for IL-12 in the pathogenesis of various arthropathies.

IL-12 and arthritis

IL-12 has been shown to play a pivotal role in the induction of various animal models of inflammatory polyarthritis, including collagen-induced arthritis (CIA), streptococcal cell wall-induced arthritis (SCWA) and *Borrelia burgdorferi*-induced arthritis.[87,88] Unbalanced production of TNF, IL-1, IL-6 and IL-12, as opposed to the Th2 cytokines IL-4 and IL-10, correlates with disease susceptibility and severity. IL-12 mRNA and protein were also found to be markedly elevated following injection of *Mycoplasma arthritidis*.[89] Furthermore, administration of IL-12 can replace adjuvant in CIA.[90–92] Expression of IL-12 by gene transfer also exacerbates disease severity in CIA.[93] Although IL-12 can play a pivotal role in the 'induction' of CIA, its pathogenic role in 'established' CIA (i.e. after onset of arthritis) can be more variable; indeed low doses of IL-12 can exacerbate CIA whereas high doses can ameliorate it.[94–96] These dualistic actions of IL-12 are also consistent with the complicated effects of IFN-γ in models of arthritis. In vivo neutralization of IFN-γ can prevent arthritis in IL-12-treated mice. Surprisingly though, IFN-γ knockout mice have an increased predisposition to CIA and IFN-γ administration may actually be protective in established CIA.[97,98] However, in proteoglycan-induced arthritis disease is reduced in IFN-γ knockout mice.[99] Indeed, IL-12 and IFN-γ are not the only cytokines that have complicated and sometimes opposing effects on models of autoimmune disease. TNF also has well-documented inflammatory and immunosuppressive actions.[100,101]

IL-18 given in conjunction with IL-12 results in more severe disease[102] whereas in IL-18-deficient mice CIA is suppressed concomitant with reduced IL-12 levels.[103] IL-4 and IL-13 oppose Th1 differentiation and IFN-γ production. Accordingly, overexpression of IL-4, IL-10 and IL-13 through the use of viral vectors or treatment with recombinant cytokines generally attenuates CIA.[104–110]

Blockade of IL-12 with anti-IL-12 antibodies during the induction phase of arthritis has been shown to decrease the severity of murine Lyme arthritis, CIA and SCWA.[111–113] Typically this is associated with reduced levels of IFN-γ, TNF, IL-6 and IL-10. However, in another study, anti-IL-12 therapy initiated after the onset of clinical symptoms accelerated disease in chronic relapsing homologous CIA in DBA/1 mice.[114] Additionally, administration of anti-IL12 antibodies to mice with severe combined immunodeficiency increased the severity of acute Lyme arthritis.[115]

Surprisingly little work has been done using IL-12, IL-12 receptor and STAT4 knockout mice in various arthritis models. In CIA, some IL-12p40-deficient animals developed severe disease in a single paw in spite of the minimized Th1 response.[116] In proteoglycan-induced arthritis disease is significantly suppressed in STAT4 knockout mice. However, over an extended period of time mice develop milder disease (authors' unpublished observations). B10.Q/J mice, a substrain of the normally CIA-susceptible B10.Q mice, have a heritable, but undefined defect in IL-12 signaling resulting in absent STAT4 phosphorylation. These mice are resistant to the induction of CIA.[97,98] Parenthetically, IL-18 knockout DBA/1 mice have also been shown to have a markedly decreased susceptibility to CIA.[103]

IL-12 and human arthropathies

A variety of clinical studies have demonstrated that IL-12 plays an important role in the patho-genesis of rheumatoid arthritis (RA), psoriatic arthritis and juvenile chronic arthritis (JCA).[117–127] Elevated levels of IL-12 and IFN-γ have also been detected in serum of patients with various arthropathies. In patients with RA, IL-12 is expressed by infiltrating macrophages and cells in the synovial lining. IL-12 levels in the synovial fluid of patients with RA are higher than the circulating serum levels, which, in turn, are elevated compared to normal controls. Patients with elevated IL-12 levels were more likely to have an increased joint involvement and acute phase reactants and patients responsive to therapy were found to have decreased levels of IL-12 compared to those who failed to respond. These IL-12 changes correlated with changes in IFN-γ, TNF, IL-2 and IL-6 but were inversely related to changes in IL-10.[128] Furthermore, improvement of synovitis with standard therapies is reflected by suppressed levels of IL-12 and a shift from a Th1 cytokine profile to that of a Th2 cytokine profile supporting a causal relationship between IL-12 and arthritis. Severe RA exacerbation has also been associated with IL-12 administration for metastatic cervical cancer.[129] Interestingly, one study showed increased IL-12 p40 but not p70 in the serum samples from active JCA, implying perhaps, a pathogenic role for IL-23.[130]

As with the animal studies, several studies in RA patients suggest a synergistic role for IL-18. IL-18 mRNA expression is increased in synovial tissue monocytes from RA patients as compared to OA controls.[131] Furthermore, IL-18 protein is elevated in the synovial fluid and blood from RA patients.[132] IL-18 has also been shown to synergistically enhance IL-12-induced IFN-γ production by RA synovial tissue cells.[133]

In contrast to the consistently shown predominant Th1 cytokine profile in RA joints, a more prominent Th2 immune response was present in the joints of reactive arthritis patients.[134] Synovial fluid samples from a small group of patients with reactive arthritis following infection with *Chlamydia trachomatis*, *Yersinia enterocolitica* and *Salmonella enteritidis*, were found to have high levels of IL-10 and low levels of IFN-γ and TNF. Immunohistochemical analysis of synovial membranes revealed high levels of IL-4 compared to the number of IFN-γ-secreting cells. Perhaps the suppression of the Th1 immune response might aid the persistence of bacteria.

IL-12 and inflammatory bowel disease

In parallel with the studies of RA, IL-12 has been implicated in the inflammation of other autoimmune diseases. A notable example of this is Crohn's disease, which is clearly associated with increased production of IL-12 by antigen-presenting cells in the lamina propria of the gut, as well as downstream Th1 cytokines induced by IL-12, IFN-γ and TNF-α.[135–137] This is in contrast to the situation in ulcerative colitis, a second form of inflammatory bowel disease, where IL-12 and IFN-γ are not increased and the inflammation has been presumed to be due to Th2 cytokines.[137]

The role of IL-12 in Crohn's disease but not in ulcerative colitis is reflected in the fact that in the many murine models of colitis that resemble Crohn's disease histopathologically, a Th1 inflammation is invariably present whereas in those that resemble ulcerative colitis, a Th2 inflammation is the rule.[138] This is perhaps best illustrated in two models of colitis induced by intra-rectal application of contactant agents, trinitrobenzene sulfonate (TNBS) and oxazalone. In the former case, i.e. in TNBS colitis (induced in SJL/J or C57BL/10 mice), the colonic inflammation resembles Crohn's disease and is a 'pure' Th1 response associated with high IL-12 and IFN-γ response.[139] Consequently, this inflammation is dramatically blocked even after the disease is well established by administration of monoclonal anti-IL-12 antibodies. In contrast, in the latter case, i.e. oxazalone colitis, the colonic inflammation resembles ulcerative colitis and is due to an IL-4-mediated Th2 response that is blocked by anti-IL-4 antibody administration.[140] The relation of IL-12 to the Th1 colitis in TNBS colitis is mirrored in numerous other Th1 models where again anti-IL-12 antibody administration ameliorates disease.[138] The only apparent exception to this generaliza-

tion proves the rule: while anti-IL-12 is an effective treatment of the colitis associated with IL-10 deficiency early on, it has a diminished effect late or after the disease is well established.[141] In this case, however, it has been shown that while Th1 cytokine mediates the initial phase of the inflammation, Th2 cytokines mediate the later phases. Similarly, in a mouse model of intestinal inflammation resembling Crohn's disease both histologically (by the presence of granulomas) and distributionally (by the presence of skip lesions scattered throughout the small intestine), anti-IL-12 has not been proven to be a fully effective treatment perhaps due to the fact that in this model Th2 response also becomes prominent as the disease progresses (F. Cominelli, personal communication).

The mechanism of action of anti-IL-12 in the treatment of Th2 models of colitis is due to several factors. Perhaps the most important is the fact that Th1 cells deprived of IL-12 undergo apoptosis.[142] This is shown by the fact that anti-IL-12 administered to mice with TNBS colitis is followed by the appearance of numerous TUNEL-positive (apoptotic) cells in the inflamed lamina propria. Apparently this apoptosis is related to increased susceptibility to FAS-mediated cell lysis since it is blocked by co-administration of FAS-Fc, an agent that blocks FAS activation.

Another mechanism of anti-IL-12 activity probably relates to the fact that IL-12 is necessary for chemokine or selectin ligand expression and thus the homing of cells to the site of inflammation.[79,80] Thus, while mucosal inflammation is due to antigen loading of APCs in the mucosal tissues proper, the actual activation of effector T cells probably occurs in draining lymph nodes;[143] thus, the inflammation is dependent on adequate recirculation of activated T cells back to the lamina propria. Evidence that anti-IL-12 treatment interferes with T cell traffic comes from the fact that anti-IL-12 treatment is associated with spleen cell enlargement; and in addition, in a model of psoriasis (another IL-12-mediated inflammation), Th1 cells would accumulate in lymph nodes upon anti-IL-12 administration.[144]

Finally, it is possible that anti-IL-12 ameliorates disease by simply removing the drive for the production of Th1 cytokines. This is seen most dramatically in the case of mucosal inflammation due to a mutation in the TNF-α gene leading to defective degradation of TNF mRNA and over-production of TNF-α (the TNF$^{\Delta ARE}$ defect).[145] In this case, the disease is ameliorated by anti-IL-12 presumably because the T cells producing the TNF-α require an IL-12 drive to activate the defective TNF production mechanism.

TARGETING IL-12

The efficacy of anti-IL-12 in murine models of mucosal inflammation and, indeed, in other types of autoimmune inflammation such as RA has prompted a therapeutic trial with anti-IL-12 in Crohn's disease and in RA. The antibody currently being tested is a human immunoglob-ulin mutated in its variable region so as to bind to IL-12 with high affinity. So far a phase I/II trial has been initiated and the results have not yet been reported. The expectation, however, is that anti-IL-12 will be an effective treatment of patients and one that will have a considerable duration, given the ability of anti-IL-12 to induce apoptosis of Th1 cells.

While anti-IL-12 is the most obvious treatment mediating a blockade of IL-12 activity in Crohn's disease and other Th1-mediated inflammation, other treatments to accomplish a similar end can also be envisioned.[146] This relates to the fact that IL-12 production by antigen-presenting cells can be influenced by a wide variety of agents includ-ing β$_2$ agonists, pentoxyfylline, thalidomide, angiotensin-converting enzyme inhibitors, a variety of bacterial products, immune complexes, ADP-ribosylating agents, the CR3 receptor chemoattractants, and a host of cytokines including IL-10, TGF-β and the Th2 cytokines IL-4 and IL-13.[147] Any or all of these substances could conceivably be used to treat IL-12-mediated inflammations and indeed studies in humans evaluating some of these substances are currently underway.

One form of inhibition of IL-12 that merits particular emphasis is that caused by TGF-β. The latter is a molecule synthesized by many cells that has been shown to downregulate immune responses. This is best appreciated in TGF-β1-deficient mice who manifest inflamma-tion in many organs and rarely survive beyond 6 weeks of age.[148] The particular relation of TGF-β to inflammation is best understood in the context of our evolving understanding of exper-imental/clinical mucosal inflammation. It is now generally believed that such inflammation results from an imbalance between mucosal effector T cells reacting to antigens in the mucosal microflora that are capable of mediat-ing Th1- or Th2-type inflammation and regula-tory T cells reacting to similar antigens and producing TGF-β or IL-10. This formulation of mucosal inflammation is, in turn, a reflection of the fact that mucosal responses in general are regulated by the phenomenon of oral tolerance which oral antigen administration elicits in unresponsiveness and are due to induction of cellular antigen or induction of suppressor cells producing TGF-β. This understanding of mucosal inflammation leads to the possibility that such inflammation can be controlled/prevented by the judicious administration of TGF-β.

On this basis, investigators have recently created DNA plasmids encoding TGF-β and have introduced this DNA into cells migrating to the gastrointestinal tract by administration of the DNA via intranasal inflammation.[149] They went on to show that such TGF-β-secret-ing cells can either prevent or treat TNBS colitis. As to the mechanism of this effect they showed that TGF-β induces IL-10 production, a cytokine that downregulates IL-12 production. In addition, they showed that TGF-β down-regulates the IL-12Rβ2 chain and interferes with IL-12 signaling. These studies thus demonstrate that the appropriate application of a regulatory cytokine can also be used to regulate IL-12 production and thus treat Th1-mediated inflammation.

REFERENCES

1. Gately MK, Desai BB, Wolitzky AG et al. Regulation of human lymphocyte proliferation by a heterodimeric cytokine, IL-12 (cytotoxic lymphocyte maturation factor). *J Immunol* 1991; **147**(3): 874–82.

2. Gubler U, Chua AO, Schoenhaut DS et al. Coexpression of two distinct genes is required to generate secreted bioactive cytotoxic lymphocyte maturation factor. *Proc Natl Acad Sci USA* 1991; **88**(10): 4143–7.

3. Wolf SF, Temple PA, Kobayashi M et al. Cloning of cDNA for natural killer cell stimulatory factor, a heterodimeric cytokine with multiple biologic effects on T and natural killer cells. *J Immunol* 1991; **146**(9): 3074–81.

4. Trinchieri G, Scott P. Interleukin-12: a proinflammatory cytokine with immunoregulatory functions. *Res Immunol* 1995; **146**(7–8): 423–31.

5. Trinchieri G, Scott P. Interleukin-12: basic principles and clinical applications. *Curr Top Microbiol Immunol* 1999; **238**: 57–78.

6. Esche C, Shurin MR, Lotze MT. IL-12. In: Oppenheim JJ, Feldmann M, eds. *Cytokine Reference* (San Diego: Academic Press, 2000) 189–201.

7. Ma X, Trinchieri G. Regulation of interleukin-12 production in antigen-presenting cells. *Adv Immunol* 2001; **79**: 55–92.

8. Weinmann AS, Plevy SE, Smale ST. Rapid and selective remodeling of a positioned nucleosome during the induction of IL-12 p40 transcription. *Immunity* 1999; **11**(6): 665–75.

9. Weinmann AS, Mitchell DM, Sanjabi S et al. Nucleosome remodeling at the IL-12 p40 promoter is a TLR-dependent, Rel-independent event. *Nat Immunol* 2001; **2**(1): 51–7.

10. Smale ST, Fisher AG. Chromatin structure and gene regulation in the immune system. *Ann Rev Immunol* 2002; **20**: 427–62.

11. Murphy TL, Cleveland MG, Kulesza P, Magram J, Murphy KM. Regulation of interleukin 12 p40 expression through an NF-kappa B half- site. *Mol Cell Biol* 1995; **15**(10): 5258–67.

12. Ma X, Chow JM, Gri G et al. The interleukin 12 p40 gene promoter is primed by interferon gamma in monocytic cells. *J Exp Med* 1996; **183**(1): 147–57.

13. Ma X, Neurath M, Gri G, Trinchieri G. Identification and characterization of a novel Ets-2-related nuclear complex implicated in the activation of the human interleukin-12 p40 gene promoter. *J Biol Chem* 1997; **272**(16): 10389–95.

14. Plevy SE, Gemberling JH, Hsu S et al. Multiple control elements mediate activation of the murine and human interleukin 12 p40 promoters: evidence of functional synergy between C/EBP and Rel proteins. *Mol Cell Biol* 1997; **17**(8): 4572–88.

15. Wang IM, Contursi C, Masumi A et al. An IFN-gamma-inducible transcription factor, IFN consensus sequence binding protein (ICSBP), stimulates IL-12 p40 expression in macrophages. *J Immunol* 2000; **165**(1): 271–9.

16. Medzhitov R. Toll-like receptors and innate immunity. *Nature Rev Immunol* 2001; **1**(2): 135–45.

17. Barton GM, Medzhitov R. Control of adaptive immune responses by Toll-like receptors. *Curr Opin Immunol* 2002; **14**(3): 380–3.

18. Akira S, Takeda K, Kaisho T. Toll-like receptors: critical proteins linking innate and acquired immunity. *Nat Immunol* 2001; **2**(8): 675–80.

19. Scanga CA, Aliberti J, Jankovic D et al. Cutting edge: MyD88 is required for resistance to Toxoplasma gondii infection and regulates parasite-induced IL-12 production by dendritic cells. *J Immunol* 2002; **168**(12): 5997–6001.

20. D'Andrea A, Ma X, Aste-Amezaga M et al. Stimulatory and inhibitory effects of interleukin (IL)-4 and IL-13 on the production of cytokines by human peripheral blood mononuclear cells: priming for IL-12 and tumor necrosis factor alpha production. *J Exp Med* 1995; **181**(2): 537–46.

21. Takenaka H, Maruo S, Yamamoto N et al. Regulation of T cell-dependent and -independent IL-12 production by the three Th2-type cytokines IL-10, IL-6, and IL-4. *J Leukoc Biol* 1997; **61**(1): 80–7.

22. Hochrein H, O'Keeffe M, Luft T et al. Interleukin (IL)-4 is a major regulatory cytokine governing bioactive IL-12 production by mouse and human dendritic cells. *J Exp Med* 2000; **192**(6): 823–33.

23. Marshall JD, Robertson SE, Trinchieri G, Chehimi J. Priming with IL-4 and IL-13 during HIV-1 infection restores in vitro IL-12 production by mononuclear cells of HIV-infected patients. *J Immunol* 1997; **159**(11): 5705–14.

24. Major J, Fletcher JE, Hamilton TA. IL-4 pretreatment selectively enhances cytokine and chemokine production in lipopolysaccharide-stimulated mouse peritoneal macrophages. *J Immunol* 2002; **168**(5): 2456–63.

25. Koch F, Stanzl U, Jennewein P et al. High level IL-12 production by murine dendritic cells: upregulation via MHC class II and CD40 molecules and downregulation by IL-4 and IL-10. *J Exp Med* 1996; **184**(2): 741–6.

26. Snijders A, Hilkens CM, van der Pouw Kraan TC et al. Regulation of bioactive IL-12 production in lipopolysaccharide-stimulated human monocytes is determined by the expression of the p35 subunit. *J Immunol* 1996; **156**(3): 1207–12.

27. Schindler H, Lutz MB, Rollinghoff M, Bogdan C. The production of IFN-gamma by IL-12/IL-18-activated macrophages requires STAT4 signaling and is inhibited by IL-4. *J Immunol* 2001; **166**(5): 3075–82.

28. Aliberti J, Sher A. Positive and negative regulation of pathogen induced dendritic cell function by G-protein coupled receptors. *Mol Immunol* 2002; **38**(12–13): 891–3.

29. Oppmann B, Lesley R, Blom B et al. Novel p19 protein engages IL-12p40 to form a cytokine, IL-23, with biological activities similar as well as distinct from IL-12. *Immunity* 2000; **13**(5): 715–25.

30. Pflanz S, Timans J, Cheung J et al. IL-27, a heterodimeric cytokine composed of EBI3 and p28 protein, induces proliferation of naive CD4⁺ T cells. *Immunity* 2002; **16**: 779–90.

31. Devergne O, Birkenbach M, Kieff E. Epstein–Barr virus-induced gene 3 and the p35 subunit of interleukin 12 form a novel heterodimeric hematopoietin. *Proc Natl Acad Sci USA* 1997; **94**(22): 12041–6.

32. Devergne O, Hummel M, Koeppen H et al. A novel interleukin-12 p40-related protein induced by latent Epstein–Barr virus infection in B lymphocytes. *J Virol* 1996; **70**(2): 1143–53.

33. Chua AO, Chizzonite R, Desai BB et al. Expression cloning of a human IL-12 receptor component. A new member of the cytokine receptor superfamily with strong homology to gp130. *J Immunol* 1994; **153**(1): 128–36.

34. Chua AO, Wilkinson VL, Presky DH, Gubler U. Cloning and characterization of a mouse IL-12 receptor-beta component. *J Immunol* 1995; **155**(9): 4286–94.

35. Presky DH, Yang H, Minetti LJ et al. A functional interleukin 12 receptor complex is composed of two beta-type cytokine receptor subunits. *Proc Natl Acad Sci USA* 1996; **93**(24): 14002–7.

36. Esche C, Shurin MR, Lotze MT. IL-12 receptor. In: Oppenheim JJ, Feldmann M, eds. *Cytokine Reference* (San Diego: Academic Press, 2000).

37. Naeger LK, McKinney J, Salvekar A, Hoey T. Identification of a STAT4 binding site in the interleukin-12 receptor required for signaling. *J Biol Chem* 1999; **274**(4): 1875–8.

38. Grohmann U, Belladonna ML, Bianchi R et al. IL-12 acts directly on DC to promote nuclear localization of NF-kappaB and primes DC for IL-12 production. *Immunity* 1998; **9**(3): 315–23.

39. Lighvani AA, Frucht DM, Jankovic D et al. T-bet is rapidly induced by interferon-gamma in lymphoid and myeloid cells. *Proc Natl Acad Sci USA* 2001; **98**(26): 15137–42.

40. Afkarian M, Sedy JR, Yang J et al. T-bet is a Stat1-induced regulator of IL-12 receptor expression in naive CD4⁺ T cells. *Nat Immunol* 2002; **3**(6): 549–57.

41. Szabo SJ, Dighe AS, Gubler U, Murphy KM. Regulation of the interleukin (IL)-12R beta 2 subunit expression in developing T helper 1 (Th1) and Th2 cells. *J Exp Med* 1997; **185**(5): 817–24.

42. Rogge L, Barberis-Maino L, Biffi M et al. Selective expression of an interleukin-12 receptor component by human T helper 1 cells. *J Exp Med* 1997; **185**(5): 825–31.

43. Sinigaglia F, D'Ambrosio D, Panina-Bordignon P, Rogge L. Regulation of the IL-12/IL-12R axis: a critical step in T-helper cell differentiation and effector function. *Immunol Rev* 1999; **170**: 65–72.

44. Nishikomori R, Gurunathan S, Nishikomori K, Strober W. BALB/c mice bearing a transgenic IL-12 receptor beta 2 gene exhibit a nonhealing phenotype to Leishmania major infection despite intact IL-12 signaling. *J Immunol* 2001; **166**(11): 6776–83.

45. Nishikomori R, Ehrhardt RO, Strober W. T helper type 2 cell differentiation occurs in the presence of interleukin 12 receptor beta2 chain expression and signaling. *J Exp Med* 2000; **191**(5): 847–58.

46. Parham C, Chirica M, Timans J et al. A receptor for the heterodimeric cytokine IL-23 is composed of IL-12Rbeta1 and a novel cytokine receptor subunit, IL-23R. *J Immunol* 2002; **168**(11): 5699–708.

47. Yoshida H, Hamano S, Senaldi G et al. WSX-1 is required for the initiation of Th1 responses and resistance to L. major infection. *Immunity* 2001; **15**(4): 569–78.

48. Chen Q, Ghilardi N, Wang H et al. Development of Th1-type immune responses requires the type I cytokine receptor TCCR. *Nature* 2000; **407**(6806): 916–20.

49. Dong C, Flavell RA. Th1 and Th2 cells. *Curr Opin Hematol* 2001; **8**(1): 47–51.

50. Glimcher LH. Lineage commitment in lympho-cytes: controlling the immune response. *J Clin Invest* 2001; **108**(7): s25–s30.

51. O'Shea JJ, Gadina M, Schreiber RD. Cytokine signaling in 2002: new surprises in the Jak/Stat pathway. *Cell* 2002; **109**(Suppl): S121–31.

52. O'Shea JJ, Paul WE. Regulation of T(H)1 differen-tiation controlling the controllers. *Nat Immunol* 2002; **3**(6): 506–8.

53. Farrar JD, Asnagli H, Murphy KM. T helper subset development: roles of instruction, selec-tion, and transcription. *J Clin Invest* 2002; **109**(4): 431–5.

54. Ho IC, Glimcher LH. Transcription: tantalizing times for T cells. *Cell* 2002; **109**(Suppl): S109–20.

55. Lawless VA, Zhang S, Ozes ON et al. Stat4 regulates multiple components of IFN-gamma-inducing signaling pathways. *J Immunol* 2000; **165**(12): 6803–8.

56. Fukao T, Frucht DM, Yap G et al. Inducible expression of Stat4 in dendritic cells and macro-phages and its critical role in innate and adaptive immune responses. *J Immunol* 2001; **166**(7): 4446–55.

57. Frucht DM, Fukao T, Bogdan C et al. IFN-gamma production by antigen-presenting cells: mecha-nisms emerge. *Trends Immunol* 2001; **22**(10): 556–60.

58. Belladonna ML, Renauld JC, Bianchi R et al. IL-23 and IL-12 have overlapping, but distinct, effects on murine dendritic cells. *J Immunol* 2002; **168**(11): 5448–54.

59. Bacon CM, McVicar DW, Ortaldo JR et al. Interleukin 12 (IL-12) induces tyrosine phospho-rylation of JAK2 and TYK2: differential use of Janus family tyrosine kinases by IL-2 and IL-12. *J Exp Med* 1995; **181**(1): 399–404.

60. Zou J, Presky DH, Wu CY, Gubler U. Differential associations between the cytoplasmic regions of the interleukin-12 receptor subunits beta1 and beta2 and JAK kinases. *J Biol Chem* 1997; **272**(9): 6073–7.

61. Bacon CM, Petricoin EF, 3rd, Ortaldo JR et al. Interleukin 12 induces tyrosine phosphorylation and activation of STAT4 in human lymphocytes. *Proc Natl Acad Sci USA* 1995; **92**(16): 7307–11.

62. Jacobson NG, Szabo SJ, Weber-Nordt RM et al. Interleukin 12 signaling in T helper type 1 (Th1) cells involves tyrosine phosphorylation of signal transducer and activator of transcription (Stat)3 and Stat4. *J Exp Med* 1995; **181**(5): 1755–62.

63. Gollob JA, Schnipper CP, Murphy EA et al. The

64. functional synergy between IL-12 and IL-2 involves p38 mitogen-activated protein kinase and is associated with the augmentation of STAT serine phosphorylation. *J Immunol* 1999; **162**(8): 4472–81.

64. Zhang S, Kaplan MH. The p38 mitogen-activated protein kinase is required for IL-12-induced IFN-gamma expression. *J Immunol* 2000; **165**(3): 1374–80.

65. Visconti R, Gadina M, Chiariello M et al. Importance of the MKK6/p38 pathway for inter-leukin-12-induced STAT4 serine phosphoryla-tion and transcriptional activity. *Blood* 2000; **96**(5): 1844–52.

66. Mattner F, Magram J, Ferrante J et al. Genetically resistant mice lacking interleukin-12 are suscepti-ble to infection with Leishmania major and mount a polarized Th2 cell response. *Eur J Immunol* 1996; **26**(7): 1553–9.

67. Magram J, Connaughton SE, Warrier RR et al. IL-12-deficient mice are defective in IFN gamma production and type 1 cytokine responses. *Immunity* 1996; **4**(5): 471–81.

68. Wu C, Ferrante J, Gately MK, Magram J. Characterization of IL-12 receptor beta1 chain (IL-12Rbeta1)-deficient mice: IL-12Rbeta1 is an essential component of the functional mouse IL-12 receptor. *J Immunol* 1997; **159**(4): 1658–65.

69. Wu CY, Gadina M, Wang K et al. Cytokine regulation of IL-12 receptor beta2 expression: differential effects on human T and NK cells. *Eur J Immunol* 2000; **30**(5): 1364–74.

70. Decken K, Kohler G, Palmer-Lehmann K et al. Interleukin-12 is essential for a protective Th1 response in mice infected with Cryptococcus neoformans. *Infect Immun* 1998; **66**(10): 4994–5000.

71. Piccotti JR, Li K, Chan SY et al. Alloantigen-reactive Th1 development in IL-12-deficient mice. *J Immunol* 1998; **160**(3): 1132–8.

72. Camoglio L, Juffermans NP, Peppelenbosch M et al. Contrasting roles of IL-12p40 and IL-12p35 in the development of hapten-induced colitis. *Eur J Immunol* 2002; **32**(1): 261–9.

73. Frucht DM. IL-23: a cytokine that acts on memory T cells. *Sci STKE* 2002; **2002**(114): PE1.

74. de Jong R, Altare F, Haagen IA et al. Severe mycobacterial and Salmonella infections in inter-leukin-12 receptor-deficient patients. *Science* 1998; **280**(5368): 1435–8.

75. Doffinger R, Dupuis S, Picard C et al. Inherited disorders of IL-12- and IFNgamma-mediated

immunity: a molecular genetics update. *Mol Immunol* 2002; **38**(12–13): 903–9.

76. Thierfelder WE, van Deursen JM, Yamamoto K et al. Requirement for Stat4 in interleukin-12-mediated responses of natural killer and T cells. *Nature* 1996; **382**(6587): 171–4.

77. Kaplan MH, Sun YL, Hoey T, Grusby MJ. Impaired IL-12 responses and enhanced development of Th2 cells in Stat4-deficient mice. *Nature* 1996; **382**(6587): 174–7.

78. Nakahira M, Tomura M, Iwasaki M et al. An absolute requirement for STAT4 and a role for IFN-gamma as an amplifying factor in IL-12 induction of the functional IL-18 receptor complex. *J Immunol* 2001; **167**(3): 1306–12.

79. Iwasaki M, Mukai T, Nakajima C et al. A mandatory role for STAT4 in IL-12 induction of mouse T cell CCR5. *J Immunol* 2001; **167**(12): 6877–83.

80. Lim YC, Xie H, Come CE et al. IL-12, STAT4-dependent up-regulation of CD4(+) T cell core 2 beta-1,6-n-acetylglucosaminyltransferase, an enzyme essential for biosynthesis of P-selectin ligands. *J Immunol* 2001; **167**(8): 4476–84.

81. White SJ, Underhill GH, Kaplan MH, Kansas GS. Cutting edge: differential requirements for Stat4 in expression of glycosyltransferases responsible for selectin ligand formation in Th1 cells. *J Immunol* 2001; **167**(2): 628–31.

82. Nakahira M, Ahn HJ, Park WR et al. Synergy of IL-12 and IL-18 for IFN-gamma gene expression: IL-12-induced STAT4 contributes to IFN-gamma promoter activation by up-regulating the binding activity of IL-18-induced activator protein 1. *J Immunol* 2002; **168**(3): 1146–53.

83. Neubauer H, Cumano A, Muller M et al. Jak2 deficiency defines an essential developmental checkpoint in definitive hematopoiesis. *Cell* 1998; **93**(3): 397–409.

84. Parganas E, Wang D, Stravopodis D et al. Jak2 is essential for signaling through a variety of cytokine receptors. *Cell* 1998; **93**(3): 385–95.

85. Shimoda K, Kato K, Aoki K et al. Tyk2 plays a restricted role in IFN alpha signaling, although it is required for IL-12-mediated T cell function. *Immunity* 2000; **13**(4): 561–71.

86. Karaghiosoff M, Neubauer H, Lassnig C et al. Partial impairment of cytokine responses in Tyk2-deficient mice. *Immunity* 2000; **13**(4): 549–60.

87. Joe B, Wilder RL. Animal models of rheumatoid arthritis. *Mol Med Today* 1999; **5**(8): 367–9.

88. Joe B, Griffiths MM, Remmers EF, Wilder RL. Animal models of rheumatoid arthritis and related inflammation. *Curr Rheumatol Rep* 1999; **1**(2): 139–48.

89. Mu HH, Sawitzke AD, Cole BC. Modulation of cytokine profiles by the Mycoplasma superantigen Mycoplasma arthritidis mitogen parallels susceptibility to arthritis induced by M. arthritidis. *Infect Immun* 2000; **68**(3): 1142–9.

90. Germann T, Szeliga J, Hess H et al. Administration of interleukin 12 in combination with type II collagen induces severe arthritis in DBA/1 mice. *Proc Natl Acad Sci USA* 1995; **92**(11): 4823–7.

91. Germann T, Hess H, Szeliga J, Rude E. Characterization of the adjuvant effect of IL-12 and efficacy of IL-12 inhibitors in type II collagen-induced arthritis. *Ann N Y Acad Sci* 1996; **795**: 227–40.

92. Szeliga J, Hess H, Rude E et al. IL-12 promotes cellular but not humoral type II collagen-specific Th 1-type responses in C57BL/6 and B10.Q mice and fails to induce arthritis. *Int Immunol* 1996; **8**(8): 1221–7.

93. Parks E, Strieter RM, Lukacs NW et al. Transient gene transfer of IL-12 regulates chemokine expression and disease severity in experimental arthritis. *J Immunol* 1998; **160**(9): 4615–19.

94. Kasama T, Yamazaki J, Hanaoka R et al. Biphasic regulation of the development of murine type II collagen-induced arthritis by interleukin-12: possible involvement of endogenous interleukin-10 and tumor necrosis factor alpha. *Arthritis Rheum* 1999; **42**(1): 100–9.

95. Hess H, Gately MK, Rude E et al. High doses of interleukin-12 inhibit the development of joint disease in DBA/1 mice immunized with type II collagen in complete Freund's adjuvant. *Eur J Immunol* 1996; **26**(1): 187–91.

96. Joosten LA, Lubberts E, Helsen MM, van den Berg WB. Dual role of IL-12 in early and late stages of murine collagen type II arthritis. *J Immunol* 1997; **159**(8): 4094–102.

97. Ortmann RA, Shevach EM. Susceptibility to collagen-induced arthritis: cytokine-mediated regulation. *Clin Immunol* 2001; **98**(1): 109–18.

98. Ortmann R, Smeltz R, Yap G et al. A heritable defect in IL-12 signaling in B10.Q/J mice. I. In vitro analysis. *J Immunol* 2001; **166**(9): 5712–19.

99. Kaplan C, Valdez JC, Chandrasekaran R et al. Th1 and Th2 cytokines regulate proteoglycan-specific autoantibody isotypes and arthritis. *Arthritis Res* 2002; **4**(1): 54–8.

100. Cope AP. Regulation of autoimmunity by proin-flammatory cytokines. *Curr Opin Immunol* 1998; **10**(6): 669–76.

101. O'Shea JJ, Ma A, Lipsky P. Cytokines and autoimmunity. *Nature Rev Immunol* 2002; **2**(1): 37–45.

102. Leung BP, McInnes IB, Esfandiari E et al. Combined effects of IL-12 and IL-18 on the induction of collagen-induced arthritis. *J Immunol* 2000; **164**(12): 6495–502.

103. Wei XQ, Leung BP, Arthur HM et al. Reduced incidence and severity of collagen-induced arthritis in mice lacking IL-18. *J Immunol* 2001; **166**(1): 517–21.

104. Lubberts E, Joosten LA, Chabaud M et al. IL-4 gene therapy for collagen arthritis suppresses synovial IL-17 and osteoprotegerin ligand and prevents bone erosion. *J Clin Invest* 2000; **105**(12): 1697–710.

105. Woods JM, Tokuhira M, Berry JC et al. Interleukin-4 adenoviral gene therapy reduces production of inflammatory cytokines and prostaglandin E2 by rheumatoid arthritis synovium ex vivo. *J Investig Med* 1999; **47**(6): 285–92.

106. Woods JM, Katschke KJ Jr, Tokuhira M et al. Reduction of inflammatory cytokines and prostaglandin E2 by IL-13 gene therapy in rheumatoid arthritis synovium. *J Immunol* 2000; **165**(5): 2755–63.

107. Woods JM, Katschke KJ, Volin MV et al. IL-4 adenoviral gene therapy reduces inflammation, proinflammatory cytokines, vascularization, and bony destruction in rat adjuvant-induced arthritis. *J Immunol* 2001; **166**(2): 1214–22.

108. Woods JM, Amin MA, Katschke KJ Jr et al. Interleukin-13 gene therapy reduces inflammation, vascularization, and bony destruction in rat adjuvant-induced arthritis. *Hum Gene Ther* 2002; **13**(3): 381–93.

109. Joosten LA, Lubberts E, Durez P et al. Role of interleukin-4 and interleukin-10 in murine collagen-induced arthritis. Protective effect of interleukin-4 and interleukin-10 treatment on cartilage destruction. *Arthritis Rheum* 1997; **40**(2): 249–60.

110. Finnegan A, Mikecz K, Tao P, Glant TT. Proteoglycan (aggrecan)-induced arthritis in BALB/c mice is a Th1-type disease regulated by Th2 cytokines. *J Immunol* 1999; **163**(10): 5383–90.

111. Anguita J, Persing DH, Rincon M et al. Effect of anti-interleukin 12 treatment on murine lyme borreliosis. *J Clin Invest* 1996; **97**(4): 1028–34.

112. Malfait AM, Butler DM, Presky DH et al. Blockade of IL-12 during the induction of collagen-induced arthritis (CIA) markedly attenuates the severity of the arthritis. *Clin Exp Immunol* 1998; **111**(2): 377–83.

113. Joosten LA, Helsen MM, van Den Berg WB. Blockade of endogenous interleukin 12 results in suppression of murine streptococcal cell wall arthritis by enhancement of interleukin 10 and interleukin 1Ra. *Ann Rheum Dis* 2000; **59**(3): 196–205.

114. Malfait AM, Williams RO, Malik AS et al. Chronic relapsing homologous collagen-induced arthritis in DBA/1 mice as a model for testing disease-modifying and remission-inducing therapies. *Arthritis Rheum* 2001; **44**(5): 1215–24.

115. Anguita J, Samanta S, Barthold SW, Fikrig E. Ablation of interleukin-12 exacerbates Lyme arthritis in SCID mice. *Infect Immun* 1997; **65**(10): 4334–6.

116. McIntyre KW, Shuster DJ, Gillooly KM et al. Reduced incidence and severity of collagen-induced arthritis in interleukin-12-deficient mice. *Eur J Immunol* 1996; **26**(12): 2933–8.

117. Bucht A, Larsson P, Weisbrot L et al. Expression of interferon-gamma (IFN-gamma), IL-10, IL-12 and transforming growth factor-beta (TGF-beta) mRNA in synovial fluid cells from patients in the early and late phases of rheumatoid arthritis (RA). *Clin Exp Immunol* 1996; **103**(3): 357–67.

118. Schlaak JF, Pfers I, Meyer Zum Buschenfelde KH, Marker-Hermann E. Different cytokine profiles in the synovial fluid of patients with osteoarthritis, rheumatoid arthritis and seronegative spondylarthropathies. *Clin Exp Rheumatol* 1996; **14**(2): 155–62.

119. Morita Y, Yamamura M, Nishida K et al. Expression of interleukin-12 in synovial tissue from patients with rheumatoid arthritis. *Arthritis Rheum* 1998; **41**(2): 306–14.

120. Sakkas LI, Johanson NA, Scanzello CR, Platsoucas CD. Interleukin-12 is expressed by infiltrating macrophages and synovial lining cells in rheumatoid arthritis and osteoarthritis. *Cell Immunol* 1998; **188**(2): 105–10.

121. Kim W, Min S, Cho M et al. The role of IL-12 in inflammatory activity of patients with rheumatoid arthritis (RA). *Clin Exp Immunol* 2000; **119**(1): 175–81.

122. Spadaro A, Rinaldi T, Riccieri V et al. Interleukin 13 in synovial fluid and serum of patients with psoriatic arthritis. *Ann Rheum Dis* 2002; **61**(2): 174–6.

123. Yilmaz M, Kendirli SG, Altintas D et al. Cytokine levels in serum of patients with juvenile rheumatoid arthritis. *Clin Rheumatol* 2001; **20**(1): 30–5.

124. Scola MP, Thompson SD, Brunner HI et al. Interferon-gamma: interleukin 4 ratios and associated type 1 cytokine expression in juvenile rheumatoid arthritis synovial tissue. *J Rheumatol* 2002; **29**(2): 369–78.

125. Ribbens C, Andre B, Kaye O et al. Increased synovial fluid levels of interleukin-12, sCD25 and sTNF- RII/sTNF-RI ratio delineate a cytokine pattern characteristic of immune arthropathies. *Eur Cytokine Netw* 2000; **11**(4): 669–76.

126. Miyata M, Ohira H, Sasajima T et al. Significance of low mRNA levels of interleukin-4 and -10 in mononuclear cells of the synovial fluid of patients with rheumatoid arthritis. *Clin Rheumatol* 2000; **19**(5): 365–70.

127. Morita Y, Yang J, Gupta R et al. Dendritic cells genetically engineered to express IL-4 inhibit murine collagen-induced arthritis. *J Clin Invest* 2001; **107**(10): 1275–84.

128. Kotake S, Schumacher HR, Jr, Yarboro CH et al. In vivo gene expression of type 1 and type 2 cytokines in synovial tissues from patients in early stages of rheumatoid, reactive, and undifferentiated arthritis. *Proc Assoc Am Physicians* 1997; **109**(3): 286–301.

129. Peeva E, Fishman AD, Goddard G et al. Rheumatoid arthritis exacerbation caused by exogenous interleukin-12. *Arthritis Rheum* 2000; **43**(2): 461–3.

130. Gattorno M, Picco P, Vignola S et al. Serum interleukin 12 concentration in juvenile chronic arthritis. *Ann Rheum Dis* 1998; **57**(7): 425–8.

131. Gracie JA, Forsey RJ, Chan WL et al. A proinflammatory role for IL-18 in rheumatoid arthritis. *J Clin Invest* 1999; **104**(10): 1393–401.

132. Yamamura M, Kawashima M, Taniai M et al. Interferon-gamma-inducing activity of interleukin-18 in the joint with rheumatoid arthritis. *Arthritis Rheum* 2001; **44**(2): 275–85.

133. Tanaka M, Harigai M, Kawaguchi Y et al. Mature form of interleukin 18 is expressed in rheumatoid arthritis synovial tissue and contributes to interferon-gamma production by synovial T cells. *J Rheumatol* 2001; **28**(8): 1779–87.

134. Yin Z, Braun J, Neure L et al. Crucial role of interleukin-10/interleukin-12 balance in the regulation of the type 2 T helper cytokine response in reactive arthritis. *Arthritis Rheum* 1997; **40**(10): 1788–97.

135. Monteleone G, Biancone L, Marasco R et al. Interleukin 12 is expressed and actively released by Crohn's disease intestinal lamina propria mononuclear cells. *Gastroenterology* 1997; **112**(4): 1169–78.

136. Camoglio L, Te Velde AA, Tigges AJ et al. Altered expression of interferon-gamma and interleukin-4 in inflammatory bowel disease. *Inflamm Bowel Dis* 1998; **4**(4): 285–90.

137. Fuss IJ, Neurath M, Boirivant M et al. Disparate CD4⁺ lamina propria (LP) lymphokine secretion profiles in inflammatory bowel disease. Crohn's disease LP cells manifest increased secretion of IFN-gamma, whereas ulcerative colitis LP cells manifest increased secretion of IL-5. *J Immunol* 1996; **157**(3): 1261–70.

138. Strober W, Fuss IJ, Blumberg RS. The immunology of mucosal models of inflammation. *Ann Rev Immunol* 2002; **20**: 495–549.

139. Neurath MF, Fuss I, Kelsall BL et al. Antibodies to interleukin 12 abrogate established experimental colitis in mice. *J Exp Med* 1995; **182**(5): 1281–90.

140. Boirivant M, Fuss IJ, Chu A, Strober W. Oxazolone colitis: a murine model of T helper cell type 2 colitis treatable with antibodies to interleukin 4. *J Exp Med* 1998; **188**(10): 1929–39.

141. Spencer DM, Veldman GM, Banerjee S et al. Distinct inflammatory mechanisms mediate early versus late colitis in mice. *Gastroenterology* 2002; **122**(1): 94–105.

142. Fuss IJ, Marth T, Neurath MF et al. Anti-interleukin 12 treatment regulates apoptosis of Th1 T cells in experimental colitis in mice. *Gastroenterology* 1999; **117**(5): 1078–88.

143. Malmstrom V, Shipton D, Singh B et al. CD134L expression on dendritic cells in the mesenteric lymph nodes drives colitis in T cell-restored SCID mice. *J Immunol* 2001; **166**(11): 6972–81.

144. Hong K, Berg EL, Ehrhardt RO. Persistence of pathogenic CD4⁺ Th1-like cells in vivo in the absence of IL-12 but in the presence of autoantigen. *J Immunol* 2001; **166**(7): 4765–72.

145. Kontoyiannis D, Pasparakis M, Pizarro TT et al. Impaired on/off regulation of TNF biosynthesis in mice lacking TNF AU-rich elements: implications for joint and gut-associated immunopathologies. *Immunity* 1999; **10**(3): 387–98.

146. van Deventer SJ. Small therapeutic molecules for the treatment of inflammatory bowel disease. *Gut* 2002; **50**(Suppl 3): III47–53.

147. Braun MC, Kelsall BL. Regulation of interleukin-12 production by G-protein-coupled receptors. *Microbes Infect* 2001; **3**(2): 99–107.

148. Shull MM, Ormsby I, Kier AB et al. Targeted disruption of the mouse transforming growth factor-beta 1 gene results in multifocal inflammatory disease. *Nature* 1992; **359**(6397): 693–9.

149. Kitani A, Fuss IJ, Nakamura K et al. Treatment of experimental (trinitrobenzene sulfonic acid) colitis by intranasal administration of transforming growth factor (TGF)-beta1 plasmid: TGF-beta1-mediated suppression of T helper cell type 1 response occurs by interleukin (IL)-10 induction and IL-12 receptor beta2 chain downregulation. *J Exp Med* 2000; **192**(1): 41–52.

15

Interleukin-15

Iain B McInnes and Foo Y Liew

Introduction • Interleukin-15 – molecule, receptor and function • IL-15 in immune-mediated pathology • IL-15 expression beyond inflammatory synovitis • Conclusions • Acknowledgments • References

INTRODUCTION

There is considerable interest in understanding those mechanisms whereby innate and acquired immune responses interact in the context of chronic inflammation. In rheumatoid arthritis (RA) patients, the synovial membrane exhibits features suggesting that components of both compartments of the immune response are of functional importance.[1,2] Most cytokines present within synovium are of macrophage and synovial fibroblast derivation.[3,4] In particular, interleukin-15 (IL-15) is a cytokine with quaternary structural similarities to IL-2,[5,6] that is produced primarily by macrophages. We have recently focused upon the activities of IL-15, which is characteristically expressed during the early stages of innate immune responses. We have explored the hypothesis that IL-15 expression in the synovial membrane can promote and sustain T-cell responses that in turn contribute directly to tumor necrosis factor alpha (TNF-α) production. Recent data suggest that relevant bioactivities of IL-15 extend beyond this to include neutrophil, natural killer (NK) cell, macrophage and dendritic cell activation. In this chapter, we will review evidence which indicates that IL-15 represents an intriguing therapeutic target.

INTERLEUKIN-15 – MOLECULE, RECEPTOR AND FUNCTION

Biology of IL-15 and its receptor

IL-15 mRNA is broadly expressed throughout numerous normal human tissues and cell types, including activated monocytes, dendritic cells and fibroblasts[5,7] (Table 15.1). IL-15 mRNA expression, however, is not synonymous with protein detection in tissues, reflecting tight regulatory control of translation and secretion.[8] IL-15 is subject to significant post-transcriptional regulation. IL-15 mRNA 5'-untranslated region (UTR) contains 12 AUG triplets that significantly reduce the efficiency of translation. Deletion of this AUG-rich 5-UTR sequence in the HuT-102 cell line permits significant constitutive IL-15 secretion.[9] Similarly, replacement of the 48 amino acid signal peptide with that of IL-2 or CD33 induces significantly higher levels of IL-15 production in transfected cells.[8,10] A third regulatory element in the C-terminal region has also been proposed, since FLAG fusion proteins exhibit higher levels of secretion than native constructs.[7,8] Two isoforms of IL-15 are generated through this process. Secreted IL-15 is derived from a long signalling peptide (LSP) containing a 48 amino acid leader sequence,

Table 15.1   Expression of IL-15 in tissues.

Cell types in which IL-15 identified

Macrophage/monocyte
Dendritic cells
T lymphocytes
Bone marrow stromal cells – primary culture/lines
Thymic epithelium
Epithelial tissues
  Fetal intestine
  Kidney
  Keratinocytes
  Fetal skin
  Retinal pigment
Renal proximal tubule cells
Fibroblasts
Chondrocytes
Astrocytes

whereas a second isoform which contains a short signalling peptide (SSP) of 21 amino acids is retained within the cell and has been localized to non-endoplasmic regions in both cytoplasmic and nuclear compartments.[10–14] Altered glycosylation of the IL-15 48 amino acid isoform may further regulate intracellular trafficking.[7] Ultimately, cell membrane expression may be crucial in mediating extracellular function rather than secretion (see below). The physiological implications of this regulatory structure are still unclear.

Factors that drive endogenous IL-15 release are as yet poorly understood. The IL-15 promoter contains a variety of transcription sites in its 5' regulatory region that are typical of many proinflammatory cytokines, including NFκB, NF-IL-6, GC-binding factor (GCF), interferon regulatory factor-E (IRF-E) and interferon response element (γ-IRE).[7,15,16] However, to establish consistent IL-15 secretion in vitro has proven difficult in most systems thus far investi-

gated. Factors demonstrated thus far to induce IL-15 secretion by human cells are diverse and include human herpesvirus 6 and 7, *Mycobacterium leprae*, *Mycobacterium tuberculosis*, *Staphylococcus aureus*, lipopolysaccharide and ultraviolet irradiation.[17–22]

IL-15 binds a specific heterotrimeric receptor (IL-15R) that is widely distributed and which consists of a β-chain (shared with IL-2) and the common γ-chain, together with a unique α-chain (IL-15α). IL-15Rα is alternatively spliced to yield eight isoforms; those that lack exon 2 are unable to bind IL-15.[5–7,23–26] Intriguingly, IL-15Rα (probably via an exon 2 coding region) and SSP-IL-15 localize to the nuclear membrane/nucleus; the functional implications of this are as yet unknown. The IL-15Rαβγ complex signals through JAK1/3 and STAT3/5.[7,25,27] Additional signalling through *src*-related tyrosine kinases and Ras/Raf/MAPK to fos/jun activation is also proposed. Whether IL-15Rα in the absence βγ-chain expression transduces signal is unclear. The cytoplasmic tail of IL-15Rα contains regions homologous to TRAF2-binding domains, analogous to CD40, and may compete with TNFRI for TRAF2 binding.[28] Irrespective of signalling potential, the high affinity (10^{11} M^{-1}) and slow off-rate of IL-15Rα in soluble form provides for a useful and specific inhibitor in biological systems.

Bioactivities of IL-15

Commensurate with the broad expression of IL-15R, diverse proinflammatory activities have been attributed to IL-15 (Table 15.2). Key effects are discussed below.

T cells

T cells upregulate IL-15Rα as an early feature of activation. IL-15 induces proliferation of mitogen-activated CD4+ and CD8+ T cells, T-cell clones and γδ T cells, with release of soluble IL-2Rα, and enhances cytotoxicity in both CD8+ T cells and lymphokine-activated killer cells.[5,6,29–31] Induction of numerous membrane activation markers, including CD69, FasL, CD40L, TNFRII and CD25, has been observed,[32,33] primarily on CD45RO+ but not CD45RA+ T-cell subsets.[32] IL-

Table 15.2 Biological effects of IL-15.

Cell type	Key effects
T lymphocyte	Activation/proliferation
	Cytokine production Th/c1 and Th/c2
	Cytotoxicity
	Chemokinesis
	Cytoskeletal rearrangement
	Adhesion molecule expression
	Reduced apoptosis
B lymphocyte	Ig production
	Proliferation
NK cell	Cytotoxicity
	Cytokine production
	Reduced apoptosis
	Lineage development
Macrophage	Dose-dependent effect on activation
	Membrane expression – ?costimulation
Osteoclast	Maturation
	Calcitonin receptor
Dendritic cell	Maturation
	Activation
Neutrophil	Activation
	Cytoskeletal rearrangement
	Cytokine release
	Reduced apoptosis

15 exhibits T-cell chemokinetic activity[34,35] and induces adhesion molecule (e.g. intercellular adhesion molecule (ICAM)-3) redistribution.[36] It further induces chemokine (CC-, CXC- and C-type) and chemokine receptor (CC but not CXC) expression on T cells.[37] Thus, IL-15 can recruit T cells and, thereafter, modify homo- or heterotypic cell–cell interactions within inflammatory sites.

IL-15 is generally considered to favour differentiation of type 1 responses. IL-15 primes naive CD4+ T cells from T-cell receptor (TCR)-transgenic mice for subsequent interferon gamma (IFN-γ) expression, but not IL-4 production.[38] Antigen-specific responses in T cells from human immunodeficiency virus (HIV)-infected patients in the presence of high-dose IL-15 exhibit increased IFN-γ production.[39] Similarly, IL-15 induces IFN-γ/IL-4 ratios which favour Th1 dominance in mitogen-stimulated human T cells.[40] However, IL-15 induces IL-5 production from allergen-specific human T-cell clones, implying a positive role in Th2-mediated allergic responses.[41] Moreover, administration of soluble IL-15-IgG2b fusion protein in murine hypersensitivity models clearly implicates IL-15 in Th2 lesion development.[42] In contrast, IL-15 expression in type 2-associated atopic dermatitis patients was significantly lower than that in normal or psoriasis patients.[43] Formal analysis of functional T-cell maturation in IL-15- and IL-15R-targeted mice will be informative.

A prominent role in T-cell memory is emerging. IL-15 induces CD8+ T-cell expansion in vivo.[44] IL-15Rα-deficient mice exhibit lymphopenia due to reduced proliferation and homing of mature lymphocytes, particularly of the CD8+ subset. A key role in the development of several cell lineages, such as NK cells, of the innate immune response was also confirmed.[45] Similar abnormalities are observed in IL-15-deficient mice.[46] T-cell-independent hematopoietic IL-15Rα signals are vital for poly-I:C-induced bystander responses in CD8+ T cells, further suggesting a vital role in maintaining memory responses.[47] Studies in IL-15-transgenic mice infected with *Listeria monocytogenes* further support a role for IL-15 in generating long-term antigen-specific memory in the CD8+ compartment.[48] Recent reports have extended these observations to include CD4+ T cells,[49,50] suggesting that such effects may have broader consequences.

NK cells

IL-15 plays a fundamental role in thymic development of T-cell and, particularly, NK cell lineages. Thus, IL-15, IL-15Rα, IL-15Rβ, IRF-1 and JAK3 gene targeted mouse strains all exhibit either deficiency or absence of NK cell development and function. IL-15 induces NK cell activation, measured by direct cytotoxicity, by antibody-dependent cellular cytotoxicity, or by production of cytokines.[20,51–53] IL-15 acts as an NK cell survival factor in vivo by maintaining Bcl-2 expression.[54–57] It has recently been directly implicated in promoting NK cell-mediated shock in mice.[58] The effects of IL-15 in the NK cell compartment have recently been comprehensively reviewed.[59]

Macrophages
Macrophages bind IL-15 with high affinity via expression of IL-15Rα/β/γ. IL-15 may function as an autocrine regulator of macrophage activation, such that low levels of IL-15 suppress whereas higher levels enhance proinflammatory monokine production.[60] The latter includes TNF-α, IL-1 and IL-6, together with the chemokines IL-8 and membrane cofactor protein-7 (MCP-1).[60,61] Moreover, since human macrophages constitutively express bioactive membrane-bound IL-15, such autocrine effects are probably of early importance during macrophage activation.[61] Lipopolysacharide (LPS) or granulocyte–macrophage colony-stimulating factor (GM-CSF) rapidly induce translocation of preformed IL-15 to the plasma membrane of blood-derived CD14+ macrophages, where it is able to sustain T-cell proliferation.[62] This membrane expression may represent a major effector pathway for IL-15. Thus, IL-15–LSP that is secreted only at low levels is more efficient in viral host defence than is IL-15 engineered to be secreted at high levels.[63]

Dendritic cells
IL-15, together with GM-CSF, has recently been shown to support the maturation of monocytes into dendritic cells (DCs) (CD1a+, DR+, CD14-) that could be further matured by LPS, TNF-α or CD-40L into CD83+, DC-LAMP+ cells.[64] A proportion of these cells expressed E-cadherin and CCR6, reminiscent of Langerhans cells. Moreover, DCs from common γ-chain-deficient

mice exhibit reduced IL-12 and NO release that was shown in IL-15-deficient mice to be dependent primarily upon IL-15.[65] Together, these data suggest that IL-15 may operate at an early stage to promote DC maturation and functional activation.

Neutrophils
Neutrophils expressing IL-15Rα and IL-15 can induce neutrophil activation and cytoskeletal rearrangement.[66,67] Thus, IL-15 enhances neutrophil phagocytosis, increases de novo protein mRNA and protein synthesis (e.g. cytokines and chemokines) and resists progression of apoptosis. These effects have functional relevance, since growth inhibition of *Candida albicans* is enhanced.

Osteoclasts
Addition of IL-15 to rat bone marrow cultures induces osteoclast development and upregulates calcitonin receptor expression.[68]

IL-15 and its receptor are expressed on a wide range of haemopoietic and non-haemopoietic cell types. IL-15 thus provides a pathway whereby host tissues can contribute to the early phase of immune responses, providing enhancement of polymorphonuclear and NK cell responses, and subsequently T-cell responses. Such activity may facilitate chronic, rather than self-limiting, inflammation should IL-15 synthesis be dysregulated.

IL-15 IN IMMUNE-MEDIATED PATHOLOGY

IL-15 expression in inflammatory arthritis

The pleiotropic effects of IL-15 documented above clearly render it a candidate cytokine in the pathogenesis of inflammatory arthritis. IL-15 mRNA and protein have now been detected in RA synovial membrane by a number of investigators. IL-15 mRNA levels are higher in RA than in reactive arthritis synovial biopsies.[69] Although cautious interpretation of mRNA data is required, it is of interest that levels are higher in patients prior to commencement of immune suppressive therapy.[69] Several ELISAs are now available, all of which detect IL-15 in around 60% of RA, but not osteoarthritis, synovial fluids (SF). Levels correlate directly with TNF-α and remain constant after removal of rheumatoid factor, which probably interfered with earlier efforts to quantify IL-15, leading to overestimation of the concentrations present. Concentrations present are similar to levels of TNF-α or IL-12 detected in parallel assays,[70] but are lower than those of other monokines, e.g. IL-6 and IL-18. These observations have recently been confirmed.[71–74] Lower or absent levels have also been reported, perhaps reflecting the assay systems employed or the presence of inhibitory factors within SF that can interfere with IL-15 detection. IL-15 has also been measured in RA SF using soluble IL-15Rα chain in a novel receptor capture assay,[70] in which IL-15 levels in RA SF correlate closely with those detected by ELISA. Moreover, recombinant soluble IL-15Rα interferes with the detection of IL-15 by ELISA (J. A. Gracie, unpublished observations). Finally, we recently detected IL-15 in SF derived from patients with psoriatic arthritis (H. Wilson, J. A. Gracie and I. B. McInnes, unpublished observations), suggesting that IL-15 may be present in a broad range of inflammatory arthropathies.

Low levels of IL-15 are also present in sera of up to 40% of RA patients, although variable levels have been reported in distinct populations.[75–78] Serum IL-15 expression does not apparently correlate with the disease subsets thus far recognized. Whereas RA serum TNF-α levels correlate with the presence of germinal centres in parallel synovial biopsies, IL-15 levels were elevated in patents in whom either germinal centres or diffuse lymphocytic infiltrative patterns were observed.[76] IL-15 has also been detected in rheumatoid pleural effusions.[79]

IL-15 expression in inflamed synovium is found in lining-layer macrophages, together with synovial fibroblasts and endothelial cells.[80–82] Whether synovial T cells also express IL-15 remains unclear;[81] low-level IL-15 expression in peripheral blood T cells is now recognized, and IL-15 itself was originally cloned from a T-cell lymphoma line. The distribution of IL-15 is similar in psoriatic arthritis (PsA) and reactive arthritis (ReA) synovial membranes, but expression is at reduced levels as compared to RA.[81,83] Of interest, both PsA and ReA synovium contain IL-2, with which IL-15 may exhibit counter-regulatory activities. IL-15 expression has also recently been detected in synovial membrane derived from juvenile RA patients,[84] associated with IL-18, IL-12 and IFN-γ expression.

IL-15 expression in synovial tissues in vitro

Spontaneous production of IL-15 by primary RA synovial membrane cultures and by isolated synovial fibroblasts has been reported.[71,85] Such release is sensitive to the cyclosporin (and FK-506) tractable pathway operating through cAMP.[85] In similar studies, we have observed upregulation of IL-15 mRNA and intracellular IL-15 protein expression in purified synovial fibroblasts, although we have been unable to consistently detect IL-15 secretion thus far. In long-term cultures of mixed synovial tissues, outgrowth of tissues was found to be dependent upon the presence of T cells, which in turn lead to local release of IL-15, IL-17 and fibroblast growth factor-1 (FGF-1).[86] Nevertheless, it has proven difficult to consistently achieve IL-15 secretion in in vitro systems, and studies characterizing the regulation of intracellular processing events leading to IL-15–LSP production in synovial membrane are urgently required, as is formal comparison of LSP and SSP isoform expression.[7]

Factors that in turn drive synovial IL-15 expression are unclear (Figure 15.1). We have recently found that activated T cells can induce IL-15 expression in macrophages via cognate interactions (see below). Exposure of synovial fibroblasts to TNF-α or IL-1β also induces high levels of IL-15 expression, although we have rarely detected this in secreted form. Recent studies in dermal fibroblasts similarly demonstrated that TNF-α but not IFN-γ induces membrane expression of IL-15, which in turn can sustain T-cell growth.[87] A further pathway promoting IL-15 production has been suggested in studies of synovial embryonic growth factor expression. Overexpression of the wingless

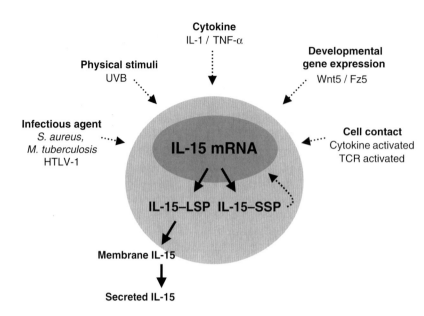

Figure 15.1 Various stimuli increase expression of IL-15 mRNA, which is the dominant species since translation is tightly regulated (see text). Protein expression is in two forms – IL-15 long signalling peptide (IL-15–LSP) and IL-15 short signalling peptide (IL-15–SSP) which traffic in distinct pathways within the cell. Membrane IL-15 expression is reported primarily on macrophages, where it probably has functional activity. Secreted IL-15 is found in only a limited set of culture conditions, usually in primary cultures from cells activated in vivo, e.g. RA synovial tissues.

(*Wnt5*) and frizzled (*Fz5*) ligand pair is associated with increased production and secretion of IL-15 by RA synovial fibroblasts, together with IL-6 and IL-8.[88] Furthermore, suppression of *Wnt5* or *Fz5* using antisense, dominant negative mutants or neutralizing antibodies led to a reduction in IL-15 expression.[89] Thus a variety of stimuli including cellular feedback loops, may promote IL-15 release in synovium (Figure 15.1).

Bioactivities of IL-15 in inflammatory arthritis

The biological effects of IL-15 previously elucidated (Table 15.2) suggest numerous potential pathological effects in RA. Data will be discussed that indicate an important role for IL-15, in synergy with other locally expressed cytokines such as IL-12 and IL-18, in recruitment and activation of synovial T cells, which in turn promote macrophage cytokine release, primarily via cell contact-dependent interactions. An important consequence of these studies has been to establish the central importance of synovial T cells in promoting chronic inflammation in the joint, via persistent macrophage activation and TNF-α release.

Promotion of synovial T-cell effector function
TNF-α blockade is effective in ameliorating clinical signs and symptoms of RA and in reducing radiographic progression, suggesting true disease-modifying effects.[90,91] There is now considerable interest in identifying mechanisms that in turn drive TNF-α production.[92] Histological studies suggest that TNF-α in synovial membrane is predominantly macrophage derived.[93,94] Data consistent with a central role for T cells in driving such TNF-α expression have recently been provided in vivo and in vitro. Anti-CD2-mediated T-cell depletion in synovial grafts in NOD-SCID mice leads to suppression of TNF-α and IL-15 levels and to matrix metalloproteinase (MMP) expression.[95] Similarly, T-cell depletion from primary RA synovial cultures reduces the capacity for TNF-α release.[96] A critical observation has been that cytokines within the synovium can sustain this T-cell-dependent process.

Whereas IL-15 can mediate direct effects on macrophages,[60] we hypothesized that IL-15 is more likely to drive cognate interactions between T cells and macrophages, which clearly lie in juxtaposition within RA synovial membrane. Using IL-1/IL-1Ra release in

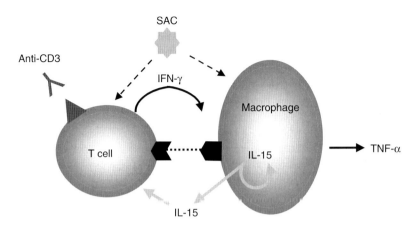

SAC

Anti-CD3

IFN-γ

Macrophage

T cell

IL-15

TNF-α

IL-15

Figure 15.2 IL-15 neutralization with soluble IL-15Rα suppresses TNF-α release by human macrophages following interaction with T cells activated by anti-CD3/anti-CD28, by cytokine (IL-15 itself) or by mitogen (PHA/PMA [phytohemagglutin/phorbol myristate acetate]). Direct macrophage stimulation with IFN-γ and *S. aureus* Cowan (SAC) also induces TNF-α release that is reduced by addition of sIL-15Rα.

macrophages, Isler et al first showed that T cell–macrophage contact could favour pro- versus anti-inflammatory cytokine expression.[97] Thus, mitogen-activated T cells and T-cell clones induce proinflammatory cytokine production by macrophages and synovial fibroblasts.[98–100]. Neutralization studies implicate at least CD69, CD40L/CD40 and LFA-1/ICAM-1 ligand pairs in T cell–macrophage activation and membrane cytokines in T-cell–fibroblast interactions.[98,101] Addition of IL-15 to RA synovial membrane cultures induces TNF-α secretion, which is localized by intracellular fluorescence-activated cell sorting (FACS) analysis primarily in macrophages (J. A. Gracie and I. B. McInnes, unpublished data). We demonstrated that freshly isolated synovial fluid T cells can induce TNF-α synthesis by blood- or synovial-derived macrophages through cell membrane contact, with no requirement for secretory factor synthesis.[98] This activity is maintained in vitro by addition of IL-15 alone, although combinations of cytokines including IL-15, IL-2, IL-6 and TNF-α may be more effective.[101] This was consistent with prior studies demonstrating antigen-independent, cytokine-mediated bystander activation of human CD4+ memory T cells.[102] This capacity for contact-induced macrophage activation has recently been demonstrated in synovial membrane-derived T cells.[96] Importantly, synovial T cells induce signalling events

in target macrophages that are identical to those induced by cytokine-activated T cells, but distinct from those induced by conventionally activated T cells (via anti-CD3/C28). These data suggest that cytokine-mediated activation may predominate in RA synovial tissues to promote effector function.[96]

We recently demonstrated that IL-15-activated T cells induce synovial macrophages to release IL-15 in vitro via cell contact, and that addition to these cultures of soluble IL-15Rα significantly suppresses TNF-α release (Gracie et al, unpublished observations). These data suggest that T-cell–macrophage interactions could themselves induce IL-15 release and that TNF-α production is sensitive to such IL-15 expression (Figure 15.2). Moreover, IL-15 neutralization reduced TNF-α release after a variety of stimuli, including *S. aureus* and anti-CD3/anti-CD28 (Figure 15.2). Similarly, IFN-γ production in T-cell–monocyte co-cultures is suppressed by IL-15 neutralization, indicating cooperative activity of IL-12 and IL-15 through effects on IL-12Rβ1 expression, enhanced CD40 expression and direct effects on CD4+ T-cell cytokine production.[103] It is of interest that secreted IL-15 was not detected in such cultures, indicating that functionally active membrane IL-15 may be involved. Complex networks involving secreted and cognate pathways are therefore predicted in which cytokine secretion and adhesion molecule expression interact to sustain chronic macrophage activation.[104] IL-15 apparently operates as a critical factor in these pathways.

Direct effects on T-cell function

IL-15 can promote secretory activity in synovial T cells. Purified SF, but not peripheral blood (PB) T lymphocytes, produce cytokines in vitro in response to IL-15, including TNF-α together with IFN-γ and IL-10, suggesting that direct effects of IL-15 on T cells may contribute to synovial cytokine production. IL-15 induces high levels of IL-17 release. IL-17 is a recently described Th1-associated cytokine that is expressed in RA synovial tissues.[105] IL-17 overexpression induces erosive disease, whereas neutralization suppresses inflammatory parameters in vivo.[106] IL-17 induces fibroblast activation and, via modulation of receptor activator of nuclear factor kappaB ligand (RANKL) expression, provides a link to bone resorption. Together with its capacity to activate osteoclast activation, this suggests that IL-15 targeting could suppress articular destructive pathways. Commensurate with this, elevated IL-15 mRNA expression at the cartilage pannus junction in RA and PsA patients has recently been observed (D. Kane, personal communication). It is of interest that IL-15, but not IL-2, is also expressed in implant interface tissues obtained following revision of failed arthroplasty,[107] in macrophages, multinucleated giant cells and endothelial cells. In these studies, IL-15 expression was upregulated in U937 cells by retrieved metal particles, providing a direct link between initiating agent and an IL-15-mediated pathology that is locally erosive. Finally, we recently detected Toll-like receptor (TLR) 2 expression in inflammatory synovitis (H. Wilson H, J. A. Gracie and I. B. McInnes, unpublished observations). IL-15 upregulates TLR2 expression on T cells, providing an important link to innate response recognition pathways.[108] Since bacterial peptidoglycans that are present in synovial tissues[109] represent a critical TLR2 ligand, this provides a further mechanism whereby IL-15 could promote synovial inflammation.

T-cell recruitment

Many chemokine activities have been detected in RA synovial membrane.[110,111] Antibody neutralization studies indicate that IL-15 represents part of this chemokinetic activity, in combination with at least IL-8, MCP-1 and MIP-1α (MIP, macrophage inflammatory protein).[35,80] That IL-15 also upregulates chemokine receptors may be of prime importance. For example, IL-15-mediated CXCR4 expression promotes stromal-derived factor-1 (SDF-1)-induced synovial T-cell migration.[112] IL-15 simultaneously upregulates CD69 and leukocyte function-associated antigen-1 (LFA-1)[98,99] and induces redistribution of adhesion molecules, including ICAMs 1–3, CD43 and CD44, to uropods to further facilitate migration.[36] Injection of IL-15 into the footpad of either *Corynebacterium parvum* primed or type II collagen-primed mice induces a sustained local inflammatory infiltrate, consisting primarily of CD3+ lymphocytes, associated with local lymphadenopathy, indicating that such in vitro observations are probably of in vivo relevance.[80] Subsequent studies have demonstrated IL-15 expression on synovial endothelial cells, where it mediates activated, memory T-cell migration into synovial membrane tissues transplanted into SCID mice.[82] Conversely, IL-15 may feed-back on endothelial cells, since IL-15 upregulates endothelial cell hyaluronan expression and promotes intraperitoneal migration of T cells through a CD44-dependent pathway.[113]

T-cell survival in situ

Numerous pathways provide for longevity of T cells in the synovial compartment including interactions with the extracellular matrix and adjacent inflammatory leukocyte populations. Signalling studies indicate that the predominant pathways that account for rescue from apoptosis in RA SF seem independent of IL-15 signalling,[114] but rather reflect the activities of type I interferons. Thus, although IL-15 retards apoptosis in vivo and in vitro in T and B lymphocytes induced by cytokine withdrawal, by anti-Fas or anti-antigen receptor antibody or by dexamethasone,[7,114,115] this property is not

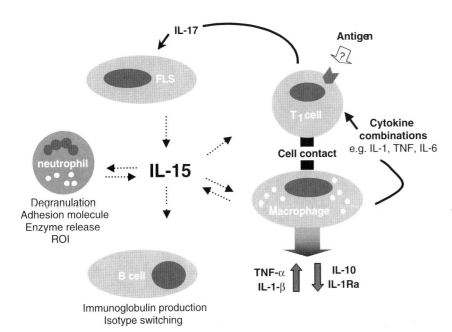

Figure 15.3 Data support a role for IL-15 in synovial inflammation through T-cell–macrophage interactions, T-cell cytokine release (IL-17), direct effects on neutrophil activation, and fibroblast activation. Synergy with other proinflammatory cytokines, including IL-12 and IL-18, is necessary for optimal responses. Potential effects on dendritic cells and endothelial cell function remain to be explored. FLS, fibroblast-like synoviocytes; ROI, reactive oxygen intermediates.

prominent in RA. This may reflect complex pro- and anti-inflammatory cytokine networks in SF, or simply illustrate that IL-15 present in SF (low picogram range[70]) is quantitatively less important than interferon (low nanogram range[114]).

Activation of other inflammatory synovial cells

Neutrophils can be activated by IL-15.[66,67] Moreover, in studies investigating chemokine, cytokine and CD11b expression and f-MLP-induced chemiluminescence (MLP, N-formyl-methionyl-leucyl-phenylalanine), enhanced responsiveness to IL-15 is detected in RA compared with normal control-derived neutrophils.[116] Neutrophil activation directly by RA SF may be partially ameliorated by addition of anti-IL-15 antibodies, providing further evidence that bioactive IL-15 is present in SF. Whereas the role of NK cells in RA synovitis remains poorly understood, the potent effect of IL-15 on NK cell biology indicates that this is also a plausible synovial target for IL-15.[59] We have previously demonstrated that IL-15 can promote granzyme A and B release in synovial cultures.[117] Detailed analysis of synovial NK cell activation by IL-15 is awaited.

In summary, IL-15 has now been shown to mediate a variety of proinflammatory activities in the context of synovial inflammation. These are summarized in Figure 15.3.

Synergy with other proinflammatory cytokines

It is now clear that IL-15 mediates many biological functions intracellularly or in paracrine loops through membrane-bound expression.[7,12,14,61] Accordingly, absolute levels detected in biological solutions, including SF and culture supernatants, may underestimate its net contribution. Consistent with this, IL-15 blockade in vitro and in vivo by specific moieties modulates inflammatory models in which detection of significant IL-15 levels has proven elusive. Nevertheless, there have been suggestions that since the absolute concentrations of secreted IL-15 detected are often low, there may not be sufficient IL-15 to sustain independent activity. Several recent studies indicating that IL-15, even at very low concentrations, possesses potent activities when operating in synergy with other innate response cytokines such as IL-12 and IL-18 provide a robust response to this criticism.

IL-18 is a recently described member of the IL-1 cytokine family that is highly expressed in RA synovial membrane.[118] In synergy with IL-15, IL-18 can promote synovial macrophage activation either directly, via IFN-γ/IL-17 release, or via enhancement of T-cell cognate interactions (see Figure 15.3).[119] Similar synergistic effects of IL-15 have been observed with IL-12.[118] We have observed that in the presence of IL-12, ambient IL-15 down to 1 pg/ml can promote synovial TNF-α release in vitro. IL-6 and TNF-α may similarly contribute directly to cytokine-mediated 'bystander' T-cell activation in combination with IL-15.[101] We therefore hypothesize that amplification of synovial inflammation by T cells is driven synergistically by combinations of cytokines. Cytokine-mediated non-specific activation of T cells is increasingly recognized to be of importance in several immune activities, particularly memory compartment maintenance.[47] Polyclonal T-cell activation follows injection of type I IFN or IL-15 in vivo in mice, and resting human CD4+ T cells can be activated to produce cytokines and provide B-cell help in vitro by a combination of IL-2, IL-1β and TNF-α.[102,120] Moreover, soluble cytokines further modify the effects of cognate interactions with target cells. GM-CSF enhances cytokine-activated, T-cell-induced TNF-α synthesis by blood-derived monocytes, whereas IL-10 is inhibitory.[101] By this means, the cooperative action of soluble or cell-bound cytokine products of cognate interactions may feed back to 'fine-tune' macrophage activation. T-cell-mediated inflammation need not therefore be perpetuated primarily by local recognition of antigen. (It should be noted, however, that these pathways are compatible with parallel 'arthritogen'-specific responses.)

Strategies to target IL-15 in vivo

The functional activities of IL-15 and its demonstrable effects in synovial inflammation clearly indicate that effective neutralization could confer significant benefits in RA. However, the complexities of IL-15 physiology pose considerable difficulties in determining what should be the optimal therapeutic strategy. Thus far, three approaches have been considered, namely, neutralizing antibodies (none reported thus far), soluble IL-15Rα and mutated IL-15 species, usually generated as fusion proteins. Several studies utilizing these diverse approaches have been attempted, or are currently ongoing.

Administration of IL-15 during priming with type II collagen in incomplete Freund's adjuvant induces development of an erosive inflammatory arthritis in DBA/1 mice. Co-administration of IL-12 or IL-18 synergistically enhances onset of arthritis, suggesting that combinations of 'innate' cytokines can promote onset of erosive inflammatory arthritis (B. P. Leung, unpublished observations). We have used full-length soluble IL-15Rα administration to manipulate IL-15 bioactivities in vivo. When sIL-15Rα is injected daily following antigen challenge, the development of collagen-induced arthritis (CIA) is suppressed, associated with delayed development of anti-collagen-specific antibodies (IgG$_{2a}$) and with reduced antigen-specific IFN-γ and TNF-α production in vitro.[121] On discontinuation of sIL-15Rα administration, CIA developed to levels comparable with controls, suggesting that the anti-inflammatory effects are transient. In subsequent studies, we have generated targeted mutants of IL-15Rα and identified the sushi domain as essential for functional cytokine neutralization.[122] Selected deletion of cysteine residues similarly disrupted folding to abrogate binding and function. Studies are ongoing to determine whether small molecule derivatives of sIL-15Rα are of therapeutic utility in the CIA model. This also provides opportunities to investigate the potential for dual targeting of synergistic cytokine activities, e.g. IL-15 and IL-18.

An alternative approach has been to generate mutant IL-15 forms that can specifically modify IL-15 activities. An IL-15/Fcγ2a fusion protein that antagonizes the activities of IL-15 in vitro, suppresses the onset of delayed-type hypersensitivity (DTH) responses in vivo, associated with reduction in CD4+ T-cell infiltration.[122] This fusion protein has also proven effective in vivo in preventing rejection of murine islet cell allografts in combination with CTLA4/Fc.[124] Studies in CIA are ongoing at this time.

IL-15 EXPRESSION BEYOND INFLAMMATORY SYNOVITIS

IL-15 expression in the context of immune-mediated pathology has now been reported in several disease states. Elevated serum concentrations of IL-15 are reported in several rheumatic diseases, including systemic lupus erythematosis,[75] and inflammatory myositis. IL-15 mRNA and protein levels are also elevated in peripheral blood mononuclear cells and in inflamed colon from ulcerative colitis (UC) and, to a lesser extent, Crohn's disease (CD) patients.[125] Within colonic lesions, IL-15 is expressed not only in macrophages but also in intestinal epithelial cells, upon which IL-15 exerts autocrine effects.[126] Intraepithelial lymphocytes exhibit enhanced proliferative, cytotoxic and cytokine secretory responses to IL-15, compared with IL-2. We recently observed elevated secretion of IL-15 from explant cultures of colonic tissues from UC but not CD patients, and found that such IL-15 production correlated with spontaneous TNF-α release. Elevated serum IL-15 expression is described also in chronic hepatic diseases, in which it correlates with disease activity,[127] in cerebrospinal fluid and serum of multiple sclerosis patients,[128,129] and in myasthenia gravis. In the latter, myocytes expressed IL-15 in response to anti-acetylcholine receptor antibody.[130] Finally, IL-15 has been detected at high levels in alveolar macrophages from pulmonary sarcoid patients.[131] IL-15 promotes IFN-γ production and CD28 expression on CD4$^+$ T cells isolated from sarcoid T-cell alveolitis lesions and further enhances costimulatory molecule expression on alveolar macrophages.[132] Increased expression has also been reported in *M. tuberculosis*.[133] Thus, the significance of the biological activities elucidated for IL-15 in RA synovitis can likely be extended to include several important human inflammatory diseases.

CONCLUSIONS

IL-15 represents an intriguing cytokine activity with pleiotropic effects in RA synovial membrane. Recent studies suggest broader expression in a range of autoimmune diseases. Many data now support a proinflammatory role. The success of TNF-α blockade clearly illustrates the potential in effective targeting of regulatory cytokines. Those patients in whom either a partial or absent response occurs, however, demonstrate the need for further studies to determine factors that in turn regulate TNF-α production, operate in synergy with TNF-α or, indeed, operate independently of TNF-α. The data presented above provide compelling evidence to support such a role for IL-15 in synovial inflammation. Further studies will be required to determine what the optimal targeting mechanisms may be, given the complex membrane and intracellular expression of IL-15 in a number of tissues. Nevertheless, it clearly represents a target worthy of exploration, either alone or as a component of combination cytokine targeting approaches.

ACKNOWLEDGMENTS

The support of the Nuffield Foundation (Oliver Bird Fund), the Wellcome Trust and the Arthritis Research Campaign (UK) is acknowledged. Bernard P. Leung, J. Alastair Gracie, Ros Forsey, Morag Prach, Holger Ruchatz, Xiao Qing Wei, Max Field, Peter Wilkinson and Roger D. Sturrock provided invaluable contributions. Clinical support from Hilary Capell, John Hunter, Duncan Porter, Andy Kininmonth and Rajan Madhok is acknowledged.

REFERENCES

1. Fox DA. The role of T cells in the immunopathogenesis of rheumatoid arthritis: new perspectives. *Arthritis Rheum* 1997; **40**: 598–609.

2. Panayi GS, Lanchbury JS, Kingsley GH. The importance of the T-cell in initiating and maintaining the chronic synovitis of rheumatoid arthritis. *Arthritis Rheum* 1992; **35**: 729–35.

3. Feldmann M, Brennan FM, Maini RN. Role of cytokines in rheumatoid arthritis. *Annu Rev Immunol* 1996; **14**: 397–440.

4. Arend WP, Dayer JM. Inhibition of the production and effects of interleukin-1 and tumor necrosis factor alpha in rheumatoid arthritis. *Arthritis Rheum* 1995; **38**: 151–60.

5. Grabstein KH, Eisenman J, Shanebeck K et al. Cloning of a T-cell growth factor that interacts with the beta chain of the interleukin-2 receptor. *Science* 1994; **264**: 965–8.

6. Bamford R, Grant A, Burton J et al. The interleukin (IL) 2 receptor {beta} chain is shared by IL-2 and a cytokine, provisionally designated IL-T, that stimulates T-cell proliferation and the induction of lymphokine-activated killer cells. *Proc Natl Acad Sci USA* 1994; **91**: 4940–4.

7. Waldmann TA, Tagaya Y. The multifaceted regulation of interleukin-15 expression and the role of this cytokine in NK cell differentiation and host response to intracellular pathogens. *Annu Rev Immunol* 1999; **17**: 19–49.

8. Bamford RN, DeFilippis AP, Azimi N et al. The 5' untranslated region, signal peptide and the coding sequence of the carboxyl terminus of IL-15 participate in its multifaceted translational control. *J Immunol* 1998; **160**: 4418–26.

9. Bamford RN, Battiata AP, Burton JD et al. Interleukin (IL) 15/IL-T production by the adult T-cell leukemia cell line HuT-102 is associated with a human T-cell lymphotrophic virus type I R region/IL-15 fusion message that lacks many upstream AUGs that normally attenuate IL-15 mRNA translation. *Proc Natl Acad Sci USA* 1996; **93**: 2897–902.

10. Onu A, Pohl T, Krause H, Bulfone-Paus S. Regulation of IL-15 secretion via the leader peptide of two IL-15 isoforms. *J Immunol* 1997; **158**: 255–62.

11. Meazza R, Verdiani S, Biassoni R et al. Identification of a novel interleukin-15 (IL-15) transcript isoform generated by alternative splicing in human small cell lung cancer cell lines. *Oncogene* 1996; **12**: 2187–92.

12. Tagaya Y, Kurys G, Thies TA et al. Generation of secretable and nonsecretable interleukin 15 isoforms through alternate usage of signal peptides. *Proc Natl Acad Sci USA* 1997; **94**: 14444–9.

13. Nishimura H, Washizu J, Nakamura N et al. Translational efficiency is up-regulated by alternative exon in murine IL-15 mRNA. *J Immunol* 1998; **160**: 936–42.

14. Gaggero A, Azzarone B, Andrei C et al. Differential intracellular trafficking, secretion and endosomal localization of two IL-15 isoforms. *Eur J Immunol* 1999; **29**: 1265–74.

15. Azimi N, Brown K, Bamford RN et al. Human T-cell lymphotropic virus type I Tax protein transactivates interleukin 15 gene transcription through an NF-kappa B site. *Proc Natl Acad Sci USA* 1998; **95**: 2452–7.

16. Washizu J, Nishimura H, Nakamura N et al. The NF-kappaB binding site is essential for transcriptional activation of the IL-15 gene. *Immunogenetics* 1998; **48**: 1–7.

17. Flamand L, Stefanescu I, Menezes J. Human herpesvirus-6 enhances natural killer cell cytotoxicity via IL-15. *J Clin Invest* 1996; **97**: 1373–81.

18. Atedzoe BN, Ahmad A, Menezes J. Enhancement of natural killer cell cytotoxicity by the human herpesvirus-7 via IL-15 induction. *J Immunol* 1997; **159**: 4966–72.

19. Jullien D, Sieling PA, Uyemura K et al. IL-15, an immunomodulator of T-cell responses in intracellular infection. *J Immunol* 1997; **158**: 800–6.

20. Carson WE, Ross ME, Baiocchi RA et al. Endogenous production of interleukin 15 by activated human monocytes is critical for optimal production of interferon-gamma by natural killer cells in vitro. *J Clin Invest* 1995; **96**: 2578–82.

21. Chehimi J, Marshall JD, Salvucci O et al. IL-15 enhances immune functions during HIV infection. *J Immunol* 1997; **158**: 5978–87.

22. Mohamadzadeh M, Takashima A, Dougherty I et al. Ultraviolet B radiation up-regulates the expression of IL-15 in human skin. *J Immunol* 1995; **155**: 4492–6.

23. Giri JG, Kumaki S, Ahdieh M et al. Identification and cloning of a novel IL-15 binding protein that is structurally related to the alpha chain of the IL-2 receptor. *EMBO J* 1995; **14**: 3654–63.

24. Waldmann T, Tagaya Y, Bamford R. Interleukin-

2, interleukin-15 and their receptors. *Int Rev Immunol* 1998; **16**: 205–26.

25. Tagaya Y, Bamford RN, DeFilippis AP, Waldmann TA. IL-15: a pleiotropic cytokine with diverse receptor/signaling pathways whose expression is controlled at multiple levels. *Immunity* 1996; **4**: 329–36.

26. Anderson DM, Kumaki S, Ahdieh M et al. Functional characterization of the human interleukin-15 receptor alpha chain and close linkage of IL15RA and IL2RA genes. *J Biol Chem* 1995; **270**: 29862–9.

27. Tagaya Y, Burton ID, Miyamoto Y, Waldmann TA. Identification of a novel receptor/signal transduction pathway for IL-15/T in mast cells. *EMBO J* 1996; **15**: 4928–39.

28. Bulfone-Paus S, Bulanova E, Pohl T et al. Death deflected: IL-15 inhibits TNF-alpha-mediated apoptosis in fibroblasts by TRAF2 recruitment to the IL-15Ralpha chain. *FASEB J* 1999; **13**: 1575–85.

29. Nishimura H, Hiromatsu K, Kobayashi N et al. IL-15 is a novel growth factor for murine gamma delta T cells induced by Salmonella infection. *J Immunol* 1996; **156**: 663–9.

30. Korholz D, Banning U, Bonig H et al. The role of interleukin-10 (IL-10) in IL-15-mediated T-cell responses. *Blood* 1997; **90**: 4513–21.

31. Treiber-Held S, Stewart DM, Kurman CC, Nelson DL. IL-15 induces the release of soluble IL-2Ralpha from human peripheral blood mononuclear cells. *Clin Immunol Immunopathol* 1996; **79**: 71–8.

32. Kanegane H, Tosato G. Activation of naive and memory T cells by interleukin-15. *Blood* 1996; **88**: 230–5.

33. Mottonen M, Isomaki P, Luukkainen R et al. Interleukin-15 up-regulates the expression of CD154 on synovial fluid T cells. *Immunology* 2000; **100**: 238–44.

34. Wilkinson PC, Liew FY. Chemoattraction of human blood T lymphocytes by interleukin-15. *J Exp Med* 1995; **181**: 1255–9.

35. Al-Mughales J, Blyth TH, Hunter JA, Wilkinson PC. The chemoattractant activity of rheumatoid synovial fluid for human lymphocytes is due to multiple cytokines. *Clin Exp Immunol* 1996; **106**: 230–6.

36. Nieto M, del Pozo MA, Sanchez-Madrid F. Interleukin-15 induces adhesion receptor redistribution in T lymphocytes. *Eur J Immunol* 1996; **26**: 1302–7.

37. Perera LP, Goldman CK, Waldmann TA. IL-15 induces the expression of chemokines and their receptors in T lymphocytes. *J Immunol* 1999; **162**: 2606–12.

38. Seder RA. High-dose IL-2 and IL-15 enhance the in vitro priming of naive CD4 T cells for IFN-gamma but have differential effects on priming for IL-4. *J Immunol* 1996; **156**: 2413–22.

39. Seder RA, Grabstein KH, Berzofsky JA, McDyer JF. Cytokine interactions in human immunodeficiency virus-infected individuals: roles of interleukin (IL)-2, IL-12 and IL-15. *J Exp Med* 1995; **182**: 1067–77.

40. Borger P, Kauffman HF, Postma DS et al. Interleukin-15 differentially enhances the expression of interferon-gamma and interleukin-4 in activated human (CD4) T lymphocytes. *Immunology* 1999; **96**: 207–14.

41. Mori A, Suko M, Kaminuma O et al. IL-15 promotes cytokine production of human T helper cells. *J Immunol* 1996; **156**: 2400–5.

42. Ruckert R, Herz U, Paus R et al. IL-15–IgG2b fusion protein accelerates and enhances a Th2 but not a Th1 immune response in vivo, while IL-2–IgG2b fusion protein inhibits both. *Eur J Immunol* 1998; **28**: 3312–20.

43. Ong PY, Hamid QA, Travers JB et al. Decreased IL-15 may contribute to elevated IgE and acute inflammation in atopic dermatitis. *J Immunol* 2002; **168**: 505–10.

44. Tough DF, Zhang X, Sprent J. An ifn-gamma-dependent pathway controls stimulation of memory phenotype cd8() t cell turnover in vivo by il-12, il-18 and ifn-gamma. *J Immunol* 2001; **166**: 6007–11.

45. Lodolce JP, Boone DL, Chai S et al. IL-15 receptor maintains lymphoid homeostasis by supporting lymphocyte homing and proliferation. *Immunity* 1998; **9**: 669–76.

46. Kennedy MK, Glaccum M, Brown SN et al. Reversible defects in natural killer and memory CD8 T-cell lineages in interleukin 15-deficient mice. *J Exp Med* 2000; **191**: 771–80.

47. Lodolce JP, Burkett PR, Boone DL et al. T cell-independent interleukin 15R{alpha} signals are required for bystander proliferation. *J Exp Med* 2001; **194**: 1187–94.

48. Yajima T, Nishimura H, Ishimitsu R et al. Overexpression of IL-15 in vivo increases antigen-driven memory CD8+ T cells following a microbe exposure. *J Immunol* 2002; **168**: 1198–203.

49. Geginat J, Sallusto F, Lanzavecchia A. Cytokine-driven proliferation and differentiation of human

naive, central memory and effector memory CD4+ T cells. *J Exp Med* 2001; **194**: 1711–20.

50. Niedbala W, Wei X, Liew FY. IL-15 induces type 1 and type 2 CD4(+) and CD8(+) T cells proliferation but is unable to drive cytokine production in the absence of TCR activation or IL-12/IL-4 stimulation in vitro. *Eur J Immunol* 2002; **32**: 341–7.

51. Carson WE, Giri JG, Lindemann MJ et al. Interleukin (IL) 15 is a novel cytokine that activates human natural killer cells via components of the IL-2 receptor. *J Exp Med* 1994; **180**: 1395–403.

52. Bluman EM, Bartynski KJ, Avalos BR, Caligiuri MA. Human natural killer cells produce abundant macrophage inflammatory protein-1 alpha in response to monocyte-derived cytokines. *J Clin Invest* 1996; **97**: 2722–7.

53. Warren HS, Kinnear BF, Kastelein RL, Lanier LL. Analysis of the costimulatory role of IL-2 and IL-15 in initiating proliferation of resting (CD56dim) human NK cells. *J Immunol* 1996; **156**: 3254–9.

54. Cavazzana-Calvo M, Hacein-Bey S, de Saint Basile G et al. Role of interleukin-2 (IL-2), IL-7 and IL-15 in natural killer cell differentiation from cord blood hematopoietic progenitor cells and from gamma c transduced severe combined immunodeficiency X1 bone marrow cells. *Blood* 1996; **88**: 3901–9.

55. Mrozek E, Anderson P, Caligiuri MA. Role of interleukin-15 in the development of human CD56 natural killer cells from CD34 hematopoietic progenitor cells. *Blood* 1996; **87**: 2632–40.

56. Yu H, Fehniger TA, Fuchshuber P et al. Flt3 ligand promotes the generation of a distinct CD34() human natural killer cell progenitor that responds to interleukin-15. *Blood* 1998; **92**: 3647–57.

57. Carson WE, Fehniger TA, Haldar S et al. A potential role for interleukin-15 in the regulation of human natural killer cell survival. *J Clin Invest* 1997; **99**: 937–43.

58. Carson WE, Yu H, Dierksheide J et al. A fatal cytokine-induced systemic inflammatory response reveals a critical role for NK cells. *J Immunol* 1999; **162**: 4943–51.

59. Fehniger TA, Caligiuri MA. Interleukin 15: biology and relevance to human disease. *Blood* 2001; **97**: 14–32.

60. Alleva DG, Kaser SB, Monroy MA et al. IL-15 functions as a potent autocrine regulator of macrophage proinflammatory cytokine production: evidence for differential receptor subunit utilization associated with stimulation or inhibition. *J Immunol* 1997; **159**: 2941–51.

61. Musso T, Calosso L, Zucca M et al. Human monocytes constitutively express membrane-bound, biologically active and interferon-gamma-upregulated interleukin-15. *Blood* 1999; **93**: 3531–9.

62. Neely GG, Robbins SM, Amankwah EK et al. Lipopolysaccharide-stimulated or granulocyte–macrophage colony-stimulating factor-stimulated monocytes rapidly express biologically active IL-15 on their cell surface independent of new protein synthesis. *J Immunol* 2001; **167**: 5011–17.

63. Perera LP, Goldman CK, Waldmann TA. Comparative assessment of virulence of recombinant vaccinia viruses expressing IL-2 and IL-15 in immunodeficient mice. *Proc Natl Acad Sci USA* 2001; **98**: 5146–51.

64. Mohamadzadeh M, Berard F, Essert G et al. Interleukin 15 skews monocyte differentiation into dendritic cells with features of Langerhans cells. *J Exp Med* 2001; **194**: 1013–20.

65. Ohteki T, Suzue K, Maki C et al. Critical role of IL-15–IL-15R for antigen-presenting cell functions in the innate immune response. *Nat Immunol* 2001; **2**: 1138–43.

66. Girard D, Paquet ME, Paquin R, Beaulieu AD. Differential effects of interleukin-15 (IL-15) and IL-2 on human neutrophils: modulation of phagocytosis, cytoskeleton rearrangement, gene expression and apoptosis by IL-15. *Blood* 1996; **88**: 3176–84.

67. Girard D, Boiani N, Beaulieu AD. Human neutrophils express the interleukin-15 receptor alpha chain (IL-15Ralpha) but not the IL-9Ralpha component. *Clin Immunol Immunopathol* 1998; **88**: 232–40.

68. Ogata Y, Kukita A, Kukita T et al. A novel role of IL-15 in the development of osteoclasts: inability to replace its activity with IL-2. *J Immunol* 1999; **162**: 2754–60.

69. Kotake S, Schumacher HR Jr, Yarboro CH et al. In vivo gene expression of type 1 and type 2 cytokines in synovial tissues from patients in early stages of rheumatoid, reactive and undifferentiated arthritis. *Proc Assoc Am Physicians* 1997; **109**: 286–301.

70. McInnes IB, Leung BP, Feng GJ et al. A role for IL-15 in rheumatoid arthritis – reply. *Nat Med* 1998; **4**: 643.

71. Harada S, Yamamura M, Okamoto H et al. Production of interleukin-7 and interleukin-15 by fibroblast-like synoviocytes from patients with rheumatoid arthritis. *Arthritis Rheum* 1999; **42**: 1508–16.

72. Shah MH, Hackshaw KV, Caligiuri MA. A role for IL-15 in rheumatoid arthritis? *Nat Med* 1998; **4**: 643.

73. Ortiz AM, Garcia-Vicuna R, Sancho D et al. Cyclosporin A inhibits CD69 expression induced on synovial fluid and peripheral blood lymphocytes by interleukin 15. *J Rheumatol* 2000; **27**: 2329–38.

74. Ziolkowska M, Koc A, Luszczykiewicz G et al. High levels of IL-17 in rheumatoid arthritis patients: IL-15 triggers in vitro IL-17 production via cyclosporin A-sensitive mechanism. *J Immunol* 2000; **164**: 2832–8.

75. Aringer M, Stummvoll GH, Steiner G et al. Serum interleukin-15 is elevated in systemic lupus erythematosus. *Rheumatology* 2001; **40**: 876–81.

76. Klimiuk PA, Sierakowski S, Latosiewicz R et al. Serum cytokines in different histological variants of rheumatoid arthritis. *J Rheumatol* 2001; **28**: 1211–17.

77. Cordero OJ, Salgado FJ, Mera-Varela A, Nogueira M. Serum interleukin-12, interleukin-15, soluble CD26 and adenosine deaminase in patients with rheumatoid arthritis. *Int Rheumatol* 2001; **21**: 69–74.

78. Hidaka T, Suzuki K, Kawakami M et al. Dynamic changes in cytokine levels in serum and synovial fluid following filtration leukocytapheresis therapy in patients with rheumatoid arthritis. *J Clin Apheresis* 2001; **16**: 74–81.

79. Yanagawa H, Takeuchi E, Miyata J et al. Rheumatoid pleural effusion with detectable level of interleukin-15. *J Intern Med* 1998; **243**: 331–2.

80. McInnes IB, al-Mughales J, Field M et al. The role of interleukin-15 in T-cell migration and activation in rheumatoid arthritis. *Nat Med* 1996; **2**: 175–82.

81. Thurkow EW, van der Heijden IM, Breedveld FC et al. Increased expression of IL-15 in the synovium of patients with rheumatoid arthritis compared with patients with Yersinia-induced arthritis and osteoarthritis. *J Pathol* 1997; **181**: 444–50.

82. Oppenheimer-Marks N, Brezinschek RI, Mohamadzadeh M et al. Interleukin 15 is produced by endothelial cells and increases the transendothelial migration of T cells in vitro and in the SCID mouse–human rheumatoid arthritis model in vivo. *J Clin Invest* 1998; **101**: 1261–72.

83. Danning CL, Illei GG, Hitchon C et al. Macrophage-derived cytokine and nuclear factor kappaB p65 expression in synovial membrane and skin of patients with psoriatic arthritis. *Arthritis Rheum* 2000; **43**: 1244–56.

84. Scola MP, Thompson SD, Brunner HI et al. Interferon-gamma:interleukin 4 ratios and associated type 1 cytokine expression in juvenile rheumatoid arthritis synovial tissue. *J Rheumatol* 2002; **29**: 369–78.

85. Cho ML, Kim WU, Min SY et al. Cyclosporine differentially regulates interleukin-10, interleukin-15 and tumor necrosis factor a production by rheumatoid synoviocytes. *Arthritis Rheum* 2002; **46**: 42–51.

86. Wakisaka S, Suzuki N, Nagafuchi H et al. Characterization of tissue outgrowth developed in vitro in patients with rheumatoid arthritis: involvement of T cells in the development of tissue outgrowth. *Int Arch Allergy Immunol* 2000; **121**: 68–79.

87. Rappl G, Kapsokefalou A, Heuser C et al. Dermal fibroblasts sustain proliferation of activated T cells via membrane-bound interleukin-15 upon long-term stimulation with tumor necrosis factor-alpha. *J Invest Dermatol* 2001; **116**: 102–9.

88. Sen M, Lauterbach K, El-Gabalawy H et al. Expression and function of wingless and frizzled homologs in rheumatoid arthritis. *Proc Natl Acad Sci USA* 2000; **97**: 2791–6.

89. Sen M, Chamorro M, Reifert J et al. Blockade of Wnt-5A/frizzled 5 signaling inhibits rheumatoid synoviocyte activation. *Arthritis Rheum* 2001; **44**: 772–81.

90. Lipsky PE, van der Heijde DM, St Clair EW et al. Infliximab and methotrexate in the treatment of rheumatoid arthritis. Anti-Tumor Necrosis Factor Trial in Rheumatoid Arthritis with Concomitant Therapy Study Group. *N Engl J Med* 2000; **343**: 1594–602.

91. Bathon JM, Martin RW, Fleischmann RM et al. A comparison of etanercept and methotrexate in patients with early rheumatoid arthritis. *N Engl J Med* 2000; **343**: 1586–93.

92. Gracie JA, Leung BP, McInnes IB. Novel pathways that regulate necrosis factor-alpha production in rheumatoid arthritis. *Curr Opin Rheumatol* 2002; **14**: 270–5.

93. Chu CQ, Field M, Feldmann M, Maini RN. Localization of tumor necrosis factor alpha in

synovial tissues and at the cartilage–pannus junction in patients with rheumatoid arthritis. *Arthritis Rheum* 1991; **34**: 1125–32.

94. Deleuran BW, Chu CQ, Field M et al. Localization of tumor necrosis factor receptors in the synovial tissue and cartilage–pannus junction in patients with rheumatoid arthritis. Implications for local actions of tumor necrosis factor alpha. *Arthritis Rheum* 1992; **35**: 1170–8.

95. Klimiuk PA, Yang H, Goronzy JJ, Weyand CM. Production of cytokines and metalloproteinases in rheumatoid synovitis is T-cell dependent. *Clin Immunol* 1999; **90**: 65–78.

96. Brennan FM, Hayes AL, Ciesielski CJ et al. Evidence that rheumatoid arthritis synovial T cells are similar to cytokine-activated T cells: involvement of phosphatidylinositol 3-kinase and nuclear factor kappaB pathways in tumor necrosis factor alpha production in rheumatoid arthritis. *Arthritis Rheum* 2002; **46**: 31–41.

97. Isler P, Vey E, Zhang JH, Dayer JM. Cell surface glycoproteins expressed on activated human T cells induce production of interleukin-1 beta by monocytic cells: a possible role of CD69. *Eur Cytokine Netw* 1993; **4**. 15–23.

98. McInnes IB, Leung BP, Sturrock RD et al. Interleukin-15 mediates T cell-dependent regulation of tumor necrosis factor-alpha production in rheumatoid arthritis. *Nat Med* 1997; **3**: 189–95.

99. Kasyapa CS, Stentz CL, Davey MP, Carr DW. Regulation of IL-15-stimulated TNF-alpha production by rolipram. *J Immunol* 1999; **163**: 2836–43.

100. Rezzonico R, Burger D, Dayer JM. Direct contact between T lymphocytes and human dermal fibroblasts or synoviocytes down-regulates types I and III collagen production via cell-associated cytokines. *J Biol Chem* 1998; **273**: 18720–8.

101. Sebbag M, Parry SL, Brennan FM, Feldmann M. Cytokine stimulation of T lymphocytes regulates their capacity to induce monocyte production of tumor necrosis factor-alpha, but not interleukin-10: possible relevance to pathophysiology of rheumatoid arthritis. *Eur J Immunol* 1997; **27**: 624–32.

102. Unutmaz D, Pileri P, Abrignani S. Antigen-independent activation of naive and memory resting T cells by a cytokine combination. *J Exp Med* 1994; **180**: 1159–64.

103. Avice MN, Demeure CE, Delespesse G et al. IL-15 promotes IL-12 production by human monocytes via T cell-dependent contact and may contribute to IL-12-mediated IFN-gamma secretion by CD4 T cells in the absence of TCR ligation. *J Immunol* 1998; **161**: 3408–15.

104. McInnes IB, Leung BP, Liew FY. Cell–cell interactions in synovitis. Interactions between T lymphocytes and synovial cells. *Arthritis Res* 2000; **2**: 374–8.

105. Chabaud M, Durand JM, Buchs N et al. Human interleukin-17: a T cell-derived proinflammatory cytokine produced by the rheumatoid synovium. *Arthritis Rheum* 1999; **42**: 963–70.

106. Lubberts E, Joosten LAB, Oppers B et al. IL-1-independent role of IL-17 in synovial inflammation and joint destruction during collagen-induced arthritis. *J Immunol* 2001; **167**: 1004–13.

107. Saeed S, Revell PA. Production and distribution of interleukin 15 and its receptors (IL-15Ralpha and IL-R2beta) in the implant interface tissues obtained during revision of failed total joint replacement. *Int J Exp Pathol* 2001; **82**: 201–9.

108. Musikacharoen T, Matsuguchi T, Kikuchi T, Yoshikai Y. Nf-kappab and stat5 play important roles in the regulation of mouse toll-like receptor 2 gene expression. *J Immunol* 2001; **166**: 4516–24.

109. Schrijver IA, Melief MJ, Markusse HM et al. Peptidoglycan from sterile human spleen induces T-cell proliferation and inflammatory mediators in rheumatoid arthritis patients and healthy subjects. *Rheumatology (Oxford)* 2001; **40**: 438–46.

110. Szekanecz Z, Strieter RM, Kunkel SL, Koch AE. Chemokines in rheumatoid arthritis. *Springer Semin Immunopathol* 1998; **20**: 115–32.

111. Szekanecz Z, Koch AE. Chemokines and angiogenesis. *Curr Opin Rheumatol* 2001; **13**: 202–8.

112. Nanki T, Hayashida K, El-Gabalawy HS et al. Stromal cell-derived factor-1–CXC chemokine receptor 4 interactions play a central role in CD4 T-cell accumulation in rheumatoid arthritis synovium. *J Immunol* 2000; **165**: 6590–8.

113. Estess P, Nandi A, Mohamadzadeh M, Siegelman MH. Interleukin 15 induces endothelial hyaluronan expression in vitro and promotes activated T-cell extravasation through a CD44-dependent pathway in vivo. *J Exp Med* 1999; **190**: 9–19.

114. Pilling D, Akbar AN, Girdlestone J et al. Interferon-beta mediates stromal cell rescue of T cells from apoptosis. *Eur J Immunol* 1999; **29**: 1041–50.

115. Bulfone-Paus S, Ungureanu D, Pohl T et al. Interleukin-15 protects from lethal apoptosis in vivo. *Nat Med* 1997; **3**: 1124–8.

116. Leung BP, Chaudhuri K, Forsey RJ et al.

Interleukin-15 induces cytokine production by rheumatoid arthritis (RA) synovial neutrophils. *Arthritis Rheum* 1997; **40** (suppl 274): 1457.

117. McInnes IB, Leung BP, Forsey RJ et al. Interleukin-15 (IL-15) induces granzyme synthesis by rheumatoid arthritis (RA) synovial T cells. *Arthritis Rheum* 1997; **40** (suppl 274): 1458.

118. Gracie JA, Forsey RJ, Chan WL et al. A proinflammatory role for IL-18 in rheumatoid arthritis. *J Clin Invest* 1999; **104**: 1393–401.

119. McInnes IB, Gracie JA, Leung BP et al. Interleukin 18: a pleiotropic participant in chronic inflammation. *Immunol Today* 2000; **21**: 312–15.

120. Sprent J, Zhang X, Sun S, Tough D. T-cell turnover in vivo and the role of cytokines. *Immunol Lett* 1999; **65**: 21–5.

121. Ruchatz H, Leung BP, Wei XQ et al. Soluble IL-15 receptor alpha-chain administration prevents murine collagen-induced arthritis: a role for IL-15 in development of antigen-induced immunopathology. *J Immunol* 1998; **160**: 5654–60.

122. Wei X, Orchardson M, Gracie JA et al. The sushi domain of soluble IL-15 receptor alpha is essential for binding IL-15 and inhibiting inflammatory and allogenic responses in vitro and in vivo. *J Immunol* 2001; **167**: 277–82.

123. Kim YS, Maslinski W, Zheng XX, Kim YS et al. Targeting the IL-15 receptor with an antagonist IL-15 mutant/Fc gamma2a protein blocks delayed-type hypersensitivity. *J Immunol* 1998; **160**: 5742–8.

124. Ferrari-Lacraz S, Zheng XX, Kim YS et al. An antagonist IL-15/Fc protein prevents costimulation blockade-resistant rejection. *J Immunol* 2001; **167**: 3478–85.

125. Kirman I, Nielsen OH. Increased numbers of interleukin-15-expressing cells in active ulcerative colitis. *Am J Gastroenterol* 1996; **91**: 1789–94.

126. Sakai T, Kusugami K, Nishimura H et al. Interleukin 15 activity in the rectal mucosa of inflammatory bowel disease. *Gastroenterology* 1998; **114**: 1237–43.

127. Kakumu S, Okumura A, Ishikawa T et al. Serum levels of IL-10, IL-15 and soluble tumour necrosis factor-alpha (TNF-alpha) receptors in type C chronic liver disease. *Clin Exp Immunol* 1997; **109**: 458–63.

128. Kivisakk P, Matusevicius D, He B et al. IL-15 mRNA expression is up-regulated in blood and cerebrospinal fluid mononuclear cells in multiple sclerosis (MS). *Clin Exp Immunol* 1998; **111**: 193–7.

129. Pashenkov M, Mustafa M, Kivisakk P, Link H. Levels of interleukin-15-expressing blood mononuclear cells are elevated in multiple sclerosis. *Scand J Immunol* 1999; **50**: 302–8.

130. Stegall T, Krolick KA. Myocytes respond in vivo to an antibody reactive with the acetylcholine receptor by upregulating interleukin-15: an interferon-gamma activator with the potential to influence the severity and course of experimental myasthenia gravis. *J Neuroimmunol* 2001; **119**: 377–86.

131. Agostini C, Trentin L, Facco M et al. Role of IL-15, IL-2 and their receptors in the development of T-cell alveolitis in pulmonary sarcoidosis. *J Immunol* 1996; **157**: 910–18.

132. Agostini C, Trentin L, Perin A et al. Regulation of alveolar macrophage–T cell interactions during Th1-type sarcoid inflammatory process. *Am J Physiol* 1999; **277**: L240–50.

133. Muro S, Taha R, Tsicopoulos A et al. Expression of IL-15 in inflammatory pulmonary diseases. *J Allergy Clin Immunol* 2001; **108**: 970–5.

16

Interleukin-18

Charles A Dinarello

Introduction • **IL-18 and its functions** • **IL-18 production** • **IL-18 binding protein** • **Role of IL-12 in the induction of IFNγ by IL-18** • **Role of IL-18 in models of autoimmune disease** • **References**

INTRODUCTION

Although interleukin-18 (IL-18) is a member of the IL-1 family of ligands (Table 16.1), IL-18 appears to have unique characteristics, some of which are important for its role in rheumatoid arthritis. The most salient biological property of IL-18 that distinguishes this cytokine from IL-1 is its ability to induce IFNγ in the presence of IL-12. IL-18 was originally identified as an IFNγ-inducing factor. Because IL-18 appears to be essential for IFNγ production, the role of IL-18 in disease must consider its role in regulating IFNγ production. IFNγ is itself unlike other pro-inflammatory cytokines because it has been administered in thousands of humans with a variety of diseases, including rheumatoid arthritis. IFNγ was also administered to patients with bur injuries to improve intracellular killing of bacteria, particularly by mononuclear phagocytes. There are also reports of IFNγ treatment in cancer. Overall, there has not been a worsening of disease with the exception of reports on exacerbation of CNS lesions in multiple sclerosis. Therefore, unlike the systemic inflammatory response of humans injected with IL-1 or TNFα, IFNγ appears to be tolerated by humans, and in some disease states can be considered therapeutic. For example, in patients with chronic granulomatous disease or atypical mycobacterium infections (including leprosy), IFNγ is used in conjunction with specific antibiotic therapies.

As with any cytokine, its role in a particular disease process is best assessed using specific blockade or neutralization in a complex disease

Table 16.1 IL-1 gene superfamily.

New name	Former name(s)	Property
IL-1F1	IL-1α	Agonist
IL-1F2	IL-1β	Agonist
IL-1F3	IL-1Ra	Antagonist
IL-1F4	IL-18; IFNγ inducing factor	Agonist
IL-1F5	IL-1Hy1, FIL1δ, IL-1H3, IL-1RP3, IL-1L1, IL-1δ	Unknown
IL-1F6	FIL-1ε, IL-1ε	Unknown
IL-1F7	FIL-1ζ, IL-1H4, IL-1RP1	Unknown
IL-1F8	FIL-1ν, IL-1H2	Unknown
IL-1F9	IL-1H1, IL-1RP2	Unknown
IL-1F10	IL-1Hy2, FKSG75	Unknown

model such as adjuvant or collagen-induced arthritis. If a single cytokine or receptor is blocked, and there is a dramatic reduction in the severity of the model, then that cytokine or receptor plays a critical role. The difficulty arises when one can show that blocking other cytokines, for example, blocking IL-1, IL-15, IL-17 or TNFα, results in the same reduction in the severity of the model. The dilemma is then: which cytokine is best to block or neutralize clinically? In general, the cytokine to block or neutralize is the cytokine with the least role in normal cell function, repair or host defense. The issue is also not which cytokine is 'better' or 'best' to neutralize but which one has the greatest safety parameter while being efficacious. Another approach is the use of combinations of two or more anticytokines. This increases efficacy but the inherent danger is overzealous use of high doses. In general the best approach is to reduce the dose of each to gain efficacy without increasing risks.

IL-18 neutralization, IL-18-deficient mice or mice deficient in IL-18 receptor-α chain reveal varying degrees of reduced severity in models of systemic and local disease. In fact, there is considerable overlap in blocking IL-1, IL-18, IFNγ and TNFα in models of endotoxemia. For the treatment of humans with rheumatoid arthritis using antibodies against IL-18, antibodies that block the IL-18 receptor or the IL-18 binding protein (IL-18BP), the relevant models are collagen-induced arthritis (CIA), streptococcal wall (SCW) arthritis and to a lesser extent adjuvant arthritis. However, because IL-18 regulates IFNγ, primary immunization with collagen in mice deficient in IL-18 or deficient in the IL-18 receptor is problematic as low titers of anti-collagen antibodies may affect the disease model. Nevertheless, IL-18 neutralization in wild-type DBA-1 mice is effective in reducing CIA.[1]

IL-18 AND ITS FUNCTIONS

The discovery of IL-18 and its role in models of systemic inflammation

IL-18 was first described as an IFNγ-inducing factor found in the circulation during endotoxemia.[2] In those experiments mice had been preconditioned with a prior infection of *Propionibacterium acnes*. Because of its property of inducing IFNγ, IL-18 is by default a member of the T-cell helper type I (Th1)-inducing family of cytokines (IFNγ, IL-2, IL-12, IL-15). However, because antibodies to IL-18 also reduced the hepatotoxicity of endotoxemia,[3] IL-18 was considered to possess other biological properties beyond that of inducing IFNγ. Like all cytokine responses to infections, there are two sides to the coin. IL-18 functions to protect the host in that its ability to induce IFNγ and other immunostimulatory cytokines assists the immune system in a specific T- and B-cell-mediated response. However, the other pathological consequences of infection are, in part, also mediated by IL-18 and in somewhat the same fashion are mediated by IL-1 and TNFα. These include the increases in cell adhesion molecules and chemokines, inflammatory mediators such as nitric oxide (NO) and neutrophil activation.

The support for a role for IL-18 in the pathological processes of systemic inflammation is derived from animal studies in which specific blockade of IL-18 reduces the impact on organ damage or improves the survival of the host. The first experiments showed that mice deficient in caspase-1, failure to process the IL-18 and IL-1β precursors survived lethal endotoxemia[4,5] whereas mice deficient in IL-1β died.[6] In fact, specific antibodies against mouse IL-18 also protected against the hepatic toxicity of endotoxemia.[3,7] On the other hand, in naive mice not preconditioned with a prior infection of *P. acnes*, IL-18 neutralization also reduces lethal endotoxemia. Moreover, this protection is observed in mice deficient in IFNγ.[8] Thus, one may conclude that preconditioning with a prior infection of *P. acnes* is needed for an IFNγ-sensitive animal model.

Since IL-18 induces synthesis of the proinflammatory cytokines TNFα, IL-1β and the chemokines IL-8 and macrophage inflammatory protein-1α, neutralization of IL-18 would have a beneficial effect in lethal endotoxemia in naive mice. Anti-IL-18 antibodies protected mice against a lethal injection of *E. coli* or *S. typhimurium*.[8] Anti-IL-18 also reduced myelo-

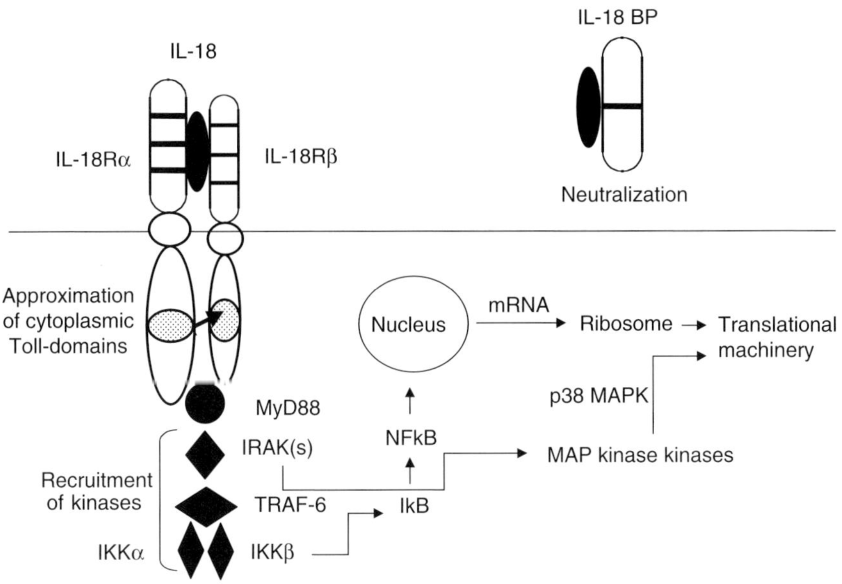

Figure 16.1 Signal transduction of IL-18.

peroxidase levels in the liver and lungs.[8] An increased survival was accompanied by decreased levels of IFNγ and macrophage inflammatory protein-2 in anti-IL-18-treated animals challenged with *E. coli* LPS, whereas IFNγ and TNFα concentrations were decreased in treated mice challenged with *S. typhimurium*.

IL-18 receptors and signal transduction

The activity of IL-18 begins with the formation of a heterodimeric complex comprised of two chains of the IL-18 receptor (IL-18R) complex plus IL-18. The ligand binding chain is termed IL-18Rα. It was reported using amino acid sequencing of a purified protein using ligand affinity purification.[9] IL-18Rα is a member of the IL-1 receptor family, previously identified as the IL-1R related protein (IL-1Rrp).[10] Following the binding of IL-18 to the IL-18Rα chain, a second chain is recruited to the complex (Figure 16.1). This second chain, termed IL-18Rβ chain, is a different gene product but is structurally related to IL-18Rα; however, the IL-18Rβ chain does not bind to IL-18 unless IL-18 is already bound to the α-chain. Because the IL-18Rβ chain is struc-

turally related to the IL-1 signal-transducing chain, IL-1R accessory protein, the IL-18Rβ chain was initially termed the IL-18R accessory protein-like (AcPL) chain.[11] The binding of IL-18 to the IL-18Rα chain is a low-affinity binding (20–40 nM)[9] but the formation of the tricomplex with the IL-18Rβ chain forms a high-affinity complex (600 nM). These two distinct binding affinities can be observed experimentally on T-cells.[12]

Recruitment of MyD88 and IL-1 receptor-activating kinases

After the formation of the high-affinity complex, the IL-18R recruits a cytosolic protein termed MyD88. This small protein has many of the characteristics of cytoplasmic domains of receptors but it lacks any known extracellular or trans-membrane structure. Mice deficient in MyD88 do not respond to IL-1 or IL-18.[13] It is unclear exactly how MyD88 functions since it does not have any known kinase activity. However, it may assist in the binding of the IL-1 receptor-activating kinases (IRAKs) to the complex and hence MyD88 appears to function as an adapter or anchoring molecule.[14] Like IL-1 signaling, MyD88 has a role in IL-18 signaling. MyD88-deficient mice do not produce acute phase proteins and have diminished cytokine responses. Recently, Th1-developing cells from MyD88-deficient mice were found to be unresponsive to IL-18-induced activation of NFκB and c-Jun N-terminal kinase (JNK).[13] Thus, MyD88 is an essential component in the signaling cascade that follows IL-1 receptor binding as well as IL-18 receptor binding. It appears that there is a well-established cascade of sequential recruitment of MyD88, IRAK and then TNF receptor-associated factor 6 (TRAF-6). Although some reports show that IL-1 and IL-18 activate NFκB-inducing kinases (NIKs), cells from mice deficient in NIKs respond to IL-1 and TNFα.[15] NIK is required for signaling of lymphotoxin-β receptor but not TNF receptors.

Degradation of IκBK and release of NFκB are nearly identical for IL-1 as well as for IL-18. Indeed, in cells transfected with IL-18Rα and then stimulated with IL-18, translocation of NFκB is observed using electromobility shift assay.[9] In U1 macrophages, which already express the gene for IL-18Rα, there is translocation of NFκB and stimulation of the human immunodeficiency virus-type 1 (HIV-1) production.[16]

IRAK and IL-18

Similar to IL-1 signal transduction, the recruitment of MyD88 to the IL-18 receptor complex phosphorylates a series of kinases, most notably the IRAKs. Although IRAKs have been discovered and studied as part of the IL-1 and Toll-like receptor signal-transducing processes, IRAK is also an essential component of IL-18 signaling. The IL-18 receptor complex contains IRAK.[17] Moreover, mice deficient in IRAK lack responsiveness to IL-18.[18] In cells from IRAK-deficient mice, there is a significant reduction in the activation of NFκB by IL-18.[18]

IRAK-1 associates with the IL-18R complex.[19,20] This was demonstrated using IL-12-stimulated T-cells followed by immunoprecipitation with anti-IL-18R or anti-IRAK.[19] Furthermore, IL-18-triggered cells also recruited TRAF-6.[19] IRAK is structurally related to the Drosophila Pelle protein. There are presently four isoforms of IRAK.[21] Each IRAK is a serine–threonine kinase. Deletion of IRAK-1 results in a partial reduction in IL-1 signaling. In mice with a deletion in IRAK-4, there is reduced endotoxin response (via Toll-like receptor-4) as well as IL-1 signaling.[21] In fact, mice with a targeted disruption in IRAK-4 are resistant to lethal endotoxemia.[21] The response to CpG (bacterial DNA via TLR-9), peptidoglycan (via TLR-2) and poly I:C (via TLR-3) was also decreased in IRAK-4-deficient mice compared to wild-type controls. Although cell signaling by IL-18 was not directly tested in IRAK-4-deficient mice, IFNγ induction by infection with lymphocytic choriomenigitis virus was absent,[21] strongly suggesting that IL-18 signaling is equally as dependent on IRAK-4 as is IL-1 and TLR-2, -3, -4 and -9.

It is likely that the binding of IRAKs to the IL-18R complex is as critical a step in the activation by IL-18 as it is for IL-1.[22] Like IL-1, the IL-18Rβ chain is essential for the recruitment and activation of IRAK.[18,23,24] For IL-1, the deletion of specific amino acids in the IL-1R-AcP cytoplasmic domain results in loss of IRAK-1 association and decreased NFκB activation.[23] For IL-18, a similar reduction in NFκB as well as Jun kinase was observed.[18] There was a marked decrease in IFNγ production in IRAK-1-deficient mice in IL-18-dependent models.[18] The critical step in the activation of IRAK appears to be the docking of MyD88 to the IL-18 receptor complex allowing IRAK to become phosphorylated as takes place following IL-1.[22,25]

IRAK then dissociates from the IL-18R complex and associates with TRAF-6.[26] TRAF-6 then phosphorylates NIK,[27] although studies in NIK-deficient mice show intact IL-1 and TNFα signaling.[15] NIK is known to phosphorylate the inhibitory κB kinases (IKK-1 and IKK-2).[28] Once phosphorylated, IκB is rapidly degraded by a ubiquitin pathway liberating NFκB which translocates to the nucleus for gene transcription. Some studies suggest that NIK is not necessary for IL-1 signaling, although specific testing for IL-18 responses in NIK-deficient mice has not been reported to date. However, in mice deficient in TRAF-6, there is no IL-1 signaling in thymocytes and the phenotype exhibits severe osteopetrosis and defective formation of osteo-clasts.[29]

Activation of MAP kinases following IL-18 receptor binding

Multiple phosphorylations take place during the first 15 minutes following IL-18 receptor binding. Most consistently, IL-18 activates protein kinases, which phosphorylate serine and threonine residues, targets of the MAP kinase family. Similar to IL-1 signaling, IL-18 activation of serine–threonine kinases likely results in the phosphorylation of tyrosine residues on upstream MAP kinases.[30,31] Tyrosine phosphory-lation induced by IL-18 is likely due to activation of MAP kinase kinase, which then phosphory-lates tyrosine and threonine on MAP kinases.

IL-18 PRODUCTION

In general, macrophage stimulators such as LPS, exotoxins from Gram-positive bacteria and a variety of microbial products induce each of the macrophage cytokines. These include IL-1, TNF, IL-6, IL-10 and several others. Thus, it is not surprising that these same activators also stimu-late IL-18 production. With few exceptions, stimulation of IL-18 production by Toll-like receptors is caspase-1 dependent. However, in a model of Fas ligand-induced liver damage, which is IL-18 dependent, mice deficient in caspase-1 also experienced liver damage.[32] Granulocyte-macrophage colony-stimulating factor (GM-CSF) was used to induce human blood monocytes into macrophages, which were then infected with influenza A virus. The result-ing supernatant induced T-cells to release IFNγ, which was prevented using a neutralizing antibody to IFNα/β.[33] IFNα and IL-18 acted synergistically to increase IFNγ production yet there was no demonstrable role for IL-12 in these cultures.

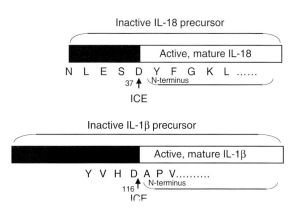

Figure 16.2 Caspase-1 processing of the IL-18 and IL-1β precursors. IL-1β converting enzyme (ICE) cleaves the IL-18 and IL-1β precursors at the aspartic acid P1 position.

Caspase-1 processing of the IL-18 precursor

As shown in Figure 16.2, caspase-1 processing of the IL-18 precursor is similar to that of IL-1β. Caspase-1 is constitutively expressed in various cells as a primary transcript of 45 kDa (inactive precursor) requiring two internal cleavages before becoming the enzymatically active heterodimer comprised of a 10 and 20 kD chain. The active site cysteine is located on the 20 kD chain. Caspase-1 itself contributes to autopro-cessing of the caspase-1 precursor by undergo-ing oligomerization with itself or homologs of caspase-1. In the presence of specific inhibitors of caspase-1, the generation and secretion of mature IL-1β is reduced and precursor IL-1β accumulates mostly inside but the precursor is also found outside the cell. This latter finding supports the concept that precursor IL-1β can be released from a cell independent of processing by caspase-1. Due to alternate RNA splicing, there are five isoforms of human caspase-1 (α, β, γ, δ and ε); caspase-1α cleaves the caspase-1 precursor and the IL-1β precursor. It is presumed that caspase-1β and γ also process precursor caspase-1. Caspase-1ε is a truncated form of caspase-1, which may inhibit caspase-1 activity by binding to the p20 chain of caspase-1 to form an inactive caspase-1 complex.

The secretion of mature IL-1β is facilitated by a reduction in the intracellular levels of potassium, which takes place when a cell is exposed to high levels of ATP.[34] This has, however, not been observed with the IL-18 precursor. Treatment of stimulated macrophages with millimolar concentrations of ATP also results in the processing and release of IL-1β but not IL-18.[35] The effect of ATP or nigericin is due to a net decrease in the intracellular levels of potassium. Increasing the extracellular level of potassium also results in the inhibition of caspases by preventing the formation of a large intracellular complex associated with activation of caspases.[36]

The P2X-7 receptor and secretion of IL-1β and IL-18

Since ATP results in the rapid release of mature IL-1β within minutes, a receptor-mediated event has been proposed. For ATP, a purinergic receptor (since adenosine is a purine) is found on monocytes and macrophages and is designated P2X-7. When triggered by millimolar concentrations of ATP, reversible pores form in the plasma membrane, and due to ion fluxes the electrical potential of the membrane is transiently lost. In the presence of LPS, this activation by ATP triggers the release of mature IL-1β.[37] A monoclonal antibody to the P2X-7 receptor prevents the release of mature IL-1β from activated macrophages.[38] Importantly, the secretion of IL-1β via activation of the P2X-7 receptor by ATP is independent of caspase-1, since highly specific inhibitors of caspase-1 prevent processing of the IL-1β and IL-18 precursors but have no effect on release of the IL-1β precursor or the release of lactic dehydrogenase in cells stimulated with ATP.[39] Triggering of the P2X-7 receptor is specific for the release of mature IL-1β and also IL-18, but does not result in the release of TNFα. ATP or nigericin also stimulate the release of IL-1 and IL-18 in LPS-stimulated whole blood cultures.[40] Convincing evidence for a role of the P2X-7R receptor in the post-translational processing and secretion of IL-1β is found in mice deficient in this receptor. Similar to wild-type macrophages, P2X-7R-deficient macrophages synthesize PGE2 and the IL-1β precursor in response to endotoxins. However, when activated by ATP, P2X-7R-deficient macrophages do not process or release IL-1β.[41] Similar results have been observed with IL-18. In vivo, wild-type and P2X-7R-deficient mice release the same amounts of IL-6 into the peritoneal cavity, but there is no release of mature IL-1β from P2X-7R-deficient mice.

Production of IL-18 from monocytes/macrophages

In the mouse, the production of IL-18 is derived from experiments in mice preconditioned by *Propionibacterium acnes* and then challenged with LPS 4–6 days later. Compared to non-preconditioned mice, LPS induces in preconditioned mice a more rapid and higher level of IFNγ. When preconditioned mice are passively immunized with a neutralizing antibody to IL-18, markedly reduced circulating levels of IFNγ are observed.[7] The preconditioning results in a dramatic increase in the number and activity of liver Kupffer cells and splenic macrophages. Therefore, the role of IL-18 in LPS-induced IFNγ production is likely to be exaggerated. Similar to other activators of the reticuloendothelial system, preconditioning in this model does not provide information on the role of IL-18 under 'normal' conditions.

Production of IL-18 from human dentritic cells

Like human blood monocytes,[35] human dendritic cells constitutively produce IL-18.[42] For comparison, IL-1β is not expressed constitutively in these same cells. However, because dendritic cells readily interact with T-cells, this interaction contributes to the processing and secretion of mature IL-18. Dendritic cells incubated with all-specific T-cells release mature IL-18 into the supernatant but not when incubated with autologous T-cells. The stimulation and secretion of IL-18 is mediated via a CD-40 signal since anti-CD40 agonist antibody also stimulates secretion of IL-18.[42] Similar to IL-1β, the IL-18 precursor is found diffusely in the cytosol but approximately 20% is co-localized to the lyosomal compartment. Following sub-cellular fractionations, the IL-18 precursor co-localizes with the endolysosomes.[43] The precursor of IL-1β is also found diffusely in the cytosol and co-localizes with these specialized endolysosomes.[44] Whereas stimulation with LPS results in release of mature IL-1β from monocytes via caspase-1 cleavage, there is little if any secretion of mature IL-18.[35] A similar lack of LPS-induced secretion of IL-18 is observed in dendritic cells.[43] However, upon contact with activated, alloreactive T-cells, dendritic cells release the IL-18 precursor via the endolysosomal pathway. As a result, the levels of constitutive IL-18 precursor inside the cell rapidly decrease.[43] It is well established that exocytosis of these specialized lysosomes is a calcium-dependent mechanism. In fact, increasing the extracellular calcium flux results in release of the IL-18 precursor.[43] Interestingly, increasing the intracellular release of calcium affects the secretion of the IL-18 precursor. It has been proposed that the low level of recovery of mature IL-18 may be due to the rapid uptake by activated T-cells.[43] If the IL-18 precursor is rapidly released by exocytosis upon contact with activated, immunospecific T-cells, then how is post-translational and post-secretory IL-18 processed into an active cytokine?

Non-caspase processing of IL-18

Extracellular processing of the IL-1β precursor has been reported and is a caspase-1-independent mechanism. The enzyme that seems most associated with the processing of both the IL-1β precursor as well as the IL-18 precursor is proteinase-3.[45] The IL-18 precursor is constitutively expressed in primary human oral epithelial cells and several epithelial cell lines. When primed by IFNγ and then stimulated with proteinase-3 in the presence of LPS, these cells release active IL-18 into the supernatant.[46] Since lactate dehydrogenase activity is not released, the appearance of active IL-18 is not due to cell leakage or death. The release of active IL-18 is independent of caspase-1 activity. Injecting mice

with recombinant Fas-ligand results in hepatic damage, which is IL-18 dependent. However, the same results are observed by Tsutsui et al.[32] Therefore, IL-18 processing seems to take place in the absence of caspase-1.

IL-18 BINDING PROTEIN

IL-18BP is a naturally occurring, secreted protein, which possesses a high-affinity binding to IL-18 (dissociation constant of 400 pM) and therefore neutralizes the biological activity of IL-18.[47,48] IL-18BP is specific for mature IL-18 and does not bind the IL-18 precursor when assessed by ELISA[49] or BiaCore binding.[48] IL-18BP was discovered using ligand affinity chromatography, which had been used to isolate soluble (extracellular domain) receptors for other cytokines,[50,51] including TNF receptors p55 and p75.[52,53] However, IL-18BP is not the soluble receptor for IL-18 and is only distantly related structurally to IL-18Rα.[48] Unlike all members of the IL-1 receptor family, which have three Ig-like domains in the extracellular receptor segment, IL-18BP has only one Ig-like domain. It seems that the transmembrane and the first two extracellular domains of the ancestoral IL-18 receptor were deleted during evolution. The only amino acid identity with the IL-18Rα chain and IL-18BP is found in the third Ig domain of the α chain.[54] There is limited amino acid homology between IL-18BP and the IL-1 receptor type II, also known as the IL-1 decoy receptor. In fact, IL-18 is similar biologically to the IL-1 decoy receptor in that its function is primarily to bind and neutralize the ligand rather than act as a ligand passer.

The human IL-18BP gene is located on chromosome 11q13. Using Northern blot analysis, IL-18BP is highly expressed in spleen and the intestinal tract, both immunologically active tissues. There are four isotypes of human IL-18BP and two isotypes of murine IL-18BP.[47] These isotypes are formed by alternate mRNA splicing of the respective genes. A single copy of IL-18BP exists for humans, mice and rats.[55] Only those isoforms that retain the intact Ig domain are biologically functional by neutralizing IL-18.[48] For example, human IL-18BP has four isotypes termed IL-18BPa, b, c and d. Only IL-18BPa and IL-18BPc have the intact Ig domain and neutralize IL-18.[48] The other two isoforms, although they are produced in humans, do not bind and do not neutralize IL-18. However, the mRNA splicing that creates these isoforms is not a haphazard event in that the spliced mRNA has an open reading frame, which results in the same carboxyl terminal for all isoforms. It is possible that IL-18BP isoform b and d bind another member of the IL-1 family. The mouse has two isoforms, IL-18BPc and IL-18BPd. Murine IL-18BPc and IL-18BPd isoforms, possessing the identical Ig domain, also neutralize >95% murine IL-18. However, murine IL-18BPd, which shares a common C-terminal motif with human IL-18BPa, also neutralizes human IL-18.[48]

The binding sites for IL-1 to the IL-1 receptor type I were used to model the binding of IL-18 to IL-18BP.[48] Modeling predicted a large mixed electrostatic and hydrophobic binding site in the Ig domain of IL-18BP, which could account for its high-affinity binding to the ligand. In the site, the binding of IL-18 glutamic acid at position 35 and lysine at position 89 to oppositely charged amino acids in IL-18BP were thought to participate. If correct, mutations in these amino acids would alter two properties of IL-18: binding to the IL-18Rα chain and binding to IL-18BP. Therefore, biological activity as well as the ability to be neutralized by IL-18BP would be affected. In fact, mutational analysis established that these two amino acids are functionally important for biological activity[54,56] as well as for neutralization.[54]

Seven amino acids of the human IL-18BPa isoform have been mutated to alanine resulting in an 8–750-fold decrease in binding affinity, associated with increased off-rates using BiaCore affinity studies.[57] The mutations were located in the strands that comprise the Ig-like domain.

A divalent fusion protein of human IL-18BP-linked human IgG1 Fc (IL-18BP:Fc) binds and neutralizes human, mouse and rat IL-18 with a dissociation constant of 0.3–5 nM. Using E. coli-derived LPS with a lethal dose of 90%, IL-18BP:Fc administered 10 minutes prior to the LPS significantly reduced mortality.[58] IFNγ levels were also reduced in these mice. Because of the long plasma half-life of Fc fusion protein, IL-18BP:Fc reduced LPS-induced IFNγ when administered 6 days before the LPS challenge. IL-18BP:Fc reduced hepatic injury as well as expression of Fas.[58] IL-18BP:Fc also decreased granuloma formation, macrophage-inflammatory protein-1-α and macrophage-inflammatory protein-2 production. As shown previously using anti-mouse IL-18,[59] IL-18 mediates the hepatic damage caused by intravenously injected Concanavalin-A.[58] Fas ligand expression as well as liver damage induced by Pseudomonas aeruginosa exotoxin A or by anti-Fas agonistic Ab were also reduced by IL-18BP.[58]

Viral IL-18BP: a natural experiment for the importance of IL-18 in inflammatory and immune responses

The human sequence for IL-18BP is found in various members of the pox viruses. The greatest homology is found in Molluscum contagiosum,[47] a common infection of the skin that is characterized by a large number of viral particles in the epithelial cells without a significant presence of inflammatory or immunologically active cells. The viral genes encoding for IL-18BP-like proteins have been expressed and the recombinant proteins neutralize mammalian IL-18 activity.[60] The ability of viral IL-18BP to reduce the activity of mammalian IL-18 may explain the blandness of the inflammatory and immune response of the viral infection. The viral genes encoding for the IL-18BP-like proteins also exhibit signal peptides, N-glycosylation sites and cysteine residues similar to those in human IL-18BP.[61] The ability of human IL-18BP to neutralize human and murine IL-18 was compared to the ability of pox viral IL-18BP to neutralize human and murine IL-18. The dissociation constants of the viral IL-18BP for murine IL-18 were 12–50-fold lower than that for human IL-18.[62]

There are three M. contagiosum genes that are homologous to human IL-18BP: MC54L, MC51L and MC53L. The amino acid identities are in the range 20–35%.[63] MC54L binds and neutralizes human IL-18 and contains five of the seven amino acids that provide stability to the Ig domain of human IL-18BP. However, the mutation in MC54L from a nonconserved valine to phenylalanine increased the affinity of the viral IL-18BP for human IL-18 ten-fold.[63] Although the absolute amino acid sequence identity between MC54L and human IL-18BPa is low, the viral IL-18BP possesses functional binding sites for human IL-18 that are highly similar to those of human IL-18BP. The conclusions of these mutational studies support the concept that viral IL-18BP and specifically the MC54L gene functions as an anti-inflammatory and immunosuppressive product enabling the virus to avoid triggering the host defense mechanisms that target viral elimination.

IL-18BP levels in health and disease

The serum levels of IL-18BP isoform 'a' in a cohort of healthy subjects as determined by a specific ELISA are 2.15 ± 0.15 ng/ml (range 0.5–7 ng/ml).[49] In patients with sepsis and acute renal failure the levels rose to 21.9 ± 1.44 ng/ml (range 4–132 ng/ml) but this rise was due to increased production and not to renal retention since there was no correlation with creatinine levels. Using the law of mass action and knowing the dissociation constant of IL-18BP to IL-18, total IL-18 and free IL-18 were calculated. Total IL-18 in healthy individuals was 64 ± 17 pg/ml and approximately 85% was in the free form.[49] Total IL-18 and IL-18BPa were both elevated in sepsis patients upon admission (1.5 ± 0.4 and 28.6 ± 4.5 ng/ml, respectively). At these levels, most of the IL-18 is bound to IL-18BPa; however, the remaining free IL-18 in sepsis patients is still higher than in healthy individuals. One can conclude from these studies that IL-18BPa considerably inhibits circulating IL-18 in sepsis. Nevertheless, exogenous administration of IL-18BP may further reduce circulating IL-18 activity.

The relative gene expression of the IL-18 neutralizing (a and c isoforms) and non-neutralizing (b and d isoforms) of IL-18BP was studied in Crohn's disease during active phases of the disease.[64] Intestinal endothelial cells and macrophages were the major source of IL-18BP within the submucosa. These findings were similar to those for IL-18BP in cultures of human endothelial cells and peripheral blood monocytes. Gene expression as measured by steady-state mRNA levels for IL-18BP as well as the IL-18BP protein were elevated in intestinal biopsies from patients with active disease.[64] A control group was assessed for comparison. Unbound IL-18BP isoforms a and c and inactive isoform d were present in specimens from patients with active disease as well as from tissues from control patients. The IL-18BP isoform b was not detected.

The regulation of IL-18BP gene expression appears to be via IFNγ.[65] In a human colon carcinoma epithelial cell line, IFNγ induced gene expression and release of IL-18BPa. The increase in IL-18BP was also observed in a variety of intestinal cell lines and in the human keratinocyte cell line HaCaT. The histone deacetylase inhibitor sodium butyrate suppressed IFNγ-induced IL-18BP.[65]

Comparison of soluble IL-18 receptor α and β chains

Although the β chain of IL-18R is required for signaling, the soluble (extracellular) form does not bind IL-18, and its role in inhibiting IL-18 is unclear. Neutralization of IL-18 by soluble receptors was compared with that of IL-18BP. At an equimolar concentration IL-18BP to IL-18, inhibition of 90% of IL-18 activity was observed, whereas a 4-fold molar excess of the soluble IL-18Rα had no effect.[66] A dimeric construct of soluble IL-18R linked to the Fc domain of IgG1 increased IL-18 activity 2.5-fold. In PBMC stimulated with LPS or in whole blood stimulated with *Staphylococcus epidermidis*, 3 nM IL-18BP reduced IFNγ by 80%, whereas IL-18Rα:Fc had no effect. A construct of the soluble IL-18Rβ linked to Fc did not affect IL-18-induced IFNγ even at 80-fold molar excess of IL-18. However, the combination of both soluble receptors reduced IFNγ by 80%. In KG-1 macrophage-like cells, a 50% reduction in IL-18 activity was observed using an 80-fold molar excess of soluble IL-18Rα:Fc but only in the presence of soluble IL-18Rβ:Fc. These studies reveal that the combination of the ligand- and the nonligand-binding extracellular domains of IL-18R is needed to inhibit IL-18, whereas IL-18BP neutralizes at an equimolar concentration.

ROLE OF IL-12 IN THE INDUCTION OF IFNγ BY IL-18

IL-18 as an IFNγ-inducing factor

In general, IL-18 alone does not induce IFNγ. Although IL-12 induces IFNγ, this may be due to the fact that IL-18 is constitutively expressed in human and mouse tissues.[35] Until the discovery of IL-18, the dominant IFNγ-inducing factor from the macrophage was the heterodimeric cytokine IL-12.[67] In some studies, IL-1 can also be shown to augment IFNγ production,[68] but compared to IL-12 and IL-18 the induction of IFNγ is not a dominant biological property of IL-1. Once IL-12 binds to its cell surface receptor, nuclear translocation of 'signal tranducer and activator of transcription' (STAT) 3 and STAT4 takes place triggering promoter regions of the IFNγ gene. Mice deficient in the p40 chain of IL-12 manifest decreased IFNγ production. However, upon closer examination, the induction of IFNγ by IL-12 was, in fact, a co-induction. IL-12 itself induces only a small increase in IFNγ production from primary human CD4+ T-cells;[69] however, in the presence of co-stimulants such as anti-CD3/CD28, mitogens or specific antigens, large amounts of IFNγ are produced. The role of these co-stimulants in IL-12-augmented IFNγ production now appears to be related to activation pathways for the production of IL-18. Until the generation of IL-18-deficient mice,[70] the precise role of IL-18 in endotoxin-induced IFNγ production by IL-12 was uncertain because macrophage (or other cell) production of IL-18 could not be ruled out. As discussed below, little or no IFNγ is produced from mice or cells deficient in IL-18[70] or deficient in caspase-1.[4,5,71] Importantly, the lack of IFNγ production in these experiments takes place with ample IL-12 present.[71] It should be noted here that mitogens such as concanavalin A and phytohemagglutinin induce IFNγ production in caspase-deficient mice.[72]

IL-18 induction of IFNγ is similar to that of IL-12 in that as a sole cytokine, IL-18 induces low levels of IFNγ but, in the presence of co-stimulants, IFNγ production is greatly enhanced. When LPS is used as a co-stimulant, macrophages present in the culture produce IL-18 and it is likely that the endogenous IL-18 acts as the co-factor. In the absence of a co-stimulant, primary human CD4+ T-cells produce a small amount of IFNγ (four-fold increase over background) but in the same cultures IL-12 has no effect.[69] These findings were confirmed using a human IFNγ promoter linked to a luciferase reporter transiently transfected into human CD4+ T-cells. IL-18 alone stimulated strong promoter activity whereas IL-12 only did so when added with the co-stimulants anti-CD3 and anti-CD28. IL-18 appeared to activate the IFNγ promoter at an AP-1 site whereas IL-12 resulted in the binding to a STAT4 site; the combination of a co-stimulant and IL-12 resulted in activation of both sites. By supershift, IL-18 activated the binding of c-jun to the AP-1 site.[69] The conclusions made from these studies resolve basic issues regarding the relative roles of IL-18 and IL-12 in the production of IFNγ in CD4+ primary human T-cells. IFNγ promoter activation can take place by binding of c-jun to the AP-1 site, whereas in the same cells STAT4 binding takes place by IL-12. The activation of AP-1 in the IFNγ promoter is sufficient for IFNγ gene expression and synthesis but IL-12 activation of STAT4 does not trigger the IFNγ promoter unless another signal is provided, such as anti-CD3/anti-CD28.

The synergism between IL-18 and IL-12 for IFNγ production

Although T-cells are the major source of IFNγ, IL-18 and IL-12 act synergistically to increase IFNγ production from murine bone marrow-derived macrophages.[73] Similar to several studies in T-cells, the combination of IL-18 and IL-12 was far more effective in inducing IFNγ from these macrophagic cells than either cytokine alone. In fact, the most consistent conclusion that can be made about IFNγ production is that IL-12 is needed for IL-18-induced IFNγ production and that IL-18 induces IFNγ only when its receptor is unregulated by IL-12. Hence synergism with these two IFNγ-inducing factors is reported in each study to date. There are some exceptions: KG-1 cells[74] and U1 macrophagic cells[16] respond to IL-18 without a need for IL-12 but it is likely that in these cell lines IL-18Rβ is already expressed. However, in primary cells both cytokines are required for IFNγ production.

IFNγ production in IL-18-deficient mice

Mice with a null mutation for IL-18 were preconditioned with *P. acnes* and after 4 days injected with LPS. Circulating levels of IL-18 were not detectable compared to the wild-type controls similarly preconditioned and injected. In another experiment, mice were preconditioned with *P. acnes* for 7 days and then injected with LPS; circulating IFNγ levels in IL-18-deficient mice were one-fifth those in wild-type controls.[70] The levels of IL-12 in the IL-18-deficient mice were nearly the same as in wild-type controls. Hence, IL-18 deficiency is associated with a near but not absolute absence of IFNγ production. These findings are similar to those reported for mice injected with neutralizing antibodies to IL-18[3] and in mice deficient in caspase-1, as discussed above.

IFNγ production in caspase-1-deficient mice

Mice preconditioned with *P. acnes* and then injected with LPS have markedly elevated circulating levels of IFNγ compared to non-preconditioned mice. However, in preconditioned mice deficient in caspase-1, circulating IFNγ was markedly reduced.[4,5] In vitro, production of IFNγ using non-endotoxin stimulants such as zymosan or *Staphylococcus epidermidis* in spleen cells from caspase-1-deficient mice was also significantly decreased (>75%).[71] In the latter case, IL-12 levels were elevated demonstrating the requirement for IL-18 in LPS-induced IFNγ production even in the presence of high levels of IL-12. In contrast to microbial stimulants, mitogen-stimulated IFNγ production was unaffected in spleen cell cultures from caspase-1-deficient mice.[71] In addition to a deficiency in caspase-1, specific inhibitors of caspase-1 added to spleen cell cultures from wild-type mice also produce less IFNγ.[71] Also, antibodies to murine IL-18 suppress LPS-induced IFNγ in vitro.[71]

Other effects of IL-18 on T-cells

IL-18 activates T-cells to synthesize IL-2, GM-CSF and TNFα. There are also reports that IL-18 suppresses the production of IL-10 and does not induce the production of IL-1Ra. In general, the ability of IL-18 to induce different cytokines depends on the cellular targets. Mouse spleen cells and human PBMC are mixed populations of T-cells and monocytic cells. Frequently used, freshly obtained human PBMC are mostly (70–80%) T-cells. Of these, approximately 50% are CD4[+] cells. The percentage of monocytes in PBMC populations varies from 10 to 30%. In addition, there are NK cells and some basophils but, in general, PBMC are predominantly T-cells. Therefore, the response of PBMC to IL-18 should be made using cultures of selected cells. Each cell type is separated using magnetic beads coated with specific antibodies. In PBMC stimulated with IL-18 for 24 hours, the production of cytokines IL-1β, TNFα and IL-8 is observed but, in fact, the cell that responds to the IL-18 is the resting T-cell and the NK cell.[75]

Role of IL-18 in NK activity

IFNγ is the dominant cytokine activating NK for killing various tumor cells and therefore, not surprisingly, stimulation of NK cells with exogenous IL-18 enhances NK activity.[3,7,76] Endogenous NK activity, however, is reduced but not absent in IL-18-deficient mice.[70] Intraperitoneal administration of exogenous IL-18 to these IL-18-deficient mice not only restored NK function but also actually enhanced the lytic activity over that of the wild-type control. The combination of IL-18 and IL-12 increased NK activity in both knockout as well as wild-type controls.[70] The enhancement of NK activity by exogenous IL-18 in the IL-18R-deficient mice was due to an increase in gene expression of IL-18Rβ, which was particularly elevated in mice preconditioned with *P. acnes*. IL-12 was also administered to IL-18-deficient mice in an attempt to restore NK activity. At 5 and 10 ng/mouse no increase in NK activity was observed in the IL-18-deficient mice, but after 2 days of 100 ng of IL-12 per mouse (8000 ng/kg) spleen cell NK activity was equal to that of the wild-type mice. These latter results suggest that at high doses of exogenous IL-12 NK activity can be restored in IL-18-deficient mice. These results are somewhat difficult to reconcile with the finding that NK activity in IL-18-deficient mice is only one-third that of the wild-type mice despite the same level of IL-12 production in both mouse strains.

Th1 responses and IL-18

The role of IL-18 in the Th1 response has been studied primarily in T-cells from the BALB/C mouse strain. Subsets of T-cells exhibit a differential responsiveness to IFNγ production by IL-12. This seems to be due to a reciprocal regulation of the IL-12 receptor β2 chain, in that IL-4 suppresses the expression of this receptor whereas IFNγ increases its expression and counteracts the inhibitory effect of IL-4.[77] Since the BALB/C mouse strain is a high producer of IL-4, it tends to develop a Th2 response to various antigens. In BALB/C mice, IL-18 is clearly a cofactor with IL-12 for the development of the Th1 response. This is likely because of the IFNγ-inducing nature of IL-18. In contrast, C57BL6 mice do not exhibit a requirement for IL-18 for the development of the Th1 response. Any role of IL-18 in the Th1 response appears to be via the production of IFNγ, which counters the suppressive effect of IL-4 on the expression of the IL-12Rβ2 chain. The addition of anti-IL-4 antibodies reduces the effect of IL-18 presumably because the requirement for IFNγ is reduced.[20]

Using ovalbumin-sensitized T-cell receptor overexpressing CD4 cells, Robinson et al demonstrated that IL-18 potentiated the IL-12-induced development of the Th1 response by measuring increased production of IFNγ after 48 hours.[20] This observation of IL-12 synergy with IL-18 is consistent with the observations of others who claimed that IL-18 alone was able to drive the Th1 response independent of IL-12.[3,78] However, it is unlikely that the effect of IL-18 in those studies was truly without IL-12 because the presence of small numbers of macrophages could have contributed IL-12 in the culture. However, in a macrophage-free culture where endogenous IL-12 production was excluded, a marked synergism was observed with IL-12 and IL-18 in both BALB/C and C57BL6 mice.[20] The addition of IL-18 in the secondary stimulation of T-cells revealed that the Th1 response can take place in the absence of IL-12.

It seems consistent with the current studies to conclude that there is an absolute requirement for IL-12 in the developing Th1 response. It is well established that IL-12 induces naive CD4+ cells to develop into Th1 cells by their ability to secrete IFNγ. On the other hand, IL-18 itself does not shift naive T-cells into the Th1 phenotype. Although one can propose that in both in vivo and in vitro settings small amounts of IL-18 are co-produced, IL-12-driven development of naive T-cells into Th1 cells was observed in mice deficient in IL-18.[70]

IL-12 increases the responsiveness to IL-18 via an increase in IL-18Rα and IL-18Rβ chain expression

The hallmark of IL-18 induction of IFNγ is the near absolute requirement for a second signal provided by LPS and other stimuli, but particularly by IL-12. Since these other stimuli are themselves inducers of IL-12, it is likely that IFNγ production is the result of an IL-18/IL-12 effect. In general, in mouse and human cells, IL-12 itself even at nanomolar concentrations does not induce IFNγ, but in the presence of low picomolar concentrations of IL-12, IL-18 becomes essential for the production of IFNγ. This has been shown using LPS induction of IFNγ in caspase-1-deficient mice[71] and in mice deficient in IL-18.[70] In both models, IL-12 is present in normal to even high levels. However, in IL-12-deficient mice, IFNγ production is also absent. The explanation for these observations is that IL-12 is needed to upregulate the receptor for IL-18.

Initial studies indicated that there was increased responsiveness to IL-18 following exposure of T-cells to IL-12 in Th1-committed clones.[79] Data clearly demonstrate that IL-12 increases gene expression and surface expression of the IL-18Rα chain.[12] In cells not responsive to IL-18 but expressing the IL-18Rα chain, transfection of the IL-18Rβ chain restores responsiveness to IL-18.[80] The effect of IL-12 on IL-18 responsiveness is, in fact, due to upregulation of both chains of the IL-18R.[80] Both chains increase steady-state mRNA in a time- and concentration-dependent fashion.

IL-12 and IL-18 have different signaling pathways in Th1 cells

IL-12 binding to its specific receptors triggers a cascade of phosphorylations of which nuclear translocation of two transcription factors STAT3 and STAT4 takes place.[81] IL-12-deficient and STAT4-deficient mice have an impaired Th1 response.[82,83] Unlike IL-12, IL-18 does not activate STAT4. In fact, using a supershift assay, IL-18 on Th1 clones does not appear to activate any of the STAT transcription factors associated with Th1 development.[20] Using transfection with the IFNγ promoter linked to a luciferase reporter, IL-18 directly induced IFNγ promoter activity,[69] whereas for IL-12 activation of this promoter, co-stimulation with anti-CD3 was required. Either IL-12 or IL-18 plus anti-CD3 activated 'activation protein-1' (AP-1). Mutation of the AP-1 site reduced both IL-12 and IL-18-mediated promoter activity. However, mutation of the STAT4 site only affected IL-12 activity. The conclusions of these studies suggest that both AP-1 and STAT4 sites are required for IL-12-dependent IFNγ promoter activity but IL-18 induces a direct activation pathway via the AP-1 site.

ROLE OF IL-18 IN MODELS OF AUTOIMMUNE DISEASE

Models of arthritis

Studies were carried out using SCW-induced arthritis.[84] Using C57BL/6 or BALB/c mice, a neutralizing rabbit anti-murine IL-18 antibody was injected shortly before induction of arthritis by intra-articular injection of SCW fragments into the right knee joint. Significant (>60%) suppression of joint swelling was noted on days 1 and 2 of SCW arthritis after blockade of endogenous IL-18 and joint TNFα and IL-1 levels were also decreased. Severe inhibition of chondrocyte proteoglycan synthesis is a prominent component of SCW-induced arthritis but a near complete reversal of the inhibition of chondrocyte proteoglycan synthesis was observed in the anti-IL-18-treated animals. Although these studies clearly established the pathological role for endogenous IL-18 in this model, the effect of IL-18 is apparently independent of IFNγ since mice deficient in IFNγ showed similar results using anti-IL-18 antibodies.[84]

IL-18 also plays a role in CIA. IL-18 was injected into DBA-1 mice immunized with collagen in incomplete Freund's adjuvant. There was an increase in the erosive and inflammatory component of the arthritis.[85] Using mice deficient in IL-18, CIA was less severe compared to wild-type controls.[86] Histologically, there was evidence of decreased joint inflammation and the destructive component of the model. Levels of bovine collagen-induced IFNγ, TNFα, IL-6 and IL-12 from spleen cell cultures were decreased in IL-18-deficient mice. However, there was a significant reduction in serum anti-collagen antibody levels in the IL-18-deficient mice, raising the perennial issue that gene deletions on immunologically active cytokines can obscure the role of a cytokine in CIA. Nevertheless, from these studies, there is likely a pathological role for IL-18 in CIA.

Other studies in CIA used wild-type DBA-1 mice treated with either neutralizing antibodies to IL-18 or IL-18BP after clinical onset of disease. The therapeutic efficacy of neutralizing endogenous IL-18 was assessed using different pathological parameters of disease progression. The clinical severity in mice undergoing CIA was significantly reduced after treatment with either IL-18-neutralizing antibodies or IL-18BP.[1] Attenuation of the disease was associated with reduced cartilage erosion evident on histology. The decreased cartilage degradation was further documented by a significant reduction in the levels of circulating cartilage oligomeric matrix protein (an indicator of cartilage turnover). Both strategies efficiently slowed disease progression, but only anti-IL-18 antibody treatment significantly decreased an established synovitis. Serum levels of IL-6 were significantly reduced with both neutralizing strategies. In vitro, neutralizing IL-18 resulted in a significant inhibition of TNF-α, IL-6 and IFNγ secretion by macrophages.[1]

Models of inflammatory bowel disease

Several studies have shown that IL-18 is expressed in the affected intestinal tissues of patients with Crohn's disease.[87–90] In general, the cytokine is found in both intestinal epithelial cells as well as in the mononuclear cells of the lamina propria cells. The finding of constitutively expressed IL-18 in intestinal mucosa is not unusual since epithelial cells express IL-18 in health. However, there seems to be a pathological role in the expression of IL-18 in the mononuclear cell population in this disease. As with all cytokine-associated diseases, the role of IL-18 in inflammatory bowel disease is best revealed using specific blockade as described below.

The role of IL-18 was examined in intestinal inflammation using a neutralizing anti-murine IL-18 antiserum in dextran sulfate sodium (DSS)-induced colitis in either BALB/c or C57BL/6 mice.[91] Using increasing doses or oral DSS, levels of colonic IL-18 increased parallel with clinical worsening. With the use of confocal laser microscopy, the increased IL-18 was localized to the intestinal epithelial layer. Anti-IL-18 antibody treatment resulted in a dose-dependent reduction of the severity of colitis in both BALB/c and C57BL/6 mice. Colon shortening following DSS-induced colitis, a marker of severity in this model, was partially prevented in the anti-IL-18 treatment groups. In the colon tissue homogenates, IFNγ concentrations were lower in the anti-IL-18-treated DSS-fed mice compared with untreated DSS-fed mice. This suppressive effect of anti-IL-18 administered in vivo was also observed on spontaneous TNFα, IL-18 and IFNγ

production from ex vivo colon organ cultures. Similar to spleen cells, the stimulation of lamina propria mononuclear cells by IL-18 plus IL-12 resulted in a synergistic increase in IFNγ synthesis. Using this model, IL-18 appears to be a pivotal mediator in experimental colitis.

The role of IL-18 was also studied in the trinitrobenzene sulfonic acid (TNBS)-induced colitis model in which the activity of endogenous IL-18 was neutralized using human IL-18BP isoform 'a'.[92] Daily injection of IL-18BP resulted in less severe clinical score, less body weight loss and a stabilization of colon weight when compared with saline-treated mice. In IL-18BP-treated mice, the intensity of the colitis as assessed histologically was reduced. Similar to anti-IL-18 antibody treatment in DSS-induced colitis, there was a decrease in colonic levels of TNFα, IL-6 and IL-1β in mice treated with IL-18BP. However, there was no reduction in IFNγ levels in these same tissues, a finding which contrasts with the effect of anti-IL-18 antibody treatment in DSS-induced colitis.

The systemic administration of daily injections of IL-12 plus IL-18 to BALB/c mice results in a severe wasting syndrome with intestinal inflammation and fatty liver.[93] Intestinal mucosal inflammation is prominent in this model with bloody diarrhea and weight loss. There are high levels of serum IFNγ in these mice associated with elevated serum NO levels. In mice deficient in inducible NO, the disease failed to develop. Moreover, the disease was also induced in mice deficient in Fas. The disease did not develop in mice deficient in IFNγ.

In this study, IL-18 is strongly expressed by intestinal epithelial cells in a murine model of Crohn's disease which takes place by the transfer of a population of CD62+ and CD4+ T-cells into SCID mice. The activity of endogenous IL-18 was reduced using an adenovirus expressing IL-18 antisense mRNA.[94] Local administration of the anti-sense adenovirus to mice with established colitis resulted in expression of the vector in the intestinal epithelial cells. In these mice there was a reduction in the severity of the colitis as assessed histologically. In addition, IFNγ production from mucosal but not spleen cells was observed with the use of the anti-sense adenovirus.

In acute DSS-induced colitis, mice deficient in caspase-1 exhibited a greater than 50% decrease of the clinical scores of weight loss, diarrhea, rectal bleeding and colon length, whereas daily treatment with IL-1 receptor antagonist revealed a modest reduction in colitis severity.[95] To further characterize the function of caspase-1 and its role in intestinal inflammation, chronic colitis was induced over a 30-day time period. During this chronic time course, caspase-1-deficient mice exhibited a near complete protection, as reflected by significantly reduced clinical scores and almost absent histological signs of colitis. Consistently, colon shortening occurred only in DSS-exposed wild-type mice but not in caspase-1-deficient mice. Protection was accompanied by reduced spontaneous release of the proinflammatory cytokines IL-18, IL-1β and IFNγ from total colon cultures. In addition, flow cytometric analysis of isolated mesenteric lymph node cells revealed evidence of reduced cell activation in caspase-1-deficient mice as evaluated by surface expression of CD3, CD69 and CD4/CD25.

IL-18 in models of brain inflammation

Since IL-1 is a sleep-inducing factor, IL-18 was examined for its ability to induce sleep in rats and rabbits.[96] IL-18 injected intracerebroventricularly into rabbits increased non-rapid eye movement sleep. The sleep effects of IL-18 introduced directly into the brain coincided with increases in brain temperature.[96] Similar results were obtained after intracerebroventricular injection of IL-18 into rats. Intraperitoneal IL-18 failed to induce fever in mice[97] and rats.[96] Anti-human IL-18 antibody significantly attenuated muramyl dipeptide-induced sleep. These data are consistent with a role for IL-18 in mechanisms of sleep responses to infection.

In caspase-1-deficient mice, experimental autoimmune encephalomyelitis was studied.[98] This is the animal model for multiple sclerosis. Steady-state levels of caspase-1 are elevated in this model and correlate with disease severity as well as the upregulation of cytokines such as TNFα, IL-1β, IL-6 and IFNγ. In caspase-1-deficient mice, there was a reduction in the severity of the disease, although this was dependent on the amount of the encephalitogenic myelin oligodendrocyte glycoprotein antigen used to induce the disease. The administration of the tetrapeptide inhibitor of caspase-1 to mice with the developed disease did not alter the severity index, although pretreatment was effective. It was concluded that inhibition of caspase-1, perhaps via reduction in the processing of the IL-1β as well as the IL-18 precursors, is a potential treatment possibility for relapsing remitting multiple sclerosis. The importance of IFNγ in brain inflammation is supported by studies in mice showing a spontaneous neurodegenerative disease using overexpression of IFNγ in the brain with a glial promoter.[99]

Jander et al studied the expression of caspase-1 and IL-18 in focal brain ischemia induced in rats either by permanent middle cerebral artery occlusion or by photothrombosis of cortical microvessels. In this study,[100] steady-state IL-18 mRNA levels increased starting at 48 hours after the injury and reached maximal levels from day 7 to day 14. Similar to other studies using the same model,[101,102] IL-1β was upregulated within a few hours after the injury.[100] IL-18 was expressed on microglia surrounding the necrotic lesion, although these were likely macrophages from the blood as well as CNS microglia. These studies are consistent with a delayed expression of IL-18 in focal brain ischemia.

Models of hepatic injury

The administration of Con A or of *Pseudomonas aeruginosa* exotoxin A (PEA) results in an acute hepatic injury. In both models, leptin-deficient (ob/ob) mice were protected from liver damage and showed lower induction of TNFα and IL-18 compared with their lean littermates.[59] Neutralization of TNFα reduced induction of IL-18 by either Con A (70% reduction) or PEA (40% reduction). Pretreatment of lean mice with either soluble TNF receptors or with an anti-IL-18 antiserum significantly reduced Con A- and

PEA-induced liver damage. The simultaneous neutralization of TNFα and IL-18 fully protected the mice against liver toxicity. However, neutralization of either IL-18 or TNFα did not inhibit Con A-induced production of IFNγ.[59] Thymus atrophy and alterations in the number of circulating lymphocytes and monocytes were observed in ob/ob mice. Exogenous leptin replacement restored the responsiveness of ob/ob mice to Con A and normalized their lymphocyte and monocyte populations. These results demonstrate that leptin deficiency leads to reduced production of TNFα and IL-18 associated with reduced T-cell-mediated hepatotoxicity. In addition, both TNFα and IL-18 appear to be essential mediators of T-cell-mediated liver injury.

The daily injection of IL-12 plus IL-18 results in prominent intestinal mucosal inflammation and fatty liver changes.[93] The effects on the liver, however, are both IFNγ and NO dependent. Administration of recombinant soluble Fas ligand to mice preconditioned with *P. acnes* induced elevated serum liver enzyme levels. This Fas-ligand-induced liver injury did not develop in IL-18-deficient mice. The disease also did not develop in caspase-1-deficient mice.[32]

Table 16.2 lists the role of IL-18 in various disease processes using specific neutralization of IL-18 by either anti-IL-18 antiserum or IL-18BP.

Table 16.2   Reduction in disease severity reported with neutralization of endogenous IL-18.

DSS-induced colitis
TNBS-induced colitis
CD69 transfer-induced colitis
Streptococcal wall-induced arthritis
Collagen-induced arthritis
Con-A-induced hepatitis
Pseudomonas exotoxin-A-induced hepatitis damage
IL-12-induced intestinal inflammation
LPS-induced hepatic necrosis
LPS-induced lethality
LPS-induced pulmonary neutrophils
Melanoma hepatic metastasis
Melanoma-induced VCAM-1 expression
Ischemia-induced acute renal failure
Ischemia-induced myocardial dysfunction
LPS-induced myocardial dysfunction

In addition, the IL-18-deficient mouse or the mouse deficient in the IL-18Rα chain have been used.

REFERENCES

1. Plater-Zyberk C, Joosten LA, Helsen MM et al. Therapeutic effect of neutralizing endogenous IL-18 activity in the collagen-induced model of arthritis. *J Clin Invest* 2001; **108**: 1825–32.
2. Nakamura K, Okamura H, Wada M et al. Endotoxin-induced serum factor that stimulates gamma inteferon production. *Infect Immun* 1989; **57**: 590–5.
3. Okamura H, Nagata K, Komatsu T et al. A novel costimulatory factor for gamma interferon induction found in the livers of mice causes endotoxic shock. *Infect Immun* 1995; **63**: 3966–72.
4. Gu Y, Kuida K, Tsutsui H et al. Activation of interferon-γ inducing factor mediated by interleukin-1β converting enzyme. *Science* 1997; **275**: 206–9.

5. Ghayur T, Banerjee S, Hugunin M et al. Caspase-1 processes IFN-gamma-inducing factor and regulates LPS-induced IFN-gamma production. *Nature* 1997; **386**: 619–23.
6. Fantuzzi G, Zheng H, Faggioni R et al. Effect of endotoxin in IL-1β-deficient mice. *J Immunol* 1996; **157**: 291–6.
7. Okamura H, Tsutsui H, Komatsu T et al. Cloning of a new cytokine that induces interferon-γ. *Nature* 1995; **378**: 88–91.
8. Netea MG, Fantuzzi G, Kullberg BJ et al. Neutralization of IL-18 reduces neutrophil tissue accumulation and protects mice against lethal Escherichia coli and Salmonella typhimurium endotoxemia. *J Immunol* 2000; **164**: 2644–9.

9. Torigoe K, Ushio S, Okura T et al. Purification and characterization of the human interleukin-18 receptor. *J Biol Chem* 1997; **272**: 25737–42.

10. Parnet P, Garka KE, Bonnert TP et al. IL-1Rrp is a novel receptor-like molecule similar to the type I interleukin-1 receptor and its homologues T1/ST2 and IL-1R AcP. *J Biol Chem* 1996; **271**: 3967–70.

11. Born TL, Thomassen E, Bird TA, Sims JE. Cloning of a novel receptor subunit, AcPL, required for interleukin-18 signaling. *J Biol Chem* 1998; **273**: 29445–50.

12. Yoshimoto T, Takeda K, Tanaka T et al. IL-12 upregulates IL-18 receptor expression on T cells, Th1 cells and B cells: synergism with IL-18 for IFNγ production. *J Immunol* 1998; **161**: 3400–7.

13. Adachi O, Kawai T, Takeda K et al. Targeted disruption of the MyD88 gene results in loss of IL-1- and IL-18-mediated function. *Immunity* 1998; **9**: 143–50.

14. Medzhitov R, Preston-Hurlburt P, Kopp E et al. MyD88 is an adaptor protein in the hToll/IL-1 receptor family signaling pathways. *Mol Cell* 1998; **2**: 253–8.

15. Yin L, Wu L, Wesche H et al. Defective lymphotoxin-beta receptor-induced NF-kappaB transcriptional activity in NIK-deficient mice. *Science* 2001; **291**: 2162–5.

16. Shapiro L, Puren AJ, Barton HA et al. Interleukin-18 stimulates HIV type 1 in monocytic cells. *Proc Natl Acad Sci USA* 1998; **95**: 12550–5.

17. Thomassen E, Bird TA, Renshaw BR et al. Binding of interleukin-18 to the interleukin-1 receptor homologous receptor IL-1Rrp1 leads to activation of signaling pathways similar to those used by interleukin-1. *J Interferon Cytokine Res* 1998; **18**: 1077–88.

18. Kanakaraj P, Ngo K, Wu Y et al. Defective interleukin (IL)-18-mediated natural killer and T helper cell type 1 responses in IL-1 receptor-associated kinase (IRAK)-deficient mice. *J Exp Med* 1999; **189**: 1129–38.

19. Kojima H, Takeuchi M, Ohta T et al. Interleukin-18 activates the IRAK-TRAF6 pathway in mouse EL-4 cells. *Biochem Biophys Res Commun* 1998; **244**: 183–6.

20. Robinson D, Shibuya K, Mui A et al. IGIF does not drive Th1 development but synergizes with IL-12 for interferon-γ production and activates IRAK and NFκB. *Immunity* 1997; **7**: 571–81.

21. Suzuki N, Suzuki S, Duncan GS et al. Severe impairment of interleukin-1 and Toll-like receptor signalling in mice lacking IRAK-4. *Nature* 2002; **416**: 750–6.

22. Croston GE, Cao Z, Goeddel DV. NFkB activation by interleukin-1 requires an IL-1 receptor-associated protein kinase activity. *J Biol Chem* 1995; **270**: 16514–17.

23. Wesche H, Korherr C, Kracht M et al. The interleukin-1 receptor accessory protein is essential for IL-1-induced activation of interleukin-1 receptor-associated kinase (IRAK) and stress-activated protein kinases (SAP kinases). *J Biol Chem* 1997; **272**: 7727–31.

24. Huang J, Gao X, Li S, Cao Z. Recruitment of IRAK to the interleukin 1 receptor complex requires interleukin 1 receptor accessory protein. *Proc Natl Acad Sci USA* 1997; **94**: 12829–32.

25. Cao Z. Signal transduction of interleukin-1. *Eur Cytokine Netw* 1998; **9**: 378 (abs).

26. Cao Z, Xiong J, Takeuchi M et al. Interleukin-1 receptor activating kinase. *Nature* 1996; **383**: 443–6.

27. Malinin NL, Boldin MP, Kovalenko AV, Wallach D. MAP3K-related kinase involved in NF-kappaB induction by TNF, CD95 and IL-1. *Nature* 1997; **385**: 540–4.

28. DiDonato JA, Hayakawa M, Rothwarf DM. A cytokine-responsive I kappaB kinase that activates the transcription factor NF-kappaB. *Nature* 1997; **388**: 548–54.

29. Lomaga MA, Yeh WC, Sarosi I et al. TRAF6 deficiency results in osteopetrosis and defective interleukin-1, CD40, and LPS signaling. *Genes Dev* 1999; **13**: 1015–24.

30. Freshney NW, Rawlinson L, Guesdon F et al. Interleukin-1 activates a novel protein cascade that results in the phosphorylation of hsp27. *Cell* 1994; **78**: 1039–49.

31. Kracht M, Truong O, Totty NF et al. Interleukin-1a activates two forms of p54α mitogen-activated proetin kinase in rabbit liver. *J Exp Med* 1994; **180**: 2017–27.

32. Tsutsui H, Kayagaki N, Kuida K et al. Caspase-1-independent, Fas/Fas ligand-mediated IL-18 secretion from macrophages causes acute liver injury in mice. *Immunity* 1999; **11**: 359–67.

33. Sareneva T, Matikainen S, Kurimoto M, Julkunen I. Influenza A virus-induced IFN-alpha/beta and IL-18 synergistically enhance IFN-gamma gene expression in human T cells. *J Immunol* 1998; **160**: 6032–8.

34. Perregaux D, Barberia J, Lanzetti AJ et al. IL-1β maturation: evidence that mature cytokine

formation can be induced specifically by nigercin. *J Immunol* 1992; **149**: 1294–303.

35. Puren AJ, Fantuzzi G, Dinarello CA. Gene expression, synthesis and secretion of IL-1β and IL-18 are differentially regulated in human blood mononuclear cells and mouse spleen cells. *Proc Natl Acad Sci USA* 1999; **96**: 2256–61.

36. Thompson GJ, Langlais C, Cain K et al. Elevated extracellular K inhibits death-receptor and chemical-mediated apoptosis prior to caspase activation and cytochrome c release. *Biochem J* 2001; **357**: 137–45.

37. Ferrari D, Chiozzi P, Falzoni S et al. Extracellular ATP triggers IL-1 beta release by activating the purinergic P2Z receptor of human macrophages. *J Immunol* 1997; **159**: 1451–8.

38. Buell G, Chessell IP, Michel AD et al. Blockade of human P2X7 receptor function with a monoclonal antibody. *Blood* 1998; **92**: 3521–8.

39. Perregaux DG, Gabel CA. Post-translational processing of murine IL-1: evidence that ATP-induced release of IL-1 alpha and IL-1 beta occurs via a similar mechanism. *J Immunol* 1998; **160**: 2469–77.

40. Perregaux DG, McNiff P, Laliberte R et al. ATP acts as an agonist to promote stimulus-induced secretion of IL-1 beta and IL-18 in human blood. *J Immunol* 2000; **165**: 4615–23.

41. Solle M, Labasi J, Perregaux DG et al. Altered cytokine production in mice lacking P2X(7) receptors. *J Biol Chem* 2001; **276**: 125–32.

42. Gardella S, Andrei C, Costigliolo S et al. Interleukin-18 synthesis and secretion by dendritic cells are modulated by interaction with antigen-specific T cells. *J Leukoc Biol* 1999; **66**: 237–41.

43. Gardella S, Andrei C, Poggi A et al. Control of interleukin-18 secretion by dendritic cells: role of calcium influxes. *FEBS Lett* 2000; **481**: 245–8.

44. Andrei C, Dazzi C, Lotti L et al. The secretory route of the leaderless protein interleukin 1beta involves exocytosis of endolysosome-related vesicles. *Mol Biol Cell* 1999; **10**: 1463–75.

45. Coeshott C, Ohnemus C, Pilyavskaya A et al. Converting enzyme-independent release of TNFα and IL-1β from a stimulated human monocytic cell line in the presence of activated neutrophils or purified proteinase-3. *Proc Natl Acad Sci USA* 1999; **96**: 6261–6.

46. Sugawara S, Uehara A, Nochi T et al. Neutrophil proteinase 3-mediated induction of bioactive IL-18 secretion by human oral epithelial cells. *J Immunol* 2001; **167**: 6568–75.

47. Novick D, Kim S-H, Fantuzzi G et al. Interleukin-18 binding protein: a novel modulator of the Th1 cytokine response. *Immunity* 1999; **10**: 127–36.

48. Kim S-H, Eisenstein M, Reznikov L et al. Structural requirements of six naturally occurring isoforms of the interleukin-18 binding protein to inhibit interleukin-18. *Proc Natl Acad Sci USA* 2000; **97**: 1190–5.

49. Novick D, Schwartsburd B, Pinkus R et al. A novel IL-18BP ELISA shows elevated serum il-18bp in sepsis and extensive decrease of free IL-18. *Cytokine* 2001; **14**: 334–42.

50. Novick D, Engelmann H, Wallach D, Rubinstein M. Soluble cytokine receptors are present in normal human urine. *J Exp Med* 1989; **170**: 1409–14.

51. Novick D, Engelmann H, Wallach D et al. Purification of soluble cytokine receptors from normal human urine by ligand-affinity and immunoaffinity chromatography. *J Chromat* 1990; **510**: 331–7.

52. Engelmann H, Aderka D, Rubinstein M et al. A tumor necrosis factor-binding protein purified to homogeneity from human urine protects cells from tumor necrosis factor toxicity. *J Biol Chem* 1989; **264**: 11974–80.

53. Engelmann H, Novick D, Wallach D. Two tumor necrosis factor-binding proteins purified from human urine. Evidence for immunological cross-reactivity with cell surface tumor necrosis factor receptors. *J Biol Chem* 1990; **265**: 1531–6.

54. Kim SH, Azam T, Novick D et al. Identification of amino acid residues critical for biological activity in human interleukin-18. *J Biol Chem* 2002; **14**: 14.

55. Im SH, Kim SH, Azam T et al. Rat interleukin-18 binding protein: cloning, expression, and characterization. *J Interferon Cytokine Res* 2002; **22**: 321–8.

56. Kim SH, Azam T, Yoon DY et al. Site-specific mutations in the mature form of human IL-18 with enhanced biological activity and decreased neutralization by IL-18 binding protein. *Proc Natl Acad Sci USA* 2001; **98**: 3304–9.

57. Xiang Y, Moss B. Determination of the functional epitopes of human interleukin-18-binding protein by site-directed mutagenesis. *J Biol Chem* 2001; **276**: 17380–6.

58. Faggioni R, Cattley RC, Guo J et al. IL-18-binding protein protects against lipopolysaccharide-induced lethality and prevents the development of Fas/Fas ligand-mediated models of liver disease in mice. *J Immunol* 2001; **167**: 5913–20.

59. Faggioni R, Jones-Carson J, Reed DA et al. Leptin-

deficient (ob/ob) mice are protected from T cell-mediated hepatotoxicity: role of tumor necrosis factor alpha and IL-18. *Proc Natl Acad Sci USA* 2000; **97**: 2367–72.

60. Xiang Y, Moss B. IL-18 binding and inhibition of interferon gamma induction by human poxvirus-encoded proteins. *Proc Natl Acad Sci USA* 1999; **96**: 11537–42.

61. Xiang Y, Moss B. Identification of human and mouse homologs of the MC51L-53L-54L family of secreted glycoproteins encoded by the Molluscum contagiosum poxvirus. *Virology* 1999; **257**: 297–302.

62. Calderara S, Xiang Y, Moss B. Orthopoxvirus IL-18 binding proteins: affinities and antagonist activities. *Virology* 2001; **279**: 22–6.

63. Xiang Y, Moss B. Correspondence of the functional epitopes of poxvirus and human interleukin-18-binding proteins. *J Virol* 2001; **75**: 9947–54.

64. Corbaz A, ten Hove T, Herren S et al. IL-18-binding protein expression by endothelial cells and macrophages is up-regulated during active Crohn's disease. *J Immunol* 2002; **168**: 3608–16.

65. Paulukat J, Bosmann M, Nold M et al. Expression and release of IL-18 binding protein in response to IFN-gamma. *J Immunol* 2001; **167**: 7038–43.

66. Reznikov LL, Kim SH, Zhou L et al. The combination of soluble IL-18Rα and IL-18Rβ chains inhibits IL-18-induced IFN-γ. *J Interferon Cytokine Res* 2002; **22**: 593–601.

67. Trinchieri G. Interleukin-12: a proinflammatory cytokine with immuno-regulatory functions that bridge innate resistance and antigen-specific adaptive immunity. *Ann Rev Immunol* 1995; **13**: 251–74.

68. Hunter CA, Chizzonite R, Remington JS. IL-1b is required for IL-12 to induce the production of IFN-γ by NK cells. *J Immunol* 1995; **155**: 4347–54.

69. Barbulescu K, Becker C, Schlaak JF et al. IL-12 and IL-18 differentially regulate the transcriptional activity of the human IFN-γ promotor in primary CD4+ T lymphocytes. *J Immunol* 1998; **160**: 3642–7.

70. Takeda K, Tsutsui H, Yoshimoto T et al. Defective NK cell activity and Th1 response in IL-18-deficient mice. *Immunity* 1998; **8**: 383–90.

71. Fantuzzi G, Puren AJ, Harding MW et al. IL-18 regulation of IFN-γ production and cell proliferation as revealed in interleukin-1β converting enzyme-deficient mice. *Blood* 1998; **91**: 2118–25.

72. Fantuzzi G, Reed DA, Dinarello CA. IL-12-induced IFNγ is dependent on caspase-1 processing of the IL-18 precursor. *J Clin Invest* 1999; **104**: 761–7.

73. Munder M, Mallo M, Eichmann K, Modolell M. Murine macrophages secrete interferon gamma upon combined stimulation with interleukin (IL)-12 and IL-18: a novel pathway of autocrine macrophage activation. *J Exp Med* 1998; **187**: 2103–8.

74. Ohtsuki T, Micallef MJ, Kohno K et al. Interleukin-18 enhances Fas ligand expression and induces apoptosis in Fas-expressing human myelomonocytic KG-1 cells. *Anticancer Res* 1997; **17**: 3253–8.

75. Puren AJ, Fantuzzi G, Gu Y et al. Interleukin-18 (IFN-γ-inducing factor) induces IL-1β and IL-8 via TNFα production from non-CD14+ human blood mononuclear cells. *J Clin Invest* 1998; **101**: 711–24.

76. Ushio S, Namba M, Okura T et al. Cloning of the cDNA for human IFN-γ-inducing factor, expression in Escherichia coli, and studies on the biologic activities of the protein. *J Immunol* 1996; **156**: 4274–9.

77. Szabo S, Dighe AS, Gubler U, Murphy KM. Regulation of the interleukin-12Rb2 subunit expression in developing T helper (Th1) and Th2 cells. *J Exp Med* 1997; **185**: 817–24.

78. Micallef MJ, Tanimoto T, Kohno K et al. Interleukin-18 induces the sequential activation of natural killer cells and cytotoxic T lymphocytes to protect syngeneic mice from transplantation with Meth A sarcoma. *Cancer Res* 1997; **57**: 4557–63.

79. Kohno K, Kataoka J, Ohtsuki T et al. IFN-γ-inducing factor (IGIF) is a co-stimulatory factor on the activation of Th1 but not Th2 cells and exerts its effect independently of IL-12. *J Immunol* 1997; **158**: 1541–50.

80. Kim SH, Reznikov LL, Stuyt RJ et al. Functional reconstitution and regulation of IL-18 activity by the IL-18R beta chain. *J Immunol* 2001; **166**: 148–54.

81. Jacobson NG, Szabo SJ, Weber-Nordt RM et al. Interleukin 12 signaling in T helper type 1 (Th1) cells involves tyrosine phosphorylation of signal transducer and activator of transcription (Stat)3 and Stat4. *J Exp Med* 1995; **181**: 1755–62.

82. Kaplan MH, Sun YL, Hoey T, Grusby MJ. Impaired IL-12 responses and enhanced development of Th2 cells in Stat4-deficient mice. *Nature* 1996; **382**: 174–7.

83. Thierfelder WE, van Deursen JM, Yamamoto K et al. Requirement for Stat4 in interleukin-12-

mediated responses of natural killer and T cells. *Nature* 1996; **382**: 171–4.

84. Joosten LA, van De Loo FA, Lubberts E et al. An IFN-gamma-independent proinflammatory role of IL-18 in murine streptococcal cell wall arthritis. *J Immunol* 2000; **165**: 6553–8.

85. Gracie JA, Forsey RJ, Chan WL et al. A proinflammatory role for IL-18 in rheumatoid arthritis. *J Clin Invest* 1999; **104**: 1393–401.

86. Wei XQ, Leung BP, Arthur HM et al. Reduced incidence and severity of collagen-induced arthritis in mice lacking IL-18. *J Immunol* 2001; **166**: 517–21.

87. Pizarro TT, Michie MH, Bentz M et al. IL-18, a novel immunoregulatory cytokine, is up-regulated in Crohn's disease: expression and localization in intestinal mucosal cells. *J Immunol* 1999; **162**: 6829–35.

88. Kanai T, Watanabe M, Okazawa A et al. Interleukin-18 and Crohn's disease. *Digestion* 2001; **63**: 37–42.

89. Monteleone G, Trapasso F, Parrello T et al. Bioactive IL-18 expression is up-regulated in Crohn's disease. *J Immunol* 1999; **163**: 143–7.

90. Pages F, Berger A, Lebel Binay S et al. Proinflammatory and antitumor properties of interleukin-18 in the gastrointestinal tract. *Immunol Lett* 2000; **75**: 9–14.

91. Siegmund B, Fantuzzi G, Rieder F et al. Neutralization of interleukin-18 reduces severity in murine colitis and intestinal IFN-γ and TNF-α production. *Am J Physiol Regul Integr Comp Physiol* 2001; **281**: R1264–73.

92. Ten Hove T, Corbaz A, Amitai H et al. Blockade of endogenous IL-18 ameliorates TNBS-induced colitis by decreasing local TNF-alpha production in mice. *Gastroenterology* 2001; **121**: 1372–9.

93. Chikano S, Sawada K, Shimoyama T et al. IL-18 and IL-12 induce intestinal inflammation and fatty liver in mice in an IFN-gamma dependent manner. *Gut* 2000; **47**: 779–86.

94. Wirtz S, Becker C, Blumberg R et al. Treatment of T cell-dependent experimental colitis in SCID mice by local administration of an adenovirus expressing IL-18 antisense mRNA. *J Immunol* 2002; **168**: 411–20.

95. Siegmund B, Lehr HA, Fantuzzi G, Dinarello CA. IL-1beta-converting enzyme (caspase-1) in intestinal inflammation. *Proc Natl Acad Sci USA* 2001; **98**: 13249–54.

96. Kubota T, Fang J, Brown RA, Krueger JM. Interleukin-18 promotes sleep in rabbits and rats. *Am J Physiol Regul Integr Comp Physiol* 2001; **281**: R828–38.

97. Gatti S, Beck J, Fantuzzi G et al. Effect of interleukin-18 on mouse core body temperature. *Am J Physiol Regul Integr Comp Physiol* 2002; **282**: R702–9.

98. Furlan R, Martino G, Galbiati F et al. Caspase-1 regulates the inflammatory process leading to autoimmune demyelination. *J Immunol* 1999; **163**: 2403–9.

99. Horwitz MS, Evans CF, McGavern DB et al. Primary demyelination in transgenic mice expressing interferon-γ. *Nat Med* 1997; **3**: 1037–41.

100. Jander S, Schroeter M, Stoll G. Interleukin-18 expression after focal ischemia of the rat brain: association with the late-stage inflammatory response. *J Cereb Blood Flow Metab* 2002; **22**: 62–70.

101. Loddick SA, Rothwell NJ. Neuroprotective effects of human recombinant interleukin-1 receptor antagonist in focal cerebral ischaemia in the rat. *J Cerebral Blood Flow* 1996; **16**: 932–40.

102. Loddick SA, MacKenzie A, Rothwell NJ. An ICE inhibitor, z-VAD-DCB attenuates ischaemic damage in the rat. *NeuroReport* 1996; **7**: 1465–8.

17

Th1/Th2 balance in experimental models of rheumatological diseases

Roberto G Baccala, Dwight H Kono and Argyrios N Theofilopoulos

Introduction • Th1 and Th2 cytokines • Th1/Th2 balance in mouse models of rheumatological diseases • Conclusions • References

INTRODUCTION

Cytokines are critical regulators of the immune system, affecting the differentiation, survival, activation and function of lymphoid cells. Because of these characteristics, cytokines have received considerable attention, particularly in their role as effector molecules in inflammatory and autoimmune disorders. Significant advances have been made following the observation that CD4 T cells polarize during immune responses into at least two subsets, T-helper 1 (Th1) and Th2, with distinct functions and cytokine secretion patterns.[1] Subsequent studies have shown that similar polarization also occurs for other cell types, including CD8 and γδ T cells, B cells, natural killer (NK) cells, dendritic cells (DCs), macrophages, mast cells, and eosinophils.[2] This chapter will review the role of type 1 and type 2 cytokines in mouse models of lupus and collagen-induced arthritis, focusing on how their balance deviates during disease progression and the effects of therapeutic interventions using agonists and antagonists.

TH1 AND TH2 CYTOKINES

It has been clearly established that, following antigen recognition, most helper T cells differen-

tiate into either Th1 or Th2 cells, depending on the cytokines present at the site of priming as well as on factors such as the type of antigen-presenting cells, antigen dose and affinity, duration of exposure, and costimulatory signals.[3–5] The functional differences between Th1 and Th2 cells are, at least in part, a reflection of their particular programs of cytokine production. Th1 cells produce interferon-γ (INF-γ), interleukin-2 (IL-2), TNF-β and lymphotoxin-α (LT-α), protect against intracellular pathogens, activate phagocytes, induce IgG$_{2a}$ antibodies, and promote delayed-type hypersensitivity responses. A recent study showed that Th1 cells also secrete various chemokines, including macrophage inflammatory protein (MIP)-1α, MIP-1β, Regulated upon Activation Normal T cell Expressed and Secreted (RANTES) and ATAC/lymphotactin (ATAC, activation-induced, T cell-derived and chemokine-related cytokine).[6] Th2 cells secrete IL-4, IL-5, IL-6, IL-9, IL-10 and IL-13, protect against extracellular pathogens, activate eosinophils, induce IgE-mediated allergic reactions, and promote humoral responses in which IgG$_1$ predominates. Several cell surface molecules have been reported to be differentially expressed by these two subsets. For example, Th1 cells express the cytokine receptors IL-12Rβ2, IL-18R and IFN-γRβ,[7-10] the chemokine receptors CCR5, CXCR3 and CCR1,[11] and the recently described Tim-3, a molecule that contains immunoglobulin- and mucin-like domains, and thought to play a significant role in autoimmune diseases by regulating macrophage activation and/or function.[12] Th2 cells primarily express the IL-1-like T1/ST2 and the chemokine receptors CCR3, CCR4 and CCR8, although they can also express low levels of CCR5 and CXCR3.[11,13-15]

The molecular events leading to helper T-cell polarization have not been fully clarified, but a prominent role is played by cytokines, particularly IL-12 for Th1 cells and IL-4 for Th2 cells. IL-12 is primarily produced by CD8α+ lymphoid-like DCs and other antigen-presenting cells following stimulation by microbial products through their pattern-recognition receptors, including Toll-like receptors.[16] Upon binding its receptor on CD4 T cells, IL-12 drives Th1 differentiation by activating the signal transducer and activator of transcription 4 (STAT4) and inducing IFN-γ expression. IL-12 production is increased by the T-cell factor Eta1/osteopontin,[17] and induction of IFN-γ is potentiated by IL-18, which activates IL-1 receptor associated kinase (IRAK) and NF-κB.[18] In humans, type I interferons (IFN-α/β) have also been shown to play a role in promoting IFN-γ production and Th1 differentiation by activating STAT2, which, in turn, activates STAT4.[19,20] This pathway is impaired in mice due to a minisatellite insertion into the mouse STAT2 gene.[21] However, evidence has been provided for the existence of STAT4-independent pathways to IFN-γ expression. Indeed, Th1 polarization can be induced in mice lacking STAT4 (and STAT6),[22] and this signaling molecule is not required for IFN-γ expression by T-cell receptor-stimulated CD8 T cells[23] and Th1 cells.[24] In addition, IFN-αβ enhances IL-12-dependent IFN-γ expression by mouse cells in vitro,[25] increases IL-12-independent IFN-γ production by CD8 T cells in virus-infected mice in vivo, and potently induces IFN-γ expression by mouse T cells lacking STAT1.[26] Other factors involved in Th1 maturation are β-chemokines

binding to CCR5,[27] and IL-23.[28] Downstream of STAT4 is T-bet, a member of the T-box family of transcription factors preferentially expressed in Th1 and NK cells. T-bet is critically involved in regulating Th1 differentiation by inducing IFN-γ expression and repressing Th2 cytokines such as IL-4 and IL-5.[29] Moreover, T-bet was recently shown to play a role not only in the production of IFN-γ, but also in its function. Thus, in B cells, T-bet seems to regulate IgG class switching in response to IFN-γ, promoting the Th1-dependent IgG_{2a} isotype.[30] Additional pathways activated during Th1 polarization include the p38 MAP kinase and Jun N-terminal kinase (JNK) pathways,[31] and induction of interferon regulatory factor 1 (IRF-1).[32]

Th2 cell differentiation is controlled primarily by IL-4, which is produced by subsets of T cells, mast cells, basophils and eosinophils.[3] IL-4 signals through the IL-4R to activate STAT6 and, as a result, activates several IL-4-dependent pathways, including IgE gene switch recombination[33] and expression of Th2-specific transcription factors, such as the c-Maf proto-oncogene,[34] and the zinc finger factors GATA-3[35,36] and SKAT2.[37] In particular, GATA-3 is considered to play a primary role in Th2 maturation by inhibiting T-bet expression and inducing type 2 cytokines.

Th1/Th2 BALANCE IN MOUSE MODELS OF RHEUMATOLOGICAL DISEASES

Lupus models

Systemic lupus erythematosus (SLE) is the prototypic systemic autoimmune disease, characterized by increased production of autoantibodies to various self-constituents, particularly of nuclear origin, including chromatin components, such as nucleosomes, histones and DNA. Although kidney disease due to immune complex deposition is the most prominent clinical manifestation, SLE generally involves multiple organs, including joints. Inbred animal models that consistently develop a disorder closely matching human SLE include New Zealand Black (NZB) mice, NZB crossed with New Zealand White (NZB × NZW) F1 mice, (NZB × SWR) F1 mice, MRL mice homozygous for the lymphoproliferation (*lpr*)-associated Fas gene mutation (MRL-*lpr*), and BXSB mice carrying the disease-accelerating, Y chromosome-associated *Yaa* gene, which has not yet been fully defined.[38] These mice, and their genetic variants obtained through transgenic and gene-knockout technologies, have significantly helped in clarifying the role of cytokines in SLE. As reviewed below, and summarized in Table 17.1, several studies have implicated both Th1 and Th2 cytokines, particularly IFN-γ, IL-4, IL-6 and IL-10, as well as other cytokines such as TNF-α, IL-1 and transforming growth factor beta (TGF-β).

Th1 cytokines

The primary role of IFN-γ in lupus pathogenesis has been clearly established. Studies using various methods have shown elevated IFN-γ levels in lymphoid organs and affected tissues of mice with advanced disease, particularly in the MRL-*lpr* strain.[39–41] Acceleration of disease occurs in (NZB × NZW) F1 mice treated with IFN-γ,[42,43] and a lupus-like syndrome and inflammatory skin disease develop in mice of normal background overexpressing an IFN-γ transgene in the epidermis.[44] A long-lived subline of MRL-*lpr* mice with reduced disease showed lower IFN-γ levels compared to the parental strain,[45] and disease is delayed and early mortality prevented in lupus mice lacking the IFN-γ[46,47] or IFN-γR[48,49] genes, and even in mice carrying a single copy of the IFN-γ gene.[47] Therapeutic interventions targeting IFN-γ and its receptor resulted in disease amelioration. Thus, significant reduction in lupus characteristics was observed in (NZB × NZW) F1 mice receiving either anti-IFN-γ antibodies[50,51] or soluble recombinant IFN-γR,[51] and in MRL-*lpr* mice treated with intramuscular injections of a non-viral plasmid vector encoding an IFN-γR/IgG$_1$Fc fusion molecule.[52] It is of note that the latter study showed amelioration even when the treatment was initiated at an advanced disease stage, which is an unprecedented result. The increased efficiency of this treatment might be due to the higher expression of antagonist produced by intramuscularly delivered plasmid constructs, particularly after electroporation, and to the longer half-life and avidity of the dimeric IFN-γR/IgG$_1$Fc molecule compared to the monomeric IFN-γR. The highly pleiotropic properties of IFN-γ make it difficult to precisely identify the mechanism(s) by which this cytokine mediates pathological manifestations in lupus. Among the possibilities, IFN-γ could act by increasing expression of various molecules on immunocytes and target organs, including MHC class I, MHC class II, intercellular adhesion molecule-1 (ICAM-1) and membrane cofactor protein-1 (MCP-1), thereby facilitating presentation of, and immune responses to, self-antigens.[47,52] Another possibility is that IFN-γ might act, in part, by driving Ig class switching preferentially towards the pathogenic, complement-fixing, IgG$_{2a}$ isotype, a process recently shown to be mediated by T-bet expression in B cells.[30] Interestingly, MRL-*lpr* mice lacking T-bet showed dramatic reductions in B-cell-dependent autoimmune manifestations, including autoantibody production, hypergammaglobulinemia and immune complex renal disease.[30]

Early reports indicated defective IL-2 production and function in most lupus mouse strains.[53,54] The relationship of this abnormality to lupus pathogenesis remains unclear, but could be connected to the more recent observation that normal-background mice with forced deletion of the IL-2 and IL-2R genes develop generalized autoimmune manifestations with uncontrolled T-cell activation.[55–57] In line with these studies, several reports have shown correction of the defective in vitro proliferation and apoptosis of *lpr* T cells by exogenous IL-2,[58–60] and reduced disease in MRL-*lpr* mice infected either with a vaccinia virus-IL-2 construct[61] or with attenuated *Salmonella typhimurium* transfected with the IL-2 gene.[62] A recent study suggested that such effects could be due to a genetic polymorphism that renders IL-2 hypoactive in some autoimmune mice, including MRL.[63] In contrast, other reports have shown increased disease in MRL-*lpr* mice injected intramuscularly with an IL-2 expression vector,[64] no

Table 17.1 Summary of studies showing effects of cytokine agonists and antagonists in murine lupus.

Cytokine type	Mouse strain	Treatment/modification	Suggested role in disease	References
Th1	(NZB × NZW) F1	IFN-γ	IFN-γ promotes	42,43
	(NZB × NZW) F1	IFN-γR$^{-/-}$	IFN-γ promotes	48
	(NZB × NZW) F1	Anti-IFN-γ Ab	IFN-γ promotes	50,51
	(NZB × NZW) F1	Soluble IFN-γR	IFN-γ promotes	51
	MRL-*lpr*	IFN-γ$^{-/-}$	IFN-γ promotes	46,47
	MRL-*lpr*	IFN-γ$^{+/-}$	IFN-γ promotes	47
	MRL-*lpr*	IFN-γR$^{-/-}$	IFN-γ promotes	49
	MRL-*lpr*	IFN-γR-IgG$_1$Fc, plasmid	IFN-γ promotes	52
	Normal	IFN-γ, transgene	IFN-γ promotes	44
	MRL-*lpr*	IL-2, plasmid	IL-2 promotes	64
	(NZB × NZW) F1	Anti-IL-2R Ab	IL-2 promotes	66
	Normal	IL-2$^{-/-}$	IL-2 inhibits	55
	Normal	IL-2R$^{-/-}$	IL-2 inhibits	56,57
	MRL-*lpr*	IL-2, vaccinia virus	IL-2 inhibits	61
	MRL-*lpr*	IL-2, *Salmonella typhimurium*	IL-2 inhibits	62
	(NZB × NZW) F1	IL-2, human	IL-2 has no effect	65
	MRL-*lpr*	IL-12, implanted epithelial cells	IL-12 promotes	69
	MRL-*lpr*	IL-12	IL-12 promotes	67
	MRL-*lpr*	IL-12, plasmid	IL-12 promotes	71
	MRL-*lpr*	Anti-IL-12 Ab	IL-12 promotes	71
	MRL-*lpr*	IL-12, plasmid	IL-12 inhibits	72
	MRL-*lpr*	IL-12p40, transgene	IL-12 has no effect	73
	(NZB × NZW) F1	Anti-IL-12 Ab	IL-12 has no effect	74
	MRL-*lpr*	IL-18	IL-18 promotes	75
Th2	MRL-*lpr*	Anti-IL-4	IL-4 promotes	77
	MRL-*lpr*	Soluble IL-4R	IL-4 promotes	77
	MRL-*lpr*	IL-4$^{-/-}$	IL-4 promotes	46
	(NZW × B6.Yaa)F1	IL-4$^{-/-}$	IL-4 inhibits	79
	BXSB	IL-4$^{-/-}$	IL-4 is not required	78
	(NZB × NZW) F1	IL-6	IL-6 promotes	84
	(NZB × NZW) F1	Anti-IL-6 and anti-CD4 Ab	IL-6 promotes	85
	MRL-*lpr*	Anti-IL-6R Ab	IL-6 promotes	86
	(NZB × NZW) F1	IL-10	IL-10 promotes	87
	(NZB × NZW) F1	Anti-IL-10 Ab	IL-10 promotes	87
	(NZB × NZW) F1	AS101, IL-10 inhibitor	IL-10 promotes	88
Other	(NZB × NZW) F1	TNF-α, low dose, late	TNF-α promotes	100
	Normal	TNF-α, increased in zfp36$^{-/-}$ mice	TNF-α promotes	101
	(NZB × TNF$^{-/-}$)F1	TNF-α $^{+/-}$	TNF-α inhibits	93

Table 17.1 continued

Cytokine type	Mouse strain	Treatment/modification	Suggested role in disease	References
	(NZB × NZW) F1	TNF-α, induced by anti-IL-10 Ab	TNF-α inhibits	87
	(NZB × NZW) F1	TNF-α, high dose, early	TNF-α inhibits	89,98
	(NZB × NZW) F1	TNF-α, high dose, late	TNF-α has no effect	89,98,99
	(NZB × NZW) F1	TNF-α, intermediate dose	TNF-α has no effect	100
	(NZB × NZW) F1	TNF-α, low dose, early	TNF-α has no effect	100
	(NZB × NZW) F1	IL-1	IL-1 promotes	100
	MRL-*lpr*	IL-1R	IL-1 promotes	113
	MRL-*lpr*	IL-1R	IL-1 has no effect	114
	MRL-*lpr*	Anti-TGF-β Ab	TGF-β promotes	117
	MRL-*lpr*	TGF-β, plasmid	TGF-β inhibits	64
	MRL-*lpr*	TGF-β, *Salmonella typhimurium*	TGF-β has no effect	62

Ab, antibody.

effects in (NZB × NZW) F1 mice treated with human recombinant IL-2,[65] and disease suppression in (NZB × NZW) F1 receiving anti-IL-2R antibodies.[66] These contradictory results may be due to differences in route, timing and dose of IL-2, which could affect levels of this cytokine in the specific microenvironments of tissues and lymphoid organs.

The role of the Th1-promoting IL-12 and IL-18 was also investigated. It was shown that peritoneal macrophages of MRL-*lpr* mice hyperproduce IL-12 after stimulation in vitro, and that these mice exhibit high IL-12 concentrations in serum and kidney.[67,68] In addition, MRL-*lpr* mice implanted under the kidney capsule with IL-12-producing tubular epithelial cells showed accumulation of IFN-γ-producing T cells at sites adjacent to the implant and increased pathology even in the contralateral, unimplanted, kidney.[69] Interestingly, acceleration of kidney disease in this model was IFN-γ dependent, since it was not observed in kidneys from mice lacking IFN-γR. Other studies showed that daily injections of recombinant IL-12 in MRL-*lpr* mice resulted in increased serum levels of IFN-γ and nitric oxide (NO) metabolites, and accelerated glomerulonephritis,[67] whereas NO synthase inhibitors ameliorated autoimmune manifestations.[70] Similarly, administration of IL-12p40- or IL-12p70-encoding plasmids to young MRL-*lpr* mice increased, whereas anti-IL-12 antibodies decreased, the typical lymphoaccumulation of the double-negative (CD4⁻CD8⁻) T cells,[71] further suggesting that excessive production of, and response to, IL-12 may play a significant role in this model. Nevertheless, not all reports concur with this conclusion. Intramuscular delivery of IL-12-encoding plasmids inhibited most disease manifestations in MRL-*lpr* mice in one study.[72] Furthermore, transgenic expression of IL-12p40, a potent antagonist for IL-12, decreased IFN-γ levels and IgG₂ₐ anti-DNA antibodies, but not glomerulonephritis, in MRL-*lpr* mice,[73] while treatment of (NZB × NZW) F1 mice with antibodies to IL-12 had no effect on kidney disease.[74]

With regard to IL-18, studies have shown that MRL-*lpr* mice display increased serum concentrations of this cytokine, and that daily injections of IL-18 accelerate proteinuria and glomerulonephritis.[75] Moreover, in vitro experiments have shown hyperproliferation of lymph node cells from MRL-*lpr* mice, possibly due to increased expression of the IL-18Rβ chain by these cells.[76]

Th2 cytokines

Although IL-4 levels were found to be reduced in MRL-*lpr* and (NZB × NZW) F1 mice,[40] several studies have suggested a role for this cytokine in these models. In (NZB × NZW) F1 mice, transfer of IL-4-stimulated splenocytes from 5-month-old donors into syngeneic recipients increased anti-DNA antibody production, whereas treatment with anti-IL-4 antibodies before disease onset inhibited this production and prevented kidney disease.[74] In MRL-*lpr* mice, administration of anti-IL-4 antibodies or recombinant IL-4R led to significantly reduced lymphadenopathy and end-organ diseases,[77] as did genomic deletion of the IL-4 gene.[46] In contrast, a similar deletion had no effect in BXSB mice,[78] while transgenic overexpression of IL-4 in (NZW × B6.Yaa) F1 mice reduced the nephritogenic IgG$_3$ anti-DNA antibodies (but not other IgG anti-DNA) and abrogated glomerulonephritis.[79]

IL-6 levels were either increased or unchanged in lupus mice compared to normal controls.[41,80–82] Studies in vitro showed that depletion of macrophages from splenic cells of (NZB × NZW) F1 mice resulted in decreased production of both IL-6 and anti-DNA autoantibodies.[83] Administration of recombinant IL-6 to (NZB × NZW) F1 mice increased expression of MHC class II on mesangial cells and ICAM-1 on glomerular cells, and accelerated glomerulonephritis.[84] Moreover, treatment of these mice with a rat anti-IL-6 antibody together with anti-CD4 antibodies to induce tolerance to heterologous Ig reduced disease manifestations.[85] Similarly, administration of anti-IL-6R antibodies was reported to be beneficial in MRL-*lpr* mice.[86]

IL-10 production also appears to be increased in lupus mice,[41] and administration of IL-10 accelerated disease onset in (NZB × NZW) F1 mice. Conversely, disease in these mice was reduced upon repeated injections of anti-IL-10 antibodies, an effect apparently mediated by upregulation of endogenous TNF-α,[87] and upon administration of AS101, an IL-10-inhibiting immunomodulator.[88]

Other cytokines

Early studies showed that lipopolysaccharide (LPS)-activated macrophages from NZW mice produced low levels of TNF-α compared to normal mice,[89] a defect later found to correlate with a three-base-pair insertion disrupting the AU-rich motif of the 3'-untranslated region of the TNF-α gene.[90] Reduced TNF-α production was also found in experiments using macrophages from MRL[+/+] mice.[91,92] A more direct demonstration that low TNF-α expression can contribute to lupus disease was suggested by the finding that F1 mice resulting from crosses of NZB mice and TNF-α-deficient normal mice develop enhanced autoimmunity and severe renal disease similar to that of (NZB × NZW) F1 mice.[93] Other studies, however, showed that low TNF-α levels are neither sufficient nor required to induce lupus. Thus, (NZB × NZW.PL) F1 mice, displaying increased expression of the TNF-α gene (d/d haplotype), develop delayed, but still severe, disease.[94] Increased TNF-α expression was also found in affected kidneys of (NZB × NZW) F1 and MRL-*lpr* mice.[95,96] In the latter strain, a biphasic increase in circulating TNF-α was observed with an initial peak early after birth and a second increase after the age of 2 months, which appeared progressive and proportional to the severity of renal disease.[97] In addition, it was reported that TNF-α was detected only in tubular epithelial cells of young mice, while later in life expression was more ubiquitous and also detectable in glomeruli and perivascular infiltrating cells.[97] Additional reports suggested that increased TNF-α levels might have either beneficial or detrimental effects in lupus. Studies with the low-TNF-α-producing (NZB × NZW) F1 mice showed that TNF-α replacement therapy at relatively high doses (10 μg, three times per week) efficiently delayed disease when started at ages of up to 4 months, although it was ineffective when started at the age of 6.5 months[89,98] and could not prevent the eventual development of severe renal disease.[99] In addition, sustained anti-IL-10 therapy inhibited disease, apparently by increasing TNF-α levels, since simultaneous administration of anti-TNF-α antibodies abolished the effect.[87] Similar TNF-α replacement therapy at intermediate doses (2 μg, three times per week) had no effect, while lower doses (0.2 μg, three times per week) accelerated disease when started at the age of 4 months, but not when administered between 2 and 4 months of age.[100]

Increased TNF-α levels in mice lacking the *zfp36*-encoded tristetraprolin (a component of the TNF-α negative-feedback loop that acts by destabilizing TNF-α transcripts) led to a systemic autoimmune syndrome that could be inhibited by anti-TNF-α antibodies.[101] Conversely, treatment with anti-TNF-α antibodies prevented development of pulmonary inflammatory lesions,[102] and administration of a transcriptional inhibitor of TNF-α reduced superantigen-induced inflammatory arthritis[103] in MRL-*lpr* mice. Similarly, infusion of a soluble, dimeric TNF receptor (TNFR) reduced systemic autoimmune disease in motheaten mice.[104]

Although apparently contradictory, these results, showing TNF-α as having either beneficial or detrimental functions, could be explained in part by the diverse effects produced by different doses, times and duration of treatment. Thus, low doses and/or short duration may promote autorecognition by, for example, upregulating MHC[105] or ICAM-1 and VCAM-1 (VCAM, vascular cell adhesion molecule),[106] or increasing expression of autoantigens.[107] Conversely, higher TNF-α doses and/or chronic exposure could inhibit autoimmunity, either through immunosuppressive effects, such as lymphopenia,[108] or by reducing various T-cell responses, including proliferation and cytokine production.[109,110]

Most lupus mice were found to express high IL-1 levels.[41,106,111,112] Recombinant IL-1 given to (NZB × NZW) F1 mice increased nephritis, whereas recombinant IL-1R given to MRL-*lpr* mice reduced disease in one study,[113] although no effects were reported in a second study.[114]

Surprisingly, in vitro experiments indicated that both IL-1 and IL-1R suppressed IgG production by B cells from MRL-*lpr* mice with advanced disease.[111,115,116]

TGF-β was found to be increased in both BXSB and MRL-*lpr* mice.[41] In the latter strain, this cytokine impaired defense against bacterial infections by delaying migration of polymorphonuclear leukocytes to the site of infection.[117,118] The role of TGF-β in lupus is suggested by the observation that direct intramuscular injections of a TGF-β-encoding expression vector reduced autoantibody levels in MRL-*lpr* mice.[64] In contrast, no effect was observed when TGF-β was administered by infecting MRL-*lpr* mice with a non-pathogenic strain of *Salmonella typhimurium* expressing the TGF-β gene.[62]

Arthritis models

Rheumatoid arthritis (RA) is a chronic joint disease of unknown etiology, characterized by progressive inflammation of synovia and, less frequently, extra-articular organs, finally leading to erosion and destruction of cartilage and bone. Several animal models that resemble human RA to varying degrees have been described.[119] Among them, collagen-induced arthritis (CIA), elicited in predisposed rodents upon intradermal injection of heterologous native type II collagen emulsified in complete Freund's adjuvant, is the most commonly used, and studies pertaining to the role of cytokines have largely been confined to this model. Overall, as summarized in Table 17.2, IL-12, IL-18, IL-6, TNF-α, IL-1, IL-15 and IL-17 were found to exhibit disease-promoting effects, IFN-γ plays a complex, sometimes contradictory role, whereas IL-4, IL-10 and TGF-β seem to attenuate disease characteristics.

Th1 cytokines

Several studies have addressed the participation of IFN-γ in CIA, some of which suggest that it has disease-promoting effects. Production of IFN-γ by cultured draining lymph node cells increased following immunization with collagen, reaching higher levels at the time of disease

Table 17.2   Summary of studies showing effects of cytokine agonists and antagonists in murine collagen-induced arthritis.

Cytokine type	Treatment/modification	Suggested role in disease	References
Th1	IFN-γ	IFN-γ promotes	122,123
	Anti-IFN-γ Ab	IFN-γ promotes	124
	IFN-γ, induced by IL-12 or IL-18	IFN-γ promotes	125–130
	IFN-γ, reduced by anti-IL-12 or anti-IL18	IFN-γ promotes	127,132–135
	IFN-γ, reduced in IL-12$^{-/-}$ or IL-18$^{-/-}$ mice	IFN-γ promotes	136,130
	IFN-γ, induced by anti-CD40 Ab	IFN-γ promotes	131
	IFN-γR$^{-/-}$	IFN-γ promotes	137
	IFN-γ	IFN-γ inhibits	138
	Anti-IFN-γ Ab	IFN-γ inhibits	139,140
	IFN-γR$^{-/-}$	IFN-γ inhibits	139,141
	IFN-γ$^{-/-}$	IFN-γ inhibits	142
	IL-12, low doses, before onset	IL-12 promotes	125,126,128,145
	IL-12, adenovirus	IL-12 promotes	127
	Anti-IL-12 Ab	IL-12 promotes	126,127,132–134
	IL-12p40, retrovirus	IL-12 promotes	146
	IL-12$^{-/-}$	IL-12 promotes	136
	IL-12, high doses, after onset	IL-12 inhibits	147,126
	IL-18	IL-18 promotes	128,129
	Anti-IL-18 Ab	IL-18 promotes	135
	IL-18-binding protein	IL-18 promotes	135
	IL-18$^{-/-}$	IL-18 promotes	130
Th2	IL-6$^{-/-}$	IL-6 promotes	150,151
	Anti-IL-6R Ab	IL-6 promotes	149
	IL-4R/IL-2R, transgene	IL-4 promotes	160
	IL-4	IL-4 inhibits	152,153
	Anti-IL-4 Ab	IL-4 inhibits	154
	IL-4, adenovirus	IL-4 inhibits	155,156
	IL-4, dendritic cells	IL-4 inhibits	157
	IL-4, B cells	IL-4 inhibits	158
	IL-4, macrophages	IL-4 inhibits	158
	IL-4$^{-/-}$, mice tolerized by collagen II, IV	IL-4 inhibits	159
	Anti-IL-4, mice tolerized by collagen II, IV	IL-4 inhibits	159
	IL-10	IL-10 inhibits	161,162
	IL-10, adenovirus	IL-10 inhibits	163,164
	IL-10, cationic liposomes	IL-10 inhibits	165
	IL-10, plasmid	IL-10 inhibits	166
	Viral IL-10, adenovirus	IL-10 inhibits	167–169
Other	TNF-α	TNF-α promotes	174

Table 17.2   continued

Cytokine type	Treatment/modification	Suggested role in disease	References
	Anti-TNF-α Ab	TNF-α promotes	134,174–176
	Anti-TNF-α Ab, induced by immunization	TNF-α promotes	178
	TNFR–IgG$_1$, before onset	TNF-α promotes	179
	TNFR–IgG$_1$, after onset	TNF-α has transient effect	180
	TNFR–IgG$_1$, adenovirus, after onset	TNF-α has transient effect	180
	TNF-$\alpha^{-/-}$	TNF-α is not required	181
	Anti-IL-1 Ab	IL-1 promotes	142,184–187
	IL-1R, osmotic pump	IL-1 promotes	185
	IL-1R, implanted fibroblasts	IL-1 promotes	188
	IL-1R, type II decoy, implanted keratinocytes	IL-1 promotes	189
	Inhibitors of IL-1b-converting enzyme	IL-1 promotes	190
	Soluble IL-15Rα	IL-15 promotes	191
	IL-17	IL-17 promotes	192
	Anti-IL-17 Ab	IL-17 promotes	192
	TGF-β	TGF-β inhibits	173,193
	Anti-TGF-β Ab	TGF-β inhibits	193

Ab, antibody; IV, intravenous.

onset and declining thereafter.[120,121] Moreover, during the initial phases of disease induction, treatments with IFN-γ accelerated onset and increased the incidence of arthritis,[122,123] whereas intraperitoneal injections of anti-IFN-γ antibodies reduced disease severity.[124] Increased IFN-γ production and acceleration of disease also occurred following administration of either IL-12,[125–128] IL-18[128–130] or stimulatory anti-CD40 antibodies,[131] while decreased IFN-γ production and disease characteristics were observed in mice treated with antibodies to IL-12[127,132–134] or IL-18,[135] as well as in mice lacking IL-12[136] or IL-18.[130] Further, in one report, predisposed mice lacking IFN-γR showed decreased incidence and severity of CIA and reduced levels of IgG$_{2a}$ antibodies to collagen II.[137] Other studies, however, yielded opposite results, suggesting

that IFN-γ can also have beneficial effects. Indeed, therapeutic as well as prophylactic treatments with IFN-γ inhibited CIA and suppressed anti-collagen antibody production.[138] Additionally, neutralizing anti-IFN-γ monoclonal antibodies, given either before or after disease manifestation, accelerated onset[139] and increased the number of arthritic lesions,[140] although not consistently.[124] Finally, predisposed DBA/1 mice lacking IFN-γR showed earlier disease and higher incidence of arthritis,[139,141] while CIA could be induced in non-susceptible C57BL/6 mice lacking the IFN-γ gene.[142] It should be noted that although the effects of IFN-γ often differed from one study to another, the results were primarily interpreted as supporting the role of Th1 cells in CIA.[120,132,137,139,141] Thus, depending on dose, timing and site of production, IFN-γ may exert proinflammatory actions and aggravate disease, or promote immunoregulatory effects, e.g. by suppressing expansion and inducing apoptosis of activated CD4 T cells, as observed in other experimental systems.[143,144]

Most studies indicate that IL-12 exhibits disease-promoting effects on CIA. In fact, administration of IL-12 increased the incidence and severity of arthritis, particularly when given in relatively low doses and before disease was established.[125,126,128,145] Similarly, increasing IL-12 levels using a non-replicating adenoviral vector accelerated progression and disease characteristics,[127] while disease reduction was observed when IL-12 function was inhibited by specific antibodies[126,127,132–134] or collagen-specific T cells transduced with a retroviral vector encoding the antagonist IL-12p40,[146] or through inactivation of the IL-12 gene.[136] Nevertheless, IL-12 was also shown to inhibit CIA, particularly when given at high doses[147] and/or at advanced disease stages.[126]

A pivotal role in the development of CIA has also been shown for IL-18, since injection of this cytokine increased disease in collagen-immunized DBA/1 mice,[128,129] whereas treatment with either anti-IL-18 antibodies or with a recombinant IL-18-binding protein decreased the severity and progression of CIA in the same mice.[135] In addition, DBA/1 mice lacking IL-18 gene expression showed reduced incidence and severity of disease, an effect completely reversed through administration of recombinant IL-18.[130]

Th2 cytokines

Among Th2 cytokines, IL-6 is the only cytokine consistently reported to have disease-promoting effects in CIA. IL-6 levels were found to correlate with disease activity, with peaks observed within 24 h after immunization, at onset and during exacerbation.[148–150] Moreover, disease was inhibited in collagen-immunized IL-6$^{-/-}$ DBA/1 mice,[150,151] and in mice treated with a single injection of anti-IL-6R antibodies within 3 days after immunization.[149]

In contrast, two other Th2 cytokines, IL-4 and IL-10, were found to play protective roles in this

arthritis model. Although a transient increase in IL-10 was detected shortly after immunization, both of these cytokines appeared to be profoundly suppressed during disease induction.[120] Injection of IL-4 delayed the onset, suppressed the clinical symptoms, reduced IgG$_{2a}$ anti-collagen levels and, remarkably, decreased 1000-fold the production of the disease-promoting TNF-α.[152] Similarly, systemic administration of IL-4 at high doses reduced disease activity and increased serum levels of the IL-1 receptor antagonist (IL-1Ra),[153] whereas injection of anti-IL-4 antibodies augmented the incidence and severity of CIA.[154] Also, administration of IL-4-encoding adenovirus attenuated CIA symptoms,[155,156] as did administration of dendritic cells,[157] B cells[158] or macrophages[158] engineered to produce IL-4. Moreover, the protective effect of intravenous type II collagen was ineffective in IL-4$^{-/-}$ mice and reversed by antibodies to IL-4.[159] However, CIA was exacerbated in mice transgenic for a chimeric IL-2R/IL-4R that, upon binding IL 2, transduces IL-4-specific signals.[160] In such mice, disease was associated with increases in IL-4 and other type 2 cytokines, such as IL-5 and IL-10, indicating that deviation towards Th2 responses may also have deleterious effects in this arthritis model.

Daily administration of recombinant IL-10 starting at disease onset had amelioratory effects on CIA,[161] particularly when given in combination with IL-4.[162] In addition, increasing IL-10 levels by gene delivery using recombinant adenoviral vectors,[163,164] cationic liposomes[165] or a plasmid construct[166] significantly inhibited disease incidence and progression. Similarly, amelioration was observed upon systemic or local injection of adenovirus particles encoding viral-IL-10, alone or in combination with a soluble TNFR-IgG$_1$ fusion protein.[167–169] In contrast, a higher incidence and severity of CIA were observed in predisposed mice lacking the IL-10 gene.[170,171]

Other cytokines

Several lines of evidence clearly identified TNF-α as one of the most important proinflammatory cytokines in CIA and human RA.[172] TNF-α production was found to be increased at disease onset in draining lymph nodes[120] and affected joints,[121,173] particularly in the synovial lining layer and at sites of pannus formation and erosion. Local TNF-α production began on the first day after onset and increased thereafter, preceding expression of IL-1β, which was not detected until day 3.[121] Moreover, while TNF-α injection increased CIA incidence and severity,[174] beneficial effects were observed with TNF-α-blocking reagents, such as anti-TNF-α antibodies given alone[134,174–177] or in combination with either anti-CD4,[176,177] anti-IL-12[134] or anti-IL-1[177] antibodies. Similarly, anti-TNF-α antibodies raised by immunization with a modified TNF-α molecule displaying foreign immunodominant Th epitopes ameliorated CIA.[178] Also, a TNFR-IgG$_1$ fusion protein given shortly before onset prevented CIA,[179] while only a transient effect was observed when a similar molecule, either encoded by a replication-deficient adenovirus or injected as recombinant protein, was administered to mice with established CIA.[180] Despite its importance, TNF-α does not appear to be absolutely required for CIA, since mice lacking TNF-α can develop severe joint disease, although at reduced frequency.[181] Similarly, only partial protection was observed in mice lacking TNFR1, although this could be due to compensation by the functioning TNFR2 in these mice.[179,182]

Another cytokine shown to play a prominent role in arthritis development is IL-1. Early experiments showed that administration of recombinant IL-1 through an osmotic mini-pump promoted CIA in suboptimally immunized DBA/1 mice.[183] High levels of IL-1 production were detected at disease onset in draining lymph nodes of mice with CIA,[120] while in situ analysis showed local production in the synovial lining layer and pannus.[121] IL-1-producing cells were first detected on day 3 after disease onset, i.e. shortly after TNF-α, which was detected on day 1.[121] Moreover, increased IL-1 expression was the most significant cytokine change observed in IFN-γ$^{-/-}$ C57BL/6 mice developing CIA.[142] Additional evidence in support of a disease-promoting effect of IL-1 is provided by reports

showing amelioration upon prophylactic or therapeutic administration of IL-1 blocking agents, including anti-IL-1 antibodies,[142,184–187] IL-1Rα delivered by an osmotic mini-pump[185] or by transfected fibroblasts transplanted into the knee cavity,[188] a type II decoy IL-1R expressed by engrafted keratinocytes,[189] and inhibitors of the IL-1β-converting enzyme (ICE) required to process the IL-1β precursor into proinflammatory IL-1.[190]

IL-15 and IL-17 were also found to promote inflammatory reactions in CIA. Indeed, administration of a soluble IL-15Rα resulted in significant CIA suppression in DBA/1 mice.[191] Similarly, blocking IL-17 suppressed CIA, whereas increased IL-17 expression enhanced disease, particularly upon adenovirus-mediated gene delivery into the knee joint.[192]

In contrast to the above cytokines, TGF-β exhibited protective effects in mouse CIA. Thus, systemic administration of TGF-β reduced CIA incidence and severity, and ameliorated symptoms even when started soon after disease induction, although established disease could not be reversed.[174,193] Conversely, anti-TGF-β antibodies increased disease severity.[193]

CONCLUSIONS

The findings summarized above give an impression of the degree of complexity that characterizes the highly interconnected cytokine network. The cytokines found to exhibit promoting or protecting effects in the disease models discussed herein can be classified as either Th1 or Th2, while several other cytokines also play significant agonistic or antagonistic roles. As a result, no clear conclusion can be reached as to whether these and other autoimmune diseases are strictly mediated by type 1, type 2 or other cytokines, which further emphasizes the view that the Th1/Th2 model is too simplistic for such purposes. It is also evident that the effects on disease of a given cytokine and its inhibitors frequently differ from one study to another, which could be explained by the sensitivity of such treatments in regard to timing, site, means of delivery, dose and duration. Most important, modification of one cytokine frequently has considerable, mostly unpredictable, effects on the balance of other related cytokines. While targeting one cytokine might be beneficial for prophylactic or therapeutic purposes in a particular disease, it might have deleterious ramifications for the remaining cytokine network and inadvertently promote or exacerbate another disorder. Therefore, based on these and other considerations, caution should be exercised in drawing general conclusions from individual experiments. It is also noteworthy that little is known about the mechanisms by which a given cytokine promotes or inhibits a particular disease, which severely limits the utility of cytokine therapy, an extremely promising modality. Obviously, further studies are needed to fully comprehend the complex function of, and interplay between, cytokines, and to subsequently improve therapeutic interventions that would modulate specific molecular and cellular pathways relevant to particular diseases.

REFERENCES

1. Mosmann TR, Cherwinski H, Bond MW et al. Two types of murine helper T-cell clone. I. Definition according to profiles of lymphokine activities and secreted proteins. *J Immunol* 1986; **136**: 2348–57.
2. Mosmann T. Complexity or coherence? Cytokine secretion by B cells. *Nat Immunol* 2000; **1**: 465–6.
3. Abbas AK, Murphy KM, Sher A. Functional diversity of helper T lymphocytes. *Nature* 1996; **383**: 787–93.
4. O'Garra A. Cytokines induce the development of functionally heterogeneous T helper cell subsets. *Immunity* 1998; **8**: 275–83.
5. Lanzavecchia A, Sallusto F. Dynamics of T lymphocyte responses: intermediates, effectors, and memory cells. *Science* 2000; **290**: 92–7.
6. Dorner BG, Scheffold A, Rolph MS et al. MIP-1alpha, MIP-1beta, RANTES, and ATAC/lymphotactin function together with IFN-gamma as type 1 cytokines. *Proc Natl Acad Sci USA* 2002; **99**: 6181–6.
7. Rogge L, Papi A, Presky DH et al. Antibodies to the IL-12 receptor beta 2 chain mark human Th1 but not Th2 cells in vitro and in vivo. *J Immunol* 1999; **162**: 3926–32.
8. Rogge L, Barberis-Maino L, Biffi M et al. Selective expression of an interleukin-12 receptor component by human T helper 1 cells. *J Exp Med* 1997; **185**: 825–31.
9. Szabo SJ, Jacobson NG, Dighe AS et al. Developmental commitment to the Th2 lineage by extinction of IL-12 signaling. *Immunity* 1995; **2**: 665–75.
10. Xu D, Chan WL, Leung BP et al. Selective expression and functions of interleukin 18 receptor on T helper (Th) type 1 but not Th2 cells. *J Exp Med* 1998; **188**: 1485–92.
11. Sallusto F, Mackay CR, Lanzavecchia A. The role of chemokine receptors in primary, effector, and memory immune responses. *Annu Rev Immunol* 2000; **18**: 593–620.
12. Monney L, Sabatos CA, Gaglia JL et al. Th1-specific cell surface protein Tim-3 regulates macrophage activation and severity of an autoimmune disease. *Nature* 2002; **415**: 536–41.
13. Sallusto F, Lenig D, Mackay CR, Lanzavecchia A. Flexible programs of chemokine receptor expression on human polarized T helper 1 and 2 lymphocytes. *J Exp Med* 1998; **187**: 875–83.
14. Bonecchi R, Bianchi G, Bordignon PP et al. Differential expression of chemokine receptors and chemotactic responsiveness of type 1 T helper cells (Th1s) and Th2s. *J Exp Med* 1998; **187**: 129–34.
15. Lohning M, Stroehmann A, Coyle AJ et al. T1/ST2 is preferentially expressed on murine Th2 cells, independent of interleukin 4, interleukin 5, and interleukin 10, and important for Th2 effector function. *Proc Natl Acad Sci USA* 1998; **95**: 6930–5.
16. Medzhitov R, Janeway CJ. Innate immune recognition: mechanisms and pathways. *Immunol Rev* 2000; **173**: 89–97.
17. Ashkar S, Weber GF, Panoutsakopoulou V et al. Eta-1 (osteopontin): an early component of type-1 (cell-mediated) immunity. *Science* 2000; **287**: 860–4.
18. Robinson D, Shibuya K, Mui A et al. IGIF does not drive Th1 development but synergizes with IL-12 for interferon-gamma production and

activates IRAK and NFkappaB. *Immunity* 1997; **7**: 571–81.

19. Cho SS, Bacon CM, Sudarshan C et al. Activation of STAT4 by IL-12 and IFN-alpha: evidence for the involvement of ligand-induced tyrosine and serine phosphorylation. *J Immunol* 1996; **157**: 4781–9.

20. Rogge L, D'Ambrosio D, Biffi M et al. The role of Stat4 in species-specific regulation of Th cell development by type I IFNs. *J Immunol* 1998; **161**: 6567–74.

21. Farrar JD, Smith JD, Murphy TL et al. Selective loss of type I interferon-induced STAT4 activation caused by a minisatellite insertion in mouse Stat2. *Nat Immunol* 2000; **1**: 65–9.

22. Kaplan MH, Wurster AL, Grusby MJ. A signal transducer and activator of transcription (Stat)4-independent pathway for the development of T helper type 1 cells. *J Exp Med* 1998; **188**: 1191–6.

23. Carter LL, Murphy KM. Lineage-specific requirement for signal transducer and activator of transcription (Stat)4 in interferon gamma production from CD4(+) versus CD8(+) T cells. *J Exp Med* 1999; **189**: 1355–60.

24. Ouyang W, Jacobson NG, Bhattacharya D et al. The Ets transcription factor ERM is Th1-specific and induced by IL-12 through a Stat4-dependent pathway. *Proc Natl Acad Sci USA* 1999; **96**: 3888–93.

25. Wenner CA, Guler ML, Macatonia SE et al. Roles of IFN-gamma and IFN-alpha in IL-12-induced T helper cell-1 development. *J Immunol* 1996; **156**: 1442–7.

26. Nguyen KB, Cousens LP, Doughty LA et al. Interferon alpha/beta-mediated inhibition and promotion of interferon gamma: STAT1 resolves a paradox. *Nat Immunol* 2000; **1**: 70–6.

27. Zou W, Borvak J, Marches F et al. Macrophage-derived dendritic cells have strong Th1-polarizing potential mediated by beta-chemokines rather than IL-12. *J Immunol* 2000; **165**: 4388–96.

28. Oppmann B, Lesley R, Blom B et al. Novel p19 protein engages IL-12p40 to form a cytokine, IL-23, with biological activities similar as well as distinct from IL-12. *Immunity* 2000; **13**: 715–25.

29. Glimcher LH, Murphy KM. Lineage commitment in the immune system: the T helper lymphocyte grows up. *Genes Dev* 2000; **14**: 1693–711.

30. Peng SL, Szabo SJ, Glimcher LH. T-bet regulates IgG class switching and pathogenic autoantibody production. *Proc Natl Acad Sci USA* 2002; **99**: 5545–50.

31. Yang DD, Conze D, Whitmarsh AJ et al. Differentiation of CD4+ T cells to Th1 cells requires MAP kinase JNK2. *Immunity* 1998; **9**: 575–85.

32. Coccia EM, Passini N, Battistini A et al. Interleukin-12 induces expression of interferon regulatory factor-1 via signal transducer and activator of transcription-4 in human T helper type 1 cells. *J Biol Chem* 1999; **274**: 6698–703.

33. Linehan LA, Warren WD, Thompson PA et al. STAT6 is required for IL-4-induced germline Ig gene transcription and switch recombination. *J Immunol* 1998; **161**: 302–10.

34. Ho IC, Hodge MR, Rooney JW, Glimcher LH. The proto-oncogene c-maf is responsible for tissue-specific expression of interleukin-4. *Cell* 1996; **85**: 973–83.

35. Zheng WP, Flavell RA. The transcription factor GATA-3 is necessary and sufficient for Th2 cytokine gene expression in CD4 T cells. *Cell* 1997; **89**: 587–96.

36. Zhang DH, Cohn L, Ray P et al. Transcription factor GATA-3 is differentially expressed in murine Th1 and Th2 cells and controls Th2-specific expression of the interleukin-5 gene. *J Biol Chem* 1997; **272**: 21597–603.

37. Peng SL, Gerth AJ, Ranger AM, Glimcher LH. NFATc1 and NFATc2 together control both T and B cell activation and differentiation. *Immunity* 2001; **14**: 13–20.

38. Theofilopoulos AN, Kofler R, Singer PA, Dixon FJ. Molecular genetics of murine lupus models. *Adv Immunol* 1989; **46**: 61–109.

39. Manolios N, Schrieber L, Nelson M, Geczy CL. Enhanced interferon-gamma (IFN) production by lymph node cells from autoimmune (MRL/1, MRL/n) mice. *Clin Exp Immunol* 1989; **76**: 301–6.

40. Shirai A, Conover J, Klinman DM. Increased activation and altered ratio of interferon-gamma: interleukin-4 secreting cells in MRL-lpr/lpr mice. *Autoimmunity* 1995; **21**: 107–16.

41. Prud'homme GJ, Kono DH, Theofilopoulos AN. Quantitative polymerase chain reaction analysis reveals marked overexpression of interleukin-1 beta, interleukin-1 and interferon-gamma mRNA in the lymph nodes of lupus-prone mice. *Mol Immunol* 1995; **32**: 495–503.

42. Heremans H, Billiau A, Colombatti A et al. Interferon treatment of NZB mice: accelerated progression of autoimmune disease. *Infection & Immunity* 1978; **21**: 925–30.

43. Adam C, Thoua Y, Ronco P et al. The effect of

exogenous interferon: acceleration of autoimmune and renal diseases in (NZB/W) F1 mice. *Clin Exp Immunol* 1980; **40**: 373–82.

44. Seery JP, Carroll JM, Cattell V, Watt FM. Antinuclear autoantibodies and lupus nephritis in transgenic mice expressing interferon gamma in the epidermis. *J Exp Med* 1997; **186**: 1451–9.

45. Takahashi S, Fossati L, Iwamoto M et al. Imbalance towards Th1 predominance is associated with acceleration of lupus-like autoimmune syndrome in MRL mice. *J Clin Invest* 1996; **97**: 1597–604.

46. Peng SL, Moslehi J, Craft J. Roles of interferon-gamma and interleukin-4 in murine lupus. *J Clin Invest* 1997; **99**: 1936–46.

47. Balomenos D, Rumold R, Theofilopoulos AN. Interferon-gamma is required for lupus-like disease and lymphoaccumulation in MRL-lpr mice. *J Clin Invest* 1998; **101**: 364–71.

48. Haas C, Ryffel B, Le Hir M. IFN-gamma receptor deletion prevents autoantibody production and glomerulonephritis in lupus-prone (NZB × NZW)F1 mice. *J Immunol* 1998; **160**: 3713–18.

49. Schwarting A, Wada T, Kinoshita K et al. IFN-gamma receptor signaling is essential for the initiation, acceleration, and destruction of autoimmune kidney disease in MRL-Fas(lpr) mice. *J Immunol* 1998; **161**: 494–503.

50. Jacob CO, van der Meide PH, McDevitt HO. In vivo treatment of (NZB × NZW) F1 lupus-like nephritis with monoclonal antibody to gamma interferon. *J Exp Med* 1987; **166**: 798–803.

51. Ozmen L, Roman D, Fountoulakis M et al. Experimental therapy of systemic lupus erythematosus: the treatment of NZB/W mice with mouse soluble interferon-gamma receptor inhibits the onset of glomerulonephritis. *Eur J Immunol* 1995; **25**: 6–12.

52. Lawson BR, Prud'homme GJ, Chang Y et al. Treatment of murine lupus with cDNA encoding IFN-gammaR/Fc. *J Clin Invest* 2000; **106**: 207–15.

53. Altman A, Theofilopoulos AN, Weiner R et al. Analysis of T-cell function in autoimmune murine strains. Defects in production and responsiveness to interleukin 2. *J Exp Med* 1981; **154**: 791–808.

54. Dauphinee MJ, Kipper SB, Wofsy D, Talal N. Interleukin 2 deficiency is a common feature of autoimmune mice. *J Immunol* 1981; **127**: 2483–7.

55. Sadlack B, Lohler J, Schorle H et al. Generalized autoimmune disease in interleukin-2-deficient mice is triggered by an uncontrolled activation and proliferation of CD4+ T cells. *Eur J Immunol* 1995; **25**: 3053–9.

56. Suzuki H, Kundig TM, Furlonger C et al. Deregulated T-cell activation and autoimmunity in mice lacking interleukin-2 receptor beta. *Science* 1995; **268**: 1472–6.

57. Willerford DM, Chen J, Ferry JA et al. Interleukin-2 receptor alpha chain regulates the size and content of the peripheral lymphoid compartment. *Immunity* 1995; **3**: 521–30.

58. Clements JL, Wolfe J, Cooper SM, Budd RC. Reversal of hyporesponsiveness in lpr CD4–CD8– T cells is achieved by induction of cell cycling and normalization of CD2 and p59fyn expression. *Eur J Immunol* 1994; **24**: 558–65.

59. Huang FP, Stott DI. Restoration of an early, progressive defect in responsiveness to T-cell activation in lupus mice by exogenous IL-2. *Autoimmunity* 1993; **15**: 19–29.

60. Radvanyi LG, Raju K, Spaner D et al. Interleukin-2 reverses the defect in activation-induced apoptosis in T cells from autoimmune lpr mice. *Cell Immunol* 1998; **183**: 1–12.

61. Gutierrez-Ramos JC, Andreu JL, Revilla Y et al. Recovery from autoimmunity of MRL/lpr mice after infection with an interleukin-2/vaccinia recombinant virus. *Nature* 1990; **346**: 271–4.

62. Huggins ML, Huang FP, Xu D et al. Modulation of autoimmune disease in the MRL-lpr/lpr mouse by IL-2 and TGF-beta1 gene therapy using attenuated Salmonella typhimurium as gene carrier. *Lupus* 1999; **8**: 29–38.

63. Choi Y, Simon-Stoos K, Puck JM. Hypo-active variant of IL-2 and associated decreased T-cell activation contribute to impaired apoptosis in autoimmune prone MRL mice. *Eur J Immunol* 2002; **32**: 677–85.

64. Raz E, Dudler J, Lotz M et al. Modulation of disease activity in murine systemic lupus erythematosus by cytokine gene delivery. *Lupus* 1995; **4**: 286–92.

65. Owen KL, Shibata T, Izui S, Walker SE. Recombinant interleukin-2 therapy of systemic lupus erythematosus in the New Zealand black/New Zealand white mouse. *J Biol Response Mod* 1989; **8**: 366–74.

66. Kelley VE, Gaulton GN, Hattori M et al. Anti-interleukin 2 receptor antibody suppresses murine diabetic insulitis and lupus nephritis. *J Immunol* 1988; **140**: 59–61.

67. Huang FP, Feng GJ, Lindop G et al. The role of interleukin 12 and nitric oxide in the develop-

ment of spontaneous autoimmune disease in MRL/MP-lpr/lpr mice. *J Exp Med* 1996; **183**: 1447–59.

68. Fan X, Oertli B, Wuthrich RP. Up-regulation of tubular epithelial interleukin-12 in autoimmune MRL-Fas(lpr) mice with renal injury. *Kidney Int* 1997; **51**: 79–86.

69. Schwarting A, Tesch G, Kinoshita K et al. IL-12 drives IFN-gamma-dependent autoimmune kidney disease in MRL-Fas(lpr) mice. *J Immunol* 1999; **163**: 6884–91.

70. Weinberg JB, Granger DL, Pisetsky DS et al. The role of nitric oxide in the pathogenesis of spontaneous murine autoimmune disease: increased nitric oxide production and nitric oxide synthase expression in MRL-lpr/lpr mice, and reduction of spontaneous glomerulonephritis and arthritis by orally administered NG-monomethyl-L-arginine. *J Exp Med* 1994; **179**: 651–60.

71. Xu H, Kurihara H, Ito T et al. IL-12 enhances lymphoaccumulation by suppressing cell death of T cells in MRL-lpr/lpr mice. *J Autoimmun* 2001; **16**: 87–95.

72. Hagiwara E, Okubo T, Aoki I et al. IL-12-encoding plasmid has a beneficial effect on spontaneous autoimmune disease in MRL/MP-lpr/lpr mice. *Cytokine* 2000; **12**: 1035–41.

73. Yasuda T, Yoshimoto T, Tsubura A, Matsuzawa A. Clear suppression of Th1 responses but marginal amelioration of autoimmune manifestations by IL-12p40 transgene in MRL-FAS(lprcg)/FAS(lprcg) mice. *Cell Immunol* 2001; **210**: 77–86.

74. Nakajima A, Hirose S, Yagita H, Okumura K. Roles of IL-4 and IL-12 in the development of lupus in NZB/W F1 mice. *J Immunol* 1997; **158**: 1466–72.

75. Esfandiari E, McInnes IB, Lindop G et al. A proinflammatory role of IL-18 in the development of spontaneous autoimmune disease. *J Immunol* 2001; **167**: 5338–47.

76. Neumann D, Del Giudice E, Ciaramella A et al. Lymphocytes from autoimmune MRL lpr/lpr mice are hyperresponsive to IL-18 and overexpress the IL-18 receptor accessory chain. *J Immunol* 2001; **166**: 3757–62.

77. Schorlemmer HU, Dickneite G, Kanzy EJ, Enssle KH. Modulation of the immunoglobulin dysregulation in GvH- and SLE-like diseases by the murine IL-4 receptor (IL-4–R). *Inflamm Res* 1995; **44** (suppl 2): S194–6.

78. Kono DH, Balomenos D, Park MS, Theofilopoulos AN. Development of lupus in BXSB mice is independent of IL-4. *J Immunol* 2000; **164**: 38–42.

79. Santiago ML, Fossati L, Jacquet C et al. Interleukin-4 protects against a genetically linked lupus-like autoimmune syndrome. *J Exp Med* 1997; **185**: 65–70.

80. McMurray RW, Hoffman RW, Nelson W, Walker SE. Cytokine mRNA expression in the B/W mouse model of systemic lupus erythematosus – analyses of strain, gender, and age effects. *Clin Immunol Immunopathol* 1997; **84**: 260–8.

81. Chen SY, Takeoka Y, Pike-Nobile L et al. Autoantibody production and cytokine profiles of MHC class I (beta2–microglobulin) gene deleted New Zealand black (NZB) mice. *Clin Immunol Immunopathol* 1997; **84**: 318–27.

82. Ohteki T, Okamoto S, Nakamura M et al. Elevated production of interleukin 6 by hepatic MNC correlates with ICAM-1 expression on the hepatic sinusoidal endothelial cells in autoimmune MRL/lpr mice. *Immunol Lett* 1993; **36**: 145–52.

83. Alarcon-Riquelme ME, Moller G, Fernandez C. Macrophage depletion decreases IgG anti-DNA in cultures from (NZB × NZW) F1 spleen cells by eliminating the main source of IL-6. *Clin Exp Immunol* 1993; **91**: 25.

84. Ryffel B, Car BD, Gunn H et al. Interleukin-6 exacerbates glomerulonephritis in (NZB × NZW) F1 mice. *Am J Pathol* 1994; **144**: 927–37.

85. Finck BK, Chan B, Wofsy D. Interleukin 6 promotes murine lupus in NZB/NZW F1 mice. *J Clin Invest* 1994; **94**: 585–91.

86. Kiberd BA. Interleukin-6 receptor blockage ameliorates murine lupus nephritis. *J Am Soc Nephrol* 1993; **4**: 58–61.

87. Ishida H, Muchamuel T, Sakaguchi S et al. Continuous administration of anti-interleukin 10 antibodies delays onset of autoimmunity in NZB/W F1 mice. *J Exp Med* 1994; **179**: 305–10.

88. Kalechman Y, Gafter U, Da JP et al. Delay in the onset of systemic lupus erythematosus following treatment with the immunomodulator AS101 – association with IL-10 inhibition and increase in TNF-α levels. *J Immunol* 1997; **159**: 2658–67.

89. Jacob CO, McDevitt HO. Tumour necrosis factor-alpha in murine autoimmune 'lupus' nephritis. *Nature* 1988; **331**: 356–8.

90. Jacob CO, Lee SK, Strassmann G. Mutational analysis of TNF-alpha gene reveals a regulatory role for the 3'-untranslated region in the genetic

predisposition to lupus-like autoimmune disease. *J Immunol* 1996; **156**: 3043–50.

91. Alleva DG, Kaser SB, Beller DI. Intrinsic defects in macrophage IL-12 production associated with immune dysfunction in the MRL/++ and New Zealand Black/White F1 lupus-prone mice and the Leishmania major-susceptible BALB/c strain. *J Immunol* 1998; **161**: 6878–84.

92. Alleva DG, Kaser SB, Beller DI. Aberrant cytokine expression and autocrine regulation characterize macrophages from young MRL+/+ and NZB/W F1 lupus-prone mice. *J Immunol* 1997; **159**: 5610–19.

93. Kontoyiannis D, Kollias G. Accelerated autoimmunity and lupus nephritis in NZB mice with an engineered heterozygous deficiency in tumor necrosis factor. *Eur J Immunol* 2000; **30**: 2038–47.

94. Fujimura T, Hirose S, Jiang Y et al. Dissection of the effects of tumor necrosis factor-alpha and class II gene polymorphisms within the MHC on murine systemic lupus erythematosus (SLE). *Int Immunol* 1998; **10**: 1467–72.

95. Boswell JM, Yui MA, Burt DW, Kelley VE. Increased tumor necrosis factor and IL-1 beta gene expression in the kidneys of mice with lupus nephritis. *J Immunol* 1988; **141**: 3050–4.

96. Moore KJ, Yeh K, Naito T, Kelley VR. TNF-alpha enhances colony-stimulating factor-1-induced macrophage accumulation in autoimmune renal disease. *J Immunol* 1996; **157**: 427–32.

97. Yokoyama H, Kreft B, Kelley VR. Biphasic increase in circulating and renal TNF-alpha in MRL-lpr mice with differing regulatory mechanisms. *Kidney Int* 1995; **47**: 122–30.

98. Jacob CO, Hwang F, Lewis GD, Stall AM. Tumor necrosis factor alpha in murine systemic lupus erythematosus disease models: implications for genetic predisposition and immune regulation. *Cytokine* 1991; **3**: 551–61.

99. Gordon C, Ranges GE, Greenspan JS, Wofsy D. Chronic therapy with recombinant tumor necrosis factor-alpha in autoimmune NZB/NZW F1 mice. *Clin Immunol Immunopathol* 1989; **52**: 421–34.

100. Brennan DC, Yui MA, Wuthrich RP, Kelley VE. Tumor necrosis factor and IL-1 in New Zealand Black/White mice. Enhanced gene expression and acceleration of renal injury. *J Immunol* 1989; **143**: 3470–5.

101. Taylor GA, Carballo E, Lee DM et al. A pathogenetic role for TNF alpha in the syndrome of cachexia, arthritis, and autoimmunity resulting from tristetraprolin (TTP) deficiency. *Immunity* 1996; **4**: 445–54.

102. Deguchi Y, Kishimoto S. Tumour necrosis factor/cachectin plays a key role in autoimmune pulmonary inflammation in lupus-prone mice. *Clin Exp Immunol* 1991; **85**: 392–5.

103. Edwards CK III, Zhou T, Zhang J et al. Inhibition of superantigen-induced proinflammatory cytokine production and inflammatory arthritis in MRL-lpr/lpr mice by a transcriptional inhibitor of TNF-α. *J Immunol* 1996; **157**: 1758–72.

104. Su X, Zhou T, Yang P et al. Reduction of arthritis and pneumonitis in motheaten mice by soluble tumor necrosis factor receptor. *Arthritis Rheum* 1998; **41**: 139–49.

105. Watanabe Y, Jacob CO. Regulation of MHC class II antigen expression. Opposing effects of tumor necrosis factor-alpha on IFN-gamma-induced HLA-DR and Ia expression depends on the maturation and differentiation stage of the cell. *J Immunol* 1991; **146**: 899–905.

106. McHale JF, Harari OA, Marshall D, Haskard DO. TNF-alpha and IL-1 sequentially induce endothelial ICAM-1 and VCAM-1 expression in MRL/lpr lupus-prone mice. *J Immunol* 1999; **163**: 3993–4000.

107. Dorner T, Hucko M, Mayet WJ et al. Enhanced membrane expression of the 52 kDa Ro(SS-A) and La(SS-B) antigens by human keratinocytes induced by TNF alpha. *Ann Rheum Dis* 1995; **54**: 904–9.

108. Gordon C, Wofsy D. Effects of recombinant murine tumor necrosis factor-alpha on immune function. *J Immunol* 1990; **144**: 1753–8.

109. Cope AP, Liblau RS, Yang XD et al. Chronic tumor necrosis factor alters T-cell responses by attenuating T-cell receptor signaling. *J Exp Med* 1997; **185**: 1573–84.

110. Cope AP. Regulation of autoimmunity by proinflammatory cytokines. *Curr Opin Immunol* 1998; **10**: 669–76.

111. Lebedeva TV, Singh AK. Increased responsiveness of B cells in the murine MRL/lpr model of lupus nephritis to interleukin-1 beta. *J Am Soc Nephrol* 1995; **5**: 1530–4.

112. Mao C, Singh AK. IL-1 beta gene expression in B cells derived from the murine MRL/lpr model of lupus. *Autoimmunity* 1996; **24**: 71–9.

113. Schorlemmer HU, Kanzy EJ, Langner KD, Kurrle R. Immunoregulation of SLE-like disease by the IL-1 receptor: disease modifying activity on BDF1 hybrid mice and MRL autoimmune mice. *Agents Actions* 1993; **39**: C117–20.

114. Kiberd BA, Stadnyk AW. Established murine lupus nephritis does not respond to exogenous interleukin-1 receptor antagonist; a role for the endogenous molecule? *Immunopharmacology* 1995; **30**: 131–7.

115. Singh AK, Lebedeva TV. Interleukin-1 contributes to high level IgG production in the murine MRL/lpr lupus model. *Immunol Invest* 1994; **23**: 281–92.

116. Singh AK, Mao C, Lebedeva TV. In vitro role of IL-1 in heightened IgG, anti-DNA, and nephrito-genic idiotype production by B cells derived from the murine MRL/lpr lupus model. *Clini Immunol Immunopathol* 1994; **72**: 410–15.

117. Lowrance JH, O'Sullivan FX, Caver TE et al. Spontaneous elaboration of transforming growth factor beta suppresses host defense against bacterial infection in autoimmune MRL/lpr mice. *J Exp Med* 1994; **180**: 1693–703.

118. Caver TE, O'Sullivan FX, Gold LI, Gresham HD. Intracellular demonstration of active TGF-β1 in B cells and plasma cells of autoimmune mice – IgG-bound TGF-β1 suppresses neutrophil function and host defense against Staphylococcus aureus infection. *J Clin Invest* 1996; **98**: 2496–506.

119. Holmdahl R, In: Experimental animal models of rheumatoid arthritis. Theofilopoulos AN, Bona CA, eds. *The Molecular Pathology of Autoimmune Diseases*, 2nd edn. (Taylor & Francis: New York, 2002) 23, pp. 402–17.

120. Mauri C, Williams RO, Walmsley M, Feldmann M. Relationship between Th1/Th2 cytokine patterns and the arthritogenic response in collagen-induced arthritis. *Eur J Immunol* 1996; **26**: 1511–18.

121. Marinova-Mutafchieva L, Williams RO, Mason LJ et al. Dynamics of proinflammatory cytokine expression in the joints of mice with collagen-induced arthritis (CIA). *Clin Exp Immunol* 1997; **107**: 507–12.

122. Cooper SM, Sriram S, Ranges GE. Suppression of murine collagen-induced arthritis with mono-clonal anti-Ia antibodies and augmentation with IFN-gamma. *J Immunol* 1988; **141**: 1958–62.

123. Mauritz NJ, Holmdahl R, Jonsson R et al. Treatment with gamma-interferon triggers the onset of collagen arthritis in mice. *Arthritis Rheum* 1988; **31**: 1297–304.

124. Boissier MC, Chiocchia G, Bessis N et al. Biphasic effect of interferon-gamma in murine collagen-induced arthritis. *Eur J Immunol* 1995; **25**: 1184–90.

125. Germann T, Szeliga J, Hess H et al. Administration of interleukin 12 in combination with type II collagen induces severe arthritis in DBA/1 mice. *Proc Natl Acad Sci USA* 1995; **92**: 4823–7.

126. Joosten LA, Lubberts E, Helsen MM, Van den Berg WB. Dual role of IL-12 in early and late stages of murine collagen type II arthritis. *J Immunol* 1997; **159**: 4094–102.

127. Parks E, Strieter RM, Lukacs NW et al. Transient gene transfer of IL-12 regulates chemokine expression and disease severity in experimental arthritis. *J Immunol* 1998; **160**: 4615–19.

128. Leung BP, McInnes IB, Esfandiari E et al. Combined effects of IL-12 and IL-18 on the induction of collagen-induced arthritis *J Immunol* 2000; **164**: 6495–502.

129. Gracie JA, Forsey RJ, Chan WL et al. A proinflammatory role for IL-18 in rheumatoid arthritis. *Journal of Clinical Investigation* 1999; **104**: 1393–401.

130. Wei XQ, Leung BP, Arthur HM et al. Reduced incidence and severity of collagen-induced arthritis in mice lacking IL-18. *J Immunol* 2001; **166**: 517–21.

131. Tellander AC, Michaelsson E, Brunmark C, Andersson M. Potent adjuvant effect by anti-CD40 in collagen-induced arthritis. Enhanced disease is accompanied by increased production of collagen type-II reactive IgG$_{2a}$ and IFN-gamma. *J Autoimmun* 2000; **14**: 295–302.

132. Matthys P, Vermeire K, Mitera T et al. Anti-IL-12 antibody prevents the development and progression of collagen-induced arthritis in IFN-gamma receptor-deficient mice. *Eur J Immunol* 1998; **28**: 2143–51.

133. Malfait AM, Butler DM, Presky DH et al. Blockade of IL-12 during the induction of collagen-induced arthritis (CIA) markedly attenuates the severity of the arthritis. *Clin Exp Immunol* 1998; **111**: 377–83.

134. Butler DM, Malfait AM, Maini RN et al. Anti-IL-12 and anti-TNF antibodies synergistically suppress the progression of murine collagen-induced arthritis. *Eur J Immunol* 1999; **29**: 2205–12.

135. Plater-Zyberk C, Joosten LA, Helsen MM et al. Therapeutic effect of neutralizing endogenous IL-18 activity in the collagen-induced model of arthritis. *J Clin Invest* 2001; **108**: 1825–32.

136. McIntyre KW, Shuster DJ, Gillooly KM et al. Reduced incidence and severity of collagen-induced arthritis in interleukin-12-deficient mice. *Eur J Immunol* 1996; **26**: 2933–8.

137. Kageyama Y, Koide Y, Yoshida A et al. Reduced susceptibility to collagen-induced arthritis in

mice deficient in IFN-gamma receptor. *J Immunol* 1998; **161**: 1542–8.

138. Nakajima H, Takamori H, Hiyama Y, Tsukada W. The effect of treatment with interferon-gamma on type II collagen-induced arthritis. *Clin Exp Immunol* 1990; **81**: 441–5.

139. Vermeire K, Heremans H, Vandeputte M et al. Accelerated collagen-induced arthritis in IFN-gamma receptor-deficient mice. *J Immunol* 1997; **158**: 5507–13.

140. Williams RO, Williams DG, Feldmann M, Maini RN. Increased limb involvement in murine collagen-induced arthritis following treatment with anti-interferon-gamma. *Clin Exp Immunol* 1993; **92**: 323–7.

141. Manoury-Schwartz B, Chiocchia G, Bessis N et al. High susceptibility to collagen-induced arthritis in mice lacking IFN-gamma receptors. *J Immunol* 1997; **158**: 5501–6.

142. Guedez YB, Whittington KB, Clayton JL et al. Genetic ablation of interferon-gamma up-regulates interleukin-1beta expression and enables the elicitation of collagen-induced arthritis in a nonsusceptible mouse strain. *Arthritis Rheum* 2001; **44**: 2413–24.

143. Dalton DK, Haynes L, Chu CQ et al. Interferon gamma eliminates responding CD4 T cells during mycobacterial infection by inducing apoptosis of activated CD4 T cells. *J Exp Med* 2000; **192**: 117–22.

144. Chu CQ, Wittmer S, Dalton DK. Failure to suppress the expansion of the activated CD4 T-cell population in interferon gamma-deficient mice leads to exacerbation of experimental autoimmune encephalomyelitis. *J Exp Med* 2000; **192**: 123–8.

145. Kasama T, Yamazaki J, Hanaoka R et al. Biphasic regulation of the development of murine type II collagen-induced arthritis by interleukin-12: possible involvement of endogenous interleukin-10 and tumor necrosis factor alpha. *Arthritis Rheum* 1999; **42**: 100–9.

146. Nakajima A, Seroogy CM, Sandora MR et al. Antigen-specific T cell-mediated gene therapy in collagen-induced arthritis. *J Clin Invest* 2001; **107**: 1293–301.

147. Hess H, Gately MK, Rude E et al. High doses of interleukin-12 inhibit the development of joint disease in DBA/1 mice immunized with type II collagen in complete Freund's adjuvant. *Eur J Immunol* 1996; **26**: 187–91.

148. Sugita T, Furukawa O, Ueno M et al. Enhanced expression of interleukin 6 in rat and murine arthritis models. *Int J Immunopharmacol* 1993; **15**: 469–76.

149. Takagi N, Mihara M, Moriya Y et al. Blockage of interleukin-6 receptor ameliorates joint disease in murine collagen-induced arthritis. *Arthritis Rheum* 1998; **41**: 2117–21.

150. Sasai M, Saeki Y, Ohshima S et al. Delayed onset and reduced severity of collagen-induced arthritis in interleukin-6-deficient mice. *Arthritis Rheum* 1999; **42**: 1635–43.

151. Alonzi T, Fattori E, Lazzaro D et al. Interleukin 6 is required for the development of collagen-induced arthritis. *J Exp Med* 1998; **187**: 461–8.

152. Horsfall AC, Butler DM, Marinova L et al. Suppression of collagen-induced arthritis by continuous administration of IL-4. *J Immunol* 1997; **159**: 5687–96.

153. Joosten LA, Lubberts E, Helsen MM et al. Protection against cartilage and bone destruction by systemic interleukin-4 treatment in established murine type II collagen-induced arthritis. *Arthritis Res* 1999; **1**: 81–91.

154. Yoshino S. Effect of a monoclonal antibody against interleukin-4 on collagen-induced arthritis in mice. *Br J Pharmacol* 1998; **123**: 237–42.

155. Cottard V, Mulleman D, Bouille P et al. Adeno-associated virus-mediated delivery of IL-4 prevents collagen-induced arthritis. *Gene Ther* 2000; **7**: 1930–9.

156. Kim SH, Evans CH, Kim S et al. Gene therapy for established murine collagen-induced arthritis by local and systemic adenovirus-mediated delivery of interleukin-4. *Arthritis Res* 2000; **2**: 293–302.

157. Morita Y, Yang J, Gupta R et al. Dendritic cells genetically engineered to express IL-4 inhibit murine collagen-induced arthritis. *J Clin Invest* 2001; **107**: 1275–84.

158. Guery L, Chiocchia G, Batteux F et al. Collagen II-pulsed antigen-presenting cells genetically modified to secrete IL-4 down-regulate collagen-induced arthritis. *Gene Ther* 2001; **8**: 1855–62.

159. Myers LK, Tang B, Stuart JM, Kang AH. The role of IL-4 in regulation of murine collagen-induced arthritis. *Clin Immunol* 2002; **102**: 185–91.

160. Chen Y, Rosloniec E, Goral MI et al. Redirection of T-cell effector function in vivo and enhanced collagen-induced arthritis mediated by an IL-2R beta/IL-4R alpha chimeric cytokine receptor transgene. *J Immunol* 2001; **166**: 4163–9.

161. Walmsley M, Katsikis PD, Abney E et al. Interleukin-10 inhibition of the progression of

established collagen-induced arthritis. *Arthritis Rheum* 1996; **39**: 495–503.

162. Joosten LA, Lubberts E, Durez P et al. Role of interleukin-4 and interleukin-10 in murine collagen-induced arthritis. Protective effect of interleukin-4 and interleukin-10 treatment on cartilage destruction. *Arthritis Rheum* 1997; **40**: 249–60.

163. Lubberts E, Joosten LA, van den Bersselaar L et al. Intra-articular IL-10 gene transfer regulates the expression of collagen-induced arthritis (CIA) in the knee and ipsilateral paw. *Clin Exp Immunol* 2000; **120**: 375–83.

164. Quattrocchi E, Dallman MJ, Dhillon AP et al. Murine IL-10 gene transfer inhibits established collagen-induced arthritis and reduces adenovirus-mediated inflammatory responses in mouse liver. *J Immunol* 2001; **166**: 5970–8.

165. Fellowes R, Etheridge CJ, Coade S et al. Amelioration of established collagen induced arthritis by systemic IL-10 gene delivery. *Gene Ther* 2000; **7**: 967–77.

166. Miyata M, Sasajima T, Sato H et al. Suppression of collagen induced arthritis in mice utilizing plasmid DNA encoding interleukin 10. *J Rheumatol* 2000; **27**: 1601–5.

167. Kim KN, Watanabe S, Ma Y et al. Viral IL-10 and soluble TNF receptor act synergistically to inhibit collagen-induced arthritis following adenovirus-mediated gene transfer. *J Immunol* 2000; **164**: 1576–81.

168. Apparailly F, Verwaerde C, Jacquet C et al. Adenovirus-mediated transfer of viral IL-10 gene inhibits murine collagen-induced arthritis. *J Immunol* 1998; **160**: 5213–20.

169. Whalen JD, Lechman EL, Carlos CA et al. Adenoviral transfer of the viral IL-10 gene periarticularly to mouse paws suppresses development of collagen-induced arthritis in both injected and uninjected paws. *J Immunol* 1999; **162**: 3625–32.

170. Johansson AC, Hansson AS, Nandakumar KS et al. IL-10-deficient B10.Q mice develop more severe collagen-induced arthritis, but are protected from arthritis induced with anti-type II collagen antibodies. *J Immunol* 2001; **167**: 3505–12.

171. Cuzzocrea S, Mazzon E, Dugo L et al. Absence of endogenous interleukin-10 enhances the evolution of murine type-II collagen-induced arthritis. *Eur Cytokine Netw* 2001; **12**: 568–80.

172. Feldmann M, Brennan FM, Maini RN. Role of cytokines in rheumatoid arthritis. *Annu Rev Immunol* 1996; **14**: 397–440.

173. Mussener A, Litton MJ, Lindroos E, Klareskog L. Cytokine production in synovial tissue of mice with collagen-induced arthritis (CIA). *Clin Exp Immunol* 1997; **107**: 485–93.

174. Thorbecke GJ, Shah R, Leu CH et al. Involvement of endogenous tumor necrosis factor alpha and transforming growth factor beta during induction of collagen type II arthritis in mice. *Proc Natl Acad Sci USA* 1992; **89**: 7375–9.

175. Williams RO, Feldmann M, Maini RN. Anti-tumor necrosis factor ameliorates joint disease in murine collagen-induced arthritis. *Proc Natl Acad Sci USA* 1992; **89**: 9784–8.

176. Williams RO, Mason LJ, Feldmann M, Maini RN. Synergy between anti-CD4 and anti-tumor necrosis factor in the amelioration of established collagen-induced arthritis. *Proc Natl Acad Sci USA* 1994; **91**: 2762–6.

177. Williams RO, Marinova-Mutafchieva L, Feldmann M, Maini RN. Evaluation of TNF-alpha and IL-1 blockade in collagen-induced arthritis and comparison with combined anti-TNF-alpha/anti-CD4 therapy. *J Immunol* 2000; **165**: 7240–5.

178. Dalum I, Butler DM, Jensen MR et al. Therapeutic antibodies elicited by immunization against TNF-alpha. *Nature Biotechnol* 1999; **17**: 666–9.

179. Mori L, Iselin S, De Libero G, Lesslauer W. Attenuation of collagen-induced arthritis in 55-kDa TNF receptor type 1 (TNFR1)-IgG1-treated and TNFR1-deficient mice. *J Immunol* 1996; **157**: 3178–82.

180. Quattrocchi E, Walmsley M, Browne K et al. Paradoxical effects of adenovirus-mediated blockade of TNF activity in murine collagen-induced arthritis. *J Immunol* 1999; **163**: 1000–9.

181. Campbell IK, O'Donnell K, Lawlor KE, Wicks IP. Severe inflammatory arthritis and lymphadenopathy in the absence of TNF. *J Clin Invest* 2001; **107**: 1519–27.

182. Tada Y, Ho A, Koarada S et al. Collagen-induced arthritis in TNF receptor-1-deficient mice: TNF receptor-2 can modulate arthritis in the absence of TNF receptor-1. *Clin Immunol* 2001; **99**: 325–33.

183. Hom JT, Bendele AM, Carlson DG. In vivo administration with IL-1 accelerates the development of collagen-induced arthritis in mice. *J Immunol* 1988; **141**: 834–41.

184. Van den Berg WB, Joosten LA, Helsen M, van de Loo FA. Amelioration of established murine collagen-induced arthritis with anti-IL-1 treatment. *Clin Exp Immunol* 1994; **95**: 237–43.

185. Joosten LA, Helsen MM, van de Loo FA, Van den Berg WB. Anticytokine treatment of established type II collagen-induced arthritis in DBA/1 mice. A comparative study using anti-TNF alpha, anti-IL-1 alpha/beta, and IL-1Ra. *Arthritis Rheum* 1996; **39**: 797–809.

186. Joosten LA, Helsen MM, Saxne T et al. IL-1 alpha beta blockade prevents cartilage and bone destruction in murine type II collagen-induced arthritis, whereas TNF-alpha blockade only ameliorates joint inflammation. *J Immunol* 1999; **163**: 5049–55.

187. Geiger T, Towbin H, Cosenti-Vargas A et al. Neutralization of interleukin-1 beta activity in vivo with a monoclonal antibody alleviates collagen-induced arthritis in DBA/1 mice and prevents the associated acute-phase response. *Clin Exp Rheumatol* 1993; **11**: 515–22.

188. Bakker AC, Joosten LA, Arntz OJ et al. Prevention of murine collagen-induced arthritis in the knee and ipsilateral paw by local expression of human interleukin-1 receptor antagonist protein in the knee. *Arthritis Rheum* 1997; **40**: 893–900.

189. Bessis N, Guery L, Mantovani A et al. The type II decoy receptor of IL-1 inhibits murine collagen-induced arthritis. *Eur J Immunol* 2000; **30**: 867–75.

190. Ku G, Faust T, Lauffer LL et al. Interleukin-1 beta converting enzyme inhibition blocks progression of type II collagen-induced arthritis in mice. *Cytokine* 1996; **8**: 377–86.

191. Ruchatz H, Leung BP, Wei XQ et al. Soluble IL-15 receptor alpha-chain administration prevents murine collagen-induced arthritis: a role for IL-15 in development of antigen-induced immunopathology. *J Immunol* 1998; **160**: 5654–60.

192. Lubberts E, Joosten LA, Oppers B et al. IL-1-independent role of IL-17 in synovial inflammation and joint destruction during collagen-induced arthritis. *J Immunol* 2001; **167**: 1004–13.

193. Kuruvilla AP, Shah R, Hochwald GM et al. Protective effect of transforming growth factor beta 1 on experimental autoimmune diseases in mice. *Proc Natl Acad Sci USA* 1991; **88**: 2918–21.

18

Th1/Th2 balance in human disease

Sergio Romagnani, Andrea Matucci and Oliviero Rossi

Definition, properties and functions of human Th1 and Th2 cells • Role of Th1/Th2 cells in rheumatologic disorders • Concluding remarks • References

DEFINITION, PROPERTIES AND FUNCTIONS OF HUMAN Th1 AND Th2 CELLS

In 1986, Mosmann et al provided evidence that repeated stimulation of murine CD4[+] T-helper (Th) lymphocytes in vitro with given antigens results in the development of restricted and stereotyped patterns of lymphokine production. Type 1 or Th1 cells produce interferon (IFN)-γ, interleukin (IL)-2 and tumor necrosis factor (TNF)-β, whereas type 2 or Th2 cells produce IL-4, IL-5, IL-6, IL-9 and IL-13.[1] The first clear-cut demonstration of the existence of human Th1 and Th2 cells similar to those described in mice was provided by establishing T-cell clones specific for *Toxocara canis* excretory/secretory (TES) antigens and purified protein derivative (PPD) of *Myobacterium tuberculosis* from normal donors. TES-specific clones exhibited a Th2-like profile of cytokine secretion (production of IL-4 and IL-5, but no or low production of IFN-γ and IL-2), whereas the great majority of PPD-specific T-cell clones derived from the same donors showed a clear-cut Th1 profile (production of IL-2 and IFN-γ, but no IL-4 and IL-5).[2,3] In general, however, human T-cell clones exhibit a less restricted cytokine profile than murine T cells. IL-2, IL-6 and IL-10 tend to segregate less clearly among human CD4[+] subsets than in the mouse.[4]

In subsequent years, it has become clear that murine Th1 cells promote not only the activation of macrophages, but also the production of IgG_{2a} opsonizing, complement-fixing antibodies and antibodies involved in antibody-dependent cell cytotoxicity.[5] For these reasons, Th1 cells can be considered to be responsible for phagocyte-dependent host responses rather than simply cell-mediated immunity.[6,7] On the other hand, Th2 cells provide optimal help not only for humoral immune responses, including IgE and IgG_1 isotype switching, but also mucosal immunity, through production of mast cell and eosinophil growth and differentiation factors (Figure 18.1). Moreover, some Th2-derived cytokines, such as IL-4, IL-10 and IL-13, inhibit several macrophage functions. Therefore, Th2 cells can be considered to be responsible for phagocyte-independent host responses.[6,7] Other cytokines, such as IL-3, granulocyte–macrophage colony-stimulating factor (GM-CSF) and TNF-α, are produced by both Th1 and Th2 cells.[1] Moreover, Th1 and Th2 are not the only cytokine patterns possible, but rather strongly polarized forms of a much more heterogeneous T-cell effector response. T cells expressing cytokines of both patterns have been designated type O (ThO), and usually mediate intermediate effects depending upon the ratio of lymphokines

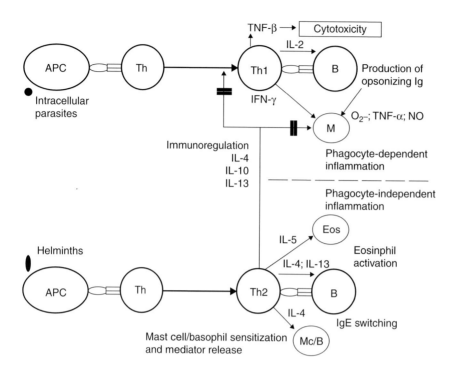

Figure 18.1 Properties and functions of Th1- and Th2-polarized responses. APC, antigen-presenting cell; Th, T-helper cell; Th1, type 1 Th; Th2, type 2 Th; B, B lymphocyte; M, macrophage; Eos, eosinophil; Mc/B, mast cell/basophil; IFN, interferon; TNF, tumor necrosis factor; IL, interleukin.

produced and the nature of the responding cells. T cells producing large amounts of transforming growth factor (TGF)-β have been termed type 3 (Th3), and additional patterns have been described among long-term clones. ThO cells probably represent a heterogeneous population of partially differentiated effector cells consisting of multiple discrete subsets which can secrete both Th1 and Th2 cytokines.[8] The cytokine response at the effector level can remain mixed or can be induced to further differentiate into the Th1 or Th2 pathway under the influence of signals received from the microenvironment. Some studies, however, have demonstrated heterogeneity of cytokine synthesis at the single-cell level, even in polarized Th1 and Th2 responses.[9] Moreover, each of the cytokine genes seems to be under unique control, with distinct tendencies for concordance (e.g. IL-4 and IL-5) or discordance (e.g. IL-4 and IFN-γ).[10] Thus, a more likely possibility is that cytokine profiles are largely random at the clonal level and that the exogenous signals which appear to direct T cells to differentiate into Th1 and Th2 cells (see below) act by increas-

ing the probability of expression of certain cytokine genes at the population level, rather than by activating the expression of a cassette of transcriptionally linked genes in the individual cell.[11]

Regardless of whether the variation in cytokine synthesis by T cells represents a continuum or discrete subsets, there is no doubt that many T-cell clones and in vivo immune responses show a dramatic Th1 or Th2 polarization. Thus, although Th1 and Th2 cells are certainly not the result of a pre-existing functional dichotomy of CD4+ T cells, they can be regarded as polarized forms of the specific immune response that frequently develop under the combined action of genetic and environmental factors. At present, the majority of authors define Th2 or Th2-like cells as CD4+ T cells that have been differentiated to produce IL-4 but not IFN-γ, and Th1 or Th1-like cells as CD4+ T cells that produce IFN-γ but not IL-4, without considering the other set of Th1 or Th2 cytokines. Moreover, it has also been suggested that CD4+ T-effector lymphocytes that maintain the ability to produce IL-4 should be considered as Th2

Table 18.1 Surface molecules preferentially expressed by human Th1 or Th2 cells.	
Th1	**Th2**
CD26	CD30
LAG-3	CD62L
Membrane IFN-γ	CCR4
IL-12Rβ2 chain	CCR8
CCR5	CRTH2
CXCR3	
Tim-3	

cells, and that CD4+ effectors that have lost this ability should be considered as Th1 cells.[12] Taking all these points in mind, the Th1/Th2 paradigm may provide a useful model for understanding the pathogenesis of several pathophysiologic conditions and possibly for the development of novel immunotherapeutic strategies. The possibility that the Th1 or Th2 polarization of the effector response is associated with expression of distinctive molecules on the cell surface has also been investigated in both mice and humans. Although specific markers for a given cell type probably do not exist, several molecules showing preferential association with Th1 or Th2 cells have been described in humans (Table 18.1). This may occur because their expression is dependent upon, or upregulated by, the production of a given cytokine. For example, lymphocyte activation gene 3 (LAG-3) expression is upregulated by IFN-γ, CD30 is dependent upon the production of IL-4, and the IL-12R β-chain is upregulated by IFN-γ and downregulated by IL-4. Membrane IFN-γ is a prototypic component of Th1 cells. The preferential association of CD62L, CCR3, CCR4, CCR8 and CRTH2 with Th2 cells and of CCR5 and CXCR3 with Th1 cells is due to the fact that they represent chemoattractant receptors or adhesion molecule ligands involved in the attraction and permanence of Th1 or Th2 cells at the level of inflamed tissues.[13] A trans-

membrane protein, Tim-3, which contains an immunoglobulin and mucin-like domain and is expressed on differentiated Th1 cells, has been recently described.[14]

Mechanisms responsible for Th1 or Th2 polarization

The factors responsible for the polarization of the specific immune response into a predominant Th1 or Th2 profile have been extensively investigated. There is conclusive evidence that Th1 and Th2 cells do not derive from distinct lineages, but rather develop from the same Th cell precursor under the influence of both environmental and genetic factors acting at the level of antigen presentation. Among the environmental factors, roles for the route of antigen entry, the physical form of immunogen, the type of adjuvant and the dose of antigen have been suggested. The genetic mechanisms responsible for controlling the type of Th cell differentiation still remain elusive. The environmental and genetic factors mixed together can influence Th1/Th2 differentiation, mainly by modulating: (1) a group of contact-dependent factors; and (2) the predominance of a given cytokine in the microenvironment of the responding Th cell. Among contact-dependent factors, the most important are: (1) the extent of T-cell receptor (TCR) ligation; and (2) the signals delivered by OX4OL–OX4O and B7–CD28 interactions. IL-4 production by naive T cells appears to be highly dependent on B7 molecules. Naive CD4 T cells seem to be receptive to CD28-dependent IL-4 production only if they receive a weak TCR signal. Thus, naive Th cells themselves are able to produce small amounts of IL-4 from their initial activation, and the concentration of IL-4 at the level of the Th cell response increases with increasing lymphocyte activation. The inducing effect of IL-4 dominates over other cytokines, so that if IL-4 levels reach a necessary threshold, differentiation of the Th cell into the Th2 phenotype occurs. Under certain circumstances, another IL-4 source may be a small subset of CD4+ NK1.1+ cells capable of recognizing antigens presented in association with the non-

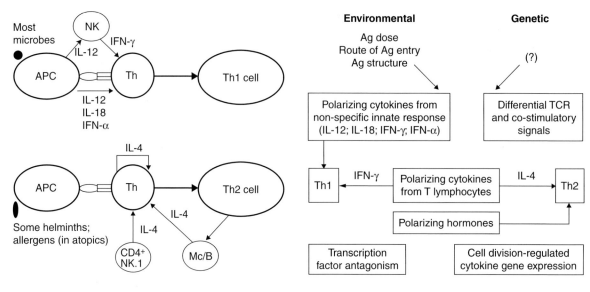

Figure 18.2 Cytokines involved in Th1 and Th2 differentiation and their sources. NK, natural killer; TCR, T-cell receptor.

Figure 18.3 Network of factors involved in Th1 and Th2 polarization. Ag, antigen.

polymorphic β_2-microglobulin-associated molecule, CD1.

In contrast to IL-4, the early production of IL-12, IL-18 and IFNs favors Th1 development. IL-12, which is the most powerful Th1-inducing agent, is mainly produced by dendritic cells (DCs) under the stimulation provided by exogenous signals and is upregulated by both CD40L–CD40 interaction and the presence of IFN-γ. It is of interest that IFN-γ but not IFN-α plays an important role in mice, whereas both IFN-γ and IFN-α promote Th1 differentiation in humans, the latter upregulating the expression of the IL-12 receptor β-chain. Prostaglandin E_2 (PGE_2) and IL-10, which can also be produced by DCs, inhibit IL-12 production, thus biasing naive Th cell development towards the Th2 pathway. Thus, different signals from pathogens or other antigens can modulate the type and the amount of cytokines produced by DCs, or, more likely, may stimulate functionally distinct DC subsets. Hormones have also been found to play some role in Th cell differentiation; glucocorticoids, calcitriol and progesterone favor Th2 cell development, while androgen steroids and relaxin favor Th1 cell development. Recently,

it has been shown that Th cell fate is not only dependent on differentiative signals delivered to CD4 T cells by TCR ligation, costimulatory molecules, cytokines and hormones, but is also regulated by cell cycle expression. Cell cycle progression and cytokine signaling appear to act in concert to relieve epigenetic repression.[13] The main mechanisms responsible for Th1/Th2 differentiation are summarized in Figures 18.2 and 18.3.

ROLE OF Th1/Th2 CELLS IN RHEUMATOLOGIC DISORDERS

The predominance of Th1 or Th2 polarization in the specific CD4[+] T-helper cell-mediated immune response has been shown to play an important pathogenic role in different human pathophysiologic conditions (Table 18.2).[15] Among these conditions, even some rheumatologic disorders may be included.

Reactive arthritis

Reactive arthritis is an excellent model for understanding the predominance and role of Th1/Th2

Table 18.2 Human pathophysiologic conditions characterized by Th1 or Th2 predominance.

Th1	Th2
Hashimoto's thyroiditis	Omen's syndrome
Grave's ophthalmopathy	Vernal conjunctivitis
Multiple sclerosis	Atopic disorders
Type 1 diabetes mellitus	Progressive systemic sclerosis
Crohn's disease	Cryptogenic fibrosing alveolitis
Rheumatoid arthritic	Chronic periodontitis
Lyme arthritis	Progression to AIDS in HIV infection
Reactive arthritis	Tumor progression
Acute allograft rejection	
Unexplained recurrent abortions	
Helicobacter pylori-induced peptic ulcer	
Sarcoidosis	
Atherosclerosis	

---

cells in the inflammatory process, since the etiologic agent responsible for reactive arthritis is generally recognizable. The most classic forms of reactive arthritis are sustained by bacterial agents, such as *Borrelia burgdorferi*, *Chlamydia trachomatis* and *Yersinia enterocolitica*. *B. burgdorferi* is a gram-negative spirochete that can cause Lyme disease (also called Lyme borreliosis) in humans. *B. burgdorferi*-reactive Th1-type CD4[+] T cells seem to be involved in the pathogenesis of Lyme disease. Indeed, CD4[+] T-cell clones generated from the synovial fluid of patients with Lyme arthritis produce IFN-γ, but not IL-4 or IL-5. This initial finding was subsequently confirmed by examining the intracellular cytokine secretion profile of T lymphocytes freshly isolated from the synovial fluid of subjects with Lyme arthritis.[16] Moreover, the severity of the disease was found to be correlated with the ratio of Th1/Th2 cells,[16] but also with reduced production of TNF-α.[17] The latter finding suggests that a state of relative immunodeficiency in the context of the Th1 response to *B. burgdorferi* may contribute to the bacterial persistence in the disease.[18] It is of note that treat-ment-resistant chronic Lyme arthritis patients contained *B. burgdorferi* antigen-specific Th1 cells localized to the synovial fluid,[16] suggesting that Th1 responses to *B. burgdorferi* may not only be important in the protection against the infectious agent, but also involved in the pathogenesis of Lyme disease. In agreement with the results obtained by studies investigating the cytokine profile of T-cell clones generated from the synovial fluid from patients with *B. burgdorferi*-induced reactive arthritis, T-cell clones generated from the synovial fluid from patients with *C. trachomatis*-induced arthritis were also found to exhibit a prevalent Th1 profile.[19]

Y. enterocolitica is a gram-negative enterobacterium which causes enteritis, lymphadenitis or sepsis, and restive arthritis in genetically selected (HLA-B27) individuals. Reactive arthritis develops after *Y. enterocolitica* infection has cleared; that is, in resistant individuals and *Y. enterocolitica*-reactive T-cell clones from the inflamed joints of patients with reactive arthritis produce IFN-γ but no IL-4, i.e. they are of the Th1 type.[20] Thus, like *B. burgdorferi*-specific Th1 cells, *Y. enterocolitica*-reactive Th1 cells seem to be not only protective against the pathogen, but also responsible for the immunopathologic reaction at the joint level in susceptible individuals.

Rheumatoid arthritis (RA) and juvenile RA (JRA)

RA is an autoimmune chronic synovitis which often leads to joint destruction. It is well established that proinflammatory cytokines, such as TNF-α, IL-1, GM-CSF and IL-6, as well as chemokines, such as IL-8, regulated upon activation normal T cell expressed and secreted (RANTES) and macrophage inflammatory protein 1 (MIP-1), are produced by the synovial membrane in RA and play an important role in the pathophysiology of the disease. In fact, these cytokines can both induce bone resorption and cartilage destruction, and can stimulate PG_2 release and collagenase production. In contrast to the abundance of monocyte-derived cytokines, T-cell-derived cytokine proteins have often proven difficult to detect in RA synovium, despite the fact that synovial membrane-infiltrating T cells appear to be phenotypically activated. This has led to the suggestion that the pathogenesis of RA is mediated solely by macrophages and their effector cytokines.[21] An alternative view is that T-cell cytokines may be important, but are expressed at levels too low for easy detection by conventional methods.[22] In favor of this possibility, both epidemiologic observations and experimental findings have been reported.

There are two main epidemiologic findings suggesting Th1 predominance in RA. First, a mutual antagonism of RA and hay fever, a mainly Th2-mediated disorder,[13] has been observed.[23] Second, remission of RA in normal pregnancy has been attributed to the Th1/Th2 switch,[24] which has been suggested to occur in order to avoid acute rejection of the fetal hemiallograft.[25] With regard to the experimental findings, mRNA for IFN-γ and IL-2 has been demonstrated by either PCR or in situ hybridization in synovial tissue of RA patients, whereas IL-4 mRNA was detectable in only a few cases.[26–28] Moreover, most T-cell clones derived from the RA synovium are of the Th1 type.[29–31]

More recent studies performed by intracellular detection at the single-cell level of cytokines produced by freshly isolated cells[32,33] or by quantitative PCR on synovial mRNA,[34] provide convincing evidence in favor of a Th1 predominance in RA synovium. This possibility has been more recently supported by the observation that T cells present in RA synovium exhibit CXCR3 and CCR5,[35–37] two chemokine receptors which are selectively or prevalently expressed by human Th1 cells.[38] Finally, DCs and their soluble factors contained in RA synovial fluid yield a subset of myeloid DCs that preferentially activate Th1 inflammatory responses.[39] Since in some studies a decreased proportion of Th1 cells in the circulation of RA patients has been observed, the possibility that the presence of Th1 cells at the synovial level reflects selective trapping of these cells in the affected joints has been suggested[40] (Figure 18.4). This possibility has been indirectly confirmed by the observation that treatment of RA patients with anti-TNF-α antibody results in a significant increase of Th1 cells in their peripheral blood.[41] Interestingly, treatment of RA patients with a non-depleting humanized anti-CD4 antibody resulted in both clinical improvement and reduction of Th1 cell activity.[42]

In addition to proinflammatory cytokines, a compensatory anti-inflammatory response has been observed in RA synovial membranes. Thus, there is expression of high levels of IL-1RA, soluble TNF receptors (of both the 55- and 75-kDa receptor), TGF-β and IL-10 in the RA synovium,[43–45] and high IL-10 production by T-cell clones generated from RA synovium,[46] which suggests that homeostatic mechanisms exist in the rheumatoid joint by which the immune system attempts to contain inflammation and limit joint destruction. IL-10 may function as an endogenous regulatory molecule in rheumatoid synovium.[47] Indeed, blocking IL-10 in synovial membrane cultures resulted in increases in both TNF-α and IL-1β.[48] Likewise, treatment of RA patients with cyclosporin A induced both clinical improvement and a strong increase of IL-10 production, as well as correction of the Th1/Th2 balance. Owing to the

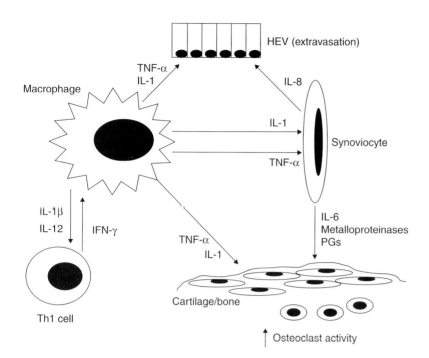

Figure 18.4 Cytokines involved in the pathogenesis of rheumatoid arthritis. HEV, high endothelial venule; PGs, prostaglandins.

powerful inhibitory activity of IL-10 on Th1 cytokine production,[49,50] it is reasonable to suggest that IL-10 represents the (or one of the) reason(s) for the 'elusiveness' of Th1-derived cytokines in RA. Indeed, the frequency of CD4+ regulatory T cells producing IL-10 in RA synovium appeared to be inversely related to the frequency of Th1 cells and the markers of disease activity.[51] However, IL-4 was found to be more effective than IL-10 or TGF-β, at least in vitro, in reducing the number of IFN-γ-producing T cells.[52] The predominant Th1 response in RA patients appears to be related to high IL-12 production,[53] IL-12 being the most powerful Th1-inducing agent in humans.[54] A possible role for IL-15 and IL-18 in T-cell migration and activation in RA has also been suggested.[55,56]

Despite the lower number of studies, data obtained in subjects with JRA are also in favor of a dominant Th1 profile in the specific immune response,[57] or at least of lowered IL-4-producing T cells and decreased IL-4 production[58] in JRA patients.

Sjogren's syndrome (SS)

SS is a chronic autoimmune disease clinically defined by the simultaneous presence of kerato-conjuctivitis sicca and xerostomia, and immuno-logically by a hyperactivity expressed by hypergammaglobulinemia, multiple organ and non-organ-specific autoantibodies and focal lymphocytic infiltration of the exocrine glands, in patients not fulfilling criteria for any other chronic inflammatory connective tissue disease.[59,60] Although not yet conclusive, the results of different studies suggest a predominant activation of Th1 cells in patients with SS. First, the cytokines IL-1, IL-6, TNF-α and IFN-γ were identified in labial salivary gland specimens from patients with SS.[61–63] Second, increased levels of IL-2, IL-6, TNF-α and IFN-γ have been found in the serum of SS patients.[64,65] Finally, spontaneous IFN-γ mRNA in freshly isolated unstimulated T cells from SS patients has been observed. In addition, the two main Th1-inducer cytokines, IL-12 and IL-18, were

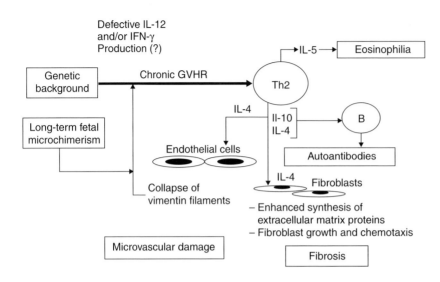

Figure 18.5 Hypothetical model of pathogenetic mechanisms of progressive systemic sclerosis. GVHR, graft-versus-host reaction.

equally and highly expressed in all oral mucosa biopsy samples from SS patients.[66] Increased production of IL-10 by stimulated, and spontaneous IL-10 mRNA expression by freshly isolated, peripheral blood mononuclear cells (PBMC) from SS patients has also been reported,[67] which may reflect, as in RA, the attempt to downregulate the inflammatory reaction induced by Th1 cytokines.

Progressive systemic sclerosis (PSS)

PSS is a disorder characterized by inflammatory, vascular and fibrotic changes of the skin (scleroderma) and a variety of internal organs, such as the gastrointestinal tract, lungs, heart, kidney and joints. Although this not a pure rheumatic disorder, the possible role of Th1/Th2 cells in its pathogenesis is of interest, since a Th2 rather than a Th1 predominance appears to be involved in the genesis of inflammation and in subsequent complications. TGF-β and IL-4 seem to be the cytokines mainly responsible for the intense fibrotic process which is characteristic of this syndrome. IL-4 does indeed induce human fibroblasts to synthesize elevated levels of extracellular matrix proteins, as well as to stimulate the growth of subconfluent fibroblasts and

induce chemotaxis of these cells.[68] Interestingly, PBMCs from patients with PSS produce higher amounts of IL-2 and IL-4 than controls.[69] Likewise, IL-2, IL-4 and IL-6, but not IFN-γ, were each found more frequently in sera from PSS patients than in sera from normal individuals.[70,71] More recently, analysis by RT–PCR of PBMCs from PSS patients showed spontaneous IL-4 and IL-5, but no IFN-γ or IL-10, mRNA expression. The great majority of T-cell clones generated from the skin cellular infiltrates of PSS patients were Th2. Accordingly, by in situ hybridization, large numbers of CD4⁺ T cells present in the perivascular infiltrates of skin biopsy specimens of the same patients expressed IL-4, but not IFN-γ, mRNA.[72]

PSS has clinical features similar to those of chronic graft-versus-host-disease (GVHD),[73] a chimeric disorder that occurs in recipients of allogenic stem cell transplants, where Th2-type responses also predominate.[74,75] Recently, fetal DNA and cells have been observed in skin lesions and blood of women with PSS.[76] In a more recent study, we found that male offspring T cells reactive with maternal MHC antigens were present in the blood and skin of women with PSS that showed a cytokine production profile (high IL-4, poor or no IFN-γ production) similar to the profile of T cells present in patients with chronic GVHD.[77] These findings support the hypothesis that a long-term fetal microchimerism may play a pathogenic role in PSS via the induction of a chronic Th2-mediated inflammatory process which may be responsible for several pathophysiologic manifestations of this syndrome (Figure 18.5).

CONCLUDING REMARKS

Data so far available suggest that the so-called Th1/Th2 paradigm[78] can be conveniently used for understanding the pathogenesis of at least some human rheumatic disorders. Th1 responses, which are highly protective against infectious agents, such as *B. burgdorferi*, *C. trachomatis* and *Y. enterocolitica*, may also sustain in some individuals the inflammatory processes at the joint level that

are responsible for reactive arthritis. Th1 responses against still unknown antigens at the synovial level may also represent the initial triggering factor for joint inflammation in patients with RA or JRA, which is then maintained by the chronic production by macrophages of proinflammatory cytokines. High IL-10 production at the joint level in these patients probably reflects the occurrence of homeostatic mechanisms by which the immune system attempts to contain inflammation and limit joint destruction. Th1 predominance and production of counter regulatory cytokines has also been observed in the inflamed glands and joints of patients with PSS. By contrast, a Th2-mediated inflammation, resulting from a chronic GVHD triggered by long-term fetal microchimerism, may play an important role in the induction of several pathophysiologic manifestations in PSS.

REFERENCES

1. Mosmann TR, Cherwinski H, Bond MW et al. Two types of murine T cell clones. I. Definition according to profiles of lymphokine activities and secreted proteins. *J Immunol* 1986; **136**: 2348–57.
2. Del Prete GF, De Carli M, Mastromauro C et al. Purified protein derivative of Myobacterium tuberculosis and excretory–secretory antigen(s) of Toxocara canis expand in vitro human T cells with stable and opposite (type 1 T helper or type 2 T helper) profile of cytokine production. *J Clin Invest* 1991; **88**: 346–51.
3. Romagnani S. Human Th1 and Th2: doubt no more. *Immunol Today* 1991; **12**: 256–7.
4. Romagnani S. Lymphokine production by human T cells in disease states. *Annu Rev Immunol* 1994; **12**: 227–57.
5. Mosmann TR, Coffman RL. Th1 and Th2 cells: different patterns of lymphokine secretion lead to different functional properties. *Annu Rev Immunol* 1989; **7**: 145–73.
6. Romagnani S. Biology of human Th1 and Th2 cells. *J Clin Immunol* 1995; **15**: 121–9.
7. Abbas AK, Murphy KM, Sher A. Functional diversity of helper T lymphocytes. *Nature* 1996; **383**: 787–93.
8. Mosmann TR, Sad S. The expanding universe of

T-cell subsets: Th1, Th2 and more. *Immunol Today* 1996; **17**: 138–46.
9. O'Garra A, Murphy KM. Role of cytokines in the development of Th1 and Th2 cells. *Chem Immunol* 1996; **63**: 1–13.
10. Bucy RP, Karr L, Huang G-Q et al. Single cell analysis of cytokine gene coexpression during CD4+ T-cell phenotype development. *Proc Natl Acad Sci USA* 1995; **92**: 7565–9.
11. Kelso A. Th1 and Th2 subsets: paradigm lost? *Immunol Today* 1995; **16**: 374–9.
12. Hu-Li J, Chen H, Ben-Sasson SZ, Paul WE. IL-4 and IL-13 production in differentiated T helper type 2 cells is not IL-4 dependent. *J Immunol* 1997; **15**(159): 3731–8.
13. Romagnani S. T-cell subsets (Th1 versus Th2). *Ann Allergy Asthma* 2000; **85**: 9–18.
14. Monney L, Sabatos CA, Gaglia JL et al. Th1-specific cell surface protein Tim-3 regulates macrophase activation and severity of an autoimmune disease. *Nature* 2002; **415**: 536–41.
15. Romagnani S. The Th1/Th2 paradigm. *Immunol Today* 1997; **18**: 263–6.
16. Gross DM, Steere AC, Huber BT. T helper 1 response is dominant and localized to the synovial fluid in patients with Lyme arthritis. *J Immunol* 1998; **160**: 1022–8.

17. Braun J, Yin Z, Spiller I et al. Low secretion of tumor necrosis factor alpha, but no other Th1 or Th2 cytokines, by pheripheral blood mononuclear cells correlates with cronicity in reactive arthritis. *Arthritis Rheum* 1999; **42**: 2039–44.

18. Thiel A, Wu P, Luster R et al. Analysis of the antigen-specific T cell response in reactive arthritis by flow cytometry. *Arthritis Rheum* 2000; **43**: 2834–42.

19. Simon AK, Seipelt E, Wu P et al. Analysis of cytokine profiles in synovial T cell clones from chlamydial reactice arthritis patients: predominance of the Th1 subset. *Clin Exp Allergy* 1993; **94**: 122–6.

20. Schlaak J, Hermann E, Ringhoffer M et al. Predominance of Th1-type T cells in synovial fluid of patients with Yersinia-induced reactive arthritis. *Eur J Immunol* 1992; **22**: 2271–6.

21. Firestein GS, Zvaifler NJ. The role of T cells in rheumatoid arthritis. *Ann Rheum Dis* 1993; **52**: 765.

22. Panayi GS, Lanchbury JS, Kingsley GH. The importance of the T cell in initiating and maintaining the chronic synovitis of rheumatoid arthritis. *Arthritis Rheum* 1992; **35**: 729–35.

23. Verhoef CM, van Roon JA, Vianen ME et al. Mutual antagonism of rheumatoid arthritis and hay fever; a role for type 1/type 2 T cell balance. *Ann Rheum Dis* 1998; **57**: 275–80.

24. Russel AS, Johnston C, Chew C, Maksymowych WP. Evidence for reduced Th1 function in normal pregnancy: a hypothesis for the remission of rheumatoid arthritis. *J Rheumatol* 1997; **24**: 1045–50.

25. Piccinni M-P, Beloni L, Maggi E et al. Defective production of both leukemia inhibitory factor and type 2 T-helper cytokines by decidual T cells in unexplained recurrent abortions. *Nat Med* 1998; **4**: 1020–4.

26. Firestein GS, Alvaro-Garcia JM, Maki R et al. Quantitative analysis of cytokine gene expression in rheumatoid arthritis. *J Immunol* 1990; **144**: 3347–53.

27. Simon AK, Seipelt E, Sieper J. Divergent T-cell cytokine patterns in inflammatory arthritis. *Proc Natl Acad Sci USA* 1999; **96**: 5668–73.

28. Miyata M, Ohira H, Sasajima T et al. Significance of low mRNA levels of interleukin-4 and -10 in mononuclear cells of the synovial fluid of patients with rheumatoid arthritis. *Clin Rheumatol* 2000; **19**: 365–70.

29. Miltenburg AMM, Van Laar JM, De Kniper R et al. T cell clones from human rheumatoid synovial membrane functionally represent the Th1 subset. *Scand J Rheumatol* 1992; **35**: 603–10.

30. Quayle AJ, Chomarat P, Miossec P et al. Rheumatoid inflammatory T-cell clones express mostly Th1 but also Th2 and mixed (ThO-like) cytokine patterns. *Scand J Rheumatol* 1993; **38**: 75–82.

31. Dolhain RJ, van der Heiden AN, ter Haar NT et al. Shift toward T lymphocytes with a T helper 1 cytokine-secretion profile in the joints of patients with rheumatoid arthritis. *Arthritis Rheum* 1996; **39**: 1961–9.

32. Kusaba M, Honda J, Fukuda T, Oizumi K. Analysis of type 1 and type 2 T cells in synovial fluid and peripheral blood of patients with rheumatoid arthritis. *J Rheumatol* 1998; **25**: 1466–71.

33. van der Graff WL, Prins AP, Niers T et al. Quantitation of inteferon gamma- and interleukin-4-producing T cells in synovial fluid and peripheral blood of arthritis patients. *Rheumatology* 1999; **38**: 214–20.

34. Canete JD, Martinez SE, Farres J et al. Differential Th1/Th2 cytokine patterns in chronic arthritis. interferon gamma is highly expressed in synovium of rheumatoid arthritis compared with seronegative spondyloarthropathies. *Arthritis Rheum Dis* 2000; **43**: 175–83.

35. Suzuki N, Nakajima A, Yoshino S et al. Selective accumulation of CCR5+ T lymphocytes into inflamed joints of rheumatoid arthritis. *Int Immunol* 1999; **11**: 553–9.

36. Wedderburn LR, Robinson N, Patel A et al. Selective recruitment of polarized T cells expressing CCR5 and CXCR3 to the inflamed joints of children with juvenile idiopathic arthritis. *Arthritis Rheum* 2000; **43**: 765–74.

37. Patel DD, Zachariah JP, Whichard LP. CXCR3 and CCR5 ligands in rheumatoid arthritis synovium. *Clin Immunol* 2001; **98**: 39–45.

38. Loetscher M, Loetscher P, Brass N et al. Lymphocyte-specific chemokine receptor CXCR3: regulation, chemokine binding and gene localization. *Eur J Immunol* 1998; **28**: 3696–705.

39. Santiago-Schwarz F, Anand P, Liu S, Carsons SE. Dendritic cells (DCs) in rheumatoid arthritis (RA): progenitor cells and soluble factors contained in RA synovial fluid yield a subset of myeloid DCs that preferntially activate Th1 inflammatory-type responses. *J Immunol* 2001; **167**: 1758–68.

40. Mangge H, Felsner P, Herrmann J et al. Early rheumatoid arthritis is associated with diminished numbers of TH1 cells in stimulated peripheral blood. *Immunobiology* 1999; **200**: 290–4.

41. Maurice MM, van der Graaff WL, Leow A et al. Treatment with monoclonal anti-tumor necrosis factor alpha antibody results in an accumulation of Th1 CD4+ T cells in the peripheral blood of patients with rheumatoid arthritis. *Arthritis Rheum* 1999; **42**: 2166–73.

42. Schulze-Koops H, Davis LS, Haverty TP et al. Reduction of Th1 cell activity in the peripheral circulation of patients with rheumatoid arthritis after treatment with a non-depleting humanized monoclonal antibody to CD4. *J Rheumatol* 1998; **25**: 2065–76.

43. Deleuran B, Chu C-Q, Field M et al. Localization of interleukin Ia (IL-1a), type 1 IL-1 receptor and interleukin 1 receptor antagonist protein in the synovial membrane and cartilage/pannus junction in rheumatoid arthritis. *Br J Rheumatol* 1992; **91**: 801–9.

44. Brennan FM, Chantry D, Turner M et al. Detection of transforming growth factor-beta in rheumatoid arthritis synovial tissue: lack of effect on spontaneous cytokine production in joint cell cultures. *Clin Exp Immunol* 1990; **81**: 278–85.

45. Katsikis PD, Chu C-Q, Brennan FM, Maini R, Feldmann M. Immunoregulatory role of interleukin 10 in rheumatoid arthritis. *J Exp Med* 1994; **179**: 1517–27.

46. Cohen SB, Katsikis PD, Chu CQ et al. High level of interleukin-10 production by the activated T cell population within the rheumatoid synovial membrane. *Arthritis Rheum* 1995; **38**: 946–52.

47. Isomaki P, Luukkainen R, Saario R et al. Interleukin-10 functions as an antiinflammatory cytokine in rheumatoid synovium. *Arthritis Rheum* 1996; **39**: 286–95.

48. Kim WU, Cho ML, Kim SI et al. Divergent effect of cyclosporine on Th1/Th2 type cytokines in patients with severe, refractory rheumatoid arthritis. *J Rheumatol* 1999; **27**: 324–31.

49. Del Prete GF, De Carli M, Almetigogna F et al. Human IL-10 is produced by both type 1 helper (Th1) and type 2 helper (Th2) T cell clones and inhibits their antigen-specific proliferation and cytokine production. *J Immunol* 1993; **150**: 1–8.

50. Fiorentino DE, Bond MW, Mosmann TR. Two types of mouse T helper cell. Th2 clones secrete a factor that inhibits cytokine production by Tl clones. *J Exp Med* 1989; **150**: 1–8.

51. Yudoh K, Matsuno H, Nakazawa F et al. Reduced expression of the regulatory CD4+ T cell subset is related to Th1/Th2 balance and disease severity in rheumatoid arthritis. *Arthritis Rheum* 2000; **43**: 617–27.

52. Yin Z, Siegert S, Neure L et al. The elevated ratio of interferon gamma-/interleukin-4-positive T cells found in synovial fluid and synovial membrane of rheumatoid arthritis patients can be changed by interleukin-4 but not by interleukin-10 or transforming growth factor beta. *Rheumatology* 1999; **38**: 1058–67.

53. Park SH, Min DJ, Cho ML et al. Shift toward T helper 1 cytokines by type II collagen-reactive T cells in patients with rheumatoid arthritis. *Arthritis Rheum* 2000; **44**: 561–9.

54. Manetti R, Parronchi P, Guiudizi M-G et al. Natural killer cell stimulatory factor (interleukin-12) induces T helper type 1 (Th1)-specific immune responses and inhibits the development of IL-4-producing Th cells. *J Exp Med* 1993; **177**: 1199–204.

55. McInnes IB, al-Mughales J, Field M et al. The role of interleukin-15 in T-cell migration and activation in rheumatoid arthritis. *Nat Med* 1996; **2**: 175–82.

56. Gracie JA, Forsey RJ, Chan WL et al. A proinflammatory role for IL-18 in rheumatoid arthritis. *J Clin Invest* 1999; **104**: 1393–401.

57. Grom AA, Hirsch R. T-cell and T-cell receptor abnormalities in the immunopathogenesis of juvenile rheumatoid arthritis. *Curr Opin Rheumatol* 2000; **12**: 420–4.

58. Huang JL, Kuo ML, Hung IJ et al. Lowered IL-4-producing T cells and decreased IL-4 secretion in peripheral blood from subjects with juvenile rheumatoid arthritis. *Chang Gung Med J* 2001; **24**: 77–83.

59. Skopouli FN, Dorsos AA, Papaioannu T, Moutsopoulos HM. Preliminary diagnostic criteria for Sjogren's syndrome. *Scand J Rheumatol* 1986; **61** (suppl): 22–5.

60. Fox RI, Kang H-I. Pathogenesis of Sjogren's syndrome. *Rheum Dis Clin North Am* 1992; **18**: 517–38.

61. Roxe D, Griffith M, Stewart J, Novick D, Beverley PCL, Isenberg DA. HLA class I and class II, interferon, interleukin-2, and the interleukin-2 receptor expression on labial biopsy specimens from patients with Sjogren's syndrome. *Ann Rheum Dis* 1987; **46**: 580–6.

62. Oxholm P, Daniels TE, Bendtzen K. Cytokine

expression in labial salivary glands from patients with primary Sjogren's syndrome. *Autoimmunity* 1992; **12**: 185–91.

63. Konttinen YT, Kemppinen P, Koski H et al. Th1 cytokines are produced in labial salivary glands in Sjogren's syndrome, but also in healthy individuals. *Scand J Rheumatol* 1999; **28**: 106–12.

64. Al-Janadi M, Al-Balla S, Al-Dalaan A et al. Cytokine profile in systemic lupus erythematosus, rheumatoid arthritis, and other rheumatic diseases. *J Clin Immunol* 1993; **13**: 58–67.

65. Garcic-Carrasco M, Font J, Filella X et al. Circulating levels of Th1/Th2 cytokines in patients with primary Sjogren's syndrome: correlation with clinical and immunological features. *Clin Exp Rheumatol* 2001; **19**: 411–15.

66. Kolkowski EC, Reth P, Pelusa F et al. Th1 predominance and performin expression in minor salivary glands from patients with primary Sjogren's syndrome. *J Autoimmunity* 1999; **13**: 155–62.

67. Villareal GM, Alcocer-Varela J, Llorente L. Cytokine gene and CD25 antigen expression by pheripheral blood T cells from patients with primary Sjogren's syndrome. *Autoimmunity* 1995; **20**: 223–9.

68. Gillery P, Fertin C, Nicolas JF et al. Interleukin-4 stimulates collagen gene expression in human fibroblast monolayer cultures. Potential role in fibrosis. *FEBS Lett* 1992; **302**: 231–4.

69. Famulario G, Procopio A, Giacomelli R et al. Soluble interleukin-2 receptor, interleukin-2 and interleukin-4 in sera and supernatants from patients with progressive systemic sclerosis. *Clin Exp Immunol* 1990; **81**: 368–72.

70. Needleman BW, Wigley FM, Stair RW. Interleukin 2, interleukin 4, interleukin 6, tumor necrosis factor α, and interferon γ levels in sera from scleroderma patients. *Arthritis Rheum* 1992; **35**: 67–72.

71. Sato IH, Fujimoto S, Kikuchi M, Takehara K. Demonstration of IL-2, IL-4, IL-6 in sera from patients with scleroderma. *Arch Dermatol Res* 1995; **287**: 193–7.

72. Mavilia C, Scaletti C, Romagnani P et al. Type 2 helper T (Th2) cell predominance and high CD30 expression in systemic sclerosis. *Am J Pathol* 1997; **6**: 1751–8.

73. Chosidow O, Bagot M, Vernant JP et al. Sclerodermatous chronic graft-versus-host disease. Analysis of seven cases. *J Am Acad Dermatol* 1992; **26**: 49–55.

74. de Wit D, Van Mechelen M, Zanin C et al. Preferential activation of Th2 cells in chronic graft-versus-host reaction. *J Immunol* 1993; **150**: 361–3.

75. Sakurai J, Ohata J, Saito K et al. Blockade of CTLA-4 signals inhibits Th2-mediated murine chronic graft-versus-host disease by an enhanced expansion of regulatory CD8$^+$ T cells. *J Immunol* 2000; **164**: 664–9.

76. Artlett CM, Smith JB, Jimenez SA. Identification of fetal DNA and cells in skin lesions from women with systemic sclerosis. *N Engl J Med* 1998; **338**: 1186–91.

77. Scaletti C, Vultaggio A, Bonifacio S et al. Type 2 helper (Th2)-oriented profile of male offspring T cells present in women with systemic sclerosis and reactive with maternal MHC antigens. *Arthritis Rheum* 2002; **46**: 445–50.

78. Romagnani S. *Molecular Biology Intelligence Unit. The Th1/Th2 Paradigm in Disease* (Springer: Heidelberg/R.G. Landes Company: Austin, 1997).

19

The balance between pro- and anti-inflammatory cytokines

Danielle Burger and Jean-Michel Dayer

Summary • Introduction • Levels of control of IL-1 and TNF-α action • Levels of control of TNF-α and IL-1 production • Control of T-cell activation/differentiation stage • Blockade of T-cell contact-mediated cytokine induction in monocyte–macrophages • Modulation of IL-1β and TNF-α production in monocyte–macrophages • Intracellular control of IL-1β and TNF-α production • Conclusions • References

SUMMARY

Many chronic immuno-inflammatory diseases are characterized by the influx into the target tissue of peripheral blood cells such as T and B lymphocytes, neutrophils, and mononuclear phagocytes. This influx is associated with the proliferation of invading and resident tissue cells, along with destruction and remodeling of the extracellular matrix. Tissue destruction is carried out by proteases, mainly matrix metalloproteinases (MMPs). The expression of these proteases and their inhibitors is controlled by soluble factors (i.e. cytokines, chemokines, hormones), cell–cell interactions and contact with matrix or breakdown products. In pathologic conditions, the production of cytokines by infiltrating and resident tissue cells escapes regulatory mechanisms. The cytokine network is a homeostatic system that is ruled by subtle balances. The biological significance of cytokines in biological fluids can be interpreted correctly only by taking into account the levels of other synergistic or antagonistic cytokines, their respective inhibitors (i.e. soluble receptors, binding proteins, autoantibodies), and the expression and affinity of their receptors. Owing to their potent activities in many different processes, including cell growth and differentiation, development, repair and other processes leading to the restoration of homeostasis, the cytokine activities have to be tightly controlled by natural inhibitory mechanisms. Since one of the main functions of cytokines is to mediate interactions between the immune and inflammatory systems, it is thought that chronic immuno-inflammatory diseases such as rheumatoid arthritis (RA) might be caused in part by the uncontrolled production of the prototypic proinflammatory and 'pro-destructive' cytokines interleukin-1 (IL-1) and tumor necrosis factor alpha (TNF-α). This chapter aims to summarize some important mechanisms that control cytokine production in RA and that might possibly constitute targets for specific, biological therapeutic intervention.

INTRODUCTION

RA is a chronic inflammatory disease of unknown etiology, characterized by synovial inflammation and joint destruction. Numerous observations support the contention that tissue destruction and resulting disability in RA are partly the result of extracellular matrix degradation by proteolytic enzymes including MMP, the release of the mineral phase (Ca^{2+} release) by prostaglandin E$_2$ (PGE$_2$), and the maturation of promonocytes into osteoclasts by the receptor activator of NFκB ligand (RANKL). The production of MMP and PGE$_2$ by fibroblast-like synoviocytes and chondrocytes is essentially induced by the proinflammatory cytokines IL-1 and TNF-α, which play a major role in RA pathogenesis according to in vitro and in vivo experiments with cultured cells and in animal models, as well as clinical trials (see Chapters 11 and 12). However, many other cytokines can synergize with IL-1 and TNF-α in processes leading to tissue destruction and impairment of repair, e.g. IL-17 and growth factors.[1] IL-1 and TNF-α are mainly produced by monocyte–macrophages, which, in non-infectious conditions, are mainly activated by direct contact with stimulated T cells at the inflammatory site.[2,3] Indeed, based on the premise that T lymphocytes play a pivotal role in the pathogenesis of

chronic inflammatory diseases, we demonstrated that direct cell–cell contact with stimulated T lymphocytes is a major stimulus triggering the production of large amounts of TNF-α and IL-1β in monocytes.[4,2,3] However, the identity of the ligands on plasma membrane of stimulated T cells that trigger the signaling of monocyte–macrophages as well as that of the counter-ligands on monocytes is still elusive. In the human system some of the signaling may be attributed to CD69, β2-integrins (CD11b, CD11c), CD23, CD40–CD40L and lymphocyte activation antigen-3 (LAG-3),[5–9] as summarized in Table 19.1. Membrane-associated TNF-α and IL-1 do not play a crucial part in this particular cellular interaction, contrasting with their significant role in activation processes induced by stimulated T cells in human fibroblasts–synoviocytes or microvascular endothelial cells.[2,3,10,11]

LEVELS OF CONTROL OF IL-1 AND TNF-α ACTION

The therapeutic strategy of blocking IL-1 and TNF-α biological action is by now well established and approved for clinical use. Both approaches had their origin in clinical observations. For IL-1, it was observed that IL-1 biological activity was masked by an inhibitor present in urine of patients with severe diseases such as monocytic leukemia, where a large number of activated monocytes are present,[12–14] and in the presence of remitting fever (i.e. juvenile rheumatoid arthritis).[15] A similar inhibitory activity towards IL-1 was observed in supernatants of monocyte–macrophages.[16–18] This led to the elucidation of the mechanism of action of the inhibitor that acts as competitor by blocking ligand (IL-1) binding, thus acting as an IL-1 receptor antagonist (IL-1Ra).[18,19] Numerous studies have focused on the factors that can preferentially induce IL-1Ra over IL-1, and these include IL-4, transforming growth factor beta (TGF-β) and IL-10. It is of interest that intravenous immunoglobulins (IVIg) promote circulating IL-1Ra in the human system.[20] TNF-α-specific inhibitors were also first observed in urine of febrile patients and proven to be TNF soluble receptors.[21–23] The shedding of these soluble receptors is controlled

---

Table 19.1 Possible ligands and counter-ligands involved in T-cell contact-mediated induction of IL-1 and TNF-α production in monocyte–macrophages.

Ligands on T cells	Counter-ligands on monocyte–macrophages
sCD23[a], CD54[a]	CD11b[a], CD11c[a],
(CD102, CD242?)	CD47–vitronectin receptor[a]
CD40L[a]	CD40[a]
CD69[a]	?
Sialo-lectin?	CD45[a]
LAG-3[a]	MHC class II?
Apo A-I ligand	?

[a]Ligands and counter-ligands that have been shown to be involved in contact-mediated induction of cytokines. Putative ligands or counter-ligands are labeled with '?'.

by specific proteases. However, the same proteases can also cleave and release TNF-α. Therefore, the impact of protease inhibitors on these ambivalent functions is still elusive.[24] In addition, soluble IL-1RII can be released by metalloproteases.[25] An important functional difference exists between the two receptors for IL-1. Indeed, in contrast to IL-1RI, which transduces the signal, IL-1RII acts as a 'decoy' receptor and inactivates IL-1α and IL-1β.[26] Thus, factors increasing the expression of IL-1RII may be beneficial.[27,28] When solubilized, the two IL-1 receptors also display significant functional differences. Indeed, both IL-1sRI and IL-1sRII are able to bind IL-1Ra, but IL-1sRI diminishes the inhibitory capacity of IL-1Ra, whereas IL-1sRII synergizes with IL-1Ra in inhibiting IL-1 activity.[29] Preliminary clinical trials with the latter compound are currently in progress. Finally, the presence of natural blocking autoantibodies to IL-1α may also play a role in some patients.[30] In addition to blocking the binding of cytokines to their functional receptor, theoretically there are still many other possibilities for interfering with IL-1 and TNF-α activity as listed in Table 19.2.

Table 19.2   Possible levels of inhibition of IL-1 and TNF-α activity.

Use of interfering agents	Modulation of regulatory pathway
• TNFsRI/II[a] • Blocking antibodies to TNF-α[a] • IL-1Ra[a] • IL-1sRII • Blocking antibodies to receptors	• Overexpression of IL-1 'decoy' receptor (IL-1RII) • Downregulation of TNFRs and IL-1RI • Cleavage of surface receptors • Interference with specific transduction pathways or nuclear factors involved in TNF-α and IL-1 expression

[a]Approved for clinical use.

In contrast with TNF-α, which is predominantly detected in the early stages of disease, both IL-1α and IL-1β are detected long after the onset of RA.[31,32] Furthermore, TNF-α and IL-1 display synergistic effects, including the triggering of MMP, PGE$_2$ and RANKL production, warranting the use of both TNF-α and IL-1 blocking therapies. The importance of TNF and IL-1 as key mediators of inflammation, bone resorption and cartilage destruction in RA has been well established. However, we still do not know the precise reasons why such treatments work very well in some patients and not in others. Moreover, when the treatment is stopped, the inflammatory processes start again.

LEVELS OF CONTROL OF TNF-α AND IL-1 PRODUCTION

The blockade of TNF-α and IL-1 activity is actually downstream of the immuno-inflammatory cascade (Figure 19.1). This implies that, in addition to direct targeting of prototypical pro-inflammatory cytokines, attempts at restoring cytokine homeostasis with more proximal anti-inflammatory cytokines or inducers of anti-inflammatory cytokines are attractive. Indeed, the blockade of both IL-1 and TNF-α might be envisioned at several levels, one being the triggering level on monocyte–macrophages. As shown in Figure 19.1, several mechanisms might be targeted to inhibit the production of pro-inflammatory cytokines, including: (1) the stage of T-cell activation; (2) the blockade of contact-mediated activation of monocyte–macrophages; (3) the stage of monocyte–macrophage activation; (4) intracellular pathways leading to TNF and IL-1 production; and (5) the enhancement of the production of anti-inflammatory cytokines and cytokine inhibitors.

CONTROL OF T-CELL ACTIVATION/DIFFERENTIATION STAGE

RA is thought to be a Th1-mediated disease.[33,34] This is strengthened by the premise that Th2 cytokines such as IL-4 and IL-13 are expressed at very low levels when detected in the synovium,

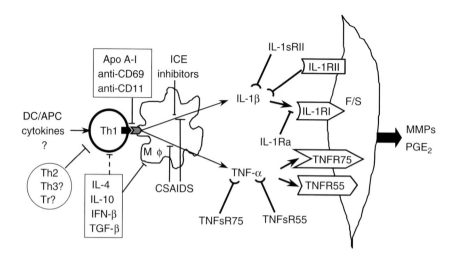

Figure 19.1 Possible levels of IL-1 and TNF-α blockade in the RA inflammatory cascade. Depending on the stimulus (cytokines or antigen-presenting cells (APCs), dendritic cells (DCs)), T cells (Th1) may induce different products in monocyte–macrophages (Mφ). IL-4, IL-10, TGF-β and interferon beta (IFN-β) can modulate the activation of T cells and the expression of surface molecules that activate Mφ. The presence of T cells from other subsets (Th2, T-regulatory cells (Tr), and Th3) might also modulate the activity of Th1 cells. The triggering of IL-1 and TNF-α production may be inhibited by apolipoprotein A-I (Apo A-I), anti-CD11 and anti-CD69 antibodies that block their induction by direct contact with stimulated T cells. IL-4, IL-10, TGF-β and IFN-β inhibit the production of IL-1 and TNF-α in Mφ. IFN-β also induces the production of IL-1Ra in Mφ. Blocking its processing by ICE inhibits the production of soluble IL-1β. The production of both IL-1 and TNF-α can be inhibited by the p38 kinase inhibitors (cytokine-suppressing anti-inflammatory drugs (CSAIDS)). IL-1 activity may be inhibited by binding to either soluble receptor II (IL-1sRII) or decoy receptor (IL-1RII) and by binding of IL-1Ra to IL-1RI, thus impeding signal transduction. TNF-α activity can be inhibited by both soluble receptors (TNFsR55 and TNFsR75). F/S, fibroblast/synoviocytes.

although IL-10 is present in most samples.[35,36] IL-4 and IL-13 are typically produced by Th2 cells, but IL-10 can also be produced by other cells present in RA synovium, including synovial macrophages and a subset of CD4+ T cells that do not produce IL-4 and IL-2.[37–40] This suggests that, unlike IL-4, IL-10 might be involved in the endogenous anti-inflammatory response in the RA synovium. IL-10 is also an important product of T-regulatory cells (Tr1).[41] IL-13 displays similarities with IL-4 but it does not act on T cells.[42] Both exogenous IL-10 and IL-4 have been assessed for their anti-arthritic properties. Although IL-4 is a major inducer of T-helper cell differentiation into Th2 cells, it succeeded in overcoming the Th2 differentiation defect in less than 50% of RA patients.[43] This implies that T

cells do not represent an important target for IL-4 anti-inflammatory therapy in RA. Interestingly, both Th1 and Th2 cells are able to induce cytokine (IL-1) production in monocyte–macrophages upon direct cell–cell contact,[44] although Th1 cells preferentially induce IL-1β while Th2 cells mostly induce IL-1Ra production.[45] Among many effects on T cells, IL-10 strongly inhibited cytokine production and proliferation of T cells and T-cell clones activated in the presence of antigen-presenting cells (APCs), although this effect was mainly due to its downregulatory effects on APC functions.[39] However, IL-10 also directly modulates T-cell functions, since the latter express IL-10 receptor.[46] In T cells stimulated in the absence of APCs, IL-10 inhibits cell proliferation and the production of IL-2, IL-5 and TNF-α, but not that of IL-4 and interferon gamma (IFN-γ).[47–49] Furthermore, IL-10 might play a part in the induction and maintenance of non-responsiveness or anergy in CD4+ T cells.[39] In contrast, in vitro IL-10 displays both anti- and proinflammatory effects on CD8+ T cells.[50,51] As in the case of IL-4, the anti-inflammatory effects of IL-10 administered to animal models of arthritis are unlikely to be due to its effect on T cells.[52]

As recently reviewed,[3] most T-cell types including T-cell clones, freshly isolated T lymphocytes and T-cell lines such as HUT-78 cells, induce IL-1 and TNF-α in monocyte–macrophages when stimulated by phytohemagglutinin (PHA) and phorbol myristate acetate (PMA). Various stimuli other than PHA/PMA induce T lymphocytes to activate monocytes by direct cellular contact: (1) crosslinking of CD3 by immobilized anti-CD3 monoclonal antibody (mAb) with or without crosslinking of the costimulatory molecule CD28;[45,53,54] (2) antigen recognition on antigen-specific T-cell clones;[45] and (3) cytokines.[55–57] This suggests that the expression of activating factors at the surface of T cells is elicited as soon as T cells are activated. It follows that the modulation of this activity might be of great interest in RA therapy. We established that therapeutic agents administered to RA patients, i.e. leflunomide (LF)[58] and IFN-β,[59,60] affect the contact-mediated activation of monocytes. This was due, at least in part, to the inhibitory activity of the latter products on T cells. The activation of T cells in the presence of LF inhibits their ability to trigger IL-1β production in monocytes, resulting in an enhancement of the IL-1Ra/IL-1β molar ratio.[61] Similar results were obtained with IFN-β, in that T cells stimulated in the presence of IFN-β displayed a reduced capacity to induce cytokine production in monocytes.[62] However, surface molecules of T lymphocytes that are likely to be involved in contact signaling of monocytes (i.e. TNF-α, CD69, CD18, CD11a, CD11b, CD11c, CD40L and LAG-3) were not modulated by IFN-β or LF, suggesting that other surface activators on T lymphocytes are involved in the contact-mediated activation of monocytes by stimulated T lymphocytes. Furthermore, IFN-β modulates

cytokine production of T lymphocytes by diminishing TNF-α, IFN-γ and IL-4 and enhancing IL-10 production.[62] IFN-β might also decrease T-cell activation by diminishing IFN-γ and TNF-α binding to lymphocytes.[63,64] However, the sum of these effects might justify clinical trials in RA, although IFN-β effects could be boosted by other therapeutic agents.[59,60]

Depending on the stimulus, T cells induce different products in monocyte–macrophages upon direct cellular contact. Interestingly, recent studies by Brennan et al[54] have led to the concept that, based on their effect on monocyte–macrophages, T cells can be classified as T_{ck} (cytokine-activated) or T_{TCR} (T-cell receptor-activated). Contact with T_{TCR} induced both IL-10 and TNF-α production in monocyte–macrophages, whereas contact with T_{ck} induced TNF-α in the absence of IL-10.[53,55] T cells isolated from RA synovial tissue acted like T_{ck}.[54] Since in vitro T_{ck} are obtained after 8 days of incubation with a cytokine cocktail containing TNF-α, IL-6 and IL-12, changes in the level of the latter cytokines might again influence the global cytokine homeostasis in RA synovium.

Treatment of rodents with active TGF-β during the induction phase of collagen-induced arthritis (CIA) prevents the development of disease symptoms.[65] Furthermore, intramuscular injection of a plasmid DNA encoding TGF-β suppresses chronic disease in a model of streptococcal cell wall-induced arthritis.[66] Whether these effects might be due to some extent to a direct effect of TGF-β in T cells remains to be determined. Indeed, TGF-β is an important effector of T cells which induces Th3 polarization.[67] However, in spite of the premise that TGF-β and IL-4 separately inhibit the induction of Th1 cells by IFN-γ and IL-12, together, TGF-β and IL-4 stimulate the development of Th1 cells independently of IL-12.[68]

BLOCKADE OF T-CELL CONTACT-MEDIATED CYTOKINE INDUCTION IN MONOCYTE–MACROPHAGES

Since the contact-mediated activation of monocyte–macrophages is a major pathway triggering cytokine production, the modulation of this mechanism, i.e. the blockade of IL-1 and TNF-α production at the triggering level of contact-mediated activation, would be of therapeutic interest. Different antibodies or recombinant proteins were used to block contact-mediated induction of IL-1β and TNF-α in monocyte–macrophages. In our experimental system using membranes isolated from stimulated T cells to activate either peripheral blood monocytes or THP-1 cells, we did not observe significant inhibition with blocking antibodies to CD40L, CD23, lymphotoxin β, Fas LAG-3, or blocking fusion proteins such as lymphotoxin β receptor–Fc, and cytotoxic T-lymphocyte antigen-4 (CTLA-4)–Ig (Burger and Dayer, unpublished observations). However, we recently demonstrated that contact-mediated induction of IL-1β and TNF-α in monocyte–macrophages by stimulated T cells was blocked by a plasma protein, apolipoprotein A-I (apo A-I), which is likely to interact with activating molecules expressed at the surface of stimulated T lymphocytes, thus potently inhibiting the production of both IL-1β and TNF-α[69]. The inhibition of T-cell signaling of monocytes might be important in that it would maintain a low level of monocyte activation within the bloodstream. Apo A-I, the principal protein of high-density lipoproteins (HDLs), is a 'negative acute-phase protein', that is, its plasma levels are lowered during the acute phase. In RA, the levels of circulating apo A-I and HDL cholesterol in untreated patients were lower than in normal controls.[70–72] In contrast, apo A-I was enhanced in synovial fluid of RA patients,[73] although its concentrations remained 10-fold lower in synovial fluid than in plasma. The elevation of apo A-I levels in synovial fluid of RA patients was accompanied by an increase in cholesterol levels, suggesting an infiltration of HDL particles into the inflamed joint. We recently demonstrated that apo A-I was consistently present in inflamed synovial tissue that contained infiltrating T cells and macrophages, and was absent from non-inflamed tissue samples obtained from treated patients and from normal subjects.[74] Positive apo A-I staining was particularly abundant in the perivascular

areas and extended with a halo-like aspect into the surrounding cellular infiltrate. Other circulating acute-phase proteins, including C-reactive protein and serum amyloid A (SAA), were absent from the same perivascular areas of inflamed tissues. The perivascular localization of apo A-I suggests that it might be able to fulfill its inhibitory function in zones where T lymphocytes are in close contact with monocyte–macrophages and have a tendency to form 'lymphoid microstructures'.[75] Since upon remission apo A-I is almost absent from synovium, its presence in the inflamed tissue in active RA suggests that infiltration of apo A-I following a flare of RA could inhibit the induction of proinflammatory cytokines, thus impeding the progression and maintenance of inflammation. The infiltration of apo A-I might thus explain why RA, like many other chronic inflammatory diseases, presents as a relapse-remitting disease at least in the inflammatory period of the disease. Since endogenous apo A-I is able to infiltrate the inflamed synovium, it might be a useful approach to treat RA.

MODULATION OF IL-1β AND TNF-α PRODUCTION IN MONOCYTE–MACROPHAGES

In the inflamed synovium, monocyte–macrophages are the principal producers of the proinflammatory cytokines IL-1β and TNF-α, which are themselves under the control of other cytokines that in turn may potentially be targets for therapeutic intervention. The anti-inflammatory functions of type 2 cytokines observed in vitro in RA synovium might be explained by their effects on monocyte–macrophages in addition to their effects on T cells as described above. In particular, IL-4 and IL-10 have been tested for their anti-arthritic properties, as recently reviewed.[52]

Many arthritogenic activities are downregulated by IL-4 in several experimental conditions in vivo and in vitro.[52] Therefore, the possibility exists that RA patients might benefit from treatment with this cytokine. Indeed, IL-4 has been shown to inhibit the production of IL-

1β, TNF-α, IL-6 and IL-8 in human synovial tissue cultures, isolated synovial cells, RA synovial fluid macrophages and peripheral blood mononuclear cells (PBMCs). Furthermore, the anti-inflammatory activity of IL-4 is supported by the premise that it induces the production of IL-1Ra by RA synovium.[76] However, besides its inhibitory activity in proinflammatory cytokine production, IL-4 increases antigen presentation by macrophages, which is associated with upregulation of MHC class II expression and of B7-1 (CD80) and B7-2 (CD86). IL-4 also inhibits IFN-γ secretion and proliferation of type 1 T-helper (Th1) and T-cytotoxic (Tc1) cells isolated from RA synovial fluid and peripheral blood.[77,78] As stated above, IL-4 does not display a marked effect on RA T cells; thus the latter effect is likely to be mediated indirectly by the inhibition of Th1-stimulatory cytokines, such as IL-12, which, in vitro, is produced by monocyte–macrophages from peripheral blood and synovial fluid of RA patients.[79] In vivo, IL-4 administered to mice with proteoglycan-induced arthritis (a Th1-mediated arthritis) significantly inhibits IL-1 and IL-6 production in the joints.[80] In CIA, contradictory results have been obtained following IL-4 administration.[81,82] The different results obtained with IL-4 in mice were confirmed by clinical trials in RA patients. The subcutaneous administration of IL-4 to RA patients (up to 2 μg/kg, three times a week for 6 weeks) did not result in a significant improvement of disease activity, although IL-4 was well tolerated.[83] This might be because IL-4 in association with T-cell membrane factors enhances MMP-1 production in macrophages, thus favoring tissue destruction.[84]

As recently reviewed, IL-10 strongly inhibits the production of IL-1α, IL-1β, IL-6, IL-8, IL-10 itself, IL-12, granulocyte–macrophage colony-stimulating factor (GM-CSF), granulocyte colony-stimulating factor (G-CSF), macrophage colony-stimulating factor (M-CSF), TNF-α, monocyte chemoattractant protein-1α (MIP-1α), MIP-1β, MIP-2, RANTES and leukemia inhibitory factor (LIF) by activated monocyte–macrophages.[85] The mechanism of inhibition is variable, depending on the target cytokine.

Inhibition may occur at the transcriptional and/or post-transcriptional level(s), and may involve mRNA destabilization. Interestingly, inhibition of TNF-α production is independent of the ability of IL-10 to inhibit NF-κB activation.[86] The premise that neutralization of IL-10 triggers an increase in the levels of IL-1β, TNF-α and GM-CSF[37] and that its administration to RA synovium explant cultures suppresses IL-1β, TNF-α and IL-6 production suggests that IL-10 might be a potential therapeutic agent. In animal models of RA, IL-10 administration has led to beneficial effects that might be attributed in part to the inhibition of cytokine production by monocyte–macrophages.[52] However, as in the case of IL-4, clinical trials (subcutaneous administration of up to 20 μg/kg daily for 4 weeks) did not result in significant improvement, although circulating IL-1 and TNF-α inhibitors (IL-1Ra and TNFsR) were enhanced.[87]

Like many cytokines, TGF-β can display either synergistic or antagonistic effects on other cytokines, depending on the cellular context. In resting peripheral blood monocytes, TGF-β induces mRNA expression of IL-1α, IL-1β, TNF-α, platelet-derived growth factor (PDGF)-BB and basic fibroblast growth factor (bFGF), whereas in tissue macrophages it enhances IL-1Ra production.[67] In rodent models of arthritis, it is thus difficult to attribute the beneficial effects of TGF-β to its action on monocytic cytokine homeostasis.

One cytokine that could possibly restore a balanced production of proinflammatory cytokines in monocyte–macrophages is IFN-β. Although it has mostly been used to treat multiple sclerosis patients, encouraging results have been obtained in RA patients.[59,60] Indeed, IFN-β induced IL-1Ra in the absence of IL-1β in monocyte–macrophages.[62,88] Upon contact-mediated activation of monocyte–macrophages by stimulated T cells, IFN-β not only enhanced the production of IL-1Ra but inhibited that of IL-1β and TNF-α.[62] Furthermore, IFN-β enhanced the capacity of mature monocyte-derived dendritic cells to stimulate autologous T cells to produce anti-inflammatory cytokines such as IL-13, IL-5 and IL-10, although, at early stages, it

Table 19.3 Differential control of production of IL-1β and IL-1Ra in monocyte–macrophages.

Regulatory process	IL-1β	IL-1Ra
Cellular release	ICE (caspase 1)-dependent Unknown process of 'secretion'	Existence of intracellular forms Secretion through the classical Golgi pathway
Signal transduction	Enhanced by PI3-K inhibitor and okadaic acid	Decreased by PI3-K inhibitor and okadaic acid
Cytokine modulation	Inhibited by IL-4, IL-13, IL-10, TGF-β, and IFN-β	Increased by IL-4, IL-13, IL-10, TGF-β and IFN-β
Translation	P38 MAP kinase-dependent	p38 MAP kinase-independent

inhibited the development of the latter cells.[89] However, IFN-β, together with IL-3, induced monocyte differentiation into dendritic cells that, while producing low levels of IL-12, potently stimulated T cells to produce IFN-γ and IL-5.[90] This demonstrates that, like other cytokines, IFN-β also displays 'proinflammatory' activities depending on the cytokine environment.

INTRACELLULAR CONTROL OF IL-1β AND TNF-α PRODUCTION

The generation of the active forms of IL-1β and TNF-α is tightly controlled in activated monocyte–macrophages. Depending on the type of stimulus, different intracellular pathways exist in monocyte–macrophages for the production of the same cytokine. Cellular contact with stimulated T cells as well as lipopolysaccharide (LPS) can induce the production of TNF-α, IL-1β and IL-1Ra in human monocyte–macrophages. In other cases, IL-1Ra might be induced in the absence of IL-1, but from what is known at present, all stimuli eliciting IL-1β production also trigger IL-1Ra production, at any rate in monocyte–macrophages. The balance between IL-1 and IL-1Ra is likely to be crucial for the

biological activity of IL-1. Some regulatory mechanisms ruling the latter are summarized in Table 19.3. The production of both IL-1β and TNF-α is tightly regulated at several levels, including the dissociation between transcription and translation.[91] For example, stimuli such as C5a, hypoxia, blood clotting or surface contact are not sufficient to provide a signal for translation, despite a potent signal for transcription.[91–94,91] Consequently, some stimuli might provide signals for complete cytokine gene transcription but no translational signaling. IL-1β and TNF-α translation can be blocked by pyridinyl-imidazol compounds that bind and inactivate the mitogen-activated protein (MAP) kinase p38.[95–97] These compounds are referred to as 'cytokine-suppressing anti-inflammatory drugs', or CSAIDs. Although these compounds have shown some beneficial effects in animal models of arthritis[98,99] and displayed anti-inflammatory activity in isolated chondrocytes and osteoblasts,[100,101] to our knowledge they have not been used to treat RA patients.

LPS is the stimulus most frequently used in in vitro studies performed with the objective of identifying transduction pathways underlying cytokine production in monocyte–macrophages. Components of the transduction pathways induced by toll-like receptor 4 (reviews: Beutler[102] and Aderem and Ulevitch[103]) and leading to the translocation of NFκB and AP-1, as well as protein kinase C (PKC)[104] and p44/42 (extracellular signal-regulated kinase),[105] are all likely to be involved also in cytokine gene induction by other stimuli. Other components of transcription pathways leading to cytokine synthesis have been identified after signaling by engagement of cell surface molecules. The engagement of CD45 ligand leading to TNF-α production in monocytes follows a unique signaling pathway (PI3-K) as well as pathways shared with LPS (NFκB and p38 kinase).[106] Furthermore, different products induced by the same stimulus may depend on different signaling pathways; for example, the PI3-K pathway selectively controls IL-1Ra, and not IL-1β, in 'septic' THP-1 cells.[107] Upon T-cell contact-mediated activation of monocyte–macrophages, different pathways are involved in the induction of IL-10 or TNF-α.[108,109] Interestingly, PI3-K is mainly involved in IL-10 induction, whereas NFκB is involved in TNF-α production, suggesting that PI3-K is preferentially involved in pathways controlling the production of anti-inflammatory factors. PI3-K might also represent a checkpoint signaling molecule favoring IL-1Ra synthesis over that of IL-1β, since suppression of its activity in monocytes stimulated by LPS, anti-CD11b mAb or membranes of stimulated T cells results in inhibition of IL-1Ra and upregulation of IL-1β production.[110] Furthermore, we demonstrated that upon contact with stimulated T cells, the balance between IL-1β and IL-1Ra production in monocytes was regulated by Ser/Thr phosphatase(s).[111]

In addition to activation pathways, signaling of cytokines can be regulated by suppressors of cytokine signaling (SOCS).[112–114] SOCS3 is abundantly expressed in RA synovium.[115,116] Interestingly, the periarticular injection of a recombinant adenovirus carrying the SOCS3 cDNA into the ankle joints of mice with CIA drastically reduced the severity of arthritis and joint swelling compared with control groups, and SOCS3 was more effective than the

dominant negative form of STAT3 in the CIA model.[116] These data suggest that SOCS3 induction could represent a new approach to the treatment of RA.

IL-1β is controlled by caspase-1 (interleukin-converting enzyme, ICE), whose activation by RIP-2 is prevented by ICEBERG.[117] However, the therapeutic use of intracellular protein inhibitors such as ICEBERG requires intracellular expression and is therefore premature. Furthermore, ICEBERG inhibits the production of the soluble, active form of IL-1β without affecting the production of IL-1α, whose destructive functions might persist.

The control of cytokines and cytokine inhibitors as a means of restoring balance at the level of nuclear factors is likely to be premature. Indeed, studies using LPS to activate monocyte–macrophages have demonstrated that the 5'-flanking regions of the TNF-α, IL-1β, and IL-1Ra genes all display common features.[118–120] In addition to a TATA box, consensus binding sites for various transcription factors have been identified, including NFκB, cAMP response element (CRE), and Spi-1/PU.1 (purine-rich box). Interestingly, the latter nuclear factor might impart cell/tissue specificity, since not all cells constitutively express it. Human blood monocytes constitutively express Spi-1/PU.1 and are thus highly sensitive to cytokine induction by LPS.[118–120] AP-1 consensus binding sequences have been identified on both IL-1β and TNF-α gene promoters. ATF-2, AP-2, SP-1, Krox-24, and NF-AT (nuclear factor-activated T cells) are present in the TNF-α promoter, and SBE in the IL-1Ra promoter, and NF-IL-6 (C/EBPβ) is involved in the activation of the IL-1β gene via a Spi-1/PU.1 protein–protein tether.[121] Thus much more work is required to identify nuclear factors specifically involved in the regulation of pro- or anti-inflammatory cytokine gene expression before envisioning such factors as potential targets in therapy.

CONCLUSIONS

The blockade of both IL-1 and TNF-α has afforded major beneficial effects in the therapy of RA. However, the blockade of cytokine activity, which, besides its devastating influence in chronic inflammatory diseases, is an important element in immune response, may induce immunosuppression. Although blockade of enzymes involved in intracellular pathways leading to cytokine production is efficient in vitro, the intricate cross-talk between the intracellular signaling pathways and the importance of individual kinases in many processes besides inflammation raise the question of the specific targeting of those solely involved in chronic inflammatory mechanisms. Therefore, strategies aimed at specifically inhibiting the production of proinflammatory cytokines, particularly at the triggering level, might lead to therapies that target only the uncontrolled, pathogenic production of TNF-α and IL-1.

REFERENCES

1. Chabaud M, Garnero P, Dayer JM et al. Contribution of interleukin 17 to synovium matrix destruction in rheumatoid arthritis. *Cytokine* 2000; **12**: 1092–9.
2. Dayer JM, Burger D. Cytokines and direct cell contact in synovitis: relevance to therapeutic intervention. *Arthritis Res* 1999; **1**: 17–20.
3. Burger D. Cell contact-mediated signaling of monocytes by stimulated T cells: a major pathway for cytokine induction. *Eur Cytokine Netw* 2000; **11**: 346–53.
4. Vey E, Zhang JH, Dayer J-M. IFN-gamma and 1,25(OH)2D3 induce on THP-1 cells distinct patterns of cell surface antigen expression, cytokine production, and responsiveness to contact with activated T cells. *J Immunol* 1992; **149**: 2040–6.
5. Isler P, Vey E, Zhang JH, Dayer JM. Cell surface glycoproteins expressed on activated human T-cells induce production of interleukin-1 beta by monocytic cells: a possible role of CD69. *Eur Cytokine Netw* 1993; **4**: 15–23.
6. Rezzonico R, Chicheportiche R, Imbert V, Dayer JM. Engagement of CD11b and CD11c beta2 integrin by antibodies or soluble CD23 induces IL-1 beta production on primary human monocytes through mitogen-activated protein kinase-dependent pathways. *Blood* 2000; **95**: 3868–77.
7. Hermann P, Armant M, Brown E et al. The vitronectin receptor and its associated CD47 molecule mediates proinflammatory cytokine synthesis in human monocytes by interaction with soluble CD23. *J Cell Biol* 1999; **144**: 767–75.
8. Wagner DH, Stout RD, Suttles J. Role of the CD40–CD40 ligand interaction in CD4(+) T-cell contact-dependent activation of monocyte interleukin-1 synthesis. *Eur J Immunol* 1994; **24**: 3148–54.
9. Avice MN, Sarfati M, Triebel F et al. Lymphocyte activation gene-3, a MHC class II ligand expressed on activated T cells, stimulates TNF-alpha and IL-alpha production by monocytes and dendritic cells. *J Immunol* 1999; **162**: 2748–53.
10. Burger D, Rezzonico R, Li JM et al. Imbalance between interstitial collagenase (MMP-1) and tissue inhibitor of metalloproteinases-1 (TIMP-1) in synoviocytes and fibroblasts upon direct contact with stimulated T lymphocytes: involvement of membrane-associated cytokines. *Arthritis Rheum* 1998; **41**: 1748–59.
11. Lou J, Dayer JM, Grau GE, Burger D. Direct cell/cell contact with stimulated T lymphocytes induces the expression of cell adhesion molecules and cytokines by human brain microvascular endothelial cells. *Eur J Immunol* 1996; **26**: 3107–13.
12. Balavoine JF, De Rochemonteix B, Cruchaud A, Dayer JM. Collagenase- and PGE₂-stimulating activity (interleukin-1-like) and inhibitor in urine from a patient with monocytic leukaemia. In: Kluger MJ, Oppenheim JJ, Powanda MC, eds. *The Physiologic, Metabolic, and Immunologic Actions of Interleukin-1* (Alan R. Liss: New York, 1985) 429–36.
13. Balavoine JF, De Rochemonteix B, Williamson K et al. Prostaglandin E2 and collagenase production by fibroblasts and synovial cells is regulated by urine-derived human interleukin 1 and inhibitor(s). *J Clin Invest* 1986; **78**: 1120–4.
14. Seckinger P, Lowenthal JW, Williamson K et al. A urine inhibitor of interleukin 1 activity that blocks ligand binding. *J Immunol* 1987; **139**: 1546–9.

15. Prieur AM, Kaufmann MT, Griscelli C, Dayer JM. Specific interleukin-1 inhibitor in serum and urine of children with systemic juvenile chronic arthritis. *Lancet* 1987; **2**: 1240–2.

16. Arend WP, Joslin FG, Massoni RJ. Effects of immune complexes on production by human monocytes of interleukin 1 or an interleukin 1 inhibitor. *J Immunol* 1985; **134**: 3868–75.

17. Roux-Lombard P, Modoux C, Dayer JM. Production of interleukin-1 (IL-1) and a specific IL-1 inhibitor during human monocyte–macrophage differentiation: influence of GM-CSF. *Cytokine* 1989; **1**: 45–51.

18. Galve-de Rochemonteix B, Nicod LP, Junod AF, Dayer JM. Characterization of a specific 20- to 25-kD interleukin-1 inhibitor from cultured human lung macrophages. *Am J Respir Cell Mol Biol* 1990; **3**: 355–61.

19. Mazzei GJ, Seckinger PL, Dayer JM, Shaw AR. Purification and characterization of a 26-kDa competitive inhibitor of interleukin 1. *Eur J Immunol* 1990; **20**: 683–9.

20. Aukrust P, Froland SS, Liabakk NB et al. Release of cytokines, soluble cytokine receptors, and interleukin-1 receptor antagonist after intravenous immunoglobulin administration in vivo. *Blood* 1994; **84**: 2136–43.

21. Seckinger P, Isaaz S, Dayer JM. A human inhibitor of tumor necrosis factor α. *J Exp Med* 1988; **167**: 1511–16.

22. Seckinger P, Vey E, Turcatti G et al. Tumor necrosis factor inhibitor: purification, NH2-terminal amino acid sequence and evidence for anti-inflammatory and immunomodulatory activities. *Eur J Immunol* 1990; **20**: 1167–74.

23. Seckinger P, Zhang JH, Hauptmann B, Dayer JM. Characterization of a tumor necrosis factor alpha (TNF-alpha) inhibitor: evidence of immunological cross-reactivity with the TNF receptor. *Proc Natl Acad Sci USA* 1990; **87**: 5188–92.

24. Williams LM, Gibbons DL, Gearing A et al. Paradoxical effects of a synthetic metalloproteinase inhibitor that blocks both p55 and p75 TNF receptor shedding and TNF alpha processing in RA synovial membrane cell cultures. *J Clin Invest* 1996; **97**: 2833–41.

25. Orlando S, Sironi M, Bianchi G et al. Role of metalloproteases in the release of the IL-1 type II decoy receptor. *J Biol Chem* 1997; **272**: 31764–9.

26. Re F, Muzio M, De Rossi M et al. The type II 'receptor' as a decoy target for interleukin 1 in polymorphonuclear leukocytes: characterization

27. Bessis N, Guery L, Mantovani A et al. The type II decoy receptor of IL-1 inhibits murine collagen-induced arthritis. *Eur J Immunol* 2001; **30**: 867–75.

28. Mantovani A, Locati M, Vecchi A et al. Decoy receptors: a strategy to regulate inflammatory cytokines and chemokines. *Trends Immunol* 2001; **22**: 328–36.

29. Burger D, Chicheportiche R, Giri JG, Dayer JM. The inhibitory activity of human interleukin-1 receptor antagonist is enhanced by type II interleukin-1 soluble receptor and hindered by type I interleukin-1 soluble receptor. *J Clin Invest* 1995; **96**: 38–41.

30. Garrone P, Djossou O, Fossiez F et al. Generation and characterization of a human monoclonal autoantibody that acts as a high affinity interleukin-1 alpha specific inhibitor. *Mol Immunol* 1996; **33**: 649–58.

31. Ulfgren AK, Grondal L, Lindblad S et al. Interindividual and intra-articular variation of proinflammatory cytokines in patients with rheumatoid arthritis: potential implications for treatment. *Ann Rheum Dis* 2000; **59**: 439–47.

32. Firestein GS, Alvaro-Gracia JM, Maki R. Quantitative analysis of cytokine gene expression in rheumatoid arthritis. *J Immunol* 1990; **144**: 3347–53.

33. Dolhain RJEM, Vanderheiden AN, Terhaar NT et al. Shift toward T lymphocytes with a T helper 1 cytokine-secretion profile in the joints of patients with rheumatoid arthritis. *Arthritis Rheum* 1996; **39**: 1961–9.

34. Miossec P, van den BW. Th1/Th2 cytokine balance in arthritis. *Arthritis Rheum* 1997; **40**: 2105–15.

35. Woods JM, Haines GK, Shah MR et al. Low-level production of interleukin-13 in synovial fluid and tissue from patients with arthritis. *Clin Immunol Immunopathol* 1997; **85**: 210–20.

36. Morita Y, Yamamura M, Kawashima M et al. Flow cytometric single-cell analysis of cytokine production by CD4+ T cells in synovial tissue, and peripheral blood from patients with rheumatoid arthritis. *Arthritis Rheum* 1998; **41**: 1669–76.

37. Katsikis PD, Chu CQ, Brennan FM et al. Immunoregulatory role of interleukin 10 in rheumatoid arthritis. *J Exp Med* 1994; **179**: 1517–27.

38. Cohen SB, Katsikis PD, Chu CQ et al. High level of interleukin-10 production by the activated T-cell population within the rheumatoid synovial membrane. *Arthritis Rheum* 1995; **38**: 946–52.

39. Moore KW, de Waal Malefyt R, Coffman RL, O'Garra A. Interleukin-10 and the interleukin-10 receptor. *Annu Rev Immunol* 2001; **19**: 683–765.

40. Yudoh K, Matsuno H, Nakazawa F et al. Reduced expression of the regulatory CD4+ T-cell subset is related to Th1/Th2 balance and disease severity in rheumatoid arthritis. *Arthritis Rheum* 2000; **43**: 617–27.

41. Roncarolo MG, Bacchetta R, Bordignon C et al. Type 1 T regulatory cells. *Immunol Rev* 2001; **182**: 68–79.

42. Chomarat P, Banchereau J. Interleukin-4 and interleukin-13: their similarities and discrepancies. *Int Rev Immunol* 1998; **17**: 1–52.

43. Skapenko A, Wendler J, Lipsky PE et al. Altered memory T-cell differentiation in patients with early rheumatoid arthritis. *J Immunol* 1999; **163**: 491–9.

44. Li JM, Isler P, Dayer JM, Burger D. Contact-dependent stimulation of monocytic cells and neutrophils by stimulated human T-cell clones. *Immunology* 1995; **84**: 571–6.

45. Chizzolini C, Chicheportiche R, Burger D, Dayer JM. Human Th1 cells preferentially induce interleukin (IL)-1 beta while Th2 cells induce IL-1 receptor antagonist production upon cell/cell contact with monocytes. *Eur J Immunol* 1997; **27**: 171–7.

46. Liu Y, Wei SH, Ho AS et al. Expression cloning and characterization of a human IL-10 receptor. *J Immunol* 1994; **152**: 1821–9.

47. de Waal MR, Yssel H, de Vries JE. Direct effects of IL-10 on subsets of human CD4+ T-cell clones and resting T cells. Specific inhibition of IL-2 production and proliferation. *J Immunol* 1993; **150**: 4754–65.

48. Schandene L, Alonso-Vega C, Willems F et al. B7/CD28–dependent IL-5 production by human resting T cells is inhibited by IL-10. *J Immunol* 1994; **152**: 4368–74.

49. Taga K, Tosato G. IL-10 inhibits human T-cell proliferation and IL-2 production. *J Immunol* 1992; **148**: 1143–8.

50. Groux H, Bigler M, de Vries JE, Roncarolo MG. Inhibitory and stimulatory effects of IL-10 on human CD8+ T cells. *J Immunol* 1998; **160**: 3188–93.

51. Rowbottom AW, Lepper MA, Garland RJ et al. Interleukin-10-induced CD8 cell proliferation. *Immunology* 1999; **98**: 80–9.

52. van Roon JA, Lafeber FP, Bijlsma JW. Synergistic activity of interleukin-4 and interleukin-10 in suppression of inflammation and joint destruction in rheumatoid arthritis. *Arthritis Rheum* 2001; **44**: 3–12.

53. Parry SL, Sebbag M, Feldmann M, Brennan FM. Contact with T cells modulates monocyte IL-10 production. Role of T-cell membrane TNF-alpha. *J Immunol* 1997; **158**: 3673–81.

54. Brennan FM, Hayes AL, Ciesielski CJ et al. Evidence that rheumatoid arthritis synovial T cells are similar to cytokine-activated T cells: involvement of phosphatidylinositol 3-kinase and nuclear factor kappaB pathways in tumor necrosis factor alpha production in rheumatoid arthritis. *Arthritis Rheum* 2002; **46**: 31–41.

55. Sebbag M, Parry SL, Brennan FM, Feldmann M. Cytokine stimulation of T lymphocytes regulates their capacity to induce monocyte production of tumor necrosis factor-alpha, but not interleukin-10: possible relevance to pathophysiology of rheumatoid arthritis. *Eur J Immunol* 1997; **27**: 624–32.

56. McInnes IB, Leung BP, Sturrock RD et al. Interleukin-15 mediates T cell-dependent regulation of tumor necrosis factor-alpha production in rheumatoid arthritis. *Nat Med* 1997; **3**: 189–95.

57. Ribbens C, Dayer JM, Chizzolini C. CD40–CD40 ligand (CD154) engagement is required but may not be sufficient for human T helper 1 cell induction of interleukin-2- or interleukin-15-driven, contact-dependent, interleukin-1beta production by monocytes. *Immunology* 2000; **99**: 279–86.

58. Breedveld FC, Dayer JM. Leflunomide: mode of action in the treatment of rheumatoid arthritis. *Ann Rheum Dis* 2000; **59**: 841–9.

59. Tak PP, 't Hart BA, Kraan MC et al. The effects of interferon beta treatment on arthritis. *Rheumatology* 1999; **38**: 362–9.

60. Smeets TJ, Dayer JM, Kraan MC et al. The effects of interferon-beta treatment of synovial inflammation and expression of metalloproteinases in patients with rheumatoid arthritis. *Arthritis Rheum* 2000; **43**: 270–4.

61. Déage V, Burger D, Dayer JM. Exposure of T lymphocytes to leflunomide but not to dexamethasone favors the production by monocytic cells of interleukin-1 receptor antagonist and the tissue-inhibitor of metalloproteinases-1 over that of interleukin-1beta and metalloproteinases. *Eur Cytokine Netw* 1998; **9**: 663–8.

62. Jungo F, Dayer JM, Modoux C et al. IFN-beta inhibits the ability of T lymphocytes to induce TNF-alpha and IL-1beta production in monocytes upon direct cell–cell contact. *Cytokine* 2001; **14**: 272–82.

63. Lee SH, Stehlik C, Reed JC. Cop, a caspase recruitment domain-containing protein and inhibitor of caspase-1 activation processing. *J Biol Chem* 2001; **276**: 34495–500.

64. Bongioanni P, Lombardo F, Moscato G et al. T-cell interferon gamma receptor binding in interferon beta-1b-treated patients with multiple sclerosis. *Arch Neurol* 1999; **56**: 217–22.

65. Kuruvilla AP, Shah R, Hochwald GM et al. Protective effect of transforming growth factor beta 1 on experimental autoimmune diseases in mice. *Proc Natl Acad Sci USA* 1991; **88**: 2918–21.

66. Song XY, Gu M, Jin WW et al. Plasmid DNA encoding transforming growth factor-beta1 suppresses chronic disease in a streptococcal cell wall-induced arthritis model. *J Clin Invest* 1998; **101**: 2615–21.

67. Letterio JJ, Roberts AB. Regulation of immune responses by TGF-beta. *Annu Rev Immunol* 1998; **16**: 137–61.

68. Lingnau K, Hoehn P, Kerdine S et al. IL-4 in combination with TGF-beta favors an alternative pathway of Th1 development independent of IL-12. *J Immunol* 1998; **161**: 4709–18.

69. Hyka N, Dayer JM, Modoux C et al. Apolipoprotein A-I inhibits the production of interleukin-1beta and tumor necrosis factor-alpha by blocking contact-mediated activation of monocytes by T lymphocytes. *Blood* 2001; **97**: 2381–9.

70. Park YB, Lee SK, Lee WK et al. Lipid profiles in untreated patients with rheumatoid arthritis. *J Rheumatol* 1999; **26**: 1701–4.

71. Doherty NS, Littman BH, Reilly K et al. Analysis of changes in acute-phase plasma proteins in an acute inflammatory response and in rheumatoid arthritis using two-dimensional gel electrophoresis. *Electrophoresis* 1998; **19**: 355–63.

72. Lakatos J, Harsagyi A. Serum total, HDL, LDL cholesterol, and triglyceride levels in patients with rheumatoid arthritis. *Clin Biochem* 1988; **21**: 93–6.

73. Ananth L, Prete PE, Kashyap ML. Apolipoproteins A-I and B and cholesterol in synovial fluid of patients with rheumatoid arthritis. *Metabolism* 1993; **42**: 803–6.

74. Bresnihan B, Gogarty M, Burger D et al. Localization of apolipoprotein A-1 at sites of T lymphocyte and macrophage contact in rheumatoid arthritis tissue. *Rheumatology* 2002; **41**: 65 (abstract).

75. Weyand CM, Braun A, Takemura S, Goronzy JJ. Lymphoid microstructures in rheumatoid synovitis. *Curr Dir Autoimmun* 2001; **3**: 168–87.

76. Chomarat P, Vannier E, Dechanet J et al. Balance of IL-1 receptor antagonist/IL-1β in rheumatoid synovium and its regulation by IL-4 and IL-10. *J Immunol* 1995; **154**: 1432–9.

77. van Roon JA, van Roy JL, Duits A et al. Proinflammatory cytokine production and cartilage damage due to rheumatoid synovial T helper-1 activation is inhibited by interleukin-4. *Ann Rheum Dis* 1995; **54**: 836–40.

78. Isomaki P, Luukkainen R, Lassila O et al. Synovial fluid T cells from patients with rheumatoid arthritis are refractory to the T helper type 2 differentiation-inducing effects of interleukin-4. *Immunology* 1999; **96**: 358–64.

79. Bonder CS, Finlay-Jones JJ, Hart PH. Interleukin-4 regulation of human monocyte and macrophage interleukin-10 and interleukin-12 production. Role of a functional interleukin-2 receptor gamma-chain. *Immunology* 1999; **96**: 529–36.

80. Finnegan A, Mikecz K, Tao P, Glant TT. Proteoglycan (aggrecan)-induced arthritis in BALB/c mice is a Th1–type disease regulated by Th2 cytokines. *J Immunol* 1999; **163**: 5383–90.

81. Horsfall AC, Butler DM, Marinova L et al. Suppression of collagen-induced arthritis by continuous administration of IL-4. *J Immunol* 1997; **159**: 5687–96.

82. Joosten LA, Lubberts E, Durez P et al. Role of interleukin-4 and interleukin-10 in murine collagen-induced arthritis. Protective effect of interleukin-4 and interleukin-10 treatment on cartilage destruction. *Arthritis Rheum* 1997; **40**: 249–60.

83. Van Den Bosch F, Russel A, Keystone EC et al. rHuIL-4 in subjects with active rheumatoid arthritis: a phase I dose escalating safety study. *Arthritis Rheum* 1998; **41** (suppl. 9): S56 (abstract).

84. Chizzolini C, Rezzonico R, De Luca C et al. Th2 cell membrane factors in association with IL-4 enhance matrix metalloproteinase-1 (MMP-1) while decreasing MMP-9 production by granulocyte-macrophage colony-stimulating factor-differentiated human monocytes. *J Immunol* 2000; **164**: 5952–60.

85. de Waal Malefyt R. IL-10. In: Oppenheim JJ, Feldmann M, eds. *Cytokine Reference* (Academic Press: New York, London, 2000) 165–85.

86. Clarke CJ, Hales A, Hunt A, Foxwell BM. IL-10-mediated suppression of TNF-alpha production is independent of its ability to inhibit NF kappa B activity. *Eur J Immunol* 1998; **28**: 1719–26.

87. Maini RN, Paulus H, Breedveld FC et al. rHuIL-10 in subjects with active rheumatoid arthritis: a phase I and cytokine response study. *Arthritis Rheum* 1997; **40** (suppl 9): S224 (abstract).

88. Sciacca FL, Canal N, Grimaldi LME. Induction of IL-1 receptor antagonist by interferon beta: implication for the treatment of multiple sclerosis. *J Neurovir* 2000; **6**: S33–7.

89. Wiesemann E, Sonmez D, Heidenreich F, Windhagen A. Interferon-beta increases the stimulatory capacity of monocyte-derived dendritic cells to induce IL-13, IL-5 and IL-10 in autologous T-cells. *J Neuroimmunol* 2002; **123**: 160–9.

90. Buelens C, Bartholome EJ, Amraoui Z et al. Interleukin-3 and interferon beta cooperate to induce differentiation of monocytes into dendritic cells with potent helper T-cell stimulatory properties. *Blood* 2002; **99**: 993–8.

91. Schindler R, Gelfand JA, Dinarello CA. Recombinant C5a stimulates transcription rather than translation of interleukin-1 (IL-1) and tumor necrosis factor: translational signal provided by lipopolysaccharide or IL-1 itself. *Blood* 1990; **76**: 1631–8.

92. Ghezzi P, Dinarello CA, Bianchi M et al. Hypoxia increases production of interleukin-1 and tumor necrosis factor by human mononuclear cells. *Cytokine* 1991; **3**: 189–94.

93. Schindler R, Clark BD, Dinarello CA. Dissociation between interleukin-1 beta mRNA and protein synthesis in human peripheral blood mononuclear cells. *J Biol Chem* 1990; **265**: 10232–7.

94. Mileno MD, Margolis NH, Clark BD et al. Coagulation of whole blood stimulates interleukin-1 beta gene expression. *J Infect Dis* 1995; **172**: 308–11.

95. Lee JC, Laydon JT, McDonnell PC et al. A protein kinase involved in the regulation of inflammatory cytokine biosynthesis. *Nature* 1994; **372**: 739–46.

96. McDonnell PC, DiLella AG, Lee JC, Young PR. Localization of the human stress responsive MAP kinase-like CSAIDs binding protein (CSBP) gene to chromosome 6q21.3/21.2. *Genomics* 1995; **29**: 301–2.

97. Lee JC, Young PR. Role of CSB/p38/RK stress response kinase in LPS and cytokine signaling mechanisms. *J Leukoc Biol* 1996; **59**: 152–7.

98. Badger AM, Bradbeer JN, Votta B et al. Pharmacological profile of SB 203580, a selective inhibitor of cytokine suppressive binding protein/p38 kinase, in animal models of arthritis, bone resorption, endotoxin shock and immune function. *J Pharmacol Exp Ther* 1996; **279**: 1453–61.

99. Badger AM, Blake S, Kapadia R et al. Disease-modifying activity of SB 273005, an orally active, nonpeptide alphavbeta3 (vitronectin receptor) antagonist, in rat adjuvant-induced arthritis. *Arthritis Rheum* 2001; **44**: 128–37.

100. Badger AM, Cook MN, Lark MW et al. SB 203580 inhibits p38 mitogen-activated protein kinase, nitric oxide production, and inducible nitric oxide synthase in bovine cartilage-derived chondrocytes. *J Immunol* 1998; **161**: 467–73.

101. Kumar S, Votta BJ, Rieman DJ et al. IL-1- and TNF-induced bone resorption is mediated by p38 mitogen activated protein kinase. *J Cell Physiol* 2001; **187**: 294–303.

102. Beutler B. Toll-like receptors: how they work and what they do. *Curr Opin Hematol* 2002; **9**: 2–10.

103. Aderem A, Ulevitch RJ. Toll-like receptors in the induction of the innate immune response. *Nature* 2000; **406**: 782–7.

104. Shapira L, Takashiba S, Champagne C et al. Involvement of protein kinase C and protein tyrosine kinase in lipopolysaccharide-induced TNF-alpha and IL-1 beta production by human monocytes. *J Immunol* 1994; **153**: 1818–24.

105. Liu MK, Herrera Velit P, Brownsey RW, Reiner NE. CD14-dependent activation of protein kinase C and mitogen-activated protein kinases (p42 and p44) in human monocytes treated with bacterial lipopolysaccharide. *J Immunol* 1994; **153**: 2642–52.

106. Hayes AL, Smith C, Foxwell BM, Brennan FM. CD45-induced tumor necrosis factor alpha production in monocytes is phosphatidylinositol 3-kinase-dependent and nuclear factor-kappaB-independent. *J Biol Chem* 1999; **274**: 33455–61.

107. Learn CA, Boger MS, Li L, McCall CE. The phosphatidylinositol 3-kinase pathway selectively controls sIL-1RA not interleukin-1beta production in the septic leukocytes. *J Biol Chem* 2001; **276**: 20234–9.

108. Foey AD, Green P, Foxwell B et al. Cytokine-stimulated T cells induce macrophage IL-10 production dependent on phosphatidylinositol 3-kinase and p70S6K: implications for rheumatoid arthritis. *Arthritis Res* 2002; **4**: 64–70.

109. Foxwell B, Browne K, Bondeson J et al. Efficient adenoviral infection with IkappaB alpha reveals that macrophage tumor necrosis factor alpha production in rheumatoid arthritis is NF-kappaB dependent. *Proc Natl Acad Sci USA* 1998; **95**: 8211–15.

110. Hyka N, Kaufmann MT, Chicheportiche R et al. Interferon-beta induces interleukin-1 receptor antagonist production in human monocytes through PI3-kinase-STAT1 signaling pathway. *Autoimmunity Rev* 2002; **1**: 64 (abstract).

111. Vey E, Dayer JM, Burger D. Direct contact with stimulated T cells induces the expression of IL-1 beta and IL-1 receptor antagonist in human monocytes. Involvement of serine/threonine phosphatases in differential regulation. *Cytokine* 1997; **9**: 480–7.

112. Oreopoulos GD, Bradwell S, Lu Z et al. Synergistic induction of IL-10 by hypertonic saline solution and lipopolysaccharides in murine peritoneal macrophages. *Surgery* 2001; **130**: 157–65.

113. Crespo A, Filla MB, Russell SW, Murphy WJ. Indirect induction of suppressor of cytokine signalling-1 in macrophages stimulated with bacterial lipopolysaccharide: partial role of autocrine/paracrine interferon-alpha/beta. *Biochem J* 2000; **349**: 99–104.

114. Stoiber D, Stockinger S, Steinlein P et al. Listeria monocytogenes modulates macrophage cytokine responses through STAT serine phosphorylation and the induction of suppressor of cytokine signaling 3. *J Immunol* 2001; **166**: 466–72.

115. Rottapel R. Putting the brakes on arthritis: can suppressors of cytokine signaling (SOCS) suppress rheumatoid arthritis? *J Clin Invest* 2001; **108**: 1745–7.

116. Shouda T, Yoshida T, Hanada T et al. Induction of the cytokine signal regulator SOCS3/CIS3 as a therapeutic strategy for treating inflammatory arthritis. *J Clin Invest* 2001; **108**: 1781–8.

117. Humke EW, Shriver SK, Starovasnik MA et al. ICEBERG: a novel inhibitor of interleukin-1 beta generation. *Cell* 2000; **103**: 99–111.

118. Aggarwal BB, Samanta A, Feldmann M. TNF-alpha. In: Oppenheim JJ, Feldmann M, eds. *Cytokine Reference* (Academic Press: New York, London, 2000) 413–34.

119. Dinarello CA. IL-1beta. In: Oppenheim JJ, Feldmann M, eds. *Cytokine Reference* (Academic Press: New York, London, 2000) 351–74.

120. Burger D, Dayer JM. IL-1Ra. In: Oppenheim JJ, Feldmann M, eds. *Cytokine Reference* (Academic Press: New York, London, 2000) 319–36.

121. Yang Z, Wara-Aswapati N, Chen C et al. NF-IL6 (C/EBPbeta) vigorously activates il1b gene expression via a Spi-1 (PU.1) protein–protein tether. *J Biol Chem* 2000; **275**: 21272–7.

20

Chemokines

Zoltán Szekanecz, Joon Kim and Alisa E Koch

Introduction • Chemokines • Chemokine receptors • Chemokines in rheumatoid arthritis • Chemokine receptors in rheumatoid arthritis • Regulation of chemokine production • Chemokine targeting attempts in rheumatoid arthritis and animal models of rheumatoid arthritis • Conclusions • Acknowledgments • References

INTRODUCTION

Rheumatoid arthritis (RA) is a chronic inflammatory disease often leading to the destruction of multiple joints. RA affects 1.8–3% of the population.[1] In RA, the synovial tissue (ST) is invaded by inflammatory leukocytes. These cells, as well as their products, including cytokines, play an essential role in synovitis, pannus formation, and cartilage and bone injury.[1] A distinct family of cytokines termed chemokines consists of several inflammatory mediators with structural homology. Chemokines exert chemotactic activity towards neutrophils, lymphocytes and monocytes, and they play an important role in the inflammatory, destructive and fibrovasculoproliferative phases of RA (reviews: Szekanecz et al,[2] Szekanecz and Koch,[3] Koch et al,[4] Kunkel et al,[5] Oppenheim et al,[6] Strieter et al,[7] Taub[8] and Walz et al[9]). Several of these chemokines are also involved in RA-associated angiogenesis.[2–4,10] In the RA synovium, macrophages are the main producers of chemokines.[2–6] The usual management of RA is often difficult, and includes long-term use of immunosuppressive drugs. Recently, biological therapy using anti-cytokine antibodies

and inhibitors was introduced into the therapy of RA. Most of these attempts are discussed elsewhere in this book. There have also been preliminary trials to target chemokines and their receptors in arthritis.

Here we will give a general update on chemokines (Table 20.1) and their receptors (Table 20.2). This will be followed by a more detailed overview of those chemokines and chemokine receptors which may be important in the pathogenesis of RA and thus become potential targets for anti-chemokine therapy (Table 20.3). The chemokine interleukin (IL)-8 will serve as a prototype, since it has been studied most extensively in RA, as well as in other forms of arthritis. We will then briefly summarize the regulation of chemokine production, including interactions between chemokines and other cytokines in the context of RA. Finally, we will also review current experimental data on anti-chemokine targeting in arthritis.

CHEMOKINES

Chemotactic cytokines termed chemokines are involved in the chemotaxis and migration of

Table 20.1 Chemokine families and their most relevant representatives in rheumatoid arthritis.[2,3,11]

C-X-C chemokines

    Interleukin-8 (IL-8, CXCL8)

    Epithelial-neutrophil activating protein-78 (ENA-78, CXCL5)

    Growth-related gene product α (groα, CXCL1)

    Connective tissue activating protein-III (CTAP-III, CXCL6)

    Interferon-γ-inducible protein (IP-10, CXCL10)

    Platelet factor 4 (PF4, CXCL4)

    Monokine induced by interferon-γ (MIG, CXCL9)

    Stromal cell-derived factor (SDF-1, CXCL12)

C-C chemokines

    Monocyte chemoattractant protein-1 (MCP-1, CCL2)

    Macrophage inflammatory protein-1α (MIP-1α, CCL3)

    Macrophage inflammatory protein-3α (MIP-3α, CCL20)

    Regulated upon activation normally T-cell expressed and secreted (RANTES, CCL5)

C chemokines

    Lymphotactin (XCL1)

C-X3-C chemokines

    Fractalkine (CX3CL1)

Table 20.2 Some chemokine receptors and their ligands in rheumatoid arthritis.

Chemokine receptor	Ligand with importance in RA
C-X-C chemokine receptors	
CXCR1	IL-8
CXCR2	IL-8, ENA-78, groα
CXCR3	IP-10, MÍG
CXCR4 (fusin)	SDF-1
CXCR5	
DARC (Duffy antigen receptor for chemokines)	IL-8, ENA-78, groα
C-C chemokine receptors	
CCR1	MIP-1α, RANTES
CCR2	MCP-1
CCR3	RANTES
CCR4	
CCR5	MIP-1α, RANTES
CCR6	MIP-3α
CCR7	
CCR8	
CCR10	MCP-1
C-X3-C chemokine receptors	
CX3CR1	Fractalkine

See Table 20.1 for abbreviations.

inflammatory cells through the endothelial barrier into the inflamed synovium.[1,2,5,6,11] Chemokines have been classified into at least four distinct supergene families based on their structural homology regarding the location of two of four conserved cysteine residues (Table 20.1). These chemokine families and their receptors are designated as C-X-C, C-C, C and C-X3-C chemokines, as well as CXCR, CCR, CR and CX3CR chemokine receptors, respectively.[2,3,11] Recently, a new classification system has been introduced. Now all chemokines are considered

as chemokine ligands and each chemokine has been assigned a designation of CXCL (CXCL1 to CXCL15), CCL (CCL1 to CCL27), XCL and CX3CL1[11] (Table 20.1).

In C-X-C chemokines these two conserved cysteines are separated by one unconserved amino acid (reviews: Walz et al[9] and Zlotnik and Yoshie[11]). This chemokine subfamily includes, among others, IL-8 (CXCL8), epithelial-neutrophil activating protein (ENA)-78 (CXCL5), growth-regulated oncogene α (groα) (CXCL1), connective tissue activating peptide

Table 20.3 Effects of chemokines in rheumatoid synovitis.

Chemokine	Proinflam-matory	Angio-genesis
C-X-C chemokines		
IL-8	+	+
ENA-78	+	+
groα	+	+
CTAP-III	+	+
IP-10	−	−
PF4	−	−
MIG	−	−
SDF-1	+/−	+
C-C chemokines		
MCP-1	+	+
MIP-1α	+	ND
MIP-3α	+	ND
RANTES	+	ND

+, stimulation; −, inhibition; ND, not determined. See text for additional abbreviations.

(CTAP)-III (CXCL6), platelet factor-4 (PF4) (CXCL4), monokine induced by interferon (IFN)-γ (MIG) (CXCL9), IFN-γ-inducible protein (IP-10) (CXCL10) and stromal-derived factor-1 (SDF-1) (CXCL12) (reviews: Szekanecz et al,[2] Walz et al[8] and Zlotnik and Yockie[11]) (Table 20.1). C-X-C chemokines are mostly neutrophil chemotactic factors, although PF4 and IP-10 may also chemoattract monocytes and T lymphocytes.[9] These chemokines are involved in a number of mechanisms underlying inflammation, including the stimulation of leukocyte integrin expression, L-selectin shedding, cell–matrix adhesion, cytoskeleton reorganization, neutrophil degranulation, respiratory burst and phagocytosis, as well as matrix metalloproteinase, leukotriene and platelet-activating factor (review: Waltz et al[9]). Some C-X-C chemokines promote, while others inhibit,

angiogenesis (reviews: Szekanecz and Koch[3] and Strieter et al[7,10]) (Table 20.3). In general, chemokines carrying the ELR (glutamyl-leucyl-arginyl) motif, such as IL-8, ENA-78, groα and CTAP-III, are angiogenic, while ELR-lacking chemokines, including PF4, IP-10 and MIG, are angiostatic.[7,10,12,13] However, there may be exceptions, as seen in the case of the ELR-lacking, but angiogenic, SDF-1.[3,12]

In contrast to C-X-C chemokines, the C-C chemokine subfamily members have adjacent conserved cysteine residues (reviews: Taub[8] and Zlotnik and Yoshie[11]). Both subfamilies have a number of members, but only some of them have been associated with RA. The most relevant C-C chemokines are monocyte chemoattractant protein-1 (MCP-1) (CCL2), macrophage inflammatory protein-1α (MIP-1α) (CCL3), MIP-3α (LARC, CCL20), as well as the chemokine termed 'regulated upon activation normally T-cell expressed and secreted, (RANTES) (CCL5) (reviews: Szekanecz et al,[2] Walz et al[9] and Zlotnik and Yoshie[11]) (Table 20.1). These chemokines mainly induce monocyte chemotaxis, although they may also chemoattract T lymphocytes, NK cells, basophils and eosinophils (reviews: Szekanecz et al[2] and Taub[8]).

Recently, two additional chemokine families termed C chemokines and C-X3-C chemokines have been described based on the unique position of cysteine residues.[2,3,14] The former family contains lymphotactin (XCL1), while the C-X3-C family also includes the solitary member fractalkine (CX3CL1).[2,3,11,14–16] Lymphotactin is involved in the migration of T-cell subsets to inflammatory sites.[16] Fractalkine is expressed on cytokine-activated endothelia, but, in contrast to other chemokines, not on peripheral blood (PB) leukocytes.[14,15]

CHEMOKINE RECEPTORS

There are several known receptors for C-X-C and C-C chemokines, abbreviated as CXCR and CCR, respectively. These receptors exhibit non-specific affinity for their chemokine ligands (Table 20.2). The C-X3-C chemokine, fractalkine, has its own receptor, termed C-X3-CR1.[14,15] It has been suggested recently that chemokine receptors may play a differential role in various inflammatory reactions based on Th1- or Th2-type responses. For example, CCR3 is expressed by lymphocytes exhibiting the Th2, but not the Th1, phenotype. Accordingly, CCR3 is expressed in allergic lymphocytic infiltrates. In contrast, CCR5, present on most Th1-, but not on Th2-type lymphocytes, has been detected in RA synovial fluid (SF) and ST. CXCR3, expressed by both Th1- and Th2-type cells, was detected in both allergic and arthritic infiltrates.[17] Both CCR5 and CXCR3 are preferentially expressed by CD45RO$^+$ memory T cells.[18] Regarding angiogenesis, endothelial cells express receptors for angiogenic chemokines, which is important for the initiation and maintenance of chemokine-mediated neovascularization.[2,3,9,10,19–21]

CHEMOKINES IN RHEUMATOID ARTHRITIS

C-X-C chemokines in rheumatoid arthritis

We and others have shown that IL-8, ENA-78, groα, and CTAP-III are involved in the inflammatory mechanisms underlying RA. IP-10, PF4 and MIG exert anti-inflammatory and anti-angiogenic effects in RA.[2,3,22–27] Recently, a role of SDF-1 in RA has been suggested.[28,29]

IL-8 (CXCL8)

We and other investigators have detected bioactive IL-8 in high quantities in the SF, ST and, unlike a number of other cytokines, in the sera of RA patients.[22,27,30,31] Serum IL-8 levels showed significant positive correlations with IL-8 concentrations in SF.[27] Thus, serum IL-8 levels may reflect intra-articular IL-8 levels, and thus its measurement may serve as a useful tool in monitoring the perpetuation of inflammation within the joint.

In RA ST, a number of cell types – interstitial macrophages, macrophage-derived synovial lining cells and endothelial cells – express IL-8.[27,32,33] However, the synovial macrophage seems to be the principal producer of IL-8.[27] We have also shown that isolated synovial macrophages constitutively produce IL-8 mRNA and protein in vitro, and this cannot be further stimulated by IL-1.[27] In contrast to macrophages, synovial fibroblasts produce IL-8 in vitro in the presence of IL-1 and tumor necrosis factor alpha (TNF-α).[34,35] Furthermore, IL-4 further enhanced, while IFN-γ inhibited, proinflammatory cytokine-mediated IL-8 synthesis.[36] RA synovial stromal cells produce IL-8, and these cells have the capacity to attract PB monocytes.[37] Recently, clinically involved and uninvolved joints of RA patients were compared using arthroscopy, and ST chemokine production was studied. IL-8 protein and mRNA levels were specifically increased in the involved joints compared to the uninvolved joints of patients, as confirmed by immunohistochemistry and in situ hybridization, respectively.[38]

Regarding the functions of IL-8 in arthritis, this chemokine induced synovial inflammation after a single intra-articular injection of recombinant IL-8 into the rabbit knee joint. Arthritis was associated with early entry of neutrophils into the SF, followed by the subsequent accumulation of mononuclear cells. In the ST, early neutrophil infiltration of the synovial lining and the perivascular area was observed, followed by proliferation of the synovial lining layer. The histological picture resembled the human RA synovium.[30] The onset and development of arthritis was studied by IL-8 cDNA transfer in animal models of RA. Rabbit IL-8 cDNA was transduced into rabbit synoviocytes.[39]

IL-8 regulates leukocyte adhesion molecule expression and angiogenesis in RA. SF IL-8 levels correlate with β2 integrin expression on SF neutrophils.[40] We have presented IL-8 as a mediator of angiogenesis[33,41] (Table 20.3). RA tissue homogenates exert chemotactic activity towards endothelial cells and induce angiogenesis in vivo.[33] The ELR motif-containing IL-8 is both chemotactic and mitogenic for endothelial cells in vitro and it is a potent angiogenic factor in in vivo models of angiogenesis.[7,10,41] Endothelial cells express receptors for IL-8.[19,21] Thus, IL-8 is an important chemotactic cytokine which participates in other inflammatory events such as cell adhesion and angiogenesis underlying RA.

ENA-78 (CXCL5)

ENA-78 is a potent chemotactic factor for neutrophils and is also angiogenic[9,10,33,42] (Tables 20.1 and 20.3). We have detected large amounts of ENA-78 in RA SF and ST.[26] Both RA SF mononuclear cells and ST fibroblasts produce ENA-78. ENA-78 synthesis by fibroblasts is further augmented by TNF-α. Within the ST, synovial lining cells, interstitial macrophages, endothelial cells and fibroblasts produce significant amounts of ENA-78. For diagnostic purposes, ENA-78, as well as IL-8, can be readily measured in serum samples.[26] RA ST homogenates produce high amounts of ENA-78. ENA-78 accounts for a large proportion of RA ST-induced angiogenic activity both in vitro and in vivo.[33]

We have studied the temporal expression of an ENA-78-like protein in the sera and joint homogenates of rats with adjuvant-induced arthritis (AA). Almost all animals injected with *Mycobacterium butyricum* and Freund's adjuvant developed arthritis within 2 weeks after the injection. We found significant levels of this chemokine in the sera of arthritic rats. The levels of ENA-78-like protein in ankle joint homogenates were increased in arthritic rats later in the development of the disease compared to control, sham-injected rats. Expression of this chemokine in both the sera and joint homogenates correlated with the progression of arthritis.[43]

Groα (CXCL1)

Groα stimulates the growth of fibroblasts, chemoattracts neutrophils and promotes angiogenesis[9,10] (Tables 20.1 and 20.3). We and others suggested that SF neutrophils and mononuclear cells, isolated ST fibroblasts and articular chondrocytes produce groα mRNA and protein.[23,34,35] The synthesis of fibroblast-derived groα is further stimulated by IL-1 or TNF-α.[23,35] In the ST, lining cells and subsynovial macrophages express high amounts of groα protein and mRNA.[23,44]

The relative importance of IL-8, ENA-78 and groα in RA

Since IL-8, ENA-78 and groα are all produced in large amounts in RA, it is important to know which of these chemokines plays the greatest role in leukocyte emigration into the joint. We simultaneously immunodepleted RA SF of IL-8, ENA-78 and groα, and measured the chemotactic response of normal neutrophils to these SFs. In our study, IL-8, ENA-78 and groα accounted for 36%, 34% and 28% of the chemotactic activity, respectively. These results suggest that all three chemokines are important in neutrophil recruitment into the RA joint, with IL-8 accounting for slightly more of the neutrophil chemotactic activity than the other two chemokines.[23] Certainly, further studies are needed to determine the relative importance of various chemokines in RA.

CTAP-III (CXCL6)

CTAP-III is a human platelet α-granule-derived growth factor.[45] This chemokine, as well as β-thromboglobulin (βTG) and neutrophil-activating protein-2 (NAP-2), are NH₂-truncated cleavage products of platelet basic protein.[9,10] CTAP-III is angiogenic, and affects many aspects of connective tissue metabolism, including the proliferation and proteoglycan production of human synovial fibroblasts[7,10,45,46] (Tables 20.1 and 20.3). RA sera contain high levels of CTAP-III but not βTG or NAP-2.[45] This chemokine was also detected in RA ST.[46]

IP-10 (CXCL10), PF4 (CXCL4) and MIG (CXCL9)

These C-X-C chemokines, unlike the others described above, chemoattract monocytes and T cells rather than neutrophils.[4,9] IP-10, MIG and PF4 do not contain the ELR domain in their structure and have been shown to inhibit neovascularization.[7,10]

Very little IP-10 has been detected in the sera of RA patients.[24] On the other hand, significant amounts of IP-10 were found in the SF and ST of RA patients.[47] MIG was also detected in RA SF and ST.[47] In the ST, MIG is expressed in the synovial lining layer.[44] A peptide sequence from PF4 inhibited murine type II collagen-induced arthritis (CIA).[25] These mediators, in contrast to other C-X-C chemokines discussed above, may be suppressors of arthritis-associated inflammatory and angiogenic mechanisms.

SDF-1 (CXCL12)

SDF-1 specifically binds to CXCR4 (fusin) (Tables 20.1 and 20.2). SDF-1 is expressed by synovial endothelial cells, and this chemokine is able to induce strong integrin-mediated adhesion of SF T cells to intercellular adhesion molecule-1 (ICAM-1).[28] Recently, SDF-1 has been implicated in CD4+ T-cell recruitment into the RA synovium.[29] Direct cellular contact of cytokine-stimulated T cells with synovial fibroblasts resulted in the production of SDF-1 by these fibroblasts.[48] SDF-1 may be a unique chemokine as, despite the fact that it lacks the ELR motif, it promotes angiogenesis.[12,49] Transforming growth factor beta (TGF-β) exerts dual, both pro- and anti-inflammatory, effects in RA (review: Szekanecz et al[50]). TGF-β induces persistent, SDF-1-mediated retention of T cells within the RA synovium.[28] Thus, SDF-1, as well as its inducer, TGF-β, may exert biphasic effects in RA.

C-C chemokines in rheumatoid arthritis

MCP-1 (CCL2)

MCP-1 chemoattracts monocytes, T cells, NK cells and basophils.[8] MCP-1 may be involved in angiogenesis, as in a recent study this chemokine induced endothelial chemotaxis in vitro, as well as angiogenesis in the chick chorioallantoic membrane assay in vivo.[21] We and others have shown high levels of MCP-1 in SF from RA patients.[51,52] RA synovial fibroblasts produce MCP-1 in response to IL-1, TNF-α or IFN-γ.[35,53] In the RA ST, interstitial macrophages are the major source of MCP-1.[52] The main function of MCP-1 in the joint may be the recruitment of macrophages, as injection of MCP-1 into rabbit joints resulted in marked macrophage infiltration of the ST.[51] In a recent report, RA synovial stromal cells were found to produce MCP-1 and thus have the capacity to chemoattract peripheral blood leukocyte (PBL) monocytes.[37]

MIP-1α (CCL3)

MIP-1α is chemotactic for monocytes, T, B and NK cells, basophils and eosinophils.[2,8] We found abundant MIP-1α in RA SF.[54] We and others have

reported that SF mononuclear cells and ST fibroblasts produce MIP-1α mRNA and protein.[35,54] The production of this chemokine by fibroblasts could be further stimulated by IL-1 and TNF-α. Like MCP-1, the main producers of MIP-1α in RA ST are macrophages and fibroblasts.[54]

MIP-3α (CCL20)

MIP-3α is a recently identified chemokine which chemoattracts memory T cells, naive B cells and immature dendritic cells. This chemokine binds to its specific receptor CCR6[55] (Tables 20.1 and 20.2). In a recent report, high amounts of MIP-3α were detected in RA SF and ST. In the ST, mostly synovial lining cells and infiltrating mononuclear cells expressed this chemokine. Cultured RA synovial fibroblasts were capable of producing this chemokine in response to TNF-α and IL-1.[55,56] In our hands, MIP-3α dose-dependently stimulated the chemotaxis of monocytes. In addition, RA SF contained high amounts of this chemokine. Cultured RA ST fibroblasts produced MIP-3α upon stimulation by TNF-α, IL-1 or IL-18.[56]

RANTES (CCL5)

RANTES is a chemotactic factor for monocytes, memory T lymphocytes, NK cells, eosinophils and basophils.[8,57] RA synovial fibroblasts produce RANTES mRNA upon stimulation with TNF-α or IL-1.[35,36] Articular chondrocytes also produce RANTES.[58] These effects of TNF-α or IL-1 on RANTES mRNA expression can be further increased by IFN-γ, but suppressed by IL-4.[36] RANTES mRNA has also been detected in RA PB and SF T cells, as well as in the lining layer and sites of lymphocytic infiltration in RA ST.[44,59]

C and C-X3-C chemokines in rheumatoid arthritis

There is very little information available on the role of the C chemokine lymphotactin in arthritis. In one in vitro study using a transwell system, lymphotactin stimulated the transmigration of the CD45RO+/CD45RB− T-cell subset. This subpopulation of T lymphocytes preferentially accumulates in vivo within the affected joints of RA patients.[16]

Fractalkine is a solitary member of the C-X3-C chemokine subfamily. Fractalkine is chemotactic for monocytes and lymphocytes and also serves as a cellular adhesion molecule,[14,15] We detected high levels of fractalkine in RA SF. In the PB and SF, mostly monocytes expressed this chemokine. In RA ST, macrophages, fibroblasts and endothelial and dendritic cells expressed fractalkine. In rat AA, fractalkine production increased 18 days post-adjuvant injection, in the later stage of the disease.[15]

CHEMOKINE RECEPTORS IN RHEUMATOID ARTHRITIS

CXCR3, among C-X-C chemokine receptors, and CCR5, among C-C chemokine receptors, show strong expression on RA SF T lymphocytes, as well as in T-cell-rich areas of RA ST.[17,18] Others found high expression of CCR5 and CXCR3 on synovial fluid T cells in juvenile RA associated with a high IFN-γ/IL-4 ratio, suggesting a preferential Th1 over Th2 phenotype of these T cells.[60] Among chemokines listed in Table 20.1, the main ligand for CXCR3 is IP-10, while the main ligands for CCR5 are MIP-1α and RANTES[18] (Table 20.2).

A number of studies confirmed the predominance of CCR5-expressing mononuclear cells in SF from arthritic patients.[61,62] Articular chondrocytes also express CCR5 in RA.[58,63] Recently, the frequency of the wild-type CCR5 allele in comparison to the truncated Δ32-CCR5 nonfunctional receptor allele in RA, systemic lupus erythematosus (SLE) and controls was studied. There was no difference between the frequency of wild-type CCR5 genotype in RA, SLE patients and controls. However, while none of the RA patients had the homozygous Δ32-CCR5 genotype, some SLE and control subjects expressed this genotype, supporting the functional role of CCR5 in RA.[64] Regarding the other important chemokine receptor, CXCR3, this receptor is expressed by endothelial cells, certain dendritic cell subsets and sites of lymphocytic infiltrates.[65]

We have compared chemokine receptor expression on PB, SF and ST monocytes/macrophages in RA. In our hands, RA PB monocytes expressed CCR1, CCR2, CCR3, CCR4 and CCR5. SF cells expressed CCR3 and CCR5, but very little CCR1, CCR2 and CCR4. CXCR3 was hardly detected on PB or SF monocytes. SF monocyte CCR5 expression was correlated with leukocyte count. In RA ST, CCR1-, CCR2- and CCR5-immunoreactive cells were detected and co-localized with CD68+ macrophages. We suggested that, based on the differential expression of mainly CCR chemokine receptors on PB and SF cells, some receptors may play a role in monocyte recruitment from the circulation, while others may be involved in monocyte retention in the joint.[66] Our data suggest that CCR1–CCR5 may all play a role in monocyte recruitment in RA. It is important to remember that, as discussed above, MCP-1, binding to CCR2, MIP-1α, recognized by CCR1 and CCR5, and RANTES, binding to CCR1, CCR3 and CCR5, were all found to be important in the pathogenesis of RA (Tables 20.1 and 20.2).

Apart from CCR5 and CXCR3, other chemokine receptors may also be important in RA. For example, CCR6, a receptor for MIP-3α, was detected on infiltrating leukocytes in the RA ST, but not in osteoarthritis (OA).[55] RA articular chondrocytes express CCR3 and produce its ligand, RANTES.[58,63] As discussed above, CXCR4, the only receptor for SDF-1, may play a role in the SDF-1-derived retention of T cells within the RA ST.[28,29] In a recent study, RA articular chondrocytes expressed CCR1, CCR2, CCR3, CCR5, CXCR1 and CXCR2.[63] In another study, chemokine receptor expression on synovial CD4+ cells was correlated with cytokine production by these cells. Correlations between IL-10 and CCR7, IFN-γ and CCR5, as well as TNF-related activation-induced cytokine (TRANCE) and CXCR4, was detected.[67]

Regarding the possible role of chemokine receptors in RA-associated angiogenesis, a number of these receptors may be detected on endothelial cells, and thus play a role in chemokine-induced angiogenesis. The role of endothelial IL-8 receptors in this process is mentioned above.[19,20] MCP-1-induced neovascularization was associated with abundant endothelial expression of CCR2.[21] CXCR2 may be the most important endothelial receptor for ELR-containing angiogenic CXC chemokines: CXCR2 is a major receptor for these chemokines.[9,10,20]

REGULATION OF CHEMOKINE PRODUCTION

Temporal expression of chemokines in animal models of rheumatoid arthritis

Monitoring the temporally controlled production of chemokines may help us to better understand the inflammatory events underlying the development of arthritis, as well as enable early intervention in the disease. This type of assessment is hardly feasible in humans. Therefore, we have recently assessed the temporal expression of ENA-78, MCP-1 and MIP-1α during the course of rat AA, a model for human RA, in order to differentiate between chemokines involved in the early events or later stages of the disease. The amounts of these chemokines in the sera and joint homogenates of AA and control rats were measured. The production of ENA-78 and MIP-1α showed a very early increase, preceding clinical symptoms. Correlation studies revealed that the abundant production of these chemokines was associated with early inflammatory events, including leukocyte, mainly neutrophil, ingress and the production of acute-phase reactants. In contrast, MCP-1 seems to be involved mostly in the later phase of AA.[68] In another series of experiments, treatment of AA rats with anti-ENA antibody also revealed that ENA-78 may be involved in the very early inflammatory events underlying AA.[43] Others found increased RANTES and MIP-1α production in mice with CIA compared to controls.[69]

Two-way interactions between cytokines and chemokines in rheumatoid arthritis

A regulatory network of proinflammatory cytokines, such as TNF-α and IL-1, and chemokines exists in the RA synovium.[2,3,50,70]

Both TNF-α and IL-1 are abundantly produced in the RA joint.[50,70] While, as described before, monocyte/macrophages in the RA synovium constitutively express most chemokines, including IL-8, ENA-78, groα, MCP-1 and MIP-1α,[23,26,27,52,54] resting synovial fibroblasts and articular chondrocytes produce only small amounts of chemokines. However, TNF-α and IL-1 further stimulate chemokine production by fibroblasts.[2,3,26,34,35,50,53]

The synovial microenvironment containing a mixture of various regulatory cytokines may influence the production of C-X-C and C-C chemokines, the balance between chemokines with pro- and anti-inflammatory activity, and thus the outcome of synovial inflammation. Interestingly, cytokine-mediated IL-8 secretion by RA synovial fibroblasts is upregulated by IL-4 but inhibited by IFN-γ. In contrast, cytokine-dependent RANTES production by the same cells is decreased by IL-4 but stimulated by IFN-γ.[36] IFN-γ is mostly produced by Th1-type lymphocytes, while IL-4 is secreted by Th2 cells. The major differences between Th1- and Th2-type cells are discussed above. These data suggest that the type of cellular infiltrate, namely the dominance of Th1- or Th2-type lymphocytes, as well as their characteristic cytokine production may result in a differential local chemokine pattern.

Inverse relationships between chemokines and cytokines may also exist in the RA synovium. For example, MIP-1α stimulates the synthesis of IL-1, TNF-α or IL-6 by murine macrophages, suggesting a positive-feedback mechanism between MIP-1α and these cytokines.[2,71] In our hands, treatment of rat AA with a polyclonal antibody to an ENA-78-like protein resulted in downregulation of synovial IL-1 expression, suggesting a regulatory role for ENA-78 in IL-1 production.[43]

These cytokine–chemokine interactions may be important for the perpetuation of inflammatory mediator production within the inflamed synovium. In addition, not only direct chemokine targeting, but also suppressing the production of proinflammatory cytokines, may be useful for controlling chemokine-mediated leukocyte ingress into the RA joint.

CHEMOKINE TARGETING ATTEMPTS IN RHEUMATOID ARTHRITIS AND ANIMAL MODELS OF RHEUMATOID ARTHRITIS

Chemokine production in the RA joint could be targeted in a number of ways. Disease-modifying anti-rheumatic drugs (DMARDs), currently used in the treatment of RA, may themselves influence chemokine production. Also, as described above, as there is a direct relationship between proinflammatory cytokines and chemokines, anti-TNF-α and anti-IL-1 strategies discussed by others in this book may also downregulate chemokine synthesis. Most of these approaches have already been tried in RA. Finally, preliminary trials using antibodies to chemokines or chemokine inhibitors carried out in animal models of arthritis suggest that direct, specific chemokine or chemokine receptor targeting may also be available in the near future.

Effects of anti-inflammatory agents on chemokines

Among immunosuppressive agents, corticosteroids, such as dexamethasone, effectively suppressed IL-8 production in RA.[31,72,73] In contrast, non-steroidal anti-inflammatory drugs, as well as DMARDs including gold salts and methotrexate, had mild effects or no effect on IL-8 synthesis.[72-74] MCP-1 production could be altered by dexamethasone and, to a much lesser extent, gold salts.[72] We found that sulfapyridine inhibited cytokine-stimulated endothelial cell expression of IL-8 and MCP-1.[75]

TNF-α induces chemokine production in part via generation of reactive oxygen intermediates. Antioxidants, such as N-acetyl-L-cysteine and 2-oxothiazolidine-4-carboxylate, suppressed TNF-α-induced IL-8 and MCP-1 mRNA synthesis in isolated human synovial cells.[76] These antioxidants may be useful in inhibiting chemokine production in RA.

Effects of anti-TNF-α and anti-IL-1 targeting on chemokine production

The suppression of proinflammatory cytokine production may also block the synthesis of cytokine-dependent chemokines. Anti-TNF-α and anti-IL-1 targeting strategies are discussed elsewhere in this book. For example, infliximab, an anti-TNF-α monoclonal antibody blocker, reduced synovial expression of IL-8 and MCP-1 in RA patients. This was associated with diminished inflammatory cell ingress into the synovium.[77]

Direct chemokine targeting

The inflammatory action of chemokines may be directly suppressed using specific antibodies or other inhibitors. Anti-chemokine targeting may be used in future anti-rheumatic therapy. In addition, plenty of information may be gathered on the actions of chemokines from these trials. In our hands, antibodies to IL-8, ENA-78 and groα, at least partially, neutralized RA SF-derived chemotactic activity for neutrophils in vitro.[23] In another study, we have used a neutralizing polyclonal anti-ENA-78 antibody to treat rats with AA, a model for RA. Anti-ENA-78 administered intravenously after adjuvant injection but prior to the onset of arthritis attenuated the severity of the disease as determined by joint size measurements. In addition, anti-ENA-78 significantly reduced the number of IL-1-immunoreactive cells in the synovial lining layer, indicating a possible role of ENA-78 in the maintenance of proinflammatory cytokine production in the synovium. This antibody was unable to influence the disease course when injected during the further development of arthritis.[43] These data suggest that ENA-78 is possibly involved in the early events associated with synovial neutrophil influx in AA. In addition, anti-ENA-78 antibodies administered in the very early phase of the disease may inhibit the further progression of arthritis.

Other anti-chemokine antibodies have also been tried in arthritis models. Passive immunization with anti-MIP-1α delayed the onset and reduced the severity of CIA in mice.[5,78] A neutralizing monoclonal antibody to MCP-1 reduced ankle swelling by 30% and significantly decreased the number of synovial macrophages in rat CIA.[79]

Apart from antibodies, chemokine antagonists or angiostatic, anti-inflammatory chemokines may also be used as anti-rheumatic agents. For example, a 67 amino acid sequence of MCP-1, which acts as an MCP-1 antagonist in vitro, abrogated arthritis in MRL-lpr autoimmune mice.[80] A bioactive synthetic peptide derived from the angiogenesis inhibitor chemokine PF4 suppressed murine CIA, as well as arthritis-associated angiogenesis.[25]

CONCLUSIONS

In this chapter, we have discussed the putative role of chemokines and their receptors in RA. Chemokines are involved in a number of inflammatory mechanisms, including adhesion, angiogenesis and tissue destruction, underlying the pathogenesis of arthritis. Anti-chemokine targeting may be therapeutically used in future anti-rheumatic therapies. In addition, we can learn a lot from these trials about the actions of the targeted chemokines. It is likely that clinically available specific antagonists of chemokines or their receptors will be developed and administered to patients. Future directions in chemokine, as well as cytokine, research may also include somatic gene therapy. Hopefully, these strategies will lead to the everyday use of specific immunomodulatory therapies, including anti-chemokine targeting, which will prevent joint destruction and thus will benefit RA patients.

ACKNOWLEDGMENTS

This work was supported by NIH grants HL-58695 and AI-40987 (A.E.K.), funds from the Veterans' Administration Research Service (A.E.K.), and the Gallagher Professorship for Arthritis Research (A.E.K.), grant F 025813 from the Hungarian National Scientific Research Fund (OTKA) (Z.S.), and grant No. 0018 from the Research and Development Fund for Highest Education (FKFP) (Z.S.).

REFERENCES

1. Harris ED. Rheumatoid arthritis: pathophysiology and implications for therapy. *N Engl J Med* 1990; **332**: 1277–87.

2. Szekanecz Z, Kunkel SL, Strieter RM, Koch AE. Chemokines in rheumatoid arthritis. *Springer Semin Immunopathol* 1998; **20**: 115–32.

3. Szekanecz Z, Koch AE. Chemokines and angiogenesis. *Curr Opin Rheumatol* 2001; **13**: 202–8.

4. Koch AE, Kunkel SL, Strieter RM. Chemokines in arthritis. In: Koch AE, Strieter RM, eds. *Chemokines in Disease* (RG Landes Company: Austin, 1996) 103–16.

5. Kunkel SL, Lukacs N, Kasama T, Strieter RM. The role of chemokines in inflammatory joint disease. *J Leukoc Biol* 1996; **58**: 6–12.

6. Oppenheim JJ, Zachariae COC, Mukaida N, Matsushima K. Properties of the novel proinflammatory supergene 'intercrine' cytokine family. *Annu Rev Immunol* 1991; **9**: 617–48.

7. Strieter RM, Polverini PJ, Kunkel SL et al. The functional role of the ELR motif in CXC chemokine-mediated angiogenesis. *J Biol Chem* 1995; **270**: 27348–57.

8. Taub DD. C-C chemokines – an overview. In: Koch AE, Strieter RM, eds. *Chemokines in Disease* (RG Landes Company: Austin, 1996) 27–54.

9. Walz A, Kunkel SL, Strieter RM. C-X-C chemokines – an overview. In: Koch AE, Strieter RM, eds. *Chemokines in Disease* (RG Landes Company: Austin, 1996) 1–25.

10. Strieter RM, Kunkel SL, Shanafelt AB et al. The role of C-X-C chemokines in the regulation of angiogenesis. In: Koch AE, Strieter RM, eds. *Chemokines in Disease* (RG Landes Company: Austin, 1996) 195–209.

11. Zlotnik A, Yoshie O. Chemokines: a new classification system and their role in immunity. *Immunity* 2000; **12**: 121–7.

12. Moore BB, Keane MP, Addison CL et al. CXC chemokine modulation of angiogenesis: the importance of balance between angiogenic and angiostatic members of the family. *J Invest Med* 1998; **46**: 113–20.

13. Keane MP, Strieter RM: The role of CXC chemokines in the regulation of angiogenesis. *Chem Immunol* 1999; **72**: 86–101.

14. Bazan JF, Bacon KB, Hardiman G et al. A new class of membrane bound chemokine with a X3C motif. *Nature* 1997; **385**: 640–4.

15. Ruth JH, Volin MV, Haines III GK et al. Fractalkine, a novel chemokine in rheumatoid arthritis and rat adjuvant-induced arthritis. *Arthritis Rheum* 2001; **44**: 1568–81.

16. Borthwick NJ, Akbar AN, MacCormac LP et al. Selective migration of highly differentiated primed T cells, defined by low expression of CD45RB, across human umbilical vein endothelial cells: effects of viral infection on transmigration. *Immunology* 1997; **90**: 272–80.

17. Loetscher P, Uguccioni M, Bordoli L et al. CCR5 is characteristic of Th1 lymphocytes. *Nature* 1998; **391**: 344–5.

18. Qin S, Rottman JB, Myers P et al. The chemokine receptors CXCR3 and CCR5 mark subsets of T cells with a homing predilection for certain inflammatory sites. *J Clin Invest* 1998; **101**: 746–50.

19. Rot A, Hub E, Middleton J et al. Some aspects of IL-8 pathophysiology. III. Chemokine interaction with endothelial cells. *J Leukoc Biol* 1996; **59**: 39–44.

20. Schonbeck U, Brandt E, Petersen F et al. IL-8 specifically binds to endothelial but not to smooth muscle cells. *J Immunol* 1995; **154**: 2375–83.

21. Salcedo R, Ponce ML, Young HA et al. Human endothelial cells express CCR2 and respond to MCP-1: direct role of MCP-1 in angiogenesis and tumor progression. *Blood* 2000; **96**: 34–40.

22. Hogan M, Sherry B, Ritchlin C et al. Differential expression of the small inducible cytokines groα and groβ by synovial fibroblasts in chronic arthritis: possible role in growth regulation. *Cytokine* 1994; **6**: 61–9.

23. Koch AE, Kunkel SL, Shah MR et al. Growth related gene product alpha: a chemotactic cytokine for neutrophils in rheumatoid arthritis. *J Immunol* 1995; **155**: 3660–6.

24. Narumi S, Tominaga Y, Tamaru M et al. Expression of IFN-inducible protein-10 in chronic hepatitis. *J Immunol* 1997; **158**: 5536–44.

25. Wooley PH, Schaefer C, Whalen JD et al. A peptide sequence from platelet factor 4 (CT-112) is effective in the treatment of type II collagen induced arthritis in mice. *J Rheumatol* 1997; **24**: 890–8.

26. Koch AE, Kunkel SL, Harlow LA et al. Epithelial neutrophil activating peptide-78: a novel chemotactic cytokine for neutrophils in arthritis. *J Clin Invest* 1994; **94**: 1012–18.

27. Koch AE, Kunkel SL, Burrows JC et al. Synovial tissue macrophage as a source of the chemotactic cytokine IL-8. *J Immunol* 1991; **147**: 2187–95.

28. Buckley CD, Amft N, Bradfield PF et al. Persistent induction of the chemokine receptor CXCR4 by TGF-beta 1 on synovial T cells contributes to their accumulation within the rheumatoid synovium. *J Immunol* 2000; **165**: 3423–9.

29. Nanki T, Hayashida K, El-Gabalawy HS et al. Stromal cell-derived factor-1-CXC chemokine receptor 4 interactions play a central role in CD4+ T-cell accumulation in rheumatoid arthritis synovium. *J Immunol* 2000; **165**: 6590–8.

30. Endo H, Akahoshi T, Takagishi K et al. Elevation of interleukin-8 (IL-8) levels in joint fluids of patients with rheumatoid arthritis and the induction by IL-8 of leukocyte infiltration and synovitis in rabbit joints. *Lymphokine Cytokine Res* 1991; **10**: 245–52.

31. Seitz M, Dewald B, Gerber N, Baggiolini M. Enhanced production of neutrophil-activating peptide-1/interleukin-8 in rheumatoid arthritis. *J Clin Invest* 1991; **87**: 463–9.

32. Deleuran B, Lemche P, Kristensen M et al. Localisation of interleukin 8 in the synovial membrane, cartilage–pannus junction and chondrocytes in rheumatoid arthritis. *Scand J Rheumatol* 1994; **23**: 2–7.

33. Koch AE, Volin MV, Woods JM et al. Regulation of angiogenesis by the C-X-C chemokines interleukin-8 and epithelial neutrophil activating peptide-78 in the rheumatoid joint. *Arthritis Rheum* 2001; **44**: 31–40.

34. Bedard PA, Golds EE. Cytokine-induced expression of mRNAs for chemotactic factors in human synovial cells and fibroblasts. *J Cell Physiol* 1993; **154**: 433–41.

35. Hosaka S, Akahoshi T, Wada C, Kondo H. Expression of the chemokine superfamily in rheumatoid arthritis. *Clin Exp Immunol* 1994; **97**: 451–7.

36. Rathanaswami P, Hachicha M, Sadick M et al. Expression of the cytokine RANTES in human rheumatoid synovial fibroblasts. Differential regulation of RANTES and interleukin-8 genes by inflammatory cytokines. *J Biol Chem* 1993; **268**: 5834–9.

37. Hayashida K, Nanki T, Girschick H et al. Synovial stromal cells from rheumatoid arthritis patients attract monocytes by producing MCP-1 and IL-8. *Arthritis Res* 2001; **3**: 118–26.

38. Kraan MC, Patel DD, Haringman JJ et al. The development of clinical signs of rheumatoid synovial inflammation is associated with increased synthesis of the chemokine CXCL8 (interleukin-8). *Arthritis Res* 2001; **3**: 65–71.

39. Chen Y, Davidson BL, Marks RM. Adenovirus-mediated transduction of the interleukin 8 gene into synoviocytes. *Arthritis Rheum* 1994; **37**: S304.

40. De Gendt CM, De Clerck LS, Bridts CH et al. Relationship between interleukin-8 and neutrophil adhesion molecules in rheumatoid arthritis. *Rheumatol Int* 1996; **16**: 169–73.

41. Koch AE, Polverini PJ, Kunkel SL et al. Interleukin-8 as a macrophage-derived mediator of angiogenesis. *Science* 1992; **258**: 1798–801.

42. Walz A, Burgener R, Car B et al. Structure and neutrophil-activating properties of a novel inflammatory peptide (ENA-78) with homology to interleukin 8. *J Exp Med* 1991; **174**: 1355–62.

43. Halloran MM, Woods JM, Strieter RM et al. The role of an epithelial neutrophil-activating peptide-78-like protein in rat adjuvant-induced arthritis. *J Immunol* 1999; **162**: 7492–500.

44. Konig A, Krenn V, Toksoy A et al. Mig, GRO alpha and RANTES messenger RNA expression in lining layer, infiltrates and different leucocyte populations of synovial tissue from patients with rheumatoid arthritis, psoriatic arthritis and osteoarthritis. *Virchows Arch* 2000; **436**: 449–58.

45. Castor CW, Andrews PC, Swartz RD et al. The origin, variety, distribution, and biologic fate of connective tissue activating peptide-III isoforms: characteristics in patients with rheumatic, renal, and arterial disease. *Arthritis Rheum* 1993; **36**: 1142–53.

46. Castor CW, Smith EM, Hossler PA et al. Detection of connective tissue activating peptide-III isoforms in synovium from osteoarthritis and rheumatoid arthritis patients: patterns of interaction with other synovial cytokines in cell culture. *Arthritis Rheum* 1992; **35**: 783–93.

47. Patel DD, Zachariah JP, Whichard LP. CXCR3 and CCR5 ligands in the rheumatoid arthritis synovium. *Clin Immunol* 2001; **98**: 39–45.

48. Burger D. Cell contact interactions in rheumatology. The Kennedy Institute for Rheumatology, London, UK, 1–2 June 2000. *Arthritis Res* 2000; **2**: 472–6.

49. Salcedo R, Wasserman K, Young HA et al. Vascular endothelial growth factor and basic fibroblast growth factor induce expression of CXCR4 on human endothelial cells: in vivo neovascularization induced by stromal-derived factor-1alpha. *Am J Pathol* 1999; **154**: 1125–35.

50. Szekanecz Z, Strieter RM, Koch AE. Cytokines in rheumatoid arthritis: potential targets for pharmacological intervention. *Drugs Aging* 1998; **12**: 377–90.

51. Akahoshi T, Wada C, Endo H et al. Expression of monocyte chemotactic and activating factor in rheumatoid arthritis. *Arthritis Rheum* 1993; **36**: 762–71.

52. Koch AE, Kunkel SL, Harlow LA et al. Enhanced production of monocyte chemoattractant protein-1 in rheumatoid arthritis. *J Clin Invest* 1992; **90**: 772–9.

53. Villiger PM, Terkeltaub R, Lotz M. Production of monocyte chemoattractant protein-1 by inflamed synovial tissue and cultured synoviocytes. *J Immunol* 1992; **149**: 722–7.

54. Koch AE, Kunkel SL, Harlow LA et al. Macrophage inflammatory protein-1 alpha. A novel chemotactic cytokine for macrophages in rheumatoid arthritis. *J Clin Invest* 1994; **93**: 921–8.

55. Matsui T, Akahoshi T, Namai R et al. Selective recruitment of CCR6-expressing cells by increased production of MIP 3 alpha in rheumatoid arthritis. *Clin Exp Immunol* 2001; **125**: 155–61.

56. Ruth JH, Morel JCM, Park, CC et al. MIP-3α expression in the rheumatoid joint. *Arthritis Rheum* 2000; **43** (Suppl 9): S78.

57. Schall TJ, Bacon K, Toy KJ, Goeddel DV. Selective attraction of monocytes and T lymphocytes of the memory phenotype by cytokine RANTES. *Nature* 1990; **347**: 669–71.

58. Alaaeddine N, Olee T, Hashimoto S et al. Production of the chemokine RANTES by articular chondrocytes and role in cartilage degradation. *Arthritis Rheum* 2001; **44**: 1633–43.

59. Robinson E, Keystone EC, Schall TJ et al. Chemokine expression in rheumatoid arthritis (RA): evidence of RANTES and macrophage inflammatory protein (MIP)-1 beta production by synovial T cells. *Clin Exp Immunol* 1995; **101**: 398–407.

60. Wedderburn LR, Robinson N, Patel A et al. Selective recruitment of polarized T cells expressing CCR5 and CXCR3 to the inflamed joints of children with juvenile idiopathic arthritis. *Arthritis Rheum* 2000; **43**: 765–74.

61. Mack M, Bruhl H, Gruber R et al. Predominance of mononuclear cells expressing the chemokine receptor CCR5 in synovial effusions of patients with different forms of arthritis. *Arthritis Rheum* 1999; **42**: 981–8.

62. Suzuki N, Nakajima A, Yoshino S et al. Selective accumulation of CCR5+ T lymphocytes into inflamed joints in rheumatoid arthritis. *Int Immunol* 1999; **11**: 553–9.

63. Borzi RM, Mazzetti I, Cattini L et al. Human chondrocytes express functional chemokine receptors and release matrix-degrading enzymes in response to C-X-C and C-C chemokines. *Arthritis Rheum* 2000; **43**: 1734–41.

64. Gomez-Reino JJ, Pablos JL, Carreira PE et al. Association of rheumatoid arthritis with a functional chemokine receptor, CCR5. *Arthritis Rheum* 1999; **42**: 989–92.

65. Garcia-Lopez MA, Sanchez-Madrid F, Rodriguez-Frade JM et al. CXCR3 chemokine receptor distribution in normal and inflamed tissues. *Lab Invest* 2001; **81**: 409–18.

66. Katschke KJ jr, Rottman JB, Ruth JH et al. Differential expression of chemokine receptors on peripheral blood, synovial fluid and synovial tissue monocytes/macrophages in rheumatoid arthritis. *Arthritis Rheum* 2001; **44**: 1022–32.

67. Nanki T, Lipsky PE. Cytokine, activation marker and chemokine receptor expression by individual CD4(+) memory T cells in rheumatoid arthritis synovium. *Arthritis Res* 2000; **2**: 415–23.

68. Szekanecz Z, Halloran MM, Volin MV et al. Temporal expression of inflammatory cytokines and chemokines in rat adjuvant-induced arthritis. *Arthritis Rheum* 2000; **43**: 1266–77.

69. Thornton S, Duwel LE, Boivin GP et al. Association of the course of collagen-induced arthritis with distinct patterns of cytokine and chemokine messenger RNA expression. *Arthritis Rheum* 1999; **42**: 1109–18.

70. Feldmann M, Brennan FM, Maini RN. Role of cytokines in rheumatoid arthritis. *Annu Rev Immunol* 1996; **14**: 397–440.

71. Fahey TJ, Tracey KJ, Tekamp-Olson P et al. Macrophage inflammatory protein 1 modulates macrophage function. *J Immunol* 1991; **148**: 2764–9.

72. Loetscher P, Dewald B, Baggiolini M, Seitz M. Monocyte chemoattractant protein 1 and interleukin 8 production by rheumatoid synoviocytes: effects of anti-rheumatic drugs. *Cytokine* 1994; **6**: 162–70.

73. Youssef PP, Haynes DR, Triantafillou S et al. Effects of pulse methylprednisolone on inflammatory mediators in peripheral blood, synovial fluid, and synovial membrane in rheumatoid arthritis. *Arthritis Rheum* 1997; **40**: 1400–8.

74. Seitz M, Loetscher P, Dewald B et al. Methotrexate action in rheumatoid arthritis: stimulation of cytokine inhibitor and inhibition of chemokine production by peripheral blood mononuclear cells. *Br J Rheumatol* 1995; **34**: 602–9.

75. Volin MV, Harlow LA, Woods JM et al. Treatment with sulfasalazine or sulfapyridine, but not 5-aminosalicyclic acid, inhibits basic fibroblast growth factor-induced endothelial cell chemotaxis. *Arthritis Rheum* 1999; **42**: 1927–35.

76. Sato M, Miyazaki T, Nagaya T et al. Antioxidants inhibit tumor necrosis factor-alpha mediated stimulation of interleukin-8, monocyte chemoattractant protein-1, and collagenase expression in cultured human synovial cells. *J Rheumatol* 1996; **23**: 432–8.

77. Taylor PC, Peters AM, Paleolog E et al. Reduction of chemokine levels and leukocyte traffic to joints by tumor necrosis factor alpha blockade in patients with rheumatoid arthritis. *Arthritis Rheum* 2000; **43**: 38–47.

78. Kasama T, Strieter RM, Lukacs NW et al. Interleukin-10 expression and chemokine regulation during the evolution of murine type II collagen-induced arthritis. *J Clin Invest* 1995; **95**: 2868–76.

79. Ogata H, Takeya M, Yoshimura T et al. The role of monocyte chemoattractant protein-1 (MCP-1) in the pathogenesis of collagen-induced arthritis in rats. *J Pathol* 1997; **182**: 106–14.

80. Gong JH, Ratkay LG, Waterfield JD, Clark-Lewis I. An antagonist of monocyte chemoattractant protein 1 (MCP-1) inhibits arthritis in the MRL-lpr mouse model. *J Exp Med* 1997; **186**: 131–7.

21

Osteoprotegerin

Allison R Pettit and Ellen M Gravallese

Introduction • The RANKL/RANK/OPG system – essential role in osteoclastogenesis • Osteoclastogenesis – the current paradigm • Contribution of osteoclasts to focal bone erosion in rheumatoid arthritis • OPG as a therapeutic agent in animal models of arthritis • Other potential therapeutic applications of OPG • Additional considerations in the use of OPG as a therapeutic agent • Conclusion • References

INTRODUCTION

Rheumatoid arthritis (RA) is an immune-mediated disease that leads to inflammatory synovitis with accompanying destruction of the extracellular matrices of joint cartilage and bone. Although many of the mechanisms of cartilage destruction have been elucidated, the cellular and molecular mechanisms of bone loss in RA have only recently been studied in detail. Three distinct forms of bone loss occur in patients with RA. These include marginal and subchondral focal bone erosions, juxta-articular osteopenia in trabecular bone adjacent to inflamed joints, and generalized osteopenia/osteoporosis of the axial and appendicular skeleton.[1–3] Protection from bone erosion is one important goal of therapeutic intervention, as radiologic damage of large and small joints is associated with disease severity and disability.[4,5] Thus far, therapeutic approaches in RA have not directly targeted the process of marginal and subchondral focal bone erosion.

Recent research has demonstrated that osteoclasts play an important role in the pathogenesis of focal bone erosion,[6–15] and possibly also in juxta-articular osteopenia.[16,17] This finding is not unexpected, since osteoclasts are the cells responsible for bone resorption in physiologic bone remodeling. Osteoprotegerin (OPG) is a recently identified member of the tumor necrosis factor (TNF) receptor superfamily which blocks the differentiation, activation and survival of osteoclasts.[18–22] Therefore, OPG is being studied in animal models of RA as a potential therapy to block bone destruction. This chapter reviews the scientific evidence for the role of OPG in the inhibition of osteoclastogenesis, osteoclast activation and osteoclast survival in physiologic and pathologic bone resorption, and discusses the potential therapeutic benefit of OPG treatment in RA and in other diseases in which pathologic bone destruction is a prominent feature.

THE RANKL/RANK/OPG SYSTEM – ESSENTIAL ROLE IN OSTEOCLASTOGENESIS

OPG was originally identified and cloned as a novel soluble factor that was instrumental in regulating bone mass.[18] This factor is identical to osteoclastogenesis inhibitory factor (OCIF),[19,20] follicular dendritic cell receptor-1 (FDCR-1)[21]

and TNF receptor superfamily member 1 (TR-1).[22] Human OPG is a 55-kDa glycoprotein that, unlike most other members of the TNF receptor superfamily, lacks a hydrophobic membrane sequence and is therefore expressed as a secreted protein.[18,19] OPG is predominantly produced as a homodimer but is also functional in its monomeric form.[18] OPG mRNA is expressed in many human tissues, including bone, lung, heart, kidney and immune organs.[18,19]

The ligand for OPG was identified as receptor activator of NFκB ligand (RANKL). The ability of OPG to bind RANKL with high affinity facilitated the discovery of this ligand as the essential factor for osteoclastogenesis.[23,24] The ligand-binding domain of OPG consists of four highly conserved cysteine-rich TNF receptor-like domains located near the N-terminus of the protein.[25] Specific binding of the OPG receptor to RANKL prevents ligation of RANKL to the signaling receptor, receptor activator of NFκB (RANK – also identified as TRANCE receptor (TRANCER) and osteoclast differentiation and activation receptor (ODAR)).[26–28] Therefore, OPG acts as a non-signaling decoy receptor for RANKL and is thus a negative regulator of osteoclastogenesis.[23,29–34]

RANKL was identified independently by several research groups and was termed osteoclast differentiation factor (ODF)[24] and osteoprotegerin ligand (OPGL).[23] RANKL was also cloned and identified as TNF-related activation-induced cytokine (TRANCE),[26] a factor that is upregulated after T-cell receptor stimulation and participates in cooperative T-cell–dendritic cell interactions.[27,35] As recommended by the American Society for Bone and Mineral Research (ASBMR) President's Committee on Nomenclature, we will refer to these factors as RANKL, RANK and OPG for the purposes of this chapter.[36,37]

RANKL, a member of the TNF-ligand superfamily of cytokines, can be expressed as a membrane-bound ligand, a membrane-cleaved soluble product and as a distinct secreted soluble product, all of which are potent stimulators of RANK.[13,38–41] RANKL is required for the differentiation of osteoclasts from their precursor cells in the presence of macrophage colony-stimulating factor (M-CSF) and is also a potent stimulator of osteoclast activity and survival.[23,28,29,31,32,42–44] The antagonist interaction of OPG with RANKL provides a naturally occurring mechanism that could be manipulated with the goal of regulating osteoclast number and activity. Growing evidence supports the hypothesis that the relative expression levels of RANKL and OPG (often represented as the RANKL/OPG expression ratio), rather than the absolute level of expression of either factor, determines the degree of osteoclast-mediated bone resorption.[42,45–47]

Recently, the crystal structure of the murine RANKL extracellular domain was resolved, demonstrating that it forms a homotrimer with each monomer containing the conserved structural scaffold of the TNF-ligand superfamily (β-sandwich or β-strand jellyroll – two, flat, anti-parallel β-pleated sheets). RANKL has four unique surface loops, distinguishing it from TNF-β and TNF-related apoptosis-inducing ligand (TRAIL), also members of the TNF-ligand superfamily.[40,48] One of these unique loops (AA') is necessary for RANK activation, as analysis of the activity of homotrimers with the AA' loop either deleted or replaced by an analogous loop from TNF-β failed to support osteoclastogenesis in vitro.[40] These observations lend weight to the potential of small molecule drug design based on the structurally distinct regions of RANKL, providing novel therapeutic approaches for targeted regulation of osteoclastogenesis.

RANK, the signaling receptor for RANKL, was originally described as a receptor on T cells and dendritic cells. RANK is a type I transmembrane protein and is structurally distinct from OPG. It is expressed on many cell types, including osteoclasts and their precursor cells, dendritic cells, and certain B and T cells.[27,28,49] Binding of RANKL to RANK ultimately leads to activation of NFκB (prompting the nomenclature) and AP-1 transcription factors via the IκB kinase, JNK (c-Jun N-terminal kinase) and p38 kinase signaling pathways.[28,32,50–54] Several

Table 21.1 Factors regulating osteoclast differentiation and activity: function based on knockout and transgenic mice.

Mouse	Bone phenotype	Immune phenotype	Other phenotypes
RANKL[-/-] [42,59]	Defective tooth eruption Severe osteopetrosis No osteoclasts Chondroplasia and growth plate defects	Absence of peripheral LN Defects in T- and B-cell maturation Altered splenic B-cell follicle structure Thymic hypoplasia	Failure to form lactating mammary gland[156]
RANK[-/-] [56,57]	Defective tooth eruption Severe osteopetrosis No osteoclasts	Absence of peripheral LN B-cell deficiency Intact thymic development	Failure to form lactating mammary gland[156]

RANKL[-/-]/RANKL T-cell Tg[58,59]	Partial rescue of osteopetrosis in long bones
	Persistence of:
	  club-shaped bones
	  chondroplasia and growth plate defects
	  defective tooth eruption
		Predominantly restored LN organogenesis	NR

CTLA-4[-/-] [13]	Osteoporosis	Constitutive systemic T-cell activation Lymphoproliferative disease	NR
OPG Tg[18,46]	Osteopetrosis Decreased osteoclast number	Splenomegaly in high expressing lines only	NR
RANK-Fc Tg[28]	Osteopetrosis Decreased osteoclast number	Splenomegaly	NR
OPG[-/-] [61,62]	Osteoporosis	Pro-B-cell accumulation Impaired IgG isotype switching Enhanced DC stimulatory capacity	Arterial calcification

Tg, transgenic; NR, not reported; LN, lymph node; DC, dendritic cell.

animal models in which these signaling components are absent demonstrate osteopetrosis due to impaired osteoclast differentiation, supporting the importance of an intact RANK signaling pathway for osteoclastogenesis.[55]

The essential role of the RANKL/RANK/OPG system in osteoclast-mediated bone resorption is definitively illustrated by the phenotype of mice in which these genes have been deleted (Table 21.1). Both the RANKL[-/-] and RANK[-/-] mice exhibit defective tooth eruption and display severe osteopetrosis, including short club-shaped long bones and growth retardation, that is associated with a complete absence of osteoclasts.[42,56–58] In the RANK[-/-] mice, the absence of osteoclasts is due to an intrinsic defect in maturation of hematopoietic precursors, as reconstitution of RANK[-/-] mice with bone marrow from recombination activation gene (RAG)[-/-] mice, or transfection of RANK[-/-] hematopoietic precursors with RANK cDNA, restores the capacity for osteoclastogenesis in these mice.[57] Conversely, hematopoietic precursors from RANKL[-/-] mice have normal osteoclastogenic potential in vitro in the presence of M-CSF and RANKL,[42] indicating that the defect in maturation of these cells is due to the absence of non-hematopoietic RANKL expression.

Both RANK[-/-] and RANKL[-/-] mice demonstrate immune-related defects, supporting a role for these factors in the immune system. These mice display an absence of lymph node organogenesis and defects in lymphocyte maturation.[42,56,57,59,60] The absence of lymph nodes appears to be related to defects in CD45[+]CD4[+]CD3[-] cell colonization and cluster formation in developing lymph nodes.[59] The B-cell defect results from a failure of progression from pro- to pre-B cells.[42,56] Altered splenic B-cell follicle structure has been described in RANKL[-/-] mice.[59] The RANKL[-/-] mice also have defects in T-cell maturation and display thymic hypoplasia.[42] Kim et al demonstrated partial rescue of the osteopetrotic phenotype in the RANKL[-/-] mice by transgenically expressing RANKL specifically in lymphocytes in the RANKL[-/-] background.[58] Along these lines, CTLA-4[-/-] mice, in which T cells are constitutively active and express high levels of membrane-bound RANKL, have an osteoporotic phenotype that is dependent on RANKL signaling.[13] Taken together, these studies suggest that T-cell RANKL expression may have a significant impact on bone homeostasis and pathologic osteolysis.

Overexpression of OPG in transgenic animals also results in an osteopetrotic phenotype by interfering with the osteoclast-inducing activity of endogenous RANKL.[18,46] However, in contrast to the RANK and RANKL osteopetrotic phenotype, tooth eruption as well as bone elongation and shape were normal in OPG transgenic mice. Min et al demonstrated that endosteal osteoclast activity is absent in OPG transgenic mice but that, in periosteal sites, osteoclasts are present and show evidence of bone-resorbing activity.[46] These finding are consistent with previous observations demonstrating that local RANKL expression levels are relatively high on periosteal bone surfaces in comparison to endosteal trabecular sites, and suggest that overexpression of OPG in transgenic mice is sufficient to effectively block RANKL activity only in endosteal trabecular bone.[23,46] The severity of the phenotype correlates with the amount of OPG expressed in three different OPG transgenic mouse lines expressing low, medium and high levels of OPG, demonstrating a gene dosage effect.[46] Splenomegaly is the only reported abnormality in lymphoid tissues in OPG transgenic mice and is present only in high OPG-expressing lines.[18,46] A transgenic mouse overexpressing a RANK–Fc fusion protein, which also acts as a soluble decoy for RANKL, phenotypically resembles OPG transgenic mice.[28]

Conversely, OPG[-/-] mice develop severe osteoporosis, as a result of unopposed osteoclastogenesis induced by endogenous RANKL.[61,62] In addition, OPG[-/-] mice develop arterial calcification and immune abnormalities,[62,63] including enhanced proliferative responses of pro-B cells ex vivo, accumulation of pro-B cells in vitro, compromised antibody responses to T-dependent antigens, defects in IgG class switching, and increased stimulatory capacity of dendritic cells. Interestingly, activated B cells have recently been shown to express both RANKL and OPG and to have the capacity to stimulate osteoclastogenesis in vitro.[21,64] The osteoporotic phenotype in the OPG[-/-] mice can be rescued by systemic delivery of OPG.[46] Additionally, a gene dosage effect is again evident, as OPG[+/-] littermates display a similar but less severe phenotype than OPG[-/-] mice.[61] The dosage effects observed in both the OPG[-/-] and transgenic mice are a further indication that it is the RANKL/OPG expression ratio that is critical in determining osteoclast differentiation and activation.

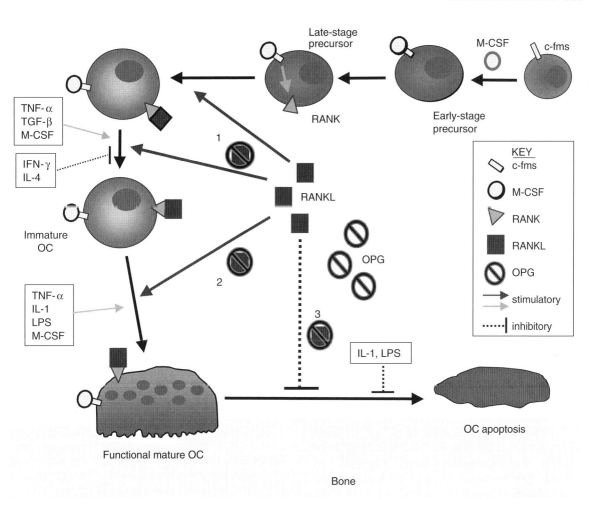

Figure 21.1 Model of osteoclastogenesis. Osteoclasts (OC) are derived from hematopoietic precursor cells of the monocyte–macrophage lineage. Early osteoclast precursors express c-fms, the receptor for M-CSF, binding of which results in expression of RANK. (1) Differentiation of c-fms+RANK+ late precursor cells into mononuclear immature osteoclasts requires RANKL. Osteoclast differentiation is also stimulated by TNF-α, TGF-β and M-CSF, but inhibited by IFN-γ. (2) Continued stimulation of immature osteoclasts by RANKL drives cell fusion and activation, resulting in fully functional mature osteoclasts with bone-resorption capability. TNF-α, interleukin-1 (IL-1), lipopolysaccharide (LPS) and M-CSF also directly enhance the activity of osteoclasts, and IL-1 and LPS can stimulate osteoclast fusion. (3) Exposure of mature osteoclasts to RANKL, IL-1 and LPS prolongs their survival. OPG is an effective antagonist of RANKL at all stages (1, 2 and 3) of RANKL activity.

OSTEOCLASTOGENESIS – THE CURRENT PARADIGM

The current model of osteoclastogenesis is represented in Figure 21.1. Osteoclasts are derived from hematopoietic precursor cells of the monocyte–macrophage lineage, although the exact point(s) of diversion of these cells to the osteoclast pathway have not been definitively identified.[65,66] Early osteoclast precursors express c-fms, the receptor for M-CSF, binding of which is required for survival and expansion of early precursor cells and for expression of RANK.[67–69] Engagement of RANK by RANKL on c-fms+RANK+ late precursor cells is required for diversion from the monocyte–macrophage differentiation pathway and is the earliest described initiation point for differentiation into mononuclear immature osteoclasts.[65] Continued stimulation of these immature osteoclasts by RANKL drives cell fusion and activation, resulting in fully functional mature osteoclasts with bone-resorption capability.[32,70] Exposure of mature osteoclasts to RANKL also enhances their bone-resorbing activity and prolongs their survival.[23,29,32,71] OPG is an effective antagonist of RANKL activity in vitro and in vivo at all stages of RANKL-induced osteoclast differentiation, activation and survival (Figure 21.1).[23,29–34]

Several factors have been shown to have direct effects on osteoclasts or their precursor cells (Figure 21.1). M-CSF stimulates the proliferation of osteoclast precursor cells, and M-CSF and TNF-α promote osteoclast differentiation. Additionally, M-CSF, TNF-α and interleukin (IL)-1 enhance osteoclast activity and survival by acting directly on osteoclasts.[51,65,67,68,72–76] Recent studies suggest that RANKL and TNF-α act synergistically in their activation of osteoclast differentiation and function.[51,72,74–78] There is, however, continued debate regarding whether or not permissive levels of RANKL are required for the direct action of TNF-α on osteoclast precursor cells,[51,75,76] or whether TNF-α can act in this regard independent of RANKL.[72,74] IL-1 stimulates osteoclast fusion and activates mature osteoclasts in a RANKL-independent manner.[79] TGF-β, a factor abundant in bone, also acts directly on osteoclast precursors to enhance RANKL- and M-CSF-stimulated osteoclastogenesis.[69,80] This is in contrast to the action of TGF-β on osteoblast stromal cells, which results in enhanced OPG expression.[80,81] The bacterial product lipopolysaccharide (LPS) may directly promote the activation, fusion and survival of osteoclasts independent of RANKL, IL-1 or TNF-β.[82] Interferon gamma (IFN-γ) and IL-4, activated T-cell products, are negative regulators of osteoclastogenesis, acting directly on osteoclast precursor cells by interfering with the RANKL signaling cascade.[83,84] Similarly, recent studies suggest that IFN-β may be an important

Stimulation of osteoclastogenesis

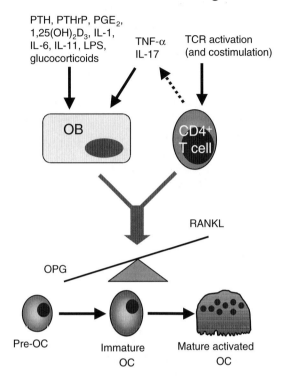

Figure 21.2 Factors that stimulate osteoclastogenesis indirectly. Many of the factors associated with increased osteoclastic bone resorption exert their effects indirectly by acting predominantly on osteoblast/bone lining cells (OB) or activated T cells to increase the RANKL/OPG expression ratio, subsequently increasing osteoclast (OC) differentiation and activity. Parathyroid hormone (PTH), PTH-related peptide (PTHrP), prostaglandin E$_2$ (PGE$_2$), 1,25(OH)$_2$ vitamin D$_3$ (1,25(OH)$_2$D$_3$), glucocorticoids and TNF-α simultaneously upregulate RANKL and downregulate OPG expression in OB.[24,86–94,96] IL-1, IL-6, IL-11 and IL-17 increase RANKL expression in OB, while either not affecting or minimally increasing OPG expression.[86,92,93,95,125] LPS increases the RANKL expression in both OB and leukocytes.[157,158] Activation of CD4$^+$ T cells through the TCR and costimulation pathways increases the RANKL/OPG expression ratio in these cells.[13,97,98] The net effect of these pro-resorptive factors is an increased RANKL/OPG expression ratio that is sufficient to drive osteoclast differentiation and activation.

autoregulatory factor in osteoclast precursor cells, interfering with RANKL-induced c-Fos production and activity.[85] It has yet to be determined whether IFN-β is also an inhibitor of RANKL osteoclast activity and survival in immature and mature osteoclasts.

Therefore, a complex system of stimulatory and suppressive factors for osteoclast differentiation and activity is emerging, with the RANKL/RANK/OPG system being a central and required component. In vitro and in vivo studies indicate that many of the factors associated with increased osteoclastic bone resorption exert their effects on osteoclast differentiation and activity indirectly by converging on the RANKL/RANK/OPG system. As summarized in Figure 21.2, calcitropic hormones and pro-resorptive signals stimulate RANKL expression primarily on osteoblasts/bone lining cells. Additionally, many of these factors simultaneously downregulate (or do not alter) OPG expression, resulting in an increased RANKL/OPG ratio and subsequent promotion of osteoclast differentiation and activation.[24,86–96] Activation of CD4+ T cells via the T-cell receptor (TCR) also contributes to the shift in the RANKL/OPG ratio by inducing RANKL production.[13,97,98] Similarly, many factors that suppress bone erosion (Figure 21.3) also act indirectly on osteoblast/bone lining cells or CD4+ T cells to decrease the RANKL/OPG ratio and inhibit osteoclastogenesis.[81,99–104] OPG is present in detectable levels in adult human serum,[105] suggesting that suppression of osteoclastogenesis may be an ongoing process.

CONTRIBUTION OF OSTEOCLASTS TO FOCAL BONE EROSION IN RHEUMATOID ARTHRITIS

The role of osteoclasts in marginal and subchondral focal bone erosion in RA has been suspected for many years, based on several studies indirectly implicating these cells in the process of bone erosion.[6,7,9–12,98,106] Further evidence for the role of osteoclasts in bone resorption in RA came from studies examining the potential role

Suppression of osteoclastogenesis

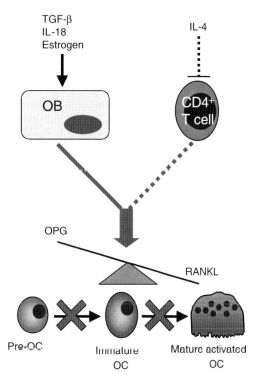

Figure 21.3 Factors that suppress osteoclastogenesis indirectly. Many factors that suppress bone resorption act indirectly on osteoblast/bone lining cells (OB) or on CD4+ T cells to decrease the RANKL/OPG ratio and inhibit osteoclastogenesis. TGF-β, IL-18 and estrogens increase OPG expression in OB,[99–103] and TGF-β also suppresses RANKL expression.[81] IL-4 inhibits RANKL induction in CD4+ T cells.[104,159] The net effect of these suppressive factors is a decreased RANKL/OPG expression ratio, resulting in suppression of osteoclastogenesis. OC, osteoclast.

of RANKL in this process. It was first demonstrated that mRNA[98,107] and protein[107] for RANKL are expressed in synovial fibroblasts cultured from patients with RA. In addition, RANKL mRNA is expressed by T lymphocytes in RA synovial tissues[13,97] and by activated CD4+ lymphocytes derived from these tissues.[98]

Activated T lymphocytes not only express membrane-bound RANKL, but also secrete soluble RANKL, as detected in culture supernatants of CD4+ T lymphocytes activated by anti-CD3 plus anti-CD28.[13] Furthermore, co-culture experiments were performed using RA synovial fibroblasts and peripheral blood mononuclear cells as a source of osteoclast precursors. In the presence of 1,25-dihydroxy vitamin D_3, multinucleated cells with the phenotypic features of osteoclasts were generated, and their generation was inhibited by the addition of OPG.[107,108] Human T cells activated by con-canavalin A (mimicking TCR activation) were co-cultured with murine adherent spleen cells, leading to the formation of cells with phenotypic markers of osteoclasts, a process that was enhanced by the addition of IL-1α and TGF-β.[97] Similarly, activated RANKL-expressing T cells induced osteoclastogenesis from autologous peripheral blood monocytes, a process that was inhibited in a dose-dependent fashion by OPG.[109] It was also demonstrated that macrophages isolated from RA synovial tissues have the capability of differentiating into osteoclasts in the presence of osteoblast-like cells, 1,25-dihydroxy vitamin D_3, and M-CSF,[110] or in the presence of M-CSF plus RANKL.[111] In the latter study, OPG inhibited osteoclast formation from RA synovial macrophages in a dose-dependent fashion. Osteoclasts can also be generated from bone marrow derived from the iliac bone of patients with RA.[112]

Recent studies have extended these observations on the potential role for the RANKL/RANK/OPG system in osteoclastogenesis in RA. Tissue samples from RA patients undergoing orthopedic surgery were taken either from synovium remote from bone or from pannus tissue. Cells digested from these tissues were placed in culture, and generated tartrate-resistent acid phosphatase-positive (TRAP+) multinucleated cells with the capacity to form resorption pits on dentine slices.[113,114] Pit formation was completely inhibited by the addition of OPG. Furthermore, a strong positive correlation was demonstrated between ratios of RANKL/OPG mRNA levels in these tissues and the number of resorption pits produced.[113] In an additional study, a soluble form of RANKL (sRANKL) was detected in the synovial fluid of patients with RA, and the ratio of sRANKL/OPG in synovial fluids, as detected by ELISA assay, was significantly higher in RA samples as compared with samples from patients with OA, gout or trauma.[109] Fibroblast-like synovial cells from patients with RA have also been found to be a source of OPG.[115] Taken together, these studies support a role for the RANKL/RANK/OPG system in the process of osteoclastic bone resorption in RA, as well as demonstrating that cells within the synovial environment and/or within bone marrow from RA patients can provide a source of osteoclast precursors.

Many of the cytokines and growth factors that influence osteoclast formation, activity and/or survival are produced by inflamed synovial tissues in RA.[116–120] Some of these factors may act indirectly on osteoclastogenesis and activity by increasing the RANKL/OPG expression ratio in the local bone environment (see Figures 21.2 and 21.3), while others, including TNF-α, M-CSF, and IL-1α and IL-1β (see Figure 21.1),[116–120] may have a direct action, promoting osteoclast differentiation and/or activation. Therapeutic blockade of IL-1 and TNF-α in RA can modulate both inflammation and bone erosion.[121,122] Additionally, recruitment and activation of T cells may also contribute to osteoclast-mediated bone resorption due to expression by activated T cells of RANKL and other pro-resorptive T-cell-derived cytokines such as IL-15 and IL-17.[123–125] IL-17 is a potent stimulator of osteoclastogenesis by indirect mechanisms.[125,126] Conversely, the inflamed synovium is also a source of factors that are negative regulators of osteoclastogenesis, including IFN-β and -γ, IL-4, IL-10 and IL-18.[83–85,99,127–129]

OPG AS A THERAPEUTIC AGENT IN ANIMAL MODELS OF ARTHRITIS

The first definitive demonstration of the critical role of RANKL in the pathogenesis of osteoclast-mediated bone resorption, and of the potential role of OPG as an agent to block bone erosion in inflammatory arthritis, was reported in studies using the rat in an adjuvant-induced arthritis (AA) model.[13] Arthritic rats were shown to express RANKL mRNA in synovial cells and in inflammatory cells within synovial tissues. In addition, activated T cells in this model expressed RANKL protein. Treatment using a soluble form of OPG was initiated at disease onset. OPG-treated rats demonstrated only minimal loss of cortical and trabecular bone, as compared with severe bone loss in the untreated control animals. Accordingly, osteoclast numbers were also dramatically decreased in the joints of treated animals. Protection from cartilage destruction was also demonstrated in OPG-treated arthritic rats. These observations have been extended in a preliminary kinetic study examining various OPG doses and treatment schedules, and evaluating inflammation by clinical and histopathologic scoring methods, and bone damage by quantitative dual energy X-ray absorptiometry (DEXA) analysis, histopathology and quantitation of osteoclast numbers. No OPG dose had any effect on inflammation. However, OPG dramatically decreased the number of intralesional osteoclasts, and protected articular bone from destruction in a dose-dependent manner. OPG treatment was most effective when given early in the course of disease, when erosions could be prevented from occurring.[130]

AA is a T-cell-driven experimental arthritis, and therefore it is useful to examine other animal models of arthritis to determine whether blockade of osteoclastogenesis and osteoclast activity may provide protection from bone erosion induced by other pathogenic mechanisms. An important role for B cells and their products in inflammatory arthritis is suggested from studies depleting B cells in RA patients.[131] A useful animal model that clearly demonstrates the ability of antibody to provoke arthritis is the T-cell transgenic K/BxN spontaneous arthritis model.[132–134] This spontaneous arthritis is dependent upon T-cell–B-cell interactions, resulting in the production of pathogenic anti-glucose-6-phosphate isomerase (GPI) antibody.[132–135] Transfer of serum containing anti-GPI antibody from arthritic mice results in the development of

arthritis in recipient mice (serum transfer arthritis).[136] However, T cells and B cells are not required for the serum transfer variant, as, once produced, the anti-GPI antibodies are sufficient to confer disease.[134] The serum transfer arthritis model provides an opportunity to investigate the role of RANKL in osteoclastogenesis and bone erosion, independent of its role in immune responses, as the generation of serum transfer arthritis is independent of cooperative T-cell–dendritic cell interactions. To further substantiate the role of RANKL-driven osteoclastogenesis in focal bone erosion in arthritis, inflammatory arthritis was generated in the RANKL$^{-/-}$ by mice using the serum transfer model.[14]

The degree of bone erosion in RANKL$^{-/-}$ mice with serum transfer arthritis was dramatically reduced compared to arthritic control mice, despite comparable levels of ongoing inflammation. As expected, multinucleated TRAP$^+$ osteoclast-like cells were completely absent in the RANKL$^{-/-}$ mice, but present in large numbers at sites of bone erosion in arthritic control mice, demonstrating the absolute requirement for RANKL in osteoclastogenesis in this model of inflammatory arthritis. Cartilage erosion was present in both control mice and in RANKL$^{-/-}$ mice, although a trend toward milder cartilage damage was noted in RANKL$^{-/-}$ mice. This was due at least in part to protection of subchondral bone. This study confirmed the central role of RANKL, and of osteoclasts, in the pathogenesis of focal bone erosion in an antibody-driven arthritis model.

Given the central role of TNF-α in the pathogenesis of RA in humans, it is important to examine the role of osteoclast-mediated bone erosion in an arthritis model driven by TNF-α. The opportunity to do so was provided by studies of Keffer et al,[137] who generated mice bearing a human TNF-α transgene, leading to deregulated expression of this cytokine. These mice develop a spontaneous, chronic, destructive polyarthritis at an early age, consistent with the hypothesis that TNF-α is a key cytokine in the initiation and perpetuation of inflammatory arthritis. TNF-α transgenic mice were treated

Table 21.2   Osteoclast-targeted treatment in animal models of arthritis.

Arthritis model	Treatment/ blockade	Treatment initiated	Outcome compared to controls		
			Gross inflammation	Bone erosion	Cartilage destruction
AA	sOPG	Disease onset	Continued and equivalent	Dramatic protection	Dramatic protection
Serum transfer	RANKL$^{-/-}$	NA	Continued and equivalent	Dramatic protection	Attenuated
TNF-α Tg	Fc–OPG	Disease onset	Continued and equivalent	56% reduction in size of erosions	NDA
	Pamidronate	Disease onset	Continued and equivalent	53% reduction in size of erosions	NDA
	Fc–OPG + pamidronate	Disease onset	Continued and equivalent	81% reduction in size of erosions	NDA
CIA	Fc–OPG	Disease onset	Continued and equivalent	Dramatic protection	Dramatic protection

sOPG, soluble OPG; Tg, transgenic; NA, not applicable; NDA, not directly assessed.

with osteoclast-targeted therapies, and inflammation and tissue destruction was assessed.[15] Mice treated with Fc–OPG alone, pamidronate alone or Fc–OPG plus pamidronate failed to show improvement in parameters of inflammation. However, quantitative histologic analysis revealed a 56% reduction in the size of bone erosions in the Fc–OPG-treated mice, a 53% reduction in the pamidronate-treated mice, and an 81% reduction in mice treated with the combination of Fc–OPG and pamidronate. Osteoclast numbers were also assessed, and there was a significant reduction of osteoclast numbers in animals treated with Fc–OPG alone, and a further reduction in those animals treated with the combination of Fc–OPG and pamidronate. Osteoclasts were not entirely eliminated, however, even in the Fc–OPG plus pamidronate treatment arm, leaving open the question of whether these osteoclasts mediate

the low level of continued bone erosion or whether other cell types may also be contributing. Other cell types present at the pannus–bone interface that may contribute to focal bone erosion include activated macrophages and synovial fibroblasts. Synovial fibroblasts express cathepsin K,[9,138] which may allow these cells to contribute to the degradation of bone matrix and bone dissolution. The contribution of cell types other than osteoclasts to focal bone erosion is actively being investigated.

Romas et al have preliminarily reported treatment of rats with CIA using an Fc–OPG fusion protein to target osteoclast-mediated bone erosion.[16,17,139] Treatment with Fc–OPG was initiated at the onset of inflammation. The study demonstrated that paw swelling was unchanged in Fc–OPG-treated arthritic rats compared to IgG$_1$-treated arthritic control rats. However, there was a greater than 75% reduction in osteoclast numbers in juxta-articular bone, an absence of osteoclasts at the synovial–bone attachment, protection from bone erosion and preservation of cartilage integrity in the Fc–OPG-treated rats. Table 21.2 provides a summary of animal models of arthritis in which osteoclasts have been targeted by treatment regimens. These data support the hypothesis that RANKL-driven osteoclastogenesis is a critical mechanism of bone erosion in inflammatory arthritis, and that OPG treatment may have a protective effect on bone in patients with RA.

OPG and protection of cartilage in inflammatory arthritis

It is clear from the studies of OPG treatment or equivalent RANKL blockade in animal models of arthritis that this intervention is protective to cartilage. It appears that this results in large part from protection from subchondral bone erosion, with 'secondary' protection of attached cartilage. However, RANKL blockade may also have a lesser direct protective effect on cartilage,[13,14,139] suggesting that the RANKL/RANK/OPG system may play a modulatory role in cartilage destruction. RANKL, RANK and OPG are expressed by articular chondrocytes, and the level of expression of these factors may be increased in osteoarthritis.[140] However, RANKL did not activate NFκB in chondrocytes in vitro, suggesting an absence of signaling through the RANK receptor, and it did not alter chondrocyte production of the proinflammatory mediators collagenase or nitric oxide.[140] Further investigation into mechanisms of primary protection of cartilage by RANKL blockade is required.

OTHER POTENTIAL THERAPEUTIC APPLICATIONS OF OPG

Other conditions in which the RANKL/RANK/OPG system has been implicated in pathologic bone loss include osteoporosis, tumor metastases to bone, osteolysis associated with prosthetic joint loosening, and alveolar bone loss in periodontal infection. Given the role of OPG in suppression of osteoclastogenesis, the admin-

istration of genetically engineered Fc–OPG has been tested in humans as a means of decreasing bone resorption. In a pilot study, Fc–OPG was administered to 52 healthy postmenopausal women to determine its effect on bone resorption. After a single subcutaneous injection, levels of urinary N-telopeptide (NTX), a biochemical marker indicating collagen degradation in bone, decreased within 12 h, with a mean decrease of 80% 4 days after OPG administration. The effects on suppression of NTX levels were sustained for up to 6 weeks,[141] suggesting that the effect of OPG in humans is prolonged and includes blockade of osteoclast differentiation. In rodent models of osteopenia induced by ovariectomy[18] and tail suspension,[142] treatment with OPG has been shown to increase bone mineral density. These studies suggest that OPG treatment could be effective in humans in diseases characterized by generalized bone resorption, such as osteoporosis.

The RANKL/RANK/OPG system has also been implicated in the pathogenesis of tumor metastasis to bone in breast cancer,[143] prostate cancer[144] and myeloma,[145] among others. TGF-β has been shown to induce breast cancer cell production of parathyroid hormone-related peptide (PTHrP), which in turn promotes local osteoclastogenesis by upregulation of RANKL production and downregulation of OPG production in cells of the osteoblast lineage in the bone microenvironment.[143] Myeloma cells themselves have been shown to express RANKL, which may contribute to their osteolytic potential.[145] Additionally, myeloma cells can increase the RANKL/OPG ratio expressed by osteoblast/bone lining cells.[146] OPG therapy in animal models of bony metastasis has been shown to block osteoclastogenesis and osteolysis associated with certain tumor metastases.[144,147,148] Osteolysis associated with loosening of prosthetic joints may also be mediated at least in part by the RANKL/RANK/OPG system. Joint fluid from patients with failed total hip replacements induced marked osteoclastogenesis when added in murine co-culture systems containing osteoblasts and bone marrow-derived osteoclast precursor cells, an effect that was inhibited by the addition of OPG.[149,150] Finally, in a murine model of periodontal infection, local CD4+ T cells were implicated as mediators of alveolar bone destruction. These cells were shown to express RANKL upon exposure to *Actinobacillus actinomycetemcomitans*, a microorganism identified as an etiologic agent in periodontitis. Alveolar bone destruction was inhibited by treatment of mice with a recombinant human Fc–OPG fusion protein.[151] This inhibition, however, was not complete, suggesting that either drug dose or delivery was insufficient or that other cell types may be contributing to alveolar bone destruction in this setting.

ADDITIONAL CONSIDERATIONS IN THE USE OF OPG AS A THERAPEUTIC AGENT

Evidence in animal models highlights OPG as a promising therapeutic agent in the treatment of bone erosion in RA and other diseases characterized by pathologic bone loss. Certain potential drawbacks of OPG as a therapeutic agent, however, remain to be considered and fully investigated. The RANKL/RANK/OPG system does play a role in immune responses, as reviewed earlier. Studies using OPG treatment in animal models of arthritis demonstrate little effect on gross inflammation. However, more subtle effects on the inflammatory response, such as changes in cytokine expression or antibody responses that could occur in the setting of RANKL blockade,[27,104,152] have not been assessed. In one study, OPG-/- mice challenged with a T-dependent antigen had defects in immune responses.[63] Therefore, the effects of OPG therapy on these aspects of immune responses need to be further investigated. The potential role of OPG in inhibition of apoptosis also needs to be considered. Recent studies have demonstrated that OPG is a decoy receptor for TRAIL.[153] OPG was demonstrated to inhibit TRAIL-induced apoptosis of Jurkat T cells,[153] and was shown to be a survival factor for prostate cancer cells through its interaction with TRAIL.[154] The potential for OPG as a survival factor for malignant cells, if confirmed, would have implications

for its therapeutic application as an anti-resorptive agent. Finally, the impact of OPG therapy on fracture healing and bone structural integrity needs to be further elucidated. A recent study by Childs et al suggested that blockade of RANKL using a RANK–Fc fusion protein has no deleterious effects on fracture healing in a murine model of closed tibia fracture. Additionally, RANK signaling was not found to be required for fracture healing, as 25% of RANK-/- mice with fractures healed normally.[155] These studies suggest that osteoclasts may not be absolutely required for fracture healing. However, normal instances of repair of micro-damage may require osteoclast-mediated remodeling of bone.

CONCLUSION

Several lines of evidence now support the theory that osteoclasts play an important role in the pathogenesis of focal bone erosions in RA, and that RANKL is a critical cytokine in this process. The degree of bone resorption in physiologic states is predominantly regulated by the ratio RANKL/OPG, with high ratios favoring bone resorption, and it is likely that a similar relationship exists in pathologic states. OPG treatment in animal models of arthritis provides initial evidence that therapeutic approaches targeting osteoclast differentiation, activity and/or survival can provide protection from bone erosion. These studies suggest that OPG therapy is most effective when given early in the course of the erosive process. Currently available therapies that target osteoclasts, including OPG, however, have not been demonstrated to block inflammation. Therefore, these therapies would need to be used in combination with disease-modifying agents that specifically block inflammation. The potential negative effects of OPG administration on the immune system and on bone have been discussed. The ultimate goal in the treatment of patients with RA is to improve functional status and prevent the destruction of cartilage and bone. In the absence of a cure for RA, therapies such as OPG that target bone destruction represent a rational addition to our therapeutic armamentarium.

REFERENCES

1. Goldring SR. Osteoporosis and rheumatic diseases. In: Favus MJ, ed. *Primer on the Metabolic Bone Diseases and Disorders of Mineral Metabolism*, 3rd edn. (Lippincott-Raven: Philadelphia, 1996) 299–301.

2. Deodhar AA, Woolf AD. Bone mass measurement and bone metabolism in rheumatoid arthritis: a review. *Br J Rheumatol* 1996; **35**: 309–22.

3. Goldring SR, Polisson RP. Bone disease in rheumatological disorders. In: Avioli L, Krane SM, eds. *Metabolic Bone Disease*, 2nd edn. (Academic Press: San Diego, 1998) 621–35.

4. Drossaers-Bakker KW, Kroon HM, Zwinderman AH et al. Radiographic damage of large joints in long-term rheumatoid arthritis and its relation to function. *Rheumatology (Oxford)* 2000; **39**: 998–1003.

5. van Zeben D, Hazes JMW, Zwinderman AH et al. Factors predicting outcome of rheumatoid arthritis: results of a followup study. *J Rheumatol* 1993; **20**: 1288–96.

6. Leisen JCC, Duncan H, Riddle JM et al. The erosive front: a topographic study of the junction between the pannus and the subchondral plate in the macerated rheumatoid metacarpal head. *J Rheumatol* 1988; **15**: 17–22.

7. Bromley M, Woolley DE. Chondroclasts and osteoclasts at subchondral sites of erosion in the rheumatoid joint. *Arthritis Rheum* 1984; **27**: 968–75.

8. Gravallese EM, Goldring SR. Cellular mechanisms and the role of cytokines in bone erosions in rheumatoid arthritis. *Arthritis Rheum* 2000; **43**: 2143–51.

9. Hummel KM, Petrow PK, Franz JK et al. Cysteine proteinase cathepsin K mRNA is expressed in synovium of patients with rheumatoid arthritis and is detected at sites of synovial bone destruction. *J Rheumatol* 1998; **25**: 1887–94.

10. Suzuki Y, Nishikaku F, Nakatuka M et al. Osteoclast-like cells in murine collagen induced arthritis. *J Rheumatol* 1998; **25**: 1154–60.

11. Kuratani T, Nagata K, Kukita T et al. Induction of abundant osteoclast-like multinucleated giant cells in adjuvant arthritic rats with accompanying disordered high bone turnover. *Histol Histopathol* 1998; **13**: 751–9.

12. Romas E, Bakharevski O, Hards DK et al. Expression of osteoclast differentiation factor at sites of bone erosion in collagen-induced arthritis. *Arthritis Rheum* 2000; **43**: 821–6.

13. Kong YY, Feige U, Sarosi I et al. Activated T cells regulate bone loss and joint destruction in adjuvant arthritis through osteoprotegerin ligand. *Nature* 1999; **402**: 304–9.

14. Pettit AR, Ji H, von Stechow D et al. TRANCE/RANKL knockout mice are protected from bone erosion in a serum transfer model of arthritis. *Am J Pathol* 2001; **159**: 1689–99.

15. Redlich K, Hayer S, Maier A et al. Tumor necrosis factor alpha-mediated joint destruction is inhibited by targeting osteoclasts with osteoprotegerin. *Arthritis Rheum* 2002, **46**. 785 92.

16. Romas E, Sims NA, Hards D et al. Fc–osteoprotegerin fusion protein (Fc–OPG) reduces osteoclast numbers and prevents bone destruction in rats with collagen-induced arthritis. *Arthritis Rheum* 2001; **44**: S47.

17. Romas E, Sims NA, Hards D et al. Fc–osteoprotegerin (Fc–OPG) fusion protein reduces osteoclast numbers and prevents bone destruction in rats with collagen-induced arthritis. *J Bone Miner Res* 2001; **16**: S270.

18. Simonet WS, Lacey DL, Dunstan CR et al. Osteoprotegerin: a novel secreted protein involved in the regulation of bone density. *Cell* 1997; **89**: 309–19.

19. Yasuda H, Shima N, Nakagawa N et al. Identity of osteoclastogenesis inhibitory factor (OCIF) and osteoprotegerin (OPG): a mechanism by which OPG/OCIF inhibits osteoclastogenesis in vitro. *Endocrinology* 1998; **139**: 1329–37.

20. Tsuda E, Goto M, Mochizuki S et al. Isolation of a novel cytokine from human fibroblasts that specifically inhibits osteoclastogenesis. *Biochem Biophys Res Commun* 1997; **234**: 137–42.

21. Yun TJ, Chaudhary PM, Shu GL et al. OPG/FDCR-1, a TNF receptor family member, is expressed in lymphoid cells and is up-regulated by ligating CD40. *J Immunol* 1998; **161**: 6113–21.

22. Kwon BS, Wang S, Udagawa N et al. TR1, a new member of the tumor necrosis factor receptor superfamily, induces fibroblast proliferation and inhibits osteoclastogenesis and bone resorption. *FASEB J* 1998; **12**: 845–54.

23. Lacey DL, Timms E, Tan HL et al. Osteoprotegerin ligand is a cytokine that regulates osteoclast differentiation and activation. *Cell* 1998; **93**: 165–76.

24. Yasuda H, Shima N, Nakagawa N et al. Osteoclast differentiation factor is a ligand for

osteoprotegerin/osteoclastogenesis-inhibitory factor and is identical to TRANCE/RANKL. *Proc Natl Acad Sci USA* 1998; **95**: 3597–602.

25. Yamaguchi K, Kinosaki M, Goto M et al. Characterization of structural domains of human osteoclastogenesis inhibitory factor. *J Biol Chem* 1998; **273**: 5117–23.

26. Wong BR, Josien R, Lee SY et al. TRANCE (tumor necrosis factor [TNF]-related activation-induced cytokine), a new TNF family member predominantly expressed in T cells, is a dendritic cell-specific survival factor. *J Exp Med* 1997; **186**: 2075–80.

27. Anderson DM, Maraskovsky E, Billingsley WL et al. A homologue of the TNF receptor and its ligand enhance T-cell growth and dendritic-cell function. *Nature* 1997; **390**: 175–9.

28. Hsu H, Lacey DL, Dunstan CR et al. Tumor necrosis factor receptor family member RANK mediates osteoclast differentiation and activation induced by osteoprotegerin ligand. *Proc Natl Acad Sci USA* 1999; **96**: 3540–5.

29. Lacey DL, Tan HL, Lu J et al. Osteoprotegerin ligand modulates murine osteoclast survival in vitro and in vivo. *Am J Pathol* 2000; **157**: 435–48.

30. Udagawa N, Takahashi N, Yasuda H et al. Osteoprotegerin produced by osteoblasts is an important regulator in osteoclast development and function. *Endocrinology* 2000; **141**: 3478–84.

31. Shalhoub V, Faust J, Boyle WJ et al. Osteoprotegerin and osteoprotegerin ligand effects on osteoclast formation from human peripheral blood mononuclear cell precursors. *J Cell Biochem* 1999; **72**: 251–61.

32. Jimi E, Akiyama S, Tsurukai T et al. Osteoclast differentiation factor acts as a multifunctional regulator in murine osteoclast differentiation and function. *J Immunol* 1999; **163**: 434–42.

33. Hakeda Y, Kobayashi Y, Yamaguchi K et al. Osteoclastogenesis inhibitory factor (OCIF) directly inhibits bone-resorbing activity of isolated mature osteoclasts. *Biochem Biophys Res Commun* 1998; **251**: 796–801.

34. Akatsu T, Murakami T, Nishikawa M et al. Osteoclastogenesis inhibitory factor suppresses osteoclast survival by interfering in the interaction of stromal cells with osteoclast. *Biochem Biophys Res Commun* 1998; **250**: 229–34.

35. Wong BR, Rho J, Arron J et al. TRANCE is a novel ligand of the tumor necrosis factor receptor family that activates c-Jun N-terminal kinase in T cells. *J Biol Chem* 1997; **272**: 25190–4.

36. The American Society for Bone and Mineral Research President's Committee on Nomenclature. Proposed standard nomenclature for new tumor necrosis factor family members involved in the regulation of bone resorption. *J Bone Miner Res* 2000; **15**: 2293–6.

37. The American Society for Bone and Mineral Research President's Committee on Nomenclature. Proposed standard nomenclature for new tumor necrosis factor members involved in the regulation of bone resorption. *Bone* 2000; **27**: 761–4.

38. Lum L, Wong BR, Josien R et al. Evidence for a role of a tumor necrosis factor-alpha (TNF-alpha)-converting enzyme-like protease in shedding of TRANCE, a TNF family member involved in osteoclastogenesis and dendritic cell survival. *J Biol Chem* 1999; **274**: 13613–18.

39. Miyamoto N, Higuchi Y, Mori K et al. Human osteosarcoma-derived cell lines produce soluble factor(s) that induces differentiation of blood monocytes to osteoclast-like cells. *Int Immunopharmacol* 2002; **2**: 25–38.

40. Lam J, Nelson CA, Ross FP et al. Crystal structure of the TRANCE/RANKL cytokine reveals determinants of receptor-ligand specificity. *J Clin Invest* 2001; **108**: 971–9.

41. Nagai M, Kyakumoto S, Sato N. Cancer cells responsible for humoral hypercalcemia express mRNA encoding a secreted form of ODF/TRANCE that induces osteoclast formation. *Biochem Biophys Res Commun* 2000; **269**: 532–6.

42. Kong YY, Yoshida H, Sarosi I et al. OPGL is a key regulator of osteoclastogenesis, lymphocyte development and lymph-node organogenesis. *Nature* 1999; **397**: 315–23.

43. Udagawa N, Takahashi N, Jimi E et al. Osteoblasts/stromal cells stimulate osteoclast activation through expression of osteoclast differentiation factor/RANKL but not macrophage colony-stimulating factor: receptor activator of NF-kappaB ligand. *Bone* 1999; **25**: 517–23.

44. Burgess TL, Qian Y, Kaufman S et al. The ligand for osteoprotegerin (OPGL) directly activates mature osteoclasts. *J Cell Biol* 1999; **145**: 527–38.

45. Fazzalari NL, Kuliwaba JS, Atkins GJ et al. The ratio of messenger RNA levels of receptor activator of nuclear factor kappaB ligand to osteoprotegerin correlates with bone remodeling indices in normal human cancellous bone but not in osteoarthritis. *J Bone Miner Res* 2001; **16**: 1015–27.

46. Min H, Morony S, Sarosi I et al. Osteoprotegerin

reverses osteoporosis by inhibiting endosteal osteoclasts and prevents vascular calcification by blocking a process resembling osteoclastogenesis. *J Exp Med* 2000; **192**: 463–74.

47. Gori F, Hofbauer LC, Dunstan CR et al. The expression of osteoprotegerin and RANK ligand and the support of osteoclast formation by stromal–osteoblast lineage cells is developmentally regulated. *Endocrinology* 2000; **141**: 4768–76.

48. Ito S, Wakabayashi K, Ubukata O et al. Crystal structure of the extracellular domain of mouse RANK ligand at 2.2-A resolution. *J Biol Chem* 2002, **277**. 6631 6.

49. Nakagawa N, Kinosaki M, Yamaguchi K et al. RANK is the essential signaling receptor for osteoclast differentiation factor in osteoclastogenesis. *Biochem Biophys Res Commun* 1998; **253**: 395–400.

50. Wong BR, Besser D, Kim N et al. TRANCE, a TNF family member, activates Akt/PKB through a signaling complex involving TRAF6 and c-Src. *Mol Cell* 1999; **4**: 1041–9.

51. Zhang YH, Heulsmann A, Tondravi MM et al. Tumor necrosis factor-alpha (TNF) stimulates RANKL-induced osteoclastogenesis via coupling of TNF type 1 receptor and RANK signaling pathways. *J Biol Chem* 2001; **276**: 563–8.

52. Darnay BG, Ni J, Moore PA et al. Activation of NF-kappaB by RANK requires tumor necrosis factor receptor-associated factor (TRAF) 6 and NF-kappaB-inducing kinase. Identification of a novel TRAF6 interaction motif. *J Biol Chem* 1999; **274**: 7724–31.

53. Franzoso G, Carlson L, Xing L et al. Requirement for NF-kappaB in osteoclast and B-cell development. *Genes Dev* 1997; **11**: 3482–96.

54. Matsumoto M, Sudo T, Saito T et al. Involvement of p38 mitogen-activated protein kinase signaling pathway in osteoclastogenesis mediated by receptor activator of NF-kappa B ligand (RANKL). *J Biol Chem* 2000; **275**: 31155–61.

55. Gravallese EM, Galson DL, Goldring SR et al. The role of TNF-receptor family members and other TRAF-dependent receptors in bone resorption. *Arthritis Res* 2001; **3**: 6–12.

56. Dougall WC, Glaccum M, Charrier K et al. RANK is essential for osteoclast and lymph node development. *Genes Dev* 1999; **13**: 2412–24.

57. Li J, Sarosi I, Yan XQ et al. RANK is the intrinsic hematopoietic cell surface receptor that controls osteoclastogenesis and regulation of bone mass and calcium metabolism. *Proc Natl Acad Sci USA* 2000; **97**: 1566–71.

58. Kim N, Odgren PR, Kim DK et al. Diverse roles of the tumor necrosis factor family member TRANCE in skeletal physiology revealed by TRANCE deficiency and partial rescue by a lymphocyte-expressed TRANCE transgene. *Proc Natl Acad Sci USA* 2000; **97**: 10905–10.

59. Kim D, Mebius RE, MacMicking JD et al. Regulation of peripheral lymph node genesis by the tumor necrosis factor family member TRANCE. *J Exp Med* 2000; **192**: 1467–78.

60. Manabe N, Kawaguchi H, Chikuda H et al. Connection between B lymphocyte and osteoclast differentiation pathways. *J Immunol* 2001; **167**: 2625–31.

61. Bucay N, Sarosi I, Dunstan CR et al. Osteoprotegerin-deficient mice develop early onset osteoporosis and arterial calcification. *Genes Dev* 1998; **12**: 1260–8.

62. Mizuno A, Amizuka N, Irie K et al. Severe osteoporosis in mice lacking osteoclastogenesis inhibitory factor/osteoprotegerin. *Biochem Biophys Res Commun* 1998; **247**: 610–15.

63. Yun TJ, Tallquist MD, Aicher A et al. Osteoprotegerin, a crucial regulator of bone metabolism, also regulates B-cell development and function. *J Immunol* 2001; **166**: 1482–91.

64. Choi Y, Woo KM, Ko SH et al. Osteoclastogenesis is enhanced by activated B cells but suppressed by activated CD8(+) T cells. *Eur J Immunol* 2001; **31**: 2179–88.

65. Arai F, Miyamoto T, Ohneda O et al. Commitment and differentiation of osteoclast precursor cells by the sequential expression of c-Fms and receptor activator of nuclear factor kappa B (RANK) receptors. *J Exp Med* 1999; **190**: 1741–54.

66. Miyamoto T, Arai F, Ohneda O et al. An adherent condition is required for formation of multinuclear osteoclasts in the presence of macrophage colony-stimulating factor and receptor activator of nuclear factor kappa B ligand. *Blood* 2000; **96**: 4335–43.

67. Quinn JM, Elliott J, Gillespie MT et al. A combination of osteoclast differentiation factor and macrophage-colony stimulating factor is sufficient for both human and mouse osteoclast formation in vitro. *Endocrinology* 1998; **139**: 4424–7.

68. Tanaka S, Takahashi N, Udagawa N et al. Macrophage colony-stimulating factor is indispensable for both proliferation and differentiation of osteoclast progenitors. *J Clin Invest* 1993; **91**: 257–63.

69. Kaneda T, Nojima T, Nakagawa M et al. Endogenous production of TGF-beta is essential for osteoclastogenesis induced by a combination of receptor activator of NF-kappa B ligand and macrophage-colony-stimulating factor. *J Immunol* 2000; **165**: 4254–63.

70. Takami M, Woo JT, Nagai K. Osteoblastic cells induce fusion and activation of osteoclasts through a mechanism independent of macrophage-colony-stimulating factor production. *Cell Tissue Res* 1999; **298**: 327–34.

71. Tsukii K, Shima N, Mochizuki S et al. Osteoclast differentiation factor mediates an essential signal for bone resorption induced by 1 alpha,25-dihydroxyvitamin D3, prostaglandin E2, or parathyroid hormone in the microenvironment of bone. *Biochem Biophys Res Commun* 1998; **246**: 337–41.

72. Kobayashi K, Takahashi N, Jimi E et al. Tumor necrosis factor alpha stimulates osteoclast differentiation by a mechanism independent of the ODF/RANKL–RANK interaction. *J Exp Med* 2000; **191**: 275–85.

73. Fuller K, Owens JM, Jagger CJ et al. Macrophage colony-stimulating factor stimulates survival and chemotactic behavior in isolated osteoclasts. *J Exp Med* 1993; **178**: 1733–44.

74. Fuller K, Murphy C, Kirstein B et al. TNF-alpha potently activates osteoclasts, through a direct action independent of and strongly synergistic with RANKL. *Endocrinology* 2002; **143**: 1108–18.

75. Lam J, Takeshita S, Barker JE et al. TNF-alpha induces osteoclastogenesis by direct stimulation of macrophages exposed to permissive levels of RANK ligand. *J Clin Invest* 2000; **106**: 1481–8.

76. Komine M, Kukita A, Kukita T et al. Tumor necrosis factor-alpha cooperates with receptor activator of nuclear factor kappaB ligand in generation of osteoclasts in stromal cell-depleted rat bone marrow cell culture. *Bone* 2001; **28**: 474–83.

77. Zou W, Hakim I, Tschoep K et al. Tumor necrosis factor-alpha mediates RANK ligand stimulation of osteoclast differentiation by an autocrine mechanism. *J Cell Biochem* 2001; **83**: 70–83.

78. Azuma Y, Kaji K, Katogi R et al. Tumor necrosis factor-alpha induces differentiation of and bone resorption by osteoclasts. *J Biol Chem* 2000; **275**: 4858–64.

79. Jimi E, Nakamura I, Duong LT et al. Interleukin 1 induces multinucleation and bone-resorbing activity of osteoclasts in the absence of osteoblasts/stromal cells. *Exp Cell Res* 1999; **247**: 84–93.

80. Quinn JM, Itoh K, Udagawa N et al. Transforming growth factor beta affects osteoclast differentiation via direct and indirect actions. *J Bone Miner Res* 2001; **16**: 1787–94.

81. Thirunavukkarasu K, Miles RR, Halladay DL et al. Stimulation of osteoprotegerin (OPG) gene expression by transforming growth factor-beta (TGF-beta). Mapping of the OPG promoter region that mediates TGF-beta effects. *J Biol Chem* 2001; **276**: 36241–50.

82. Suda K, Woo JT, Takami M et al. Lipopolysaccharide supports survival and fusion of preosteoclasts independent of TNF-alpha, IL-1, and RANKL. *J Cell Physiol* 2002; **190**: 101–8.

83. Takayanagi H, Ogasawara K, Hida S et al. T-cell-mediated regulation of osteoclastogenesis by signalling cross-talk between RANKL and IFN-gamma. *Nature* 2000; **408**: 600–5.

84. Abu-Amer Y. IL-4 abrogates osteoclastogenesis through STAT6-dependent inhibition of NF-kappaB. *J Clin Invest* 2001; **107**: 1375–85.

85. Takayanagi H, Kim S, Matsuo K et al. RANKL maintains bone homeostasis through c-Fos-dependent induction of interferon-beta. *Nature* 2002; **416**: 744–9.

86. Horwood NJ, Elliott J, Martin TJ et al. Osteotropic agents regulate the expression of osteoclast differentiation factor and osteoprotegerin in osteoblastic stromal cells. *Endocrinology* 1998; **139**: 4743–6.

87. Lee S, Lorenzo JA. Parathyroid hormone stimulates TRANCE and inhibits osteoprotegerin messenger ribonucleic acid expression in murine bone marrow cultures: correlation with osteoclast-like cell formation. *Endocrinology* 1999; **140**: 3552–61.

88. Li X, Okada Y, Pilbeam CC et al. Knockout of the murine prostaglandin EP2 receptor impairs osteoclastogenesis in vitro. *Endocrinology* 2000; **141**: 2054–61.

89. Iida-Klein A, Zhou H, Lu SS et al. Anabolic action of parathyroid hormone is skeletal site specific at the tissue and cellular levels in mice. *J Bone Miner Res* 2002; **17**: 808–16.

90. Itoh K, Udagawa N, Matsuzaki K et al. Importance of membrane- or matrix-associated forms of M-CSF and RANKL/ODF in osteoclastogenesis supported by SaOS-4/3 cells expressing recombinant PTH/PTHrP receptors. *J Bone Miner Res* 2000; **15**: 1766–75.

91. Ma YL, Cain RL, Halladay DL et al. Catabolic effects of continuous human PTH (1-38) in vivo is associated with sustained stimulation of RANKL and inhibition of osteoprotegerin and gene-associated bone formation. *Endocrinology* 2001; **142**: 4047–54.

92. Brandstrom H, Bjorkman T, Ljunggren O. Regulation of osteoprotegerin secretion from primary cultures of human bone marrow stromal cells. *Biochem Biophys Res Commun* 2001; **280**: 831–5.

93. Hofbauer LC, Lacey DL, Dunstan CR et al. Interleukin-1beta and tumor necrosis factor-alpha, but not interleukin-6, stimulate osteoprotegerin ligand gene expression in human osteoblastic cells. *Bone* 1999; **25**: 255–9.

94. Hofbauer LC, Dunstan CR, Spelsberg TC et al. Osteoprotegerin production by human osteoblast lineage cells is stimulated by vitamin D, bone morphogenetic protein-2, and cytokines. *Biochem Biophys Res Commun* 1998; **250**: 776–81.

95. Weitzmann MN, Cenci S, Rifas L et al. Interleukin-7 stimulates osteoclast formation by up-regulating the T-cell production of soluble osteoclastogenic cytokines. *Blood* 2000; **96**: 1873–8.

96. Thomas RJ, Guise TA, Yin JJ et al. Breast cancer cells interact with osteoblasts to support osteoclast formation. *Endocrinology* 1999; **140**: 4451–8.

97. Horwood NJ, Kartsogiannis V, Quinn JMW et al. Activated T lymphocytes support osteoclast formation in vitro. *Biochem Biophys Res Commun* 1999; **265**: 144–50.

98. Gravallese EM, Manning C, Tsay A et al. Synovial tissue in rheumatoid arthritis is a source of osteoclast differentiation factor. *Arthritis Rheum* 2000; **43**: 250–8.

99. Makiishi-Shimobayashi C, Tsujimura T, Iwasaki T et al. Interleukin-18 up-regulates osteoprotegerin expression in stromal/osteoblastic cells. *Biochem Biophys Res Commun* 2001; **281**: 361–6.

100. Hofbauer LC, Khosla S, Dunstan CR et al. Estrogen stimulates gene expression and protein production of osteoprotegerin in human osteoblastic cells. *Endocrinology* 1999; **140**: 4367–70.

101. Lindberg MK, Erlandsson M, Alatalo SL et al. Estrogen receptor alpha, but not estrogen receptor beta, is involved in the regulation of the OPG/RANKL (osteoprotegerin/receptor activator of NF-kappa B ligand) ratio and serum interleukin-6 in male mice. *J Endocrinol* 2001; **171**: 425–33.

102. Saika M, Inoue D, Kido S et al. 17beta-estradiol stimulates expression of osteoprotegerin by a mouse stromal cell line, ST-2, via estrogen receptor-alpha. *Endocrinology* 2001; **142**: 2205–12.

103. Viereck V, Grundker C, Blaschke S et al. Phytoestrogen genistein stimulates the production of osteoprotegerin by human trabecular osteoblasts. *J Cell Biochem* 2002; **84**: 725–35.

104. Josien R, Wong BR, Li HL et al. TRANCE, a TNF family member, is differentially expressed on T-cell subsets and induces cytokine production in dendritic cells. *J Immunol* 1999; **162**: 2562–8.

105. Yano K, Tsuda E, Washida N et al. Immunological characterization of circulating osteoprotegerin/osteoclastogenesis inhibitory factor: increased serum concentrations in postmenopausal women with osteoporosis. *J Bone Miner Res* 1999; **14**: 518–27.

106. Gravallese EM, Harada Y, Wang JT et al. Identification of cell types responsible for bone resorption in rheumatoid arthritis and juvenile rheumatoid arthritis. *Am J Pathol* 1998; **152**: 943–51.

107. Takayanagi H, Iizuka H, Juji T et al. Involvement of receptor activator of nuclear factor kappa-B ligand/osteoclast differentiation factor in osteoclastogenesis from synoviocytes in rheumatoid arthritis. *Arthritis Rheum* 2000; **43**: 259–69.

108. Shigeyama Y, Pap T, Kunzler P et al. Expression of osteoclast differentiation factor in rheumatoid arthritis. *Arthritis Rheum* 2000; **43**: 2523–30.

109. Kotake S, Udagawa N, Hakoda M et al. Activated human T cells directly induce osteoclastogenesis from human monocytes: possible role of T cells in bone destruction in rheumatoid arthritis patients. *Arthritis Rheum* 2001; **44**: 1003–12.

110. Fujikawa Y, Sabokbar A, Neale S et al. Human osteoclast formation and bone resorption by monocytes and synovial macrophages in rheumatoid arthritis. *Ann Rheum Dis* 1996; **55**: 816–22.

111. Itonaga I, Fujikawa Y, Sabokbar A, Murray DW, Athanasou NA. Rheumatoid arthritis synovial macrophage-osteoclast differentiation is osteoprotegerin ligand-dependent. *J Pathol* 2000; **192**: 97–104.

112. Toritsuka Y, Nakamura N, Lee SB et al. Osteoclastogenesis in iliac bone marrow of patients with rheumatoid arthritis. *J Rheumatol* 1997; **24**: 1690–6.

113. Haynes DR, Crotti TN, Loric M et al. Osteoprotegerin and receptor activator of nuclear

factor kappaB ligand (RANKL) regulate osteoclast formation by cells in the human rheumatoid arthritic joint. *Rheumatology (Oxford)* 2001; **40**: 623–30.

114. Suzuki Y, Tsutsumi Y, Nakagawa M et al. Osteoclast-like cells in an in vitro model of bone destruction by rheumatoid synovium. *Rheumatology (Oxford)* 2001; **40**: 673–82.

115. Yano K, Nakagawa N, Yasuda H et al. Synovial cells from a patient with rheumatoid arthritis produce osteoclastogenesis inhibitory factor/osteoprotegerin: reciprocal regulation of the production by inflammatory cytokines and basic fibroblast growth factor. *J Bone Miner Metab* 2001; **19**: 365–72.

116. Feldmann M, Brennan FM, Maini RN. Role of cytokines in rheumatoid arthritis. *Annu Rev Immunol* 1996; **14**: 397–440.

117. Feldmann M, Brennan F, Paleolog E et al. Anti-tumor necrosis factor alpha therapy of rheumatoid arthritis. Mechanism of action. *Eur Cytokine Network* 1997; **8**: 297–300.

118. Chu CQ, Field M, Feldmann M et al. Localization of tumor necrosis factor alpha in synovial tissues and at the cartilage pannus junction in patients with rheumatoid arthritis. *Arthritis Rheum* 1991; **34**: 1125–32.

119. Deleuran BW, Chu CQ, Field M et al. Localization of interleukin-1 alpha, type 1 interleukin-1 receptor and interleukin-1 receptor antagonist in the synovial membrane and cartilage/pannus junction in rheumatoid arthritis. *Br J Rheumatol* 1992; **31**: 801–9.

120. Romas E, Martin TJ. Cytokines in the pathogenesis of osteoporosis. *Osteoporos Int* 1997; **7**: S47–53.

121. Jiang Y, Genant HK, Watt I et al. A multicenter, double-blind, dose-ranging, randomized, placebo-controlled study of recombinant human interleukin-1 receptor antagonist in patients with rheumatoid arthritis: radiologic progression and correlation of Genant and Larsen scores. *Arthritis Rheum* 2000; **43**: 1001–9.

122. Lipsky PE, van der Heijde DM, St Clair EW et al. Infliximab and methotrexate in the treatment of rheumatoid arthritis. Anti-Tumor Necrosis Factor Trial in Rheumatoid Arthritis with Concomitant Therapy Study Group. *N Engl J Med* 2000; **343**: 1594–602.

123. McInnes IB, Leung BP, Sturrock RD et al. Interleukin-15 mediates T cell-dependent regulation of tumour necrosis factor-alpha production in rheumatoid arthritis. *Nat Med* 1997; **3**: 189–95.

124. Ogata Y, Kukita A, Kukita T et al. A novel role of IL-15 in the development of osteoclasts: inability to replace its activity with IL-2. *J Immunol* 1999; **162**: 2754–60.

125. Kotake S, Udagawa N, Takahashi N et al. IL-17 in synovial fluids from patients with rheumatoid arthritis is a potent stimulator of osteoclastogenesis. *J Clin Invest* 1999; **103**: 1345–52.

126. Chabaud M, Lubberts E, Joosten L et al. IL-17 derived from juxta-articular bone and synovium contributes to joint degradation in rheumatoid arthritis. *Arthritis Res* 2001; **3**: 168–77.

127. Horwood NJ, Udagawa N, Elliott J et al. Interleukin 18 inhibits osteoclast formation via T-cell production of granulocyte macrophage colony-stimulating factor. *J Clin Invest* 1998; **101**: 595–603.

128. Owens JM, Gallagher AC, Chambers TJ. IL-10 modulates formation of osteoclasts in murine hemopoietic cultures. *J Immunol* 1996; **157**: 936–40.

129. Hong MH, Williams H, Jin CH et al. The inhibitory effect of interleukin-10 on mouse osteoclast formation involves novel tyrosine-phosphorylated proteins. *J Bone Miner Res* 2000; **15**: 911–18.

130. Koch A, Campagnuolo G, Bolon B et al. Kinetics of bone protection by recombinant osteoprotegerin (OPG) therapy in Lewis rats with mycobacteria-induced adjuvant arthritis. *Arthritis Rheuma* 2001; **44**: S267.

131. Edwards J. Sustained improvement in rheumatoid arthritis following a protocol designed to deplete B lymphocytes. *Rheumatology* 2001; **40**: 205–11.

132. Matsumoto I, Staub A, Benoist C et al. Arthritis provoked by linked T and B-cell recognition of a glycolytic enzyme. *Science* 1999; **286**: 1732–5.

133. Kouskoff V, Korganow AS, Duchatelle V et al. Organ-specific disease provoked by systemic autoimmunity. *Cell* 1996; **87**: 811–22.

134. Korganow AS, Ji H, Mangialaio S et al. From systemic T-cell self-reactivity to organ-specific autoimmune disease via immunoglobulins. *Immunity* 1999; **10**: 451–61.

135. Matsumoto I, Maccioni M, Lee DM et al. How antibodies to a ubiquitous cytoplasmic enzyme may provoke joint-specific autoimmune disease. *Nat Immunol* 2002; **3**: 360–5.

136. Korganow A, Weber JC, Martin T. Animal models and autoimmune diseases. *Rev Med Int* 1999; **20**: 283–6.

137. Keffer J, Probert L, Cazlaris H et al. Transgenic mice expressing human tumour necrosis factor: a predictive genetic model of arthritis. *EMBO J* 1991; **10**: 4025–31.

138. Hou WS, Li W, Keyszer G et al. Comparison of cathepsins K and S expression within the rheumatoid and osteoarthritic synovium. *Arthritis Rheum* 2002; **46**: 663–74.

139. Romas E, Gillespie MT, Martin TJ. Involvement of receptor activator of NFkappaB ligand and tumor necrosis factor-alpha in bone destruction in rheumatoid arthritis. *Bone* 2002; **30**: 340–6.

140. Komuro H, Olee T, Kuhn K et al. The osteoprotegerin/receptor activator of nuclear factor kappaB/receptor activator of nuclear factor kappaB ligand system in cartilage. *Arthritis Rheum* 2001; **44**: 2768–76.

141. Bekker PJ, Holloway D, Nakanishi A et al. The effect of a single dose of osteoprotegerin in postmenopausal women. *J Bone Miner Res* 2001; **16**: 348–60.

142. Bateman TA, Dunstan CR, Ferguson VL et al. Osteoprotegerin mitigates tail suspension-induced osteopenia. *Bone* 2000; **26**: 443–9.

143. Guise TA. Molecular mechanisms of osteolytic bone metastases. *Cancer* 2000; **88**: 2892–8.

144. Zhang J, Dai J, Qi Y et al. Osteoprotegerin inhibits prostate cancer-induced osteoclastogenesis and prevents prostate tumor growth in the bone. *J Clin Invest* 2001; **107**: 1235–44.

145. Croucher PI, Shipman CM, Lippitt J et al. Osteoprotegerin inhibits the development of osteolytic bone disease in multiple myeloma. *Blood* 2001; **98**: 3534–40.

146. Giuliani N, Bataille R, Mancini C et al. Myeloma cells induce imbalance in the osteoprotegerin/osteoprotegerin ligand system in the human bone marrow environment. *Blood* 2001; **98**: 3527–33.

147. Morony S, Capparelli C, Sarosi I et al. Osteoprotegerin inhibits osteolysis and decreases skeletal tumor burden in syngeneic and nude mouse models of experimental bone metastasis. *Cancer Res* 2001; **61**: 4432–6.

148. Honore P, Luger NM, Sabino MA et al. Osteoprotegerin blocks bone cancer-induced skeletal destruction, skeletal pain and pain-related neuro-chemical reorganization of the spinal cord. *Nat Med* 2000; **6**: 521–8.

149. Kim KJ, Kotake S, Udagawa N et al. Osteoprotegerin inhibits in vitro mouse osteoclast formation induced by joint fluid from failed total hip arthroplasty. *J Biomed Mater Res* 2001; **58**: 393–400.

150. Goater JJ, O'Keefe RJ, Rosier RN et al. Efficacy of ex vivo OPG gene therapy in preventing wear debris induced osteolysis. *J Orthop Res* 2002; **20**: 169–73.

151. Teng YT, Nguyen H, Gao X et al. Functional human T-cell immunity and osteoprotegerin ligand control alveolar bone destruction in periodontal infection. *J Clin Invest* 2000; **106**: R59–67.

152. Josien R, Li HL, Ingulli E et al. TRANCE, a tumor necrosis factor family member, enhances the longevity and adjuvant properties of dendritic cells in vivo. *J Exp Med* 2000; **191**: 495–502.

153. Emery JG, McDonnell P, Burke MB et al. Osteoprotegerin is a receptor for the cytotoxic ligand TRAIL. *J Biol Chem* 1998; **273**: 14363–7.

154. Holen I, Croucher PI, Hamdy FC et al. Osteoprotegerin (OPG) is a survival factor for human prostate cancer cells. *Cancer Res* 2002; **62**: 1619–23.

155. Childs LM, Ulrich-Vinther M, Abuzzahab F et al. Effects of RANK blockadE on fracture healing. *Arthritis Rheum* 2001; **44**: S267.

156. Fata JE, Kong YY, Li J et al. The osteoclast differentiation factor osteoprotegerin-ligand is essential for mammary gland development. *Cell* 2000; **103**: 41–50.

157. Jiang Y, Mehta CK, Hsu TY et al. Bacteria induce osteoclastogenesis via an osteoblast-independent pathway. *Infect Immun* 2002; **70**: 3143–8.

158. Kikuchi T, Matsuguchi T, Tsuboi N et al. Gene expression of osteoclast differentiation factor is induced by lipopolysaccharide in mouse osteoblasts via Toll-like receptors. *J Immunol* 2001; **166**: 3574–9.

159. Lubberts E, Joosten LA, Chabaud M et al. IL-4 gene therapy for collagen arthritis suppresses synovial IL-17 and osteoprotegerin ligand and prevents bone erosion. *J Clin Invest* 2000; **105**: 1697–710.

Section III

Transcription factors and signaling molecules

22

NF-κB

Keith Brown, Estefania Claudio and Ulrich Siebenlist

Introduction • Structure of NF-κB polypeptides • Structure and modes of action of IκB inhibitors • Activation mechanisms I: degradation of classical IκBs • Activation mechanisms II: processing of p100/NF-κB2 and p105/NF-κB1 • Distinct molecular mechanisms involved in release of NF-κB from inhibitors • Signaling pathways regulating NF-κB activity • Activation via modulation of transactivating functions • Biological functions and targets, deduced primarily from knockout studies • Possible therapeutic strategies • Acknowledgments • References

INTRODUCTION

NF-κB transcription factors are central regulators and coordinators of immune and inflammatory processes, and of stress responses in general.[1-7] Given the large number of host defense mediators that are transcriptionally regulated by NF-κB in response to pathogens, including not only anti-pathogenic agents but also mediators of migration, adhesion, activation, proliferation and survival,[8] it is not surprising that NF-κB is often intimately involved in driving inflammatory reactions in disease.[4,7] In addition, its cell survival activity appears to contribute to tumorigenesis.[4,6] Consequently, NF-κB factors and their regulators/activators have taken center stage as potential targets for therapeutic interventions in a large number of inflammatory diseases and cancers.

This review introduces basic concepts of NF-κB structure, general biological function and regulation. Such information is necessary to help illuminate how NF-κB may be inappropriately activated in disease, and how it may contribute to initiation and progression of disease. In addition, knowledge of normal functions of NF-κB and its regulators/activators provides the basis for identifying the most specific targets for therapeutic intervention in a given disease. To better appreciate the roles and regulation of NF-κB factors in a biological context, we discuss important inflammatory signaling pathways and biological roles of NF-κB factors. Insights into in vivo function were gained primarily by analyses of knockout mice. We direct the reader to other chapters in this book in which some of NF-κB's roles are described in the context of various inflammatory diseases. Due to space constraints not all of the relevant research is discussed. Also references to original papers are necessarily limited and reviews have been referred to wherever feasible. Apologies are extended to the original authors.

STRUCTURE OF NF-κB POLYPEPTIDES

NF-κB refers to a family of dimeric transcription factors, composed of members of the Rel/NF-κB family of polypeptides, which in mammals are

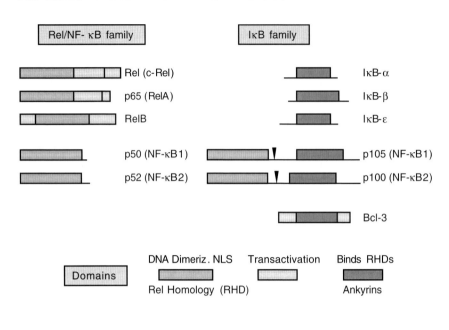

Figure 22.1 The mammalian families of Rel/NF-κB and IκB polypeptides. Characteristic domains and their primary functions are indicated: DNA, DNA binding; Dimeriz., dimerization domain; RHD, Rel homology domain; NLS, nuclear localization sequence; Transactivation, transactivating domain, functions at nuclear target sites; Ankyrins, ankyrin repeat domain, functions by binding and inhibiting RHDs (Bcl-3 is an exception since it does not inhibit).

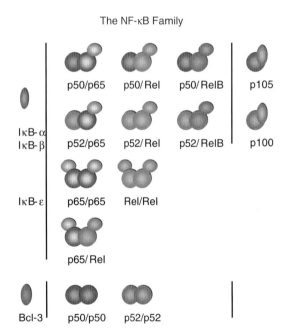

Figure 22.2 The family of dimeric NF-κB transcription factors. The various Rel/NF-κB polypeptides combine as dimers to form functional transcription factors. Most but not all combinations are permitted. Also shown are which dimers are targeted by the various IκB family members.

p50/NF-κB1, p52/NF-κB2, RelA (p65), RelB and c-Rel (Rel) (Figure 22.1).[1,9,10] Through combinatorial power the various polypeptides can form a larger set of distinct homo- and heterodimeric NF-κB dimers. All combinations are possible except in the case of RelB, which seems to only dimerize with p50 or p52 (Figure 22.2). In the past, the term NF-κB has also been used to denote p50/p65 heterodimers only, presumably because these dimers are generally most abundant and often dominate rapidly inducible κB-DNA-binding activity. However in this review NF-κB refers to the entire repertoire of dimeric complexes, in agreement with common usage now.

NF-κB dimers can be traced back in evolution to insects, where Dorsal, Dif and Relish make up the corresponding family in Drosophila Rel/NF-κB-like proteins.[3,11,12] As in mammals, the Drosophila members of this family, and in particular Dif and Relish, function as critical regulators of immune responses in Drosophila. Dorsal has an additional unique role as the essential morphogen responsible for the establishment of the dorsal–ventral axis during development, a role not associated with any of the mammalian NF-κB proteins.[13]

All Rel/NF-κB proteins share a fairly well conserved so-called Rel homology domain

(RHD) of approximately 300 amino acids in length (Figure 22.1).[10] RHDs encode DNA binding domains in their N-terminal halves and dimerization domains in their C-terminal halves, with the edge of the dimerization regions contributing to non-specific DNA binding as well. The C-terminal ends of the RHDs contain a nuclear localization sequence (NLS). The structures of p50/p50, p52/p52 and c-Rel homodimers and p50/p65 heterodimers have been elucidated.[5,14] A consensus DNA binding site for NF-κB complexes reads 5'-GGGRNNYYCC-3'. In the case of p50/p65 heterodimers, the 5' end of this consensus site binds to the p50 subunit, while the 3' end binds to p65.

The p50 and p52 subunits are composed of just RHDs, harboring no known transactivation domains, while the larger Rel, RelA (p65) and RelB proteins each contain non-homologous transactivation domains located C-terminal to their RHDs (Figure 22.1). p50 and p52 are generated by proteolytic processing during or after synthesis of the much larger p105/NF-κB1 and p100/NF-κB2 proteins, as discussed in the following sections.

STRUCTURE AND MODES OF ACTION OF IκB INHIBITORS

In most cells a specific signal is required to activate NF-κB. Without such a signal, NF-κB dimers are held in an inactive form in the cytoplasm by association with IκB inhibitors. Release of NF-κB dimers follows the signal-induced proteolytic degradation of the inhibitors. All IκB family members share a domain consisting of several ankyrin repeats, which mediates binding to NF-κB dimers (Figure 22.2). Structures of IκB proteins have been solved.[5,15]

The 'classic' or small IκB inhibitors are the closely related IκBα, IκBβ and IκBε proteins. These proteins bind to NF-κB dimers and fully or partially shield the NLSs in the dimers, thus helping to retain the complexes in the cytoplasm. In the case of IκBα and the p50/p65(RelA) heterodimer, the inhibitor fully shields the NLS of p65, but not that of p50. Consequently, some complexes are thought to enter nuclei, but are rapidly returned to the cytoplasm due to nuclear

export signals (NESs) present on both IκBα and p65. In contrast, IκBβ more effectively shields both NLSs of p50/p65 and itself lacks an NES, apparently preventing shuttling between cytoplasm and nucleus,[5] although some evidence suggests that even this factor may enter nuclei in some circumstances, possibly related to its phosphorylation status.[16] It remains unclear why complexes bound by IκBα shuttle between the cytoplasm and nucleus, since this inhibitor also blocks DNA binding of the associated dimers. Interestingly, the IκBβ inhibitor does not block DNA binding in in vitro assays.[17] The importance of these differences are called into question by gene targeting experiments in which the gene for IκBα, but not its regulatory region was replaced by IκBβ. Mice altered in such a way did not appear to have any defects.[18]

All three IκBs inhibit p65-containing complexes, much more strongly than they do RelB complexes, while they are essentially unable to keep p50 or p52 homodimers out of the nucleus (the latter are not usually observed in gel shift experiments). Thus, the relatively abundant p50 homodimers usually localize to cell nuclei even in the absence of signal. RelB appears to be regulated differently, independently of the classical IκBs (see below).

In addition to the small, classical IκBs, this family of proteins also includes p105 and p100, the long forms of NF-κB1 and NF-κB2, respectively (Figure 22.2). These proteins encode the p50 and p52 subunits in their N-terminal halves, respectively, while bearing IκB-like ankyrin domains in their C-terminal halves. The p105 and p100 proteins can inhibit dimerized NF-κB partners with their C-terminal domains that act as built-in IκBs. This appears to be the primary way in which RelB is inhibited. The p105 and p100 IκB domains may also inhibit existing NF-κB dimers much like small IκBs would, thus forming trimers or even higher-order complexes, should p105/p100 also be partnered with other NF-κB proteins via their RHDs.[19] While most NF-κB activation occurs by degradation of the classical small IκB inhibitors, an alternative activation path involves liberation of dimers via processing and/or complete degradation of the p105 and p100 inhibitors (see below).

Another member of the IκB family is Bcl-3 (Figure 22.2). This protein is unusual in that it does not function as a classical inhibitor. Bcl-3 is not degraded in response to activation signals, is frequently found in the nucleus and preferentially binds p50 and p52 homodimers. When complexed with p52 homodimers in transfection experiments (and to a lesser extent when complexed with p50 homodimers), Bcl-3 is able to transactivate κB reporters. Thus Bcl-3 may help to induce rather than inhibit NF-κB activity, but its precise physiologic roles remain somewhat elusive. Bcl-3's actions may be modulated or even changed by phosphorylation

events that are not understood at this time.[10,15,20,21]

The most recently identified member of the IκB family of proteins is termed IκB-ζ or MAIL. This protein is inducible and nuclear, but its function remains to be determined.[22,23]

ACTIVATION MECHANISMS I: DEGRADATION OF CLASSICAL IκBs

Activation of NF-κB proceeds primarily via signal-induced, ubiquitin-dependent proteolytic destruction of inhibitor proteins, an event that uncovers nuclear localization signals on the

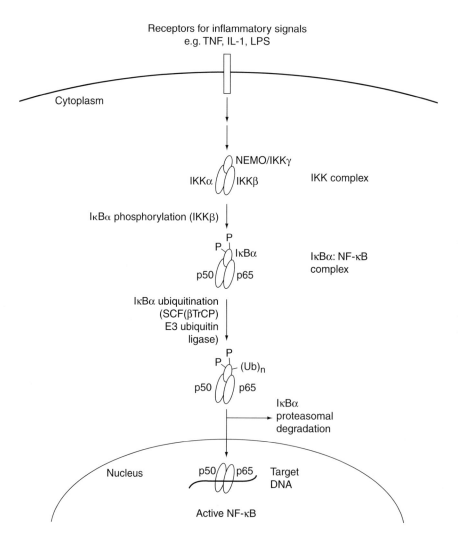

Figure 22.3 Canonical pathway of NF-κB activation via IκB degradation. In this scheme, inflammatory signals induce phosphorylation of IκBα bound to cytosolic NF-κB. Phosphorylation is carried out by the IKK complex composed of NEMO/IKKγ and two catalytic subunits, IKKα and IKKβ. Phosphorylation tags the IκB for ubiquitination by the SCF(βTrCP) E3 ubiquitin ligase complex and ultimate proteasomal degradation, liberating NF-κB for translocation to the nucleus (where further activation may occur) and transactivation of target genes.

previously bound NF-κB dimers and leads to their translocation into the nucleus.[2,5,24] There, the dimers bind to cognate DNA sites to transcriptionally regulate target genes. As discussed later, an additional layer of control over transactivation is exercised by signal-dependent modulation of the transactivation potential of the NF-κB dimers released into the nucleus

Signal-induced proteolytic degradation of the 'classical' inhibitors IκB-α, -β, and -ε is initiated by phosphorylation of two conserved serines that lie within the N-terminal domains of these proteins. Phosphorylation is carried out by the IκB kinase complex (IKK), which is composed of a regulatory subunit, NEMO/IKKγ, and two catalytic subunits, IKKα and IKKβ. NEMO is required to receive upstream signals, while IKKβ appears to be the primary kinase involved in phosphorylation of small IκBs in response to inflammatory signals (Figure 22.3). Phosphorylation by IKKs (primarily IKKβ) marks the IκB inhibitors for recognition and polyubiquitination by the SCF(βTrCP) E3 ubiquitin ligase complex, and thereby ultimately for destruction by proteasomes. A recent unexpected finding suggests that ubiquitination of the inhibitor, but not phosphorylation, may occur in the nucleus, since the βTrCP protein is largely nuclear. If so, the phosphorylated IκB proteins bound to NF-κB complexes would have to shuttle to the nucleus prior to degradation, but this remains to be demonstrated.[2,5,24]

IκBα and IκBβ differ somewhat in terms of how readily they are degraded in response to a given signal – IκBβ is usually less responsive, potentially related to its association with κB-Ras proteins[25] – but probably more importantly, these proteins differ in terms of their expression. Once NF-κB has been activated, it strongly induces expression of IκB-α and IκB-ε, but not IκB-β.[18] Induced expression of IκB-α constitutes an immediate negative feedback loop that delimits activation of the NF-κB transcription factors. Although relatively unstable when not complexed, the newly induced IκB-α can readily enter nuclei to recapture previously liberated NF-κB complexes, even when bound to DNA.

Due to NESs, IκB-α and any associated dimers then promptly return to the cytoplasm, thus terminating the activation phase.[5]

ACTIVATION MECHANISMS II: PROCESSING OF p100/NF-κB2 AND p105/NF-κB1

Proteolytic processing/degradation of the p105/NF-κB1 and p100/NF-κB2 inhibitory proteins in response to signals can represent an alternative pathway to activation of NF-κB, independent of degradation of the small IκBs. However, most p50 is generated constitutively and thus does not require a known signal, although smaller amounts of p105 may be subject to signal-induced processing/degradation. On the other hand, p52 is generated primarily via signal-induced processing of p100.

Constitutive processing may occur primarily via a cotranslational, ubiquitin- and proteasome-assisted mechanism, in which the protein is never fully synthesized. In this model, which is particularly relevant for generation of p50, the nascent polypeptide chain is recognized by ubiquitin ligases, polyubiquitinated and progressively degraded by proteasomes, which remove parts of the chain extending past the N-terminal p50 domains. A glycine-rich stretch just C-terminal to the RHD (at the end of the p50 domain) appears to function as a direct or indirect stop signal for the advancing proteasome. An indirect mechanism might involve proteolytic cleavage of the accessible glycine stretch. Cotranslational processing of NF-κB2 to p52 appears to be inefficient[26] possibly due to only weak recognition of the nascent chain by E3-ubiquitin ligases.

With appropriate signals, however, significant amounts of p52 can be generated by p100 processing, signals that may also lead to low levels of processing and/or total degradation of p105 (see below). Signal-activated IKK kinases have been reported to phosphorylate two serines within C-terminal motifs of both p105 and p100, which closely resemble critical phosphorylation motifs found in the classical, small IκBs.[27,28] Similar to what happens with the small IκBs, the SCF(βTrCP) E3 ubiquitin ligase then binds the phosphorylated p105 and p100 proteins, polyubiquitinates them and thereby initiates their proteasome-mediated processing/degradation.[27,29] To generate p50 or p52, rather than to degrade the entire precursor, the advancing proteasome must be stopped – directly or indirectly – by the glycine-rich stretch located just C-terminal to the RHDs, as discussed above for constitutive processing. In the case of p105, however, phosphorylation by IKK may instead lead to its complete degradation (including the p50 domain).[27] Clearly, many aspects of processing/degradation of NF-κB1/2 remain to be determined.

Importantly, processing or complete degradation of p105 and processing of p100 would release NF-κB proteins that were sequestered in the cytoplasm by the inhibitory ankyrin domains of these proteins. If not rapidly captured by small IκBs, these complexes could directly enter nuclei to transactivate genes. This may be especially true for RelB, since RelB dimers are not well inhibited by small IκBs in any case. Therefore, NF-κB activation may not always have to depend on release from small IκB inhibitory proteins, and, as discussed below, some activation signals specifically effect signal-induced processing of p100.

DISTINCT MOLECULAR MECHANISMS INVOLVED IN RELEASE OF NF-κB FROM INHIBITORS

Many diverse signals can activate NF-κB, albeit to various degrees. Most inflammatory signals appear to target the small IκB inhibitors for proteolytic destruction via phosphorylation by the canonical IκB kinase complex (IKK: IKKα–IKKβ–NEMO/IKKγ). IKK-mediated signals can release large amounts of NF-κB dimers into the nucleus. Although some reports suggest that other kinases may exist that can phosphorylate these inhibitors, including an IKKi/IKKε-associated kinase,[30] numerous activation signals have been shown to converge at the canonical IKKα–β–γ complex.[31,32] IKKα and IKKβ are tightly associated with each other and with NEMO/IKKγ and they are reportedly able to

auto- or transphosphorylate, which may be a mechanism for activating them.

Despite their similarities, each kinase subunit can have distinct functions. IKKβ, together with the regulatory subunit NEMO/IKKγ but independent of IKKα, is necessary and sufficient to rapidly phosphorylate small IκBs in response to inflammatory stimuli, leading to activation of NF-κB[32] (Figure 22.4). The IKKα kinase, on the other hand, is both necessary and sufficient for the signal-induced processing of p100 to p52 (see below). In addition to their distinct substrate preferences, these kinases may also be distinctly targeted by upstream signals. A recent report suggests that RANK-receptor-mediated activation of NF-κB in mammary epithelial cells is mediated via IKKα, an event critical to mammary development during pregnancy.[33] Surprisingly, the primary role of IKKα in this situation appears to be to bring about the degradation of the small inhibitor IκBα, rather than the proteolytic processing of p100, although this occurs as well. It is not known, however, if IKKα directly phosphorylates IκB downstream of RANK or if it functions indirectly by first activating IKKβ.

Signal-induced phosphorylation/processing of p100 appears to represent an activation mode distinct from degradation of small IκBs. As discussed above, IKKα, but not IKKβ, is necessary for inducible p52 generation, based on analyses of IKKα-deficient mutant cells.[34] Furthermore our recent results indicate that IKKα-dependent processing of p100 can occur in the absence of NEMO/IKKγ. Therefore an IKKα kinase activity independent of the canonical IKK complex must exist (Figure 22.4). This IKKα activity may target p100 only, since IKKβ is reportedly able to phosphorylate p105.[27] The MAP3 kinase NIK binds to p100[28] and has been demonstrated to phosphorylate and activate IKKα and to induce processing of p100,[34] while phosphorylation of p105 (possibly by IKKβ) in response to TNF may involve the MAP3 kinase Tpl-2 (COT), which has been shown to bind to this precursor.[35] Tpl-2 has also been proposed to lie in a pathway leading to activation of IKKs/NF-κB in response to stimulation of T cells

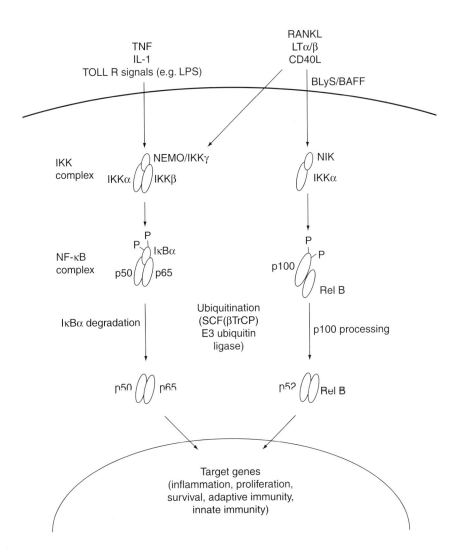

Figure 22.4 Signal transduction pathways for NF-κB activation. The canonical pathway phosphorylates small IκBs (largely mediated by IKKβ) in response to inflammatory stimuli. This leads to their proteasomal degradation and release of NF-κB, which migrates to the nucleus where it activates target genes. The second pathway is activated by several signals, including BAFF, CD40L, RANKL and LTα/β. Some of these (with the possible exception of BAFF) are also known to activate the canonical pathway. The second pathway proceeds via IKKα, independently of the classical IKK complex and leads to processing of p100/NF-κB2, generating predominantly p52/RelB heterodimers, which migrate to the nucleus.

via CD3 and CD28.[36,37] Recent data from our laboratory have identified several signals that can induce processing of p100, including the TNF family members BAFF, CD40, RANKL and lymphotoxin α/β (see also below).

The regulation of NF-κB activity via two distinct classes of IκB proteins (the small 'classical' IκBs versus p100 and to a lesser degree probably p105) is already present in Drosophila, where these two regulatory pathways appear to serve somewhat distinct biological roles.[3,12,13] Drosophila has only one small IκB protein named Cactus, which inhibits the Drosophila Rel/NF-κB proteins Dorsal and Dif. Activation of Dorsal via proteasome-dependent degradation of Cactus is particularly important in early embryos, where Dorsal serves as the ventral morphogen. Activation of Dif via degradation of Cactus is particularly important in immune responses to fungal pathogens. Many responses to gram-negative bacterial pathogens, by contrast, require the Drosophila Relish protein. This protein structurally resembles the p100 and p105 precursors, and it can be inducibly processed to a p50/p52-like form that enters nuclei. Signal-induced processing of Relish requires phosphorylation by an IKK-like Drosophila kinase, which therefore behaves much like the mammalian IKKα, including the fact that it is largely dispensable for phosphorylation/degradation of Cactus. This Drosophila IKK is associated with a Drosophila NEMO homolog called Kenny. Curiously, a Drosophila kinase for Cactus has not yet been identified. Unlike p100, Relish processing is not mediated by proteasomes, but instead may be mediated via a pathway involving the caspase, Dredd. Therefore, despite remarkable similarities between Drosophila and mammals in terms of mechanisms of activation and functions of their respective NF-κB complexes, there are also many significant differences.

In addition to the well-documented proteolytic degradation of the small IκBs initiated by the IKK-dependent phosphorylation of two closely spaced N-terminal serine residues, the IκBα inhibitor may also be functionally inactivated via phosphorylation of an N-terminal tyrosine residue. However, the exact mechanism for how tyrosine phosphorylation interferes with the inhibitory activity of IκBα remains unclear. With respect to the physiologic relevance, a recent report suggests that direct tyrosine phosphorylation of IκBα by the JAK2 kinase may contribute to activation of NF-κB by erythropoeitin in neurons.[38] Such a pathway was suggested to contribute to the protection erythropoietin administration affords neurons challenged with apoptotic insults.

Finally, a proteasome-independent, but calcium-calmodulin-dependent pathway leading to degradation of IκBα has been reported to contribute to constitutive activation of NF-κB in some B cells.[39] In potentially related studies, proteasome-independent, but casein kinase II (CK2)- and calpain-protease-dependent IκBα degradation was reported to contribute to constitutive NF-κB activation in breast cancer cell lines.[40,41] Casein kinase II has been implicated in phosphorylation of IκBα, especially its C-terminal PEST domain,[42] the domain responsible for the relatively rapid turnover of this protein, a process that may involve calpain proteases.[43] Thus, the aforementioned observations could be related and may reflect mechanisms by which the normal

turnover rate of IκBα can be increased, which in turn may contribute to the maintenance of constitutive NF-κB activity. However, the physiologic significance of such mechanisms remains to be determined.

SIGNALING PATHWAYS REGULATING NF-κB ACTIVITY

The precise molecular steps by which the classical IKK complex is activated are not yet known. It remains unclear if IKKs are activated by specific kinases or if complexes are assembled in ways which permit activation by auto- or transphosphorylation. NEMO/IKKγ has been shown to be required for activation of the IKK complex in response to many signals, but exactly how NEMO functions or what proteins it may associate with in specific signaling paths has remained a mystery.

Incontinentia pigmenti is an X-linked disease in females in which one of the NEMO alleles is truncated. Such severe mutations are lethal to males in utero, as is the complete lack of NEMO in mice. In contrast, the pathology associated with incontinentia pigmenti in females, which develops after birth, may be lethal or may eventually resolve, similar to heterozygous knockout female mice. Females develop with a mixture of NEMO-containing and NEMO-deficient cells, depending on which X-chromosome has been lyonized. It has been proposed that NEMO-deficient cells may be highly sensitive to apoptosis, which may induce massive inflammation mediated by NEMO-containing cells, in particular in skin.[44,45] If the deficient cells are eliminated in time before the animals succumb, the disease may resolve. Missense mutations in NEMO have been linked to the disease anhydrotic ectodermal dysplasia associated with immunodeficiency (EDA-ID). Many but not all of these mutations have been localized to the C-terminal zinc finger domain, which is thus implicated in transmitting at least some signals, a fact supported by transfection studies involving mutations. Anhydrotic ectodermal dysplasia (without immune deficiency) is also caused by mutations in the paired TNF ligand/receptor family members EDA/EDAR, which therefore can be assumed to signal important functions via NEMO and NF-κB. The immunodeficiencies of EDA-ID associated also with hyper-IgM have been suggested to result from some defects in CD40L signaling, and possibly also IL-1, IL-18 and TNF signaling, although this is not fully understood at this time.[46,47]

A few proteins have been shown to interact with NEMO, but their exact roles in activation of IKK remain largely unknown. The HTLV-1 TAX protein has been shown to activate NF-κB via interaction with the C-terminus of NEMO.[48] A cellular protein termed CIKS or Act1 has been shown to interact with NEMO and it was suggested to play a role in CD40-induced NF-κB activation, but its mechanisms of action are not known.[49,50] The kinase RIP also appears to bind NEMO after TNF stimulation, as discussed below.

While it remains unclear precisely how the IKK complex becomes activated, signaling cascades leading up to this particular step are coming into focus, especially in the cases of activation via TNF- and IL-1/Toll receptors.[51–53] Upon ligation of these particular model receptors, death-domain containing adaptors are recruited: TRADD in the case of TNF receptor I, and MyD88 in the case of IL-1 or Toll receptors (some Toll receptors can also recruit a MyD88-related protein termed MAL or Tirap). Both the TRADD and MyD88 adaptors mediate dual and opposing functions: they can activate apoptotic pathways and they can activate NF-κB, which generally has anti-apoptotic survival functions. To activate apoptosis, TRADD and MyD88 couple to the FADD adaptor that binds procaspase 8. To activate NF-κB, TRADD recruits the TRAF2 adaptor as well the serine/threonine kinase RIP (Figure 22.5). According to recent reports, the serine/threonine kinase RIP specifically interacts

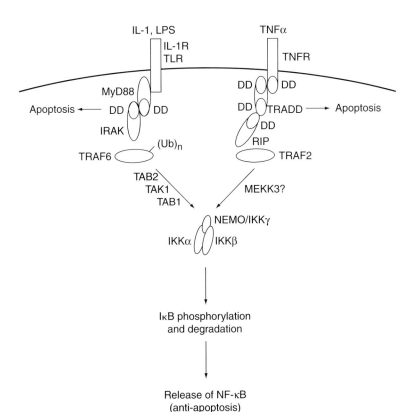

Figure 22.5 The TNF and IL-1/Toll signal cascades. Engagement of ligand with its cognate receptor triggers ligation of these receptors and death domain (DD) adaptor proteins are recruited: TRADD and MyD88. These can activate apoptotic pathways as well as NF-κB. TRADD recruits the RIP kinase and the TRAF2 adaptor protein. This results in activation of the classic IKK complex and NF-κB activation. A fraction of the IKK complexes may be recruited to the receptor, where the NEMO/IKKγ subunit may interact with RIP. MEKK3 may also play a role in activating the IKK complex in this pathway. MyD88 recruits IRAK, which is phosphorylated and then dissociates from the receptor. IRAK then associates with TRAF6 in the cytoplasm. TRAF6 may then activate NF-κB by several routes, including via association with TAB2/TAK1, which is thought to target IKKs. The activation of TAK1 may require ubiquitination of TRAF6.

with NEMO/IKKγ within the receptor complex. The role of TRAF2 in this process is controversial, with one study suggesting that TRAF2 recruits IKKs to the ligand-activated receptor by interaction with the kinase subunits.[51,54,55] As discussed, these interactions activate the IKK kinases by unknown mechanisms, but, surprisingly, independent of the RIP kinase activity. It also remains to be established how activation of relatively few IKKs at the receptor leads to activation of a much larger fraction of the cellular IKKs. There may be additional kinases required for activation of the IKKs by RIP and, according to one report, MEKK3 may function to phosphorylate and thus activate IKKs.[56] Alternatively, RIP together with NEMO may lead to multimerization of the IKKs and thus activation via transphosphorylation.

In the case of the IL-1 and Toll receptors, MyDD 88, once complexed to these receptors, then recruits the serine/threonine kinase, IRAK, along with its binding partner Tollip (MAL, the MyD 88-related adaptor may recruit IRAK2, a relative of IRAK), leading to the phosphorylation of IRAK by an unknown kinase.[53] Recently it has been demonstrated that IRAK4 is also required for proper signal transduction in response to IL-1 as well as several Toll receptors.[57] The function of Tollip may be to inhibit IRAK activity in the absence of stimulation, since phosphorylated IRAK apparently dissociates from both Tollip and the receptor. The kinase activity of IRAK is not essential for activation of NF-κB, which is reminiscent of the role of RIP in TNF signaling. After IRAK phosphorylation and dissociation from the receptor and Tollip, IRAK transiently associates with TRAF6, possibly to guide this adaptor from a membrane location to the cytoplasm.[52,53] Similarly, phosphorylated IRAK may also transiently associate with and bring TAB2 to the cytoplasm, where this adaptor is conjectured to bridge a transient association between TRAF6 and the TAK1 kinase/TAB1 adaptor complex.[58] TAB2, TAB1 and TAK1 become phosphorylated and the activated TAK1 serine/threonine kinase is presumed to phosphorylate and activate the IKKs directly. TRAF6 has been shown to cause

the activation of the IKKs in partially purified cellular fractions in vitro and this activation depends on two activities: an unusual E3 ubiquitin ligase activity encoded by the ring finger motif of TRAF6 and the TAK1/TAB2 kinase complex discussed above.[59] In concert with a non-standard E2 ubiquitin dimer, the TRAF6 containing E3 ligase reportedly forms uncommon polyubiquitin chains with lysine (K)-63, possibly on oligomerized TRAF6 itself. Such chains are not recognized by proteasomes and thus are likely modifiers of protein activity instead. The so-modified TRAF6 may activate the TAK1 kinase (linked to TRAF6 via TAB2), although how this might be accomplished is not known. Once activated, TAK1 could then directly phosphorylate and activate IKKα/β, dependent on NEMO/IKKγ (Figure 22.5). The authors of this study further suggested that a similar K-63-ubiquitin-dependent mechanism is involved in the TRAF2-mediated activation of NF-κB downstream of the TNF receptor. Recently it has been reported that TAK1 can also become activated via direct association with the RANK receptor and TRAF6, bypassing IRAK altogether.[60]

There are many other signaling paths that result in activation of the IKKs, but in no case is it fully understood how the IKKs are activated or what exact role the required NEMO/IKKγ subunit plays. It is known from studies with NEMO/IKKγ-deficient or -impaired cells that this regulatory IKK subunit is absolutely required for signal transduction to the IKK kinases α and β downstream of most extracellular signals tested to date (see exceptions below).[44,45] In addition to the already discussed upstream mediators RIP, IRAK (IRAK2), TAK1/TAB2, the TRAFs (in addition to TRAF2 and TRAF6, TRAF5 in particular can mediate NF-κB activation downstream of several members of the TNF receptor family), CIKS (Act-1), TAX, Tpl-2/COT, NIK and MEKK3, many other kinases and adaptors have been implicated as direct or at least proximal activators of the IKKs, and thus of NF-κB.[5,61] Additional kinases implicated in this way include MEKK1, MEKK2, aPKC together with p62 (which can bind RIP),

AKT/PKB, RNA-dependent PKR, DNA protein kinase, RICK (RIP-2, CARDIAK, a RIP-related kinase with a Card domain) together with Nod1 (Card4) or Nod2 (part of intracellular LPS-sensing receptors), IKKε (IKKi), and TBK1 together with TANK and possibly also TRAF2 (TBK1 (NAK/TK2) and IKKε/i are most similar to each other and distantly related to IKKα,β). Additional adaptor-like proteins implicated in activation of IKKs (without a specifically associated known kinase), include the Card protein complexes Card9/Bcl-10, Bimp1 (Card10)/Bcl-10/MALT1, Card11/Bcl-10 and Card14/Bcl-10.[5,61–66]

Bcl-10 was reported necessary for activation of NF-κB in mature T and B cells stimulated via their respective antigen receptors (TCR and BCR). The TCR-initiated signaling to NF-κB in mature T cells also requires the TCR complex-associated PKCθ kinase.[67] The corresponding BCR-initiated signaling in mature B cells may depend on novel PKCs (including PKCθ) and/or PKCβ. PKCβ is a known target of the BCR-associated Bruton's tyrosine kinase (BTK), a kinase that has been shown to be necessary for activation of NF-κB in mature B cells.[68]

Mutations in Nod2 have been linked to susceptibility to Crohn's disease (CD), a chronic inflammatory bowel disease.[7,61] The Nod2 Card-containing protein is expressed in monocytes and appears to be involved in activation of NF-κB in response to bacterial lipopolysaccharides together with the Card- and death-domain-containing kinase RICK/RIP2/CARDIAK. RICK can associate with IKKγ/NEMO and the IKK complex. Nod2 mutants in CD may cause disease by altering the recognition of bacterial components and/or over-activating NF-κB in monocytes. Thus the Nod/RICK/IKK pathway may provide a link between an innate immune response to microbial pathogens and disease.

While most signals and pathways only target the classical, NEMO-dependent IKK complex, some signals activate IKKα to induce processing of p100.[34] The B cell factor BAFF (BLyS) acts primarily as a survival factor during generation and maintenance of mature B cells. When overexpressed in animals by way of an inserted transgene, BAFF leads to increased numbers of B cells and autoimmune-like conditions.[69–72] As shown in our laboratory recently, BAFF induces processing of p100/NF-κB2 to p52 in maturing and mature B cells, dependent on the BAFF receptor (along with BCMA and TACI, one of three receptors BAFF may interact with) and dependent on the kinase NIK. As discussed, NIK binds to p100 and can phosphorylate and activate IKKα. A natural mutation in NIK, dubbed aly for alymphoplasia, as well as a NIK knockout show defects in secondary lymphoid architecture due to defects in stromal cells and probably also B cells.[73,74] Similar defects were seen in NF-κB2 knockout mice[75] and in mice lacking lymphotoxin β receptors (present on stromal cells) or their ligands (LTα/LTβ₂, expressed on, for example, B cells).[76] Consistent with this, agonists of LTβR on fibroblasts also induce processing of p100 dependent on NIK and IKKα, but not IKKβ or NEMO, as recently shown in our laboratory. The LTβR also activates the classical pathway and thus degradation of small IκBs. Induction of p100 processing is slow – it takes several hours – and is dependent on protein synthesis, possibly because continued synthesis of the very poorly expressed NIK protein is required. Preliminary evidence from our laboratory further suggests that CD40 and RANK receptors can induce processing as well.

ACTIVATION VIA MODULATION OF TRANSACTIVATING FUNCTIONS

Beyond the IKK-mediated liberation of NF-κB from its inhibitors, it is increasingly appreciated that the activity of NF-κB is importantly controlled in additional ways. Although at least some liberation from inhibitors must occur, the level of transcriptional stimulation of a given target gene can be significantly modulated via mechanisms that affect transactivation functions, presumably via modifications of the NF-κB/Rel proteins themselves and/or of their accessory proteins. Thus, the elimination of an IKK-related kinase (TBK1/NAK/TK2) that was initially reported to function upstream of the

IKK complex[77] seems to have no role in TNF- or IL-1-induced translocation and DNA binding of NF-κB, at least not in the cell types analyzed. Instead, TBK1/TK2's absence significantly impaired transactivation functions of NF-κB in these cells.[78] Intriguingly, the lack of NF-κB-mediated transactivation in TBK1 knockouts was gene specific, indicating that modulation of NF-κB activity is complex and promoter context dependent. Relatively little is known about how TBK1 might carry out such functions. Prior reports suggested that TBK1 activates NF-κB via the IKKs as part of a trimeric complex with the adaptor proteins TANK and TRAF2, but that this complex is not involved in activation in response to TNF, IL-1 or CD40L stimulation.[79] Our recent data indicate that TBK1 (and the related kinase IKKε) can synergistically interact with TANK to form a complex with IKKs via NEMO, potentially bringing this kinase in proximity to the NF-κB complex.[80] Clearly, the precise mode of action, biological function and regulation of TBK1 remains to be established.

Mice deficient in the kinase GSK3β also show defects in NF-κB-mediated transactivations, but to date no possible mechanisms for this have been reported.[81] In many instances it will be important to establish whether the various signals, kinases or adaptors presumed to be involved in NF-κB activation do so via direct or by indirect mechanisms. If direct, it will be important to determine whether these signals and mediators function to stimulate the transactivation potential or if, instead, they function to degrade small IκBs or to process/degrade NF-κB1/2 precursors.

Phosphorylation of the RelA protein in particular has been studied in more detail and appears to be important for its transactivation potential.[5] p65 (RelA) is phosphorylated on serine 276 by protein kinase A (PKA). The catalytic PKA subunit associates with p65/IκB complexes and phosphorylates p65 only after IκB is degraded, although some constitutive phosphorylation may occur as well. Another kinase reported to activate p65 in a similar fashion is casein kinase II (CKII), which can phosphorylate serine 529 following TNF-induced degradation of IκB.

While the relative importance of the different kinases that phosphorylate p65 is unkown, it appears that phosphorylation of p65 enhances κB DNA binding and facilitates its interaction with the coactivator CBP/p300. Both coactivators such as CBP/p300 and corepressors such as the histone deacetylases (HDAC) are thought to function by linking sequence-specific transcription factors including NF-κB to basal transcription factors and/or altering chromatin sites to regulate access to promoter/enhancers of target genes. Based on current knowledge it is not clear whether PKA- and CKII-mediated phosphorylations are subject to independent signal-induced regulation or if they automatically occur once IκBs are degraded. Even if automatic, however, some specificity may exist if these kinases are associated only with subsets of NF-κB complexes that are differentially targeted by various signals.

Another kinase implicated in enhancing the transactivation potential of NF-κB is AKT/PKB, a kinase within and downstream of the PI3Kinase pathway, which is activated by many cytokines and other signals, including Ras and the CD28 coreceptor on T cells.[82,83] CD28-activated AKT may enhance the transactivation of the NF-κB complexes liberated from their inhibitors downstream of TCR stimulation. Although AKT has been suggested to activate IKK-mediated phosphorylation and degradation of IκB-α directly, this is controversial and most evidence suggests instead a role in transactivation functions.[82] AKT has been shown to enhance p65 (RelA)-mediated transactivation activity by causing phosphorylation of the C-terminus of RelA (p65), apparently dependent on the activity of IKKα[84] and the mitogen-activated kinase p38, which is induced by AKT.[82] AKT has also been reported to interact and synergize with PKCθ[83] and to synergize with coactivators CBP/p300 in the activation of p65.[82] p38 has recently been implicated in the regulation of NF-κB by its phosphorylation and induced phosphoacetylation of histone H3 in response to inflammatory stimuli.[85] It was suggested that p38-dependent H3 phosphorylation marks a subset of selected cytokine and chemokine gene promoters for enhanced accessibility of NF-κB to otherwise cryptic κB binding sites.

p65 was reported to employ multiple coactivators for transactivation, including CBP/p300 and CBP associated factor (p/CAF). The histone acetyl transferase (HAT) activity of p/CAF, but not that of CBP, was found to be required.[86] HAT domains are present on many coactivator proteins; their usual function is to acetylate lysines in the amino terminal regions of core histones.[87] Only phosphorylated p65 was observed to associate with CBP/p300 in the nucleus, while unphosphorylated p65 associated with the histone deacetylase-1 (HDAC-1). Any unphosphorylated, and thus not properly activated, p65 that might find its way into the nucleus would have a repressive function on target genes instead of activating these genes. In addition, the predominantly nuclear p50 homodimers were also found to be associated with HDAC-1. In unstimulated cells, transcriptionally inactive p50 homodimers bound to HDAC-1 are proposed to repress NF-κB-dependent target genes. Upon signal-induced liberation and phosphorylation of p65-containing complexes, these complexes are then thought to associate with CBP/p300 in the nucleus and displace p50 homodimer/HDAC-1 complexes due to higher affinity for natural κB sites, thus activating transcription. This mechanism would allow for tight control of gene expression.[87]

The IκB protein Bcl-3 can help to transactivate target genes via association with p50 or p52 homodimers in the nucleus, and, consistent with such a function, Bcl-3 has been shown to interact with the histone acetylase Tip60.[20]

A further role of acetylation in NF-κB regulation has been reported.[88] p65 itself can be become acetylated following stimulation by TNFα. Acetylation appears to weaken binding to IκBα, which might be a way to prolong the presence of some p65-containing NF-κB complexes in the nucleus, even after newly induced synthesis of IκBα. Deacetylation by histone deacetylase-3 (HDAC-3) then may restore binding to IκBα, with deacetylation possibly functioning as a switch to terminate

NF-κB transactivation, although it is not known whether deacetylation is regulated. Another report describes an association of p65 with HDAC-1 and, indirectly, HDAC-2 in repression of NF-κB target genes.[89]

There is now an extensive body of literature which indicates that the interaction of NF-κB with a range of kinases and nuclear coactivators and corepressors regulates both signal-induced and basal-level transactivation of NF-κB target genes, in addition to the regulation asserted by the IκB cytoplasmic family of inhibitors. A number of important questions need to be answered regarding modulation of transactivation. What is the function of each specific phosphorylation/modification? Which of these steps is regulated, and if so, how? Finally, are the phosphorylations/modifications generally relevant for transactivation or only in the context of specific promoters? Answers to these questions are critical to determine possible targets for specific therapeutic interventions.

BIOLOGICAL FUNCTIONS AND TARGETS, DEDUCED PRIMARILY FROM KNOCKOUT STUDIES

Mice deficient in various members of the NF-κB family of proteins or their regulators were generated to define their unique and critical functions in vivo. Death in utero due to massive liver apoptosis has emerged as one of the earliest developmental and clearest phenotypes associated with NF-κB impairments. This particular phenotype is revealed in knockout mice lacking RelA, IKKβ or NEMO.[90] These proteins therefore appear to define a pathway. Interestingly, if RelA or IKKβ knockout mice also lack TNF receptor I, mice survive to birth, although they develop other immune-related defects later. Therefore, IKKβ- and NEMO-dependent activation of RelA/NF-κB in hepatocytes protects these cells from TNF-induced apoptosis during development. The fact that RelA, IKKβ and NEMO are required for a critical function downstream of an inflammatory signal is consistent with the rapid and strong activation of RelA complexes via the canonical pathway of NF-κB activation. Surprisingly, TBK1 (T2K) knockouts present with the same defect, they die in utero due to massive apoptosis in the liver.[78] As discussed above, this IKK-related kinase has been implicated in modulating the transactivation functions of liberated NF-κB complexes, but how it does so, and whether this also occurs in response to TNF in hepatocytes is not presently known.

Protection from apoptosis appears to be an oft-employed function of NF-κB complexes in vivo. B and T cells require NF-κB for optimal progression at various transition points in their development, even if this requirement is not always absolute. In addition, maintenance and survival of mature B cells is linked to NF-κB activity. Some defects in survival (as well as various other defects) may only emerge if more than one NF-κB factor is missing, indicative of redundant functions encoded by these factors. Thus, adoptively transferred fetal liver cells lacking RelA and NF-κB1 or RelA and c-Rel (or lacking IKKβ) fail to generate any lymphocytes in lethally irradiated hosts, due to early apoptosis. However, this defect is not cell-autonomous, but appears to be mediated by extrinsic factors, since mutant T and B cells can develop in the presence of wild-type hematopoietic cells.[91,92] Although T and B cells do develop in these transfers, they are not fully functional, and in the case of B cells, they fail to fully mature. IKKβ-deficient mice in addition have been demonstrated to generate T and B cells in the absence of TNF receptor I, though again ultimately impaired ones.[5] That the absence of TNF receptor I mitigates the problems indicates a role for TNF signaling in the early lymphopoietic defect, even if it is not cell-autonomous. Homeostatic mechanisms during hematopoiesis may become sufficiently disregulated in these mutant mice to result in granulocytosis, and likely as a result excess production of TNF.

Further evidence for antiapoptotic functions of NF-κB during lymphocytic development has emerged. Pre-T cells appear to be protected from apoptosis, based on analysis of mice in which NF-κB activity was specifically impaired in T cells by a transgene expressing a mutant form of IκBα that can no longer be degraded in response to signals.[93] Recent work from our laboratory has revealed that transitional B cells appear to be protected from apoptosis by NF-κB complexes. B cells missing NF-κB1 and NF-κB2 do not progress past the earliest transitional stage of development in spleen. Early transitional B cells in spleen represent recent immigrants after having exited the bone marrow. These cells do not yet respond properly to antigenic stimulation and have to undergo both positive and negative selection steps in the spleen before they become mature, naive B cells. As shown in our laboratory, BAFF-induced processing of NF-κB2 p100 is an important step for progression of these transitional B cells, because it appears to extend their lifetime, thus allowing for their proper development. Processing relieves p100-mediated general inhibition of NF-κB complexes, and it releases, in particular, RelB/p52 into the nucleus (see above). B cells lacking c-Rel and RelA are blocked during transitional stages in spleen as well, and one of the important targets may include the antiapoptotic Bcl-2 gene product.[92] NF-κB can also be critical for developmental progression and survival of other cells. NF-κB1/2-deficient mice fail to generate osteoclasts, since lack of these factors appears to block an important RANK-mediated signal in early osteoclast precursor cells.[94,95]

The ability of NF-κB complexes to help cells survive better is the likely reason why NF-κB activity is frequently constitutively high in tumor cells. This inappropriate activation has been shown to contribute to the survival and presumably generation of diffuse large-cell lymphomas, for example.[6,96] Exactly how NF-κB becomes activated in various tumors is not usually known, but in some cases signaling molecules capable of contributing to NF-κB activation appear to be altered. For example, upregulation of casein kinase II may contribute to persistent NF-κB activation and thus to tumorigenesis of breast epithelial cells.[41] Crohn's disease, a form of inflammatory bowel disease associated with persistent NF-κB activation, can be caused by mutations in Nod2 (see above) and is associated with increased risk of colorectal cancers.[6,61] In some Hodgkin's lymphomas, the IκB inhibitor itself has been mutated in such a way that it no longer serves as an effective inhibitor.[97] NF-κB proteins have been shown to be mutated or altered in their expression in various tumors.[6,98] Recurrent amplifications of c-Rel have been noted in B cell lymphomas, translocations of Bcl-3 are found in B cell lymphocytic leukemias (leading to inappropriate or high levels of expression) and chromosomal rearrangements resulting in truncations of p100 have been associated with chronic lymphocytic leukemias, multiple myelomas and T and B cell lymphomas. The truncations of p100 relieve p100 inhibition and increase levels of p52 as well as adding extra protein sequence to the end of p52. However, in none of these cases is it fully understood exactly what are the critical tumorigenic targets of these changes.

Even in much more defined systems the critical targets of NF-κB remain unclear. Mouse embryo fibroblasts lacking RelA, IKKβ or NEMO are particularly sensitive to TNF-induced apoptosis and thus these cells have been used as a model to find targets of RelA complexes that may rescue them, but even in this situation multiple targets may synergize to protect cells.[99,100] Based on studies in various cell types, a number of NF-κB target genes have been identified that encode proteins that may function to directly or indirectly inhibit apoptosis. This list includes the Bcl-2 family members Bcl-xL and A1, possibly also Bcl-2 itself, anti-apoptotic c-IAP proteins, TRAF proteins, GADD45b (which may suppress Jun kinase activity and thus apoptotic functions associated with the actions of this kinase) and FLICE, an inhibitor of, for example, FAS-induced apoptotic mechanisms.[4,90,100]

NF-κB proteins are critical for the generation and maintenance of secondary lymphoid organs. Mice deficient in NF-κB2, RelB and RelA (on TNF receptor I-deficient background, see above), and to a lesser degree Bcl-3 present with overlapping sets of phenotypes, which include impaired T/B cell separations, impaired follicular dendritic cell networks and marginal zone abnormalities in spleen, and partial or complete lack of Peyer's patches and lymph nodes.[7,92] Where analyzed, these mutant mice are also unable to form proper germinal centers in response to antigenic stimulation and their humoral immunity is impaired. RelB-deficient mice and NF-κB1/2 double knockouts also present with fairly severe defects in thymic architecture, especially in the medulla. While some of the defects are due in part to hematopoietic cell deficiencies, most of the lymphoid organ defects derive from defects in stromal, radioresistant cells. Defects similar to those observed in NF-κB- and RelB-deficient mice in particular have also been noted in mice blocked in signaling via lymphotoxin (LT) β receptors.[5,76] LTβ receptors are present on stromal cells and are known to signal via activation of NF-κB. Interestingly, preliminary evidence from our laboratory has recently shown that these receptors can activate NF-κB via the canonical pathway, as well as via processing of NF-κB2 p100 to p52. This may explain why NF-κB2-, RelB- and RelA-deficient mice have some overlapping phenotypes. In addition to LTβ receptors, signals transmitted via TNF receptors on stromal cells also appear to contribute to the structure of lymphoid organs, based on various knockout studies. The ligands of these receptors, LTα/β and TNF heterotrimers are expressed on hematopoietic cells, in particular on B cells. It is thus likely that continuous stimulation between B cells and stromal cells helps set up lymphoid organization. Some of the probable NF-κB targets in stromal cells include persistently synthesized chemokines like BLC/CXCL13, SLC/CCL21 and ELC/CCL19, which are required for proper migration and separation of lymphoid cells.

Mice deficient in one or more NF-κB proteins have been subjected to various pathogenic challenges (including LCMV, influenza, *T. gondii*, *L. major*, *S. pneumoniae* and *L. monocytogenes*) and often these mice have turned out to show enhanced susceptibility to one or more of these pathogens.[7] However, the exact causes for the increased susceptibility cannot be fully determined, since defects in multiple interacting cell types are presumably responsible. NF-κB activity is important during innate and adaptive immune responses, and in linking these responses. Cell types in which NF-κB signaling has been shown to have critical functions during immune responses include early sentinel cells such as fibroblasts and endothelial cells, disease-fighting macrophages, antigen-presenting dendritic cells and T and B cells. When studied ex vivo, such cells when isolated from mice lacking components of the NF-κB system are often impaired in expression of various cytokines, chemokines and coactivators, and in the case of mature antigen-activated lymphoid cells, also show defects in cell proliferation and/or survival.[7] For example, Bcl-3-deficient mice succumb to *T. gondii* infection at least in part due to failure to generate IFNγ-producing antigen-specific T cells.[101] Impaired production of IFNγ has also been observed in RelB knockout mice after exposure to *T. gondii*. Macrophages from mice deficient in NF-κB2 or c-Rel are defective for IL-12 production, and c-Rel has been demonstrated to directly participate in the regulation of this gene. Interestingly, while RelB may be required for production of some continuously synthesized chemokines in the spleen, RelB has been proposed to function as a feedback repressor of chemokines and cytokines produced by fibroblasts during their initial encounter with pathogens. In the absence of RelB these mediators are produced for prolonged periods, initiating multi-focal inflammatory cell infiltrations at various sites, including skin, which ultimately kill the animal. Inflammation and infiltrations by granulocytes of, in particular, skin, resembling dermatitis and psoriasis, have also been seen in mice lacking the IκBα inhibitor, which leads to higher and persistent levels of NF-κB activity. In such mutant mice B cells show enhanced proliferative capacity and may survive better, which in turn may allow autoreactive B cells to escape elimination.[102] c-Rel deficient lymphocytes are defective in mitogenesis.[92] In the case of mutant T cells this is due in part to lower production of IL-2, and in the case of B cells probably due to lower levels of the A1 survival gene as well as possible direct effects on the progression through the G1 phase

of the cell cycle. Cyclin D1 has been shown to be a direct and critical target of NF-κB activated by RANK receptors in expanding mammary epithelial cells during pregnancy.[6,33]

Mice lacking components of the NF-κB system can be seriously impaired in numerous immune responses due to defects in expression of cytokines, chemokines, coactivators and antipathogenic agents, defects in lymphoid architecture associated with lack of germinal center formation and impaired switch reactions, as well as defects in survival and proliferation of T and B cells. This is so despite the fact that the various NF-κB factors often encode redundant activities. It is possible that unique activities encoded by the various factors are responsible for the overall defects, and/or the quantitative reduction in overall NF-κB activity, even in cases where just one factor is missing. The quantity as well as quality and persistence of NF-κB activation are likely to be important for proper responses.

POSSIBLE THERAPEUTIC STRATEGIES

In order to stop inflammatory reactions or to stop cancer growth that is dependent on NF-κB activity, one would ideally want to inhibit activation of NF-κB only in the relevant cells and only downstream of a particular activation signal. A general blockade of this transcription factor is likely to have severe unwanted side-effects, at least in the long run. It remains doubtful that cell- and signal-specific inhibition can be easily achieved by interference with the well-known signaling proteins, given that so many of them are often part of several and large signaling complexes. Consequently, inhibiting any one of these factors might interfere with several different signaling pathways, not only NF-κB. The best chance for finding a specific target among signaling proteins might lie in the least well-understood part of signaling to NF-κB, namely the proteins that are presumed to interact with NEMO to help activate IKKs downstream of specific signaling paths. Such proteins might be specific to a given signaling pathway and may not have signaling functions other than activation of the IKKs. The overall best strategy may well lie in targeting two or more proteins in a given signaling pathway, but inhibiting them only partially. Specificity may result from combining two or more inhibitors. And in any case, inhibiting NF-κB only partly may be sufficient in many situations, since both quantitative and kinetic aspects of activation of this factor are important in terms of what genes are ultimately turned on. Finally, the novel mode of activation via IKKα-dependent processing of p100 may represent an important point of therapeutic attack, especially in autoimmune diseases, given the importance of processing during the formation of mature B cells and in generating inflammatory centers together with stromal cells.

ACKNOWLEDGMENTS

The authors thank members of the Siebenlist laboratory for helpful discussions and Dr Jürgen Müller for making available unpublished results for this review. Mary Rust is thanked for expert editorial assistance and Dr Anthony Fauci for continued support.

REFERENCES

1. Ghosh S, May MJ, Kopp EB. NF-kappa B and Rel proteins: evolutionarily conserved mediators of immune responses. *Annu Rev Immunol* 1998; **16**: 225–60.
2. Karin M, Ben-Neriah Y. Phosphorylation meets ubiquitination: the control of NF-[kappa]B activity. *Annu Rev Immunol* 2000, **18**. 621–63.
3. Silverman N, Maniatis T. NF-kappaB signaling pathways in mammalian and insect innate immunity. *Genes Dev* 2001; **15**: 2321–42.
4. Baldwin AS. Control of oncogenesis and cancer therapy resistance by the transcription factor NF-kappaB. *J Clin Invest* 2001; **107**: 241–6.
5. Ghosh S, Karin M. Missing pieces in the NF-kappaB puzzle. *Cell* 2002; **109**(Suppl): S81–96.
6. Karin M, Cao Y, Greten FR, Li ZW. NF-kappaB in cancer: from innocent bystander to major culprit. *Nat Rev Cancer* 2002; **2**: 301–10.
7. Caamano J, Hunter CA. NF-kappaB family of transcription factors: central regulators of innate and adaptive immune functions. *Clin Microbiol Rev* 2002; **15**: 414–29.
8. Pahl HL. Activators and target genes of Rel/NF-kappaB transcription factors. *Oncogene* 1999; **18**: 6853–66.
9. Baldwin AS Jr. The NF-kappa B and I kappa B proteins: new discoveries and insights. *Annu Rev Immunol* 1996; **14**: 649–83.
10. Siebenlist U, Franzoso G, Brown K. Structure, regulation and function of NF-kappa B. *Annu Rev Cell Biol* 1994; **10**: 405–55.
11. Khush RS, Leulier F, Lemaitre B. Drosophila immunity: two paths to NF-kappaB. *Trends Immunol* 2001; **22**: 260–4.
12. Hoffmann JA, Reichhart JM. Drosophila innate immunity: an evolutionary perspective. *Nat Immun* 2002; **3**: 121–6.
13. Belvin MP, Anderson KV. A conserved signaling pathway: the Drosophila toll-dorsal pathway. *Annu Rev Cell Dev Biol* 1996; **12**: 393–416.
14. Cramer P, Müller CW. A firm hand on NFkappaB: structures of the IkappaBalpha-NFkappaB complex. *Structure Fold Des* 1999; **7**: R1–6.
15. Michel F, Soler-Lopez M, Petosa C et al. Crystal structure of the ankyrin repeat domain of Bcl-3: a unique member of the IkappaB protein family. *EMBO J* 2001; **20**: 6180–90.
16. Suyang H, Phillips R, Douglas I, Ghosh S. Role of unphosphorylated, newly synthesized I kappa B beta in persistent activation of NF-kappa B. *Mol Cell Biol* 1996; **16**: 5444–9.
17. Tran K, Merika M, Thanos D. Distinct functional properties of IkappaB alpha and IkappaB beta. *Mol Cell Biol* 1997; **17**: 5386–99.
18. Cheng JD, Ryseck RP, Attar RM et al. Functional redundancy of the nuclear factor kappa B inhibitors I kappa B alpha and I kappa B beta. *J Exp Med* 1998; **188**: 1055–62
19. Kanno T, Franzoso U, Siebenlist U. Human T-cell leukemia virus type I Tax-protein-mediated activation of NF-kappa B from p100 (NF-kappa B2)-inhibited cytoplasmic reservoirs. *Proc Natl Acad Sci USA* 1994; **91**: 12634–8.
20. Dechend R, Hirano F, Lehmann K et al. The Bcl-3 oncoprotein acts as a bridging factor between NF-kappaB/Rel and nuclear co-regulators. *Oncogene* 1999; **18**: 3316–23.

21. Heissmeyer V, Krappmann D, Wulczyn FG, Scheidereit C. NF-kappaB p105 is a target of IkappaB kinases and controls signal induction of Bcl-3-p50 complexes. *EMBO J* 1999; **18**: 4766–78.

22. Yamazaki S, Muta T, Takeshige K. A novel IkappaB protein, IkappaB-zeta, induced by proinflammatory stimuli, negatively regulates nuclear factor-kappaB in the nuclei. *J Biol Chem* 2001; **276**: 27657–62.

23. Kitamura H, Kanehira K, Okita K et al. MAIL, a novel nuclear I kappa B protein that potentiates LPS-induced IL-6 production. *FEBS Lett* 2000; **485**: 53–6.

24. Ben-Neriah Y. Regulatory functions of ubiquitination in the immune system. *Nat Immunol* 2002; **3**: 20–6.

25. Fenwick C, Na SY, Voll RE et al. A subclass of Ras proteins that regulate the degradation of IkappaB. *Science* 2000; **287**: 869–73.

26. Heusch M, Lin L, Geleziunas R, Greene WC. The generation of nfkb2 p52: mechanism and efficiency. *Oncogene* 1999; **18**: 6201–8.

27. Heissmeyer V, Krappmann D, Hatada EN, Scheidereit C. Shared pathways of IkappaB kinase-induced SCF(betaTrCP)-mediated ubiquitination and degradation for the NF-kappaB precursor p105 and IkappaBalpha. *Mol Cell Biol* 2001; **21**: 1024–35.

28. Xiao G, Harhaj EW, Sun SC. NF-kappaB-inducing kinase regulates the processing of NF-kappaB2 p100. *Mol Cell* 2001; **7**: 401–9.

29. Fong A, Sun SC. Genetic evidence for the essential role of beta-transducin repeat-containing protein in the inducible processing of NF-kappa B2/p100. *J Biol Chem* 2002; **277**: 22111–14.

30. Peters RT, Maniatis T. A new family of IKK-related kinases may function as I kappa B kinase kinases. *Biochim Biophys Acta* 2001; **2**: M57–62.

31. Karin M, Delhase M. The I kappa B kinase (IKK) and NF-kappa B: key elements of proinflammatory signalling. *Semin Immunol* 2000; **12**: 85–98.

32. Senftleben U, Karin M. The IKK/NF-kappaB pathway. *Crit Care Med* 2002; **30**: S18–26.

33. Cao Y, Bonizzi G, Seagroves TN et al. IKKalpha provides an essential link between RANK signaling and cyclin D1 expression during mammary gland development. *Cell* 2001; **107**: 763–75.

34. Senftleben U, Cao Y, Xiao G et al. Activation by IKKalpha of a second, evolutionary conserved, NF-kappa B signaling pathway. *Science* 2001; **293**: 1495–9.

35. Belich MP, Salmeron A, Johnston LH, Ley SC. Protein TPL-2 kinase regulates the proteolysis of the NF-kappaB-inhibitory protein NF-kappaB1 p105. *Nature* 1999; **397**: 363–8.

36. Lin X, Cunningham ET Jr, Mu Y et al. The proto-oncogene Cot kinase participates in CD3/CD28 induction of NF-kappaB acting through the NF-kappaB-inducing kinase and I kappaB kinases. *Immunity* 1999; **10**: 271–80.

37. Kane LP, Mollenauer MN, Xu Z et al. Akt-dependent phosphorylation specifically regulates cot induction of NF-kappaB-dependent transcription. *Mol Cell Biol* 2002; **22**: 5962–74.

38. Digicaylioglu M, Lipton SA. Erythropoietin-mediated neuroprotection involves cross-talk between Jak2 and NF-kappaB signalling cascades. *Nature* 2001; **412**: 641–7.

39. Shumway SD, Berchtold CM, Gould MN, Miyamoto S. Evidence for unique calmodulin-dependent nuclear factor-kappaB regulation in WEHI-231 B cells. *Mol Pharmacol* 2002; **61**: 177–85.

40. Pianetti S, Arsura M, Romieu-Mourez R et al. Her-2/neu overexpression induces NF-kappaB via a PI3-kinase/Akt pathway involving calpain-mediated degradation of IkappaB-alpha that can be inhibited by the tumor suppressor PTEN. *Oncogene* 2001; **20**: 1287–99.

41. Romieu-Mourez R, Landesman-Bollag E, Seldin DC et al. Roles of IKK kinases and protein kinase CK2 in activation of nuclear factor-kappaB in breast cancer. *Cancer Res* 2001; **61**: 3810–18.

42. McElhinny JA, Trushin SA, Bren GD et al. Casein kinase II phosphorylates I kappa B alpha at S-283, S-289, S-293, and T-291 and is required for its degradation. *Mol Cell Biol* 1996; **16**: 899–906.

43. Shumway SD, Maki M, Miyamoto S. The PEST domain of IkappaBalpha is necessary and sufficient for in vitro degradation by mu-calpain. *J Biol Chem* 1999; **274**: 30874–81.

44. Courtois G, Israel A. NF-kappa B defects in humans: the NEMO/incontinentia pigmenti connection. *Sci STKE* 2000; **2000**: E1.

45. Courtois G, Smahi A, Israel A. NEMO/IKK gamma: linking NF-kappa B to human disease Trends. *Mol Med* 2001; **7**: 427–30.

46. Doffinger R, Smahi A, Bessia C et al. X-linked anhidrotic ectodermal dysplasia with immunodeficiency is caused by impaired NF-kappaB signaling. *Nat Genet* 2001; **27**: 277–85.

47. Jain A, Ma CA, Liu S et al. Specific missense mutations in NEMO result in hyper-IgM syndrome with hypohydrotic ectodermal dysplasia. *Nat Immunol* 2001; **2**: 223–8.

48. Harhaj EW, Sun SC. IKKgamma serves as a docking subunit of the IkappaB kinase (IKK) and mediates interaction of IKK with the human T-cell leukemia virus Tax protein. *J Biol Chem* 1999; **274**: 22911–14.

49. Leonardi A, Chariot A, Claudio E et al. CIKS, a connection to I kappa B kinase and stress-activated protein kinase. *Proc Natl Acad Sci USA* 2000; **97**: 10494–9.

50. Qian Y, Zhao Z, Jiang Z, Li X. Role of NFkappa B activator Act1 in CD40-mediated signaling in epithelial cells. *Proc Natl Acad Sci USA* 2002; **99**: 9386–91.

51. Chen G, Goeddel DV. TNF-R1 signaling: a beautiful pathway. *Science* 2002; **296**: 1634–5.

52. Akira S, Takeda K, Kaisho T. Toll-like receptors: critical proteins linking innate and acquired immunity. *Nat Immunol* 2001; **2**: 675–80.

53. O'Neill LA. The interleukin-1 receptor/Toll-like receptor superfamily: signal transduction during inflammation and host defense. *Sci STKE* 2000; **2000**: RE1.

54. Zhang SQ, Kovalenko A, Cantarella G, Wallach D. Recruitment of the IKK signalosome to the p55 TNK receptor: RIP and A20 bind to NEMO (IKKgamma) upon receptor stimulation. *Immunity* 2000; **12**: 301–11.

55. Devin A, Cook A, Lin Y et al. The distinct roles of TRAF2 and RIP in IKK activation by TNF-R1: TRAF2 recruits IKK to TNF-R1 while RIP mediates IKK activation. *Immunity* 2000; **12**: 419–29.

56. Yang J, Lin Y, Guo Z et al. The essential role of MEKK3 in TNF-induced NF-kappaB activation. *Nat Immunol* 2001; **2**: 620–4.

57. Suzuki N, Suzuki S, Duncan GS et al. Severe impairment of interleukin-1 and Toll-like receptor signalling in mice lacking IRAK-4. *Nature* 2002; **416**: 750–6.

58. Qian Y, Commane M, Ninomiya-Tsuji J et al. IRAK-mediated translocation of TRAF6 and TAB2 in the interleukin-1-induced activation of NFkappa B. *J Biol Chem* 2001; **276**: 41661–7.

59. Wang C, Deng L, Hong M et al. TAK1 is a ubiquitin-dependent kinase of MKK and IKK. *Nature* 2001; **412**: 346–51.

60. Mizukami J, Takaesu G, Akatsuka H et al. Receptor activator of NF-kappaB ligand (RANKL) activates TAK1 mitogen-activated protein kinase kinase kinase through a signaling complex containing RANK, TAB2, and TRAF6. *Mol Cell Biol* 2002; **22**: 992–1000.

61. Inohara N, Ogura Y, Nunez G. Nods: a family of cytosolic proteins that regulate the host response to pathogens. *Curr Opin Microbiol* 2002; **5**: 76–80.

62. D'Acquisto F, Ghosh S. PACT and PKR: turning on NF-kappa B in the absence of virus. *Sci STKE* 2001; **2001**: RE1.

63. Bertin J, Guo Y, Wang L et al. CARD9 is a novel caspase recruitment domain-containing protein that interacts with BCL10/CLAP and activates NF-kappa B. *J Biol Chem* 2000; **275**: 41082–6.

64. Bertin J, Wang Y, Guo Y et al. CARD11 and CARD14 are novel caspase recruitment domain (CARD)/membrane-associated guanylate kinase (MAGUK) family members that interact with BCL10 and activate NF-kappa B. *J Biol Chem* 2001; **276**: 11877–82.

65. McAllister-Lucas LM, Inohara N, Lucas PC et al. Bimp1, a MAGUK family member linking protein kinase C activation to Bcl10-mediated NF-kappaB induction. *J Biol Chem* 2001; **276**: 30589–97.

66. Wang L, Guo Y, Huang WJ et al. Card10 is a novel caspase recruitment domain/membrane-associated guanylate kinase family member that interacts with BCL10 and activates NF-kappa B. *J Biol Chem* 2001; **276**: 21405–9.

67. Isakov N, Altman A. Protein kinase C(theta) in T cell activation. *Annu Rev Immunol* 2002; **20**: 761–94.

68. Saijo K, Mecklenbrauker I, Santana A et al. Protein kinase C beta controls nuclear factor kappaB activation in B cells through selective regulation of the IkappaB kinase alpha. *J Exp Med* 2002; **195**: 1647–52.

69. Mackay F, Browning JL. BAFF: a fundamental survival factor for B cells. *Nat Rev Immunol* 2002; **2**: 465–75.

70. Rolink AG, Tschopp J, Schneider P, Melchers F. BAFF is a survival and maturation factor for mouse B cells. *Eur J Immunol* 2002; **32**: 2004–10.

71. Mackay F, Mackay CR. The role of BAFF in B-cell maturation, T-cell activation and autoimmunity. *Trends Immunol* 2002; **23**: 113–15.

72. Do RK, Chen-Kiang S. Mechanism of BLyS action in B cell immunity. *Cytokine Growth Factor Rev* 2002; **13**: 19–25.

73. Fagarasan S, Shinkura R, Kamata T et al. Alymphoplasia (aly)-type nuclear factor kappaB-inducing kinase (NIK) causes defects in secondary lymphoid tissue chemokine receptor signaling and homing of peritoneal cells to the gut-associated lymphatic tissue system. *J Exp Med* 2000; **191**: 1477–86.

74. Yin L, Wu L, Wesche H et al. Defective lympho-toxin-beta receptor-induced NF-kappaB transcriptional activity in NIK-deficient mice. *Science* 2001; **291**: 2162–5.

75. Franzoso G, Carlson L, Poljak L et al. Mice deficient in nuclear factor (NF)-kappa B/p52 present with defects in humoral responses, germinal center reactions, and splenic microarchitecture. *J Exp Med* 1998; **187**: 147–59.

76. Matsumoto M. Role of TNF ligand and receptor family in the lymphoid organogenesis defined by gene targeting. *J Med Invest* 1999; **46**: 141–50.

77. Tojima Y, Fujimoto A, Delhase M et al. NAK is an IkappaB kinase-activating kinase. *Nature* 2000; **404**: 778–82.

78. Bonnard M, Mirtsos C, Suzuki S et al. Deficiency of T2K leads to apoptotic liver degeneration and impaired NF-kappaB-dependent gene transcription. *Embo J* 2000; **19**: 4976–85.

79. Pomerantz JL, Baltimore D. NF-kappaB activation by a signaling complex containing TRAF2, TANK and TBK1, a novel IKK-related kinase. *EMBO J* 1999; **18**: 6694–704.

80. Chariot A, Leonardi A, Muller J et al. Association of the adaptor TANK with the I-kappaB-kinase (IKK) regulator NEMO connects IKK complexes with IKKepsilon and TBK1 kinases. *J Biol Chem* 2002; **19**: 19.

81. Hoeflich KP, Luo J, Rubie EA et al. Requirement for glycogen synthase kinase-3beta in cell survival and NF-kappaB activation. *Nature* 2000; **406**: 86–90.

82. Madrid LV, Mayo MW, Reuther JY, Baldwin AS Jr. Akt stimulates the transactivation potential of the RelA/p65 Subunit of NF-kappa B through utilization of the Ikappa B kinase and activation of the mitogen-activated protein kinase p38. *J Biol Chem* 2001; **276**: 18934–40.

83. Bauer B, Krumbock N, Fresser F et al. Complex formation and cooperation of protein kinase C theta and Akt1/protein kinase B alpha in the NF-kappa B transactivation cascade in Jurkat T cells. *J Biol Chem* 2001; **276**: 31627–34.

84. Sizemore N, Lerner N, Dombrowski N et al. Distinct roles of the Ikappa B kinase alpha and beta subunits in liberating nuclear factor kappa B (NF-kappa B) from Ikappa B and in phosphorylating the p65 subunit of NF-kappa B. *J Biol Chem* 2002; **277**: 3863–9.

85. Saccani S, Pantano S, Natoli G. p38-Dependent marking of inflammatory genes for increased NF-kappa B recruitment. *Nat Immunol* 2002; **3**: 69–75.

86. Sheppard KA, Rose DW, Haque ZK et al. Transcriptional activation by NF-kappaB requires multiple coactivators. *Mol Cell Biol* 1999; **19**: 6367–78.

87. Zhong H, May MJ, Jimi E, Ghosh S. The phosphorylation status of nuclear NF-kappa B determines its association with CBP/p300 or HDAC-1. *Mol Cell* 2002; **9**: 625–36.

88. Chen L, Fischle W, Verdin E, Greene WC. Duration of nuclear NF-kappaB action regulated by reversible acetylation. *Science* 2001; **293**: 1653–7.

89. Ashburner BP, Westerheide SD, Baldwin AS Jr. The p65 (RelA) subunit of NF-kappaB interacts with the histone deacetylase (HDAC) corepressors HDAC1 and HDAC2 to negatively regulate gene expression. *Mol Cell Biol* 2001; **21**: 7065–77.

90. Karin M, Lin A. NF-kappaB at the crossroads of life and death. *Nat Immunol* 2002; **3**: 221–7.

91. Grossmann M, Nakamura Y, Grumont R, Gerondakis S. New insights into the roles of ReL/NF-kappa B transcription factors in immune function, hemopoiesis and human disease. *Int J Biochem Cell Biol.* 1999; **31**: 1209–19.

92. Gugasyan R, Grumont R, Grossmann M et al. Rel/NF-kappaB transcription factors: key mediators of B-cell activation. *Immunol Rev* 2000; **176**: 134–40.

93. Voll RE, Jimi E, Phillips RJ et al. NF-kappa B activation by the pre-T cell receptor serves as a selective survival signal in T lymphocyte development. *Immunity* 2000; **13**: 677–89.

94. Franzoso G, Carlson L, Xing L et al. Requirement for NF-kappaB in osteoclast and B-cell development. *Genes Dev* 1997; **11**: 3482–96.

95. Xing L, Bushnell TP, Carlson L et al. NF-kappaB p50 and p52 expression is not required for RANK-expressing osteoclast progenitor formation but is essential for RANK- and cytokine-mediated osteoclastogenesis. *J Bone Miner Res* 2002; **17**: 1200–10.

96. Davis RE, Brown KD, Siebenlist U, Staudt LM. Constitutive nuclear factor kappaB activity is required for survival of activated B cell-like diffuse large B cell lymphoma cells. *J Exp Med* 2001; **194**: 1861–74.

97. Staudt LM. The molecular and cellular origins of Hodgkin's disease. *J Exp Med* 2000; **191**: 207–12.

98. Gilmore T, Gapuzan ME, Kalaitzidis D, Starczynowski D. Rel/NF-kappaB/IkappaB signal transduction in the generation and treatment of human cancer. *Cancer Lett* 2002; **181**: 1–9.

99. De Smaele E, Zazzeroni F, Papa S et al. Induction

of gadd45beta by NF-kappaB downregulates pro-apoptotic JNK signalling. *Nature* 2001; **414**: 308–13.

100. Orlowski RZ, Baldwin AS. NF-kappaB as a therapeutic target in cancer. *Trends Mol Med* 2002; **8**: 385–9.

101. Franzoso G, Carlson L, Scharton-Kersten T et al. Critical roles for the Bcl-3 oncoprotein in T cell-mediated immunity, splenic microarchitecture, and germinal center reactions. *Immunity* 1997; **6**: 479–90

102. Beg AA, Sha WC, Bronson RT, Baltimore D. Constitutive NF-kappa B activation, enhanced granulopoiesis, and neonatal lethality in I kappa B alpha-deficient mice. *Genes Dev* 1995; **9**: 2736–46.

23

Stats and Jaks

Martin Aringer, Wendy Watford and John J O'Shea

Introduction • Stats • Jaks • SOCS (CIS, JAB, SSI) molecules and their potential therapeutic role • Protein inhibitors of activated Stats • Conclusions • References

INTRODUCTION

Cytokines are essential for the regulation and coordination of the immune system. Cytokines bind specific receptors; it is these receptors that are responsible for transmitting the cytokine signal to the nucleus. Within the nucleus, transcription factors activated following cytokine binding induce or suppress the transcription of genes by binding to promoter and enhancer elements.

Many of the immunologically relevant cytokines, i.e. most of the interleukins and all interferons, bind to receptors that lack intrinsic signaling functions. Accordingly, these receptors recruit cytoplasmic kinases, namely the Janus kinases (Jaks), to transmit their signals. All these receptors also bind transcription factors of the 'signal transducer and activator of transcription' (Stat) family and employ them for their signal transduction.[1–3]

Most commonly, Jaks and Stats are shown to function together in so-called Jak–Stat pathways. Within this pathway, Jaks and Stats as well as cytokine receptors are mainly activated by the phosphorylation of specific tyrosine residues, and Jaks are thought to be responsible

for these modifications. However, there is now ample evidence that Stats may be phosphorylated by tyrosine kinases other than Jaks. Conversely, Jaks phosphorylate target proteins other than Stats. Therefore, while useful, the term Jak–Stat pathways is clearly an oversimplification. Taking this into account, our review will begin with a discussion of the Stat proteins and the current knowledge on Stats pertaining to possible therapeutic interventions. We will then address the Jaks and briefly discuss the inhibitors of Jak–Stat pathways, including the suppressor of cytokine signaling (SOCS) family of inhibitors and the PIAS molecules.

STATS

Signal transducers and activators of transcription (Stats) are transcription factors unique in that they themselves transport the signal from the cell surface receptors straight to the nucleus. Stats bind to a wide variety of cytokine and hormone receptors on tyrosine-phosphorylated binding sites.[4] Stats are then activated by tyrosine phosphorylation, dissociate from the receptor chains, dimerize and, sometimes after additional modifications, shuttle to the nucleus.

Here Stat dimers bind canonical sites and regulate gene transcription. Whereas the nuclear import of Stats is gained through the process of dimerization, detachment from DNA exposes a nuclear export signal that leads to the transport of Stats back to the cytoplasm.[5] This DNA detachment process is probably induced by nuclear tyrosine phosphatases that effect Stat dephosphorylation, and thus Stat inactivation.

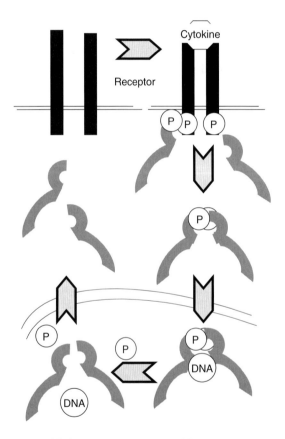

Figure 23.1 Functional cycle of Stat molecules. Upon ligand binding, specific tyrosine residues of cytokine receptor chains are phosphorylated. Stats bind these phosphorylated binding sites, whereupon they themselves undergo tyrosine phosphorylation. Following phosphorylation, they detach from the receptors and dimerize, exposing a nuclear translocation motif. In the nucleus, Stat dimers bind DNA and influence transcription. After undergoing dephosphorylation by nuclear phosphatases, they detach from DNA and display a nuclear export signal that leads to their transport back to the cytoplasm.

Stats contain SH2, DNA-binding, transcriptional activation and N-terminal protein interaction domains.[3] The SH2 domains are essential for binding receptors; domain-swapping experiments proved them to be specific for various receptor chains. In addition, in forming Stat dimers, these domains reciprocally bind their partner's phosphotyrosine just C-terminal of the SH2 domain. This phosphotyrosine–SH2 interaction is strong enough to function as the hinge in a nutcracker-shaped structure, which can then bind to DNA (in place of the nut), as crystal structure data have demonstrated[6,7] (Figure 23.1). The transcriptional activation domain is situated at the C-terminus and is essential for the full transcriptional activity of Stats.[3] Within this domain, there is a conserved serine-phosphorylation site in some Stats that appears to be important for their activity.[8] Again, as shown by resolving their crystal structure, the N-termini of Stat proteins form hook-shaped protein interaction domains.[9]

We know of seven human (and murine) Stats, namely Stat1, Stat2, Stat3, Stat4, Stat5a, Stat5b and Stat6.[2] Given that the human genome is now sequenced and that no homologous proteins have been detected, these probably constitute the complete Stat family. While most bind a variety of cytokine receptors, some of these are fairly specific (Table 23.1). For example, Stat4 binds the human interleukin-12 (IL-12) and interferon (IFN)-α receptors and plays an important role in Th1 differentiation. In contrast, Stat6 binds the receptors for IL-4 and IL-13 and is essential for the differentiation of Th2 cells.

In addition to having different receptor specificities, the Stats also bind differentially to specific DNA sequences. Stat2, which is required for IFN-α signaling, is part of a unique DNA-binding complex: Stat2 forms a heterotrimeric complex with Stat1 and another DNA-binding protein known as p48 (IRF9).[10] This Stat 1–Stat 2–IRF-9 complex, also known as IFN-stimulated gene factor 3 (ISGF3), binds to a DNA consensus sequence of AGTTTnCnTTTCC, called IFN-α stimulated response element (ISRE). This binding site significantly differs in its binding capabilities from the semipalindromic $TTCn_3GAA$ motifs to which other Stat complexes bind.

Table 23.1   Many of the most relevant cytokines associate with Stats and Jaks.

Cytokine	Stat1	Stat2	Stat3	Stat4	Stat5	Stat6	Tyk2	Jak1	Jak2	Jak3
IFN-α/β	+	+		+			+	+		
IFN-γ	+							+	+	
IL-2	+		+		+			+		+
IL-3					+				+	
IL-4			+		+	+		+		+
IL-5					+				+	
II-6			+							
IL-7			+		+			+		+
IL-9			+		+			+		+
IL-10	+		+				+	+		
IL-11			+				+	+	+	
IL-12				+			+		+	
IL-13						+		+	+	
IL-15			+		+			+		+
IL-19			+							
IL-20			+							
IL-21	+		+					+		+
IL-22	+		+		+		+			
IL-23										
EPO					+				+	
TPO					+				+	
GM-CSF					+				+	
PRL					+				+	
GH					+				+	

EPO, erythropoietin; GH, growth hormone; GM-CSF, granulocyte–macrophage colony-stimulating factor; IL, interleukin; PRL, prolactin; TPO, thrombopoietin.

In addition, the DNA-binding site of the Stat6 complex is characterized by broader spacing (TTCn$_4$GAA), whereas complexes containing Stat3 prefer narrower spacing (TTCn$_2$GAA).[11,12] However, these restrictions may not be absolute,[13] and other Stat DNA-binding sites do not obviously differ. Given the similar DNA-binding sites of some Stats, the specificity of various Stats for the transcription of different sets of genes (see below) is harder to explain.

Stat complex binding to DNA can be very complicated in many instances. Pairs of Stat dimers have been proposed to form tetramers via their N-termini, which bear interfaces suited for polar interactions on their hook-like structures.[9] Moreover, the cellular protein N-Myc interactor (Nmi) stabilizes the binding of Stats to CBP/p300 coactivator proteins and enhances transcription efficiency. A wide variety of other transcription factors bind to Stats.

In most instances, human and murine Stats are highly homologous. Therefore, the murine system is a valuable tool for determining the specificities of Stats as well as differences between them. Knockout mice in particular enable us to better understand the role of each Stat.

Stat1

Stat1-deficient mice were viable. They were born at normal frequencies, were fertile and showed no obvious physical defects. However, these mice were extremely susceptible to infections, to an extent that mice housed under normal conditions died within 48 h of weaning.[14] Moreover, even some mice housed under pathogen-free conditions succumbed to fatal infections,[15] and low dosages of *Listeria monocytogenes* or vesicular stomatitis virus killed Stat1$^{-/-}$ mice. This striking impairment in host defense was associated with an inability to respond to IFN-α/β or IFN-γ, which signal via Stat1. No other cytokines tested (among them IL-6, IL-10, epidermal growth factor (EGF), colony-stimulating factor-1 (CSF-1) and GH) were found to have impaired signaling. Presumably as a consequence of not correctly transducing IFN-γ signals, Stat1-deficient mice have also been shown to be defective in their tumor surveillance.[16] It is also interesting in this regard that a Stat1-deficient cell line failed to undergo tumor necrosis factor (TNF)-induced apoptosis, because the cells express low constitutive levels of caspases.[17] It is notable that heterozygous human Stat1 germline mutations were detected in patients with disseminated mycobacterial disease.[18] Interestingly, however, these patients showed no increase in susceptibility to viral infections.

Stat2

As for Stat1-deficient mice, normal numbers of Stat2-deficient mice were born. Under pathogen-free conditions, these Stat2$^{-/-}$ mice developed and bred normally, but in vitro tests suggested that they were highly susceptible to viral infections. As expected because of Stat2's role in the Stat1–Stat2–IRF-9 complex, they were defective in the signal transduction of IFN-α and other type I interferons.[19] Moreover, although their cells were able to respond to IFN-γ, Stat2$^{-/-}$ cells

also expressed less Stat1, which apparently is an IFN-α inducible gene. Interestingly, however, this was not true for peritoneal macrophages, which, in contrast to fibroblasts and T lymphocytes, had normal Stat1 levels and, when stimulated with IFN-α, upregulated MHC class I molecules normally.[19] Since such MHC class I upregulation did not take place in Stat1/Stat2 double-knockout macrophages, macrophage IFN-α signaling appears to use Stat1 dimers in a tissue-specific manner.

Stat3

Disruption of the Stat3 gene led to embryonic lethality between embryonic days 6.5 and 7.5.[20] Stat3 was essential for the maintenance of pluripotent embryonic stem cells, at least in part because of its importance for leukemia inhibitory factor (LIF) signaling.[21] Consequently, conditional knockout mice were made to overcome the embryonic lethality in Stat3 knockout mice. Mice with T cells lacking Stat3 grew normally and showed no defects in the development of lymphoid organs or in the amounts and distributions of T cells. However, when stimulated with IL-6, their T cells did not proliferate.[22] In fact, the anti-apoptotic potential of IL-6 was lost, and Stat3$^{-/-}$ T cells could not be rescued from apoptosis by IL-6. These knockout cells contained Bcl-2 in amounts similar to naive cells and were able to upregulate Bcl-2 when stimulated with IL-6. In addition to blocking the anti-apoptotic effect of IL-6, Stat3 deficiency also led to reduced T-cell proliferation after stimulation with IL-2. The inhibition of Stat3 also led to apoptosis in leukemic cells.[23] Experiments in which a constitutively active Stat3 molecule protected fibroblasts against apoptosis suggested that normal cells balance the effects of anti-apoptotic Stat3 and pro-apoptotic Stat1, which may partly bind the same receptor chains.[24] Ultimately, this could be resolved in Stat1/Stat3 double-knockout mice. Mice devoid of Stat3 in their macrophages and neutrophils were highly susceptible to endotoxin shock, developing chronic enterocolitis around week 20 and dying when challenged with relatively small amounts of lipopolysaccharide (LPS).[25] These mice had constitutively active macrophages; the immunosuppressive functions of IL-10 were defective in both macrophages and granulocytes, leading to a Th1 shift. Interestingly, even when keratinocyte-specific Stat3 knockout mice were generated, there were immunological effects as well.[26] The defective skin remodeling primarily found in these mice was to be expected, given the activation of Stat3 by various growth factors such as epidermal (EGF), transforming growth factor (TGF) α and hepatocyte (HGF) growth factors, which had impaired signaling in these mice.[27] Interestingly, however, the same defects were also found in thymic epithelial cells and led to hypoplasia of the thymus with clearly reduced double-positive thymocytes.[26] Thymocytes from these mice were more prone to undergo apoptosis and showed impaired proliferation. However, there were no obvious peripheral lymphocyte problems found in these mice.

Stat4

Stat4 knockout mice were normal, with the exception of their immune system. Although wild-type mice express large amounts of Stat4 in their testes, Stat4$^{-/-}$ mice had normal testicular development and fertility.[28] They also had normal lymphoid subpopulations. When stimulated with IL-12, however, their lymphocytes did not upregulate IFN-γ,[28] the IL-18 receptor β-chain[29] or the chemokine receptor CCR5,[30] as wildtype cells did. Their T cells also failed to proliferate when stimulated with IL-12, but they proliferated normally when activated by IL-2.[28] In addition, Stat4$^{-/-}$ natural killer (NK) cells caused less than 10% of normal cytotoxicity and could also not increase their cytotoxic activity when stimulated with IL-12.[28] Moreover, Stat4-deficient mice were more susceptible to *Trypanosoma* infection[31] and chemically induced lymphomas[32] than wild-type mice. Overall, lymphocytes of Stat4$^{-/-}$ mice had a clear propensity to differentiate into Th2 cells, producing more IL-4, IL-5 and IL-10 than those of wild-type mice, but very little IFN-γ and reduced amounts

of lymphotoxin.[28] However, in the absence of both Stat4 and Stat6, the Th1 phenotype prevailed.[33] Consistent with the fact that Stat4 is also expressed in human monocytes, macrophages and dendritic cells,[34] Stat4$^{-/-}$ murine dendritic cells are defective in IFN-γ and nitric oxide (NO) production.[35]

Stat5a

Stat5a$^{-/-}$ mice were born in normal numbers, developed normally, and were fertile.[36] However, Stat5a-deficient female mice exhibited defective lobuloalveolar development of their mammary glands, which is efficiently induced by prolactin (PRL) in wild-type mice.[36,37] Thymic cellularity was normal in these mice, but the splenocytes were slightly decreased in number, although they displayed normal CD4/CD8 ratios and activation markers.[38] γδ-T cells were also diminished, while B cells and monocytes were again normal.[38] Stat5a$^{-/-}$ T cells appeared to have somewhat impaired IL-2 and IL-15 signaling and diminished upregulation of the IL-2R α-chain (CD25).[38] The relevance of the latter in vitro findings has been disputed; they may be due to concomitant decreases in Stat5b expression.[39] In vivo, however, Stat5a$^{-/-}$ cells also had defective Th2 differentiation, with reduced IgE and IgG$_1$, but increased IgG$_{2a}$ production, as well as fewer CD4$^+$CD25$^+$ (immunoregulatory) T cells.[40,41] These data suggest that Stat5a and Stat5b are not entirely redundant in terms of their immunological functions.

Stat5b

Mice deficient in Stat5b lacked sexual dimorphism in body growth; male Stat5b$^{-/-}$ mice were much smaller than their wild-type counterparts and of the same size as females.[42] Their GH levels were rather elevated, but their plasma insulin-like growth factor (IGF)-1 concentrations were clearly reduced, suggesting an effect on the signal transduction of GH pulses in the liver, where IGF-1 is predominantly produced in male animals. This is not surprising given that the amount of Stat5b present in the liver of wild-type mice by far exceeds that of Stat5a.[43] Consistent with these ideas, some sexually dimorphic liver genes (e.g. MUP) were also not different between males and females among Stat5b knockouts. Female Stat5b[-/-] mice had impaired mammary gland involvement, suggestive of impaired PRL signaling, and, although their mammary glands expressed milk proteins, were not able to feed pups. Moreover, they consistently aborted between pregnancy days 8 and 17. Pregnancies could be maintained by treatment with progesterone, the levels of which suddenly fell by pregnancy day 12, consistent with defective PRL signaling[37] (see next paragraph). These mice also had modestly diminished numbers of thymocytes and splenocytes, CD8[+] and CD4[-]/CD8[-] double-negative lymphocytes in particular.[44] NK cytolytic activity was clearly impaired, as were the expression of the IL-2R β-chain and perforin, all of these probably due to signaling defects of IL-15 (and IL-2).

Stat5a/Stat5b

Stat5a/Stat5b double-knockout mice were born at normal frequencies, but a significant portion died of unknown causes within 48 h,[37] and only 5% survived for 4 weeks.[45] Mice devoid of both Stat5a and Stat5b were infertile.[37] Their ovaries did not develop functional corpora lutea, which can be attributed to defective PRL signaling and may be caused by the successive lack of p27 expression. Both male and female Stat5 double-knockout mice were small; their epidermal fat pads were reduced to one-fifth, suggesting a total loss of GH effects in these mice. Stat5a[-/-]Stat5b[-/-] embryos have been reported to be clearly anemic, which was found to be due to disturbed EPO signaling,[46] but this is a controversial issue.[2] Accordingly, it is also a matter of debate why Stat5a[-/-]Stat5b[-/-] mice developed splenomegaly and extramedullary hematopoiesis with age.[39] Detailed studies on the peripheral blood of these Stat5-deficient animals demonstrated decreases in erythrocytes, platelets and lymphocytes.[45,47] Bone marrow cells, including even granulocyte numbers in the bone marrow, and colony-forming units were also clearly reduced.[47] With reduced efficiency, bone marrow grafts from Stat5a[-/-]Stat5b[-/-] mice could also repopulate the blood cell lineages of lethally irradiated hosts. However, these grafts failed to produce significant numbers of CD4[+] T lymphocytes, consistent with their clearly decreased peripheral lymphocyte counts.[45] Moreover, competitive experiments showed that these grafts were much less tolerant to radiation and exhibited decreased cellular survival, but normal proliferation.[47] Peripheral T cells of these Stat5-deficient mice failed to proliferate when stimulated by IL-2 or T-cell receptor (TCR) crosslinking, similar to mice lacking the IL-2R β-chain.[37,39] They completely lacked NK cells and NK cytolytic activity.[39] It is pertinent that Stat5-deficient lymphocytes were unable to express cyclin D2, cyclin D3, cyclin A or cdk6 after activation with IL-2 or by TCR crosslinking, thereby preventing their cell cycle progression and proliferation.[39] Interestingly, as do IL-2[-/-] mice and mice with defective IL-2 signaling, these mice developed higher percentages of activated T lymphocytes with age, suggesting defects in negative regulation.[39] Stat5a/Stat5b double-knockout animals also have a reduction in IL-7-induced bone marrow colonies.[37] This defect in IL-7 signaling also led to an impairment in pre- and pro-B-cell development and to a significant reduction of peripheral B cells.[48]

Stat6

Mice deficient in Stat6 were viable, developed normally, and were fertile.[49–51] Their lymphocyte subpopulations were grossly normal. Functionally, however, they showed defective IL-4 and IL-13 signaling: their lymphocytes failed to increase surface markers such as Thy-1, CD23, the IL-4 receptor or surface MHC class II molecules. Moreover, Stat6-deficient lymphocytes showed clearly impaired proliferation when stimulated with IL-4, but normal proliferation in response to IL-2. In vitro, Stat6[-/-] B cells failed to undergo isotype switching to IgE production, but showed normal upregulation of

IgM and IgG$_1$ and normal or increased production of IgG$_{2a}$, IgG$_{2b}$, IgG$_3$ and IgA.[49,50] In vivo, the IgE response to parasites (*Nippostrongylus brasiliensis*) was absent, and the IgG$_1$ response was greatly reduced, whereas IgG$_2$, IgG$_3$ and IgA levels were slightly higher in knockout cells.[51] Although B cells were able to produce IgG$_1$ in vitro, this immunoglobulin class, which is typical for Th2 situations, was almost absent in vivo, suggesting deficient Th2 lymphocyte help. In line with these ideas, Stat6-deficient T lymphocytes normally differentiated into Th1 cells, but they were unable to differentiate into Th2 cells in spite of stimulation with IL-4 or IL-13.[49,50] The additional impairment of IL-13 signaling probably explains the more pronounced phenotype of Stat6$^{-/-}$ mice as compared to IL-4-deficient animals.

Stat molecules as possible therapeutic targets

Given the remarkable immunoregulatory specificity of some Stats (Table 23.2), it was not unexpected to hear advocates for the targeting of Stat proteins as therapeutic agents. For example, Epling-Burnette et al suggested targeting Stat3 in hematological malignancies, and in large granular lymphocytic (LGL) leukemia in particular.[23] Stat3 is overexpressed in rheumatoid arthritis,

Table 23.2   Various Stats are essential for different cytokines, as demonstrated in knockout mice.

Stat	Cytokine/hormone affected
Stat1	IFN-α, IFN-γ
Stat2	IFN-α (not in macrophages)
Stat3	IL-6, IL-10, LIF, EGF, TGF-α, HGF, IL-2
Stat4	IL-12
Stat5	IL-2, IL-7, IL-15, EPO, GH, PRL
Stat5a	PRL
Stat5b	IL-15, IL-2, GH (males), PRL
Stat6	IL-4, IL-13

where anti-Stat3 treatment might also be effective.[52] Moriggl et al pointed out that drugs targeting Stat5 might be used to control T-cell expansion and function,[39] although the findings of increased T-cell activation probably warrant a note of caution in this regard. Kaplan et al discussed the possibility of shifting the Th1/Th2 balance by targeting Stat4.[28] As compared to targeting other Stats, targeting Stat4 has the additional advantage of not afflicting organs outside the immune system.[53] This Stat4-directed approach may be relevant for the treatment of rheumatoid arthritis, where, in this Th1-dominated disease, monocytes in the synovial lining layer overexpress Stat4.[34] Moreover, even an as yet unknown problem leading to defective Stat4 phosphorylation made mice resistant to collagen-induced arthritis.[54] Obviously, the same approach as for Stat4 might work in the other direction by targeting Stat6 for treating allergic disease.[55] Skinnider et al recently discussed whether targeting either Stat6 or IL-13 may be helpful in the therapy of Hodgkin's disease.[56] Blocking the function of the other two Stats, namely Stat1 and Stat2, is a less likely therapeutic intervention. Stat1 activation may play a pathogenic role in diseases such as systemic lupus erythematosus (SLE), given that IFN-γ causes severe flares in such patients.[57,58] However, blocking Stat1 signaling may pose even greater risks with regard to immunosuppression, cancer and mycobacterial disease. On the other hand, an agent enhancing Stat1 transcriptional activity might be useful, e.g. in chronic hepatitis. In the case of Stat2, an activating drug might also be interesting, given the effect of IFN-β on multiple sclerosis as one example. Such drugs would, however, have to be fairly specific for single Stats in order to tailor the therapy for specific immunological diseases. Moreover, given the fact that Stats are strictly intracellular, pharmacological properties may be important in order to permit efficient transmembrane transport.

JAKS

Jaks are non-receptor tyrosine kinases essential for the signaling of most interleukins and all

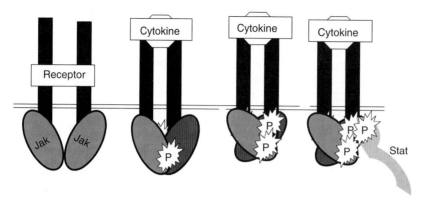

Figure 23.2 Janus kinase activation and function. Upon cytokine binding, the receptor chains of the cognate cytokine receptor bring the attached Janus kinases to close proximity, which first leads to their reciprocal tyrosine phosphorylation and full activation, then to the phosphorylation of the Stat binding motifs on the receptor chains and finally to the phosphorylation of the Stats binding these motifs.

interferons.[3] Their name derives from a structural peculiarity: adjacent to their kinase domain, Jaks have a pseudokinase domain. This side-by-side domain structure was reminiscent of the two-faced Roman god Janus, whose name they now bear.[59] We know of four mammalian Jaks, namely Tyk2 (tyrosine kinase 2), Jak1, Jak2, and Jak3, and it is unlikely by now that more will follow. These kinases specifically bind to a wide variety of cytokine receptors. Upon ligand binding, adjacent receptor chains bring the Jaks close enough together that they activate themselves by transphosphorylation.[60] After this reciprocal activation process, Jaks phosphorylate motifs on the receptor chains, and the Stats bind to these phosphorylated sites (Figure 23.2). In this way, Jaks are essential for the first steps in cytokine signaling.

In addition to cytokine receptors and Stats, Jaks also have other substrates. For example, Jak3 apparently activates Syk.[61] Moreover, the IL-2-induced phosphorylation of p98 was also absent in Jak3-deficient cells, making p98 another very probable Jak3 substrate.[62]

Unfortunately, we still lack crystallographic data on the Jaks. Therefore, their folding and the precise functions of their domains are still largely unknown. Nevertheless, both induced and naturally occurring mutations have shed some light on the functions. The (tyrosine) kinase domain, which is essential for Jak function, is situated at the C-terminus. Within

this domain, and its activation loop in particular, tyrosine residues with essentially opposing effects can be phosphorylated, thus providing a means to switch kinase activity on or off.[63] The pseudokinase domain has a complex regulatory role and, at least in vitro, it associates with the kinase domain.[64,65] The N-terminus, which comprises a FERM domain, is essential for receptor chain binding,[66,67] but the FERM domain also binds to the kinase domain and regulates its function.[68] This at least partly explains why FERM domain mutations have significant influence on kinase activity. Many of these data have led to speculations on how the Jak proteins might fold. It will be interesting to see how close we have come to the actual structure when crystallographic data become available.

As with the Stats, we can heavily rely on murine knockout data for estimating potential effects of Jak-targeted therapy (Table 23.3). For Jak3, however, there are also human mutations available for study. Although the features of Jak3-deficient mice have been studied in great detail,[69,70] the data on human mutations are as abundant, and we know of some differences in Jak3 deficiency between mice and humans. In particular, most Jak3-deficient individuals lack T cells and have functionally impaired B cells, whereas Jak3 knockout mice lack B cells but develop dysfunctional T lymphocytes.[71] Therefore, after exploring the knockout mouse data on

Table 23.3 Jaks are specifically required by different cytokines, as demonstrated in knockout mice.

Jak	Cytokine/hormone affected
Tyk2	IFN-α/β, IFN-γ, IL-12
Jak1	IFN-α/β, IFN-γ, IL-10, IL-2, IL-4, IL-7, IL-6, CNTF, LIF, OSM, CT-1
Jak2	IFN-γ, IL-3, IL-5, EPO, TPO, GM-CSF
Jak3	IL-2, IL-4, IL-7, IL-15

Tyk2, Jak1, and Jak2, we will address the function of Jak3 based on human data.

Tyk2

Tyk2-deficient mice were born in normal numbers and showed no gross abnormalities in development, fertility, and blood cell ontogeny.[72,73] Tyk2[-/-] bone marrow-derived macrophages expressed reduced Stat1 levels, but some Stat1 phosphorylation could still be detected after stimulation with IFN-α or IFN-β.[72] Stat2 levels were normal, although Stat2 phosphorylation was reduced but still present. Low concentrations of IFN-α did not lead to MHC class I upregulation on Tyk2[-/-] spleen cells.[33] Interestingly, Stat3 phosphorylation after IFN-α/β stimulation was completely absent in spite of normal Stat3 levels.[72] Moreover, Tyk2 deficiency also impaired Stat1 and Stat2 phosphorylation after IFN-γ treatment. When Tyk2[-/-] splenocytes were stimulated with IL-12, Stat3 phosphorylation was also absent,[72] and Stat4 phosphorylation was weak.[72,73] This also led to decreased IFN-γ production after IL-12 stimulation.[72,73] No IFN-γ message was detected after IL-12 stimulation,[73] but IL-12-induced proliferation was normal. Accordingly, the in vitro differentiation of naive Tyk2[-/-] CD4[+] lymphocytes into TH1 cells was less effective.[73] In contrast to IL-12 and IFN function, IL-10, IL-6, LIF, IL-3, granulocyte colony-stimulating factor

(G-CSF) and TPO function were undisturbed.[72,73] Peritoneal macrophages were clearly impaired in their NO upregulation when challenged with LPS or with IFN-α/β. Low dosages of IFN-α did not confer protection against vesicular stomatitis virus in Tyk2[-/-] spleen cells, but high concentrations did.[73] Low concentrations of IFN-γ were similarly active in wild-type and knockout cells. Approximately 20% of Tyk2 knockout mice succumbed to vesicular stomatitis virus, but all wild-type animals survived.[72] Additionally, when infected with vaccinia virus, Tyk2[-/-] mice had enhanced viral replication in the spleen. Despite these abnormalities, it should be emphasized that the phenotype associated with Tyk2 deficiency was far more modest than what was expected based on studies of deficient cell lines.

Jak1

Mice deficient in Jak1 died perinatally.[74] Although normal Mendelian proportions were preserved throughout pregnancy, not a single one of 326 Jak1[-/-] mice survived for 24 h. Newborn Jak1[-/-] pups weighed 40% less than heterozygous or wild-type ones, but they showed no other gross abnormalities. However, these mice failed to nurse. Jak1[-/-] mice had significantly lower numbers of sensory neurons than wild-type animals, and the number of neurons in newborn Jak1[-/-] mice could be partially rescued by NGF (nerve growth factor). While the gp130 ligands CNTF (ciliary neurotrophic factor), LIF, OSM (oncostatin M), CT-1 (cardiotrophin-1) and IL-6 were equally effective in rescuing wild-type neurons, they all failed to rescue those of Jak1-deficient animals. Therefore, it is likely that the defective signaling of some of these factors led to the fatal neurological condition observed. Jak1[-/-] mice also display immunological abnormalities. In contrast to their normal erythrocyte, monocyte–macrophage, neutrophil and platelet counts, the newborn animals had small thymi and severely reduced numbers of thymocytes, probably due to a primary block in thymocyte production. Moreover, B lymphocytes had a developmental block at the step between pro- and pre-B cells.

Probably explaining the latter findings, Jak1$^{-/-}$ cells proliferate neither after stimulation with IL-7 nor when stimulated with IL-2 or IL-4. Jak1$^{-/-}$ cells also exhibited clearly reduced but detectable Stat3 phosphorylation in response to stimulation with either IL-6 or LIF (both gp130 ligands). Finally, Jak1$^{-/-}$ embryonic fibroblasts and macrophages failed to react to activation with class II cytokine receptor ligands, namely IFN-α, IFN-γ, and IL-10. In contrast, signaling by TNF, IL-3, GM-CSF and EPO was unaffected.

Jak2

All Jak2-deficient animals died between embryonic days 12 and 13 due to a defect in hematopoiesis, which normally starts on day 10.[75,76] Only proerythroblasts and very few nucleated erythrocytes were seen, while enucleated fetal liver erythrocytes could never be seen.[75] These data were highly reminiscent of EPO receptor knockout mice, but Jak2$^{-/-}$ fetal livers contained even higher percentages of CD44hi and C-kit$^+$ CD34$^+$ hematopoietic cells.[75] When stimulated with IL-3, stem cell factor (SCF), GM-CSF and EPO, EPO-R$^{-/-}$ fetal liver cells developed around 10% of the normal erythroid burst- and colony-forming units. In contrast, Jak2$^{-/-}$ fetal liver cells did not develop these precursors at all.[75] Moreover, while EPO-R$^{-/-}$ fetal liver cell cultures developed hemoglobin-containing cells, those of Jak2$^{-/-}$ embryos did not.[75] Jak2$^{-/-}$ fetal liver cells were defective in their responses to IL-3, EPO and TPO, as well as IL-5 and GM-CSF.[76] In contrast, G-CSF signaling was normal and CCF-1 and SCF were functional. As expected, precursors were present and erythroid burst- and colony-forming unit formation could be rescued by retroviral Jak2 transfer.[76] B lymphopoiesis appeared largely normal,[75] and when Jak2$^{-/-}$ fetal liver cells were used to reconstitute sublethally irradiated Jak3$^{-/-}$ cells, both functional B cells and T cells developed out of these cells.[76] LIF[75] and IL-6[76] upregulated IRF-1 in embryonic stem cells, and IFN-α had the same effect on embryonic fibroblasts. However, IFN-γ was ineffective in these Jak2$^{-/-}$ cells.[75,76] Additionally, IFN-γ could not protect Jak2$^{-/-}$ cells against encephalomyocarditis virus-induced cytopathy.[76]

Jak3

Shortly after the cloning of L-Jak (leukocyte JAK),[77] the kinase, then renamed Jak3, was found to co-precipitate with the IL-2 receptor complex[78] and to be phosphorylated upon IL-2 and IL-4 stimulation.[78,79] As hypothesized,[78] Jak3 bound to the common γ-chain of the IL-2, IL-4, IL-7 and IL-9 receptors,[80,81] which, as we now know, also constitutes an essential part of the receptors for IL-15 and IL-21.[82] Moreover, mutations of the common γ-chain led to X chromosome-linked severe combined immune deficiency (X-SCID), and some of these γ-chain mutations also prevented Jak3 binding.[81] This led to the subsequent hypothesis that Jak3 mutations, like common γ-chain mutations, would lead to T$^-$B$^+$SCID (i.e. SCID with a lack of T cells in the presence of functionally impaired B cells).[81] The only difference to be expected was an autosomal trait for Jak3, given its localization on chromosome 19p13.1.[83] Indeed, such a patient was soon found,[84] and several more patients with SCID due to Jak3 mutations have added to our knowledge on the importance of Jak3 in cytokine signaling.[71,85]

Jak3 mutations in SCID patients disrupt normal signaling via several mechanisms. In many cases, Jak3 protein was not expressed or was too unstable to sustain sufficient amounts. In some patients, however, at least some Jak3 was present. Some of these patients failed to phosphorylate Jak3; others constitutively phosphorylated Jak3. All of the patients' Jak3 mutations, however, failed to effectively phosphorylate Stat5a following IL-2 stimulation. Stat6 phosphorylation was also reduced but still present after activation with IL-4.[71] Most of the patients completely lacked T lymphocytes, but one patient with impaired Stat5a phosphorylation developed T lymphocytes with an activated phenotype and suboptimal IL-2-induced proliferation at 3 months of age.[86,87] Interestingly, although Jak3 was upregulated in monocytes by IFN-γ or LPS stimulation and subsequently phosphorylated following stimulation with IL-2, IL-4, or IL-7,[88] no functional impairment could be detected in the monocytes of SCID patients.[89] Together, these findings closely fit the defects caused by impaired signaling of IL-2, IL-7, and IL-15. IL-7 is clearly essential for T lymphocytes,[90] whereas IL-15 is required for NK cell function.[91] Accordingly, where Stat5a phosphorylation could not be found, both T and NK cells were totally absent in Jak3 SCID patients. Moreover, IL-2 signaling defects led to an activated T-lymphocyte phenotype and overt autoimmunity,[97] and Jak3 deficient patients' lymphocytes had a similar phenotype. Finally, IL-4 can signal to some degree through the IL-13 receptor, which does not contain the common γ-chain and thus remains independent of Jak3.[93] This explains the only somewhat reduced phosphorylation of Stat6 following IL-4 stimulation. Consistent with this idea, IL-13-induced Stat6 phosphorylation was similar in wild-type and Jak3 SCID patient B cells, whereas IL-4-induced Stat6 phosphorylation was reduced in Jak3 patient B cells.[94] The effects of Jak3 deficiency on IL-9 and IL-21 signaling have not yet been elucidated, but the expectation is that they would be abrogated unless alternative, γ-chain-independent receptors contribute to signaling.

The data on Jak3-deficient mice are largely consistent with the findings in human Jak3 SCID patients, with the exception that Jak3$^{-/-}$ mice develop non-functional T cells but lack B cells.[95,96] Thymic reconstitution of Jak3$^{-/-}$ animals with Jak3, however, has shed some additional light on open questions.[97,98] Although thymic expression of Jak3 restored a normal T-cell phenotype, the absence of Jak3 in the peripheral T lymphocytes of older animals resulted in the same activated, dysfunctional T cells as in the Jak3-deficient animals. Therefore, Jak3 is essential for both lymphocyte proliferation and maintaining a quiescent state of peripheral T lymphocytes.

Jaks as possible therapeutic targets

Because of their vital roles in a variety of organ systems (see above), Jak1 and Jak2 are unlikely candidates for Jak-directed therapy. Tyk2 might be a somewhat better candidate, given that some autoimmune diseases probably rely on IL-12 and IFN signaling, but the extent of any therapeutic effect may be quite weak, given the moderate effects even in Tyk2 total knockouts. Among the Jaks, clearly the most likely candidate for therapeutic approaches is Jak3, an idea expressed as soon as the role of Jak3 in IL-2 and IL-4 signaling became apparent.[78] Given that constitutively active Jaks may lead to malignant transformation,[99] Jak activation is clearly undesirable. The available targets for novel therapies could thus be the removal of Jak3 or, more likely, the blockage of Jak3 function or Jak3 receptor binding. In the latter regard, substantial work has already been done to delineate the region of Jak3 that binds to the common γ-chain,[66,67] and attempts to gain crystallographic data on the actual structure of Jak3 should improve the chances of modeling drugs that block this interaction. At least three substances have already been reported to inhibit Jak3. These inhibitors are the undecylprodigiosin analog PNU156804, the tyrphostin AG-490, and the quinalzoline derivative WHI-P97, and other molecules may have similar functions.[100–103] Before any evaluation of their clinical usefulness, all these substances will have to undergo more comprehensive testing for substrate specificity and, more importantly, for toxicity. Nevertheless, these data suggest that we may soon begin to use specific Jak3 inhibitors for immunosuppression.

SOCS (CIS, JAB, SSI) MOLECULES AND THEIR POTENTIAL THERAPEUTIC ROLE

Suppressor of cytokine signaling (SOCS) proteins comprise a family of proteins that are known to inhibit Jak signaling and may be of importance in targeted therapy. These proteins all contain a domain called a SOCS box and an SH2 domain for protein interactions.[3] SOCS-1 and SOCS-3 bind Jaks, whereas SOCS-2 and cytokine inducible SH2-containing protein (CIS) do not, but rather bind to receptor subunits. Recently, knockout and transgenic mice have shed more light on the function of all four SOCS molecules. Since, however, the phenotypes of most of these mice suggest serious problems in SOCS-targeted therapies, we will just briefly comment on these findings. SOCS-1[-/-] animals died before weaning, showing fatty liver cell necrosis and immunological changes, including T-cell activation, accelerated lymphocyte apoptosis, lymphopenia, and macrophage infiltration.[104,105] Animals with a truncated SOCS-1 protein that lacks the SOCS box show a similar phenotype.[106] It appears that many of these effects are due to unchecked IFN-γ signaling,[107] but SOCS-1[-/-] IFN-γ[-/-] double-knockout animals still developed polycystic kidney disease and chronic inflammation, including pneumonia, skin ulcers and granulomas.[108] While either SOCS-1 analogs or overexpression of SOCS-1 may well turn out to be useful therapeutic targets, it will be necessary to gain a better understanding of the other cytokines and hormones involved. SOCS-2 is obviously essential for dampening growth hormone signaling, given that SOCS-2 deficiency leads to gigantism.[109] SOCS-2 activity might thus be useful in treating patients with gigantism or acromegaly where surgery is not feasible. SOCS-3 knockout mice died in utero, but it is a matter of dispute whether they suffered from extensive erythrocytosis[110] or placental defects.[111] In contrast, SOCS-3 overexpression in hematopoietic tissue led to fetal anemia, which also resulted in embryonic lethality.[110] Interestingly, periarticular adenoviral overexpression of SOCS-3 was effective in dampening antigen-induced and collagen-induced arthritis,[52] but this approach might lead to serious problems if systemic overexpression of SOCS-3 cannot be avoided. CIS transgenic mice had defects in growth hormone and presumably PRL signaling. The mice were small and had defective mammary development. The similarities between the CIS transgenic mice and the Stat5[-/-] mice suggests that CIS probably blocks Stat5 action.[112] It is less obvious why transgenic mice with CD4[+] cells overexpressing CIS showed enhanced proliferation, survival and cytokine production of these T cells.[113] There are no defects reported for mice lacking CIS. Thus, the most

likely candidate of the SOCS family for targeted therapy is probably SOCS-2, although not in an immunological context. SOCS-1 may be of interest, but our present knowledge on this protein is not yet sufficient, and its specificity is unclear. Finally, SOCS-3 has shown benefits when overexpressed locally in a mouse model of arthritis, but safety issues concerning systemic overexpression will have to be resolved.

PROTEIN INHIBITORS OF ACTIVATED STATS

A family of proteins called PIAS molecules (protein inhibitors of activated Stats) have also been identified as negative regulators of Stat signaling. The first PIAS molecule (PIAS1) was discovered by a yeast two-hybrid screen as a Stat1-binding protein.[114,115] Four other family members have also been described, including Gu/RNA helicase II binding protein (GuBP), PIAS3, PIASx, and PIASy, which share >50% sequence homology. PIAS molecules bind to activated Stat dimers and inhibit their DNA-binding and transcriptional activities. The action of the PIAS molecules appears to be very specific; for example, PIAS1 binds only Stat1 dimers,[115] and PIAS3 binds Stat3 dimers.[114] Furthermore, PIAS1–Stat1 interactions require phosphorylation of Y-701 of Stat1. Unlike the SOCS proteins, which are cytokine-inducible inhibitors of cytokine signaling, PIAS3[114] is constitutively expressed in a number of tissues. Therefore, the PIAS molecules may regulate the basal pool of activated Stats rather than act in a classical negative-feedback loop like the SOCS proteins. Recent data also suggest that PIAS family molecules may have much broader functions than regulating Stats. In particular, PIAS1 and PIASx act as small ubiquitin-like modifier (SUMO) ligases, regulating transcription factors such as p53.[116] While these findings much better explain the role of the PIAS family, therapeutic targeting of these proteins becomes much less likely when they fulfill multiple functions. More precise conclusions on potential PIAS-directed therapies will rely on in-depth knowledge of their functional repertoire.

Table 23.4 Potential effects of therapies targeting Stats, Jaks or SOCS proteins.

Stat	Action	Possible indication	Expected risks
Stat1	Activating	Chronic viral, malignancy	Fever, autoimmune side-effects
Stat2	Activating	Chronic viral, multiple sclerosis	
Stat3	Suppressing	Malignancy, leukemia, arthritis	Autoimmune side-effects (colitis)
Stat4	Activating	Chronic infection, allergy (Th2)	
Stat4	Suppressing	Th1-predominant autoimmune disease	Infections
Stat5	Suppressing	Autoimmune disease, transplantation	Possibly T-cell activation
Stat6	Suppressing	Allergy, Hodgkin's lymphoma	
Tyk2	Suppressing	Th1-driven autoimmunity?	Infections
Jak3	Suppressing	Autoimmune disease, transplantation	Infections
SOCS-2	Activating	Gigantism, acromegaly	
SOCS-3	Activating	Local arthritis treatment	Multisystem problems if systemic

CONCLUSIONS

With increasing knowledge of Stats and Jaks and the inhibitory proteins that interact with these molecules, some candidates for targeted immunotherapy clearly stand out (Table 23.4). As detailed above, these include several Stats, especially those with predominant or exclusive immune functions. Two major examples are Stat4 and Stat6, with their roles in Th1 and Th2 immune responses, respectively. Another interesting approach, albeit in oncology rather than in rheumatology, might be the use of drugs targeting Stat3 or Stat6 for the treatment of hematological malignancies. Among the Jaks, Jak3 is by far the most likely candidate, given the roles of Jak1 and Jak2 within organs other than the immune system and the mild phenotype of the Tyk2-deficient animals. With the Jak3 phenotype being severe combined immunodeficiency, Jak3-targeted therapy may be useful for immunosuppression in autoimmune disease as well as in organ transplantation, and several candidate Jak3-inhibitory substances have been reported. In contrast, most of the inhibitory proteins are much less likely to be good candidates for such therapeutic approaches. Taken together, Stat- and/or Jak-targeted therapies are likely to offer exciting prospects for more specific immunotherapy. In order to arrive there, we will undoubtedly have to learn a lot more about both the diseases and new drugs to treat them. In this spirit we look forward to a fascinating experience and – hopefully – much better tools with which to help our patients.

REFERENCES

1. Bromberg J, Darnell JE, Jr. The role of STATs in transcriptional control and their impact on cellular function. *Oncogene* 2000; **19**: 2468–73.
2. Ihle JN. The Stat family in cytokine signaling. *Curr Opin Cell Biol* 2001; **13**: 211–17.
3. O'Shea JJ, Gadina M, Schreiber RD. Cytokine signaling in 2002: new surprises in the Jak/Stat pathway. *Cell* 2002; **109**: S121–31.
4. Greenlund AC, Morales MO, Viviano BL et al. Stat recruitment by tyrosine-phosphorylated cytokine receptors: an ordered reversible affinity-driven process. *Immunity* 1995; **2**: 677–87.

5. McBride KM, McDonald C, Reich NC. Nuclear export signal located within the DNA-binding domain of the STAT1 transcription factor. *EMBO J* 2000; **19**: 6196–206.

6. Becker S, Groner B, Muller CW. Three-dimensional structure of the Stat3beta homodimer bound to DNA. *Nature* 1998; **394**: 145–51.

7. Chen X, Vinkemeier U, Zhao Y et al. Crystal structure of a tyrosine phosphorylated STAT-1 dimer bound to DNA. *Cell* 1998; **93**: 827–39.

8. Kovarik P, Mangold M, Ramsauer K et al. Specificity of signaling by STAT1 depends on SH2 and C-terminal domains that regulate Ser727 phosphorylation, differentially affecting specific target gene expression. *EMBO J* 2001; **20**: 91–100.

9. Vinkemeier U, Moarefi I, Darnell JEJ, Kuriyan J. Structure of the amino-terminal protein interaction domain of STAT-4. *Science* 1998; **279**: 1048–52.

10. Martinez-Moczygemba M, Gutch MJ, French DL, Reich NC. Distinct STAT structure promotes interaction of STAT2 with the p48 subunit of the interferon-alpha-stimulated transcription factor ISGF3. *J Biol Chem* 1997; **272**: 20070–6.

11. Seidel HM, Milocco LH, Lamb P et al. Spacing of palindromic half sites as a determinant of selective STAT (signal transducers and activators of transcription) DNA binding and transcriptional activity. *Proc Natl Acad Sci USA* 1995; **92**: 3041–5.

12. Schindler U, Wu P, Rothe M et al. Components of a Stat recognition code: evidence for two layers of molecular selectivity. *Immunity* 1995; **2**: 689–97.

13. Ehret GB, Reichenbach P, Schindler U et al. DNA binding specificity of different STAT proteins. Comparison of in vitro specificity with natural target sites. *J Biol Chem* 2001; **276**: 6675–88.

14. Durbin JE, Hackenmiller R, Simon MC, Levy DE. Targeted disruption of the mouse Stat1 gene results in compromised innate immunity to viral disease. *Cell* 1996; **84**: 443–50.

15. Meraz MA, White JM, Sheehan KC et al. Targeted disruption of the Stat1 gene in mice reveals unexpected physiologic specificity in the JAK–STAT signaling pathway. *Cell* 1996; **84**: 431–42.

16. Kaplan DH, Shankaran V, Dighe AS et al. Demonstration of an interferon gamma-dependent tumor surveillance system in immunocompetent mice. *Proc Natl Acad Sci USA* 1998; **95**: 7556–61.

17. Kumar A, Commane M, Flickinger TW et al. Defective TNF-alpha-induced apoptosis in STAT1-null cells due to low constitutive levels of caspases. *Science* 1997; **278**: 1630–2.

18. Dupuis S, Dargemont C, Fieschi C et al. Impairment of mycobacterial but not viral immunity by a germline human STAT1 mutation. *Science* 2001; **293**: 300–3.

19. Park C, Li S, Cha E, Schindler C. Immune response in Stat2 knockout mice. *Immunity* 2000; **13**: 795–804.

20. Takeda K, Noguchi K, Shi W et al. Targeted disruption of the mouse Stat3 gene leads to early embryonic lethality. *Proc Natl Acad Sci USA* 1997; **94**: 3801–4.

21. Raz R, Lee CK, Cannizzaro LA et al. Essential role of STAT3 for embryonic stem cell pluripotency. *Proc Natl Acad Sci USA* 1999; **96**: 2846–51.

22. Takeda K, Kaisho T, Yoshida N et al. Stat3 activation is responsible for IL-6-dependent T cell proliferation through preventing apoptosis: generation and characterization of T cell-specific Stat3-deficient mice. *J Immunol* 1998; **161**: 4652–60.

23. Epling-Burnette PK, Liu JH, Catlett-Falcone R et al. Inhibition of STAT3 signaling leads to apoptosis of leukemic large granular lymphocytes and decreased Mcl-1 expression. *J Clin Invest* 2001; **107**: 351–62.

24. Shen Y, Devgan G, Darnell JE Jr, Bromberg JF. Constitutively activated Stat3 protects fibroblasts from serum withdrawal and UV-induced apoptosis and antagonizes the proapoptotic effects of activated Stat1. *Proc Natl Acad Sci USA* 2001; **98**: 1543–8.

25. Takeda K, Clausen BE, Kaisho T et al. Enhanced Th1 activity and development of chronic enterocolitis in mice devoid of Stat3 in macrophages and neutrophils. *Immunity* 1999; **10**: 39–49.

26. Sano S, Takahama Y, Sugawara T et al. Stat3 in thymic epithelial cells is essential for postnatal maintenance of thymic architecture and thymocyte survival. *Immunity* 2001; **15**: 261–73.

27. Sano S, Itami S, Takeda K et al. Keratinocyte-specific ablation of Stat3 exhibits impaired skin remodeling, but does not affect skin morphogenesis. *EMBO J* 1999; **18**: 4657–68.

28. Kaplan MH, Sun YL, Hoey T, Grusby MJ. Impaired IL-12 responses and enhanced development of Th2 cells in Stat4-deficient mice. *Nature* 1996; **382**: 174–7.

29. Nakahira M, Tomura M, Iwasaki M et al. An absolute requirement for STAT4 and a role for IFN-gamma as an amplifying factor in IL-12

induction of the functional IL-18 receptor complex. *J Immunol* 2001; **167**: 1306–12.

30. Iwasaki M, Mukai T, Nakajima C et al. A mandatory role for STAT4 in IL-12 induction of mouse T cell CCR5. *J Immunol* 2001; **167**: 6877–83.

31. Tarleton RL, Grusby MJ, Zhang L. Increased susceptibility of Stat4-deficient and enhanced resistance in Stat6-deficient mice to infection with Trypanosoma cruzi. *J Immunol* 2000; **165**: 1520–5.

32. Zhang SS, Welte T, Fu XY. Dysfunction of Stat4 leads to accelerated incidence of chemical-induced thymic lymphomas in mice. *Exp Mol Pathol* 2001; **70**: 231–8.

33. Kaplan MH, Wurster AL, Grusby MJ. A signal transducer and activator of transcription (Stat)4-independent pathway for the development of T helper type 1 cells. *J Exp Med* 1998; **188**: 1191–6.

34. Frucht DM, Aringer M, Galon J et al. Stat4 is expressed in activated peripheral blood monocytes, dendritic cells, and macrophages at sites of Th1-mediated inflammation. *J Immunol* 2000; **164**: 4659–64.

35. Fukao T, Frucht DM, Yap G et al. Inducible expression of Stat4 in dendritic cells and macrophages and its critical role in innate and adaptive immune responses. *J Immunol* 2001; **166**: 4446–55.

36. Liu X, Robinson GW, Wagner KU et al. Stat5a is mandatory for adult mammary gland development and lactogenesis. *Genes Dev* 1997; **11**: 179–86.

37. Teglund S, McKay C, Schuetz E et al. Stat5a and Stat5b proteins have essential and nonessential, or redundant, roles in cytokine responses. *Cell* 1998; **93**: 841–50.

38. Nakajima H, Liu XW, Wynshaw BA et al. An indirect effect of Stat5a in IL-2-induced proliferation: a critical role for Stat5a in IL-2-mediated IL-2 receptor alpha chain induction. *Immunity* 1997; **7**: 691–701.

39. Moriggl R, Topham DJ, Teglund S et al. Stat5 is required for IL-2-induced cell cycle progression of peripheral T cells. *Immunity* 1999; **10**: 249–59.

40. Kagami S, Nakajima H, Suto A et al. Stat5a regulates T helper cell differentiation by several distinct mechanisms. *Blood* 2001; **97**: 2358–65.

41. Kagami S, Nakajima H, Kumano K et al. Both stat5a and stat5b are required for antigen-induced eosinophil and T-cell recruitment into the tissue. *Blood* 2000; **95**: 1370–7.

42. Udy GB, Towers RP, Snell RG et al. Requirement of STAT5b for sexual dimorphism of body growth rates and liver gene expression. *Proc Natl Acad Sci USA* 1997; **94**: 7239–44.

43. Ripperger JA, Fritz S, Richter K et al. Transcription factors Stat3 and Stat5b are present in rat liver nuclei late in an acute phase response and bind interleukin-6 response elements. *J Biol Chem* 1995; **270**: 29998–30006.

44. Imada K, Bloom ET, Nakajima H et al. Stat5b is essential for natural killer cell-mediated proliferation and cytolytic activity. *J Exp Med* 1998; **188**: 2067–74.

45. Bunting KD, Bradley HL, Hawley TS et al. Reduced lymphomyeloid repopulating activity from adult bone marrow and fetal liver of mice lacking expression of STAT5. *Blood* 2002; **99**: 479–87.

46. Socolovsky M, Fallon AE, Wang S et al. Fetal anemia and apoptosis of red cell progenitors in Stat5a$^{-/-}$5b$^{-/-}$ mice: a direct role for Stat5 in Bcl-X(L) induction. *Cell* 1999; **98**: 181–91.

47. Snow JW, Abraham N, Ma MC et al. STAT5 promotes multilineage hematolymphoid development in vivo through effects on early hematopoietic progenitor cells. *Blood* 2002; **99**: 95–101.

48. Sexl V, Piekorz R, Moriggl R et al. Stat5a/b contribute to interleukin 7-induced B-cell precursor expansion, but abl- and bcr/abl-induced transformation are independent of stat5. *Blood* 2000; **96**: 2277–83.

49. Kaplan MH, Schindler U, Smiley ST, Grusby MJ. Stat6 is required for mediating responses to IL-4 and for development of Th2 cells. *Immunity* 1996; **4**: 313–19.

50. Shimoda K, van Deursen J, Sangster MY et al. Lack of IL-4-induced Th2 response and IgE class switching in mice with disrupted Stat6 gene. *Nature* 1996; **380**: 630–3.

51. Takeda K, Tanaka T, Shi W et al. Essential role of Stat6 in IL-4 signalling. *Nature* 1996; **380**: 627–30.

52. Shouda T, Yoshida T, Hanada T et al. Induction of the cytokine signal regulator SOCS3/CIS3 as a therapeutic strategy for treating inflammatory arthritis. *J Clin Invest* 2001; **108**: 1781–8.

53. Waldmann TA, O'Shea J. The use of antibodies against the IL-2 receptor in transplantation. *Curr Opin Immunol* 1998; **10**: 507–12.

54. Ortmann R, Smeltz R, Yap G et al. A heritable defect in IL-12 signaling in B10.Q/J mice. I. In vitro analysis. *J Immunol* 2001; **166**: 5712–19.

55. Foster PS. STAT6: an intracellular target for the inhibition of allergic disease. *Clin Exp Allergy* 1999; **29**: 12–16.

56. Skinnider BF, Elia AJ, Gascoyne RD et al. Signal transducer and activator of transcription 6 is frequently activated in Hodgkin and Reed–Sternberg cells of Hodgkin lymphoma. *Blood* 2002; **99**: 618–26.

57. Graninger WB, Hassfeld W, Pesau BB et al. Induction of systemic lupus erythematosus by interferon-gamma in a patient with rheumatoid arthritis. *J Rheumatol* 1991; **18**: 1621–2.

58. Machold KP, Smolen JS. Interferon-gamma induced exacerbation of systemic lupus erythematosus. *J Rheumatol* 1990; **17**: 831–2.

59. Aringer M, Cheng A, Nelson JW et al. Janus kinases and their role in growth and disease. *Life Sci* 1999; **64**: 2173–86.

60. Leonard WJ, O'Shea JJ. Jaks and STATs: biological implications. *Annu Rev Immunol* 1998; **16**: 293–322.

61. Zhou YJ, Magnuson KS, Cheng TP et al. Hierarchy of protein tyrosine kinases in interleukin-2 (IL-2) signaling: activation of syk depends on Jak3; however, neither Syk nor Lck is required for IL-2-mediated STAT activation. *Mol Cell Biol* 2000; **20**: 4371–80.

62. Gadina M, Sudarshan C, O'Shea JJ. IL-2, but not IL-4 and other cytokines, induces phosphorylation of a 98-kDa protein associated with SHP-2, phosphatidylinositol 3′-kinase, and Grb2. *J Immunol* 1999; **162**: 2081–6.

63. Zhou YJ, Hanson EP, Chen YQ et al. Distinct tyrosine phosphorylation sites in JAK3 kinase domain positively and negatively regulate its enzymatic activity. *Proc Natl Acad Sci USA* 1997; **94**: 13850–5.

64. Chen M, Cheng A, Candotti F et al. Complex effects of naturally occurring mutations in the JAK3 pseudokinase domain: evidence for interactions between the kinase and pseudokinase domains. *Mol Cell Biol* 2000; **20**: 947–56.

65. Yeh TC, Dondi E, Uze G, Pellegrini S. A dual role for the kinase-like domain of the tyrosine kinase Tyk2 in interferon-alpha signaling. *Proc Natl Acad Sci USA* 2000; **97**: 8991–6.

66. Chen M, Cheng A, Chen YQ et al. The amino terminus of JAK3 is necessary and sufficient for binding to the common gamma chain and confers the ability to transmit interleukin 2-mediated signals. *Proc Natl Acad Sci USA* 1997; **94**: 6910–15.

67. Cacalano NA, Migone TS, Bazan F et al. Autosomal SCID caused by a point mutation in the N-terminus of Jak3: mapping of the Jak3-receptor interaction domain. *EMBO J* 1999; **18**: 1549–58.

68. Zhou YJ, Chen M, Cusack NA et al. Unexpected effects of FERM domain mutations on catalytic activity of Jak3: structural implication for Janus kinases. *Mol Cell* 2001; **8**: 959–69.

69. Baird AM, Thomis DC, Berg LJ. T cell development and activation in Jak3-deficient mice. *J Leukoc Biol* 1998; **63**: 669–77.

70. Thomis DC, Berg LJ. The role of Jak3 in lymphoid development, activation, and signaling. *Curr Opin Immunol* 1997; **9**: 541–7.

71. Candotti F, O'Shea JJ, Villa A. Severe combined immune deficiencies due to defects of the common gamma chain-JAK3 signaling pathway. *Springer Semin Immunopathol* 1998; **19**: 401–15.

72. Karaghiosoff M, Neubauer H, Lassnig C et al. Partial impairment of cytokine responses in Tyk2-deficient mice. *Immunity* 2000; **13**: 549–60.

73. Shimoda K, Kato K, Aoki K et al. Tyk2 plays a restricted role in IFN alpha signaling, although it is required for IL-12-mediated T cell function. *Immunity* 2000; **13**: 561–71.

74. Rodig SJ, Meraz MA, White JM et al. Disruption of the Jak1 gene demonstrates obligatory and nonredundant roles of the Jaks in cytokine-induced biologic responses. *Cell* 1998; **93**: 373–83.

75. Neubauer H, Cumano A, Muller M et al. Jak2 deficiency defines an essential developmental checkpoint in definitive hematopoiesis. *Cell* 1998; **93**: 397–409.

76. Parganas E, Wang D, Stravopodis D et al. Jak2 is essential for signaling through a variety of cytokine receptors. *Cell* 1998; **93**: 385–95.

77. Kawamura M, McVicar DW, Johnston JA et al. Molecular cloning of L-JAK, a Janus family protein-tyrosine kinase expressed in natural killer cells and activated leukocytes. *Proc Natl Acad Sci USA* 1994; **91**: 6374–8.

78. Johnston JA, Kawamura M, Kirken RA et al. Phosphorylation and activation of the Jak-3 Janus kinase in response to interleukin-2. *Nature* 1994; **370**: 151–3.

79. Witthuhn BA, Silvennoinen O, Miura O et al. Involvement of the Jak-3 Janus kinase in signalling by interleukins 2 and 4 in lymphoid and myeloid cells. *Nature* 1994; **370**: 153–7.

80. Miyazaki T, Kawahara A, Fujii H et al. Functional activation of Jak1 and Jak3 by selective association with IL-2 receptor subunits. *Science* 1994; **266**: 1045–7.

81. Russell SM, Johnston JA, Noguchi M et al.

Interaction of IL-2R beta and gamma c chains with Jak1 and Jak3: implications for XSCID and XCID. *Science* 1994; **266**: 1042–5.

82. Asao H, Okuyama C, Kumaki S et al. Cutting edge: the common gamma-chain is an indispensable subunit of the IL-21 receptor complex. *J Immunol* 2001; **167**: 1–5.

83. Riedy MC, Dutra AS, Blake TB et al. Genomic sequence, organization, and chromosomal localization of human JAK3. *Genomics* 1996; **37**: 57–61.

84. Macchi P, Villa A, Gillani S et al. Mutations of Jak-3 gene in patients with autosomal severe combined immune deficiency (SCID). *Nature* 1995; **377**: 65–8.

85. Notarangelo LD, Giliani S, Mazza C et al. Of genes and phenotypes: the immunological and molecular spectrum of combined immune deficiency. Defects of the gamma(c)-JAK3 signaling pathway as a model. *Immunol Rev* 2000; **178**: 39–48.

86. Candotti F, Oakes SA, Johnston JA et al. Structural and functional basis for JAK3-deficient severe combined immunodeficiency. *Blood* 1997; **90**: 3996–4003.

87. Brugnoni D, Notarangelo LD, Sottini A et al. Development of autologous, oligoclonal, poorly functioning T lymphocytes in a patient with autosomal recessive severe combined immunodeficiency caused by defects of the Jak3 tyrosine kinase. *Blood* 1998; **91**: 949–55.

88. Musso T, Johnston JA, Linnekin D et al. Regulation of JAK3 expression in human monocytes: phosphorylation in response to interleukins 2, 4, and 7. *J Exp Med* 1995; **181**: 1425–31.

89. Villa A, Sironi M, Macchi P et al. Monocyte function in a severe combined immunodeficient patient with a donor splice site mutation in the Jak3 gene. *Blood* 1996; **88**: 817–23.

90. Puel A, Ziegler SF, Buckley RH, Leonard WJ. Defective IL7R expression in T(–)B(+)NK(+) severe combined immunodeficiency. *Nat Genet* 1998; **20**: 394–7.

91. Lodolce JP, Boone DL, Chai S et al. IL-15 receptor maintains lymphoid homeostasis by supporting lymphocyte homing and proliferation. *Immunity* 1998; **9**: 669–76.

92. Willerford DM, Chen J, Ferry JA et al. Interleukin-2 receptor alpha chain regulates the size and content of the peripheral lymphoid compartment. *Immunity* 1995; **3**: 521–30.

93. Palmer-Crocker RL, Hughes CC, Pober JS. IL-4 and IL-13 activate the JAK2 tyrosine kinase and Stat6 in cultured human vascular endothelial cells through a common pathway that does not involve the gamma chain. *J Clin Invest* 1996; **98**: 604–9.

94. Izuhara K, Heike T, Otsuka T et al. Signal transduction pathway of interleukin-4 and interleukin-13 in human B cells derived from X-linked severe combined immunodeficiency patients. *J Biol Chem* 1996; **271**: 619–22.

95. Thomis DC, Gurniak CB, Tivol E et al. Defects in B lymphocyte maturation and T lymphocyte activation in mice lacking Jak3. *Science* 1995; **270**: 794–7.

96. Park SY, Saijo K, Takahashi T et al. Developmental defects of lymphoid cells in Jak3 kinase-deficient mice. *Immunity* 1995; **3**: 771–82.

97. Thomis DC, Berg LJ. Peripheral expression of Jak3 is required to maintain T lymphocyte function. *J Exp Med* 1997; **185**: 197–206.

98. Sohn SJ, Forbush KA, Nguyen N et al. Requirement for Jak3 in mature T cells: its role in regulation of T cell homeostasis. *J Immunol* 1998; **160**: 2130–8.

99. Aringer M, Cheng A, Nelson JW et al. Janus kinases and their role in growth and disease. *Life Sci* 1999; **64**: 2173–86.

100. Stepkowski SM, Erwin-Cohen RA, Behbod F et al. Selective inhibitor of Janus tyrosine kinase 3, PNU156804, prolongs allograft survival and acts synergistically with cyclosporine but additively with rapamycin. *Blood* 2002; **99**: 680–9.

101. Kirken RA. Targeting Jak3 for immune suppression and allograft acceptance. *Transplant Proc* 2001; **33**: 3268–70.

102. Malaviya R, Chen CL, Navara C et al. Treatment of allergic asthma by targeting janus kinase 3-dependent leukotriene synthesis in mast cells with 4-(3′, 5′-dibromo-4′-hydroxyphenyl)amino-6,7-dimethoxyquinazoline (WHI-P97). *J Pharmacol Exp Ther* 2000; **295**: 912–26.

103. O'Shea JJ, Visconti R, Cheng TP, Gadina M. Jaks and stats as therapeutic targets. *Ann Rheum Dis* 2000; **59**(suppl 1): 115–18.

104. Starr R, Metcalf D, Elefanty AG et al. Liver degeneration and lymphoid deficiencies in mice lacking suppressor of cytokine signaling-1. *Proc Natl Acad Sci USA* 1998; **95**: 14395–9.

105. Naka T, Matsumoto T, Narazaki M et al. Accelerated apoptosis of lymphocytes by augmented induction of Bax in SSI-1 (STAT-induced STAT inhibitor-1) deficient mice. *Proc Natl Acad Sci USA* 1998; **95**: 15577–82.

106. Zhang JG, Metcalf D, Rakar S et al. The SOCS box of suppressor of cytokine signaling-1 is important for inhibition of cytokine action in vivo. *Proc Natl Acad Sci USA* 2001; **98**: 13261–5.

107. Naka T, Tsutsui H, Fujimoto M et al. SOCS-1/SSI-1-deficient NKT cells participate in severe hepatitis through dysregulated cross-talk inhibition of IFN-gamma and IL-4 signaling in vivo. *Immunity* 2001; **14**: 535–45.

108. Metcalf D, Mifsud S, Di Rago L et al. Polycystic kidneys and chronic inflammatory lesions are the delayed consequences of loss of the suppressor of cytokine signaling-1 (SOCS-1). *Proc Natl Acad Sci USA* 2002; **99**: 943–8.

109. Metcalf D, Greenhalgh CJ, Viney E et al. Gigantism in mice lacking suppressor of cytokine signalling-2. *Nature* 2000; **405**: 1069–73.

110. Marine JC, McKay C, Wang D et al. SOCS3 is essential in the regulation of fetal liver erythropoiesis. *Cell* 1999; **98**: 617–27.

111. Roberts AW, Robb L, Rakar S et al. Placental defects and embryonic lethality in mice lacking suppressor of cytokine signaling 3. *Proc Natl Acad Sci USA* 2001; **98**: 9324–9.

112. Matsumoto A, Seki Y, Kubo M et al. Suppression of STAT5 functions in liver, mammary glands, and T cells in cytokine-inducible SH2-containing protein 1 transgenic mice. *Mol Cell Biol* 1999; **19**: 6396–407.

113. Li S, Chen S, Xu X et al. Cytokine-induced Src homology 2 protein (CIS) promotes T cell receptor-mediated proliferation and prolongs survival of activated T cells. *J Exp Med* 2000; **191**: 985–94.

114. Chung CD, Liao J, Liu B et al. Specific inhibition of Stat3 signal transduction by PIAS3. *Science* 1997; **278**: 1803–5.

115. Liu B, Liao J, Rao X et al. Inhibition of Stat1-mediated gene activation by PIAS1. *Proc Natl Acad Sci USA* 1998; **95**: 10626–31.

116. Schmidt D, Muller S. Members of the PIAS family act as SUMO ligases for c-Jun and p53 and repress p53 activity. *Proc Natl Acad Sci USA* 2002; **99**: 2872–7.

24

Inducible nitric oxide synthase

Steven B Abramson

Introduction • Regulation of nitric oxide production • Role of nitric oxide in inflammation and immunity – effects of nitric oxide on cellular constituents • iNOS in rheumatic diseases • Nitric oxide as a therapeutic target • Summary • References

INTRODUCTION

Since the identification of endothelium-derived relaxation factor (EDRF) as nitric oxide (NO) in 1987,[1,2] it has become evident that NO plays a vital role in the regulation of physiological processes, host defense, inflammation and immunity. The flashing of fireflies is one of the most recent examples of the many unanticipated functions of NO.[3] Released by cells in gaseous form as a highly reactive free radical, NO is synthesized via the oxidation of arginine by a family of nitric oxide synthases (NOS). Because of its capacity to react with a variety of targets (DNA, proteins, thiols, reactive oxygen intermediates), and the fact that its activity is strongly influenced by its concentration, NO can exert complex effects in tissues which may be toxic or protective. Physiologically, NO is essential for the regulation of blood pressure and maintains the patency of blood vessels by inhibiting the adhesion of platelets and neutrophils to the endothelium.[4] In the nervous system, NO is a neurotransmitter that mediates several functions, including the formation of memory, some forms of neurogenic vasodilatation, and various gastrointestinal, respiratory, and genitourinary tract functions.[2] In pathological states, NO mediates inflammatory processes including vasodilatation, edema and pain. NO production can also contribute to tissue destruction, either via direct cytotoxicity, or by its mediation of cytokine-dependent processes. It is not surprising, therefore, that excessive NO has been implicated in the pathogenesis of a variety of rheumatic diseases, including systemic lupus erythematosus (SLE), rheumatoid arthritis (RA) and osteoarthritis (OA). However, protective and toxic effects of NO may be observed in parallel. Thus, the production of NO in disease may serve a protective, or anti-inflammatory, function by preventing the adhesion and release of oxidants by activated neutrophils in the microvasculature, or by the direct inhibition of mast cell and T-cell activation. This chapter reviews the multifaceted role of NO in immunity and addresses potential therapeutic applications of NOS inhibitors.

REGULATION OF NITRIC OXIDE PRODUCTION

NOS isoforms

NO is synthesized via L-arginine oxidation by a family of NOS. Isomeric forms of NOS, representing at least three distinct gene products, have

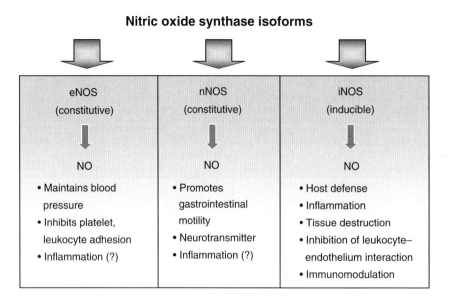

Nitric oxide synthase isoforms

eNOS (constitutive)	nNOS (constitutive)	iNOS (inducible)
NO	NO	NO
• Maintains blood pressure • Inhibits platelet, leukocyte adhesion • Inflammation (?)	• Promotes gastrointestinal motility • Neurotransmitter • Inflammation (?)	• Host defense • Inflammation • Tissue destruction • Inhibition of leukocyte–endothelium interaction • Immunomodulation

Figure 24.1 NO is synthesized by L-arginine oxidation by three known isoforms. Representative biological effects are shown.

been cloned in bovine, rat, mouse and human tissues (Figure 24.1).[5,6] NOS isoforms are either calcium-dependent and constitutively expressed (e.g. neuronal ncNOS (NOS-I)), or endothelium- (ecNOS (NOS-III)) or calcium-independent and inducible (iNOS (NOS II)). The constitutively expressed isoforms are primarily regulated by calcium fluxes and subsequent binding of calmodulin, whereas the inducible isoform is typically regulated by cytokines and requires de novo synthesis. The inducible isoform also tightly binds calmodulin following expression. Both constitutive and inducible NOS have recognition sites for NADPH, flavin-adenine dinucleotide, and flavin mononucleotide, as well as phosphorylation sites. Both types of NOS contain tetrahydrobiopterin, and the presence of this cofactor is essential for the activity of the enzyme. Constitutively expressed NOS, which are expressed in a variety of tissues, produce picomole to nanomole amounts of NO for short periods in response to receptor stimulation (e.g. acetylcholine, bradykinin) or shear stress.[7] In contrast, iNOS, expressed following exposure to diverse stimuli, such as inflammatory cytokines (e.g. interleukin-1β (IL-1β), tumor necrosis factor alpha (TNF-α)) and lipopolysaccharide (LPS),

generates significantly larger and sustained amounts of NO than do the constitutive isoforms.[5] The balance of cytokines in the microenvironment regulates the expression of iNOS; for example, transforming growth factor beta (TGF-β), IL-4 and IL-10 inhibit iNOS expression in macrophages (Table 24.1).[5] Glucocorticoids inhibit the expression of iNOS, which may account for at least some of the therapeutic actions of glucocorticoids. iNOS can be expressed in diverse cell types exposed to stimulatory cytokines, including inflammatory or immune system cells (monocyte–macrophages, natural killer (NK) cells, dendritic cells, mast cells) as well as other cells involved in immune or inflammatory reactions (endothelial cells, epithelial cells, chondrocytes, synovial cells).[8,9] Whether human neutrophils, T cells or B cells express NOS isoforms remains uncertain, since there are conflicting reports in the literature.[10–12] There is species and cell variability with regard to the regulation of iNOS expression. For example, in vitro, while iNOS is readily induced by IL-1β and TNF-α in murine leukocytes, these cytokines do not effectively induce iNOS in human leukocytes. However, interferon-alpha (IFN-α) can induce iNOS mRNA and protein in

---

Table 24.1 Regulation of iNOS expression and NO production.

Inducers	Inhibitors
Inflammatory cytokines: IL-1, IL-17, IL-18, TNF-α, interferon-γ,α	TGF-β, IL-4, IL-10
Chemokines	Arginase (depletes arginine substrate)
Immune complexes, complement fragments	Osteopontin
Microbial products	Drugs (see Table 24.5)
Mechanical stress	NO (high concentrations)
Fibronectin fragments	
NO (low concentrations)	

---

human monocytes in vitro.[13] Moreover, human monocytes and macrophages have been demonstrated to express iNOS in a variety of disease states, including RA, malaria, hepatitis C and vasculitis.[13,14] While iNOS has been the NOS isoform conventionally associated with inflammation, it is now apparent that NO production at inflammatory sites may additionally derive from ecNOS and ncNOS, and, indeed, that all known isoforms of NOS operate in the immune system.[9] For example, immunohistochemical analysis of inflamed synovium in a model of streptococcal cell wall-induced arthritis in rats revealed a distinct pattern of endothelial and neuronal NOS expression.[15] In this model, the non-specific NOS inhibitor N-monomethyl-L-arginine (L-NMMA) effectively inhibited disease, whereas the highly selective iNOS inhibitor N-iminoethyl-lysine (L-NIL) did not.

Regulation of iNOS expression and activity

Expression of the iNOS isoform is induced by inflammatory cytokines (including IFN-α, IL-1β and TNF-α), immune complexes, microbial products and mechanical stress (Table 24.1).[16,17] Activation of the iNOS gene promoter involves a number of participating transcription factors, including NFκB, AP-1, the signal transducer and activator of transcription (STAT)-1, interferon regulatory factor 1 (IRF-1), nuclear factor inter-leukin-6 (NF-IL-6), and the high-mobility group-I(Y) protein.[9,18-21] A variety of upstream signaling pathways have been described, depending on the stimulus and the cell type, including: Janus kinases Jak1, Jak2 and tyk2; Raf-1 protein kinase; mitogen-activated protein kinases p38, Erk1/2 and Jun N-kinase (JNK); and protein kinase C.[22-25] NO also regulates the transcription of iNOS, with low concentrations of NO upregulating iNOS, and high concentrations inhibiting iNOS expression.[26] IL-4, IL-10, IL-13 and TGF-β inhibit the expression of iNOS; the action of TGF-β may be due to enhanced degradation of iNOS protein.[9,27] The availability of arginine is an additional determinant of iNOS activity, particularly in high-output NO production, which depends upon extracellular uptake and transport of L-arginine.[28] Arginine concentration is modulated by arginase, an enzyme that degrades arginine to urea and ornithine. In macrophages, Th2 cytokines (e.g. IL-4, IL-10 and IL-13), and TGF-β increase arginase production, which reduces NO release by substrate depletion.[29,30]

Reactivity

NO is a gaseous free radical that is highly diffusable and, in the presence of oxygen, rapidly metabolized to nitrate and nitrite.[31] The chemistry of NO, however, involves interrelated redox forms; the most important reactions are

Table 24.2   Reactivity of NO.

Reaction with	Product/effect	Comment
Oxygen	Nitrate/nitrite	Stable metabolite, oxidant properties (?)
Superoxide anion	Peroxynitrite	Cytotoxic free radical, DNA damage, oxidant
Target proteins:		
Tyrosine residues	Nitrotyrosine	Modify, often inhibit, protein function
Sulfhydryl groups	S-Nitrosothiols	Stable NO donor, vasodilators, anti-inflammatory (?)
Heme iron:		
Guanylate cyclase	cGMP	Smooth muscle relaxation; mediates NO signaling in multiple cell types
Oxyhemoglobin	Met-hemoglobin	Major route of NO elimination
Mitochondria	Decreased ATP	Cell injury, apoptosis (?)
Actin	ADP ribosylation	Inhibition of actin stress fiber and focal adhesion formation; inhibition of 'outside-in' integrin signaling

believed to be those with oxygen, the oxygen-derived free radical superoxide anion, transitional metal ions and free thiols (Table 24.2).[31] The pleiotropic actions of NO are best understood by the recognition that NO is quickly transformed into a variety of reactive nitrogen intermediates (RNIs), which include NO free radical, NO^-, NO^+ or other conversion products, such as NO_2^-, NO_3^-, S-nitrosothiols (S-NO), peroxynitrite ($ONOO^-$) and nitrosyl–metal products (Figure 24.2) (Table 24.2).[9] The specific redox form of NO that is produced will be influenced by other factors released at the site of NO production (e.g. superoxide anion) and by the physicochemical milieu (pH, oxygen tension).[31–34] Hence, the determinants of the biologi-

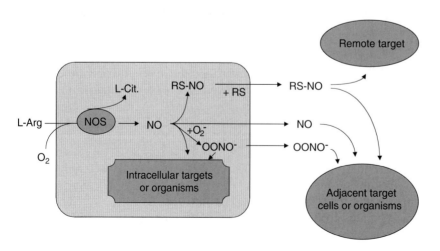

Figure 24.2 NO is produced within cells from L-arginine in the presence of oxygen. Once produced, NO may react with protein sulfhydryl groups (RS-NO) or other intracellular or extracellular targets, such as superoxide anion (O_2^-), as described in Table 24.2. Biological effects will depend upon quantity of NO produced, redox form of NO, and specific reaction products.

cal activity of NO in tissues will depend largely upon its reactivity with target molecules. The binding of NO to the heme group of soluble guanylate cyclase activates this enzyme, raising intracellular levels of cGMP in many, but not all, types of cells.[6,31] Reactivity of NO with heme-containing proteins may also account for its capacity to inhibit the leukocyte NADPH oxidase, and thereby inhibit superoxide anion generation.[35] In addition, heme reactivity may account for the capacity of NO to inhibit the mitochondrial electron transport system, recently reported in chondrocytes, which inhibits ATP production and reduces available intracellular energy stores.[32]

Another major activity of NO derives from its reaction with free thiols to form S-nitrosothiol compounds.[33] S-Nitrosothiol derivatives, formed both extra- and intracellularly, are significantly more stable than NO (e.g. $T^{1/2} > 2$ h), retain NO-like vasodilating properties, but are less cytotoxic.[33] Notable examples include S-nitroso derivatives of glutathione, cysteine and albumin, which may act as carriers or as biological sinks for NO. Thus, the activity of NO is not restricted to the site of its production, since S-nitrosothiols and S-nitrosylated proteins can circulate and liberate NO at distant sites, either spontaneously or after cleavage by ectoenzymes found on cells such as T and B lymphocytes.[9]

NO may also alter protein functions by direct nitration of tyrosine residues or by promoting ADP ribosylation, the covalent binding of ADP-ribose to acceptor amino acids.[36–38] NO induces the ADP ribosylation of G-actin in human neutrophils and inhibits actin polymerization and adhesion in neutrophils, endothelial cells and chondrocytes.[37,38] Inhibition of actin polymerization, including ADP ribosylation of actin, may be an important mechanism by which NO regulates cell adhesion, signaling from the extracellular matrix, migration and phagocytosis.[39] Finally, a key reaction that explains many injurious effects, is that between NO and superoxide anion to yield peroxynitrite, a highly toxic free radical, which nitrates proteins, and leads to the accumulation of injurious intracellular oxidants, DNA damage and apoptosis.[34,40]

ROLE OF NITRIC OXIDE IN INFLAMMATION AND IMMUNITY – EFFECTS OF NITRIC OXIDE ON CELLULAR CONSTITUENTS

To understand the divergent effects of NO in inflammation and immunity, one needs to understand local effects on cells and tissues. The diverse effects of NO on cells key to the pathogenesis of rheumatic diseases are reviewed below (Table 24.3).

Table 24.3   Effects of NO on inflammation and immunity.

Proinflammatory and tissue-damaging properties

Promotes vasodilatation and vascular leakiness

Reacts with O_2^- to form toxic peroxynitrite

Activates NFκB, JNK

Cytotoxic; promotes apoptosis of macrophages, CD4+/CD8+ thymocytes, chondrocytes

Stimulates TNF-α production

Enhances NK cell activity

In vivo, non-specific NOS inhibitors ameliorate experimental murine and canine arthritis, murine lupus, carrageenin-induced inflammation, immune complex lung injury

Anti-inflammatory and immunosuppressive properties

Inhibits mast cell degranulation

Inhibits leukocyte adhesion to endothelium, superoxide anion products, P-selectin expression

Inhibits the assembly of actin stress fibers at focal adhesion sites

Suppresses antigen-presenting cell activity

Inhibits T- and B-cell proliferation

In vivo, specific iNOS inhibitors exacerbate murine arthritis, transgenic HLA-B27 colitis, experimental allergic encephalitis

Phagocytic cells and cytotoxicity

NO formation may have originated as a first-line defense against invading microbial organisms, including parasites, bacteria and viruses.[5,41,42] Produced by phagocytic cells, NO exerts microbicidal and cytotoxic actions via the generation of peroxynitrite as well as by the reaction with iron-containing moieties in key enzymes of the respiratory cycle and DNA synthesis in target cells. The induction of iNOS and NO production by phagocytic cells is increased in a variety of experimental models of inflammation, the manifestations of which can be attenuated by NOS inhibitors. These include carrageenin-induced vascular permeability in rat skin, immune complex lung injury in rats, and the capillary leak syndrome following IL-2 administration in mice.[43] Excessive levels of NO can promote tissue injury in these models, and injury is attenuated by NOS inhibitors. Indeed, the findings that inhibition of NO production attenuates experimental animal models of SLE, inflammatory arthritis and OA provide compelling evidence that NO should be considered as a potential therapeutic target in human disease.[44–46]

Protective effects of endothelial cell-derived nitric oxide

While NO released by phagocytes may promote tissue injury, a paradoxical observation has been that NO exerts anti-inflammatory, or inhibitory, effects on phagocytic cells. For example, NO constitutively produced by endothelium is believed to play a protective role in the microvasculature by inhibiting the adhesion of platelets and leukocytes.[33,43] In in vitro studies of endothelial cell monolayers, NO donors significantly impede the rolling, adherence and/or transmigration of leukocytes.[47,48] In vivo, this effect can be shown in murine models to be due to NO derived from ecNOS and ncNOS.[43,49] The mechanism of the anti-adhesive effect is unknown, although NO has been demonstrated to downregulate the endothelial expression of members of different adhesion molecule families, such as vascular cell adhesion molecule-1 (VCAM-1), intercellular adhesion molecule-1 (ICAM-1), E-selectin and P-selectin.[48] We have demonstrated that NO donors, as well as endogenous NO induced by acetylcholine, prevent the assembly of actin stress fibers following ligation of endothelial ICAM-1.[37] This inhibitory effect on actin polymerization may be a mechanism by which constitutive NO production by ecNOS confers anti-adhesive properties to endothelial cells. Finally, in addition to its capacity to inhibit leukocyte adhesion, NO also inhibits the production of superoxide anion by activated leukocytes.[35,43] This effect may be due to the inhibition of a membrane component of the NADPH oxidase, possible via the iron nitrosylation of cytochrome b_{558}.[35]

The vascular protective properties of NO have been demonstrated in vivo by means of intravital microscopy studies, which demonstrate that NOS inhibitors increase neutrophil adherence, protein extravasation and microvascular injury following the infusion of endotoxin.[43] Moreover, in experimental myocardial ischemia reperfusion injury, endotoxic shock and the adult respiratory distress syndrome (ARDS), NOS inhibitors increased organ injury.[43] Recently, protective effects of NO production were reported in rats transgenic for HLA-B27/human β_2-microglobulin that develop a spontaneous multisystem inflammatory disorder that mimics human spondyloarthropathies.[50] In those studies, treatment with the selective iNOS inhibitor L-NIL effectively inhibited iNOS activity, but resulted in an increase in colitis. Whether this protective effect of NO was due to effects on the microvasculature or to the capacity of NO to inhibit the activation of inflammatory cells (e.g. mast cell degranulation, leukocyte oxidant production, lymphocyte proliferation) is not known.

Modulation of lymphocyte activity

Low levels of NO promote lymphocyte activation and proliferation. NO donors such as sodium nitroprusside increase lymphocyte uptake of glucose (an early event during lymphocyte activation), and stimulate TNF-α production and NFκB binding activity; NO also enhances activity of the tyrosine kinase, p56, which is implicated in lymphocyte signaling events. L-Arginine depletion and NOS inhibitors also impair phytohemagglutinin (PHA)-stimulated proliferation, while dietary L-arginine supplementation in humans increases lymphocyte mitogenic responses to concanavalin A and PHA.[51] L-Arginine has also been shown both in vitro and in vivo to enhance NK- and lymphokine-activated killer activity. In contrast, high concentrations of NO suppress antigen-presenting cell activity and T-cell proliferation.[52] There is evidence that NO exerts different effects on discrete subpopulations of T cells, inhibiting secretion of IL-2 by murine Th1 cells while increasing the secretion of IL-4 in Th2 cells. These observations may differ in humans, where the production of Th1- and Th2-associated cytokines by activated human T cells and human T-cell clones may be equally impaired by NO donors. The modulation of the immune response by NO, including effects on Th1/Th2 lymphocyte-derived cytokine production, requires further elucidation and was recently reviewed.[53]

The effects of NO on apoptosis represent additional mechanisms by which NO may dysregulate the immune system. NO promotes apoptosis in macrophages, CD4+/CD8+ thymocytes and chondrocytes.[54,55] The mechanism appears to require activation of poly-(ADP-ribose) polymerase (PARS) and nitrotyrosine formation, and is opposed by the anti-apoptotic protein BCL-2. Alternatively, NO, at lower concentrations ($< 1 \mu M$), has been reported to inhibit apoptosis of hepatocytes, B lymphocytes and eosinophils.[56] Because of its capacity to induce apoptosis, it has been speculated that NO may play a role in selection and deletion of T cells in the thymus.[57] Epithelial and dendritic cells in the thymus express iNOS, which is further upregulated after contact with self-antigens or alloantigens or with thymocytes activated by T-cell receptor (TCR) stimulation.[9,58] There is evidence that NO-derived peroxynitrite is responsible for the killing of TCR-activated double-positive thymocytes.[58]

Effects on synovial cells and chondrocytes

NO exerts a number of effects on synovial cells and chondrocytes which may contribute to tissue injury in arthritis, including: (1) inhibition of collagen and proteoglycan synthesis;[32,59] (2) activation of metalloproteinases;[60] and (3) increased susceptibility to oxidant injury and apoptosis (Figure 24.3).[55,61,62] In addition,

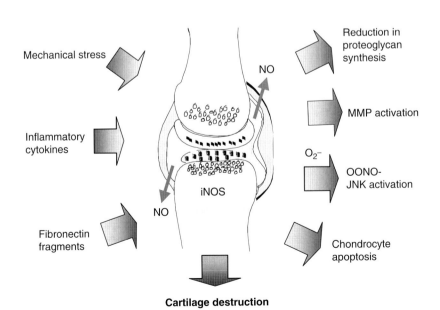

Cartilage destruction

Figure 24.3 Mechanisms of iNOS-mediated tissue damage in osteoarthritis. iNOS is induced and NO is produced by chondrocytes in osteoarthritis cartilage. Potential inducers of iNOS are shown to the left and the consequences of excessive NO production are shown on the right.

chondrocytes in arthritic cartilage respond poorly to insulin-like growth factor 1 (IGF-1) stimulation of proteoglycan synthesis. Studies with iNOS knockout mice suggest that NO is responsible for part of the cartilage insensitivity to IGF-1.[63] Studer et al have reported that chondrocyte insensitivity to the anabolic effects of IGF-1 is due to NO-dependent inhibition of IGF-1 receptor autophosphorylation.[63]

As is indicated from the above, NO, and its derivative peroxynitrite, promote what may be termed a 'catabolic phenotype' in chondrocytes. To better understand the cellular mechanisms that mediate these actions, recent studies have focused upon NO signaling through three intra-cellular mitogen-activated protein kinase (MAPK) pathways: c-Jun NH_2-terminal kinase (JNK; also called stress-activated protein kinase), extracellular signal-regulated protein kinase (ERK)-1/2, and p38 kinase.[40,64] Clancy et al have demonstrated activated JNK in the cytoplasm of OA, but not normal, chondrocytes.[40] JNK activa-tion in chondrocytes is attenuated by the NOS inhibitor L-NMMA, can be induced by exposure to peroxynitrite, and is associated with increased collagenase production and apoptosis.[40] NO-dependent activation of stress-related proteins in chondrocytes has also been shown by Tomita et al.[32] These authors report that NO inhibits chondrocyte mitochondrial respiration and ATP synthesis, effects which result in the suppression of proteoglycan synthesis. Kim et al examined the role of ERK-1/2 and p38 kinase in NO-induced apoptosis of rabbit articular chondro-cytes.[64] In these studies, NO caused inhibition of type II collagen expression and proteoglycan synthesis, apoptosis, p53 accumulation and caspase-3 activation. The authors provide evidence that NO-induced p38 kinase acts as a signal for apoptosis, whereas ERK activity provides an anti-apoptotic signal.

Firestein and coworkers have shown that JNK is highly activated in RA, but not OA, fibroblast like synoviocytes and synovium.[65] Using JNK knockout mice, these authors provide evidence that JNK is a critical MAPK pathway for IL-1-induced collagenase gene expression in synovio-cytes and is therefore a potential therapeutic

target for RA. In comparing studies of RA and OA, it is of interest that JNK activation, demon-strable in OA chondrocytes,[40] was not observed in OA synovium.[65] Similarly, van't Hof et al examined RA and OA synovial tissue for evidence of iNOS production and apoptosis.[62] The numbers of apoptotic cells were greatly increased in rheumatoid synovium compared with OA synovium. Immunohistochemistry showed co-localization of iNOS staining and apoptosis in the RA synovial lining layer. The NOS inhibitor L-NMMA strongly inhibited apoptosis in explant cultures of RA synovium. This study indicates that NO acts as a mediator of apoptosis in RA and suggests that NOS inhibitors reverse this process. Finally, in RA there is evidence that mutations in the tumor suppressor gene p53 may contribute to the trans-formed-appearing phenotype of synovial fibrob-lasts. It has been proposed that the production of NO and other reactive oxidant species in the RA synovium accounts for mutations in the p53 tumor suppressor gene.[66] An additional conclu-sion regarding target tissues in OA and RA needs to be drawn from these and other studies: namely, in OA, the absence or inconsistent detec-tion of inflammatory mediators in synovial tissue belies the striking production of these same molecules by activated chondrocytes in cartilage.[67,68]

INOS IN RHEUMATIC DISEASES

Animal models: is iNOS a treatment target?

In general, iNOS-derived NO has been viewed as a tissue-damaging free radical produced by activated macrophages infiltrating affected tissues.[69] Early reports of the beneficial effects of NOS inhibitors in experimental models of inflammatory arthritis, OA and SLE[44–46,70–72] reinforced the notion that NO exerted deleteri-ous effects in rheumatic diseases, and was a clear target for therapeutic intervention (Table 24.4).

Experimental models of inflammatory arthri-tis, including collagen-induced arthritis, adjuvant-induced arthritis and streptococcal cell

Table 24.4   Role of NO in selected rheumatic diseases.

Disease	Animal models	Human disease
Rheumatoid arthritis	L-NMMA attenuates disease; exacerbated by iNOS inhibitor, L-NIL, and in NOS$^{-/-}$ animals	Synovial fibroblasts spontaneously produce NO; increased expression of blood mononuclear cell iNOS; ex vivo peripheral mononuclear cell nitrite production correlates with disease; contributes to p53 mutation in synovial cells; induces TNF-α in synoviocytes
Osteoarthritis	iNOS inhibitors attenuate canine and murine OA; iNOS$^{-/-}$ mice protected	Spontaneously produced by OA cartilage; expression in chondrocytes promotes catabolic phenotype and apoptosis
SLE	L-NMMA attenuates glomerulonephritis and arthritis in MRL-lpr mice; iNOS$^{-/-}$ MRL-lpr mice not protected from the development of nephritis and arthritis, but vasculitis decreased	Serum elevations of nitrate, nitroso-proteins during active disease; elevated circulating endothelial cells, which express nitrotyrosine; iNOS induction in endothelium and keratinocytes

L-NMMA, *N*-monomethyl-L-arginine, a non-specific NOS inhibitor; L-NIL, *N*-iminoethyl-lysine, a specific iNOS inhibitor.

wall arthritis, can each be suppressed by the non-specific NOS inhibitor L-NMMA.[44,45] In the adjuvant-induced arthritis animals, the onset of symptoms was preceded by elevated production of nitrates and nitrites. L-NMMA blocked NO biosynthesis, paw swelling, and histopathological changes in ankle joints. Van den Berg et al have studied the development of experimental OA in iNOS-deficient mice induced by the local injection of bacterial collagenase.[73] iNOS deficiency prevented chondrocyte proteoglycan synthesis inhibition in the arthritic cartilage and restored normal responsiveness to IGF-1. Osteoarthritic joint pathology was also significantly reduced, including diminished cartilage lesions and osteophyte formation in iNOS-deficient mice. Similarly, iNOS inhibition has been shown to attenuate the course of experimental OA in dogs.[72]

However, recent studies have provided evidence that iNOS inhibition may prove less feasible for systemic inflammatory disease than had previously been anticipated. McCartney-Francis et al observed that the selective inhibition of iNOS exacerbated erosive joint disease in the streptococcal cell wall model.[15] In these studies, while the authors confirmed their prior observations that the non-specific NOS inhibitor L-NMMA attenuated synovitis, they unexpectedly observed that the iNOS-specific inhibitor, L-NIL, increased the chronic inflammatory response. Immunohistochemical analyses revealed endothelial and neuronal NOS expression in the inflamed synovium. Consistent with these findings, Veihelmann et al have reported the exacerbation of antigen-induced arthritis (AIA) in iNOS-deficient mice.[74] Swelling of the knee joint and leukocyte infiltration were enhanced in the iNOS$^{-/-}$ arthritic animals compared with iNOS$^{+/+}$ mice with AIA. AIA-associated leukocyte–endothelial cell interaction in synovial postcapillary venules was more pronounced in iNOS$^{-/-}$, compared with iNOS$^{+/+}$, arthritic mice. Strong expression of P-selectin and VCAM-1 was observed in the iNOS$^{-/-}$ arthritic mice only. These data suggest that NO production by iNOS in vivo has anti-inflammatory effects in experimental arthritis, by mediating a reduction in leukocyte adhesion and infiltration. Exacerbation of disease by iNOS inhibitors has also been observed in other experimental models of systemic inflammatory or autoimmune disease, including encephalomyelitis (EAE), myasthenia gravis-like autoimmune disease, colitis in HLA-B27 transgenic rats, and TNF-induced shock of mice.[9,73–77]

In summary, animal studies illustrate that iNOS plays a complex role in autoimmunity and tissue injury that may be summarized as follows: (1) iNOS-derived NO can contribute to cytotoxic tissue injury at local sites; (2) constitutive isoforms of NOS, ecNOS and ncNOS, can represent alternate sources of tissue-injuring NO in chronic inflammatory states; (3) iNOS exerts complex effects on immunoregulatory cells – namely, iNOS-derived NO may function as a negative feedback regulator of autoimmunity, perhaps via preferential inhibition of Th1 cells, or T-cell deletion, and may thereby protect the host against immunopathological injury;[9,78] and (4) NO exerts anti-inflammatory effects in the microcirculation by inhibiting leukocyte–endothelial cell interactions. These divergent effects of NO, which depend upon the redox form of NO produced in the microenvironment, the target cells in tissue, and immune cell regulation, make it difficult to predict the consequences of systemic iNOS inhibition as a treatment strategy in autoimmune diseases. While it is very likely that the excessive local production of NO contributes to injury of target tissues in rheumatic disease (e.g. joints, kidney, blood vessel, central nervous system (CNS)), studies in animals indicate that there are complex effects of NO on lymphocyte proliferation, Th1/Th2 balance, apoptosis and tolerance that need further elucidation.[53]

Human disease

Systemic lupus erythematosus

Excessive NO production in patients with SLE has been reported by this and other laboratories.[8] Serum nitrite is elevated in SLE patients and correlates with both SLEDAI (DAI, disease activity index) and titers of antibodies to double-stranded DNA.[8,79] Serum 3–nitrotyrosine levels are also elevated in SLE, particularly in patients with renal disease.[79] iNOS is induced in a variety of cell types during active disease. In murine studies, for example, peritoneal macrophages and splenic and renal tissue are sites of increased NOS expression.[46] Similarly, studies by Oates et al demonstrated the expression of iNOS in kidney biopsies of SLE patients with active proliferative nephritis.[79] Studies by Brundin et al[80] in neuropsychiatric SLE have demonstrated elevated cerebrospinal fluid (CSF) levels of nitrite, suggesting CNS expression of iNOS. In a related study, these authors also reported that increased levels of CSF nitrite and nitrate were associated with more severe neurological symptoms. We have demonstrated in biopsies of non-lesional skin that endothelial cells and keratinocytes express the inducible isoform of NOS during periods of active SLE.[8] Increased expression by endothelial cells of iNOS correlated with evidence of increased disease activity (SLEDAI, anti-DNA, C3a).[8] The upregulation of endothelial iNOS in vivo was consistent with our prior demonstration that histologically normal appearing vascular endothelium in active SLE exhibits increased expression of the adhesion molecules E-selectin, ICAM-1 and VCAM-1. Immune stimuli, which may account for endothelial cell activation in SLE, include immune complexes, complement components (e.g. C5a, C5b-9, C1q,), anti-endothelial cell antibodies, anti-cardiolipin antibodies, and cytokines such as IL-1 or TNF. While the effect of endothelial iNOS overexpression is uncertain, we speculate that it is associated with endothelial cell injury, peroxynitrite production, apoptosis and detachment from the basement membrane. Support for this hypothesis derives from our recent observation that flares of SLE are accompanied by elevated levels of circulating endothelial cells, a proxy for vascular injury, and that these circulating cells express iNOS and have detectable nitrotyrosine by fluorescence-activated cell sorting (FACS) analysis.[81] The potential for circulating endothelial cells to participate in microinfarction has been previously suggested in studies of sickle cell anemia and acute myocardial infarction.[81]

Rheumatoid arthritis

Increased concentrations of nitrites have been demonstrated within the joint fluids of patients with OA and RA. iNOS expression has been demonstrated in both RA and OA synoviocytes and chondrocytes by in situ hybridization and immunohistochemistry.[82] McInnes et al demonstrated that cultures of rheumatoid synovial tissue spontaneously produce NO, with immunochemical staining indicating that the majority of cells expressing iNOS are fibroblasts.[83] These authors also reported that synoviocytes, and macrophage cell lines, cultured with the NO donor S-nitroso-acetylpenicillamine, produced high concentrations of TNF-α, suggesting that NO may mediate pathology in RA through the induction of TNF-α production.[83] St Clair et al examined patients with RA and reported increased expression of blood mononuclear cell iNOS in RA patients.[14] In these studies, the degree of peripheral mononuclear cell nitrite production ex vivo correlated with disease activity, leading the authors to suggest that increased iNOS expression and NO generation may be important in the pathogenesis of RA. Subsequently, this group demonstrated that increased peripheral blood mononuclear cell (PBMC) expression of iNOS and iNOS enzyme activity were reduced following treatment with the anti-TNF monoclonal antibody infliximab. Changes in NOS activity following treatment correlated significantly with changes in the number of tender joints.

Osteoarthritis

NO production by joint tissues has been reported in both OA and RA. In OA, iNOS upregulation is predominantly observed in the chondrocytes of articular cartilage; in RA, both synovial tissue fibroblasts and articular chondrocytes express iNOS. Cartilage obtained at surgery from OA and RA patients undergoing joint replacement surgery expresses inducible NOS and spontaneously produces micromolar concentrations of NO when cultured ex vivo.[84] Normal cartilage does not produce NO or express NOS unless stimulated with cytokines such as IL-1. The chondrocyte NOS induced in both OA and RA cartilage is of particular interest, since its expression is not inhibited by either TGF-β or hydrocortisone.[84] The spontaneous production of NO by OA cartilage explants is sustained for up to 2 weeks ex vivo, but ceases if chondrocytes are released and grown in monolayer culture, indicating the importance of the diseased extracellular matrix (ECM) in maintaining the catabolic phenotype of the chondrocyte.

Several factors have been elucidated that modulate the induction of iNOS and other inflammatory mediators in OA cartilage. These include: (1) gene induction following mechanical stress; (2) catabolic cytokines produced by chondrocytes; and (3) abnormally expressed ECM proteins, particularly fibronectin fragments and osteopontin (Figure 24.3).[85–89] The induction of inflammatory gene products in response to altered biomechanical stress is an important concept in the emerging paradigm of disease perpetuation in OA. Fermor et al examined the the effects of static and intermittent compression on NOS activity, NO production, and NOS antigen expression by porcine articular cartilage explants.[17] Immunoblot analysis showed stress-induced upregulation of iNOS, but not ecNOS or nNOS. In related studies, this group[90] has investigated the relationship between mechanical stress and the production of leukotriene B$_4$ (LTB$_4$) and NO in explants of porcine articular cartilage subjected to mechanical stress in the presence or absence of the NOS2 inhibitor 1400W. Dynamic compression significantly increased LTB$_4$ and lipoxygenase (LOX) protein production in the presence of 1400W. The data suggest that LOX induction can be downregulated by concomitantly induced NO.

Altered biomechanical factors may induce the initial expression and perpetuate the release of inflammatory mediators in OA chondrocytes. However, since cartilage explants spontaneously produce inflammatory mediators ex vivo for up to 2 weeks in culture, there must be additional stimuli within diseased cartilage that sustain the activated state. Among these, perhaps the most central is IL-1.[68] OA chondrocytes in cartilage explants express IL-1β mRNA and spontaneously release detectable amounts of IL-1β protein.[67] Gene array analysis of human (normal and OA-affected) cartilage also reveals mRNA expression of IL-1 receptor accessory protein (IL-1RAcp) and IL-1 type I receptor (IL-1RI), but not IL-1 antagonist (IL-1ra) and IL-1 type II decoy receptor (IL-1RII).[91] The addition of types I and II recombinant soluble IL-1β receptor (sIL-1RI, sIL-1RII) significantly attenuates the spontaneous release of NO in OA cartilage explants,[67,91] consistent with an autocrine/paracrine action of secreted IL-1β. It is important to note that while IL-1β is among the key stimuli for iNOS induction in OA chondrocytes, it is induced NO that mediates selected IL-1 effects, such as apoptosis and inhibition of proteoglycan synthesis.[44,67] Moreover, to further amplify the process, NO promotes the production of IL-1, via its capacity to activate MAPκ and NFκB signaling pathways.[67,72,91,92] IL-1β also upregulates the expression of the chemokine RANTES by chondrocytes, which has been demonstrated to also induce the expression of iNOS and stimulates the release of matrix metalloproteinase.[93]

One consequence of this inflammatory cascade in OA cartilage is the activation of metalloproteinases with associated degradation and altered expression of ECM proteins. Increased expression of ECM proteins such as fibronectin, fibronectin fragments, collagen fragments, osteonectin and osteopontin is characteristic of OA cartilage, and it is now believed that these proteins exert effects on cartilage homeostasis.[87,94,95] For example, fibronectin fragments promote matrix degradation via the induction of metalloproteinases, in a process that depends upon IL-1 and involves the production of NO.[86-88] Signal transduction studies reveal that fibronectin fragments induce NO and IL-1 production in association with activation of focal adhesion kinase (FAK) and the MAP kinases ERK, p38 kinase and JNK.[94]

The expression of the ECM protein osteopontin is upregulated in OA cartilage compared to controls.[89] Functional analysis of the role of osteopontin in OA cartilage showed that: (1) recombinant osteopontin inhibited spontaneous and IL-1β-induced NO and prostaglandin E_2 (PGE_2) production by human OA explant cultures; and (2) neutralization of intra-articular osteopontin with anti-osteopontin antiserum augmented NO production. These data indicate that one of the functions of osteopontin in OA cartilage is to act as an innate inhibitor of IL-1, NO and PGE_2 production. Such observations, however, need to be reconciled with those of Petro et al, who have reported that osteopontin is produced by RA synovial tissue and that its effect on chondrocytes is to enhance collagenase 1 production.[96]

We have also examined the effects of ligation of the receptors for fibronectin and osteopontin, $\alpha_5\beta_1$ and $a_v\beta_3$, respectively.[85] Ligation of $\alpha_5\beta_1$ using activating monoclonal antibody (JBS7) induced the production of NO and PGE_2 as well as the cytokines, IL-1, IL-6 and IL-8. Upregulation of these proinflammatory mediators by $\alpha_5\beta_1$ integrin ligation was dependent upon autocrine production of IL-1, since type II soluble IL-1 decoy receptor inhibited their production. In contrast, an activating monoclonal antibody (LM609) to the integrin $\alpha_v\beta_3$ mimicked the effects of the natural ligand osteopontin, attenuating the production of IL-1, NO and PGE_2 in response to a variety of stimuli, including ligation of $\alpha_5\beta_1$ or stimulation with IL-1, IL-18 or TNF. These data demonstrate cross-talk in signaling mechanisms among integrins and show that integrin-mediated 'outside in' signaling very probably influences cartilage homeostasis, including the production of IL-1 and NO. Alterations of ECM, therefore, in OA may contribute to the progression of disease by sustaining the catabolic phenotype of the chondrocyte.

NITRIC OXIDE AS A THERAPEUTIC TARGET

NO, because of its potential cytotoxic effects, represents a potential novel target for pharmacological intervention in selected rheumatic diseases. Until recently, it was generally held that the ideal NOS inhibitors would target the iNOS isoform in order to spare the physiological functions of constitutively expressed NOS in vessels, brain and other tissues. However, recent animal studies, using iNOS inhibitors and iNOS-deficient mice, have unexpectedly shown enhanced tissue injury in several different models of systemic autoimmune diseases. These in vivo models have indicated that iNOS expression in the microcirculation protects against leukocyte mediated endothelial injury, and that other NOS isoforms (ecNOS and ncNOS) may be expressed at inflammatory sites. Thus, specific iNOS inhibitors may be problematic for the treatment of complex systemic diseases. It is more likely, in the near term, that iNOS inhibitors could be of greater value in the treatment of OA, where in vitro and in vivo studies consistently indicate a catabolic role for NO production in progressive disease.

It should be noted that agents currently employed in the treatment of rheumatic diseases have been reported to inhibit NO activity (Table 24.5). Glucocorticoids and cyclosporins inhibit the induction of iNOS in several tissues (although chondrocyte iNOS expression is resistant to corticosteroids). Non-steroidal anti-inflammatory drugs such as aspirin and sodium salicylate inhibit the expression of iNOS protein in murine macrophages; aspirin also inhibits the specific activity of iNOS in cell-free extracts, suggesting direct acetylation of the enzyme.[97] These effects are not shared by indomethacin, thus indicating that effects on NOS are independent of the capacity to inhibit prostaglandin production. We and others have reported that tetracyclines inhibit NO production by both chondrocytes and macrophages.[98,99] Finally, several agents used in the treatment of OA,

including hyaluronan, glucosamine and diacerein, have been shown to inhibit NO production by activated chondrocytes in vitro.[100–103] Whether any of the therapeutic benefits of the above currently available agents derive from their capacity to inhibit NO production is unknown at present.

SUMMARY

In summary, the overproduction of NO has been demonstrated in a wide variety of rheumatic diseases. When it is produced by activated leukocytes at inflammatory sites, the predominant effects of NO are to react with locally produced oxidants to form peroxynitrite and promote tissue injury and apoptosis. Similarly, the predominant effects of NO overproduction by chondrocytes in arthritic cartilage are deleterious, decreasing proteoglycan synthesis, enhancing its degradation, promoting apoptosis and mediating selected IL-1 effects. In contrast, the effects of NO in systemic disease are complex, since NO is produced and exerts pleiotroic actions at multiple sites. Thus, while cytotoxic effects may prevail in joint tissue, the potential immunomodulatory effects of NO on Th1/Th2 cells and tolerance, or upon leukocyte–endothelial cell interactions, may be protective. Future progress in targeting NO as a therapeutic strategy will depend upon better insights into the actions of NO at specific sites, elucidation of the redox forms of NO produced, and developing NOS isoform-specific, tissue-targeted approaches to treatment.

ACKNOWLEDGMENTS

I would like to thank Ms Maddy Rios for her assistance in the preparation of this manuscript.

REFERENCES

1. Ignarro LJ, Buga GM, Wood KS, Byrns RE, Chaudhuri G. Endothelium-derived relaxing factor produced and released from artery and vein is nitric oxide. *Proc Natl Acad Sci USA* 1987; **84**: 9265–9.

2. Moncada S, Higgs A. The L-arginine–nitric oxide pathway . *N Engl J Med* 1993; **329**(27): 2002–12.

3. Trimmer BA, Aprille JR, Dudzinski DM et al. Nitric oxide and the control of firefly flashing. *Science* 2001; **292**: 2486–8.

4. Clancy RM, Amin AR, Abramson SB. The role of nitric oxide in inflammation and immunity. *Arthritis Rheum* 1998; **41**:1141–52.

5. Nathan C. Perspectives Series: Nitric oxide and nitric oxide synthases. Inducible nitric oxide synthase: what difference does it make? *J Clin Invest* 1997; **100**: 2417–23.

6. Christopherson KS, Bredt DS. Perspectives Series: Nitric oxide and nitric oxide synthases. Nitric oxide in excitable tissues: physiological roles and disease. *J Clin Invest* 1997; **100**: 2424–9.

7. Stuehr DJ. Mammalian nitric oxide synthases. *Biochim Biophys Acta* 1999; **1411**: 217–30.

8. Belmont HM, Levartovsky D, Goel A et al. Increased nitric oxide production accompanied by the up-regulation of inducible nitric oxide synthase in vascular endothelium from patients with systemic lupus erythematosus. *Arthritis Rheum* 1997; **40**: 1810–16.

9. Bogdan C. Nitric oxide and the immune response. *Nat Immunol* 2001; **2**: 907–16.

10. Taylor-Robinson AW, Liew FY, Severn A et al. Regulation of the immune response by nitric oxide differentially produced by T helper 1 and T helper type 2 cells. *Eur J Immunol* 1994; **24**: 980–4.

11. Thuring H, Stenger S, Gmehling D, Rollinghoff M, Bogdan C. Lack of inducible nitric oxide synthase activity in T cell clones and T lymphocytes from naive and Leishmania major-infected mice. *Eur J Immunol* 1995; **25**: 3229–34.

12. Bauer H, Jung T, Tsikas D, Stichtenoth DO, Frolich JC, Neumann C. Nitric oxide inhibits the secretion of T-helper 1- and T-helper 2-associated cytokines in activated human T cells. *Immunology* 1997; **90**: 205–11.

13. Sharara AI, Perkins DJ, Misukonis MA, Chan SU, Dominitz JA, Weinberg JB. Interferon (IFN)-alpha activation of human blood mononuclear cells in vitro and in vivo for nitric oxide synthase (NOS) type 2 mRNA and protein expression: possible relationship of induced NOS2 to the anti-hepatitis C effects of IFN-alpha in vivo. *J Exp Med* 1997; **186**: 1495–502.

14. St Clair EW, Wilkinson WE, Lang T et al. Increased expression of blood mononuclear cell nitric oxide synthase type 2 in rheumatoid arthritis patients. *J Exp Med* 1996; **184**: 1173–8.

15. McCartney-Francis NL, Song X, Mizel DE, Wahl SM. Selective inhibition of inducible nitric oxide synthase exacerbates erosive joint disease. *J Immunol* 2001; **666**: 2734–40.

16. MacMicking J, Zie Q-w, Nathan C. Nitric oxide and macrophage function. *Annu Rev Immunol* 1997; **15**: 323–50.

17. Fermor B, Weinberg JB, Pisetsky DS, Misukonis MA, Banes AJ, Guilak F. The effects of static and intermittent compression on nitric oxide production in articular cartilage explants. *J Orth Res* 2001; **19**: 729–37.

18. Kleinert H, Wallerath T, Fritz G et al. Cytokine induction of NO synthase II in human DLD-1 cells: roles of the JAK-STAT, AP-1 and NF-B-signaling pathways. *Br J Pharmacol* 1998; **125**: 193–201.

19. Dlaska M, Weiss G. Central role of transcription factor NF-IL6 for cytokine and iron mediated regulation of murine inducible nitric oxide synthase expression. *J Immunol* 1999; **162**: 6171–7.

20. Pellacani A, Wiesel P, Razavi S et al. Down-regulation of high mobility group-I(Y) protein contributes to the inhibition of nitric oxide synthase 2 by transforming growth factor-1. *J Biol Chem* 2001; **276**: 1653–9.

21. Ganster RW, Taylor BS, Shao L, Geller DA. Complex regulation of human iNOS gene transcription by Stat1 and NF-B. *Proc Natl Acad Sci USA* 2001; **98**: 8638–43.

22. Karaghiosoff M, Neubauer H, Lassnig C et al. Partial impairment of cytokine responses in Tyk2-deficient mice. *Immunity* 2000; **13**: 549–60.

23. Chakravortty D, Kato Y, Sugiyama T et al. The inhibitory action of sodium arsenite on lipopolysaccharide-induced nitric oxide production in RAW 267.4 macrophage cells: a role of Raf-1 in lipopolysaccharide signaling. *J Immunol* 2001; **166**: 2011–17.

24. Chan ED, Morris KR, Belisle JT et al. Induction of inducible nitric oxide synthase-NO by lipoarabionomannan of mycobacterium tuberculosis is mediated by the MEK1-ERK, MKK7 JNK and NF-B signaling pathways. *J Biol Chem* 2001; **276**: 8445–52.

25. Kristof AS, Marks-Konczalik J, Moss J. Mitogen-activated protein kinases mediate activator protein-1 dependent human inducible nitric oxide synthase promotor activation. *J Biol Chem* 2001; **276**: 8445–52.

26. Connelly L, Palacios-Calender M, Ameixa C, Moncada S, Hobbs AJ. Biphasic regulation of NF-B activity underlies the pro- and anti-inflammatory actions of nitric oxide. *J Immunol* 2001; **166**: 3873–81.

27. Musial A, Eissa NT. Inducible nitric oxide synthase is regulated by the proteasome degradation pathway. *J Biol Chem* 2001; **276**: 24268–73.

28. Nicholson B, Manner CK, Kleeman J, MacLeod CL. Sustained nitric oxide production in macrophages requires the arginine transporter CAT2. *J Biol Chem* 2001; **276**: 15881–5.
29. Gotoh T, Mori M. Arginase II downregulates nitric oxide (NO) production and prevents NO-mediated apoptosis in murine macrophage-derived RAW264.7 cells. *J Cell Biol* 1999; **144**: 427–34.
30. Munder M, Eichmann K, Moran JM, Centeno F, Soler G, Modolell M. Th1/Th2-regulated expression of arginase isoforms in murine macrophages and dendritic cells. *J Immunol* 1999; **163**: 3771–7.
31. Stamler JS, Singel DJ, Loscalzo J. Biochemistry of nitric oxide and its redox-activated forms. *Science* 1992; **258**: 1898–902.
32. Tomita M, Sato EF, Nishikawa M, Yamano Y, Inoue M. Nitric oxide regulates mitochondrial respiration and functions of articular chondrocytes. *Arthritis Rheum* 2001; **44**: 96–104.
33. Myers PR, Minor Jr RL, Guerra Jr R, Bates JN, Harrison DG. Vasorelaxant properties of the endothelium-derived relaxing factor more closely resemble S-nitrosocysteine than nitric oxide. *Nature* 1990; **345**: 161–3.
34. Pryor WA, Squadrito GL. The chemistry of peroxynitrite: a product from the reaction of nitric oxide with superoxide. *Am J Physiol* 1995; **268**: L-699–722.
35. Clancy RM, Leszczynska-Piziak J, Abramson SB. Nitric oxide, an endothelial cell relaxation factor, inhibits neutrophil superoxide anion production via a direct action on the NADPH oxidase. *J Clin Invest* 1992; **90**: 1116–21.
36. Hausladen A, Privalle CT, Keng T, DeAngelo J, Stamler JS. Nitrosative stress: activation of the transcription factor *OxyR*. *Cell* 1996; **86**: 719–29.
37. Clancy RM, Abramson SB. Acetylcholine prevents intercellular adhesion molecule 1 (CD54)-induced focal adhesion complex assembly in endothelial cells via a ntric oxide-cGMP dependent pathway. *Arthritis Rheum* 2000; **43**: 2260–4.
38. Clancy R, Rediske J, Tang X et al. Outside-in signaling in the chondrocyte: nitric oxide disrupts fibronectin-induced assembly of a subplasmalemmal actin/Rho A/focal adhesion kinase signaling complex. *J Clin Invest* 1997; **100**: 1789–96.
39. Parkinson JF, Mitrovic B, Merrill JE. The role of nitric oxide in multiple sclerosis. *J Mol Med* 1997; **75**: 174–86.
40. Clancy R, Rediske J, Koehne C, Stoyanovsky D, Iyama K-i, Abramson SB. Activation of stress activated protein kinase in ostearthritic cartilage: evidence for nitric oxide dependence. *Osteoarth Cartilage* 2001; **9**: 294–9.
41. Fang FC. Perspective Series: First host/pathogen interactions. Mechanisms of nitric oxide related antimicrobial activity. *J Clin Invest* 1997; **99**: 2818–25.
42. DeGroote MA, Fang FC. Antimicrobial properties of nitric oxide. In: Fang FC, ed. *Nitric Oxide and Infection*. (Kluwer Academic/Plenum Publishers, New York, 1999) 231–61.
43. Kubes PM, Suzuki M, Granger DN. Nitric oxide: an endogenous modulator of leukocyte adhesion. *Proc Natl Acad Sci USA* 1991; **88**: 4651–5.
44. Stefanovic-Racic M, Stadler J, Evans CH. Nitric oxide and arthritis. *Arthritis Rheum* 1993; **36**: 1036–44.
45. McCartney-Francis N, Allen JB, Mizel DE et al. Suppression of arthritis by an inhibitor of nitric oxide synthase. *J Exp Med* 1993; **178**: 749–54.
46. Weinberg JB, Granger DL, Pisetsky DS et al. The role of nitric oxide in the pathogenesis of spontaneous murine autoimmune disease: increased nitric oxide production and nitric oxide synthase expression in MRL-lpr/lpr mice, and reduction of spontaneous glomerulonephritis and arthritis by orally administered NG-Monomethyl-L-Arginine. *J Exp Med* 1994; **179**: 651–60.
47. Grisham MB, Granger DN, Lefer DJ. Modulation of leukocyte–endothelial interactions by reactive metabolites of oxygen and nitrogen: relevance to ischemic heart disease. *Free Rad Biol Med* 1998; **25**: 404–33.
48. Spiecker M, Darius H, Kaboth K, Hubner F, Liao JK. Differential regulation of endothelial cell adhesion molecule expression by nitric oxide donors and antioxidants. *J Leukocyte Biol* 1998; **63**: 732–9.
49. Lefer DJ, Jones SP, Girod WG et al. Leukocyte–endothelial cell interactions in nitric oxide synthase-deficient mice. *Am J Physiol* 1999; **276**: H1943–50.
50. Blanchard HS, Dernis-Labous E, Lamarque D et al. Inducible nitric oxide synthase attenuates chronic colitis in human histocompatibility antigen HLA-B27/human b2 microglobulin transgenic rats. *Eur Cytokine Netw* 2001; **12**: 111–18.
51. Efron DT, Kirk SJ, Regan MC, Wasserkrug H, Barbul A. Nitric oxide generation from L arginine

is required for optimal human peripheral blood lymphocyte DNA synthesis. *Surgery* 1991; **110**: 327–34.

52. Merryman PF, Clancy RM, He XH, Abramson SB. Modulation of human T cell responses by nitric oxide and its derivative, S-nitrosoglutathione. *Arthritis Rheum* 1993; **36**: 1414–22.

53. Singh VK, Mehrotra S, Narayan P, Pandey CM, Agarwal SS. Modulation of autoimmune diseases by nitric oxide. *Immunol Res* 2000; **22**: 1–19.

54. Albina JE, Cui S, Mateo RB, Reichner JS. Nitric oxide-mediated apoptosis in murine peritoneal macrophages. *J Immunol* 1997; **150**: 5080–5.

55. Lotz M. The role of nitric oxide in articular cartilage damage. *Rheum Dis Clin North Am* 1999; **25**: 269–82.

56. Kim Y-M, Talanian RV, Billiar R. Nitric oxide inhibits apoptosis by preventing increases in caspase-3-like activity via two distinct mechanisms. *J Biol Chem* 1997; **272**: 31138–48.

57. Brune B, von Knethen A, Sandau KB. Nitric oxide (NO): an effector of apoptosis. *Cell Death Differ* 1999; **6**: 969–75.

58. Moulian N, Truffault F, Gaudry-Talarmain YM, Serraf A, Berrih-Aknin S. In vivo and in vitro apoptosis of human thymocytes are associated with nitrotyrosine formation. *Blood* 2001; **97**: 3521–30.

59. Taskiran D, Stefanovic-Racic M, Georgescu H, Evans C. Nitric oxide mediates suppression of cartilage proteoglycan synthesis by interleukin-1. *Biochem Biophys Res Commun* 1994; **200**: 142–8.

60. Hirai Y, Migita K, Honda S et al. Effects of nitric oxide on matrix metalloproteinase-2 production by rheumatoid synovial cells . *Life Sci* 2001; **68**: 913–20.

61. Clancy R, Abramson SB, Kohne C, Rediske J. Nitric oxide attenuates cellular hexose monophosphate shunt response to oxidants in articular chondrocytes and acts to promote oxidant injury. *J Cell Physiol* 1997; **172**: 183–91.

62. Van't Hof RJ, Hocking L, Wright PK, Ralston SH. Nitric oxide is a mediator of apoptosis in the rheumatoid joint. *Rheumatology (Oxford)* 2000; **39**: 1004–8.

63. Studer RK, Levicoff E, Georgescu H, Miller L, Jaffurs D, Evans CH. Nitric oxide inhibits chondrocyte response to IGF-I: inhibition of IGF-IRbeta tyrosine phosphorylation. *Am J Physiol* 2000; **279**: C961–9.

64. Kim SJ, Ju JW, Oh CD et al. ERL-1/2 and p38 kinase oppositely regulate nitric oxide induced apoptosis of chondrocytes in association with p53, caspase-3, and differentiation status. *J Biol Chem* 2002; **277**: 1332–9.

65. Han Z, Boyle DL, Chang L, Yang L, Manning AM, Firestein GS. c-Jun N-terminal kinase is required for metalloproteinase expression and joint destruction in inflammatory arthritis. *J Clin Invest* 2001; **108**: 73–81.

66. Tak PP, Zvaifler NJ, Green DR, Firestein GS. Rheumatoid arthritis and p53: how oxidative stress might alter the course of inflammatory diseases. *Immunol Today* 2000; **21**: 8–82.

67. Attur MG, Patel IR, Patel RN, Abramson SB, Amin AR. Autocrine production of IL-1 by human osteoarthritis-affected cartilage and differential regulation of endogenous nitric oxide, IL-6, prostaglandin E2 and IL-8. *Proc Assoc Amer Phys* 1998; **110**: 1–8.

68. Pelletier J-P, Martel-Pelletier J, Abramson SB. Osteoarthritis, an inflammatory disease. Potential implication of new therapeutic targets. *Arthritis Rheum* 2001; **44**: 1237–47.

69. Kroncke KD, Fehsel K, Kolb-Bachofen V. Inducible nitric oxide synthase in human diseases. *Clin Exp Immunol* 1998; **113**: 147–56.

70. Keng T, Privalle CT, Gilkeson GS, Weinberg JB. Peroxynitrite formation and decreased catalase activity in autoimmune MRL-lpr/lpr mice. *Mol Med* 2000; **6**: 779–92.

71. Gilkeson G, Mudgett JS, Seldin MF et al. Clinical and serologic manifestations of autoimmune disease in MRL-1pr/lpr mice lacking nitric oxide synthase type 2. *J Exp Med* 1997; **186**: 365–73.

72. Pelletier J-P, Jovanovic V, Lascau-Coman V et al. Selective inhibition of inducible nitric oxide synthase reduces progression of experimental osteoarthritis in vivo: possible link with the reduction in chondrocyte apoptosis and caspase 3 level. *Arthritis Rheum* 2000; **43**: 1290–9.

73. van den Berg WB, van de Loo F, Joosten LA, Arntz OJ. Animal models of arthritis in NOS2-deficient mice. *Osteoarth Cartilage* 1999; **7**: 413–15.

74. Veihelmann A, Landes J, Hofbauer A et al. Exacerbation of antigen-induced arthritis in inducible nitric oxide synthase-deficient mice. *Arthritis Rheum* 2001; **44**: 1420–7.

75. Shi F-D, Flodstrom M, Kim HK et al. Control of the autoimmune response by type 2 nitric oxide synthase. *J Immunol* 2001; **167**: 3000–6.

76. Cauwels A, Van Molle W, Janssen B et al. Protection against TNF-induced lethal shock by soluble guanylate cyclase inhibition requires

functional inducible nitric oxide synthase. *Immunity* 2000; **13**: 223–31.

77. Tarrant TK, Silver PB, Wahlsten JL et al. Interleukin-12 protects from a Th1-mediated autoimmune disease, experimental autoimmune uveitis, through a mechanism involving IFN-, nitric oxide and apotosis. *J Exp Med* 1999; **189**: 219–30.

78. Bogdan C. The multiplex function of nitric oxide in (auto)immunity. *J Exp Med* 1998; **187**: 1361–5.

79. Oates JC, Christensen EF, Reilly CM, Self SE, Gilkeson GS. Prospective measure of serum 3-nitrotyrosine levels in systemic lupus erythematosus: correlation with disease activity. *Proc Assoc Amer Phys* 1999; **111**: 611–21.

80. Brundin L, Svenungsson E, Morcos E et al. Central nervous system nitric oxide formation in cerebral systemic lupus erythematosus. *Ann Neurol* 1998; **44**: 704–6.

81. Clancy R, Marder G, Martin V, Belmont HM, Abramson SB, Buyon J. Circulating activated endothelial cells in systemic lupus erythematosus: further evidence for diffuse vasculopathy. *Arthritis Rheum* 2001; **44**: 1203–8.

82. Sakurai H, Kohsaka H, Liu M-F et al. Nitric oxide production and inducible nitric oxide synthase expression in inflammatory arthritides. *J Clin Invest* 1996; **96**: 2357.

83. McInnes IB, Leung BP, Field M et al. Production of nitric oxide in the synovial membrane of rheumatoid and osteoarthritis patients. *J Exp Med* 1996; **184**: 1519–24.

84. Amin AR, Di Cesare PE, Vyas P et al. The expression and regulation of nitric oxide synthase in human osteoarthritis-affected chondrocytes: evidence for up-regulated neuronal nitric oxide synthase. *J Exp Med* 1995; **182**: 2097.

85. Attur M, Dave M, Abramson SB, Amin AR. Functional genomic analysis in arthritis affected cartilage: Yin-Yang regulation of inflammatory mediators by a5b1 and avb3. *J Immunol* 2000; **164**: 2684–91.

86. Homandberg GA, Meyers R, Williams JM. Intra-articular injection of fibronectin fragments causes severe depletion of cartilage proteoglycans in vivo. *J Rheumatol* 1993; **20**: 1378–82.

87. Homandberg GA, Hui F, Wen C et al. Fibronectin-fragment-induced cartilage chondrolysis is associated with release of catabolic cytokines. *Biochem J* 1997; **321**: 751–7.

88. Arner EC, Tortorella MD. Signal transduction through chondrocyte integrin receptors induces matrix metalloproteinase synthesis and synergizes with interleukin-1 . *Arthritis Rheum* 1995; **38**: 1304–14.

89. Attur MG, Dave M, Stuchin S et al. Osteopontin: an intrinsic inhibitor of inflammation in cartilage. *Arthritis Rheum* 2001; **44**: 578–84.

90. Fermor B, Haribabu B, Weinberg JB, Pisetsky DS, Guilak F. Mechanical stress and nitric oxide influence leukotriene production in cartilage. *Biochem Biophys Res Commun* 2001; **285**: 806–10.

91. Attur MG, Dave M, Cipoletta C et al. Reversal of autocrine and paracrine effects of IL-1 in human arthritis by type II IL-1 receptor: potential for pharmacological intervention. *J Biol Chem* 2000; **22**(275): 40307–15.

92. Pelletier J-P, Lascau-Coman V, Jovanovic D et al. Selective inhibition of inducible nitric oxide synthase in experimental osteoarthritis is associated with reduction in tissue levels of catabolic factors. *J Rheumatol* 1999; **26**: 2002–14.

93. Alaaeddine N, Olee T, Hashimoto S, Creighton-Achermann L, Lotz M. Production of the chemokine RANTES by articular chondrocytes and role in cartilage degradation. *Arthritis Rheum* 2001; **44**: 1633–43.

94. Gemba T, Valbracht J, Alsalameh S, Lotz M. Focal adhesion kinase and mitogen-activated protein kinases are involved in chondrocyte activation by the 29-kDa amino-terminal fibronectin fragment. *J Biol Chem* 2002; **277**: 907–11.

95. Attur MG, Patel RN, Patel PD, Abramson SB, Amin AR. Tetracycline up-regulates COX-2 expression and prostaglandin E2 production independent of its effect on nitric oxide. *J Immunol* 1999; **162**: 3160–7.

96. Petro PK, Hummel KM, Schedel J et al. Expression of osteopontin messenger RNA and protein in rheumatoid arthritis: effects of osteopontin on the release of collagenase 1 from articular chondrocytes and synovial fibroblasts. *Arthritis Rheum* 2001; **43**: 1597–605.

97. Amin AR, Vyas P, Attur M et al. The mode of action of aspirin-like drugs: effect on inducible nitric oxide synthase. *Proc Natl Acad Sci USA* 1995; **92**: 7926–30.

98. Amin AR, Attur MG, Thakker GD et al. A novel mechanism of action of tetracyclines: effects on nitric oxide synthases. *Proc Natl Acad Sci USA* 1996; **93**: 14014–19.

99. Sadowski T, Steinmeyer J. Minocycline inhibits the production of inducible nitric oxide synthase in articular chondrocytes. *J Rheumatol* 2001; **28**: 336–40.

100. Takahashi K, Hashimoto S, Kubo T, Hirasawa Y, Lotz M, Amiel D. Hyaluronan suppressed nitric oxide production in the miniscus and synovium of rabbit osteoarthritis model. *J Orth Res* 2001; **19**: 500–3.

101. Meininger CJ, Kelly KA, Li H, Haune TE, Wu G. Glucosamine inhibits inducible nitric oxide synthesis . *Biochem Biophys Res Commun* 2000; **279**: 234–9.

102. Shikhman AR, Kuhn K, Alaaeddine N, Lotz M. N-acetylglucosamine prevents IL-1beta mediated activation of human chondrocytes. *J Immunol* 2001; **166**: 5155–60.

103. Smith GN Jr, Myers SL, Brandt KD, Mickler EA, Albrecht MD. Diacerhein treatment reduces the severity of osteoarthritis in the canine cruciate-deficiency model of osteoarthritis. *Arthritis Rheum* 1999; **42**: 545–55.

25

Cyclooxygenase and prostaglandin synthase

Leslie J Crofford

Introduction • Prostaglandin biology • Cyclooxygenase • Prostaglandin E synthase (PGES) • Summary • References

INTRODUCTION

Prostaglandins (PGs) are central mediators of the cardinal signs of inflammation – pain (dolor), swelling (tumor), erythema (rubor), and warmth (calor). Therapeutic strategies that inhibit PG production have been used in the treatment of pain and inflammation for centuries, beginning with botanical treatments in both Western and Eastern medical traditions.[1] Aspirin and non-steroidal anti-inflammatory drugs (NSAIDs) share anti-iflammatory, analgesic and antipyretic properties due to inhibition of PG synthesis, demonstrating conclusively that PGs play an important role in mediating symptoms of arthritis. The field of PG biology was revolutionized with the discovery that certain isoforms of the synthetic enzymes are highly regulated during inflammation.[2] This chapter will discuss the discovery and characterization of these novel targets for anti-inflammatory therapy in the rheumatic diseases. One such target, cyclooxygenase (COX)-2, has led to the development of specific inhibitors whose pharmacology will also be discussed.

PROSTAGLANDIN BIOLOGY

Prostaglandin biosynthesis

PGs are members of a family of lipid mediators, termed eicosanoids (eicosa = 20), derived from the 20-carbon-containing polyunsaturated fatty acid containing four double bonds (C20:4ω6) called eicosatetraenoic or arachidonic acid (AA).[3] PGs were initially characterized in the 1930s by their physiologic functions. In vitro synthesis was accomplished in 1964 using AA and an enzyme preparation of ram seminal vesicles.[4]

Generation of PGs requires the action of three synthetic enzymes (Figure 25.1). PG synthesis is initiated when phospholipase enzymes, most commonly a phospholipase A_2 (PLA$_2$), release AA from cell membranes.[5] There are multiple different PLA$_2$ enzymes, but it is likely that the cytosolic form (cPLA$_2$) is most important during inflammation.[6] AA can be metabolized to a number of stable bioactive lipid modulators of inflammation, the most abundant being PGs and leukotrienes (LTs).

The first committed step in PG biosynthesis is the insertion of oxygen and formation of a cyclopentane ring to form PGG$_2$. PGG$_2$ subsequently undergoes a two-electron reduction of a hydroperoxyl to a hydroxyl group to form PGH$_2$ (Figure 25.2).[7] Both the cyclooxygenase and peroxidase reactions are catalyzed by one of the isoforms of prostaglandin H synthase (PGH synthase) also called cyclooxygenase or COX. There is strong evidence that these reactions occur at distinct catalytic sites.[7] PGH$_2$ is an

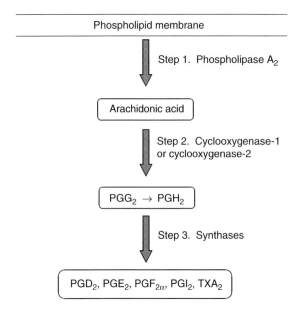

Figure 25.1 Prostaglandin (PG) and thromboxane (TX) synthetic pathway. Synthesis of PGs and TX requires the action of three different enzymes. There are different families of phospholipase A_2s, secretory (sPLA$_2$) and cytoplasmic (cPLA$_2$) being the best characterized. Either of the two cyclooxygenase enzymes, COX-1 or COX-2, catalyze the first committed step towards PG synthesis. Both PGG$_2$ and PGH$_2$ are unstable intermediates, but stable PGs or TX are formed by several cell-specific synthases.

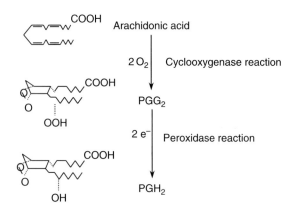

Figure 25.2 Reactions catalyzed by prostaglandin H synthase. The first committed step to PG synthesis is the insertion of two molecules of oxygen to form the cyclopentane ring of PGG$_2$, the cyclooxygenase reaction. The subsequent peroxidase reaction, a two-electron reduction of the hydroperoxyl to a hydroxyl group at carbon 15, results in the formation of PGH$_2$. Both reactions are carried out by a single enzyme, PGH synthase, that is also called cyclooxygenase (COX). Both isoforms of the COX enzyme perform identical reactions, though the COX-2 enzyme can use alternative substrates and can form different products after it has been acetylated by aspirin. (Reproduced with permission from the *Annual Review of Biochemistry*, volume 69 © 2000 by Annual Reviews, www.annualreviews.org.)

unstable intermediate that is further converted to one of a series of possible PGs by a synthase enzyme. In general, the process is cell specific, with cells producing only one or two prostanoids in abundance. PGs are released outside the cell and are believed to work locally, near their site of production. Certain PGs may also have intracellular targets, leading to direct effects on gene expression.

Prostaglandin receptors

The major PG subclasses are thromboxane A_2 (TXA$_2$), prostacyclin (PGI$_2$), PGF$_{2\alpha}$, PGD$_2$, and PGE$_2$. In biological fluids, PGD$_2$ and PGE$_2$ are slowly dehydrated to yield the cyclopentanone

PGs, PGA$_2$ and PGJ$_2$.[8] The cyclopentanone PGs contain a highly reactive α,β-unsaturated ketone moiety that may be important to their action.

A family of G-protein-coupled cell surface receptors (GPCRs) with seven transmembrane domains mediates PG actions, though there is evidence suggesting nuclear receptors, particularly for the cyclopentanone PGs.[8] The number of receptors and their different G-protein associations mediate the diversity of PG actions (Table 25.1). Several cell surface PG receptors have been cloned and characterized, some of which have splice variants affecting the C-terminal cytoplasmic tails.[9] There are four receptors for PGE$_2$ (EP receptors) with different G-protein-linked signaling pathways. Molecular evolution

Table 25.1 Prostaglandin receptors.

Receptor	Splice variants?	Natural ligands	G protein coupling[a]	Selected actions[b]
DP	No	PGD_2	G_s; increased cAMP	Mast cell function, sleep–wake cycles, body temperature
EP1	Yes	PGE_2	G_q; Ca^{2+} moblization	Smooth muscle contraction
EP2	No	PGE_2	G_s; increased cAMP	Smooth muscle relaxation, reproduction, renal function, bone homeostasis
EP3	Yes	PGF_2	G_i; reduced cAMP G_o; Ca^{2+} mobilization and increased cAMP	Fever, gastrointestinal mucosal integrity
EP4	No	PGE_2	G_s; increased cAMP	Vasodilator, closure of patent ductus arteriosus, bone remodeling
FP	Yes	$PGF_{2\alpha}$[c]	G_q; Ca^{2+} moblization	Parturition
IP	No	PGI_2[c]	G_s; increased cAMP	Nociception, antithrombosis, vasodilation
TP	Yes	TXA_2	G_q; Ca^{2+} mobilization	Platelet aggregation; smooth muscle contraction and proliferation
CRTH2	No	PGD_2	G_i; reduced cAMP	Chemotaxis of T-helper lymphocytes

[a]Coupling may change as a function of ligand concentration.[8]
[b]Based on targeted deletion experiments, use of agonists and antagonists, and receptor expression experiments.[8,9]
[c]Permissive receptor will bind many prostanoids.

studies demonstrate several receptor clusters, all containing receptors for PGE_2.[10] The earliest divergence is between clusters associated with an increase of cAMP via a G protein containing a stimulatory subunit (G_s) for adenyl cyclase (EP2, EP4, IP and DP) or a decrease of cAMP via G_i (one isoform of EP3). The ancestral EP1 receptor diverged from an EP3 receptor isoform and functions to increase intracellular Ca^{2+}, along with the FP and TP receptors. A second receptor for PGD_2, chemoattractant receptor-homologous molecule expressed on Th2 (CRTH2), has recently been identified and couples to G_i.[11]

There is considerable interest in potential nuclear actions of PGs. These may occur by interaction with nuclear receptors or by interac-

tion with intracellular proteins. The peroxisome proliferator-activated receptors (PPARs) are putative receptors for PGJ_2 (PPARγ) and PGI_2 (PPARδ). However, there is some controversy surrounding the suggested biological role of this interaction.[8] As previously noted, the cyclopentanone PGs are highly reactive nucleophiles. It has been suggested that covalent modification of certain transcription factors, such as NFκB, by cyclopentanone PGs may lead to immune response modulation.[11-14] These novel actions of PGs are exciting, but their relevance remains to be definitively determined. Nevertheless, it has been suggested that cyclopentanone PGs may be anti-inflammatory as physiologic or pharmacologic agents.[15-17]

CYCLOOXYGENASE

Discovery of COX-2

Increased local PG production has long been understood to be a feature of inflammation. Before 1990, it was thought that the rate-limiting step for increased PG production was release of AA, and the mechanism for glucocorticoid-mediated anti-inflammatory action to reduce PGs involved induction of lipocortin (annexin-1) with inhibition of PLA_2 activity.[18] The hypothesis of a regulated COX activity that was induced during inflammatory stimuli and inhibited by glucocorticoids was proposed by Masferrer et al in 1990.[19] These authors proposed that different pools of COX activity might arise from different gene products. This prediction proved true when three groups cloned a transcript with significant homology to COX-1. Kujubu et al identified a transcript induced after treatment of Swiss 3T3 cells with phorbol ester tumor promoter.[20] Xie et al cloned a mitogen-responsive gene from chicken embryo fibroblasts infected with *v*-src.[21] O'Banion et al described a transcript induced by serum and inhibited by glucocorticoids.[22] An explosion of subsequent investigation resulted in the appreciation of the molecular and structural characteristics of COX-2, as well as its potential as a therapeutic target in arthritis.

Regulation of COX-2 expression in inflammation and arthritis

COX-2 expression is particularly responsive to mediators of inflammation, such as interleukin (IL)-1β, tumor necrosis factor (TNF)-α, lipopolysaccharide (LPS), and the phorbol ester 12-O-tetradecanyolphorbol 13–acetate (TPA) in vitro.[7,23] Glucocorticoids and some anti-inflammatory cytokines inhibit COX-2 expression.

In virtually all in vivo models, COX-2 expression increases in response to inflammatory stimuli and other types of tissue damage. Markedly increased COX-2 expression was seen in animal models of inflammatory arthritis and the rat carrageenan- or lipopolysaccharide-stimulated air pouch models that paralleled increased PG production.[24–26] Pharmacologic compounds that specifically inhibit COX-2 reversed inflammation in these models.[25,26] In the air pouch models, a specific inhibitor of COX-1 had no effect on PGE_2 production.[27] In COX-1, but not COX-2, knockout animals, LPS stimulates PG production.[28,29] Mice with genetic ablation of COX-2 are protected from development of experimental arthritis.[30] These data support the notion that the COX-2 isoform is most critical for PG production during subacute and chronic inflammation.

However, both COX-1 and COX-2 are capable of PG production, depending on the type and timing of the stimulus. In a dermal Arthus reaction model, a specific inhibitor of COX-1 decreased production of PGs while a specific inhibitor of COX-2 had no effect.[27] Injection of AA into a mouse ear results in acute inflammation and PG production in COX-2 knockout mice, but not in mice deficient in COX-1.[28,29] In some models of inflammation, such as carrageenan or TPA, that can cause acute release of AA but also lead to upregulation of COX-2, both isoforms contribute to inflammation, as shown by genetic and inhibitor studies.[27–29]

Anti-inflammatory activity after inhibition of COX-2 is correlated with decreased cerebrospinal fluid PG levels.[27] There is constitutive expression of COX-2 in the spinal cord that is upregulated during inflammation.[31,32] Studies have also demonstrated that intrathecal administration of a specific COX-2 inhibitor blocks the initiation of thermal hyperalgesia after carrageenan.[33] These data suggest the possibility that some anti-inflammatory as well as the analgesic effects of COX-2 inhibition may result from blocking PG production in the central nervous system. Fever also occurs in response to inflammation and induction of cytokines. PGs have long been known to mediate fever. COX-2 expression is induced in the brain vasculature with temporal correlation to the development of fever.[34] Moreover, COX-2 knockout mice fail to develop fever in response to inflammatory stimuli.[35]

Since NSAIDs are effective in the treatment of arthritis and other forms of acute and chronic inflammation in humans, examination of the relative expression of COX-1 and COX-2 in these disorders provides some insight into potential roles for the isoforms and potential therapeutic benefits of specific COX-2 inhibition. Both COX-1 and COX-2 are expressed in synovial tissues of patients with arthritis. COX-1 is localized at the synovial lining layer and there is no difference in the level of expression in inflammatory versus non-inflammatory arthritidies.[36] COX-2 is localized to the sub-lining layers, particularly the vascular endothelial cells, infiltrating mononuclear inflammatory cells and fibroblast-like synoviocytes. COX-2 expression is increased in inflammatory forms of arthritis such as rheumatoid arthritis and ankylosing spondylitis.[36,37] These basic observations form the basis for developing specific inhibitors of COX-2 (COXIBs) as a treatment for arthritis.

COX-2-derived prostaglandins in normal physiology

There is a clear physiologic role of constitutive and inducible COX-2. Full discussion is beyond the scope of this chapter; however, in some organ systems, the physiologic role of COX-2-derived PGs is important to the understanding of the clinical effects of COXIBs in the treatment of arthritis. In the kidney, COX-2 is constitutively expressed in the renal vasculature, glomerulus, macula densa, thick ascending limb of the loop of Henle, and interstitium.[38] In animals, COX-2 is clearly inducible in the glomerulus, macula densa, and thick ascending limb of the loop of Henle.[38] Owing to expression in the macula densa, COX-2-derived PGs are important to the regulation of the renin–angiotensin system in animal models.[39,40] A similar role for COX-2 in humans is illustrated in patients with Bartter's syndrome, a disorder of abnormal salt reabsorption in the thick ascending limb of the loop of Henle associated with increased activity of the renin–angiotensin–aldosterone system. In Bartter's syndrome, volume contraction leads to upregulated PG production in the macula densa, stimulating renin secretion.[40,41] Renal biopsy of a patient with

Bartter's syndrome reveals increased COX-2 expression in the macula densa (M. Breyer, personal communication). It has recently been reported that treatment of a child with Bartter's syndrome with rofecoxib resulted in a marked reduction of plasma renin activity, urinary aldosterone with reduced fractional excretion of potassium, and reduced urinary PGs.[42] Observations regarding the expression and regulation of the COX isoforms and the demonstration of the physiologic importance of renal PGs provide the basis for the renal effects of NSAIDs and COXIBs.

COX-1- and COX-2-derived PGs play contrasting roles in the vasculature.[43] Activated platelets synthesize TXA_2 via a COX-1-dependent pathway. TXA_2 is a potent platelet aggregant and vasoconstrictor. Opposing the actions of TXA_2 is PGI_2, which is synthesized by endothelial cells, inhibits platelet activation, and causes vasodilatation. In syndromes of platelet activation, biosynthesis of PGI_2 is elevated along with TXA_2, perhaps as a modulatory mechanism.[44] In support of this concept, it has been shown that TP agonists induce PGI_2 release from endothelial cells in vitro.[45] In addition, platelet-derived endoperoxides or AA may be used by endothelial cells for transcellular metabolism to PGI2.[46,47] Inhibition of the TXA_2 synthase enhances formation of other endoperoxides, such as PGI_2, in vivo.[48] Furthermore, IP- and TP-dependent signaling pathways may interact via cross-desensitization.[49,50]

Since both COX-1 and COX-2 exist in endothelial cells, PGI_2 could be synthesized by either isoform. In vitro overexpression studies have demonstrated that the PGI_2 synthase couples preferentially with COX-2 rather than COX-1.[51] Furthermore, it has been shown that COX-2 is the primary isoform responsible for the systemic biosynthesis of PGI_2 in humans.[52,53] In a canine model of coronary artery thrombosis, specific inhibition of COX-2 results in blockade of vasodilatation in response to infused AA.[54] These findings are in agreement with in vitro data showing that laminar, but not turbulent, shear stress induced selective and sustained upregulation of COX-2 in macrovascular endothelial cells.[55] These data demonstrate that COX-2 is the isoform primarily responsible for PG production in arteries. The relative roles of the COX isoforms in PGI_2 production in the venous circulation and normal microvasculature have not been directly demonstrated. COX-2 is clearly induced in microvascular endothelial cells in arthritis and other forms of inflammation.[24,36,56]

Endogenous PGI_2 has anti-thrombotic properties, as demonstrated in mice genetically deficient in the IP receptor.[57,58] IP knockout mice have enhanced injury-induced vascular proliferation and platelet activation and are more susceptible to thrombosis.[57,58] Furthermore, IP knockout mice exhibit enhanced TXA_2 formation, supporting the hypothesis that PGI_2 modulates platelet activation in vivo.[58] These observations support the importance of a balance between TXA_2 and PGI_2 in the control of thrombosis. Selective inhibition of TXA_2 production or action in platelets, either by low-dose aspirin or by knockout of the TP, inhibits thrombosis and blood vessel narrowing in response to injury.[58,59] Whether COXIBs, by virtue of inhibition of PGI_2, are prothrombotic remains controversial.[43,60–64] Early evidence suggests that patients at higher risk for cardiovascular events are more likely to have adverse events associated with COXIBs, if indeed there is a risk at all.[60,63]

COX-2 in cancer and angiogenesis

A role for COX-2 in oncogenesis is suggested by its upregulation in many different types of malignancies.[65,66] Several mechanisms have been proposed to explain the association of COX-2 and cancer.[67] COX-2 expression is induced in neoplastic, preneoplastic, and perineoplastic cells by mutation of oncogenes (such as ras), tumor promoters, mitogens, cytokines, and certain infectious agents associated with malignancy (such as *Helicobacter pylori*). Cells overexpressing COX-2 escape apoptosis, have abnormal cell–cell interactions, and acquire invasive phenotypes.[67] Angiogenesis plays a key role in the development of malignant tumors. Both in vitro and in vivo studies indicate that

COX-2 overexpression upregulates angiogenic factors in neoplastic cells and promotes tumor angiogenesis. COX-2 expression upregulates angiogenic factors, such as vascular endothelial growth factor (VEGF), in connective tissue cells surrounding neoplastic cells, markedly affecting neovascularization and tumor growth.[68] VEGF is induced in synovial cells by PGs, and it is possible that sustained upregulation of COX-2 in synovial tissues may contribute to angiogenesis, though it has never been shown that inhibition of COX-2 modifies the progression of arthritis.[69]

Specific COX-2 inhibitors in the treatment of arthritis

COXIBs were introduced into clinical practice in the USA in 1999. These agents were predicted to have equal efficacy and reduced gastrointestinal (GI) toxicity compared with non-specific NSAIDs.[2] The definition of a COXIB for the purposes of this discussion is an agent that inhibits COX-2 without inhibiting platelet COX-1 across the entire therapeutic range in the ex vivo whole blood assay.[23,70] Celecoxib, rofecoxib, valdecoxib and etoricoxib meet this definition and are currently approved for use in osteoarthritis, rheumatoid arthritis, and pain (indications and approvals vary among specific agents). Parecoxib is a parenteral formulation likely to be targeted for use in acute pain. Efficacy superior to placebo and similar to that of non-selective NSAIDs has been demonstrated for these agents in all published clinical trials for treatment of arthritis.[71–78]

Decreased GI toxicity compared with NSAIDs may also be eventually required in the evolving definition of a COXIB. Two very large studies, CLASS (celecoxib long-term safety study) and the VIGOR (VIOXX GI outcome research) trial, have addressed the relative GI toxicity of COXIBs versus NSAIDs.[61,79] While CLASS did not meet the primary outcome measure of significantly reduced perforations, obstructions and bleeds (POBs), there was a reduction in perforations, symptomatic ulcers and ulcer-related GI bleeds (PUBs).[79] Several study issues, such as low-dose aspirin use and a high number

Table 25.2   GI risk reduction (PUBs) for COXIBs compared with NSAIDs.

	RR	ARR (rate/100 patient years)	NNT
CLASS[a]	0.6	1.5	67
VIGOR	0.5	2.4	41

[a]Includes all subjects, including those taking aspirin.
RR, relative risk; ARR, absolute risk reduction; NNT, number needed to treat to avoid one event in a 1-year period.[61,79]

of subjects who failed to complete the study, may have contributed to the failure of CLASS to achieve significant reduction of ulcer complications. The VIGOR study demonstrated reduction in both PUBs and POBs. It is not possible to compare the two trials directly, since the study populations were different and VIGOR subjects were not allowed to use aspirin. The relative risk (RR), absolute risk reduction (ARR) and the number needed to treat (NNT) to prevent one symptomatic ulcer or ulcer complication in CLASS and VIGOR are shown in Table 25.2. Special note should be made that patients on low-dose aspirin are at high risk of GI bleeding due to the aspirin itself. In the CLASS study, there was no significant difference in POBs between COXIBs and NSAIDs in the aspirin-treated patients.[79] However, this study may have had insufficient power to definitively address the question, and further studies are needed.

Tolerability of NSAIDs is most influenced by GI symptoms, such as nausea, abdominal pain, and diarrhea. These symptoms are reduced in patients on COXIBs compared to some NSAIDs, but these side-effects still occur in a substantial number of patients. Agents that are effective for treatment of dyspeptic symptoms but do not significantly reduce ulcer risk, such as H_2-blockers, may be useful in patients using COXIBs and are inexpensive. However, if patients require proton pump inhibitors (PPIs) to control GI symptoms or to treat other disorders, such as gastroesophageal reflux disease, it is currently unclear that COXIBs further reduce the risk of ulcers and their complications. PPIs reduce endoscopic ulcers to a similar extent as COXIBs, as well as reducing clinically significant ulcers.[80,81]

As previously noted, COXIBs share with NSAIDs renal toxicity and a propensity to cause or aggravate hypertension.[38] The issue of whether the pharmacologic profiles of the individual COXIBs alters the side-effect profile remains unclear. Studies comparing agents have been industry sponsored and have yielded conflicting results.[71,82] The controversy surrounding the issue of cardiovascular effects unique to COXIBs by virtue of unbalanced inhibition of PGs is not yet settled. Patients in the rofecoxib arm of the VIGOR study had a higher risk of myocardial infarction than those on naproxen.[61] A protective role for naproxen has been proposed and is supported by some recent data.[83–85]

Adverse events affecting other organ systems remain uncommon with COXIBs, as with NSAIDs. Aseptic meningitis has been reported with rofecoxib.[86] A lack of cross-reactivity between COX-2 inhibitors and aspirin and other NSAIDs in patients with aspirin-sensitive asthma has been reported.[87] It has also been demonstrated that COXIBs impair fracture healing in animal models, although this has not been demonstrated in humans.[88]

PROSTAGLANDIN E SYNTHASE (PGES)

Cloning, characterization, and regulation of the PGES isoforms

Until recently, the ability to study regulation of terminal synthase enzymes was hampered by the fact that the PGES enzyme(s) had not been purified. However, two isoforms of the terminal synthase involved in the production of PGE_2 were recently cloned and characterized.[89–92] Similar to the COX enzymes, one isoform is constitutively expressed and unresponsive to

Table 25.3   MAPEG (membrane-associated proteins involved in eicosanoid and glutathione metabolism) superfamily.

Name	Function
FLAP (5-lipoxygenase activating protein)	Facilitates transfer of arachidonic acid to 5–lipoxygenase for LT synthesis[93,95]
LTC$_4$ synthase	Enzyme that converts LTA$_4$ to LTC$_4$, to form the cysteinyl LTs (slow-reacting substance of anyphylaxis)
Microsomal glutathione transferase (MGST) 1	Cellular detoxification, conjugates glutathione to xenobiotics
MGST 2	Conjugates glutathione to LTA$_4$ or xenobiotics; glutathione-dependent peroxidase activity with hydroperoxy fatty acid substrates
MGST 3	Conjugates glutatione to LTA$_4$; glutathione-dependent peroxidase activity with hydroperoxy fatty acid substrates
Microsomal PGE synthase (mPGES)	Inducible form of synthase that converts PGH$_2$ to PGE$_2$

proinflammatory stimuli, while the other isoform is inducible. The constitutive PGES is expressed in the cytosol (cPGES), and is expressed under basal conditions in a wide variety of mammalian cell lines and rat tissues.[91] Expression is generally unaltered by stimulation with bacterial LPS.

The inducible PGES is localized to the microsomal compartment and is hence termed mPGES.[89,92] The enzyme was identified as a member of the membrane-associated proteins involved in eicosanoid and glutathione metabolism (MAPEG) family of enzymes and was originally called microsomal glutathione S-transferase 1-like 1 (mGST1–L1).[93] The MAPEG superfamily consists of six human proteins (Table 25.3).[93] Two of the family members are involved in LT synthesis. These include 5-lipoxygenase (5-LO) activating protein (FLAP), which facilitates transfer of AA to 5-LO, and the LTC$_4$ synthase.[93,94] LTC$_4$ specifically conjugates glutathione to LTA$_4$, creating the cysteinyl LTs. Other members of the family can conjugate glutathione to lipophilic substrates, are involved in the cellular detoxification of xenobiotics, and/or possess glutathione-dependent peroxidase activity with hydroperoxy fatty acid substrates.[95] mPGES is unable to conju-

gate glutathione to either LTA$_4$ or 1-chloro-2,4-dinitrobenzene, the classical substrate for glutathione transferase activity.[89] It is of interest that the same sequence was also identified as a gene induced by p53, p53-inducible gene (PIG)-12.[96] The significance of this finding for mPGES biology remains to be fully evaluated.

mPGES is inducible by IL-1β and inhibited by glucocorticoids in human cell lines, including human synovial cells.[89,97,98] Induced PGES activity in LPS-stimulated and glucocorticoid-inhibited rat macrophages is also due to mPGES.[92] Rat mPGES exhibited a high degree of sequence homology to the human mPGES, and a mouse homolog has also been cloned.[56,92,95]

In vivo, LPS has been shown to increase expression of mPGES RNA in a number of tissues with a similar pattern to COX-2.[95] In addition, treatment of rats with IL-1β was found to induce mPGES RNA in cerebral blood vessels.[56] Blood vessel endothelial cells expressing mPGES also express IL-1 type I receptors and COX-2.[56]

mPGES and COX-2 are both inducible enzymes, suggesting a functional linkage.[97,98] Indeed, using co-transfection experiments, coupling between constitutive cPGES and COX-

1, and between inducible mPGES and COX-2, was shown.[91,92] Evidence of preferential coupling between COX-2 and certain terminal synthases has also been observed with the PGI_2 synthase.[51]

Despite certain similarities between mPGES and COX-2 regulation, the promoter of the mPGES gene lacks many of the elements usually associated with cytokine-inducible genes like COX-2, such as the TATAA box, CAAT box, NFκB and AP-1 binding sites.[90] Examination of a 651 base pair promoter region revealed the presence of GC-boxes, barbie-boxes, and an aryl hydrocarbon regulatory (AHR) element, an element seen in other members of the MAPEG family. There is transcriptional stimulation of a promoter–reporter construct by IL-1β, and also enhanced transcription in response to 2,3,7,8-tetrachlorodibenzo-*p*-dioxin, known to stimulate transcription via AHR elements. Transcription was inhibited by phenobarbital, presumably acting via the barbie boxes.[90]

COX-2 expression is regulated by post-transcriptional mechanisms.[99–101] However, the mPGES gene lacks the 3-AUUA sequences that mediate degradation of mRNA transcripts.[90] mPGES mRNA persists at high levels for up to 48 h and protein for up to 72 h after stimulation with IL-1β in synovial cells in vitro.[98] However, injection of IL-1β in rats resulted in a rapid increase in mPGES mRNA, with a peak by 3 h and a return to baseline by 5 h.[56] The reason for the discrepancy may be related to the types of cell examined (synoviocytes versus endothelial cells) or active downregulation of mPGES in vivo related to a systemic factor such as glucocorticoids.

PGES and PGE_2 in arthritis

Among the stable PGs produced in rheumatoid synovia, PGE_2 plays an important role. Injection of PGE_2 recapitulates the cardinal signs of inflammation via vasodilatation with plasma extravasation and sensitization of nociceptors.[102] Furthermore, PGE_2 stimulates production of matrix metalloproteinases and angiogenesis, and inhibits apoptosis of T lymphocytes.[69,103,104] PGE_2 is specifically implicated in the symptoms of arthritis, since neutralizing antibodies against PGE_2 are able to inhibit acute and chronic inflammation in the rat adjuvant arthritis model.[105] Previous data point to a selective induction of PGE_2 in inflammation.[106–109]

Increased production of PGE_2 in arthritis is probably due to specific induction of mPGES. mPGES expression is increased in human synoviocytes after treatment with IL-1β and TNF-α.[98] In addition, mPGES mRNA and protein are increased in the paws of rats treated with mycobacterial adjuvant.[95] The therapeutic potential of inhibiting mPGES remains untested. Furthermore, the physiologic role of the PGES isoforms has not yet been determined.

SUMMARY

The concept of a regulated PG production pathway including both COX-2 and mPGES has important implications for understanding inflammation in arthritis. This pathway could lead to the marked increase in PGE_2 in preference to other PGs observed in inflammatory arthritis. Specific COX-2 inhibitors have decreased GI toxicity compared with traditional NSAIDs; however, it is clear that there are adverse effects due to inhibition of COX-2. The therapeutic potential for agents that specifically target PG synthases or specific receptors, if effective, offer the advantage of preserving the production of COX-2-derived PGs that are important in normal physiology.

REFERENCES

1. Vane JR, Botting RM. The history of anti-inflammatory drugs and their mechanism of action. In: Bazan N, Botting J, Vane J, eds. *New Targets in* *Inflammation: Inhibitors of COX-2 or Adhesion Molecules* (Kluwer Academic Publishers and William Harvey Press: London, 1996) 1–12.

2. Crofford LJ. COX-1 and COX-2 tissue expression: implications and predictions. *J Rheumatol* 1997; **24**(suppl 49): 15–19.

3. Crofford LJ. Prostaglandin biology. *Gastroenterol Clin North Am* 2001; **30**: 863–76.

4. Vane JR, Botting RM. Formation and actions of prostaglandins and inhibition of their synthesis. In: Vane JR, Botting RM, eds. *Therapeutic Roles of Selective COX-2 Inhibitors* (William Harvey Press: London, 2001) 1–47.

5. Dennis EA. The growing phospholipase A2 superfamily of signal transduction enzymes. *Trends Biochem Sci* 1997; **22**: 1–2.

6. Leslie CC. Properties and regulation of cytosolic phospholipase A2. *J Biol Chem* 1997; **272**: 16709–12.

7. Smith WL, DeWitt DL, Garavito RM. Cyclooxygenases: structural, cellular, and molecular biology. *Ann Rev Biochem* 2000; **69**: 145–82.

8. Narumiya S, FitzGerald GA. Genetic and pharmacological analysis of prostanoid receptor function. *J Clin Invest* 2001; **108**: 25–30.

9. Breyer RM, Bagdassarian CK, Myers SA et al. Prostanoid receptors: subtypes and signaling. *Annu Rev Pharmacol Toxicol* 2001; **41**: 661–90.

10. Toh H, Ichikawa A, Narumiya S. Molecular evolution of receptors for eicosanoids. *FEBS Lett* 1995; **361**: 17–21.

11. Tilley SL, Coffman TM, Koller BH. Mixed messages: modulation of inflammation and immune responses by prostaglandins and thromboxanes. *J Clin Invest* 2001; **108**: 15–23.

12. Lawrence T, Gilroy DW, Colville-Nash PR et al. Possible new role for NF-kappaB in the resolution of inflammation. *Nat Med* 2001; **7**: 1291–7.

13. Rossi A, Kapahi P, Natoli G et al. Anti-inflammatory cyclopentenone prostaglandins are direct inhibitors of IkappaB kinase. *Nature* 2000; **403**: 103–8.

14. Straus DS, Pascual G, Li M et al. 15-deoxy-delta 12,14-prostaglandin J2 inhibits multiple steps in the NF-kappa B signaling pathway. *Proc Natl Acad Sci USA* 2000; **97**: 4844–9.

15. Gilroy DW, Colville-Nash PR, Willis D et al. Inducible cyclooxygenase may have anti-inflammatory properties. *Nat Med* 1999; **5**: 698–701.

16. Kawahito Y, Kondo M, Tsubouchi Y et al. 15-deoxy-Δ12,14-PGJ2 induces synoviocyte apoptosis and suppresses adjuvant-induced arthritis in rats. *J Clin Invest* 2000; **106**: 189–97.

17. Tsubouchi Y, Kawahito Y, Kohno M et al. Feedback control of the arachidonate cascade in rheumatoid synoviocytes by 15-deoxy-delta (12,14)-prostaglandin J2. *Biochem Biophys Res Commun* 2001; **283**: 750–5.

18. Flower RJ. Lipocortin. *Prog Clin Biol Res* 1990; **349**: 11–25.

19. Masferrer JL, Zweifel BS, Seibert K et al. Selective regulation of cellular cyclooxygenase by dexamethasone and endotoxin in mice. *J Clin Invest* 1990; **86**: 1375–9.

20. Kujubu DA, Fletcher BS, Varnum BC et al. TIS10, a phorbol ester tumor promoter-inducible mRNA from Swiss 3T3 cells, encodes a novel prostaglandin synthase/cyclooxygenase homologue. *J Biol Chem* 1991; **266**: 12866–72.

21. Xie W, Chipman JG, Robertson DL et al. Expression of a mitogen-responsive gene encoding prostaglandin synthase is regulated by mRNA splicing. *Proc Natl Acad Sci USA* 1991; **88**: 2692–6.

22. O'Banion MK, Sadowski HB, Winn V et al. A serum- and glucocorticoid-regulated 4-kilobase mRNA encodes a cyclooxygenase-related protein. *J Biol Chem* 1991; **266**: 23261–7.

23. Crofford LJ, Lipsky PE, Brooks P et al. Basic biology and clinical application of specific COX-2 inhibitors. *Arthritis Rheum* 2000; **43**: 4–13.

24. Sano H, Hla T, Maier JAM et al. In vivo cyclooxygenase expression in synovial tissues of patients with rheumatoid arthritis and osteoarthritis and rats with adjuvant and streptococcal cell wall arthritis. *J Clin Invest* 1992; **89**: 97–108.

25. Anderson GD, Hauser SD, Bremer ME et al. Selective inhibition of cyclooxygenase-2 reverses inflammation and expression of COX-2 and IL-6 in rat adjuvant arthritis. *J Clin Invest* 1996; **97**: 2672–9.

26. Seibert K, Zhang Y, Leahy K et al. Pharmacological and biochemical demonstration of the role of cyclooxygenase 2 in inflammation and pain. *Proc Natl Acad Sci USA* 1994; **91**: 12013–17.

27. Smith CJ, Zhang Y, Koboldt CM et al. Pharmacological analysis of cyclooxygenase-1 in inflammation. *Proc Natl Acad Sci USA* 1998; **95**: 13313–18.

28. Langenbach R, Morham SG, Tiano HF et al. Prostaglandin synthase 1 gene disruption in mice reduces arachidonic acid-induced inflammation and indomethacin-induced gastric ulceration. *Cell* 1995; **83**: 483–92.

29. Morham SG, Langenbach R, Loftin CD et al. Prostaglandin synthase 2 gene disruption causes severe renal pathology in the mouse. *Cell* 1995; **83**: 473–82.

30. Myers LK, Kang AH, Postlethwaite AE et al. The genetic ablation of cyclooxygenase 2 prevents the development of autoimmune arthritis. *Arthritis Rheum* 2000; **43**: 2687–93.

31. Beiche F, Scheuerer S, Brune K et al. Up-regulation of cyclooxygenase-2 mRNA in the rat spinal cord following peripheral inflammation. *FEBS Lett* 1996; **390**: 165–9.

32. Samad TA, Moore KA, Sapirstein A et al. Interleukin-1beta-mediated induction of COX-2 in the CNS contributes to inflammatory pain hypersensitivity. *Nature* 2001; **410**: 471–5.

33. Dirig DM, Isakson PC, Yaksh TL. Effect of COX-1 and COX-2 inhibition on induction and maintenance of carrageenan-evoked thermal hyperalgesia. *J Pharmacol Exp Ther* 1998; **285**: 1031–8.

34. Cao C, Matsumura K, Yamagata K et al. Induction by lipopolysaccharide of cyclooxygenase-2 mRNA in rat brain; its possible role in the febrile response. *Brain Res* 1995; **697**: 187–96.

35. Li S, Wang Y, Matsumura K et al. The febrile response to lipopolysaccharide is blocked in cyclooxygenase-2(−/−), but not in cyclooxygenase-1(−/−) mice. *Brain Res* 1999; **825**: 86–94.

36. Siegle I, Klein T, Backman JT et al. Expression of cyclooxygenase 1 and cyclooxygenase 2 in human synovial tissue. Differential elevation of cyclooxygenase 2 in inflammatory joint diseases. *Arthritis Rheum* 1998; **41**: 122–9.

37. Crofford LJ, Wilder RL, Ristimaki AP et al. Cyclooxygenase-1 and -2 expression in rheumatoid synovial tissues: effects of interleukin-1β, phorbol ester, and corticosteroids. *J Clin Invest* 1994; **93**: 1095–101.

38. Brater DC, Harris C, Redfern JS et al. Renal effects of COX-2 selective inhibitors. *Am J Nephrol* 2001; **21**: 1–15.

39. Harris RC, McKanna JA, Aiai Y et al. Cyclooxygenase-2 is associated with the macula densa of rat kidney and increases with salt restriction. *J Clin Invest* 1994; **94**: 2504–10.

40. Traynor TR, Smart A, Briggs JP et al. Inhibition of macula densa-stimulated renin secretion by pharmacological blockade of cyclooxygenase-2. *Am J Physiol* 1999; **277**: F706–10.

41. Castrop H, Hartner A, Goppelt-Strube M et al. Inhibition of the renin–angiotensin system upregulates cyclooxygenase-2 expression in the macula densa. *Hypertension* 1999; **34**: 503–7.

42. Kleta R, Basoglu C, Kuwertz-Broking E. New treatment options for Bartter's syndrome. *N Engl J Med* 2000; **343**: 661–2.

43. Catella-Lawson F, Crofford LJ. Cyclooxygenase inhibition and thrombogenicity. *Am J Med* 2001; **110**: 28S–32S.

44. FitzGerald GA. Mechanisms of platelet activation: thromboxane A2 as an amplifying signal for other agonists. *Am J Cardiol* 1991; **68**: 11B–15B.

45. Nicholson NS, Smith SL, Fuller GC. Effect of the stable endoperoxide analog U-46619 on prostacyclin production and cyclic AMP levels in bovine endothelial cells. *Thrombosis Res* 1984; **35**: 183–92.

46. Marcus AJ, Weksler BB, Jaffe EA et al. Synthesis of prostacyclin from platelet-derived endoperoxides by cultured human endothelial cells. *J Clin Invest* 1980; **66**: 979–86.

47. Barry OP, Pratico D, Lawson JA et al. Transcellular activation of platelets and endothelial cells by bioactive lipids in platelet microparticles. *J Clin Invest* 1998; **99**: 2118–27.

48. Nowak J, FitzGerald GA. Redirection of prostaglandin endoperoxide metabolism at the platelet–vascular interface in man. *J Clin Invest* 1989; **83**: 380–5.

49. Murray R, Shipp E, FitzGerald GA. Prostaglandin endoperoxide/thromboxane A2 receptor desensitization. Cross-talk with adenylate cyclase in human platelets. *J Biol Chem* 1990; **265**: 21670–5.

50. Walsh MT, Foley JF, Kinsella BT. The alpha, but not the beta, isoform of the human thromboxane A2 receptor is a target for prostacyclin-mediated desensitization. *J Biol Chem* 2000; **275**: 20412–23.

51. Ueno N, Murakami M, Tanioka T et al. Coupling between cyclooxygenase, terminal prostanoid synthase, and phospholipase A2. *J Biol Chem* 2001; **276**: 34918–27.

52. Catella-Lawson F, McAdam B, Morrison BW et al. Effects of specific inhibition of cyclooxygenase-2 on sodium balance, hemodynamics and vasoactive eicosanoids. *J Pharm and Exp Ther* 1999; **298**: 735–41.

53. McAdam BF, Catella-Lawson F, Mardini IA et al. Systemic biosynthesis of prostacyclin by cyclooxygenase (COX)-2: the human pharmacology of a selective inhibitor of COX-2. *Proc Natl Acad Sci USA* 1999; **96**: 272–7.

54. Hennan JK, Huang J, Barrett TC et al. Effects of selective cyclooxygenase-2 inhibition on vascular responses and thrombosis in canine coronary arteries. *Circulation* 2001; **104**: 820–5.

55. Topper JN, Cai J, Falb D et al. Identification of vascular endothelial genes differentially responsive to fluid mechanical stimuli: cyclooxygenase-

2, manganese superoxide dismutase, and endothelial cell nitric oxide synthase are selectively up-regulated by steady laminar shear stress. *Proc Natl Acad Sci USA* 1996; **93**: 10417–22.

56. Ek M, Engblom D, Saha S et al. Inflammatory response: pathway across the blood–brain barrier. *Nature* 2001; **410**: 430–1.

57. Murata T, Ushikubi F, Matsuoka T et al. Altered pain perception and inflammatory response in mice lacking prostacyclin receptor. *Nature* 1997; **388**: 678–82.

58. Cheng Y, Austin SC, Rocca B et al. Role of prostacyclin in the cardiovascular response to thromboxane A2. *Science* 2002; **296**: 539–41.

59. Antiplatelet Trialists' Group. Collaborative meta-analysis of randomised trials of antiplatelet therapy for prevention of death, myocardial infarction, and stroke in high risk patients. *BMJ* 2002; **324**: 71–86.

60. Crofford LJ, Oates JC, McCune WJ et al. Thrombosis in patients with connective tissue diseases treated with specific COX-2 inhibitors: a report of four cases. *Arthritis Rheum* 2000; **43**: 1891–6.

61. Bombardier C, Laine L, Reicin A et al. Comparison of upper gastrointestinal toxicity of rofecoxib and naproxen in patients with rheumatoid arthritis. *N Engl J Med* 2000; **343**: 1520–8.

62. Mukherjee D, Nissen SE, Topol EJ. Risk of cardiovascular events associated with selective COX-2 inhibitors. *JAMA* 2001; **286**: 954–9.

63. Konstam MA, Weir MR, Reicin A et al. Cardiovascular thrombotic events in controlled, clinical trials of rofecoxib. *Circulation* 2001; **104**: 2280–8.

64. White WB, Faich G, Whelton A et al. Comparison of thromboembolic events in patients treated with celecoxib, a cyclooxygenase-2 specific inhibitor, versus ibuprofen or diclofenac. *Am J Cardiol* 2002; **89**: 425–30.

65. Williams CS, Mann M, DuBois RN. The role of cyclooxygenases in inflammation, cancer, and development. *Oncogene* 1999; **18**: 7908–16.

66. Howe LR, Subbaramaiah K, Brown AM et al. Cyclooxygenase-2: a target for the prevention and treatment of breast cancer. *Endocrine Rel Cancer* 2001; **8**: 97–114.

67. Tsujii S, Tsujii M, Kawano S et al. Cyclooxygenase-2 upregulation as a perigenetic change in carcinogenesis. *Exp Clin Cancer Res* 2001; **20**: 117–29.

68. Williams CS, Tsujii M, Reese J et al. Host

cyclooxygenase-2 modulates carcinoma growth. *J Clin Invest* 2000; **105**: 1589–94.

69. Ben-Av P, Crofford LJ, Wilder RL et al. Induction of vascular endothelial growth factor expression in synovial fibroblasts by prostaglandin E and interleukin-1: a potential mechanism for inflammatory angiogenesis. *FEBS Lett* 1995; **372**: 83–7.

70. Patrignani P, Panara MR, Greco A. Biochemical and pharmacological characterization of the cyclooxygenase activity of human blood prostaglandin endoperoxide synthases. *J Pharmacol Exp Ther* 1994; **271**: 1705–12.

71. Geba GP, Weaver AL, Polis AB et al. Efficacy of refecoxib, celecoxib, and acetaminophen in osteoarthritis of the knee. *JAMA* 2002; **287**: 64–71.

72. Cannon G, Caldwell J, Holt P et al. Rofecoxib, a COX-2 specific inhibitor, has clinical efficacy comparable with diclofenac sodium: results of a one-year randomized clinical trial in patients with osteoarthritis of the knee and hip. *Arthritis Rheum* 2000; **43**: 978–87.

73. Bensen WG, Fiechtner JJ, McMillen JI et al. Treatment of osteoarthritis with celecoxib, a cyclooxygenase-2 inhibitor: a randomized controlled trial. *Mayo Clin Proc* 1999; **74**: 1095–105.

74. Day R, Morrison B, Luza M et al. A randomized trial of the efficacy and tolerability of the COX-2 inhibitor rofecoxib vs ibuprofen in patients with osteoarthritis. *Arch Intern Med* 2000; **160**: 1781–7.

75. Simon LS, Lanza FL, Lipsky PE et al. Preliminary study of the safety and efficacy of SC-58635, a novel cyclooxygenase 2 inhibitor: efficacy and safety in two placebo-controlled trials in osteoarthritis and rheumatoid arthritis, and studies of gastrointestinal and platelet effects. *Arthritis Rheum* 1998; **41**: 1591–602.

76. Simon LS, Weaver AL, Graham DY et al. Anti-inflammatory and upper gastrointestinal effects of celecoxib in rheumatoid arthritis. A randomized controlled trial. *JAMA* 1999; **282**: 1921–8.

77. Schnitzer TJ, Truitt K, Fleischmann R et al. The safety profile, tolerability, and effective dose range of rofecoxib in the treatment of rheumatoid arthritis. *Clin Ther* 1999; **21**: 1688–702.

78. Emery P, Zeidler H, Kvien TK et al. Celecoxib versus diclofenac in long-term management of rheumatoid arthritis: randomised double-blind comparison. *Lancet* 1999; **354**: 2106–11.

79. Silverstein FE, Faich G, Goldstein JL et al. Gastrointestinal toxicity with celecoxib vs nonsteroidal anti-inflammatory drugs for osteoarthritis and rheumatoid arthritis. The

CLASS study: a randomized controlled trial. *JAMA* 2000; **284**: 1247–55.

80. Lanza FL. A guideline for the prevention and treatment of NSAID-induced ulcers. *Am J Gastroenterol* 1998; **93**: 2037–46.

81. Chan FKL, Chung SCS, Suen BY et al. Preventing recurrent upper gastrointestinal bleeding in patients with helicobacter pylori infection who are taking low-dose aspirin or naproxen. *N Engl J Med* 2001; **344**: 967–73.

82. Whelton FJG, Puma JA, Normandin D et al. Cyclo-oxygenase-2–specific inhibitors and cardiorenal function: a randomized, controlled trial of celecoxib and rofecoxib in older hypertensive osteoarthritis patients. *Am J Ther* 2001; **8**: 85–95.

83. Solomon DH, Glynn RJ, Levin R et al. Nonsteroidal anti-inflammatory drug use and acute myocardial infarction. *Arch Intern Med* 2002; **162**: 1099–104.

84. Watson DJ, Rhodes T, Cai B et al. Lower risk of thromboembolic cardiovascular events with naproxen among patients with rheumatoid arthritis. *Arch Intern Med* 2002; **162**: 1105–10.

85. Rahme E, Pilote L, LeLorier J. Association between naproxen use and protection against acute myocardial infarction. *Arch Intern Med* 2002; **162**: 1111–15.

86. Bonnel RA, Villalba ML, Karwoski CB et al. Aseptic meningitis associated with rofecoxib. *Arch Intern Med* 2002; **162**: 713–15.

87. Stevenson DD, Simon RA. Lack of cross-reactivity between rofecoxib and aspirin in aspirin-sensitive patients with asthma. *J Allergy Clin Immunol* 2001; **108**: 47–51.

88. Simon AM, Manigrasso MB, O'Connor JP. Cyclo-oxygenase 2 function is essential for bone fracture healing. *J Bone Miner Res* 2002; **17**: 963–76.

89. Jakobsson P-J, Thoren S, Morgenstern R et al. Identification of human prostaglandin E synthase: a microsomal, glutathione-dependent, inducible enzyme, constituting a potential novel drug target. *Proc Natl Acad Sci USA* 1999; **96**: 7220–5.

90. Forsberg L, Leeb L, Thoren S et al. Human glutathione dependent prostaglandin E synthase: gene structure and regulation. *FEBS Lett* 2000; **471**: 78–82.

91. Tanioko T, Nakatani Y, Semmyo N et al. Molecular identification of cytosolic prostaglandin E2 synthase that is functionally coupled with cyclooxygenase-1 in immediate prosta-glandin E2 biosynthesis. *J Biol Chem* 2000; **42**: 32775–82.

92. Murakami M, Naraba H, Tanioka T et al. Regulation of prostaglandin E2 biosynthesis by inducible membrane-associated prostaglandin E2 synthase that acts in concert with cyclooxygenase-2. *J Biol Chem* 2000; **42**: 32783–92.

93. Jakobsson P-J, Morgenstern R, Mancini J et al. Common structural features of MAPEG – a widespread superfamily of membrane associated proteins with highly divergent functions in eicosanoid and glutathione metabolism. *Protein Sci* 1999; **8**: 689–92.

94. Mancini JA, Abramovitz M, Cox ME et al. 5-Lipoxygenase-activating protein is an arachidonate binding protein. *FEBS Lett* 1993; **318**: 277–81.

95. Mancini JA, Blood K, Guay J et al. Cloning, expression, and up-regulation of inducible rat prostaglandin E synthase during lipopolysaccharide-induced pyresis and adjuvant-induced arthritis. *J Biol Chem* 2001; **276**: 4469–75.

96. Polyak K, Xia Y, Zweier JL et al. A model for p53-induced apoptosis. *Nature* 1997; **389**: 300–5.

97. Thoren S, Jakobsson P-J. Coordinate up- and down-regulation of glutathione dependent prostaglandin E synthase and cyclooxygenase-2 in A549 cells. Inhibition by NS-398 and leukotriene C4. *Eur J Biochem* 2000; **267**: 6428–34.

98. Stichtenoth DO, Thoren S, Bian H et al. Microsomal prostaglandin E synthase is regulated by pro-inflammatory cytokines and glucocorticoids in primary rheumatoid synovial cells. *J Immunol* 2001; **167**: 469–74.

99. Ristimaki A, Garfinkel S, Wessendorf J et al. Induction of cyclooxygenase-2 by interleukin-1 alpha. Evidence for post-transcriptional regulation. *J Biol Chem* 1994; **269**: 11769–75.

100. Ristimaki A, Narko K, Hla T. Down-regulation of cytokine-induced cyclo-oxygenase-2 transcript isoforms by dexamethasone: evidence for post-transcriptional regulation. *Biochem J* 1996; **318**: 325–31.

101. Dixon DA, Kaplan CD, McIntyre TM et al. Post-transcriptional control of cyclooxygenase-2 gene expression. The role of the 3'-untranslated region. *J Biol Chem* 2000; **275**: 11750–7.

102. Vane JR, Botting RM. Anti-inflammatory drugs and their mechanism of action. *Inflam Res* 1997; **47**(Suppl 2): S78–S87.

103. Mehindate K, Al-Daccak R, Dayer J-M et al. Superantigen-induced collagenase gene expres-

sion in human IFN-γ-treated fibroblast-like synoviocytes involves prostaglandin E2. *J Immunol* 1995; **155**: 3570–7.

104. Goetzl EJ, An S, Zeng L. Specific suppression by prostaglandin E2 of activation-induced apoptosis of human CD4+CD8+ T lymphocytes. *J Immunol* 1995; **154**: 1041–7.

105. Portanova JP, Zhang Y, Anderson GD et al. Selective neutralization of prostaglandin E2 blocks inflammation, hyperalgesia, and interleukin 6 production in vivo. *J Exp Med* 1996; **184**: 883–91.

106. Murakami M, Matsumoto R, Austen KF. Prostaglandin endoperoxide synthase-1 and -2 couple to different transmembrane stimuli to generate prostaglandin D2 in mouse bone marrow-derived mast cells. *J Biol Chem* 1994; **269**: 22269–75.

107. Stichtenoth DO, Selve N, Tsikas D et al. Increased total body synthesis of prostacyclin in rats with adjuvant arthritis. *Prostaglandins* 1995; **50**: 331–40.

108. Matsumoto H, Naraba H, Murakami M et al. Concordant induction of prostaglandin E2 synthase with cyclooxygenase-2 leads to preferred production of prostaglandin E2 over thromboxane and prostaglandin D2 in lipopolysaccharide-stimulated rat peritoneal macrophages. *Biochem Biophys Res Commun* 1997; **230**: 110–14.

109. Fournier T, Fadok V, Henson PM. Tumor necrosis factor-alpha regulates prostaglandin D2 and prostaglandin E2 production in murine macrophages. Synergistic action of cyclic AMP on cyclooxygenase-2 expression and prostaglandin E2 synthesis. *J Biol Chem* 1997; **272**: 31065–72.

26

Complement inhibition

M Kathryn Liszewski and John P Atkinson

Introduction • Principles of complement activation • Inhibition of complement activation • Summary • References

INTRODUCTION

The complement system provides an innate defense against microbes and a 'complement' to antibody-mediated humoral immunity (reviews: Holers[1] and Volanakis and Frank[2]). Complement is a double-edged sword, since deficiencies of its proteins predispose the host to infectious diseases and autoimmunity, especially systemic lupus erythematosus (SLE), while undesirable or uncontrolled activation damages tissue. In the setting of autoantibodies, complement components unwittingly serve as 'inappropriately' guided missiles.

Also, diseases mediated by immune complexes (ICs) activate complement and produce inflammation and tissue damage if ICs lodge in locations such as a vessel wall, synovium, skin or glomerulus. The complement system may also contribute to tissue damage in ischemia–reperfusion injury, adult respiratory distress syndrome (ARDS), cardiopulmonary bypass, and Alzheimer's disease. Currently, no therapeutic agent is commercially available to block complement activation. Two plasma-based therapies, though, are undergoing clinical trials (Table 26.1). This chapter will focus on these two agents.

Table 26.1 Complement activation inhibitors undergoing clinical trials.

Product	Description	Actions	Company
TP10	Soluble recombinant CR1 (sCR1)	Degrades C3b/C4b (CA) and decays C3/C5 convertases (DAA)	Avant Immunotherapeutics (Needham, MA, USA)
h5G1.1; h5G1.1-scFv	Humanized, high-affinity anti-C5 mAb; single-chain version	Blocks cleavage of C5 by C5 convertases	Alexion Pharmaceuticals (New Haven, CT, USA)

CA, cofactor activity; DAA, decay-accelerating activity; mAb, monoclonal antibody.

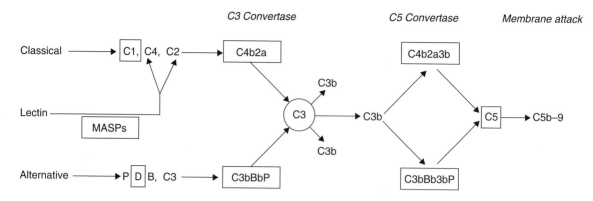

Figure 26.1 Complement pathways and sites of therapeutic intervention. The three arms of complement are the classical, lectin and alternative pathways. Current sites targeted for therapeutic intervention (boxed areas) include the initiation of the classical, lectin, and alternative pathways (C1, MASPs and factor D), formation of convertases (both C3 and C5 convertases), and commencement of the membrane attack complex (C5 component).

PRINCIPLES OF COMPLEMENT ACTIVATION

Activation

The complement system developed more than 600 million years ago and preceded antibodies in evolution. A complement system similar to that of mammals has been detected in primitive fish that lack immunoglobulins. The classical pathway (CP) 'complements' humoral immunity (hence its name). In the late 1800s, complement was thought to be a single, non-specific, innate and labile substance that required a single, specific, acquired and stable material known as antibody to mediate lysis. We now know that the complement system consists of more than 30 serum and membrane proteins that can be grouped into three divisions: activating components, receptors, and regulators (both positive and negative). Given the destructive potential of this system, it is perhaps no surprise that nearly half of complement proteins serve in regulation.

The task of the complement system is to allow rapid and robust activation in response to an invading microbe, yet simultaneously minimize injury to host cells. This goal is accomplished by strictly limiting activation in time and space.

Finite activation in *time* is necessary in order to avoid excessive consumption of complement components in any one reaction. Restriction in *space* is necessary to focus the reaction on the target and thereby avoid injuring self-tissue (i.e. wrong target) or activation in the fluid phase (i.e. no target).

The complement system consists of three 'arms' or pathways, which are activated differently yet merge at a common point (Figure 26.1). The main thrust of each pathway is to form multicomponent, enzymatic 'convertases' that cleave components C3 and C5. Once initiated, the complement system can deposit millions of its fragments onto a bacterium in less than 5 min.

The CP reaction cascade is initiated when immune complexes form and the C1q subcomponent of C1 attaches to the Fc portion of IgG or IgM. This initiates an enzymatic reaction in which the subcomponent C1r (a serine protease) cleaves subcomponent C1s (another serine protease). C1s in turn cleaves and thereby activates the next two components in line, C4 and C2. The resulting larger fragment of C4, C4b, attaches covalently to the cell surface and then binds C2a (the third serine protease of the cascade) to form the CP C3 convertase (C4b2a). C3 is cleaved by this convertase to C3a and C3b.

Like C4b, activated C3b coats (opsonizes) a surface by binding covalently to available hydroxyl groups. The association of a second C3b with the C3 convertase converts it to a C5 convertase (C4b2a3b). The cleavage of C5 by this enzyme liberates C5a, while C5b continues the cascade by serving as the initial protein of the membrane attack complex (MAC).

The lectin pathway differs from the CP only in the initiation step. Here mannan-binding lectin (MBL) in plasma (comparable to C1q) attaches to an activating surface enriched in mannoses or glucosamines (i.e. microbial membranes). MBL activates C4 and C2 in the same manner as C1s but uses distinct proteases known as MBL-associated serine protease-1 and -2 (MASP-1 and MASP-2). Thus, MASPs generate the same C3 convertase as formed by the CP.

The alternative pathway (AP) was the second complement activation pathway discovered (hence its name), but it is probably the most phylogenetically ancient of the three. The AP does not require antibody. Instead, it idles like a car waiting at a stop sign, being continuously active at a low level under normal circumstances. If this 'ticking-over' C3 encounters a foreign surface such as a microbe, it binds to the surface and then serves as the nidus for the engagement of the AP. This 'shotgun' approach to host defense provides an important surveillance or sentry-like function in the non-immune host. Amplification rapidly occurs in the presence of foreign material but is blocked by endogenous regulators on host tissue and in blood.

Factor B, which is structurally and functionally homologous to C2, binds to the deposited C3b and is cleaved by the constitutively active serine protease factor D to produce Ba and Bb. Bb continues the cascade, while Ba is released into the surrounding milieu. The resulting cell-bound complex, C3bBb, is the AP C3 convertase which is stabilized by the binding of properdin. Additional C3 is cleaved to C3b, which deposits on the target. This C3b opsonizes the activating surface and, in turn, also binds additional factor B to form more C3 convertases. As the stabilized convertase cleaves more C3 to C3b, a feedback loop (i.e. auto-amplification) is set in motion,

resulting in the deposition of large amounts of C3b on a microbe. Some of this C3b binds to the C3 convertase to form the C5 convertase of the AP, C3bBbC3b. Properdin also stabilizes this convertase. C3a, an anaphylatoxin, is liberated by AP or CP C3 convertases and activates many cell types after binding to its receptor.

All three pathways converge at the level of C3 activation, and all three pathways initiate the MAC (Figure 26.1). Cleavage of C5 to C5a and C5b triggers this common terminal membrane-modifying system. The subsequent steps represent protein interactions and are not enzymatic in nature like the early steps. C5a, an anaphylatoxin of ~10 kDa, binds its receptor and thereby serves as a potent chemotaxin and activator of many cell types, including leukocytes and mast cells. The other fragment, C5b, binds to C6, which in turn binds C7 to yield fluid-phase C5b67. This complex inserts in membranes and then recruits C8. The C5b678 forms an initial pore in the membrane. Recruitment of multiple C9s yields C5b6789n, the fully formed MAC.

Regulation

The complement system is controlled 'naturally' by the instability of biologically activated fragments and the regulatory proteins (reviews: Liszewski et al[3] and Morgan and Harris[4]). The latter block endogenous complement activity at each of the major steps, namely, initiation, amplification (leading to C3 cleavage) and membrane attack (Figure 26.1). The released anaphylatoxins are inactivated by a peptidase.

Initiation
C1 inhibitor covalently binds to and inactivates C1r and C1s as well as MASP-1 and -2. This reaction does not prevent or hinder desirable C1 activation as, for example, by an IC, but prevents excessive (chronic) activation on one target or fluid-phase activation.

Amplification
At the step of C3 cleavage, regulation occurs by two control processes, termed 'decay-accelerating activity' (DAA) and 'cofactor activity' (CA).

The former refers to the ability of a regulator to disassociate or disassemble the C3/C5 convertases, while the latter refers to the proteolytic cleavage (and thereby inactivation relative to cascade-promoting capability) of the non-catalytic component of the convertase. Cofactor activity involves two proteins, the plasma serine protease factor I and a plasma or membrane cofactor protein. The two plasma regulators involved in C3 convertase control possess both DAA and CA (factor H for C3b and the AP convertase, and C4b-binding protein for C4b and the CP convertase). However, cell-anchored regulators differ from this scheme. Membrane cofactor protein (MCP; CD46) possesses only CA but for both C4b and C3b, while decay-accelerating factor (DAF; CD55) has only DAA for the convertases. Another regulator, complement receptor type 1 (CR1; CD35), possesses DAA and CA for both CP and AP convertases but it has a much more restricted pattern of expression. This broad regulatory activity, though, is one feature that makes CR1 an attractive candidate as a therapeutic agent to inhibit complement activation at the step of C3 cleavage.

Membrane attack
The terminal pathway is regulated by the plasma protein vitronectin, and the ubiquitously expressed glycosylphosphatidylinositol (GPI)-linked protein protectin (CD59). Vitronectin

(protein S) binds MAC complexes in the fluid phase and thereby prevents insertion into their host cells. Protectin blocks C8 and C9, preventing them from properly inserting into the cell on which it is expressed. Finally, carboxypeptidase-N inactivates C3a and C5a by removing a C-terminal arginine.

INHIBITION OF COMPLEMENT ACTIVATION

Soluble complement receptor type 1 (sCR1)

In its natural setting, CR1 is a type 1 transmembrane glycoprotein of 220 kDa (most common allelic form) that mediates immune adherence and, under some circumstances, phagocytosis of C4b- and C3b-opsonized targets (reviews: Birmingham and Hebert[5] and Krych-Goldberg and Atkinson[6]). It also serves as a potent regulator of C3/C5 activation, as it possesses cofactor activity for C3b and C4b and accelerates the decay of C3 and C5 convertases. CR1 is expressed on peripheral blood cells (except for platelets and most T cells) and on follicular dendritic cells, monocytes–macrophages and B lymphocytes in tissues. Functional sites lie within repeating units called complement control protein (CCP) modules that consist of ~60 amino acids with two disulfide bridges. The most common allelic size variant possesses 30

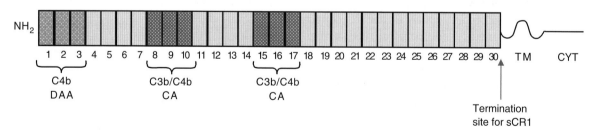

Figure 26.2 Complement receptor one (CR1) and its therapeutic analog. The most common allelic form of CR1 is shown. It consists of 30 repeating motifs termed 'complement control protein' (CCP) modules that house the functional sites for complement ligands. CR1 has three known sites for interacting with complement components C4b and C3b. The therapeutic analog, TP10, was created by placing a stop codon before the transmembrane domain. CA, cofactor activity; DAA, decay-accelerating activity.

Table 26.2 Animal models of disease in which complement inhibition with sCR1 or h5G1.1 anti-C5 has shown efficacy in vivo.[8]

Animal model	Human disease	Drug tested
Ischemia/reperfusion		
Cerebral artery ligation/release	Stroke	sCR1
Mesenteric artery ligation/release	Mesenteric ischemia	sCR1
Coronary artery ligation/release	Myocardial infarction	sCR1
Cardiopulmonary bypass	Cardiopulmonary bypass	Anti-C5/sCR1
Warm, hepatic ischemia	Microcirculatory disorders	sCR1
Organ allotransplantation		
Lung allograft	Lung transplantation	sCR1
Cardiac allograft	Heart transplantation	sCR1
Renal allograft	Kidney transplantation	sCR1
Liver allograft	Liver transplantation	sCR1
Islets of Langerhans	Diabetes	sCR1
Direct complement activation		
Pulmonary acid instillation	Aspiration pneumonitis	sCR1
Burn injury	Burn injury	sCR1
Endotoxin treatment/bacterial infection	Septic shock	Anti-C5
Remote lung injury		
Lung injury after mesenteric or hind limb ischemia	Adult respiratory distress syndrome	sCR1
Autoimmunity		
Antigen/collagen-induced arthritis	Rheumatoid arthritis	sCR1
Pulmonary IgA immune complexes	IgA-associated syndromes	sCR1
Glomerulonephritis (autoantibody)	Glomerulonephritis	sCR1
Glomerulonephritis (immune complex)	Lupus	Anti-C5
Experimental autoimmune neuritis	Guillain–Barré syndrome	sCR1
Passive antiacetylcholine receptor	Myasthenia gravis	sCR1
Experimental allergic encephalomyelitis	Multiple sclerosis	sCR1

CCP modules and binds C4b at three sites and C3b at two sites (Figure 26.2). The presence of several ligand-recognition domains indicates that each CR1 interacts with a higher affinity with complexes containing multiple (clustered) C4b and C3b molecules. A truncated form of CR1 (soluble CR1 or sCR1) was produced by placing a stop codon before the transmembrane domain (Figure 26.2). As described below, this recombinant protein is a potent plasma-based inhibitor of complement activation.

The seminal paper demonstrating the utility of sCR1 as a therapeutic agent was published in 1990.[7] Since sCR1 blocked complement activation in rats (and a few other species), it could be used, for example, in models of ischemia–reperfusion injury. In the rat model of myocardial ischemia, sCR1 produced an ~40% reduction in the magnitude of the myocardial damage. By inference, the investigators established the ability of this inhibitory protein to function in the extravascular space. On the other hand, sCR1 in this experiment was given before or simultaneously with return of coronary bloodflow.

There are now more than 100 peer-reviewed publications in which the ability of sCR1 to inhibit complement activation and thereby ameliorate tissue damage in experimental models of disease (see Table 26.2) has been assessed (reviews: Klickstein et al,[8] Kirshfink[9] and Lambris and Holers[10]). A protective effect has been demonstrated primarily in rat and dog, where the human agent blocks the complement system. In models of, for example, IgG- and IgM-mediated autoimmunity, acute lung injury syndromes, ischemia–reperfusion (acute myocardial infarction) injury, and xenografts, complement inhibition reduced tissue damage. In most reports, sCR1 was in plasma at the time of injury initiation, a situation difficult to duplicate in many of the comparable human conditions. These data, though, along with similar studies in animals lacking a complement protein, have been invaluable in further establishing a role for complement in producing tissue damage in autoantibody-mediated diseases, IC excess syndromes, and ischemia– reperfusion injury.

Soluble CR1 blocks complement activation in humans and thus proof-of-principle has been established. The most studied drug candidate, TP10, is a truncated product (i.e. without transmembrane and cytoplasmic tail domains) of CR1. It has been investigated in several phase I and II trials for indications such as ARDS, myocardial infarction, lung transplantation, pediatric cardiac surgery, and adult cardiac surgery (reviews: Klickstein et al,[8] Kirshfink[9], Lambris and Holers[10] and Rioux[11]). In these studies, sCR1 produced no unexpected side-effects. Additionally, pharmacokinetic profiles were established for complement inhibition. In general, though, these studies had limited patient numbers, and definitive claims relative to therapeutic efficacy were not possible. Only one peer-reviewed publication is available in the literature. This report is described in more detail in the next paragraph.

A phase I trial of sCR1 (TP10) was conducted to determine the safety, pharmacokinetics, biological effects, and immunogenicity in patients with acute lung injury (ALI) and ARDS.[12] The study built on earlier testing of TP10 in rat models of lung injury that demonstrated reduced vascular permeability, hemorrhage, and neutrophil infiltration.[13] The open-label, ascending-dosage phase I trial used a total of 24 patients (15 male and 9 female) diagnosed with ALI/ARDS. A single, 30-min intravenous infusion of 0.1, 0.3, 1, 3 or 10 mg/kg body weight of TP10 was administered. Patients were followed for 28 days after TP10 treatment. Plasma samples were evaluated for CH_{50} (total hemolytic complement assay), as well as levels of TP10, C3a, soluble C5b-9, and anti-TP10. The single infusion of TP10 was safe over a wide range of dosages. Serum levels of TP10 increased in proportion to the dose. TP10 half-life was ~70 h, and at doses greater than or equal to 1 mg/kg, it inhibited complement activity. The plasma clearance of TP10 after the single intravenous infusion was low (2.4 ml/kg/h) in patients with ALI compared to patients with thermal injury (18.7 ml/kg/h). Thus, the TP10 half-life of ~70 h in ALI patients contrasted with 7.9 h in patients with thermal injury. The pharmacokinetic profile in ALI correlated more closely to that in patients with a first myocardial infarction.[14]

Currently, sCR1 appears to be an effective agent for any disease process in which complement activation mediates tissue damage. The challenges are: cost (a relatively large amount of recombinantly produced protein must be given); lack of selectivity (i.e. blocks all complement pathways); intravenous administration; and potential for infectious complications. Concerning the last point, when complement is blocked, the host will probably be more susceptible to infections by bacteria such as *Staphylococcus*, *Streptococcus*, *Haemophilus*, and especially *Neisseria*. Additionally, in many of the animal models, sCR1 was given prior to or simultaneously with the insult. This, of course, will not be possible in most human diseases other than in association with procedures or operations such as hemodialysis, bypass surgery, and transplantation.

A second-generation variant, TP20, modifies the N-linked carbohydrates of TP10 by adding sialyl Lewis* (sLe*) groups.[15–17] This sugar moiety mediates binding of neutrophils to selectins. The latter appear on the surface of activated endothelial cells, an early and critical step in inducing a local inflammatory event. The goal, therefore, was to more efficiently target the complement-inhibiting activity of sCR1 to an inflammatory site and, at the same time, inhibit the leukocyte–endothelial cell adhesion process. In two animal model systems, the sLe*-modified CR1 appears to have had enhanced anti-inflammatory capability compared to TP-10.

Humanized monoclonal antibody to C5

A second therapeutic agent in clinical trials employs the straightforward strategy of blocking the function of a single component with a monoclonal antibody (mAb). The mAb designated 5G1.1 binds human C5 and blocks C5 cleavage by the C5 convertase.[18] A fully 'humanized' version has been created by grafting the complementarity-determining regions of 5G1.1 onto human framework domains, i.e. creating a specific single-chain Fv (scFv) antibody called h5G1.1scFv. A significant advantage for the mAb approach is that recombinantly produced mAbs, such as the anti-tumour necrosis factor (TNF) reagents, are already in use in clinical medicine. Recombinant mAbs also have the advantage of a relatively long half-life, and, if humanized, are usually minimally immunogenic.

Such a reagent would theoretically be ideal for a syndrome in which C5a or the MAC or both contribute substantially to tissue damage. However, the current dogma is that C3b deposition is most critical relative to dealing with microbes and, by inference, most other situations featuring complement activation. The availability of reagents like the mAb to C5a has proven extremely valuable, though, in dissecting the role of C3 versus C5 activation in producing tissue injury. Somewhat unexpectedly, many of the same, albeit more limited, conditions featuring complement activation that were inhibited via sCR1 in animal models of human disease have also been shown to be ameliorated by C5 blockade. A surprising conclusion has been that C5 activation seems to contribute more to tissue damage than would have been anticipated. Unfortunately, definitive evidence is not available in most human diseases to accurately determine how much of the tissue damage is caused by the reaction cascade through C3 versus that produced by C5a and the MAC. Of course, if the tissue damage is mediated primarily through C3 activation, inhibiting C5 would be of little value. An advantage to inhibiting C5, however, is that a selective block is obtained and the opsonic capabilities of the complement cascade remain intact. One would, therefore, envision a lower predisposition to most bacterial infections by inhibiting only C5, with the one exception of *Neisseria*. As is the case for TP10, one report is available in a peer-reviewed journal.[19]

The humanized, recombinant, single-chain antibody specific for human C5 (h5G1.1scFv) was given in a phase I trial of patients undergoing coronary artery bypass graft surgery requiring cardiopulmonary bypass (CPB).[19] The study was conducted because of evidence that complement activation during CPB probably contributes to complications. Preclinical studies determined that the mAb mediated C5 inhibition with reduced inflammation and tissue damage in models of bypass-associated bio-incompatibility[20] and myocardial ischemia followed by reperfusion.[21] For the clinical trial, the mAb was administered intravenously in one of four doses ranging from 0.2 to 2.0 mg/kg body weight before CPB. The mAb appeared to be safe. Pharmacokinetic analysis suggested a half-life of 7.0–14.5 h. At 2 mg/kg there was dose-dependent inhibition of complement hemolytic activity for up to 14 h. Generation of proinflammatory complement byproducts (sC5b-9) was inhibited in a dose-dependent fashion. Leukocyte activation was reduced in patients receiving 1 and 2 mg/kg. There was a 40% reduction in myocardial injury and an 80% reduction in new cognitive defects in patients receiving 2 mg/kg. There was also a one-unit reduction in postoperative blood loss in patients receiving 1 or 2 mg/kg. The authors concluded the single-chain mAb was a safe and effective inhibitor of pathological complement activation in CPB patients.

Many other phase I and II studies are underway and several abstracts have been produced (on file at Alexion Pharmaceuticals). In a phase I/II randomized, placebo-controlled study in patients with rheumatoid arthritis, a single dose of the antibody appeared to be safe, with no unexpected side-effects. The single-dose regimen was associated with a significant reduction in C-reactive protein. Additionally, 50% of patients were reported to meet American College of Rheumatology (ACR-20) criteria, compared to 10% of the placebo-treated patients. Preliminary results from the phase I/II trial for SLE showed a benefit as well. In this study, a single dose of mAb blocked complement activity for up to 2 weeks and may have been associated with a reduction of proteinuria. In other trials, the mAb inhibited C5 activation in patients undergoing CPB for coronary artery bypass grafting and in patients undergoing renal dialysis. The CPB study suggested that there was less blood loss, lower postoperative levels of total serum CK–MB, and a decrease in 'post-pump' cognitive deficits in treated versus placebo-controlled patients. There were no unanticipated effects in these short-term studies or an immune response to the mAb.

C1 inhibitor

C1 inhibitor (C1-INH) is the only plasma inhibitor that regulates the initiation of the classical and MBL pathways (review: Kirshfink[9]). It blocks the active site of C1r and C1s and the MASPs. A member of the 'serpin' superfamily of serine protease inhibitors, C1-INH mimics the substrate's reactive site by serving as 'bait' to bind and then trap the protease. C1-INH–protease complexes are quickly removed from the circulation by binding to the serpin–enzyme complex receptors on hepatocytes and monocytes. The wide spectrum of proteases inactivated by C1 inhibitor (activated factors XI and XII, kallikrein, plasmin

and tissue-type plasminogen activator) highlights its prominent role in controlling several proteolytic cascades. Because of this, the interpretation of results of clinical trials may be complex relative to which 'blocked' pathway is responsible for the positive or, for that matter, negative effect.

Deficiency of C1-INH produces the potentially life-threatening disease hereditary angioedema (HAE) (review: Kirshfink[9]). Replacement of C1-INH is beneficial in acute treatment of this disease. Since reduced C1-INH activity has occasionally been noted in patients with sepsis, severe burns, polytrauma, capillary leak syndrome following bone marrow transplantation, pancreatitis, urticarial reactions to contrast media, and ARDS, these patient populations have been treated with the inhibitor. However, complement activation in these conditions usually occurs in the setting of normal or augmented levels of the C1-INH. Moreover, HAE patients are not more susceptible to infection or excessive tissue damage during inflammatory reactions. Despite these data, by raising the levels to supernormal ones, the hypothesis is that C1-INH can now more effectively block one or more of these proteolytic cascades.

C1-INH is available in purified form for infusion in Europe (but not the USA) for treating attacks of HAE. In uncontrolled small trials, the treatment of septic shock, burns, reperfusion injury following revascularization, capillary leak syndrome in association with bone marrow transplantation and acute pancreatitis produced mixed but sufficiently encouraging results to suggest that this approach deserves further study. Nevertheless, it seems unlikely that this will be an efficacious means of specifically blocking complement activation in human disease. Along this line, a challenge facing the therapeutic use of C1-INH is defining an appropriate read-out to monitor the inhibitory effect of the treatment. For patients deficient in C1-INH (such as with HAE), this is straightforward, since they have low C4 levels that return to normal as adequate levels of C1-INH are established. However, for patients with normal C1-INH and C4 levels, it is less clear which proteolytic systems are affected and how to monitor a pathway in order to be certain that 'inhibition' is taking place. Thus, establishing the utility of C1-INH as a therapeutic agent to inhibit complement is not likely to be easy, and interpretations of even controlled clinical studies may prove problematic.

Other inhibitors

CAB-2

This soluble, recombinant, chimeric therapeutic is composed of two regulators of complement activation, DAF and MCP.[22,23] The 'complement activation blocker' (CAB) expresses the functional features of both proteins, namely, inactivation of both the classical and alternative C3/C5 convertases via decay activity, and factor I-mediated proteolysis of C3b/C4b. CAB-2 blocked the in vitro activation of human complement as measured by cytotoxicity assays and anaphylatoxin generation. CAB-2 inhibited both the Arthus reaction and Forssman shock in guinea pigs. The pharmacokinetics of CAB-2 protein in rats exhibited a favorable pattern of distribution and clearance. Currently, the protein is targeted for phase I trials. It would be expected to have a similar inhibitory profile as sCR1.

Small molecule inhibitors

C3 INHIBITORS

Compstatin, a synthetic C3-binding peptide inhibitor, has been utilized in animal models for C3 inhibition (reviews: Fleming and Tsokos[24] and Sahu et al[25]). Both in vitro and in vivo systems have suggested that compstatin is an effective inhibitor for the usual indications where complement activation produces tissue damage. The use of small peptides to inhibit complement activation is an attractive strategy with several potential advantages, including small size, oral delivery route, and cost. In the case of compstatin, relatively high concentra-

tions are required to bind to and block the action of native protein (1–2 mg/ml).

FACTOR D INHIBITORS

Small molecule inhibitors of and an mAb to factor D are being examined (preclinically) as specific inhibitors of the AP. Factor D is a member of the family of serine proteases, and the core of its activity resides in the three invariant residues, aspartic acid–histidine–serine, or 'catalytic triad', as it does for all serine proteases. Using structure based drug design, several serine protease inhibitors of complement, coagulation and kinin-related enzymes have been identified.[26,27] The issue of specificity has plagued this field. For this reason, a mAb approach, as was accomplished for C5, appears to be a more attractive strategy for blocking factor D and thereby the AP.[28]

C1q INHIBITION

Small molecules are also being developed that inhibit the reaction between β-amyloid and C1q in Alzheimer's disease.[29]

SUMMARY

The development of complement inhibitors and characterization of animals congenitally or genetically engineered to have a single-component complement deficiency are providing more precise information on the role of complement in disease processes. Two unanticipated observations that have already arisen from this work are: (1) complement activation contributes to tissue damage in myocardial infarctions and stroke; and (2) C5–C9 bears responsibility for more of the tissue damage during complement activation than predicted. Two inhibitors are in clinical trials, and their ability to inhibit complement activation in vivo is reasonably well established. The task ahead is that of defining via additional trials the clinical settings where complement inhibition provides therapeutic benefit.

REFERENCES

1. Holers VM. Complement as a regulatory and effector pathway in human disease. In: Lambris JD, Holers VM, eds. *Contemporary Immunology: Therapeutic Interventions in the Complement System* (Humana Press: Totowa, 2000) 1–32.

2. Volanakis JE, Frank MM. *The Human Complement System in Health and Disease* (Marcel Dekker: New York, 1998).

3. Liszewski MK, Farries TC, Lublin DM et al. Control of the complement system. *Adv Immunol* 1996; **61**: 201–83.

4. Morgan BP, Harris CL. Complement regulators in therapy. In: Morgan BP, Harris CL, eds. *Complement Regulatory Proteins* (Academic Press, Harcourt Brace & Company: San Diego, 1999) 250.

5. Birmingham DJ, Hebert LA. CR1 and CR1-like: the primate immune adherence receptors. *Immunol Rev* 2001; **180**: 100–11.

6. Krych-Goldberg M, Atkinson JP. Structure function relationships of complement receptor type 1. *Immunol Rev* 2001; **180**: 112–22.

7. Weisman HF, Bartow T, Leppo MK et al. Soluble human complement receptor type I: in vivo inhibitor of complement suppressing post ischemic myocardial inflammation and necrosis. *Science* 1990; **249**: 146–51.

8. Klickstein LB, Moore Jr FD, Atkinson JP. Therapeutic inhibition of complement activation with emphasis on drugs in clinical trials. In: Austen KF, Burakoff SJ, Strom TB, Rosen FS, eds. *Therapeutic Immunology* (Blackwell Science: Malden, MA, 2000) 287–301.

9. Kirshfink M. Targeting complement in therapy. *Immunol Rev* 2001; **180**: 177–89.

10. Lambris JD, Holers VM. *Contemporary Immunology: Therapeutic Interventions in the Complement System* (Humana Press: Totowa, NJ, 2000) 259.

11. Rioux P. TP-10. *Curr Opin Invest Drugs* 2001; **2**: 364–71.

12. Zimmerman JL, Dellinger RP, Straube RC et al. Phase I trial of the recombinant soluble complement receptor 1 in acute lung injury and acute respiratory distress syndrome. *Crit Care Med* 2000; **28**: 3149–54.

13. Mulligan MS, Yeh CG, Rudolph AR et al. Protective effects of soluble CR1 in complement- and neutrophil-mediated tissue injury. *J Immunol* 1992; **148**: 1479–85.

14. Perry GJ, Eisenberg PR, Zimmerman JI et al. Phase I safety trial of soluble complement receptor type 1 (TP10) in acute myocardial infarction. *J Am Coll Cardiol* 1998; **31**(Suppl): 411A.

15. Rittershaus CW, Thomas LJ, Miller DP et al. Recombinant glycoproteins that inhibit complement activation and also bind the selectin adhesion molecules. *J Biol Chem* 1999; **274**: 11237–44.

16. Mulligan MS, Warner RL, Rittershaus CW et al. Endothelial targeting and enhanced antiinflammatory effects of complement inhibitors possessing sialyl Lewis[x] moieties. *J Immunol* 1999; **162**: 4952–9.

17. Huang J, Kim LJ, Mealey R et al. Neuronal protection in stroke by an sLe[x]-glycosylated complement inhibitory protein. *Science* 1999; **285**: 595–9.

18. Thomas TC, Rollins SA, Rother RP et al. Inhibition of complement activity by humanized anti-C5 antibody and single-chain Fv. *Mol Immunol* 1996; **33**: 1389–401.

19. Fitch JCK, Rollins SA, Matis LA et al. Pharmacology and biological efficacy of a recombinant, humanized single-chain antibody C5 complement inhibitor in patients undergoing coronary artery bypass graft surgery utilizing cardiopulmonary bypass. *Circulation* 1999; **100**: 2499–506.

20. Rinder CS, Rinder HM, Smith BR et al. Blockage of C5a and C5b-9 generation inhibits leukocyte and platelet activation during extracorporeal circulation. *J Clin Invest* 1995; **96**: 1564–72.

21. Vakeva AP, Agah A, Rollins SA et al. Myocardial infarction and apoptosis after myocardial ischemia and reperfusion. *Circulation* 1998; **97**: 2259–67.

22. Higgins PJ, Ko J-L, Lobell R et al. A soluble chimeric complement inhibitory protein that possesses both decay-accelerating and factor I cofactor activities. *J Immunol* 1997; **158**: 2872–81.

23. Kroshus TJ, Salerno CT, Yeh CG et al. A recombinant soluble chimeric complement inhibitor composed of human CD46 and CD55 reduces acute cardiac tissue injury in models of pig-to-human heart transplantation. *Transplantation* 2000; **69**: 2282–9.

24. Fleming SD, Tsokos GC. Complement inhibitors in rheumatic diseases. In: Tsokos GC, ed. *Modern Therapeutics in Rheumatic Diseases* (Humana Press: Totowa, 2002) 443–52.

25. Sahu A, Morikis D, Lambris JD. Complement

inhibitors targeting C3, C4, and C5. In: Lambris JD, Holers VM, eds. *Contemporary Immunology: Therapeutic Interventions in the Complement System* (Humana Press: Totowa, 2000) 75–112.

26. Cole LB, Kilpatrick JM, Chu N et al. Structure of 3,4-dichloroisocoumarin-inhibited factor D. *Acta Crystallogr Sect D Biol Crystallogr* 1998; **54**: 711–17.

27. Kilpatrick JM, Babu YS, Agrawal A et al. Control of the alternative complement pathway: inhibition of factor D. In: Mazarakis H, Swart SJ, eds. *Controlling the Complement System* (International Business Communications: Southborough, MA, 1997) 203–25.

28. Fung M, Loubser PG, Undar A et al. Inhibition of complement, neutrophil, and platelet activation by an anti-factor D monoclonal antibody in simulated cardiopulmonary bypass circuits. *J Thorac Cardiovasc Surg* 2001; **122**: 113–22.

29. Pasinetti GM. Inflammatory mechanisms in neurodegeneration and Alzheimer's disease: the role of the complement system. *Neurobiol Aging* 1996; **17**: 707–16.

Section V

Matrix molecules

27

Matrix molecules

Michael Sittinger, Iris Leinhase and Gerd Burmester

What is the extracellular matrix? • Structure and classification of matrix molecules • Structure of extracellular matrix components in articular cartilage • Structure of extracellular matrix in bone • Artificial matrix for tissue regeneration • In vitro pannus model • References

WHAT IS THE EXTRACELLULAR MATRIX?

The extracellular matrix accounts for much of the actual difference in the properties of isolated human cells and is a functional tissue. It is a network of proteins, polysaccharides and proteoglycans with an impressive complexity. Extracellular matrix molecules are usually secreted by the tissue cells. However, the cells maintain extensive direct or indirect interactions with these matrix components, even when they are assembled into large macromolecular structures. Normally, this matrix resembles a relatively stable structural material, which lies underneath the epithelia and surrounds connective tissue cells. However, looking at it as just an inert supporting scaffold for these cells is no longer appropriate.[1] On the one hand, the matrix components, such as collagens, represent a source of mechanical strength for the tissue. Elastin and proteoglycans are important for matrix elasticity, and glycoproteins create a tissue network. On the other hand, matrix molecules influence gene expression, phenotype and metabolism, and control key functions in nutrition and communication between cells. The composition of the extracellular matrix varies between tissue types, but in most skeletal tissues,

such as cartilage and bone, this extracellular matrix actually determines the predominant functional properties of the tissues.

Bone and cartilage, like most other tissues, are characterized by a continuous remodeling during the entire lifespan, regulated and balanced by synthesis, assembly and degradation of matrix components. In joint diseases, this fine balance is significantly disturbed, leading to pathologic alterations or destruction of cartilage and bone. In both normal and diseased tissues, a continuous turnover of matrix releases fragments of the matrix into the surrounding environment, synovial fluids, blood and urine, where they can be detected and measured.

Further research on extracellular matrix metabolism will elucidate the complex matrix system, and additional molecules and markers of cartilage and bone matrix may be discovered. Such data may finally expand the panel of available tools and parameters to diagnose rheumatic diseases or responses to treatment options.

STRUCTURE AND CLASSIFICATION OF MATRIX MOLECULES

The essential elements of the extracellular matrix in most tissues, and specifically in connective tissues, are collagens, proteoglycans, glycosaminoglycans and non-collagenous proteins, as well as glycoproteins. Fiber-structured collagen molecules are embedded in a gel-like ground substance of polysaccharides called glycosaminoglycans (GAG). This hydrated polysaccharide gel ensures a regulated diffusion of nutrients and metabolites into the intracellular spaces between the cells.

All these matrix components fulfill essential tasks for the tissue. The collagen network provides cartilage with its form and tensile strength. Proteoglycans (Pg) and non-collagenous proteins form a hydrophilic gel system that influences the hydroelastic properties of tissues.[2] Furthermore, in bone tissue, the addition of inorganic minerals, particularly calcium phosphate molecules, provides an extremely high compressive strength.

Collagens

Collagens constitute a highly specialized family of glycoproteins. They are homo- or hetero-trimeric molecules whose subunits, the α-chains, are distinct gene products. Up to 34 different α-chains have been found and described. The different combinations of the α-chains within the superfamily of vertebral collagens constitute at least 19 different collagen types found in different tissues (Table 27.1).[3]

The biosynthesis of collagen molecules, especially their α-chains, is characterized by a normal pathway of protein synthesis followed by several co-translational and post-translational modifications, including: the hydroxylation of proline and lysine by ascorbate, iron and molecular oxygen; the glycosylation of hydroxylysine; the sulfation of tyrosine; and the insertion of carbohydrates and glycosaminoglycans.[1] The proteins are first synthesized as pro-α-chains with propeptides, which are responsible for the controlled formation of the triple helix structure to produce insoluble procollagen. The propeptides are removed extracellularly by specific proteinases during fibrillogenesis, as the procollagen molecules leave the cell.[4] The monomers align spontaneously and form collagen fibrils.

The triple helix contains three polypeptide α-chains consisting of a repeating triplet of glycine (33.5%), proline (12%) and hydroxyproline (10%).[5] Glycine is small enough to fit into the center of the helix.[4] Lysine and hydroxylysine, being desaminated by lysyloxidase, reside in specific regions, and form inter- and intramolecular covalent cross-links to the collagens, to stabilize the helical structure.[5]

The detailed structure and composition of the collagens vary among the different collagen types, among the same collagen type within the tissues, and with age.[6] Comprising about one-quarter of the total protein in the human body, the collagens represent the most significant structural extracellular matrix component. They can be subclassified into homogeneous fibril-forming collagens (types I, II, III, V and XI) and heterogeneous non-fibril-forming collagens (types IV, VI, VII, VIII, IX, X and XII).[4] According to this distinction, several subfamilies of the non-fibril-forming collagens can be differentiated: network-forming collagens (basement membrane collagen IV, type VIII and type X); microfibrillar collagen IV; FACIT (fibril-associated collagen with interrupted triple helix) (types IX, XII, XIV and XIX); and multiplexins (multi-triple-helix domain and interruptions) (types XV and XVIII).[3] Type I collagen, found in bone, cornea, skin as well as other tissues, is the most abundant collagen, accounting for almost 80–90% of total collagen in the body.[1] Type II collagen and small amounts of collagen types III, VI and XI are found in articular cartilage.[7]

Proteoglycans and glycosaminoglycans

Pgs and hyaluronan are major components within the extracellular matrix in addition to collagens. Most Pgs consist of a very long single hyaluronan chain, a protein core and, for the most part, more than 100 sulfated GAGs, existing either as monomers or as aggregates.[8] The GAGs consist of repeating units of disaccharides, of which one sugar is either *N*-acetylglucosamine or *N*-acetylgalactosamine, and the second is usually acidic (either glucuronic acid or iduronic acid).[9] With the exception of hyaluronan, these sugars are

Table 27.1   Distribution and function of collagens in the organism.[1,3,4,18,51–55]

Type	Tissue location	Function and comments
Type I	Bone, cornea, skin, tendon	Tensile strength, component of macrofibril
Type II	Cartilage, vitreous	Tensile strength, component of macrofibril
Type III	Skin, aorta, uterus, gut	Essential for type I collagen fibrillogenesis
Type IV	Basement membrane	Forms three-dimensional networks, microfibril, grid fiber
Type V	Placental tissue, bone, skin	Fibrils, in thin pericellular lamina, homology with collagen types I–III
Type VI	Cartilage, uterus, skin, cornea	Surrounding the chondrocytes, attachment of cells to the matrix, beaded filaments
Type VII	Amniotic membrane, skin, esophagus	Anti-parallel dimers that form anchoring fibrils
Type VIII	Descemet's membrane, basement membrane of the corneal endothelium	Hexagonal lattice
Type IX	Cartilage, vitreous	Tensile properties and fibril–interfibril connection cross-linked to the surface of macrofibrils
Type X	Calcified cartilage	Structural support, role in mineralization, associated with macrofibril, present in calcified layer
Type XI	Cartilage, intervertebral disk	Nucleates fibril formation, component of macrofibril, homology with collagen types I–III
Type XII	Skin, tendon, cartilage	FACIT collagen, part of macrofibril, homotrimeric
Type XIII	Endothelial cells, epidermis, ocular tissues, optic nerve bundles, ganglion cell layer of the retina	May be involved in cell–matrix and perhaps cell–cell interactions
Type XIV	Skin, tendon, cartilage	FACIT collagen, part of macrofibril, homotrimeric
Type XV	Placenta, kidney, heart, ovary, testis	Part of multiplexin collagen superfamily, join basement membrane to the underlying connective tissue stroma
Type XVI	Kidney, heart, smooth muscle, ovary, eye	No information on the physiologic functions available
Type XVII	Transmembranous component of hemidesmosomal cells	Functions in epithelial–basement membrane interactions
Type XVIII	Kidney, liver, lung	Part of multiplexin collagen superfamily, potently inhibits angiogenesis and tumor growth
Type XIX	Fibroblast cell lines, vascular, neuronal, mesenchymal, and some epithelial basement membrane zones	Involvement with angiogenic and pathologic processes

Table 27.2   Distribution of glycosaminoglycans.[1,3,9,56]

Type	Tissue location
Hyaluronic acid (hyaluronan)	Different connective tissues, skin, synovial tissue, cartilage
Chondroitin-4-sulfate	Cartilage, cornea, bone, skin, artery
Chondroitin-6-sulfate	Cornea, bone, skin, artery
Dermatan sulfate	Skin, heart, vascular
Heparan sulfate	Lung, artery, cell surface
Heparin	Liver, lung, skin, mastocyte
Keratin sulfate	Cartilage, cornea, intervertebral disk

modified by the addition of carboxyl and sulfate groups.[10] Compared to the glycoproteins, the GAGs are larger and have a higher carbohydrate content of 90–95%. Characterization of differences in the protein content, the molecule size, as well as the number and type of GAGs, shows that Pgs are extremely heterogeneous.[4] As the GAGs are highly negatively charged, forming hydrophilic, anionic macromolecules, the Pgs bind positively charged ions to their side-chains.[2,11] They trap water molecules to form hydrated gels, thereby providing mechanical support to the extracellular matrix. As a result, the side-chains repel each other, resulting in a distended molecule surface.[8] Newly synthesized Pgs do not form directly into stabilized aggregates; instead, they slowly develop their final form. As a consequence of this aggregation, the molecules gradually lose their mobility within the fibril meshwork, and the local concentration decreases.[1]

The distribution of GAGs is shown in Table 27.2.

Hyaluronic acid, the most important GAG present in most tissues, consists of an alternating polymer of D-glucuronic acid and N-acetylgly-cosamine, which implies a high content of sulfate and uronic acid, conferring a pronounced negative charge on GAGs and permitting them to take part in a large number of electrostatic interactions.[1,4] The molecular weight rises to above one million = 10^6.[12] Other than hyaluronic acid, all GAGs bind covalently to proteins in the tissue matrix. Chondroitin-4-sulfate consists of

D-glucuronic acid and N-acetyl-D-galac-tosamine, and keratan sulfate consists of D-galactose and N-acetyl-D-glucosamine, but both chondroitin-4-sulfate and keratan sulfate are disaccharides without side-chains.[4]

Several groups of proteoglycans which vary in size, protein cores and molecular properties are present in the extracellular matrix as shown in Table 27.3. Based on typical features a simplified classification has been proposed by different authors. This classification distinguishes the small leucine-rich Pgs, and the modular Pgs, with two subgroups, the non-hyaluron-binding and hyaluron- and lectin-binding Pgs.[3]

The major Pg in articular cartilage by mass is aggrecan, which contains keratan sulfate and chondroitin sulfate chains and a protein core filament.[9] It binds hyaluronan with specialized link proteins, giving stiffness to the cartilage.[10] The core protein is composed of three globular domains (G1, G2 and G3) and a large extended region between G2 and G3 to bind GAG chains. The N-terminus comprises the 61 globular domain of the core protein. G2, being homologous to the G1 domain and to the link protein, is basically involved in product processing. The G3 domain constitutes the C-terminus of the core protein.[13,14] Link proteins are present on the hyaluronic acid chain at the attachment side of Pg monomers (Figure 27.1).[15] Decorin, the smallest Pg, having only one dermatan sulfate chain, binds to the collagen fibrils during fibril formation and is concentrated on the surface and in pericellular

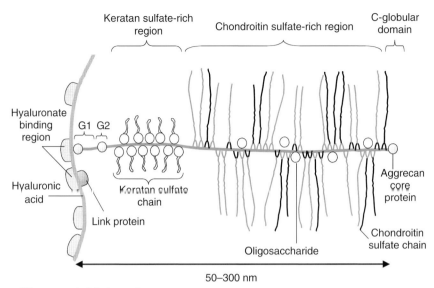

Figure 27.1 Schematic presentation of a cartilage proteoglycan aggregate. It consists of a single hyaluronic acid chain, to which proteoglycan monomers are attached by means of specific link proteins. Each Pg is composed of a central protein core, which is substituted with diverse negatively charged GAG chains and oligosaccharides. The GAGs consist mainly of keratan sulfate and chondroitin sulfate.

G2 = second globular region
G1 = binding region

Table 27.3   Function of proteoglycans.[1,3,13,18,57,58]

Type	Function and comments
Aggrecan	Compressive stiffness, binds hyaluronan, concentrated in the deep zone
Versican	Large protein core, hyaluronan-binding domain
CD44	Cell–matrix binding
Neurocan	Brain tissue specific, large protein core, hyaluronan-binding domain
Brevican	Brain tissue specific, large protein core, hyaluronan-binding domain
Perlecan	Heparan sulfate proteoglycan (HSPg), cell–matrix adhesion, located at the cell surface
Agrin	Located in the glomerular basement membrane
Testican	Located in human seminal plasma, progenitor of the unique heparan/chondroitin sulfate-bearing peptide
Decorin	Regulates the formation of macrofibrils, concentrated at articular surface and in pericellular sites
Fibromodulin	Regulates the formation of macrofibrils
Epiphycan	Leucine-rich Pg
Lumican	Regulates the formation of macrofibrils
Biglycan	Leucine-rich Pg

Table 27.4   Distribution of non-collagenous proteins and glycoproteins.[2,3,9–11,12–16,18,20]

Type	Function and comments
Fibronectin	Connective tissue, role in matrix organization and cell–matrix interaction
Tenascin	Connective tissue, role in matrix organization and cell–matrix interaction
Fibrilin-1	Connective tissue, present in pericellular sites in cartilage, forms microfibril network
Elastin	Connective tissue
Lamprin	Lamprey cartilage, related to elastin
Matrilin	Connective tissue, associated with cartilage formation and calcification
Thrombospondin	Connective tissue
Laminin	Basement membranes
Nidogen/entactin	Basement membranes
Fibulin	Basement membranes
Anchorin CII	Collagen II-binding surface protein of chondrocytes
Link protein	Homologous to part of aggrecan, stabilized binding of hyaluronan to aggrecan
Matrix-γ-carboxylglutamic acid protein	Pericellular location, inhibits calcification
Chondrocalcin	Fetal cartilage, binds to anchorin CII, role in calcification
Chondroadherin	Cell–matrix binding, bind integrin
Cartilage oligomeric protein (COMP)	Binds type II collagen, involved in macrofibril assembly, located in the territorial region
Superficial zone protein, lubricin	Also known as lubricin, synthesized by cells in superficial zone
Angiogenin	Nasal cartilage and epiphysis, may encourage the ingrowth of a vascular system prior to ossification
Chondromodulin	Fetal cartilage, unknown
Pleiotrophin	Fetal cartilage, heparin-binding, stimulates angiogenesis in tumors

sites of articular cartilage.[1] The functions of proteoglycans are summarised in Table 27.3.

Non-collagenous proteins and glycoproteins

Compared with the collagens and Pgs, the non-collagenous proteins and glycoproteins (GP) are not as well studied and understood. It has become clear that a wide variety of these proteins are responsible for cell interactions and binding of other macromolecules to the matrix.[2] In most cases, they consist of a protein framework with a few attached mono- and oligosaccharides.[9]

The distribution of non-collagenous proteins and glycoproteins is shown in Table 27.4.

STRUCTURE OF EXTRACELLULAR MATRIX COMPONENTS IN ARTICULAR CARTILAGE

Cartilage is a connective tissue derived from the mesoderm. Distinguished by form, occurrence and function, cartilage is subdivided in three main groups: hyaline, elastic and fibril-forming cartilage.[16] Hyaline cartilage is the most important type, occurring in joint cartilage, rib rudiment, nose skeleton, and tracheal cartilage. Examples of elastic cartilages are laryngeal and

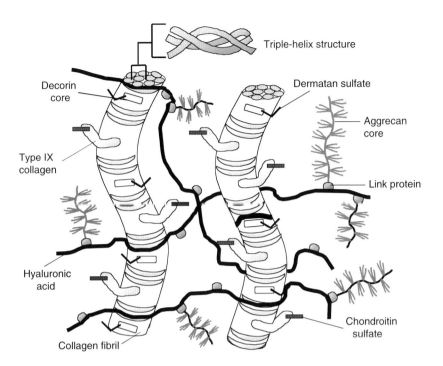

Triple-helix structure

Decorin core

Dermatan sulfate

Aggrecan core

Type IX collagen

Link protein

Hyaluronic acid

Chondroitin sulfate

Collagen fibril

Figure 27.2 Model of collagen network, showing the accumulation of the collagen fibrils as well as their connection to hyaluronic acid chains and articular proteoglycans.

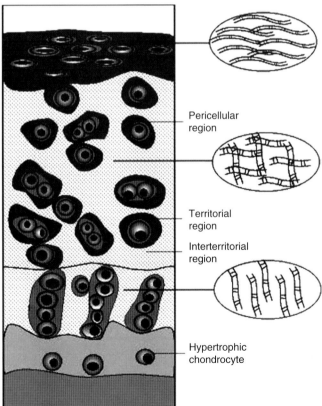

Articular surface

Superficial zone 10–20%

Pericellular region

Middle zone 40–60% (transitional)

Territorial region

Interterritorial region

Deep zone 30–40%

Calcified zone

Hypertrophic chondrocyte

Subchondral bone

Figure 27.3 Structure and zonation of articular cartilage. The schema overviews the cellular organization as well as the architecture of the matrix components and collagen fibers in the four layers or zones of cartilage tissue.

ear cartilages, whereas joint surfaces, jaw and symphyses are composed of fibril-forming cartilage.[5] The tissues are in part self-renewing, respond to mechanical forces, and provide stable movement. They vary in thickness, cell density, matrix composition and mechanical properties within the same joint, among joints and also among species.[9]

Chondrocytes comprise the only type of cell found in articular cartilage. They are embedded in a matrix macromolecular framework and an expressible fluid (matrix water), with a volume of 60–80% of its wet weight.[9] The microscopic structure of cartilage shows that the tissue consists mainly of extracellular matrix, cells representing only about 1% of the volume. Cartilage does not have a system of nerves, or blood or lymphatic vessels. The nutrient supply is supported by a complex interaction between the cells and the matrix network. Significantly, cartilage tissue appears homogeneous, but has no uniform shape.[8]

Mature articular cartilage presents a typical highly ordered zonation as described by Poole et al (Figure 27.3).[15] The so-called superficial zone of articular cartilage is lubricated by synovial fluid, and the chondrocytes are elongated and aligned parallel to the surface. The zone just below this first layer is constituted of rounded chondrocytes embedded in an extensive extracellular matrix. The so-called middle zone shows the very characteristic morphologic features of hyaline cartilage. Below that is the deep zone; where, in some joints, the cells are arranged in a column-like manner almost vertical to the cartilage surface.[17] This deep zone contains the lowest cell and collagen densities. Finally, the bottom zone is an almost calcified layer just above the subchondral bone and represents a buffer with intermediate mechanical properties. It contains hypertrophic cells able to calcify the matrix and synthesize type X collagen.[18]

Articular cartilage matrix components

As described above, the structural macromolecules in articular cartilage are collagens, Pgs and non-collagenous proteins, contributing up to 40% of its wet weight. Collagens comprise about 60%, Pgs about 25% and the non-collagenous proteins about 15–20% of the dry weight.[9] A model of a collagen network is shown in Figure 27.2.

The extracellular matrix composition of cartilage also varies between different regions in the tissue. With regard to the zonation of articular cartilage as described by Poole et al,[15] there is also significant variability in composition, organization and function of the matrix ingredients, depending on the distance from the cells (Figure 27.3).[18] Directly around the chondrocytes and covering the cell surface, a narrow layer of matrix exists. In the so-called pericellular region, the fibrillar collagen content is minimal, but the concentration of Pgs, such as decorin and aggrecan, is increased. It also contains non-collagenous proteins, such as anchorin CII and small amounts of non-fibrillar collagens, especially type VI collagen. Surrounding this first layer, in the territorial matrix, fibrillar collagen molecules form a thin network around the cells. These first two regions appear to serve the needs of chondrocytes and, furthermore, protect the cells during loading and deformation of the tissue. Further away from the cells, in the so-called interterritorial matrix, large unorganized collagen fibrils are aligned according to their distance from the joint surface. This region makes up most of the volume in mature cartilage and is responsible for the mechanical properties of the tissue.[8,9,15,18]

As described in Table 27.1, in cartilage, collagen types II, VI, IX, X and XI were found, whereas collagen types II, IX and XI mainly form the collagen fibrils. The collagen macromolecules are embedded in a hydrated polysaccharide gel mainly consisting of Pgs, finally forming a stable meshwork, providing tensile strength and stiffness to cartilage.[19] Articular cartilage contains two major classes of Pgs: large aggregating monomers such as aggrecan, attached to the protein core filament, and small Pgs such as decorin, biglycan and fibromodulin.[13] The core protein, the large Pg chains of articular cartilage, is composed of approximately 2000 amino acids and encloses about 100 chondroitin-4-sulfate

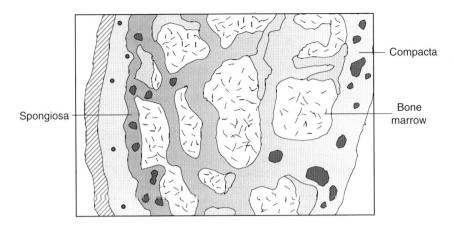

Figure 27.4 Bone architecture, showing the composition of substantia spongiosa and substantia corticalis or compacta in relation to the bone marrow.

chains, 30 keratan sulfate chains and about 40 oligosaccharides.[20] For example, the core protein of aggrecan has a molecular mass of about 230 kDa, with up to 130 GAG chains being attached to it.[19] The tissue also contains large non-aggregating Pgs that resemble aggrecan in structure and composition.

In hyaline cartilage, the Pgs are compressed by the collagen meshwork and are only partially hydrated. The molecules in situ have a volume much smaller than when in free solution.[8] Here, the large Pg aggrecan comprises about 90% of the total Pgs.[9] The remaining 20% consists of the smaller core proteins and other GAGs, such as dermatan sulfate.[19]

STRUCTURE OF EXTRACELLULAR MATRIX IN BONE

The key role of the skeleton is to provide structural support for the body, but it also serves as the body's mineral source. The mineralized structure, meaning bone structure, is fundamental for posture, supporting muscular contraction, resulting in motion; it withstands functional extensions, and protects internal organs.[21] In an unequalled manner, bone combines strength and stiffness, having a compressive strength of about 15 kg/mm and a tensile strength of 10 kg/mm; while having a minimum weight. Unfortunately, there is a general view of bone as an inert and static material. Indeed, considering bone tissue's

ability to adapt its mass and structure to functional demands, its ability to repair itself, and its capacity to rapidly mobilize mineral matrix stores, it would be better described as a dynamic biological system.[16] Within the body, bones are well suited for the structural demands made on them. They mainly consist of hollow tubes, which provide great strength and durability against axial compression forces, while at the same time minimizing the weight to keep the body unencumbered for motion.

Macroscopically, almost every bone is built in distinct layers (Figure 27.4). Substantia spongiosa, the interior layer, consists of thin lamellar structures branching in all directions and crossing each other to form a sponge-like network. Within cavities of the bone, marrow is located.[22] In contrast, substantia corticalis or compacta, the outer layer, appears solid and massive without visible cavities. With the exception of the cartilage-surrounded joint area, every bone region is covered with a tight connective tissue layer, the so-called periost.[23] The corticalis and spongiosa consist of the same cells and matrix components, but differ in structure and function. Corticalis is calcified by up to 90%, whereas spongiosa has a calcification level of only 15–25%. The remaining portion of the tissue consists of bone marrow, connective tissue and blood vessels.[24]

In contrast to articular cartilage, three clearly distinct cell types can be identified within bone. They can be classified as matrix-producing

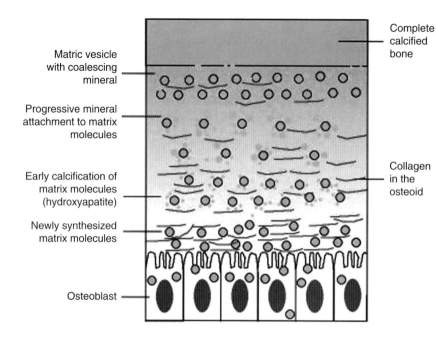

Matric vesicle with coalescing mineral

Progressive mineral attachment to matrix molecules

Early calcification of matrix molecules (hydroxyapatite)

Newly synthesized matrix molecules

Osteoblast

Complete calcified bone

Collagen in the osteoid

Figure 27.5 Schematic presentation of bone calcification. The osteoblasts secrete new matrix molecules such as GAGs and osteoid collagens, starting calcification. With the progressive attachment of minerals such as hydroxyapatite to the vesicles, the matrix begins to calcify completely.

osteoblasts, tissue-resorbing osteoclasts, and differentiated osteocytes, which account for 90% of all cells in the adult skeleton. Osteocytes can be viewed as highly specialized and fully differentiated osteoblasts 'trapped' in their own calcified matrix, changing their phenotype and reducing their cell organelles and production of matrix proteins.[25] Fibroblasts, osteoblasts, osteocytes and adipocytes derive primarily from pluripotent mesenchymal stem cells, whereas osteoclasts are of hematopoietic descent and their precursors are located in the monocytic fraction of the bone marrow.[26] Osteoblasts and bone lining cells (inactive osteoblasts) form a tight layer covering the bone surface, creating an extensive network of intercellular communication. Osteoblasts are the cells within bone that produce the extracellular matrix and regulate its mineralization.[22] The interactions between both cells and the extracellular matrix of bone are important determinants of cell proliferation and differentiation.[27] Additionally, cells of the osteoblast lineage form functional cell–cell and cell–matrix connections, and communicate with osteocytes via a variety of transmembranous proteins (integrins, connexins) and specific

receptors (for cytokines, hormones and growth factors), through cytoplasmic processes extending through canaliculi in the bone.[25] The main attribute of osteoclasts is their ability to resorb fully mineralized bone at sites called Howship's lacunae. They are highly migratory, multinucleated and polarized cells which carry a depot of lysosomal enzymes.[22]

Bone matrix components

Calcified bone contains barely 25% organic matrix, including a low content of cells (merely 2–5%), 5% matrix water, and 70% inorganic minerals (e.g. hydroxyapatite). The bone minerals are sediments of crystalline calcium phosphate (85%) and calcium carbonate (10%), appearing as hydroxyapatite crystals ($Ca_{10}(PO_4)_6(OH)_2$), with a plate-like crystal structure of length 60 nm and thickness 3–6 nm.[22,25] Because bone apatite crystals are four times smaller than geologically occurring apatites and less perfect in structure, they are more reactive and soluble, facilitating chemical turnover. Additional elements in bone are magnesium, calcium

Table 27.5 Function of non-collagenous proteins in bone.[2,3,20,25]

Type	Function and comments
Perlecan	Defining the spatial organization of the extracellular matrix, synthesis of Pgs
Biglycan	Defining the spatial organization of the extracellular matrix
Bone sioaloprotein (BSP)	Binds to hydroxyapatite
Osteocalcin	Binds to hydroxyapatite, regulatory functions in the assembly of mineralized bone
Osteonectin	Determines the orientation and organization of the bone mineral crystal, binds calcium
Osteopontin	Determines the orientation and organization of the bone mineral crystal, binds to hydroxyapatite
Matrix gla protein	Role in mineralization process
Fibromodulin	Modulates collagen fibril formation
Fibronectin	Interacts with GAGs, collagens and several bacterial cells
Thrombospondin	Binds to hydroxyapatite, calcium and several other proteins

chloride, potassium, fluorine and other trace elements.[28]

The osteoid is a freshly synthesized matrix prior to its mineralization, and consists primarily of type I collagen. Other proteins, most of them unique to bone, such as osteocalcin, are embedded in the extracellular matrix and have important signaling functions (bone morphogenic proteins, growth factors, cytokines, adhesion molecules) and play a role during the mineralization process (osteopontin, osteonectin, matrix gla protein).[25] Within a few days after the organic matrix has been secreted, the osteoid begins to mineralize. During this period, the mineral content reaches 75% of its final amount; to achieve the latter takes several months (Figure 27.5).[16] During the process of mineralization, the orientation and organization within the bone mineral matrix of the collagen fibrils, fibronectin, and the GPs, such as osteonectin and osteopontin, are determined.[22]

Most of the non-collagenous proteins in bone, such as sialoproteins and Pgs (mainly chondroitin sulfate and hyaluronan), have structural functions (Table 27.5).[29] Other GPs, such as matrix gla protein and GAGs, appear to play a role in the inhibition of excessive mineralization.[25]

ARTIFICIAL MATRIX FOR TISSUE REGENERATION

For tissue repair, the replacement of pathological tissues and even organs is one strategy.[30] The patient's immune system often causes complications of varying intensity in response to attempted repairs. These complications begin with low immune system responses, such as singe inflammation, and end with antagonizing artificial prostheses and extraneous organs. Numerous materials, such as titanium, high-grade steel, ceramics, synthetic polymers (polylactic acid, polyglycolic acid, polyethylene, polypropylene) or natural matrix components like collagen or hyaluronic acid have been tested for their biocompatibility.[12] All of these lack the renewal ability of biomaterials, and are damaged by corrosion and degradation; the decomposition products often cause toxic or allergic reactions.[31]

Autologous cell transplantation, the main approach of tissue engineering, can limit the host reactions to a minimum. Successful harvest and

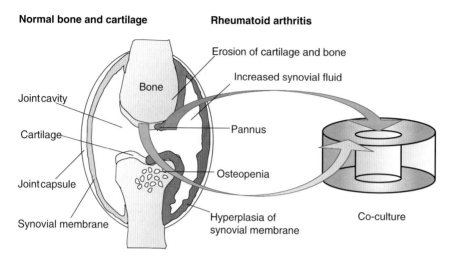

Figure 27.6 The in vitro pannus model developed by Sittinger et al. Tissue samples of articular cartilage as well as of rheumatoid synovium layer were obtained. The expanded cells were cultured interactively with a common contact zone in a co-culture system.

isolation of host cells from a small biopsy, expansion of cells in suitable culture devices and finally the re-implantation into the defect provide the potential for a biological route to restore joint, bone or connective tissue function.[32]

Various studies have shown that embedding cells in gel and a specifically designed textile scaffold allows the cells to produce an extracellular matrix, which is kept within the scaffold.[33] Such scaffolds are bioresorbable and may be sutured or glued into the defect site.[34,35] This system is able to temporarily simulate the properties of the ECM until the transplanted cells gradually reconstitute a new extracellular matrix in vivo.

Another important aspect of therapy and the development of drugs is to establish a cell–matrix system, which is able to represent the tissue functions under in vitro conditions.[36] The investigation of inflammatory joint diseases in animal models involves a variety of experimental strategies. Nevertheless, the limited comparability with the in vivo situation remains a problem, because important components of the human environment are missing. A reproducible and reliable in vitro tissue model system for destructive joint diseases would not only be able to replace certain in vivo models, but could help to overcome the limitations of conventional cell culture procedures. Results of experiments with two-dimensional monolayer cell cultures can

provide only a very poor model for processes where extracellular matrix components are involved in vivo. Thus, standard cell culture methods are not suitable for mimicking particular diseases such as rheumatoid arthritis (RA) where involvement of the extracellular matrix is implicated.

IN VITRO PANNUS MODEL

In RA, the physiologic balance between matrix composition and degradation is disturbed by chronic inflammation of the synovial joint.[37,38] Permanently activated synovial cells and infiltrated mononuclear blood cells form the hyperplastic synovial tissue (pannus), which invades cartilage and bone.[39–41] To investigate the importance of the extracellular matrix, especially to rheumatologic aspects in vitro, a so-called pannus model, which imitates the tissue matrix, was developed (Figure 27.6).

A major drawback of conventional two-dimensional cell culture is the lack of the complex network of cell–cell and cell–matrix interactions.[42–44] Therefore, it is important to develop a three-dimensional cell culture system including the formation or synthesis of an appropriate extracellular matrix. Special attention has been given to the role of the extracellular matrix and cell differentiation in artificial tissue.[32] Since chondrocytes dedifferentiate into fibroblast-like cells in monolayer cultures, neosynthesis of extracellular matrix in three-dimensional cultures is essential to study the role of matrix components in rheumatic diseases in vitro.[32,45]

The development of in vitro tissue model systems for RA which mimic the human joint microenvironment under in vitro conditions is the aim of several scientific groups. The in vitro model established by Frye et al[46] – synoviocyte-mediated cartilage invasion – allows for further molecular characterization of the invasive properties of the synoviocyte that contribute to RA. The results of D'Andrea et al[47] provide the first evidence for direct intercellular communication via calcium signaling between articular chondrocytes and synovial cells in co-culture. Kurz et al[48] found that chondrocytes establish protective mechanisms against reactive oxygen species via an interaction with synoviocytes in co-culture – a possible way to study mechanisms of inflammation in articular joints under defined conditions. Neidhart et al[49] studied distinct aspects of cartilaginous matrix destruction by RA synovial fibroblasts (RASFs) with an in vitro model of cartilage invasion by RASFs and found that interleukin-1Ra (IL-1Ra) and antibody against IL-1β could inhibit the cartilage destruction in this model.

Addressing the limitations of animal models on the one hand, and of the two-dimensional cell culture systems on the other, Schultz et al,[36] and later Smolian et al,[50] established an interactive three-dimensional in vitro model for RA (pannus model) that mimics the relevant local microenvironment in the arthritic joint, and allows us to study the destructive process in the context of the extracellular matrix and to investigate the contributions of distinct individual cell populations, such as the chondrocytes.

The model is based on special three-dimensional pellet cultures of articular chondrocytes and synovial cells cultured interactively with a common contact zone. Perfusion cell culture systems were found useful to stabilize essential culture parameters during long-term culture. Invasion of activated synovial fibroblasts and macrophages into a cartilaginous matrix formed in vitro, as well as the secretion of various proinflammatory cytokines and proteolytic enzymes, was demonstrated.

The in vitro pannus model offers several advantages compared to the previously established experimental models for RA. It offers the opportunity to supplement studies in animal systems or to even replace animal experiments and to study the effects of new therapeutic strategies in an experimental setting reflecting important features of human pathology. Furthermore, the developed pannus model opens new perspectives for the investigation of cell–cell and cell–matrix interactions in RA pathogenesis, as well as in other diseases where the extracellular matrix plays a major role in pathologic cell interactions.

REFERENCES

1. Hay ED. *Cell Biology of Extracellular Matrix*, 2nd edn. (Plenum Press: New York, 1991).
2. Neame PJ, Tapp H, Azizan A. Noncollagenous, nonproteoglycan macromolecules of cartilage. *CMLS Cell Mol Life Sci* 1999; **55**: 1327–40.
3. Aumailley M, Gayraud B. Strukture and biological activity of the extracellular matrix. *J Mol Med* 1998; **76**: 253–65.
4. Ayad S, Boot-Handford RP, Humphries MJ et al. *The Extracellular Matrix – FactsBook*, 2nd edn. (Academic Press: London, 1998).
5. Junqueiro LC, Carneiro J. *Histologie*. (Springer Verlag: Berlin, 1991).
6. Roughley PJ. Age-associated changes in cartilage matrix. *Clin Orthop* 2001; **391**: 153–60.
7. Reddi AH. Bone and cartilage differentiation. *Curr Opin Genet Dev* 1994; **4**: 737–44.
8. Newman AP. Articular cartilage repair. *Am J Sports Med* 1998; **26**: 309–24.
9. Buckwalter JA, Mankin HJ. Articular cartilage: tissue design and chondrocyte–matrix interactions. *Instr Course Lect* 1998; **47**: 477–86.
10. Guilak F, Jones WR, Ting-Beall HP et al. The deformation behavior and mechanical properties of chondrocytes in articular cartilage. *Osteoarthritis Cartilage* 1999; **7**: 59–70.

11. Wilkins RJ, Browning JA, Ellory JC. Surviving in a matrix: membrane transport in articular chondrocytes. *J Membr Biol* 2000; **177**: 95–108.

12. Noble PW. Hyaluronan and its catabolic products in tissue injury and repair. *Matrix Biol* 2002; **21**: 25–9.

13. Knudson CB, Knudson W. Cartilage proteoglycans. *Cell Dev Biol* 2001; **12**: 69–78.

14. Kiani C, Chen L, Wu YJ et al. Structure and function of aggrecan. *Cell Res* 2002; **12**: 19–32.

15. Poole AR, Pidoux I, Reiner A et al. An immuno-electron microscope study of the organisation of proteoglycan monomer, link protein, and collagen in the matrix of articular cartilage. *J Cell Biol* 1982; **93**: 921–37.

16. Geneser F. *Histologie* (Deutscher Ärtzer Verlag: Köln, 1990).

17. Meachim G. Age changes in articular cartilage. *Clin Orthop Relat Res* 2001; **391** Suppl: 6–13.

18. Poole AR, Kojima T, Yasuda T et al. Composition and structure of articular cartilage: a template for tissue repair. *Clin Orthop* 2001; **391** Suppl: 26–33.

19. Watanabe H, Yamada Y, Kimata K. Role of aggrecan, a large chondroitin sulfate proteoglycan, in cartilage structure and function. *J Biol Chem* 1998; **124**: 687–93.

20. Heinegard D, Oldberg A. Structure and biology of cartilage and bone matrix noncollagenous macromolecules. *AJEB J* 1989; **3**: 2042–51.

21. Bennet JH, Moffat S, Horton M. Cell adhesion molecules in human osteoblasts: structure and function. *Histol Histopathol* 2001; **16**: 603–11.

22. Stevens L, Lowe J. *Histologie* (VCH Verlagsgesellschaft: Weinheim, 1992).

23. Delling G, Hahn M, Vogel M. Pathomorphologische Konstruktionsprinzipien des Skelettsystems als Grundlage für das Verstaendnis der Osteoporose. *Fortschr Med* 1990; **108**: 7–9.

24. Baron B. Anatomy and ultrastructure of bone. In: Favus MJ, ed. *Primer on the Metabolic Bone Disease and Disorder of Mineral Metabolism*, 2nd edn. (Raven Press: New York, 1993) 3–9.

25. Sommerfeldt DW, Rubin CT. Biology of bone and how it orchestrates the form and function of the skeleton. *Eur Spine J* 2001; **2**: 86–95.

26. Aubin JE. Bone stem cells. *J Cell Biochem* 1998; 30–31 Suppl: 73–82.

27. Velleman SG. The role of the extracellular matrix in skeletal development. *Poult Sci* 2000; **79**: 985–9.

28. Hees H, Sinowatz F. *Histologie*, 3rd edn (Deutscher Ärtzer Verlag: Köln, 2000).

29. Garnero P, Rousseau JC, Delmas PD. Molecular basis and clinical use of biochemical markers of bone, cartilage, and synovium in joint diseases. *Arthritis Rheum* 2000; **43**: 953–68.

30. Solchaga LA, Goldberg VM, Caplan AI. Cartilage regeneration using principles of tissue engineering. *Clin Orthop* 2001; **391** Suppl: 161–70.

31. Buckwalter J, Coutts R, Hunziker E et al. Breakout Session 3: Articular cartilage. *Clin Orthop* 1999; **367**: 239–43.

32. Sittinger M, Bujia J, Rotter N et al. Tissue engineering and autologous transplant formation: practical approaches with resorbable biomaterials and new cell culture techniques. *Biomaterials* 1996; **17**: 237–42.

33. Sittinger M, Reitzel D, Dauner M et al. Resorbable polyesters in cartilage engineering: affinity and biocompatibility of polymer fiber structures to chondrocytes. *J Biomed Mater Res* 1996; **33**: 57–63.

34. Perka C, Sittinger M, Schultz O et al. Tissue engineered cartilage repair using cryopreserved and noncryopreseved chondrocytes. *Clin Orthop* 2000; **378**: 245–54.

35. Erggelet C, Sittinger M. The arthroscopic implantation of autologous chondrocytes for the treatment of full thickness cartilage defects of the knee joints. *J Arthrosc Relat Surg* (in press).

36. Schultz O, Keyszer G, Zacher J et al. Development of in vitro model systems for destructive joint diseases: novel strategies for establishing inflammatory pannus. *Arthritis Rheum* 1997; **40**: 1420–8.

37. Gay S, Gay RE, Koopman WJ. Molecular and cellular mechanisms of joint destruction in rheumatoid arthritis: two cellular mechanisms explain joint destruction? *Ann Rheum Dis* 1993; **52**: S39–47.

38. Volin MV, Koch AE. Cell cycle implications in the pathogenesis of rheumatoid arthritis. *Front Biosci* 2000; **5**: 594–601.

39. Burmester GR, Dimitriu-Bona A, Waters SJ et al. Identification of three major synovial lining cell populations by monoclonal antibodies directed to Ia antigens and antigens associated with monocytes/macrophages and fibroblasts. *Scand J Immunol* 1983; **17**: 69–82.

40. van der Laan WH, Pap T, Ronday HK et al. Cartilage degradation and invasion by rheumatoid synovial fibroblasts is inhibited by gene transfer of a cell surface-targeted plasmin inhibitor. *Arthritis Rheum* 2000; **43**: 1710–8.

41. Zvaifler NJ, Firestein GS. Pannus and pannocytes. Alternative models of joint destruction in rheumatoid arthritis. *Arthritis Rheum* 1994; **37**: 783–9.

42. Adams JC, Watt FM. Regulation of development and differentiation by the extracellular matrix. *Development* 1993; **117**: 1183–98.

43. Geiger B, Bershadsky A, Pankov R et al. Transmembrane crosstalk between the extracellular matrix – cytoskeleton crosstalk. *Nat Rev Mol Cell Biol* 2001; **2**: 793–805.

44. Kresse H, Schonherr E. Proteoglycans of the extracellular matrix and growth control. *J Cell Physiol* 2001; **189**: 266–74.

45. Schnabel M, Marlovits S, Eckhoff G et al. Dedifferentiation-associated changes in morphology and gene expression in primary human articular chondrocytes in cell culture. *Osteoarthritis Cartilage* 2002; **10**: 62–70.

46. Frye CA, Yocum DE, Tuan R et al. An in vitro model for studying mechanisms underlying synoviocyte-mediated cartilage invasion in rheumatoid arthritis. *Pathol Oncol Res* 1996; **2**: 157–66.

47. D'andrea P, Calabrese A, Grandolfo M. Intercellular calcium signalling between chondrocytes and synovial cells in co-culture. *Biochem J* 1998; **1**: 681–7.

48. Kurz B, Steinhagen J, Schunke M. Articular chondrocytes and synoviocytes in a co-culture system: influence on reactive oxygen species-induced cytotoxicity and lipid peroxidation. *Cell Tissue Res* 1999; **296**: 555–63.

49. Neidhart M, Gay RE, Gay S. Anti-interleukin-1 and anti-CD44 interventions producing significant inhibition of cartilage destruction in an in vitro model of cartilage invasion by rheumatoid arthritis synovial fibroblasts. *Arthritis Rheum* 2000; **43**: 1719–28.

50. Smolian H, Thiele S, Kolkenbrock H et al. Establishment of an in vitro model for rheumatoid arthritis as test system for therapeutical substances. *Altex* 2001; **18**: 265–80.

51. Sandberg-Lall M, Hagg PO, Wahlstrom I et al. Type XIII collagen is widely expressed in the adult and developing human eye and accentuated in the ciliary muscle, the optic nerve and the neural retina. *Exp Eye Res* 2000; **70**: 401–10.

52. Areida SK, Reinhardt DP, Muller PK et al. Properties of the collagen type XVII ectodomain. Evidence for n- to c-terminal triple helix folding. *J Biol Chem* 2001; **276**: 1594–601.

53. Myers JC, Li D, Bageris A et al. Biochemical and immunohistochemical characterization of human type XIX defines a novel class of basement membrane zone collagens. *Am J Pathol* 1997; **151**: 1729–40.

54. Myers JC, Dion AS, Abraham V et al. Type XV collagen exhibits a widespread distribution in human tissues but a distinct localization in basement membrane zones. *Cell Tissue Res* 1996; **286**: 493–505.

55. Knight DP. Unconventional collagens. *J Cell Sci* 2000; **113**: 4141–2.

56. Alberts B, Bray D, Lewis J et al. *Molecular Biology of the Cell*, 1st edn. (Garland Publishing: New York, 1983).

57. Groffen AJ, Veerkamp JH, Monnens LA et al. Recent insights into the structure and functions of heparan sulfate proteoglycans in the human glomerular basement membrane. *Nephrol Dial Transplant* 1999; **14**: 2119–29.

58. Alliel PM, Perin JP, Jolles P et al. Testican, a multidomain testicular proteoglycan resembling modulators of cell social behaviour. *Eur J Biochem* 1993; **214**: 347–50.

28

Matrix metalloproteinases

Thomas Pap, Steffen Gay and Georg Schett

Structure, nomenclature and function of matrix metalloproteinases • Regulation • Animal models • Expression of matrix metalloproteinases in rheumatoid arthritis • Matrix metalloproteinases as therapeutic targets • References

Tissue remodeling is a central feature of rheumatoid arthritis (RA). It essentially contributes to a progressive loss of joint function and leads to severe crippling that characterizes the high burden of disease. Tissue remodeling in RA is a complex mechanism and is composed of three major pathophysiological events: (1) growth, spread and invasion of inflammatory synovial tissue; (2) destruction of cartilage; and (3) bone erosion. All three processes are based on a common underlying mechanism, which is the degradation of extracellular matrix.

STRUCTURE, NOMENCLATURE AND FUNCTION OF MATRIX METALLOPROTEINASES

Matrix metalloproteinases (MMPs) comprise a family of zinc-containing enzymes involved in the degradation and remodeling of extracellular matrix proteins. The MMP protein family contains at least 16 different zinc-dependent endopeptidases.[1] All of these enzymes act extracellularly. The structure of MMPs consists of a catalytic domain containing histidine residues which form a complex with the catalytic zinc atom. The localization of this active site cleft

varies among different members of the MMP family and partly influences the substrate specificity of each of the proteins. Examples are the fibronectin type II repeats of MMP-2 and -9, which allow their binding to denatured collagen. The regulatory domain is a second essential domain of all MMPs. The regulatory domain locks the catalytic zinc site by chelating it to a cysteine residue and thus maintains the MMP in an inactive state. Upon activation of the MMP, this regulatory domain is cleaved from the protease domain, thus uncovering the active catalytic pocket. This cleavage is either autocatalytic or mediated by enzymes such as plasmin, trypsin, furin or other MMPs, especially membrane-type MMPs (MT-MMP). Except for MMP-7, which is the simplest MMP, containing a protease and a regulatory domain, other MMPs contain a variable number of structural domains. These domains determine partly substrate specificity of MMPs and are involved in the binding of matrix proteins and tissue inhibitors of metalloproteinases (TIMPs), the natural inhibitors of MMP activity.[2] Examples of structural domains are the hemopexin domains of collagenases (MMP-1, -8, -13 and -14), which allow the binding to triple-helical collagen, and the trans-

Table 28.1 Nomenclature and substrates of MMPs, including the alternative names of MMP family members.

Name	Alternative name	Major substrates	MMP substrates
MMP-1	Interstitial collagenase, collagenase 1	Collagens (I, II, III, VII, VIII, X), gelatin, aggrecan	MMP-2, -9
MMP-2	Gelatinase A, type IV collagenase	Collagens (I, IV, V, VII, X, XI, XIV), gelatin	MMP-1, -9, -13
MMP-3	Stromelysin-1	Collagens (III, IV, V, IX), gelatin, aggrecan	MMP-1, -2, -7, -8, -9, -13
MMP-7	Matrilysin	Collagens (IV, X), gelatin, aggrecan	MMP-1, -2, -9
MMP-8	Neutrophil collagenase, collagenase 2	Collagens (I, II, III, V, VII, VIII, X), gelatin, aggrecan	–
MMP-9	Gelatinase B, 92 kDa gelatinase	Collagens (IV, V, VII, X, XIV), gelatin, aggrecan	–
MMP-10	Stromelysin-2	Collagens (II, IV, V), gelatin, aggrecan	MMP-1, -8
MMP-11	Stromelysin-3	α_1-Antitrypsin, α_2-macroglobulin	–
MMP-12	Macrophage metalloelastase	Collagen (IV), gelatin, elastin	–
MMP-13	Collagenase-3	Collagens (I, II, III, IV, IX, X, XIV), gelatin, aggrecan	MMP 9
MMP-14	MT1-MMP	Collagens (I, II, III), gelatin, elastin	MMP-2, -13
MMP-15	MT2-MMP	Fibronectin, aggrecan	MMP-2
MMP-16	MT3-MMP	Collagen (III), gelatin	MMP-2
MMP-17	MT4-MMP	–	–
MMP-19	–	Gelatin	–
MMP-20	–	Amelogenin	–

membrane domains of MT-MMPs (MMP-14–17), which serve as anchors to the cell membrane.

The nomenclature of MMPs is now based on an MMP number (MMP-1, MMP-2, etc.). Earlier nomenclatures were based on the assumption that each MMP is highly substrate specific, and MMPs were named according to their capacity to degrade collagen (collagenases), denatured collagen (gelatinases) and elastin (elastases).[3] However, it was recognized that each MMP usually degrades multiple substrates and that there is substantial substrate overlap between individual MMPs. Therefore, a numerical nomenclature has become widely accepted (Table 28.1).

The function of MMPs is confined to the extracellular compartment, and MMPs act either in a soluble form outside the cells or anchored to the cell membrane (MT-MMP). First, members of the MMP family are involved in tissue remodeling under both normal and pathological conditions. Second, MMPs are necessary for the migration of normal and malignant cells through the extracellular matrix. Third, they act as regulatory molecules by processing matrix proteins, cytokines and adhesion molecules. In all these instances, MMP activity is in balance with the activity of their endogenous inhibitors TIMPs. Once activated, MMPs are substrates for TIMPs;

also, they are bound and inactivated by plasma proteins such as α_2-macroglobulin. Up to now, four different forms of TIMPs (TIMPs 1–4) have been described.[2]

Two protein families are structurally related to MMPs: the ADAMs (a desintegrin and a metalloproteinase)[4] and the ADAMTs (a desintegrin and a metalloproteinase with thrombospondin motifs).[5] The members of both families are also multidomain proteases and consist of a catalytic and a regulatory domain structurally related to MMPs. However, both families have a desintegrin domain which allows binding to cell surface integrins. Whereas ADAMs are membrane-bound molecules, ADAMTs lack a transmembrane part, but contain thrombospondin type I motifs, allowing their binding to proteoglycans. The most well-known ADAM is TACE (ADAM-17, tumor necrosis factor (TNF) converting enzyme) which cleaves membrane-bound TNF-α to a soluble form.[6,7] The most famous ADAMTs are ADAMT-4 and ADAMT-5, which are commonly known as 'aggrecanases'; they cleave aggrecan, which is the most important proteoglycan in cartilage.[8]

REGULATION

With the exception of MMP-2 and the MT-MMPs, which are constitutively expressed, MMP expression is induced (or suppressed) by extracellular signals via transcriptional activation. Three major groups of inducers can be differentiated: (1) proinflammatory cytokines; (2) growth factors; and (3) matrix molecules. Among proinflammatory cytokines, interleukin-1 (IL-1) is a central inducer of a variety of MMPs, including MMP-1, -3, -8, -13 and -14.[9–12] The effect of IL-1 on MMP expression highlights the complex nature of MMP induction: the specific effect of an extracellular signal such as IL-1 on MMP expression can be variable and depend on the type of MMP induced, the cell type, and the signal transduction pathway which is predominantly activated. Thus, for example, IL-1 differentially upregulates MMP-13, via c-Jun N-terminal kinase (JNK) and p38 protein kinase signaling,[9] and MMP-1, via signal transduction

and activation or transcription (STAT) factors,[12] in chondrocytes. Also, additive effects between IL-1 and other cytokines, such as TNF-α or oncostatin M,[12,13] or growth factors, such as fibroblast growth factor (FGF) and platelet-derived growth factor (PDGF), on the induction of MMPs are known.[14] Other cytokines pivotally involved in tissue remodeling of rheumatic diseases that induce MMP expression are TNF-α (MMP 1–3),[15] IL-17 (MMP-1 and -9),[16] and transforming growth factor (TGF)-β (MMP-13).[17] Among growth factors, FGF and PDGF are known inducers of MMPs, as they potentiate the effect of IL-1 on MMP expression.[14] Vascular endothelial growth factor (VEGF) is an inducer of MMP-13 in chondrocytes,[18] and MIP acts on MMP-9 and -13.[19] The third group of MMP inducers comprises matrix proteins (collagen, fibronectin), and especially their degradation products, which activate MMP expression in chondrocytes and fibroblasts, providing the possibility of site-specific MMP activation in regions of matrix breakdown.[20,21] Transcriptional silencers of MMPs are the anti-inflammatory and regulatory cytokines IL-4, IL-10 and IL-13,[22] as well as signaling via the p53 protein.[23]

Signaling for transcriptional activation of MMPs is mediated by several pathways. The activator protein-1 (AP-1) binding site is present in the promotor region of all MMPs (except MMP-2), suggesting a central role of jun/fos transcription factor binding. Indeed, there is much experimental evidence that all three mitogen/stress-activated protein kinase p38 mitogen/stress-activated protein kinase (MAPK/SAPK) families, extracellular regulated kinase (ERK), JNK and p38 kinase, which integrate extracellular signals upstream from jun/fos, are involved in the regulation of MMP expression. In particular, the induction of MMP-1, -9 and -13 is mediated through MAPK/SAPK signaling.[11,19,24–26] Apart from AP-1, the promoter regions of some MMPs contain NFκB,[24,25] STAT[27] and ETS[28,29] binding sites. Indeed, activation of these transcription factors has been demonstrated to occur during the induction of MMP-1, -3 and -13, which are thought to be essential for the joint damage in RA. Activation of the various

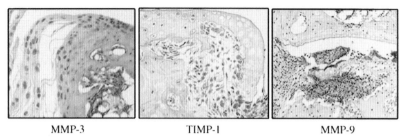

MMP-3   TIMP-1   MMP-9

Figure 28.1 MMPs and TIMPs are expressed by chondrocytes and pannocytes at site of bone and cartilage destruction. Microphotographs show the junction zone between pannus, cartilage and bone of paw sections from TNF-transgenic mice. Sections were stained for MMP-3, TIMP-1 and MMP-9 (dark colors). MMPs and TIMP are abundantly expressed by cells of the synovial membrane, the invading inflammatory synovial tissue and adjacent cartilage.

MAPK/SAPK and transcription factors, not all of which are tissue-specific signaling molecules, occurs in very distinct subcompartments of the rheumatoid joint, thus determining a specific pattern of MMP expression at each site in the synovium.[30,31] On the other hand, tissue-specific transcription factors of MMP do exist. One example is Cbfa-1 (a runx protein family member) which is essential for MMP-13 expression in cartilage and bone.[32]

ANIMAL MODELS

MMP activation has been assessed in a variety of animal models of arthritis to gain an insight into the sequence of events leading to the degeneration of articular cartilage. The increased catabolism of the cartilage proteoglycan aggrecan is a principal pathological process which leads to the degeneration of articular cartilage in arthritic joint diseases. The consequent loss of sulfated glycosaminoglycans (GAGs), which are intrinsic components of the aggrecan molecule, compromises both the functional and structural integrity of the cartilage matrix and ultimately renders the tissue incapable of resisting the compressive loads applied during joint articulation. Over time, this process leads to irreversible cartilage erosion. In situ degradation of aggrecan is a proteolytic process involving cleavage at specific peptide bonds located within the core protein. Studies on collagen-induced arthritis (CIA) and

antigen-induced arthritis (AIA) have clearly established that aggrecanases, which belong to the ADAMT protein family (ADAMT-4 and -5), are primarily responsible for the catabolism and loss of aggrecan from articular cartilage in the early stages of arthritic joint diseases that precede overt collagen catabolism and disruption of tissue integrity.[33] Cleavage of aggrecan by aggrecanases leads to the formation of specific neo-epitopes (NITEGE), which are fingerprints for the action of aggrecanase. NITEGE neo-epitopes can be stained in the cartilage of arthritic mice, appear early in the course of disease, and indicate a progressive loss of GAGs. The typical morphological result is the inability of articular cartilage to retain dyes such as toluidine blue or safranin O, which bind to GAGs. Whereas the loss of GAGs due to aggrecanase cleavage is reversible, later steps of cartilage damage are irreversible. MMPs (especially MMP-1, -3 and -13) govern the cleavage of collagen type II, which is the major matrix constituent of cartilage, and collagen type IX, which provides a link between collagen type II fibrils and GAGs.[34] When the collagen fibrils are lost, the cartilage has no effective way to retain GAGs, thus leading to irreversible damage to cartilage. Furthermore, MMPs also cleave the remaining aggrecan molecules at specific sites, leading to formation of neo-epitopes (such as VDIPEN) that differ from those induced by aggrecanases. Studies with MMP-3$^{-/-}$ mice have confirmed

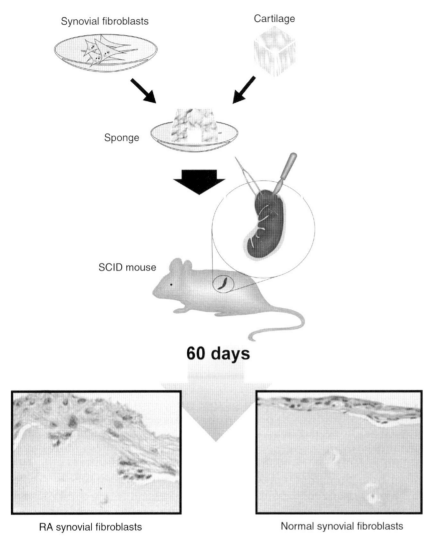

Figure 28.2 SCID mouse co-implantation model of rheumatoid arthritis (RA). Synovial fibroblasts (SFs) were isolated from RA patients (RA-SFs) or non-arthritic patients undergoing leg amputation (normal SFs). Human cartilage was obtained from cardiac surgery (rib cartilage) or non-arthritic amputations (knee cartilage). SFs and cartilage were first inserted into a cavity of inert sterile gel sponge and then co-implanted in a pocket of the surgically opened renal capsule. Sixty days after implantation histological analysis revealed cartilage invasion by RA-SFs (left) but not normal SFs (right).

these data, showing a lack of cartilage erosion as well as no formation of collagen type II or VDIPEN neo-epitopes.[34] However, the loss of GAGs was still evident in MMP-3[-/-] mice, underlining the action of aggrecanases. Thus, the expression and activation of MMPs seems to be a fateful event in irreversible damage to cartilage. Animal models of arthritis, such as AIA, have also demonstrated early upregulation of crucial MMPs, MMP-1, -3 and -13, in the course of disease.[35,36] MMPs are produced either from synovial cells invading cartilage and bone (fibroblasts, macrophages, osteoclasts) or from chondrocytes lying adjacent to cartilage and bone erosions[37] (G Schett, unpublished observations) (Figure 28.1). This suggests that cytokines synthesized by synovial cells induce a change in the expression pattern of chondrocyte proteins, shifting it from matrix synthesis to matrix degradation. Furthermore, animal models of arthritis have shown that latent MMP expression is found even in resting phases of disease, thus entailing a more rapid activation of MMPs, leading to faster and more severe cartilage resorption in flares of disease than in its primary onset.[36] The role of overexpression of MMP in cartilage resorption is also highlighted by mice transgenic for MMP-13, which develop severe cartilage damage.[38] However, knockout models of MMP have also shown that some MMPs are not crucial for soft tissue remodeling, including cartilage resorption (MMP-2[-/-] mice),[39] and others may even have key regulatory roles, like MT1-MMP (MMP-14), since the knockout mice develop arthritis.[40]

Interesting data have come also from the SCID mouse co-implantation model of RA, where synovial fibroblasts are implanted together with normal human articular cartilage into severe combined immunodeficient (SCID) mice (Figure 28.2). Owing to their lack of a functional immune system, SCID mice do not reject the human implants and allow us to study the interactions of fibroblasts and cartilage. It has been shown in a number of studies that, in the SCID mouse model, RA synovial fibroblasts (RA-SFs) attach to the co-implanted cartilage and deeply invade the cartilage matrix,[41,42] while normal synovial fibroblasts, osteoarthritis (OA) synovial fibroblasts or dermal fibroblasts do not show such invasion. It is of note that this experimental approach investigates the behavior of RA-SFs in the absence of human inflammatory cells. Therefore, the differences between RA-SFs, OA-SFs and normal SFs have been taken as evidence for the stable, intrinsic activation of RA-SFs. It has been understood that, apart from different proinflammatory cytokines, internal, cytokine-independent pathways contribute to the increased expression of MMPs and that overexpression of MMPs is closely associated with the activated phenotype of RA-SFs.[43] Conversely, inhibition of signaling pathways that are activated in RA-SFs and result in the upregulation of MMPs can reduce the invasion into the cartilage. Thus, inhibition of MAPK signaling through the delivery of dominant negative mutants of c-Raf-1 decreases the invasiveness of RA-SFs in the SCID mouse model. This is due to reduced phosphorylation of c-Jun and subsequent reduced expression of MMP-1 and MMP-13.[44] Unfortunately, there has been no precise information on how individual MMPs contribute to the invasiveness of RA-SFs, and this lack of understanding has been one major

obstacle to developing specific strategies for MMP inhibition in RA. Although data from the aforementioned MMP knockout mice indicate the particular importance of some MMPs, these models are limited by their purely immunological nature. In addition, they have demonstrated substantial overlap between different MMP family members. In this context, the SCID mouse model offers the opportunity to selectively inhibit single MMPs or MMP activation pathways in human RA-SFs and to assess their effects on the invasiveness of these cells. In this context, inhibition of plasmin – one major activator of MMPs – reduces the invasion of RA-SFs by about 30%.[45] Conversely, overexpression of TIMPs in RA-SFs through adenoviral gene transfer resulted in 50% invasion compared to control fibroblasts (unpublished observation). Other studies analyzing the role of individual MMPs in the SCID mouse model are underway and will provide more detailed insights into the concerted actions of MMP family members in rheumatoid joint destruction.

EXPRESSION OF MATRIX METALLOPROTEINASES IN RHEUMATOID ARTHRITIS

MMPs are expressed abundantly in the RA synovium, and there have been several studies correlating the expression levels of MMPs and their tissue distribution with synovial inflammation and joint destruction. In line with cell culture studies and SCID mouse experiments, RA-SFs in the lining layer constitute the major source of MMPs, underlining their role in the destruction of articular cartilage in RA.

MMP-1 (interstitial collagenase, collagenase 1) is one of the major enzymes in the rheumatoid synovium. It is found in all RA patients but in only about 55–80% of trauma samples.[46] Synovial lining cells produce most of the MMP-1 in the diseased synovium, and MMP-1 is released from these cells immediately after production (review: Sorsa et al[47]). Consequently, the expression of MMP-1 in the synovial fluid correlates positively with the degree of synovial inflammation.[48] However, it appears that serum concentrations of MMP-1 do not reflect the levels in the synovial fluid, and, therefore, the measurement of serum MMP-1 has not been used as a marker for disease activity.

As mentioned before, MMP-2 (gelatinase A) is expressed constitutively in synovial tissues from RA as well as from OA and trauma patients, but several studies have shown increased expression of MMP-2 in the rheumatoid synovium.[46] This is true also for the second member of the gelatinase family, MMP-9 (gelatinase B). MMP-9 can be found at elevated levels in the sera and synovial fluids of RA patients compared to healthy controls,[49,50] and both SFs and macrophages of the RA synovium express MMP-9. Analyzing the expression of MMP-9 in the synovial fluids of patients with RA, OA and other inflammatory arthritides, Ahrens et al found an association between increased levels of MMP-9 and inflammatory arthritis.[50] These data are of interest, because MMP-9 has also been found in osteoclasts and implicated in the resorption of bone.[51] However, despite the potential of synovial macrophages to differentiate into bone-resorbing, osteoclast-like cells, it is not clear how the expression pattern of MMP-9 correlates with erosions in RA.

Owing to its specific properties, MMP-3 plays an important role in the degradation of cartilage matrix, and early reports in the 1980s demonstrated that active MMP-1, -2 and -3 can together destroy a number of structural proteins in the synovium.[52] MMP-3 has been assigned a key role in the destruction of rheumatoid joints, because it not only degrades extracellular matrix molecules but is also involved in the activation of pro-MMPs into their active forms. It is produced abundantly by rheumatoid SFs when stimulated with macrophage-conditioned medium,[53] and, again, RA-SFs in the lining layer are the cells that predominantly express MMP-3 in the RA synovium.[54] Synovial fluids from patients with RA show about 100-fold higher concentrations of active MMP-3 than control samples.[55] Interestingly, increased levels of MMP-3 are also found in the sera of patients with RA[56–60] and correlate with systemic inflammation at the clinical[58,60] and serological[57,59,60] levels. However, the

question as to whether increased levels of circulating MMP-3 reflect radiological damage is controversial. No correlation between serum MMP-3 and radiological or functional scores was seen in the study by Manicourt at al.[59] So et al failed to establish differences in the serum levels of MMP-3 between RA patients with long standing RA (>5 years) who had low or high erosion scores.[57] In contrast, Yamanaka et al reported recently that serum MMP-3 was a predictor of joint damage in early stages of disease.[61] At present it can be concluded that the serum levels of MMP-3 reflect, at least to a certain degree, synovial inflammation and as such may correlate with ongoing joint destruction rather than past damage.

Most other MMPs have also been demonstrated in the RA synovium and particularly in RA-SFs. Among those, MMP-8, which had been described exclusively in polymorphonuclear neutrophils, is expressed also by RA-SFs,[62] and this observation was made not only in vivo but also in fibroblast cell cultures under in vitro conditions.

MMP-13 (collagenase 3) has been implicated most prominently in cartilage destruction in RA. Using degenerate primers that corresponded to highly conserved regions of the MMP gene family, Wernicke et al cloned MMP-13 from the synovium of patients with RA,[63] and subsequent studies demonstrated the expression of MMP-13, particularly in SFs but also in macrophages in the lining layer of rheumatoid synovium.[64] Owing to this localization and its substrate specificity for collagen type II, MMP-13 plays an important role in joint destruction. It is of interest that expression of MMP-13 correlates with elevated levels of systemic inflammation markers,[65] but studies in OA demonstrated clearly that the expression of MMP-13 is not specific for RA. Rather, it appears that MMP-13 is associated closely with degeneration of cartilage in different pathologies.

MT-MMPs are also expressed abundantly in cells aggressively destroying cartilage and bone in RA.[66] Although MT1-MMP is expressed constitutively in RA-SFs, elevated levels have been found in RA. This is of importance, because MT1-MMP degrades extracellular matrix components as well as activating other disease-relevant MMPs such as MMP-2 and MMP-13. In a recent study that compared the expression levels of MT-MMPs in RA, we suggested that MT1-MMP is of particular relevance to RA.[66] In this analysis, the expression of MT3-MMP mRNA was seen in fibroblasts and some macrophages, particularly in the lining layer, but expression of MT2- and MT4-MMP was characterized by scattered staining of only a few CD68-negative fibroblasts.

Collectively, all MMPs that have been associated with the remodeling of connective tissue as well as inflammatory processes can be found at elevated levels in the rheumatoid synovium. Although it appears that certain metalloproteinases (MMP-1, -3, -13 together with MT1-, MT3-MMP and aggrecanases) may contribute most significantly to the destruction of articular cartilage, no specific pattern of MMP expression has been found for RA. Specifically, the relationship of disease-induced MMP activity to normal expression in different tissues, including the synovium, needs to be established. A more detailed understanding of natural MMP inhibitors and metalloproteinase functions that are distinct from matrix degradation will help us to develop disease-specific inhibitors for RA.

MATRIX METALLOPROTEINASES AS THERAPEUTIC TARGETS

Based on these data, several strategies have been considered to interfere with the expression and activation of MMPs in the rheumatoid joint (Table 28.2).

The understanding that inflammatory stimuli contribute to the upregulation of MMPs in the rheumatoid synovium has resulted in several studies investigating the potential of anti-inflammatory and disease-modifying therapies to inhibit MMPs in the RA synovium. It was shown that drugs such as methotrexate or leflunomide, by decreasing synovial inflammation, affect also the production of MMPs and result in decreased levels of MMP-1.[67] The retardation of radiological disease progression as seen with some of these disease-modifying anti-rheumatic drugs (DMARDs), therefore, may be attributed to

Table 28.2   Current strategies to inhibit MMPs in RA.

Agents

Anti-inflammatory treatment
    DMARDs (e.g. methotrexate, leflunomide)
    Biologicals (e.g. infliximab)
Tetracyclins
    Antimicrobially effective tetracyclines (e.g. doxycycline)
    Chemically modified teracyclines (not antimicrobial)
Specific, pharmacological MMP inhibitors
    Substrate (peptide) inhibitor with alternative chelators
    Non-peptide inhibitors (e.g. sulfone hydroxamates, biaryl keto-acids)
Gene transfer
    Delivery of naturally occurring inhibitors (TIMP-1, TIMP-3)
    Generation of artificial inhibitors of MMP activation (ATF.BPTI)
    Antisense constructs (αS ODNs, αS expression constructs, ribozymes)

DMARD, disease-modifying anti-rheumatic drug; ODN, oligodeoxyribonucleotide.

decreased levels of MMPs. This notion is supported also by recent advances in the treatment of RA that have come from the use of biological agents. The use of TNF-α inhibitors such as monoclonal antibodies has offered new possibilities for treating inflammation, and early data suggest that they, at least to a certain degree, retard radiological damage. In this context, Brennan et al demonstrated that serum levels of MMP-1 and MMP-3 decrease following treatment with anti-TNF-α antibodies.[68]

Among available drugs, tetracyclines have been shown to have anti-collagenolytic effects that are due to different mechanisms, among them inhibition of MMP-1 as well as prevention of MMP activation.[69] Based on this understanding, some clinical trials have been initiated aimed at using such drugs for the treatment of RA. Nordstrom et al reported that a 3-month treatment of RA patients with daily 150 mg doxycycline had anti-collagenolytic effects.[70] This effect is not necessarily related to the antimicrobial activity of tetracyclines as there are several modified tetracyclines that are not antimicrobial but still inhibit MMPs. However, their efficacy is far less than what can be achieved with specific inhibitors of MMPs.

Based on our advanced understanding of MMP structures, low-molecular-weight pharmacological compounds have been developed by nearly all major pharmaceutical companies as well as research institutes (for a comprehensive review of their characteristics, pharmacological properties and development, see Skotnicki et al[71]). According to their structures, two strategies can be distinguished. Early but continuing efforts have started out from the structure of MMP substrates and resulted in the development of peptide and peptide-like MMP inhibitors that contained alternative chelators such as aminocarboxylates, carboxylic acids and thiol amides. Alternatively, non-peptide inhibitors of MMPs have been synthesized since Novartis disclosed its substance CGS 23161 in 1994. CGS 23161 is rather specific for MMP-3 (K_i 71 nM) and has served as a lead substance for the development of a number of sulfonamide hydroxamates and derivatives.[71,72] Both peptide and non-peptide inhibitors of MMPs are being developed continuously, and several compounds have been used in animal models of arthritis or even entered early-phase clinical studies. Thus, the peptide-type broad-spectrum MMP inhibitors BB-2516 (Marimastat) and BB-94 (Batimastat) have been evaluated for arthritis. Batimastat was demonstrated to have favorable effects in adjuvant arthritis[73] but was not investigated further due to its poor bioavailability. Marimastat, which was tested in parallel in patients with advanced cancers,[74–76] had much better pharmacokinetic properties. However, as seen in the cancer studies, Marimastat had major musculoskeletal side-effects, with muscular

pain, stiffness, and even inflammatory polyarthritis.[77,78] Notably, such musculoskeletal symptoms have also been observed with other MMP inhibitors, but their cause remains unclear. Specifically, it has not been clarified whether these side-effects are due to MMP inhibition or caused by common but non-MMP-specific features of MMP inhibitors. It has been suggested that the musculoskeletal side-effects are related to the inhibition of MMP-1, but this hypothesis has not been proven so far. Nonetheless, more selective MMP inhibitors have been tested for arthritis, such as RS-130830 (Roche Bioscience),[71] which inhibits MMP-13 much more effectively than MMP-1, and several non-peptide inhibitors with different specificities have been developed. Although the focus appears to have shifted from inflammatory arthritis to a potential application in OA, nearly all MMP inhibitors are tested for their efficacy in animal or in vitro models of RA.

In terms of clinical applications, the Roche compound Ro 32-3555l (Trocade) has been most investigated.[79,80] Trocade predominantly inhibits collagenases (MMP-1, -3 and -13) and has demonstrated its efficacy in different in vitro and in vivo models of cartilage degradation. However, no significant effects were seen in animal models of inflammatory arthritis, and early clinical data suggest that the progression of joint damage was not prevented.[79] Despite good initial data on tolerability over short periods of time,[80] long-term data from these clinical trials remain to be published. No MMP inhibitor has made its way into the clinic so far, clearly illustrating the following problem: although many pharmacological agents have been developed that inhibit MMPs with even picomolar efficacy, there seem to be conceptual difficulties with applying them in RA.[81] It appears today that inhibition of MMPs per se is less a problem than determining the specific needs for MMP inhibition in RA.

Consequently, alternative strategies have been developed that focus on the specific modulation of MMP activity through interfering with both expression and activation of MMPs. Among these, gene transfer has become one tool that

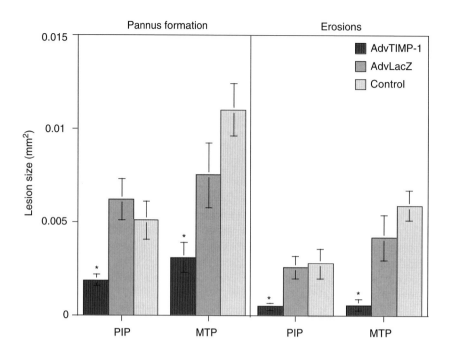

Figure 28.3 Reduction of pannus formation and erosions in TNF-transgenic mice after gene therapy with TIMP-1. Histological damage in the hindpaws of TNF-transgenic mice was quantitatively assessed at the proximal interphalangeal and the metatarsophalangeal joint compartments. Mean + Sd lesion areas and standard deviations are shown for the AdvTIMP1, AdvLacZ and PBS treatment groups. The Y-axis indicates lesion area in mm². *Significant change (P<0.01). MTP, metatarsophalangeal joints; PIP, proximal interphalangeal joints.

allows us to block distinct steps of MMP action in a highly selective manner.[82] Specific inhibition of MMPs has been associated mainly with three strategies (Table 28.2): (1) the delivery of naturally occurring inhibitors of MMPs (TIMPs); (2) the design and delivery of novel inhibitory molecules or modifications of naturally occurring inhibitors; and (3) targeting the mRNA of MMPs through different antisense strategies.

As mentioned, MMP activity is balanced by natural inhibitors (TIMPs), but in RA, the amount of MMPs produced outweighs that of the TIMPs. Therefore, it has been suggested that the delivery of functional genes for TIMPs may 'correct' for this imbalance and result in a decrease in matrix degradation. Although initial studies by Apparailly et al failed to demonstrate a significant effect of TIMP-1 gene transfer in DBA/1 mice with CIA,[83] the most recent studies in both the TNF-α transgenic animal models of RA[37] (Figure 28.3) and the SCID mouse model (unpublished data) have shown that delivery of TIMP-1 may have beneficial effects on synovial inflammation the destruction of cartilage and bone.

As an alternative approach, genes for artificial inhibitors of MMP activation can be delivered to the rheumatoid synovium. Thus, it has been proposed that delivery of a gene for a hybrid protein targeting plasmin on the surface of RA-SFs may reduce their invasive potential.[45] This is based on the aforementioned understanding that components of the plasminogen activation system are expressed at significantly higher levels in RA than in osteoarthritic and non-arthritic synovium. Therefore, a protein was constructed that consisted of the plasmin inhibitor, bovine pancreatic trypsin inhibitor (BPTI), linked to the receptor-binding N-terminal fragment of urokinase-type plasminogen activator. Adenoviral delivery of the respective gene into RA-SFs resulted in a significant reduction of cartilage degradation in vitro and in the SCID mouse model.[45] Although cartilage destruction was reduced to about 88% in vitro, cartilage degradation in vivo was reduced only by 30% in the ATF.BTPI transduced fibroblasts. These results indicate a role for plasmin in SF-dependent cartilage degradation and invasion in RA and demonstrate an effective way to inhibit this by gene transfer of a cell surface-targeted plasmin inhibitor.

Finally, several strategies have been developed that are aimed at modulating the terminal phase of MMP expression by cleaving the mRNA for these enzymes.[82] This can be achieved by different antisense strategies such as antisense ologonucleotides (ODNs), the delivery and expression of antisense expression constructs, and through ribozymes.

Ribozymes are RNA molecules that – like antisense RNA – bind to complementary mRNA but in addition are able to cleave RNA site-specifically. Such ribozymes can be used to destroy messages inside cells. RA-SFs that express ribozymes cleaving collagenase will, therefore, produce no or only limited amounts of this enzyme. The usefulness of this mode to reduce the invasiveness of RA-SFs is being currently evaluated.

REFERENCES

1. Nagase H, Woessner JF. Matrix metalloproteinases. *J Biol Chem* 1999; **274**: 21491–4.
2. Brew K, Dinakarpandian D, Nagase H. Tissue inhibitors of metalloproteinases: evolution, structure and function. *Biochim Biophys Acta* 2000; **1477**: 267–83.
3. Nagase H. Matrix metalloproteinases. In: Hooper NM, ed. *Zinc Metalloproteinases in Health and Disease* (London: Taylor and Francis, 1996) 153–204.
4. Wolfsberg TG, Primakoff P, Myles DG, White JM. ADAM, a novel family of membrane proteins containing a disintegrin and metalloprotease domain: multipotential functions in cell–cell and cell–matrix interactions. *J Cell Biol* 1995; **131**: 275–8.
5. Kaushal GP, Shah SV. The new kids on the block: ADAMTSs, potentially multifunctional metalloproteinases of the ADAM family. *J Clin Invest* 2000; **105**: 1335–7.
6. Black RA, Rauch CT, Kozlosky CJ et al. A metalloproteinase disintegrin that releases tumour-necrosis factor-alpha from cells. *Nature* 1997; **385**: 729–33.
7. Moss ML, Jin SL, Milla ME et al. Cloning of a disintegrin metalloproteinase that processes precursor tumour-necrosis factor-alpha. *Nature* 1997; **385**: 733–6.
8. Tortorella MD, Burn TC, Pratta MA et al. Purification and cloning of aggrecanase-1: a member of the ADAMTS family of proteins. *Science* 1999; **284**: 1664–6.
9. Mengshol JA, Vincenti MP, Brinckerhoff CE. IL-1 induces collagenase-3 (MMP-13) promoter activity in stably transfected chondrocytic cells: requirement for Runx-2 and activation by p38 MAPK and JNK pathways. *Nucleic Acids Res* 2001; **29**: 4361–72.
10. Gouze JN, Bianchi A, Becuwe P et al. Glucosamine modulates IL-1-induced activation of rat chondrocytes at a receptor level, and by inhibiting the NF-kappaB pathway. *FEBS Lett* 2002; **510**: 166–70.
11. Eberhardt W, Huwiler A, Beck KF et al. Amplification of IL-1 beta-induced matrix metalloproteinase-9 expression by superoxide in rat glomerular mesangial cells is mediated by increased activities of NF-kappa B and activating protein-1 and involves activation of the mitogen-activated protein kinase pathways. *J Immunol* 2000; **165**: 5788–97.
12. Catterall JB, Carrere S, Koshy PJ et al. Synergistic induction of matrix metalloproteinase 1 by interleukin-1alpha and oncostatin M in human chondrocytes involves signal transducer and activator of transcription and activator protein 1 transcription factors via a novel mechanism. *Arthritis Rheum* 2001; **44**(10): 2296–310.
13. Langdon C, Leith J, Smith F, Richards CD. Oncostatin M stimulates monocyte chemoattractant protein-1- and interleukin-1-induced matrix metalloproteinase-1 production by human synovial fibroblasts in vitro. *Arthritis Rheum* 1997; **40**: 2139–46.
14. Bond M, Fabunmi RP, Baker AH, Newby AC. Synergistic upregulation of metalloproteinase-9 by growth factors and inflammatory cytokines: an absolute requirement for transcription factor NF-kappa B. *FEBS Lett* 1998; **435**: 29–34.
15. Han YP, Tuan TL, Wu H, Hughes M, Garner WL. TNF-alpha stimulates activation of pro-MMP2 in human skin through NF-(kappa)B mediated induction of MT1-MMP. *J Cell Sci* 2001; **114**: 131–9.
16. Jovanovic DV, Martel-Pelletier J, Di Battista JA et al. Stimulation of 92-kd gelatinase (matrix metal-

loproteinase 9) production by interleukin-17 in human monocyte/macrophages: a possible role in rheumatoid arthritis. *Arthritis Rheum* 2000; **43**: 1134–44.

17. Ravanti L, Toriseva M, Penttinen R et al. Expression of human collagenase-3 (MMP-13) by fetal skin fibroblasts is induced by transforming growth factor beta via p38 mitogen-activated protein kinase. *FASEB J* 2001; **15**: 1098–100.

18. Matsubara T, Funahashi K, Umegaki Y et al. Effect of VEGF on the synthesis of metalloproteinase (MMP)-13 by human chondrocytes. *Arthritis Rheum* 2001; **44** (suppl 65): A78.

19. Onodera S, Nishihira J, Iwabuchi K et al. Macrophage migration inhibitory factor upregulates matrix metalloproteinase-9 and -13 in rat osteoblasts. *J Biol Chem*. 2002; **277**: 7865–74.

20. Loeser RF, Forsyth CB. Integrin signaling increases collagenase-3 (MMP-13) production in human articular chondrocytes. *Arthritis Rheum* 2001; **44** (suppl 45): A35.

21. Yasuda T, Shimizu M Nakagawa T et al. COOH-terminal heparin-binding fibronectin fragment induces matrix metalloproteinases in human articular cartilage. *Arthritis Rheum* 2001; **44** (suppl 63): 63.

22. Chabaud M, Garnero P, Dayer JM, Guerne PA, Fossiez F, Miossec P. Contribution of interleukin 17 to synovium matrix destruction in rheumatoid arthritis. *Cytokine* 2000; **12**: 1092–9.

23. Sun Y, Cheung JM, Wenger L et al. Rheumatoid arthritis-derived p53 mutants lose their ability to downregulate the promotors of MMP-1 and MMP-13. *Arthritis Rheum* 2001; **44** (suppl 182): 780.

24. Mengshol JA, Vincenti MP, Coon CI et al. Interleukin-1 induction of collagenase 3 (matrix metalloproteinase 13) gene expression in chondrocytes requires p38, c-Jun N-terminal kinase, and nuclear factor kappa B: differential regulation of collagenase 1 and collagenase 3. *Arthritis Rheum* 2000; **43**: 801–11.

25. Barchowsky A, Frleta D, Vincenti MP. Integration of the NF-kappaB and mitogen-activated protein kinase/AP-1 pathways at the collagenase-1 promoter: divergence of IL-1 and TNF-dependent signal transduction in rabbit primary synovial fibroblasts. *Cytokine* 2000; **12**: 1469–79.

26. Brauchle M, Gluck D, Di Padova F, Han J, Gram H. Independent role of p38 and ERK1/2 mitogen-activated kinases in the upregulation of matrix metalloproteinase-1. *Exp Cell Res* 2000; **258**: 135–44.

27. Li WQ, Dehnade F, Zafarullah M. Oncostatin M-induced matrix metalloproteinase and tissue inhibitor of metalloproteinase-3 genes expression in chondrocytes requires Janus kinase/STAT signaling pathway. *J Immunol* 2001; **166**: 3491–8.

28. Bosc DG, Goueli BS, Janknecht R. HER2/Neu-mediated activation of the ETS transcription factor ER81 and its target gene MMP-1. *Oncogene* 2001; **20**: 6215–24.

29. Westermarck J, Seth A, Kahari VM. Differential regulation of interstitial collagenase (MMP-1) gene expression by ETS transcription factors. *Oncogene* 1997; **14**: 2651–60.

30. Schett G, Tohidast-Akrad M, Smolen JS et al. Activation, differential localization, and regulation of the stress-activated protein kinases, extracellular signal-regulated kinase, c-JUN N-terminal kinase, and p38 mitogen-activated protein kinase, in synovial tissue and cells in rheumatoid arthritis. *Arthritis Rheum* 2000; **43**: 2501–12.

31. Redlich K, Kiener HP, Schett G et al. Overexpression of transcription factor Ets-1 in rheumatoid arthritis synovial membrane: regulation of expression and activation by interleukin-1 and tumor necrosis factor alpha. *Arthritis Rheum* 2001; **44**: 266–74.

32. Mengshol JA, Vincenti MP, Brinckerhoff CE. IL-1 induces collagenase-3 (MMP-13) promoter activity in stably transfected chondrocytic cells: requirement for Runx-2 and activation by p38 MAPK and JNK pathways. *Nucleic Acids Res* 2001; **29**: 4361–72.

33. van Meurs JB, van Lent PL, Holthuysen AE et al. Kinetics of aggrecanase- and metalloproteinase-induced neoepitopes in various stages of cartilage destruction in murine arthritis. *Arthritis Rheum* 1999; **42**: 1128–39.

34. van Meurs J, van Lent P, Stoop R et al. Cleavage of aggrecan at the Asn341–Phe342 site coincides with the initiation of collagen damage in murine antigen-induced arthritis: a pivotal role for stromelysin 1 in matrix metalloproteinase activity. *Arthritis Rheum* 1999; **42**: 2074–84.

35. Poole AR. Cartilage in health and disease. In: Koopmann WJ, ed. *Arthritis and Allied Conditions* (Lippincott, Williams & Wilkins: Baltimore, 2001) 226–84.

36. van Meurs JB, van Lent PL, van de Loo AA et al. Increased vulnerability of postarthritic cartilage to a second arthritic insult: accelerated MMP activity in a flare up of arthritis. *Ann Rheum Dis* 1999; **58**: 350–6.

37. Schett G, Hayer SM, Tohidast-Akrad M et al. Adenoviral-based overexpression of TIMP-1 reduces tissue damage in the joints of TNFα-transgenic mice. *Arthritis Rheum* 2001; **44**: 2888–98.

38. Neuhold LA, Killar L, Zhao W et al. Postnatal expression in hyaline cartilage of constitutively active human collagenase-3 (MMP-13) induces osteoarthritis in mice. *J Clin Invest.* 2001; **107**: 35–44.

39. Vaillant B, Chiaramonte MG, Cheever AW et al. Regulation of hepatic fibrosis and extracellular matrix genes by the th response: new insight into the role of tissue inhibitors of matrix metalloproteinases. *J Immunol* 2001; **167**: 7017–26.

40. Holmbeck K, Bianco P, Caterina J et al. MT1-MMP-deficient mice develop dwarfism, osteopenia, arthritis, and connective tissue disease due to inadequate collagen turnover. *Cell* 1999; **99**: 81–92.

41. Müller-Ladner U, Kriegsmann J, Franklin BN et al. Synovial fibroblasts of patients with rheumatoid arthritis attach to and invade normal human cartilage when engrafted into SCID mice. *Am J Pathol* 1996; **149**: 1607–15.

42. Pap T, Aupperle KR, Gay S, Firestein GS, Gay RE. Invasiveness of synovial fibroblasts is regulated by p53 in the SCID mouse in vivo model of cartilage invasion. *Arthritis Rheum* 2001; **44**: 676–81.

43. Pap T, Franz JK, Hummel KM, Jeisy E, Gay R, Gay S. Activation of synovial fibroblasts in rheumatoid arthritis: lack of expression of the tumour suppressor PTEN at sites of invasive growth and destruction. *Arthritis Res* 1999; **2**: 59–64.

44. Nawrath M, Hummel KM, Pap T et al. Effect of dominant negative mutants of raf-1 and c-myc on rheumatoid arthritis synovial fibroblasts in the SCID mouse model. *Arthritis Rheum* 1998; **41** (suppl 9): S95.

45. van der Laan WH, Pap T, Ronday HK et al. Cartilage degradation and invasion by rheumatoid synovial fibroblasts is inhibited by gene transfer of a cell surface-targeted plasmin inhibitor. *Arthritis Rheum* 2000; **43**: 1710–18.

46. Konttinen YT, Ainola M, Valleala H et al. Analysis of 16 different matrix metalloproteinases (MMP-1 to MMP-20) in the synovial membrane: different profiles in trauma and rheumatoid arthritis. *Ann Rheum Dis* 1999; **58**: 691–7.

47. Sorsa T, Konttinen YT, Lindy O et al. Collagenase in synovitis of rheumatoid arthritis. *Semin Arthritis Rheum* 1992; **22**: 44–53.

48. Maeda S, Sawai T, Uzuki M et al. Determination of interstitial collagenase (MMP-1) in patients with rheumatoid arthritis. *Ann Rheum Dis* 1995; **54**: 970–5.

49. Gruber BL, Sorbi D, French DL et al. Markedly elevated serum MMP-9 (gelatinase B) levels in rheumatoid arthritis: a potentially useful laboratory marker. *Clin Immunol Immunopathol* 1996; **78**: 161–71.

50. Ahrens D, Koch AE, Pope RM, Stein PM, Niedbala MJ. Expression of matrix metalloproteinase 9 (96-kd gelatinase B) in human rheumatoid arthritis. *Arthritis Rheum* 1996; **39**: 1576–87.

51. Okada Y, Naka K, Kawamura K et al. Localization of matrix metalloproteinase 9 (92-kilodalton gelatinase/type IV collagenase = gelatinase B) in osteoclasts: implications for bone resorption. *Lab Invest* 1995; **72**: 311–22.

52. Okada Y, Nagase H, Harris ED Jr. Matrix metalloproteinases 1, 2, and 3 from rheumatoid synovial cells are sufficient to destroy joints. *J Rheumatol* 1987; **14**: 41–2.

53. Okada Y, Takeuchi N, Tomita K, Nakanishi I, Nagase H. Immunolocalization of matrix metalloproteinase 3 (stromelysin) in rheumatoid synovioblasts (B cells): correlation with rheumatoid arthritis. *Ann Rheum Dis* 1989; **48**: 645–53.

54. Tetlow LC, Lees M, Ogata Y, Nagase H, Woolley DE. Differential expression of gelatinase B (MMP-9) and stromelysin-1 (MMP-3) by rheumatoid synovial cells in vitro and in vivo. *Rheumatol Int* 1993; **13**: 53–9.

55. Beekman B, van El B, Drijfhout JW, Ronday HK, TeKoppele JM. Highly increased levels of active stromelysin in rheumatoid synovial fluid determined by a selective fluorogenic assay. *FEBS Lett* 1997; **418**: 305–9.

56. Taylor DJ, Cheung NT, Dawes PT. Increased serum proMMP-3 in inflammatory arthritides: a potential indicator of synovial inflammatory monokine activity. *Ann Rheum Dis* 1994; **53**: 768–72.

57. So A, Chamot AM, Peclat V, Gerster JC. Serum MMP-3 in rheumatoid arthritis: correlation with systemic inflammation but not with erosive status. *Rheumatology (Oxford)* 1999; **38**: 407–10.

58. Ichikawa Y, Yamada C, Horiki T, Hoshina Y, Uchiyama M. Serum matrix metalloproteinase-3 and fibrin degradation product levels correlate with clinical disease activity in rheumatoid arthritis. *Clin Exp Rheumatol* 1998; **16**: 533–40.

59. Manicourt DH, Fujimoto N, Obata K, Thonar EJ.

Levels of circulating collagenase, stromelysin-1, and tissue inhibitor of matrix metalloproteinases 1 in patients with rheumatoid arthritis. Relationship to serum levels of antigenic keratan sulfate and systemic parameters of inflammation. *Arthritis Rheum* 1995; **38**: 1031–9.

60. Yoshihara Y, Obata K, Fujimoto N, Yamashita K, Hayakawa T, Shimmei M. Increased levels of stromelysin-1 and tissue inhibitor of metalloproteinases-1 in sera from patients with rheumatoid arthritis. *Arthritis Rheum* 1995; **38**: 969–75.

61. Yamanaka H, Matsuda Y, Tanaka M et al. Serum matrix metalloproteinase 3 as a predictor of the degree of joint destruction during the six months after measurement, in patients with early rheumatoid arthritis. *Arthritis Rheum* 2000; **43**: 852–8.

62. Hanemaaijer R, Sorsa T, Konttinen YT et al. Matrix metalloproteinase-8 is expressed in rheumatoid synovial fibroblasts and endothelial cells. Regulation by tumor necrosis factor-alpha and doxycycline. *J Biol Chem* 1997; **272**: 31504–9.

63. Wernicke D, Seyfert C, Hinzmann B, Gromnica-Ihle E. Cloning of collagenase 3 from the synovial membrane and its expression in rheumatoid arthritis and osteoarthritis. *J Rheumatol* 1996; **23**: 590–5.

64. Lindy O, Konttinen YT, Sorsa T et al. Matrix-metalloproteinase 13 (collagenase 3) in human rheumatoid synovium. *Arthritis Rheum* 1997; **40**: 1391–9.

65. Westhoff CS, Freudiger D, Petrow P et al. Characterization of collagenase 3 (matrix metalloproteinase 13) messenger RNA expression in the synovial membrane and synovial fibroblasts of patients with rheumatoid arthritis. *Arthritis Rheum* 1999; **42**: 1517–27.

66. Pap T, Shigeyama Y, Kuchen S et al. Differential expression pattern of membrane-type matrix metalloproteinases in rheumatoid arthritis. *Arthritis Rheum* 2000; **43**: 1226–32.

67. Kraan MC, Reece RJ, Barg EC et al. Modulation of inflammation and metalloproteinase expression in synovial tissue by leflunomide and methotrexate in patients with active rheumatoid arthritis. Findings in a prospective, randomized, double-blind, parallel-design clinical trial in thirty-nine patients at two centers. *Arthritis Rheum* 2000; **43**: 1820–30.

68. Brennan FM, Browne KA, Green PA, Jaspar JM, Maini RN, Feldmann M. Reduction of serum matrix metalloproteinase 1 and matrix metallo-proteinase 3 in rheumatoid arthritis patients following anti-tumour necrosis factor-alpha (cA2) therapy. *Br J Rheumatol* 1997; **36**: 643–50.

69. Greenwald RA, Golub LM, Ramamurthy NS, Chowdhury M, Moak SA, Sorsa T. In vitro sensitivity of the three mammalian collagenases to tetracycline inhibition: relationship to bone and cartilage degradation. *Bone* 1998; **22**: 33–8.

70. Nordstrom D, Lindy O, Lauhio A, Sorsa T, Santavirta S, Konttinen YT. Anti-collagenolytic mechanism of action of doxycycline treatment in rheumatoid arthritis. *Rheumatol Int* 1998; **17**: 175–80.

71. Skotnicki JS, Levin JI, Zask A, Killar LM. Matrix metalloproteinase inhibitors. In: Bottomley KMK, Bradshaw D, Nixon JS, eds. *Metalloproteinases as Targets for Anti-Inflammatory Drugs* (Birkhäuser-Verlag: Basel, 1999) 17–57.

72. MacPherson LJ, Bayburt EK, Capparelli MP et al. Discovery of CGS 27023A, a non-peptidic, potent, and orally active stromelysin inhibitor that blocks cartilage degradation in rabbits. *J Med Chem* 1997; **40**: 2525–32.

73. DiMartino MJ, High W, Galloway WA, Crimmin MJ. Preclinical antiarthritic activity of matrix metalloproteinase inhibitors. *Ann NY Acad Sci* 1994; **732**: 411–13.

74. Nemunaitis J, Poole C, Primrose J et al. Combined analysis of studies of the effects of the matrix metalloproteinase inhibitor marimastat on serum tumor markers in advanced cancer: selection of a biologically active and tolerable dose for longer-term studies. *Clin Cancer Res* 1998; **4**: 1101–9.

75. Primrose JN, Bleiberg H, Daniel F et al. Marimastat in recurrent colorectal cancer: exploratory evaluation of biological activity by measurement of carcinoembryonic antigen. *Br J Cancer* 1999; **79**: 509–14.

76. Tierney GM, Griffin NR, Stuart RC et al. A pilot study of the safety and effects of the matrix metalloproteinase inhibitor marimastat in gastric cancer. *Eur J Cancer* 1999; **35**: 563–8.

77. Drummond AH, Beckett P, Brown PD et al. Preclinical and clinical studies of MMP inhibitors in cancer. *Ann NY Acad Sci* 1999; **878**: 228–35.

78. Wojtowicz-Praga S, Torri J, Johnson M et al. Phase I trial of Marimastat, a novel matrix metalloproteinase inhibitor, administered orally to patients with advanced lung cancer. *J Clin Oncol* 1998; **16**: 2150–6.

79. Close DR. Matrix metalloproteinase inhibitors in rheumatic diseases. *Ann Rheum Dis* 2001; **60** (suppl 3): iii62–7.

80. Hemmings FJ, Farhan M, Rowland J, Banken L, Jain R. Tolerability and pharmacokinetics of the collagenase-selective inhibitor Trocade in patients with rheumatoid arthritis. *Rheumatology (Oxford)* 2001; **40**: 537–43.

81. Greenwald RA. Thirty-six years in the clinic without an MMP inhibitor. What hath collagenase wrought? *Ann NY Acad Sci* 1999; **878**: 413–19.

82. Pap T, Muller-Ladner U, Gay R, Gay S. Gene therapy in rheumatoid arthritis: how to target joint destruction? *Arthritis Res* 1999; **1**: 5–9.

83. Apparailly F, Noel D, Millet V et al. Paradoxical effects of tissue inhibitor of metalloproteinases 1 gene transfer in collagen-induced arthritis. *Arthritis Rheum* 2001; **44**: 1444–54.

Section VI

Targeted therapies in human and experimental rheumatic diseases

29

Rheumatoid arthritis

Ferdinand C Breedveld

Introduction • Tumor necrosis factor antagonists in rheumatoid arthritis • Interleukin-1 receptor antagonist in rheumatoid arthritis • Adverse reactions to tumor necrosis factor and interleukin-1 inhibitors in rheumatoid arthritis • Immunogenicity • Summary and conclusions • References

INTRODUCTION

The active search for new treatment modalities for established rheumatoid arthritis (RA) have created a dynamic period for rheumatology. Both innovative application of established disease-modifying anti-rheumatic drugs (DMARDs) and the availability of targeted interventions with products of the biotechnology industry have improved therapeutic results. As with all new therapeutic strategies, much remains to be learned about their optimal use and possible limitations. The experience at present suggests that a complex disease like RA can be brought under control and that the knowledge of the pathogenetic pathways obtained with the targeted therapies will be a stimulus for further drug development.

The motivation to develop new treatments for RA may be explained in part by three developments over the last decade: accurate description of the natural history of RA; availability of improved DMARDs; and, above all, the recognition that partial control of inflammation with an effective DMARD does not prevent joint damage.[1] Most patients with RA seen in clinical settings have persistent inflammatory symmetrical arthritis which has not responded adequately to traditional therapies. It is recog-

nized that patients monitored in the 1980s experienced poor long-term outcomes, including radiographic progression, joint deformity, functional declines, work disability, joint replacement surgery, high costs, extra-articular disease and premature mortality.[2] Furthermore, it was realized that many patients develop irreversible radiographic joint damage in the first years of the disease which necessitates preventive treatment strategies.[3]

Descriptions of the natural history of RA include the results of its therapy. Continuous treatment with DMARDs does ameliorate the course of RA, including retardation of radiographic progression, but rarely induces sustained remission. Furthermore, contemporary DMARDs such as methotrexate and sulfasalazine have considerably greater efficacy/toxicity ratios than traditional agents such as gold salts, penicillamine and azathioprine. Methotrexate emerged as a major advance during the 1990s, with long-term effectiveness and acceptable toxicities compared to other treatments.[4] Nonetheless, sustained remission is unusual, and therefore many physicians started to propose combination DMARD therapy.

The emphasis in RA clinical research has been on measures of inflammatory activity such as joint scores and acute-phase response. Control of inflammatory activity is regarded as an effective strategy to improve long-term outcome, although few studies are available to assess how completely inflammation must be controlled. Several studies reported that some improvement in joint scores, global severity scores and acute-phase response can be paralleled by significant progression of functional disability.[5] Taken together, these observations provide powerful arguments that new therapeutic principles have to be developed for RA, particularly in early disease, when drug therapy might prevent long-term damage.

During the past decade, much progress has also been made with regard to mechanisms leading to tissue destruction in RA. Based on this increasing knowledge, therapeutic principles have been developed with novel biological agents that act more specifically by targeting immune processes considered to be essential in RA. Table 29.1 gives an overview of the biological therapies already investigated in RA patients. The most precise description of the etiology of RA that can be given is that it is the interaction of a genetically susceptible host with an unidentified external inflammatory stimulus.[6] Therefore, a disease-specific therapy is not under investigation. Targeted therapies follow the most recent appreciation of the pathophysiology of a disease, which is dynamic given the fast-growing insights into cell biology and inflammation. All interventions that have been investigated in the clinic have shown efficacy in animal models of arthritis. Arthritis is mediated by a vast array of cells and soluble factors that recruit more cells at the site of inflammation. T lymphocytes, particularly those with a memory CD4+ phenotype, accumulate. Typically for an autoimmune reaction, these cells show a T-helper 1 (Th1) cytokine production profile.[7] Such cytokines activate signaling pathways in target cells, which leads to gene activation and effector functions. The end result is that resident synovial macrophages, mast cells and endothelial cells, together with blood-derived cells such as B lymphocytes and neutrophils, maintain a chronic inflammation. Activated cells produce a wide array of mediators, such as cytokines,

Table 29.1 Biological interventions investigated in rheumatoid arthritis.

Cell surface-directed therapy
  Anti-CD3 mAb, anti-CD4 mAb, anti-CD5 mAb, anti-CD7 mAb, anti-CD25 mAb, anti-CD52 mAb, anti-CD28 mAb, IL-2 fusion protein, anti-ICAM-1, CTLA-4-Ig (CD86 binding)

Cytokine-targeted therapy
  TNF antagonists (mAb, soluble TNF receptor)
  IL-1 receptor antagonist
  IL-6 antagonist (mAb against IL-6 or IL-6 receptor)
  Administration of cytokines (IL-4, IL-10, IFN-γ and IFN-β)

Tolerance induction
  Application of antigens (collagen II, HCGP-39)
  T-cell or T-cell receptor vaccination
  Interference with T-cell activation (CTLA-4-Ig)

Inhibition of chemokines

Inhibition of complement activation

High-dose intravenous immunoglobulins

Plasmapheresis, immunoadsorption column

Autologous bone marrow transplantation

mAb, monoclonal antibody; IL, interleukin; ICAM, intercellular adhesion molecule; CTLA-4, cytotoxic T-lymphocyte antigen-4; Ig, immunoglobulin; TNF, tumor necrosis factor; IFN, interferon.

chemokines and destructive enzymes, that also contribute to the hypertrophic and destructive synovial inflammation typical of RA. Observations of the presence of such components in the rheumatoid inflammation and insights into their biological significance motivated the development of new therapies.

These developments were also made possible by rapid developments in biotechnology.

Monoclonal antibodies (mAbs) are produced by a single clone of B cells, are monospecific, and therefore effective tools for therapies and diagnostics.[8] The conventional route to derive mAbs is to immunize mice and grow the selected hybridomas in laboratory animals. Various systems for in vitro mAb production are now being developed that allow large-scale production for therapeutic use. The phage display technique now allows selection and production at a high level without animals as intermediates. Furthermore, recombinant engineering techniques have emerged that permit the construction of mAbs customized with respect to the binding site, possible variations in size, and effector function. This design flexibility has resulted in the development of chimeric humanized and now fully human mAbs.

Tumor necrosis factor (TNF) and interleukin-1 (IL-1), with their broad spectra of biological activities, were, together with T cells, the first targets selected for biological therapy in RA.[8–10] Both cytokines are actively produced at the synovial site of inflammation in RA. Several biological activities of TNF overlap with those of IL-1. Both stimulate metalloproteinase and prostaglandin E_2 (PGE_2) production by synovial fibroblasts. This, together with the suppression of synthesis of matrix components by mesenchymal cells and the activation of osteoclasts, explains their capacity to promote cartilage and bone destruction. TNF and IL-1 are also potent activators of endothelial cells, with the promotion of adhesion molecule expression and subsequent leukocyte transmigration into tissue. They also stimulate the production of other cytokines and chemokines, increase the phagocytic functions of leukocytes, and stimulate proliferation of fibroblasts and endothelial cells.

TNF, IL-1 and other proinflammatory cytokines exert their effects on many cells, and their activity is controlled by many cells and molecules. When the trials on TNF and IL-1 inhibition were designed, there was a fear that blockage of one molecule would not result in substantial biological effects. However, the results of a substantial number of clinical trials have now led to the conclusion that such fears were unjustified.

TUMOR NECROSIS FACTOR ANTAGONISTS IN RHEUMATOID ARTHRITIS

Administration of a chimeric monoclonal antibody, infliximab (Remicade), which binds to TNF specifically and neutralizes its activity, was found to be of substantial clinical benefit in RA. Infliximab is a chimeric mAb that consists of the variable regions of a murine mAb linked to a human IgG_1 molecule. Infliximab has a high affinity for TNF and has been shown to inhibit both secreted and cell-associated TNF.[9] Preliminary open-label studies in patients with refractory disease visiting the Kennedy Institute of Rheumatology revealed a remarkable and direct clinical improvement and substantial improvement of biochemical and histological parameters of disease activity.[10,11] In the first randomized trial, a single infusion of 1 or 10 mg/kg infliximab was compared with placebo in 73 patients.[12] After 4 weeks, 8% of the placebo recipients fulfilled the response criteria, compared to 44% and 79% of the low- and high-dose-treated patients. The medium duration of the response in the high-dose group was 8 weeks, which could be directly related to the persistence of the circulating infliximab, with its half-life of ±10 days. In a second controlled trial, infliximab in combination with a fixed dose of methotrexate in RA patients with active disease showed an enhanced degree and duration of efficacy.[13] In the largest trial published so far, 428 patients with active RA despite treatment with methotrexate were randomized to placebo or one of four regimens of infliximab given every 4 or 8 weeks intravenously on a background of a stable dose of methotrexate. At 30 weeks, response criteria were achieved in 52–58% of patients receiving infliximab, compared with 20% of patients receiving placebo plus methotrexate.[14] The anti-inflammatory effect as well as the improvements in physical function and parameters of quality of life persisted when the patients were studied after 2 years.[15] Most remarkable was the analysis of joint X-rays taken after 1 year of treatment.[16] The median scores for joint space narrowing and bone erosion on X-rays of hands and feet progressed in the placebo- and methotrexate-treated group and were unchanged in the infliximab-treated group.

Three other TNF-binding antibodies are under clinical development. CDP571 was studied in dosages up to 10 mg/kg in 36 patients with active RA.[17] The best effects were seen in patients receiving the highest dose. CDP870 is a pegylated humanized Fab fragment produced by *Escherichia coli*. With the addition of two polyethylene glycol (PEG) chains, a half-life of 12–15 days is obtained. In a dose-finding randomized controlled trial, 200 patients with severe RA were treated with subcutaneous injections of placebo, or 50, 100, 200 or 400 mg CDP870 every 4 weeks. After 12 weeks, the percentages of ACR 20% responders were, respectively, 15%, 21%, 20%, 34% and 60%.[18] Further studies are in preparation. Adalimumab is a human anti-TNF mAb produced by means of the phage display technique. After completion of several phase II and III studies, including over 2500 patients, the dossier for the registration for RA treatment is now under review. The antibody has a half-life of 2 weeks and can be administered subcutaneously every other week. A 24-week placebo-controlled study was conducted in 271 patients with active RA receiving stable concurrent doses of methotrexate. The patients were randomized to receive placebo or subcutaneous adalimumab at doses of 20, 40 or 80 mg every other week. After 24 weeks, 14% of the placebo-treated individuals fulfilled an ACR 20% response versus 65% of the patients receiving 40 and 80 mg/2 weeks.[19] The results of phase III studies, which include X-ray and function investigations, will be presented in 2002.

Etanercept (Enbrel) was developed by linking DNA encoding the extracellular portion of the p75 TNF receptor with DNA encoding the Fc portion of human IgG$_1$.[20] The resulting fusion protein is expressed in a hamster ovary cell line and binds both soluble TNF and lymphotoxin with higher affinity than the naturally occurring monomers of soluble TNF receptors. Etanercept

was first evaluated in a double-blind, placebo-controlled, dose-evaluating study in patients with active refractory RA. Given the half-life of ±90 h, the drug was administered subcutaneously twice weekly in doses of 2, 4 or 16 mg/m^2 for 4 weeks following a single intravenous leading dose.[21] In every dose group, three received active drug and one placebo. Reductions of over 50% in individual response variables such as joint counts and acute-phase response were observed in the highest-dose group. These results were confirmed in a study where patients received placebo, or 0.25, 2 or 16 mg/m^2 etanercept, subcutaneously twice weekly for 3 months.[22] Of the patients receiving the highest dose, 75% fulfilled the ACR 20% response criterion versus only 14% of the placebo-treated patients. In another placebo-controlled trial where patients ($n = 234$) were treated for 6 months with placebo, or 10 or 25 mg of etanercept, subcutaneously twice weekly, 51% and 59% of the 10- and 25-mg-treated groups fulfilled the ACR 20% response criterion, which was significantly higher than the 11% of the placebo-treated patients.[23] To study whether the addition of etanercept to methotrexate would provide additional benefit to patients who had persistent active RA despite receiving methotrexate (15–25 mg), patients received either 25 mg etanercept or placebo injections while continuing methotrexate.[24] At 24 weeks, 71% of the patients receiving etanercept and 27% of those receiving placebo met the ACR 20% response criterion.

To study the effect of etanercept in patients in an early phase of the disease, 632 patients with a mean disease duration of 1 year received either twice-weekly subcutaneous etanercept (10 or 25 mg) or weekly oral methotrexate (mean 19 mg/week) for 12 months.[25] At 12 months, 72% of the patients in the group assigned to receive 25 mg etanercept had an ACR 20% response, as compared with 65% of those in the methotrexate group. As also noted in previous studies, the 25-mg dose was more effective than the 10-mg dose. Among patients who received the 25-mg dose of etanercept, 72% has no increase in the erosion score as compared with 60% of the patients in the methotrexate group.

INTERLEUKIN-1 RECEPTOR ANTAGONIST IN RHEUMATOID ARTHRITIS

The IL-1 gene family consists of IL-1α and IL-1β and their natural inhibitor, IL-1 receptor antagonist (IL-1Ra).[17] IL-1α and IL-1β are antagonists that exert their function via the interaction between these molecules and a receptor on target cells. The effects of IL-1α and IL-1β are blocked by the interaction of the IL-1 receptor with IL-1Ra. The production of IL-1Ra has been found to be deficient relative to the total production of IL-1 in RA patients. This led to the hypothesis that administering IL-1Ra to patients with active RA might restore the IL-1Ra/IL-1 balance. Clinical studies with a recombinant IL-1Ra, anakinra (Kineret), have substantiated this hypothesis. In a preliminary trial, 15 patients with active RA received daily subcutaneous injections of anakinra for a total of 28 days. Major reductions in the joint counts and acute-phase reactants were observed in 12 of 15 patients within 2 weeks of treatment. In a subsequent controlled trial, 175 RA patients were randomized to receive 20, 70 or 200 mg of kineret with varying dosing intervals for 3 weeks.[26] Daily dosing appeared to be most effective. Subsequently, a randomized placebo-controlled trial, in which 472 patients with relatively early and active RA were treated with daily injections of 30, 75 or 150 mg kineret or placebo for 24 weeks, was organized.[27] The clinical responses in patients receiving 150 mg/day were greater than those in the other treatment groups. An ACR 20% response was achieved in 43% of the 150 mg/day group compared to 27% of the patients in the placebo group after 24 weeks. Radiographic evaluations in this study found a statistically significant decrease in the rate of joint damage progression after treatment with kineret when compared to placebo.[28] All patients who completed the 24-week extension phase of the study were radiographically assessed after 1 year of treatment. It was reported that joint destruction was reduced even more in the second half-year of treatment.

The efficacy of anakinra plus methotrexate was evaluated in a 24-week randomized study on 419 patients who had active RA despite methotrexate treatment (12.5–25 mg/week for at least 6 months).[29] Patients were randomized to daily subcutaneous injections of placebo, or anakinra 0.04, 0.1, 1.0 or 2.0 mg/kg per day, for up to 24 weeks. The ACR 20% response at 24 weeks was seen in 42% of patients who received 1 mg/kg anakrina and in 23% of the patients in the placebo/methotrexate group.

ADVERSE REACTIONS TO TUMOR NECROSIS FACTOR AND INTERLEUKIN-1 INHIBITORS IN RHEUMATOID ARTHRITIS

Data from clinical trials with TNF and IL-1 antagonists have reported relatively low levels of toxicity of these drugs, and the incidence of adverse events during the first years of therapy seems to be acceptably low. The most common reactions in the infliximab clinical trial program in RA were headache, nausea, upper respiratory tract infections, and infusion-related reactions.[30] The latter were mild, necessitating withdrawal in <2% of the patients. Serious adverse reactions occurred in 4.4% of the infliximab recipients compared to 1.8% of the placebo recipients in a pooled analysis. These reactions included fever (0.9%), pneumonia (0.9%), dyspnea (0.4%), and rash (0.4%). About 6% of infliximab patients withdrew from treatment because of adverse events.

With etanercept, the withdrawal rate because of adverse events was also low and similar to that of placebo in randomized trials.[23,24] The most common adverse events were injection-site reactions, upper respiratory tract infections, and headache. Post-marketing studies confirm the relative safety of TNF antagonists. Among the 4794 patients enrolled in the etanercept studies and long-term open-label study, there were no increases in the rates of serious infection, malignancy, or death. Data from infliximab follow-up programs are also reassuring in this respect, but recently an increased risk of exacerbation of latent tuberculosis appeared.[31] The probability of unmasking tuberculosis may be greater with antibody therapies against TNF than with soluble receptor therapies. These observations have led to warnings in the prescribing information and to recommendations for prevention.

Wider use of TNF antagonists in RA has led to reports, largely of individual cases, of a range of serious adverse neurological, hematological, heart and serious infectious complications. It is important to realize, however, that there may be an increased risk of such complications in RA independent of treatment. It is therefore fundamentally important not just to document the occurrence of these events in a treated cohort of patients, but to compare their occurrence with what might have happened if such patients had remained on conventional therapy.

The most frequently documented side-effect of kineret therapy is injection-site reaction. In controlled trials, these were reported in 25% of patients given placebo and ±75% of patients given anakinra. These resulted in premature withdrawal from the study in 5% of anakinra-treated patients. Infections that required antibiotic therapy occurred in 12% of the placebo-treated patients and 16% of the kineret-treated patients.

IMMUNOGENICITY

Administration of large proteins can lead to the formation of antibodies against the treatment agent. In the case of mAbs, the formation of anti-idiotypic antibodies is an integral element of immunoregulation. However, the exact clinical relevance of such antibodies is currently unknown. The frequency of antibody formation against infliximab is irreversibly related to the dose and is lower when methotrexate is given concomitantly. Formation of anti-infliximab antibodies during methotrexate occurred in 15.7% and 0% of the patients treated with 1.3 and 10 mg/kg infliximab, respectively.[13] These antibodies neutralize the binding activity of infliximab to TNF. Etanercept also induces antibody formation which seems to be non-neutralizing for TNF-binding activity. Antibody formation against anakinra has not been reported.

Both infliximab and etanercept led to the formation of autoantibodies against nuclear factors in clinical trials with RA patients. The percentages were ±50% with infliximab and ±10% with etanercept. Less than 5% of these patients also developed antibodies against double-stranded DNA. Recently, there have been some case reports of RA patients being treated with either infliximab or etanercept who developed drug-induced systemic lupus erythematosus.[32,33] Further studies are necessary to clarify its prevalence and pathogenesis.

SUMMARY AND CONCLUSIONS

The concept of a targeted therapy that could affect one or more specific pathological processes in RA has enormous implications for the future. Heretofore, all the available therapies have been truly non-specific, often borrowed from other disciplines (e.g. oncology, infectious diseases), and having side-effect profiles that limit their usefulness. With the new biological agents, new therapeutic perspectives appear but many questions need to be addressed to further clarify their role. These include the following: (1) do these drugs maintain efficacy with treatments longer than 5 years; (2) do these treatments maintain the integrity of joint structures during long-term therapy; (3) are they safe with long-term therapy; (4) how can we explain non-responders; (5) how can we select patients for the different forms of targeted therapies; (6) is it justified to use the, by definition, restricted financial resources in healthcare for long-term RA treatment with biological agents?

Currently, the US Food and Drug Administration and the European Medical Agency for Drug Evaluation have approved etanercept, infliximab and anakinra for patients who have failed DMARD therapy. Whether this will change depends on more studies in early RA.

RA is a severe disease despite established treatment. The most promising therapies at present include products of biotechnology. These therapies, which have become available for many rheumatologists, may certainly be seen as breakthroughs in the treatment of RA. The optimization of TNF and IL-1 blockade through increasing experience and extended careful surveillance of patients should ensure cytokine-targeted agents a pivotal place in the therapy for RA.

REFERENCES

1. Pincus T, Breedveld FC, Emery P. Does partial control of inflammation prevent long-term joint damage? Clinical rationale for combination therapy with multiple disease-modifying antirheumatic drugs. *Clin Exp Rheumatol* 1999; **17**(suppl. 18): S2–7.
2. Pincus T, Brooks RH, Callahan LF. Prediction of long-term mortality in patients with rheumatoid arthritis according to simple questionnaire and joint count measures. *Ann Intern Med* 1994; **120**: 26–34.
3. Drossaers-Bakker KW, de Buck M, van Zeben D et al. Long-term course and outcome of functional capacity in rheumatoid arthritis. *Arthritis Rheum* 1999; **42**: 1854–60.
4. Weinblatt ME, Maier AL, Fraser PA, Coblyn JS. Longterm prospective study of methotrexate in rheumatoid arthritis: conclusion after 132 months of therapy. *J Rheumatol* 1998; **25**: 238–42.
5. Mulherin D, Fitzgerald O, Bresnihan B. Clinical improvement and radiological deterioration in rheumatoid arthritis: evidence that pathogenesis of synovial inflammation and articular erosion may differ. *Br J Rheumatol* 1996; **35**: 1263–8.
6. Feldmann M, Brennan FM, Maini RN. Rheumatoid arthritis. *Cell* 1996; **85**: 307–10.
7. Dolhain RJEM, van der Heiden AN, ter Haar NT et al. Shift toward T lymphocytes with a T helper 1 cytokine-secretion profile in the joints of patients with rheumatoid arthritis. *Arthritis Rheum* 1996; **39**: 1961–9.
8. Breedveld FC. Therapeutic monoclonal antibodies. *Lancet* 2000; **355**: 735–40.
9. Arend WP, Dayer JM. Inhibition of the production and effects of interleukin-1 and tumor necrosis factor alpha in rheumatoid arthritis. *Arthritis Rheum* 1995; **38**: 151–60.
10. Feldmann M, Elliot MJ, Woody JN, Maini RN. Anti-tumor necrosis factor-alpha therapy of rheumatoid arthritis. *Adv Immunol* 1997; **64**: 310–50.
11. Elliott MJ, Maini RN, Feldmann M et al. Treatment of rheumatoid arthritis with chimeric monoclonal antibodies to TNFα. *Arthritis Rheum* 1993; **36**: 1681–90.
12. Elliot MJ, Maini RN, Feldmann M et al. Randomised double-blind comparison of chimeric monoclonal antibody to tumour necrosis factor alpha (cA2) versus placebo in rheumatoid arthritis. *Lancet* 1994; **344**: 1105–10.
13. Maini RN, Breedveld FC, Kalden JR et al. Therapeutic efficacy of multiple intravenous infusions of anti-tumour necrosis factor α monoclonal antibody combined with low-dose weekly methotrexate in rheumatoid arthritis. *Arthritis Rheum* 1998; **41**: 1552–63.
14. Maini R, St Clair EW, Breedveld F et al. Infliximab (chimeric anti-tumour necrosis factor α monoclonal antibody) versus placebo in rheumatoid arthritis patients receiving concomitant methotrexate: a randomised phase III trial. *Lancet* 1999; **354**: 1932–9
15. Lipsky P, van der Heijde D, St Clair W et al. 102-Week clinical and radiological results from the ATTRACT trial: a 2 year, randomized, controlled, phase 3 trial of infliximab (Remicade) in patients with active RA despite MTX. *Arthritis Rheum* 2000; **43**(suppl): 269 (abstract).
16. Lipsky PE, van der Heijde DM, St Clair EW et al. Infliximab and methotrexate in the treatment of rheumatoid arthritis. Anti-tumor necrosis factor trial in rheumatoid arthritis with Concomitant Therapy Study Group. *N Engl J Med* 2000; **343**: 1594–602
17. Rankin EC, Choy EH, Kassimos D et al. The therapeutic effect on an engineered human anti-tumor-necrosis factor alpha antibody (CDP571) in rheumatoid arthritis. *Br J Rheumatol* 1995; **34**: 334–42.
18. Keystone E, Choy E, Kalden J et al. CDP870, a novel, pegylated, humanized TNF inhibitor is effective in healing rheumatoid arthritis. *Arthritis Rheum* 2001; **44**: 2946.
19. Keystone E, Weinblatt ME, Weisman M et al. The fully human anti-TNF monoclonal antibody, adalimumab (D2E7), dose ranging study: the 24-week clinical results in patients with active RA on methotrexate therapy (the Armade trial). *Ann Rheum Dis* 2001; **60**: 67 (abstract).
20. Mohler KM, Torrance DS, Smith CA et al. Soluble tumor necrosis factor (TNF) receptors are effective therapeutic agents in lethal endotoxemia and function simultaneously as both TNF carriers and TNF antagonists. *J Immunol* 1993; **151**: 1548–61.
21. Moreland LW, Margolies G, Heck LW Jr et al. Recombinant soluble tumor necrosis factor receptor (p80) fusion protein: toxicity and dose finding trial in refractory rheumatoid arthritis. *J Rheumatol* 1996; **23**: 1849–55.
22. Moreland LW, Baumgartner SW, Schiff MH et al.

Treatment of rheumatoid arthritis with recombinant human tumor necrosis factor receptor (p75)–Fc fusion protein. *N Engl J Med* 1997; **337**: 141–7.

23. Moreland LW, Schiff MH, Baumgartner SW et al. Etanercept therapy in rheumatoid arthritis: a randomized, controlled study. *Ann Intern Med* 1999; **130**: 478–86.

24. Weinblatt ME, Kremer JM, Bankhurst AD et al. A trial of Etanercept, a recombinant tumor necrosis factor receptor: Fc fusion protein, in patients with rheumatoid arthritis receiving methotrexate. *N Engl J Med* 1999; **340**: 253–9.

25. Bathon JM, Martin RW, Fleischmann RM et al. A comparison of etanercept and methotrexate in patients with early rheumatoid arthritis. *N Engl J Med* 2000; **343**: 1586–93.

26. Campion GV, Lesback ME, Lookabaugh J et al. Dose-range and dose-frequency study of recombinant human interleukin-1 receptor antagonist in patients with rheumatoid arthritis. *Arthritis Rheum* 1996; **39**: 1092–101.

27. Bresnihan B, Alvaro-Gracia JM, Cobby M et al. Treatment of rheumatoid arthritis with recombinant human interleukin-1 receptor antagonist. *Arthritis Rheum* 1998; **41**: 2196–204.

28. Jiang Y, Genant HK, Watt I et al. A multicenter, double-blind, dose-ranging, randomized and placebo controlled study of recombinant human interleukin-1 receptor antagonist in patients with rheumatoid arthritis: radiologic progression and correlation of Genant and Larsen scoring methods. *Arthritis Rheum* 2000; **43**: 1001–9.

29. Cohen S, Hurd E, Cush JJ et al. Treatment of rheumatoid arthritis with anakinra, a recombinant human interleukin-1 receptor antagonist, in combination with methotrexate: results of a twenty-four-week, multicenter, randomized, double-blind, placebo-controlled trial. *Arthritis Rheum* 2002; **46**: 574–8.

30. Hanauer SB. Safety of infliximab in clinical trials. *Aliment Pharmacol Ther* 1999; **4**(suppl. 4): 16–22.

31. Day R. Adverse reactions to TNF-α inhibitors in rheumatoid arthritis. *Lancet* 2002; **359**: 540–1.

32. Shakoor N, Michalska M, Harris CA, Block JA. Drug-induced systemic lupus erythematosus associated with etanercept therapy. *Lancet* 2002; **359**: 579–80.

33. DeBandt MJ, Descamps V, Meyer O. Two cases of etanercept-induced systemic lupus erythematosus in patients with rheumatoid arthritis. *Ann Rheum Dis* 2001; **60**: 175.

30

Early arthritis

Paul Emery

Introduction • Biological therapy • Use of etanercept in ERA • Explanation of ERA data • Infliximab in ERA • High-dose anti-TNF as potential remission-induction therapy • Preliminary results of a double-blind placebo-controlled study of infliximab in ERA • Summary • References

INTRODUCTION

For some time the management of patients with early rheumatoid arthritis (ERA) has focused on the early stage of disease. As a consequence, the management of the early phase of disease has moved from being a neglected area to being probably the most studied and important time for the care of a patient with rheumatoid arthritis (RA). The evidence supporting the importance of the early phase of disease can be summarized in the following way.

First, a body of evidence has demonstrated that untreated inflammation leads inevitably to damage of one sort or another, and that the longer a patient is left with untreated inflammation the greater the cumulative damage.[1-3] As most damage is believed to be irreversible if persistent, this damage will inevitably translate into disability, and thus a large direct cost to both the individual and society. Objective measures of damage have been developed to document these effects and include the measurement of bony erosions detected by radiology[4] and more recently evidence from high-resolution ultrasound[5] and magnetic resonance imaging (MRI).[6] Both these latter techniques show that damage occurs early in the disease

process and is much more extensive than revealed by conventional X-rays. The loss of function has also been demonstrated to occur early in the disease process and to correlate with inflammation.[7] Function is conveniently measured by the Health Assessment Questionnaire (HAQ). Finally, the use of dual-energy X-ray absorptiometry has been used as a quantitative measure of the impact of inflammation on bone and again has shown that very rapid bone loss occurs in the early phase of disease, with a close correlation between the amount of inflammation present both locally and systemically. Thus, by every assessment damage occurs early in the disease process and is associated predominantly with the amount of inflammation present.[8]

An important issue is the concept that the reversibility of damage is transitory. For example, it has been shown that the rapid treatment of inflammation can reverse functional loss in RA if done early, and that this improvement is sustained provided the inflammation remains suppressed.[7] Likewise, bone densitometry has demonstrated that bone loss can be improved in the early phases of disease when inflammation is adequately treated.[8] This (temporary?) reversibility adds urgency to the management of these patients. A final crucial and perhaps related point is the suggestion that the outcome of treatment is qualitatively different if therapy is given within a narrow therapeutic window. This concept came originally from animal models, but is supported by the evidence from an open intervention study which suggests that in patients with a diagnosis of RA with a duration of less than 12 weeks a 50% chance of remission can be obtained with early therapy.[9] Care is needed in the interpretation of these data, but by analogy with oncology even if early therapy only achieves a reduction in disease bulk, this alone can have a profound difference in outcome. The quantitative reduction in bulk may produce differences, which amount to an almost qualitative difference.

It is reasonable to conclude that the management of early disease is the crucial time for therapy and the time at which most care should be given to optimizing therapy.

BIOLOGICAL THERAPY

Biological therapy with TNF blocking agents represents the most effective therapy so far available to patients with RA. Patients experience relatively few adverse reactions and this combined with the efficacy of the therapy mean that more patients remain on active treatment. Most of the studies have been conducted in patients who had failed to respond to conventional disease-modifying anti-rheumatic drugs (DMARDs). This group of patients were thought to be largely untreatable and therefore it is important to note that these drugs were as effective in DMARD-failure patients as conventional DMARDs were in DMARD-naive patients. What these studies were not able to reveal was whether the early use of such biologicals would provide a much greater level of response than that seen with conventional DMARDs. Furthermore, there was no indication as to whether the level of improvement in an individual patient would be qualitatively different from that seen with existing treatments given early.

Despite the above caveats it was believed by most rheumatologists that early use of these agents would provide unequivocal evidence of significant advantages over existing treatments.

USE OF ETANERCEPT IN ERA

It was on this basis that a study of etanercept in patients with ERA was undertaken that compared etanercept with methotrexate in patients early in disease.[10] This study was undertaken in 632 methotrexate-naive patients who were randomized to either twice-weekly etanercept (10 or 25 mg) or oral weekly methotrexate up to 20 mg. Etanercept (25 mg) and methotrexate were equally effective in preventing joint-space narrowing and reducing the Sharpe score over one year; etanercept (25 mg) significantly slowed the erosion rates compared to methotrexate. The ACR 20 response rates at 12 months were 75 and 65% in the etanercept (25 mg) and methotrexate groups, respectively. However, the HAQ reduction was not significantly different between the groups. It was concluded that etanercept was at least as effective in preventing overall structural damage and superior in preventing erosions (the latter was not the primary end point). It was clear that etanercept produced more clinical improvement that was sustained over one year.

Importantly, follow-up has shown that at two and three years the patients who received etanercept did increasingly well compared to those who received methotrexate. Interestingly, those who later switched to etanercept never caught up in terms of the response rate with patients treated with etanercept from the outset.

EXPLANATION OF ERA DATA

The explanation for the study findings may lie in two critical areas: the methotrexate regime and the patient population. The methotrexate regime involved the use of methotrexate earlier in disease and at a higher dose than had ever previously been undertaken (starting with rapid escalation to 20 mg per week in the first three months). As these patients were 'early patients' they were much less systemically unwell, and perhaps because of this, tolerated this regime in a way that most rheumatologists would not have predicted from experience of the drug in patients with longer disease duration. This is when therapy with methotrexate is most frequently given. Therefore patients had a very effective dose of methotrexate given early and responded better than had ever previously been seen.

As the patient population was naive to methotrexate, the group contained within it a large population of responders. It is known that patients respond better to their first therapy than they do to later therapies. Interestingly, within the responder population it did not appear to make a great difference whether they were on methotrexate or etanercept. These patients appeared to do as well on methotrexate as on etanercept, and thus the effective difference between the two therapies was confined to the higher number of methotrexate non-responders. This represents a much smaller proportion of the total population than would have been predicted. Thus the above may explain the data at 12 months which did not show any significant difference in several outcome measures.

However, as is now known, over the second and third years the etanercept patients maintained their improvement, whereas more methotrexate patients failed therapy and the difference between the two groups increased with time. The implications of this study are still being assessed. However, what is clear is that therapy did not produce compelling evidence for the *blanket* use of biological therapies as first-line treatments in patients with ERA.

INFLIXIMAB IN ERA

Within the pivotal Anti-TNF Trial in Rheumatoid Arthritis with Concompitant Therapy (ATTRACT) study there were 82 patients who had a disease duration of less than three years.[11] These patients were divided into four dosing regimes; there were small numbers in each group and therefore conclusions must be limited especially as it was a retrospective analysis. The major findings were that the improvements in radiological progression seen in the whole group were also seen in this sub-group. In fact those who received methotrexate alone actually deteriorated faster than patients who had the disease of longer duration. Thus it appears that infliximab worked equally well in preventing damage in patients with early and late disease.

Currently there are two very large studies being undertaken by Centocor and Abbot that are looking at infliximab and adalimamab, respectively, compared to methotrexate (and in one case a combination of TNF blockade with methotrexate) in early disease. These studies should give much clearer evidence of the efficacy and cost-effectiveness of the early use of TNF blocking agents particularly in combination with methotrexate. Critical to these studies will be the cost-effectiveness analysis. The alternative approach would be to use the biological agents as step-up therapy to patients who have shown an incomplete response to methotrexate at an early stage of disease.

HIGH-DOSE ANTI-TNF AS POTENTIAL REMISSION-INDUCTION THERAPY

A mode of action study was undertaken in five patients with very poor prognosis RA treated at presentation.[12] This study addressed the question of whether the heterogeneous response seen in disease was due to insufficient drug, and whether a high-dose regime could induce a disease remission state, which could then be sustained without the biologicals. These patients not only received induction with a high dose (infliximab, 10 mg/kg at 0, 2, 6, and 14 weeks) but if not in imaging remission at the end of this time they were re-induced with a further induction regime of identical high-dose nature. The results showed that one patient did not respond at all and one patient achieved clinical remission; however, no patient achieved remission as judged by imaging with high-resolution ultrasound or MRI. By the protocol agreed at the outset, all patients were eligible for re-induction with a further high dose. One patient did not receive this because of side effects. The re-induction did not produce any further response either in the non-responsive patient or in the others who had not achieved remission.

It was concluded from the study that the variable response to anti-TNF was not due to insufficient drug. Furthermore, a true remission was rarely obtained with these therapies and a drug-free state could not be sustained; all patients required further TNF therapy. Finally the study demonstrated that there was a close correlation between the synovitis observed by the imaging techniques and the development of new bony defects. No new defects were seen without synovitis. Thus, it appeared that the inter-relationship between synovitis and bony damage, which had been observed in other mode of action studies with conventional DMARDs and steroids, also applied to infliximab.

PRELIMINARY RESULTS OF A DOUBLE-BLIND PLACEBO-CONTROLLED STUDY OF INFLIXIMAB IN ERA

This study was a double-blind randomized approach to patients with new untreated RA with poor prognostic features. Patients were randomized to receive methotrexate plus either placebo or infliximab. These patients received a year's treatment with frequent assessment by MRI and ultrasound in order to examine the impact of infliximab on the early phase of disease, in particular the time course of response and furthermore to establish the long-term outcome of these patients. Twenty patients were recruited, one of whom withdrew early due to a vasculitic rash. The infliximab-treated patients demonstrated an almost immediate improvement in systemic symptoms.

There was a very rapid reduction in synovitis and in swollen and tender joint count; the improvements seen at two weeks on infliximab were equivalent to those seen at 14 weeks with methotrexate. At 14 weeks a 50% greater reduction in joint count was seen in the active treated patients. Slightly delayed but also rapid was the improvement in quality of life and function. There was also a significant reversal of bony lesions demonstrated on MRI as well as synovitis. This important study which is still being assessed will provide information on how and how quickly anti-TNF therapies work.

SUMMARY

Biological therapy with anti-TNF is the most effective therapy available to patients with RA. There is no doubt that it works at least as well as DMARDs in early disease and for sub-populations unresponsive to DMARDs works considerably better. This difference appears to increase over time. Studies in progress will reveal whether there is a significant difference between patients treated with biologicals and those receiving mono-therapy or combination therapy with conventional DMARDs. However, what they may not clarify is whether this will be cost effective either in terms of direct or indirect costs both for society and to patients exposed to biologicals who may not have required them. These issues will be debated for some time. In the meantime, if costs were not an issue the most logical approach would be to treat patients initially with conventional DMARDs but rapidly to introduce biologicals if there was evidence of no or incomplete response.

REFERENCES

1. Dawes PT, Fowler PD, Clarke S et al. Rheumatoid arthritis: treatment which controls the C-reactive protein and erythrocyte sedimentation rate reduces radiological progression. *Br J Rheumatol* 1986; **25**: 44–9.
2. Fries J, Williams CA, Morfield D et al. Reduction in long-term disability in patients with rheumatoid arthritis by disease-modifying antirheumatic drug-based treatment strategies. *Arthritis Rheum* 1996; **39**: 616–22.
3. Stein CM, Pincus T. Placebo-controlled studies in rheumatoid arthritis: ethical issues. *Lancet* 1999; **353**: 400–3.
4. Abu-Shakra M, Toker R, Flusser D et al. Clinical

and radiographic outcomes of rheumatoid arthritis patients not treated with disease modifying drugs. *Arthritis Rheum* 1998; **41**: 1190–5.

5. Wakefield RJ, Gibbon W, Conaghan P et al. The value of sonography in the detection of cortical bone erosions: a comparative study with conventional radiography. *Arthritis Rheum* 2000; **43**(12): 2762–70.

6. McGonagle D, Conaghan P, O'Connor P et al. The relationship between synovitis and bone changes in early untreated RA – a controlled MRI study. *Arthritis Rheum* 1999; **42**: 1706–11.

7. Devlin J, Gough A, Huissoon A et al. The acute phase and function in early rheumatoid arthritis. CRP levels correlate with functional outcome. *J Rheum* 1997; **24**: 9–13.

8. Gough AK, Lilley J, Eyre S et al. Generalised bone loss in patients with early rheumatoid arthritis occurs early and relates to disease activity. *Lancet* 1994; **344**: 23–7.

9. Green M, Marzo-Ortega H, McGonagle D et al. Persistence of mild, early inflammatory arthritis: the importance of disease duration, rheumatoid factor, and the shared epitope. *Arthritis Rheum* 1999; **42**: 2184–8.

10. Bathon JM, Martin RW, Fleischmann RM et al. A comparison of etanercept and methotrexate in patients with early rheumatoid arthritis. *N Engl J Med* 2000; **343**(22): 1586–93.

11. Maini R, St Clair E, Breedveld F et al. Infliximab (chimeric anti-tumor necrosis factor alpha monoclonal antibody) versus placebo in rheumatoid arthritis patients receiving concomitant methotrexate: a randomised phase III trial. ATTRACT Study Group. *Lancet* 1999; **354**(9194): 1932–9.

12. Conaghan P, Quinn M, O'Connor P et al. The impact of a very high dose TNF blockade on new rheumatoid arthritis patients: a clinical and imaging pilot study. *Arthritis Rheum.* 2002; **46**(7): 1971–2.

31

Juvenile arthritis

Patricia Woo

Introduction • Impact of juvenile idiopathic arthritis • Types of juvenile idiopathic arthritis • Imbalances in cellular and cytokine networks • Genetic influences and possible targets • Therapeutic cytokine modulation • TNF-α blockade • Potential risks from TNF blockade • Other immunomodulation • Trial design and ethical considerations • Practical management of new therapies • Conclusion • References

INTRODUCTION

For children and young people with severe juvenile idiopathic arthritis (JIA), whose disease is uncontrolled by conventional disease-modifying drugs and steroids, a new group of therapies with exciting potential has emerged. Research examining cellular and cytokine control of inflammation in JIA has provided some of the scientific rationale for therapeutic agents targeting biological pathways. These biological agents include antagonists to cytokines such as tumour necrosis factor alpha (TNF-α), which have shown early promise by producing dramatic clinical benefit in many children with JIA and other autoimmune diseases. However, despite targeting specific molecules, the therapeutic actions of these new agents remain non-specific, producing variable clinical responses that raise additional ethical and administrative considerations.

IMPACT OF JUVENILE IDIOPATHIC ARTHRITIS

JIA affects 1 in 1000 children.[1] For the majority of children with polyarticular disease, methotrex-

ate and other second-line agents[2,3] have improved the prognosis of this group of diseases. However, significant numbers (approximately 30%) of children with JIA are refractory to conventional management, and suffer in addition the cumulative side-effects of long-term immunosuppressive medication. Such disease activity results in joint damage, which often necessitates joint replacement, severe growth retardation, chronic pain, and functional disability. There is also a significant impact on emotional and psychological development, lifestyle, and employment.[4,5] It is to this group of patients that biological therapy is currently targeted.

TYPES OF JUVENILE IDIOPATHIC ARTHRITIS

The classification of chronic arthritis in children has been a clinical one, attempting to separate the heterogeneous spectrum of disease into more homogeneous subgroups according to clinical features at presentation and their prognosis. There were two systems of classification in use from the 1970s, which were not identical (Table 31.1). An international taskforce convened by the International League of

Table 31.1   Comparison of the classifications of arthritis in children.

ARA: Juvenile Rheumatoid Arthritis (1977)	EULAR: Juvenile Chronic Arthritis (1977)	ILAR: Juvenile Idiopathic Arthritis (1997)
Pauciarticular (four or less joints affected, includes RF+, extended, some psoriatics and ERA as defined in ILAR)	**Pauciarticular** (four or less joints affected, includes RF+, extended, some ERA and psoriatic as defined in ILAR)	**Oligoarticular** (four or less joints affected, RF- only)
		Extended oligoarticular (RF- only)
Polyarticular (includes RF+ and RF-, some psoriatics and ERA as defined in ILAR)	**Polyarticular** (includes RF+ and RF-, some ERA and psoriatics as defined in ILAR)	**Polyarticular, RF-**
		Polyarticular, RF+
Systemic	**Systemic**	**Systemic**
Juvenile ankylosing spondyloarthritis **excluded**	**Probable and definite juvenile ankylosing spondylitis**	**Enthesitis-related arthritis** (not all would fit juvenile anklylosing spondylitis as in EULAR)
Psoriatics included in pauci/poly	Psoriatics included in pauci/poly	**Psoriatic arthritis** **Unclassified**

The categories are in bold type.
ERA, enthesis-related arthritis; RF, rheumatoid factor.

Associations of Rheumatology (ILAR) proposed and subsequently revised a unifying classification which aimed to produce clinically homogeneous subgroups that are mutually exclusive, so as to aid research into pathogenesis and therapeutic studies.[6] The discussions in this chapter will use this ILAR classification.

Since there are no obvious infectious triggers or reproducible observations of seasonality in any of these diseases, they are regarded at present as autoimmune diseases. The persistent inflammatory response is perceived by current researchers to depend on the balance of the immune and inflammatory mediators, which can be reactive to foreign antigens or self-antigens, but are also controlled genetically. Imbalances in cellular functions and interac-

tions, and in pro- and anti-inflammatory cytokines, have been found in JIA. Modulation of these imbalances is the rationale for the development of newer biological therapies, as is the case for other rheumatic diseases. In addition, the case can be strengthened in JIA, where there are genetic variations that are proinflammatory.

IMBALANCES IN CELLULAR AND CYTOKINE NETWORKS

A type 1 T-cell response (predominance of interferon (IFN)-γ-producing cells) is found in the synovial fluid and membranes of children with oligoarticular, polyarticular and enthesitis-related arthritis, but not in the peripheral blood mononuclear cells, indicating sequestration and/or in situ differentiation and polarization of T cells.[7,8] Currently, there are no data on the type of synovial T-cell response in systemic arthritis, but there is one report of a mixed type 1 and 2 response in the peripheral blood mononuclear cells.[9] Differences between rheumatoid arthritis (RA) and JIA include:

1. the lack of IgM rheumatoid factor (RF), except for the subgroup of RF-positive arthritis, which constitutes about 1% of all JIA
2. the presence of IFN-γ- and interleukin (IL)-4-producing cells in the synovial fluid and synovium of JIA
3. the variable levels of TNF-α and its soluble receptor (sTNFR) in subgroups.

Evidence that the pathological processes in JIA are cytokine dependent includes the positive correlation of serum and synovial concentrations of various cytokines with disease activity.[10–12] The effects of proinflammatory cytokines on synovial cells and osteoclasts are well described, and it is clear that the general principle of using antagonists of proinflammatory cytokines is applicable to JIA as well. The issue is whether there is a 'master cytokine' to target.

Research so far in JIA suggests that there are different cytokine imbalances in at least three areas. Systemic JIA is characterized by quotidian fevers, transient rash, enlargement of the reticuloendothelial system, serositis, and systemic vasculitis, in addition to arthritis. These patients have a vigorous acute-phase response and their serum cytokine profiles reflect excess production of IL-6 and its agonist sIL6R,[13,14] although other proinflammatory cytokines are also present.[11,15] The ratio of TNF and its natural inhibitor, sTNFR, is higher in the synovial fluid of polyarticular JIA as compared to enthesitis-related arthritis, consistent with a more aggressively erosive disease in the former.[16] The difference between oligoarticular and polyarticular JIA is that IL-4 is detected only in the synovium and fluid in oligoarticular JIA,[7,8] even though both showed type 1 T-cell responses. An additional important consideration is the genetic component of the imbalance.

GENETIC INFLUENCES AND POSSIBLE TARGETS

It is clear that HLA association studies have identified class II antigens in case–control as well as family association studies. HLA DR* 0801 has been identified as being the genetic background of early-onset JIA, in particular oligoarticular JIA.[17] The exception is systemic JIA. How these class II antigens present peptides in JIA versus controls is an active area of research, and could yield novel therapeutic approaches.

The cytokine milieu is influential in the process of antigen presentation, cellular polarization, and apoptosis. Thus, the balance of pro- and anti-inflammatory cytokines is important in the outcome of inflammation, as discussed in Chapter 19 and elsewhere in this book. Studies of genetic associations with variants of pro- and anti-inflammatory cytokines have shown interesting results in JIA. Our case–control study of the IL-10 gene has shown that the low-IL-10-producing variant is significantly associated with extended oligoarticular JIA, suggesting a genetic effect on disease severity.[18,19] This genetic variant was also shown to be a severity factor for asthma.[20] Recent studies of the TNF-α gene suggest that the −308 variant is associated with severity in a sample of Turks,[21] and a Japanese sample population.[22] This variant has been shown to influence transcription of the TNF-α gene.[23] A more comprehensive analysis of all the nucleotide variants in the regulatory region of the TNF-α gene has been reported recently for oligoarticular JIA, using a family study.[24] The function of the haplotypes remains to be characterized. Other associations include the macrophage inhibitory factor (MIF) and IL-6. MIF was found to have a genetic variant in the regulatory region which is significantly associated with all types of JIA, but its functional significance awaits further characterization.[25] The IL-6 gene has several variants in its regulatory region, and the −174 site has a dominant effect on gene expression.[26] This site controls the level of IL-6 gene expression and has been shown to be associated with early-onset systemic JIA.[27] Its biological significance is illustrated by its association with type I and II insulin-dependent diabetes, peak bone mass in adolescent young men, increased bone turnover in postmenopausal women, and survival after coronary bypass graft. Confirmation of these studies as well as analysis of the interaction of these genetic influences would provide the scientific basis for new biological therapies in each of these types of arthritis in children.

THERAPEUTIC CYTOKINE MODULATION

Cytokine modulation aims to restore homeostasis by influencing a perceived imbalance of cytokines or by promoting a particular cellular response. Established therapies have been shown to alter production of cytokines at the level of transcription and translation. Corticosteroids and cyclosporin A inhibit nuclear factors important for gene expression,[28–30] thalidomide enhances TNF-α mRNA degradation,[31] and leflunamide inhibits signal transduction pathways by blocking tyrosine phosphorylation.[32] In contrast, the principal means of TNF blockade, and of current new biologicals, is to block the molecule itself from interacting with cells, using monoclonal neutralizing antibodies or recombinant soluble cytokine receptors. Receptor interference is achieved by using naturally derived cytokine antagonists (e.g. recombinant IL-1ra) and by using monoclonal antibodies (e.g. anti IL-6R).

TNF-α BLOCKADE

Etanercept is licensed for use in children in the USA and Europe. It is a recombinant protein consisting of the binding portion of the human soluble TNF-α receptor attached to the Fc portion of human IgG (Chapter 10). It neutralizes TNF by binding with an affinity 50–1000 times that of the naturally occurring TNF receptors, and has a longer half-life. It may also exert its effect by binding other cytokines, such as lymphotoxin. It has a UK licence for use in children aged 4–17 years who show an inadequate response to, or are intolerant of,

methotrexate. Early safety and efficacy data in children less than 4 years of age are encouraging.[33] It is administered by subcutaneous injection twice-weekly, for an indefinite period, and may be used with or without methotrexate.

The most detailed trial to date enrolled 69 patients with chronic polyarthritis of variable aetiology and unresponsive to maximum conventional treatment.[34] The duration of the study was 1 year, although 5-year follow-up data are now available.[35] The initial study had a novel design, in that all patients received etanercept for the first 3 months, while all other medications, except low-dose steroids and non-steroidal anti-inflammatory drugs (NSAIDs), were stopped. Figure 31.1 shows the structure of the trial and the patient responses. Non-responders in the first 3 months were withdrawn from stage 2 of the study, as they required additional therapy. The definition of improvement was as described by Giannini et al.[36] Seventy-four per cent of all patients benefited over the first 3 months. A secondary endpoint was the time to flare of disease: during the 7 months after randomization, 77% of those receiving placebo flared at a median of 28 days, whereas only 24% of those still receiving etanercept flared at a median of 116 days. During the final, open-label phase, 74% of all patients benefited, 64% of patients improving by 50% and 36% improving by 70% (Figure 31.1). There are limitations to the interpretation of this study, but given that the patient population represents the more severe end of the disease spectrum, this is a remarkable response to treatment. At a median 2.3 years of subsequent treatment, 67% of all patients had a 70% improvement in disease activity. Other smaller studies have found similar improvements in polyarticular JIA,[37] and juvenile ankylosing spondylitis,[38] and there are reports of benefit from the simultaneous use of methotrexate.[39]

Infliximab is a chimeric human–murine monoclonal antibody that binds both soluble and cell-bound TNF-α. Infliximab is given by intravenous infusions, and combination treatment with methotrexate is recommended to avoid the development of tachyphylaxis to the

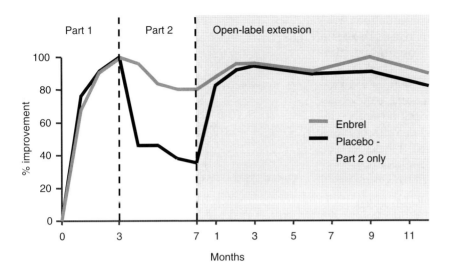

Figure 31.1 The three phases of the trial of etanercept in children with polyarticular JIA. In part 1, both groups received etanercept. In part 2, patients were blinded and randomized to receive etanercept or placebo. Part 3 was again open label, with all patients receiving the active agent.[34,35]

Table 31.2 **Comparison of etanercept and infliximab.**

	Etanercept	Infliximab
Licensed indications	Polyarticular JIA failing to respond to, or intolerant of, methotrexate	Not licensed
Half-life	70 h	200 h
Dose	0.4 mg/kg (maximum 25 mg) twice weekly	3 mg/kg at week zero, 2, 6, 14 and 8 weekly thereafter
Route of administration	Subcutaneous injection	Intravenous infusion
Side-effects	Risk of sepsis	Risk of sepsis, tachyphylaxis
Cost of vials	Four 25 mg vials – £325	100 mg vial – £451
Cost per year[a]	£4225	£4059

[a]Costs based on 30-kg child and using same vial of etanercept for both weekly doses.

murine component of the agent (Chapter 11). There is a licence for its use in adults with RA, and although there is no current license for its use in children, a multicentre phase III trial is in progress. There are anecdotal reports of its success in JIA.[40–42] High-dose anti-TNF therapy is now being piloted, showing early success in systemic JIA.[43] Table 31.2 shows a comparison of the two agents used in JIA.

POTENTIAL RISKS FROM TNF BLOCKADE

Etanercept appears to be well tolerated by children. Although headache, nausea, abdominal pain and vomiting were more common in children than were reported by adults treated with etanercept for RA, this did not result in discontinuation of treatment. Reports of skin rashes, some at the site of injection, and some vasculitic, have not led to discontinuation of the drug. There are no reports of increased risk from infection, but this remains a theoretical possibility.

There have been isolated case reports of aplastic anaemia, severe leukopenia and pancytopenia, and a possible association with demyelinating diseases of the central nervous system in adults receiving TNF blockade. The theoretical increased risk of malignancy, over that of the disease itself, has not been reflected clinically,[44] but 5 years of follow-up is still insufficient to determine the long-term risk. The risk of infection, including tuberculosis reactivation in the case of etanercept, does not appear to be greater than from the disease itself. However, there are increasing reports of reactivation of tuberculosis with the use of infliximab.[45] There are reports that adult patients receiving both types of TNF antagonist may develop antibodies to anti-nuclear antigen and dsDNA, and precipitate the clinical development of systemic lupus erythematosus (SLE) or a lupus-like syndrome.[46,47] There have been no reports of dsDNA or lupus so far in children.

OTHER IMMUNOMODULATION

IL-1 receptor antagonist (IL-1ra)

This is a non-signalling peptide of the IL-1 family, which exerts its actions by blocking the proinflammatory actions of both IL-1α and IL-1β (Chapter 12). Despite considerable natural regulation of IL-1 activity, studies have shown benefit from supra-physiological doses of recombinant IL-1ra. IL-1ra is now licensed for use in the USA and parts of Europe. Early trials in JIA have yet to complete. The rationale would be that IL-1 is more active in cartilage and bone erosions in animal models of arthritis, and should have a place in the more erosive forms of JIA.

Recombinant IL-10

This has been infused systemically to inhibit the synthesis of proinflammatory cytokines and

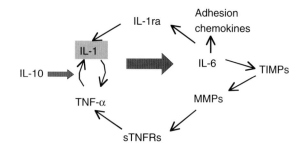

Figure 31.2 Positive and negative cytokine feedback. MMP, matrix metalloproteinase.

alter cellular differentiation and polarization. It too has a short half-life that results in poor clinical efficacy, and high systemic doses have not been well tolerated.[48] These results have led to exploration of the alternative approaches of local therapy and gene therapy.[49–51]

IL-6

This is a possible target for the treatment of systemic-onset JIA, as discussed above. Overproduction of the cytokine promotes proinflammatory cellular activity, although it also stimulates cytokine antagonists such as IL-1ra, sTNFR, and TIMP (Figure 31.2). A recombinant anti-human IL-6 receptor monoclonal antibody of the IgG$_1$ subclass, has undergone successful phase II studies in RA and is currently undergoing a phase III multicentre study in Europe. Pilot studies in Japan have shown dramatic changes in disease activity in systemic JIA and a phase II therapeutic trial is underway in the UK and Japan.

Modulation of T- and B-cell ontogeny

Direct cellular modulation using anti-CD4 antibodies is described in Chapter 1. However, inconsistent results and the observation of prolonged CD4+ T-cell depletion have been reported, thus raising anxieties about the longer-term consequences of such manipulations. Antibody targeted against CD20 markers expressed by B cells is undergoing phase II trials in RA. The rationale for its use in RA depends on the hypothesis of a clone of rheumatoid factor (RF)-producing B cells,[52] and this is unlikely to be applicable since most JIA subtypes are RF negative.

Future developments are likely to include targeting of other cytokines such as IFN-γ, combination therapy, and the use of cytokines to either divert the immune response towards tolerance, or to control apoptosis. Genetic research will also continue, not only in terms of gene therapy, but also in the identification of genetic populations most likely to respond to treatment.

TRIAL DESIGN AND ETHICAL CONSIDERATIONS

The use of anti-TNF therapy in children with chronic diseases highlights important technical and ethical considerations. The use of a novel drug in children with severe JIA must address questions of safety and efficacy in the context of a patient group previously receiving complex long-term medication. A placebo-controlled study is not ethical or appropriate in this context. Lovell et al needed to stop other disease-modifying drugs to demonstrate that beneficial effects were attributable to etanercept alone, and therefore treated all recruits with the trial medication before randomization (it being unethical to stop all disease-modifying medication in children with severe disease). Other concerns included the management of non-responders, the period of follow-up, and the interpretation of results thereafter, especially in a chronic disease characterized by relapses and remission. The open-label extension of the study addressed the problem of what to do at the end of a trial before the results were available and license obtained.

Owing to concerns about long-term safety of this new group of drugs, and to identify long-term benefit, clear guidelines and a central registry to monitor responses and side-effects is critical. This has now been established in the UK, and other European countries. The paediatric rule of the FDA in the USA has made early trials of new therapies possible in children, but other parts of the world still need to subscribe to such a policy. The pharmacokinetics and the dosages that would be efficacious are different in children, and need to be adequately assessed. It is important to acknowledge, first, that JIA comprises a group of diseases which differ from RA and should be examined separately, and second, that children require treatment during unique periods of physiological and psychological change.

PRACTICAL MANAGEMENT OF NEW THERAPIES

In addition to resources being available for supervision nationally, the success of these new drugs requires appropriate local provision. The paediatric rheumatology nurse specialist's role is to provide effective practical, educational and emotional support for the child and family. Guidance on administration, blood test monitoring, management of side-effects, which may include injection-site reactions, and appropriate response to infection are important aspects of continuing care. Effective education for both the patient and parents ensures understanding, appropriate expectations and adherence to the new drug following many years of 'ineffective' treatment and uncontrolled disease activity. Cooperation will depend on a balance between their belief that this time 'it may work', and excessive faith in a new wonder drug.

CONCLUSION

The impact of etanercept on many children and their families has been dramatic, despite uncertainty about the long-term side-effects and efficacy. Refinement of the use of TNF blockade, combination therapies, and alternative biologicals are being investigated, and in due course biologicals may be used to treat a wider cohort of children with less severe disease. To this end, vigilance and appropriate assessment of potential risks is paramount. Ultimately, these therapeutic developments may fundamentally alter our therapeutic approach to all chronic autoimmune diseases.

REFERENCES

1. Gare BA. Epidemiology. *Baillieres Clin Rheumatol* 1998; **12**: 191–208.
2. Wallace CA. The use of methotrexate in childhood rheumatic diseases. *Arthritis Rheum* 1998; **41**: 381–9.
3. Wallace CA. On beyond methotrexate: treatment of severe juvenile rheumatoid arthritis. *Clin Exp Rheum* 1999; **17**: 499–504.
4. Martin K, Woo P. Outcome in JCA. *Rev Rheum* 1997; **64**: 5242.
5. David J, Cooper C, Hickey L et al. The functional and psychological outcomes of juvenile chronic arthritis in young adulthood. *Br J Rheumatol* 1994; **33**(9): 876–81.
6. Petty RE, Southwood TR, Baum J et al. Revision of the proposed classification criteria for juvenile idiopathic arthritis: Durban, 1997. *J Rheumatol* 1998; **25**(10): 1991–4.
7. Wedderburn LR, Robinson N, Patel A et al. Selective recruitment of polarized T cells expressing CCR5 and CXCR3 to the inflamed joints of children with juvenile idiopathic arthritis. *Arthritis Rheum* 2000; **43**(4): 765–74.
8. Murray KJ, Grom AA, Thompson SD et al. Contrasting cytokine profiles in the synovium of different forms of juvenile rheumatoid arthritis and juvenile spondyloarthropathy: prominence of interleukin 4 in restricted disease. *J Rheumatol* 1998; **25**(7): 1388–98.
9. Raziuddin S, Bahabri S, Al-Dalaan A et al. A mixed Th1/Th2 cell cytokine response predominates in systemic onset juvenile rheumatoid arthritis: immunoregulatory IL-10 function. *Clin Immunol Immunopathol* 1998; **86**(2): 192–8.
10. De Benedetti F, Ravelli A, Martini A. Cytokines in juvenile rheumatoid arthritis. *Curr Opin Rheumatol* 1997; **9**(5): 428–33.
11. Rooney M, David J, Symons J et al. Inflammatory cytokine responses in juvenile chronic arthritis. *Br J Rheumatol* 1995; **34**: 454–60.
12. Grom AA, Murray KJ, Luyrink L et al. Patterns of expression of tumour necrosis factor alpha, tumor necrosis factor beta and their receptors in synovia of patients with juvenile rheumatoid arthritis and juvenile spondyloarthropathy. *Arthritis Rheum* 1996; **39**: 1703–10.
13. De Benedetti F, Massa M, Pignatti P et al. Serum soluble interleukin-6 (IL-6) receptor and IL-6/soluble IL-6 receptor complex in systemic juvenile rheumatoid arthritis. *JCI* 1994; **93**: 2114–19.
14. Keul R, Heinrich PC, Muller-Newen G et al. A possible role for soluble IL-6 receptor in the pathogenesis of systemic onset juvenile chronic arthritis. *Cytokine* 1998; **10**: 729–34.
15. Prieur AM, Roux-Lombard P, Dayer JM. Dynamics of fever and the cytokine network in systemic juvenile arthritis. *Rev Rhum Engl Ed* 1996; **63**(3): 163–70.
16. Rooney M, Varsani H, Martin K et al. Tumour necrosis factor alpha and its soluble receptors in juvenile chronic arthritis. *Rheumatology* 2000; **39**: 432–8.
17. Prahalad S, Ryan MH, Shear ES et al. Juvenile rheumatoid arthritis: linkage to HLA demonstrated by allele sharing in affected sibpairs. *Arthritis Rheum* 2000; **43**(10): 2335–8.
18. Crawley E, Kon S, Woo P. Hereditary predisposition to low interleukin-10 production in children with extended oligoarticular juvenile idiopathic arthritis. *Rheumatology* 2001; **40**(5): 574–8.
19. Crawley E, Kay R, Sillibourne J et al. Polymorphic haplotypes of the interleukin-10 5′ flanking region determine variable interleukin-10 transcription and are associated with particular phenotypes of juvenile rheumatoid arthritis. *Arthritis Rheum* 1999; **42**(6): 1101–8.
20. Lim S, Crawley E, Woo P, Barnes PJ. Haplotype associated with low interleukin-10 production in patients with severe asthma. *Lancet* 1998; **352**(9122): 113.
21. Ozen S, Alikasifoglu M, Bakkaloglu A et al. Tumour necrosis factor alpha G—>A –238 and G—>A –308 polymorphisms in juvenile idiopathic arthritis. *Rheumatology* 2002; **41**(2): 223–7.
22. Date Y, Seki N, Kamizono S et al. Identification of a genetic risk factor for systemic juvenile rheumatoid arthritis in the 5′-flanking region of the TNF alpha gene and HLA genes. *Arthritis Rheum* 1999; **42**: 2577–82.
23. Abraham LJ, Kroeger KM. Impact of the –308 TNF promoter polymorphism on the transcriptional regulation of the TNF gene: relevance to disease. *J Leukoc Biol* 1999; **66**(4): 562–6.
24. Zeggini E, Donn RP, Ollier WER et al. Linkage and association studies of single nucleotide polymorphism-tagged tumor necrosis factor haplotypes in juvenile oligoarthritis. *Arthritis Rheum* (in press).
25. Donn R, Alourfi Z, De Benedetti F et al. Mutation screening of the macrophage migration

inhibitory factor (MIF) gene: positive association of a functional polymorphism of MIF with juvenile idiopathic arthritis. *Arthritis Rheum* (in press).

26. Jeffery R, Luong L, Ogilvie E et al. The –174 polymorphism of the IL-6 alters transcription factor binding and forms functionally significant allelic associations in systemic arthritis. *Rheumatology* 2002; **41**: 10 (abstract OP28).

27. Fishman D, Faulds G, Jeffery R et al. The effect of novel polymorphisms in the interleukin-6 (IL-6) gene on IL-6 transcription and plasma IL-6 levels and an association with systemic onset juvenile chronic arthritis. *JCI* 1998; **102**: 1369–76.

28. Auphan N, DiDonato JA, Rosette C et al. Immunosuppression by glucocorticoids: inhibition of NF-kappa B activity through induction of I kappa B synthesis. *Science* 1995; **270**: 286–90.

29. Almawi WY, Beyhum HN, Rahme AA, Rieder MJ. Regulation of cytokine and cytokine receptor expression by glucocorticoids. *J Leukoc Biol* 1996; **60**: 563–72.

30. Matsuda S, Koyasu S. Mechanisms of action of cyclosporine. *Immunopharmacology* 2000; **47**(2–3): 119–25.

31. Sampaio EP, Sarno EN, Galilly R et al. Thalidomide selectively inhibits tumor necrosis factor α production by stimulating human monocytes. *J Exp Med* 1991; **173**: 699–703.

32. Xu X, Williams JW, Bremer EG et al. Inhibition of protein tyrosine phosphorylation in T cells by a novel immunosuppressive agent, leflunomide. *J Biol Chem* 1995; **270**: 12398–403.

33. Rothman D, Smith K, Kimura Y. Safety and efficacy of etanercept (enbrel) in children with JRA less than 4 years of age. *Arthritis Rheum* 2001; **44**: S293 (abstract 1435).

34. Lovell DJ, Giannini EH, Reiff A et al. Etanercept in children with polyarticular juvenile rheumatoid arthritis. *N Engl J Med* 2000; **342**: 763–9.

35. Lovell DJ, Giannini EH, Passo M et al. Long-term efficacy of etanercept (ENBREL) in children with polyarticular-course juvenile rheumatoid arthritis. PRES 2001; **60** (suppl. 2): II17–II52.

36. Giannini EH, Ruperto N, Ravelli A et al. Preliminary definition of improvement in juvenile arthritis. *Arthritis Rheum* 1997; **40**: 1202–9.

37. Kietz DA, Pepmueller PH, Moore TL. Clinical response to etanercept in polyarticular course juvenile rheumatoid arthritis. *J Rheumatol* 2001; **28**: 360–2.

38. Reiff A, Henrickson M. Prolonged efficacy of etanercept in refractory juvenile ankylosing spondylitis. *Arthritis Rheum* 2001; **44**: S292 (abstract 1434).

39. Brunner HI, Tomasi AL, Sherrard TM et al. Effectiveness and safety of etanercept for the treatment of juvenile rheumatoid arthritis (JRA) in clinical practice. *Arthritis Rheum* 2001; **44**: S292 (abstract 1436).

40. Vinje E, Obiora O, Forre O. Juvenile chronic polyarthritis treated with infliximab. *Ann Rheum Dis* 2000; **5**: 745 (abstract).

41. Billiau AD, Wouters C. Improved articular and systemic disease in a boy treated with anti-TNFa monoclonal antibody (Remicade) for refractory JIA. *Ann Rheum Dis* 2000; **59**: 744 (abstract).

42. Gerloni V, Pontikaki I, Desiati F et al. Infliximab in the treatment of persistently active refractory juvenile idiopathic arthritis. *Ann Rheum Dis* 2000; **59**: 740.

43. Kimura Y, Imundo LF, Li SC. High dose infliximab in the treatment of resistant systemic juvenile rheumatoid arthritis. *Arthritis Rheum* 2001; **44**: S272 (abstract 1316).

44. Klareskog L, Moreland LM, Cohen SB et al. Global safety and efficacy of up to five years of etanercept (Enbrel) therapy. *Arthritis Rheum* 2001; **44**: S77 (abstract 150).

45. De Rosa FG, Bonora S, Di Perri G. Tuberculosis and treatment with infliximab. *N Engl J Med* 2002; **346**(8): 623–6.

46. Shakoor N, Michalska M, Harris CA, Block JA. Drug-induced systemic lupus erythematosus associated with etanercept therapy. *Lancet* 2002; **359**: 579–80.

47. Jones RE, Moreland LW. Tumor necrosis factor inhibitors for rheumatoid arthritis. *Bull Dis Rheum* 1999; **48**: 1–3.

48. van Roon JA, Lafeber FP, Bijlsma JW. Synergistic activity of interleukin-4 and interleukin-10 in suppression of inflammation and joint destruction in rheumatoid arthritis. *Arthritis Rheum.* 2001; **44**: 3–12.

49. Fellowes R, Etheridge CJ, Coade S et al. Amelioration of established collagen induced arthritis by systemic IL-10 gene delivery. *Gene Ther* 2000; **7**: 967–77.

50. Lechman ER, Jaffurs D, Ghivizzani SC et al. Direct adenoviral gene transfer of viral IL-10 to rabbit knees with experimental arthritis ameliorates disease in both injected and contralateral control knees. *J Immunol* 1999; **163**: 2202–8.

51. Minter RM, Ferry MA, Murday ME et al. Adenoviral delivery of human and viral IL-10 in murine sepsis. *J Immunol* 2001; **167**: 1053–9.

52. Edwards JC, Cambridge G, Abrahams VM. Do self-perpetuating B lymphocytes drive human autoimmune disease? *Immunology* 1999; **97**: 188–96.

32

Psoriatic arthritis/psoriasis

Philip Mease

Introduction • Features of psoriasis and psoriatic arthritis • Pathogenesis • Conventional therapies • Studies of biological agents • Conclusions • References

INTRODUCTION

Psoriasis and psoriatic arthritis (PsA) are common disorders that can range in severity from mildly impairing to severely unsightly, painful, and disabling. Psoriasis affects approximately 2% of the population.[1] Of these patients, 7–31% develop PsA, an inflammatory arthropathy.[2,3] Patients with psoriasis experience physical discomfort, disfigurement, and, in many cases, a reduced quality of life.[4–9] Psoriatic arthritis, historically considered a benign variant of rheumatoid arthritis (RA), is now known to result in functional impairment in a large proportion of patients.[10,11] Whereas the clinical association between psoriasis and PsA is clear, the details of the immunologic association are not. However, studies of therapeutic agents that target molecules involved in the immunologic response have revealed important links in the pathophysiologic events of psoriasis and PsA. These agents may also significantly improve outcome by providing effective and relatively safe therapies for these difficult-to-treat disorders.

FEATURES OF PSORIASIS AND PSORIATIC ARTHRITIS

Plaque (vulgaris) psoriasis is the most common form of psoriasis.[12] The skin lesions of plaque psoriasis are typically thickened, erythematous, hyperkeratotic regions of epidermis, often covered by a silvery scale, characterized pathologically by elongated rete ridges resulting from the hyperproliferation and abnormal differentiation of basal keratinocytes.[13,14] These patches commonly appear over extensor surfaces, such as the elbow and/or knee, and may coalesce to cover large parts of the body. Other less common forms of psoriasis include guttate (eruptive), pustular, and erythrodermic.[12]

PsA occurs almost exclusively in patients who have psoriasis or who will develop it. The appearance of PsA is preceded by the skin manifestations of psoriasis in approximately 75% of patients. About 10–15% of patients experience simultaneous onset of psoriasis and PsA, and another 10–15% develop PsA symptoms prior to the appearance of skin lesions. Disease onset typically occurs between 30 and 55 years of age, although a juvenile form may be observed in children younger than 16 years of age.[15]

PsA is classified as a spondyloarthropathy, based on certain clinical and immunopathologic features shared with other subsets of the spondyloarthropathy family.[16] Scattered case reports suggested its association with psoriasis in the 19th and early 20th centuries.[17,18] A landmark paper by Moll and Wright in 1973 proposed an initial classification construct of five subtypes of disease.[19] These include: (1) symmetric polyarticular (similar to RA); (2) asymmetric oligoarticular; (3) spondylitic; (4) distal interphalangeal (DIP), often with associated nail dystrophy; and (5) mutilans. These varieties may overlap. Recurring enthesopathy, tenosynovitis, dactylitis, and iritis, as well as distinctive radiologic changes, help distinguish PsA from RA and ankylosing spondylitis.[20] Another feature that differentiates PsA from RA is the infrequent presence of rheumatoid factor (RF) or anti-nuclear antibodies in the serum of PsA patients.[20,21] Interestingly, 85% of PsA patients exhibit nail changes, compared with only 31% of patients with psoriasis alone.[20] PsA occurs at equal frequencies in males and females.[22]

Since PsA is a heterogeneous disorder with variable presentation and disease course, new classification criteria have been recommended in an attempt to improve diagnostic and prognostic sensitivity.[23] An international working group is beginning the process of developing updated criteria (P. Helliwell, personal communication).

PsA flares and remits, but the numbers of affected joints and the severity of joint damage tend to increase progressively over time. As a result, the disease is ultimately more serious and progressive than previously believed.[10,22] Deforming, erosive joint disease has been reported to occur in 40% of PsA patients, and polyarthritis in 61%.[22] Early disability and mortality have also been reported.[24,25]

PATHOGENESIS

Immunologic mechanisms

The role of T cells
T cells are believed to play a major role in the pathogenesis of psoriasis and PsA. Studies in which non-psoriatic skin was grafted onto immunodeficient mice have shown that purified CD4+ cells isolated from the peripheral blood of patients with psoriasis are sufficient to induce psoriatic lesions on the skin graft.[26]

Psoriatic skin lesions result from biological processes that induce abnormal cellular proliferation and inflammation.[27] Presumably, the processes are initially triggered by an endogenous or exogenous antigenic stimulus. It is thought that the presentation of this antigen, possibly by Langerhans cells, activates T-effector cells and initiates a cascade of events at the level of the T cell and the endothelial cell (Figure 32.1).[28] Activated T cells migrate from the circulation, crossing the capillary endothelium into the dermis and epidermis.[29] This transmigration appears to be facilitated by immune stimulation that triggers skin endothelial cells and keratinocytes to secrete chemotactic agents and to express leukocyte adhesion molecules on their surfaces.

The chemokines secreted by activated T cells attract leukocytes to inflammatory sites, perpetuating the inflammation (see below).[30] The proinflammatory lymphokine profiles in psoriatic skin (elevated tumor necrosis factor (TNF), interleukin (IL)-2, and interferon (IFN)-γ, and lack of IL-4)[28,31] suggest a Th1-driven process.[32–35]

The distribution of T-cell subsets changes over time in psoriatic skin lesions. CD4+ cells (helper T cells) are attracted into the dermis before the onset of keratinocyte hyperplasia and psoriatic plaque formation, and CD8+ cells (killer T cells) predominate in the epidermis of psoriatic lesions when the plaques are mature and resolving.[36,37] Whereas CD4+ T cells are involved in initiating psoriasis by inducing the release of cytokines from antigen-presenting cells and T lymphocytes, CD8+ cells may perpetuate this disease by initiating an autoimmune reaction.[38] The frequency of CD8+ T cells that are positive for the cutaneous lymphocyte antigen (CLA), a skin-homing marker, in the blood of psoriasis patients correlates closely with disease severity.[39]

T cells are also believed to be critical to the pathogenesis of PsA. As in psoriasis, the cytokine profile suggests a Th1 phenotype.[40,41] Activated, mature CD8+ T cells are the predominant cell type seen in PsA synovial fluid.[42] PsA and psoriasis thus appear to share both a predominance of CD8+ cells in evolved stages of the disease and a Th1 immune phenotype.

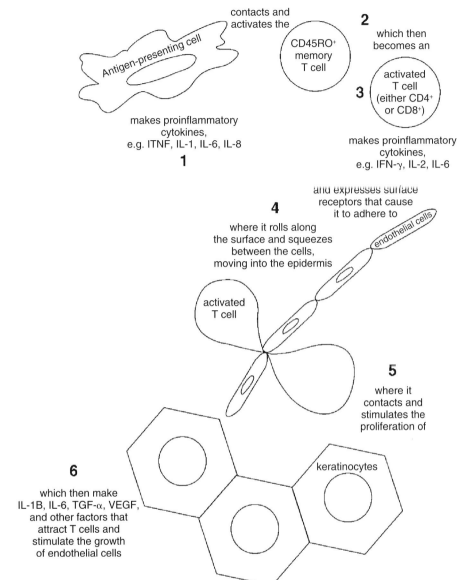

Figure 32.1
Schematic diagram of events in the formation of psoriatic plaque.

Cytokines and chemokines

A significant literature has developed cataloguing the many soluble mediators (cytokines and chemokines) that are present at abnormal levels in patients affected with psoriasis and PsA (Table 32.1). Unfortunately, reported results of assays for these molecules are not always in agreement. One apparent reason for conflicting results is that immunologic/serologic assays

may reveal the presence of a particular cytokine because specific antigenic determinants are present, but bioassays may indicate the absence of cytokine activity if the active sites are bound to receptor molecules.[43]

As might be expected, the levels of inflammatory cytokines, particularly TNF, IL-1β, and IL-8, are generally increased in psoriatic skin lesions and the joints of patients with PsA (Table 32.1).

Table 32.1   Key soluble mediators implicated in the etiology of psoriasis and PsA[a].

Cytokine/ chemokine	Observations in psoriasis	Observations in PsA	References
ESAF	Elevated in psoriatic lesions and serum, correlates with disease severity	NR	129
ET-1	Elevated in serum and psoriatic lesions, correlates with disease severity	NR	29,130
Fractalkine	Elevated in dermal blood vessels from psoriasis tissues	NR	56
IFN-γ	Elevated in psoriatic lesions and serum, produced by epidermal T cells	Elevated in skin, synovial fluid, peripheral blood mononuclear cells, and synovial T cells	45,131–134
IL-1α	Conflicting reports, probably decreased in psoriatic lesions. Negative correlation with disease activity	Elevated in basal epidermis and dermis of psoriatic lesions	54,135–137
IL-1β	Elevated in epidermal keratinocytes, seemingly inactive in some reports	Elevated in synovial fluid, basal epidermis, and dermis of psoriatic lesions, and peripheral blood mononuclear cells. Correlates with number of affected joints	54,135,136, 138–142
IL-1ra	Present in psoriatic epidermis, bound to IL-1	Elevated in serum. Correlates with joint but not skin disease	55,143,144
IL-2	Elevated in serum, correlates with disease activity	May be present in synovium (variable findings)	32,41,131, 145
IL-6	Elevated in peripheral blood mononuclear cells, serum, and keratinocytes and blister fluid of psoriatic lesions	Elevated in epidermis, synovial fluid, serum, and peripheral blood mononuclear cells	55,138,139, 141,142, 146
IL-7	Elevated in serum and psoriatic lesions, not correlated with disease activity	NR	147,148
IL-8 (CXCL8)	Elevated in neutrophils and other cell types in psoriatic lesions	Elevated in synovial fluid and peripheral blood mononuclear cells	32,35,130, 139,141, 142,149–152
IL-10	Lower in psoriatic lesions, correlated with disease activity	Elevated in serum and synovial lining	28,52–55,153
IL-12	Elevated in mononuclear cells of dermis in psoriatic lesions	Elevated in synovial fluid	154,155
IL-15	Elevated in epidermis of psoriatic lesions	Elevated in synovial lining	54,156
LT-1 (TNF-β)	NR	Elevated in skin, synovial fluid, and peripheral blood mononuclear cells	133
MCP-1	Elevated in epidermis and in infiltrating cells in the dermis	Elevated in synovial fluid and plasma	30,157

Table 32.1	continued		
Cytokine/ chemokine	**Observations in psoriasis**	**Observations in PsA**	**References**
Prostaglandin E$_2$	Increased in psoriatic blister fluid, correlates with disease severity	NR	158
RANTES	Elevated in psoriatic keratinocytes	Elevated in synovial tissues	159–161
sIL-2R	Elevated in serum, released from T cells	Elevated in synovial fluid and serum	36,43,55,162, 163
sTNFR	No increase in serum levels of p55 subunit	Both p55 and p75 elevated in synovial fluid	163,164
TNF (TNF-α)	Generally elevated in psoriatic lesions, blister fluid, and serum of patients with psoriasis, but possibly inhibited	Elevated in synovial fluid, lining and endothelial cells and in basal epidermis and dermis	28,44,45,54, 138,141,146, 165
VEGF	Produced by keratinocytes, elevated in psoriatic lesions and serum, correlates with disease activity	Elevated in synovial fluid, synovial lining, and endothelium	73,129,166

[a]This table is based mainly on reports of elevated cytokine concentrations in tissues from patients with psoriasis or PsA. Studies of cytokine production triggered in vitro are not included.

ESAF, endothelial cell stimulating angiogenesis factor; ET, endothelin; IFN, interferon; IL, interleukin; IL-1ra, interleukin-1 receptor antagonist; MCAF, monocyte chemotactic and activating factor; MCP, monocyte chemotactic protein; NR, not reported; RANTES, receptor-activated neutrophil T-cell expression and secretion; sIL-2R, soluble IL-2 receptor; sTNFR, soluble TNF receptor; TNF, tumor necrosis factor; VEGF, vascular endothelial growth factor.

Particular attention has been focused on the possible role of TNF in these diseases, as therapeutic interventions to block the activity of this cytokine are now available. This proinflammatory cytokine, which is produced by keratinocytes, mast cells, monocytes, and dendritic cells,[35] interacts with the nuclear transcription factor NFκB, thereby triggering the expression of many other molecules that promote the inflammatory response, including IL-8 and E-selectin. TNF also induces the expression of endothelial, keratinocyte and dendritic cell surface receptors involved in the trafficking of leukocytes to inflammatory lesions, such as intercellular adhesion molecule (ICAM)-1.[27,33,35,44–46] TNF mediates a number of biological processes that can result in joint damage. These include stimulation of bone resorption, inhibition of bone formation, inhibition of synthesis of proteoglycan, and induction of collagen- and cartilage-degrading metalloproteinases and prostaglandin E$_2$.[47–50]

In addition to promoting inflammation, cytokines and chemokines may play numerous other roles in psoriasis and PsA. Angiogenic cytokines such as TNF and vascular endothelial growth factor (VEGF) probably contribute to vascular proliferation. Other cytokines, such as IL-1, IL-6, and IL-8, may act as growth factors, triggering hyperproliferation of keratinocytes in psoriatic plaque.[51] Some cytokines, such as IL-10, exert anti-inflammatory activity. This cytokine is deficient in psoriatic skin lesions,[28,52,53] but, except for one conflicting report,[54] is present at

Table 32.2   Receptor–ligand pairs mediating cell–cell interactions implicated in the pathogenesis of psoriasis and PsA[a].

Cell surface molecules involved	Comments	References
E-selectin and CLA	Believed to be a major lymphocyte homing pathway in psoriasis	46,167,168
ICAM-1 (CD-54) and LFA-1 (CD11/ CD18)	Believed to be main adhesion pathway for lymphocyte homing in PsA patients	31–33,46,169–172
VCAM-1 and VLA-4	Implicated in psoriasis	31,33,46,165,173,174
LFA-3 and CD2	This interaction results in T-cell proliferation	175
B7 family and CD28, CTLA-4	Required for T-cell activation	127,176

[a]Other cell surface molecules may also be involved.

CLA, cutaneous lymphocyte antigen; ICAM, intercellular adhesion molecule; LFA, lymphocyte function-associated antigen; VCAM, vascular cell adhesion molecule; CTLA, cytotoxic T-lymphocyte antigen.

high levels in synovium and serum from patients with PsA.[40,55]

Cell–cell interactions

Altered patterns of cellular receptors and adhesion molecules are observed in patients with psoriasis and PsA. Cell surface molecules play important roles in recruiting and activating cells. These molecules may also function as chemotactic agents in their soluble forms, blurring the line between cytokines and adhesion molecules.[56] A variety of costimulatory ligand–receptor pairs may contribute to the pathogenesis of psoriasis and PsA (Table 32.2).[57]

Genetic contributions

Psoriasis and PsA have a strong familial component. Family history is positive in nearly half of patients,[13] although the concordance of PsA in identical twins is only 30–40%.[20] Psoriasis has a strong association with HLA-Cw6; the presence of this haplotype increases the risk of psoriasis at least six-fold. Other HLA antigens associated with psoriasis include HLA-B13, B17, B37, DR7, and (for Japanese patients) Cw7 and Cw11 (Table 32.3).[13] Reported HLA associations for

Table 32.3   HLA haplotypes associated with psoriasis and PsA.[13,20,32,58]

HLA allele	Associated with psoriasis	Associated with PsA
A2	✓	
B13	✓	✓
B16		✓
B27	✓	✓✓
B37	✓	
B38		✓
B39		✓
B57 (formerly B17)	✓	✓
Cw6	✓✓	✓✓
Cw7	✓ (Japanese)	
Cw11	✓ (Japanese)	
DR4		✓
DR7	✓	✓

PsA are similar (Table 32.3), although the associations are not as strong.[20,32,58] The strongest association for PsA is with the class I MHC on the short arm of chromosome 6.[59] The HLA antigens B27, B39 and DQw3 in patients with PsA are associated with more severe disease and may also be correlated with certain patterns of joint distribution in a given patient, e.g. B27 with more axial involvement.[58]

Environmental components

Infectious agents may play a role in the pathogenesis of psoriasis and PsA.[60] The presence of streptococcal RNA and antibodies to streptococcal cell wall antigens in the joints of patients with PsA suggests that certain strains of streptococci might be involved, but evidence that these bacteria play a causal role is not yet clear.[61,62] Certain viruses, including human papillomavirus 5, have been considered as triggers for psoriasis, but the evidence to date is not compelling.[61,63] The occurrence of trauma precedes disease development in some patients, but whether the traumatic event by itself acts as a trigger or whether it alters immune functioning in a way that predisposes patients to psoriasis or PsA is not known.[59]

CONVENTIONAL THERAPIES

Therapies are aimed at controlling disease symptoms and choice varies according to disease severity. Traditional therapies for psoriasis and PsA have often yielded less than satisfactory results, because of incomplete efficacy, toxicity, or both.[64] Many of the traditional therapies may exert therapeutic benefit through fortuitous effects on cytokines (Table 32.4).

Psoriasis

Mild cases of psoriasis are usually treated with topical therapies, commonly topical corticosteroids, and other therapies, such as the vitamin D analog calcipotriene or the retinoid tazarotene.[65] Phototherapy with broadband ultraviolet B is an option. Therapy with oral psoralen plus ultraviolet A (PUVA) is highly effective, but its association with cutaneous malignancies limits its use.[65] For more severe cases, systemic thera-

pies, including methotrexate (MTX) and the T-cell-suppressive agents cyclosporin A and tacrolimus, may be prescribed. In a 26-year retrospective study of long-term, low-dose MTX therapy in 157 patients with severe psoriasis, 76% of patients had a good response to MTX. However, 61% experienced side-effects, including liver function abnormalities, bone marrow suppression, and gastric complaints, and 20% discontinued treatment.[66] Cyclosporin significantly improved symptoms of psoriasis compared with placebo in a double-blind trial, with 80% of patients exhibiting clearing or near-clearing of psoriasis in the highest-dosage group (7.5 mg/kg).[67] A recent meta-analysis of cyclosporin in three major randomized studies of patients with severe psoriasis concluded that this agent is highly effective and well tolerated in the short term.[68] Tacrolimus (FK506) reduced the symptoms of severe psoriasis in a series of seven patients, but controlled trials have not been reported.[69]

Psoriatic arthritis

As with psoriasis, the therapy for PsA depends on disease severity. Mild joint symptoms may respond to physiotherapy and non-steroidal anti-inflammatory drugs (NSAIDs).[70] For more severe disease, corticosteroids or disease-modifying anti-rheumatic drugs (DMARDs) are usually required. Corticosteroids, however, are problematic in PsA, because their withdrawal can trigger impressive – even dangerous – flares of psoriasis.[32,71]

Many of the therapies used to treat PsA have been adapted based on their proven efficacy in RA, including MTX, cyclosporin A, gold, sulfasalazine, azathioprine, and antimalarials. Few of the traditional PsA therapies have actually been proven effective by rigid clinical trial criteria.[72] Trials in PsA have been small for the most part, improvements have been highly variable, and the placebo group has also improved in all trials, so that differences from placebo have been generally moderate.[72–74] A meta-analysis conducted by the Cochrane Library of all published (English-language)

Table 32.4 Effect of psoriasis and PsA therapies on key cytokines and cell surface molecules[a].

Therapy (indication)[27,152]	TNF	IL-1ra	IL-2	IL-4	ICAM-1	IL-6	IL-8 (CXCL8)	IL-10	IL-12	IFN-γ	IL-1β
Vitamin D analogs (calcitriol or calcipotriene for psoriasis)[177,178]							↓	↑		↓	
Methotrexate (for psoriasis and PsA)[73,138,179-181]		↓				↓	↓			↓	
Cyclosporin (for psoriasis and PsA)[36,51,162,178,182,183]	↓		↓	↓	↓		↓		↓	↓ (slow)	↓
Ultraviolet A with psoralen (PUVA, for psoriasis)[36]			↓								
Retinoids (e.g. etretinate for psoriasis)[178,182]	↓ (slow)			↓		↓				↓	
Tazarotene gel (for psoriasis)[184]				↓		↓					

[a]This table provides data from key papers concerning the effects of therapies on selected cytokines, but may not be fully representative of the spectrum of cytokine interactions of these drugs. In addition, some articles on this topic may have been inadvertently omitted. TNF, tumor necrosis factor; IL, interleukin; IL-1ra, IL-1 receptor antagonist; ICAM, intercellular adhesion molecule; IFN, interferon.

randomized, placebo-controlled clinical trials concluded that only high-dose MTX (at doses too toxic for current practice) and sulfasalazine produced statistically significant improvements in patients with PsA.[72]

Despite its widespread use in PsA,[75] data on MTX are fairly sparse. In a 1984 double-blind, placebo-controlled trial of low-dose pulse MTX (7.5–15.0 mg/week) in 37 patients, physician assessment of arthritis activity and skin surface area with psoriasis responded marginally more favorably to MTX therapy than to placebo in patients with PsA. However, no significant differences were found between MTX and placebo in other clinical outcomes, such as joint pain/tenderness and swelling, morning stiffness, or skin erythema, induration, or scaling.[76] A study in which low-dose MTX (up to a maximum of 15 mg/week) was compared to cyclosporin A found that both were effective in treating PsA, but that MTX was better tolerated (27.8% versus 41.2% withdrawal rate).[77]

Somewhat more data are available on sulfasalazine. In a 30-patient, double-blind, placebo-controlled trial of sulfasalazine (initial dose of 0.5 g/day, escalated by 0.5 g/day at weekly intervals to a maximum dose of 2 g/day or the highest dose that the patient could tolerate) in PsA over a period of 24 weeks, joint symptoms responded somewhat better to sulfasalazine treatment than to placebo, with a 'good' clinical response (criteria unclear) in 5 of 14 (36%) patients compared with 0 in the placebo group, but the dropout rate in the study was 40%, and skin lesions did not appear to be affected by sulfasalazine.[78] In another double-blind, placebo-controlled study of 120 patients, pain was the only primary outcome variable that showed a statistically significant difference in favor of sulfasalazine at the end of 24 weeks.[79] A 1996 Veterans Affairs Cooperative Study of 221 patients, in which sulfasalazine was compared to placebo in the treatment of PsA, concluded that sulfasalazine 2.0 g/day is well tolerated and may be more effective than placebo in the treatment of patients with this disease.[80] The overall difference in treatment response, as defined by a predetermined set of criteria, was statistically significant (sulfasalazine 57.8% versus placebo 44.6%; $P = 0.05$). However, none of the individual criteria achieved significance.[80] A subsequent study of patients with seronegative spondyloarthropathies, including 221 patients with PsA, found that sulfasalazine was effective in treating peripheral articular symptoms, but not axial manifestations.[81]

In a recent study, cyclosporin was found to be significantly more efficacious than sulfasalazine in 99 patients with PsA.[82] This study, along with the 1995 comparative study of cyclosporin and MTX, provides the strongest data in favor of the use of cyclosporin in the treatment of PsA, in the absence of a published placebo-controlled trial.

A double-blind comparison of auranofin, intramuscular gold thiomalate and placebo in 82 patients with PsA demonstrated marginally significant clinical improvements in patients receiving intramuscular gold, but no significant changes were observed in those receiving auranofin. Intramuscular gold was shown to be safe and more effective than auranofin in patients who were followed for 6 months.[83]

Although the issue of radiographic progression of joint damage has not been studied as thoroughly in PsA as it has in RA, at least one study suggests that available therapies may not have a significant impact on this parameter. This study followed 38 PsA patients who were treated with MTX for 24 months. Despite symptomatic improvement, radiographic damage scores increased in 63% of patients. No difference in the rate of radiographic progression was found between these treated patients and untreated matched controls.[84]

STUDIES OF BIOLOGICAL AGENTS

A variety of new biological agents are being investigated for psoriasis and PsA. These agents differ in their mechanisms of action but share the ability to interrupt the cascade of inflammation and immunologic cell activation, especially T-cell activation, that is involved in these diseases. The ability of at least some of these agents to mediate improvements in both skin lesions and joint symptoms provides strong evidence that

Table 32.5 Biological agents in clinical trials for the treatment of psoriasis or PsA[a].

Mechanism of action	Agent	Description	Comments
TNF inhibitors	Etanercept	Soluble TNF receptor fusion protein	FDA approved for PsA
	Infliximab	Chimeric anti-TNF monoclonal antibody	
	Onercept	Recombinant human tumor necrosis factor binding protein-1 (r-hTBP-1)	
	ISIS 104838	Antisense TNF inhibitor	Being tested as a topical preparation for psoriasis
IL-8 inhibitors	ABX IL-8	Human anti-IL-8 monoclonal antibody	
IL-2/IL-2 receptor inhibitors	Daclizumab	Humanized anti-CD25 monoclonal antibody	
	Basiliximab	Chimeric anti-CD25 monoclonal antibody	
	Denileukin deftitox	IL-2/diptheria toxin fusion protein	
Anti-inflammatory cytokines	Recombinant IL-10	Recombinant IL-10	May be more effective in treating skin lesions than joints
	Recombinant IL-11	Recombinant IL-11	
Blockade of T-cell interactions	Alefacept	Recombinant LFA-3 fusion protein	
	Siplizumab	Humanized anti-CD2 monoclonal antibody	
	Efalizumab	Humanized anti-CD11a monoclonal antibody	
	IDEC-114	Humanized anti-B7 monoclonal antibody	
	huOKT3(1(ala-ala)	Humanized anti-CD3 monoclonal antibody	
	IDEC-131	Humanized anti-CD154 (CD40 ligand)	
	ISIS 2302	Antisense ICAM-1 inhibitor	Being tested as a topical preparation for psoriasis

[a]This table covers some of the more notable compounds that have reached at least phase II clinical trials for psoriasis or PsA. Owing to the rapidly evolving nature of this field, some agents may have been inadvertently omitted.

FDA, US Food and Drug Administration; ICAM, intercellular adhesion molecule; IL, interleukin; LFA, leukocyte function-associated antigen; PsA, psoriatic arthritis; TNF, tumor necrosis factor

common pathways are involved in the pathogenesis of these two conditions. Table 32.5 lists biological agents that have reached at least phase II clinical trials for psoriasis or PsA. Because of the rapidly evolving nature of this field, the list may not be complete. Some of the major agents that have been studied are discussed in the following sections.

TNF inhibitors

The best studied of the new biological agents are the TNF inhibitors, etanercept and infliximab. These agents have been used with great success to suppress joint inflammation in RA.[85,86] Etanercept has also recently received US Food and Drug Administration (FDA) approval for use in the treatment of PsA on the basis of data from two placebo-controlled, randomized trials.

Etanercept

Etanercept is a fully human, soluble TNF receptor fusion protein. It mediates its anti-inflammatory effects by binding to TNF and preventing it from interacting with cell surface receptors. The ability of etanercept to improve symptoms and inhibit the progression of joint damage in patients with RA[87] raised the possibility that this agent might show similar activity in patients with PsA, thus leading to a placebo-controlled, randomized clinical study in which 60 patients with PsA received either etanercept (25 mg subcutaneously (SC) twice weekly) or placebo.[88] Patients in this study had long-standing disease (psoriasis for a mean of approximately 20 years and PsA for a mean of 11.5 years). Patients achieving partial benefit from MTX were allowed to continue its use in the trial; this subgroup of 47% of patients was evenly randomized to the placebo or etanercept groups. Background use of NSAIDs or prednisone ≤10 mg/day was allowed. All other DMARDs and topical medicines for psoriasis were discontinued.

The primary arthritis efficacy response measure was the Psoriatic Arthritis Response Criteria (PsARC). Four clinical improvement criteria make up this scale: an improvement of at least 1 unit (0–5 Likert scale) on the physician global assessment, an improvement of at least 1 unit (0–5 Likert scale) on the patient global assessment, and at least 30% improvement in tender and swollen joint counts. To achieve a clinical response, the patient had to improve in two of the four PsARC criteria, one of which must be tender or swollen joint score, and could not worsen in any of them. Secondary outcome measures included the proportion of patients achieving clinical response by the American College of Rheumatology preliminary criteria for improvement (ACR 20, 50 and 70 responses).[89]

At the study endpoint (12 weeks), 87% of etanercept-treated patients were responders by PsARC criteria, compared with 23% of placebo-

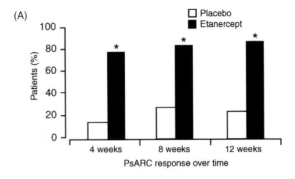

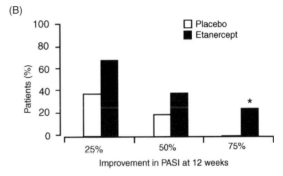

Figure 32.2 Percentage of patients with PsARC responses over time (A) and at least 25%, 50%, and 75% improvements in PASI scores at 12 weeks (B). (Reproduced with permission from Mease et al. *Lancet* 2000; **356**: 385–90.[88])

treated patients (Figure 32.2A). The effect was rapid; by 4 weeks, 77% of patients receiving etanercept qualified as responders. At 12 weeks, four patients (13%) had no tender joints and 7 patients (23%) had no swollen joints. Similar dramatic responses were noted when ACR 20, 50 and 70 criteria were applied, with 73%, 50% and 13%, respectively, showing these responses in the etanercept group, and 13%, 3% and 0% in the placebo group. Response rates between patients receiving concomitant MTX and those on etanercept monotherapy were not statistically significant.[88]

Of the 60 patients with active PsA, 38 had ≥3% body surface area involved with psoriasis, the minimum requirement for the evaluation of skin response. Evaluating dermatologists employed two skin response scoring systems, the Psoriasis Area and Severity Index (PASI) and the target lesion score. The PASI is a composite measure which assesses severity of scale, erythema and induration, weighted by lesional surface area and body region.[90] The target lesion score is derived from the amount of scale, erythema and induration of a single, preselected lesion.

The median improvement in PASI score in etanercept-treated patients (n = 19) at 3 months was 46%, compared with 9% in the placebo group (n = 19; Figure 32.2B). The corresponding median improvements in target lesion score were 50% and 0%, respectively. Twenty-six per cent of patients treated with etanercept had a 75% PASI response, representing nearly complete resolution of skin disease.

In this 3-month trial, etanercept was well tolerated. No patient in the etanercept group discontinued treatment. Twenty per cent of the etanercept-treated patients experienced mild injection-site reactions that resolved with uninterrupted, continued use. No other adverse events occurred significantly more often in the etanercept group than in the placebo group. Thus, this study demonstrated that etanercept treatment resulted in significant improvement in PsA and psoriasis and was relatively safe during this period of observation.

Patients who completed this trial (n = 58) were given etanercept during a 6-month, open-label extension.[91] The patients originally assigned to placebo had prompt and dramatic PsARC and ACR 20, 50 and 70 responses. Interestingly, the original etanercept patients demonstrated further improvement in ACR responses. Whereas 73% of patients achieved an ACR 20 response at 3 months,[88] 87% did so after an additional 6 months, and ACR 70 responses increased from 13% at 3 months to 33% after 9 months of therapy.[91] The median improvement in PASI score in patients receiving etanercept during the placebo-controlled phase of the study improved from 46% at 3 months[91] to 62% at 9

months.[92] Patients who had originally received placebo during the double-blind phase and were then switched to etanercept also achieved a 62% median improvement during the 6 months of etanercept treatment.[92] Of the 28 patients who were taking concomitant MTX at baseline, 12 (43%) decreased their MTX dose, and 7 (25%) discontinued MTX therapy. Similarly, of 18 patients taking prednisone at baseline, 12 (67%) decreased their corticosteroid dose, and 8 (44%) discontinued corticosteroid treatment. At 9 months, 28% of patients had no tender joints, 42% had no swollen joints, and 40% had a disability score of 0. Etanercept continued to be well tolerated.[91]

A phase III clinical trial of etanercept in patients with PsA confirmed and extended these observations.[93] In this double-blind, placebo-controlled study, 205 patients with PsA and psoriasis were randomized to receive 25 mg etanercept (n = 101) or placebo (n = 104) twice weekly for 24 weeks. The primary endpoint was joint response, as determined by ACR 20 criteria, at 12 weeks. At 12 weeks, 59% of patients in the etanercept group and 15% of those in the placebo group (P < 0.001) achieved an ACR 20 response. A similar difference was observed when PsARC criteria were used to assess clinical response at 12 weeks; 72% of etanercept-treated patients achieved a clinical response compared with 31% of placebo patients (P < 0.001). Significantly greater responses in the etanercept group compared with the placebo group were also observed at 24 weeks, with 50% of patients in the etanercept group achieving an ACR 20 response versus 13% in the placebo group, indicating that responses were generally maintained over the 6-month period.[93] Skin improvements were also documented. Patients with etanercept showed a 33% median improvement in target lesion score at 24 weeks versus 0% in the placebo group (P < 0.001). Of the 205 patients in this study, 66 in the etanercept group and 62 in the placebo group met criteria for evaluation by the PASI (>3% body surface area involvement). A median PASI improvement of 47% was observed in the etanercept group at 24 weeks, compared to no improvement in the placebo group (P < 0.001). Etanercept was relatively safe and well tolerated during this study, with a safety profile similar to that seen in RA.[85]

Etanercept also improves psoriatic skin lesions in patients without PsA. In a recently reported study, 112 patients with refractory chronic psoriasis and plaque psoriasis covering at least 10% of their body surface area were randomized to receive either etanercept (25 mg SC; n = 57) or placebo (n = 55) twice weekly for 24 weeks. Compared to placebo, significantly more etanercept-treated patients achieved a 75% improvement in PASI score at 12 weeks (2% for placebo versus 30% for etanercept; P < 0.0001) and at 24 weeks (5% for placebo versus 56% for etanercept; P < 0.0001). Significant differences in favor of etanercept were also observed in target lesion clearing, physician and patient global assessments, and the Dermatology Life Quality Index. As in the PsA trials, etanercept had an unremarkable adverse-event profile and was generally well tolerated.[94]

These large-scale studies are supported by many case series documenting the efficacy of etanercept in patients with PsA,[95–97] including a study of 12 patients with refractory PsA in which 10 of the patients responded to etanercept with complete resolution of skin lesions and normalization of inflammatory markers.[98]

Infliximab

Infliximab, a chimeric human–mouse anti-TNF monoclonal antibody, has been studied more extensively in psoriasis than in PsA. In a placebo-controlled study of 33 patients with moderate-to-severe psoriasis, patients were randomized to receive placebo, 5 mg/kg infliximab, or 10 mg/kg infliximab, at weeks 0, 2, and 6.[27] Clinical response was defined as a good, excellent or clear rating on the Physician's Global Assessment (PGA). Of the patients in the 5 mg/kg infliximab group, 82% showed a clinical response at 10 weeks, compared with 91% in the 10 mg/kg group and 18% in the placebo group (P < 0.01 for either dose versus placebo). A secondary endpoint was an improvement of at least 75% in the PASI score. At 10 weeks, this criterion was achieved by 9 of 11 (82%)

patients in the infliximab 5 mg/kg group, 8 of 11 (73%) patients in the infliximab 10 mg/kg group, and 2 of 11 (18%) patients in the placebo group (P < 0.05 for infliximab versus placebo). PASI scores showed a mean improvement of approximately 80% in the infliximab groups during the 10-week trial, compared with approximately 15% in the placebo group.[27] The median time to response was 4 weeks for patients in both infliximab groups. No serious adverse events occurred during this trial, and infliximab was well tolerated.[27]

An open-label study in six patients with progressive PsA and psoriasis refractory to MTX examined the effect of infliximab (5 mg/kg at weeks 0, 2, and 6) on joint symptoms as well as skin lesions. Improvement of psoriatic skin lesions was noted in all patients at 10 weeks. A marked improvement in joint symptoms was also experienced, with all six patients achieving an ACR 50 response, and five of the six achieving an ACR 70 response.[99,100] In a continuation of this study, infliximab treatment was adapted to the individual needs of the patients (typically infliximab 3–5 mg/kg at intervals of 8 weeks or greater), and four patients were added to the series. All of the patients except two were given concomitant DMARD therapy with MTX (n = 7) or sulfasalazine (n = 1). One patient stopped infliximab therapy for personal reasons at 10 weeks. Subsequently, four more patients discontinued therapy due to remission (n = 3) or a new pregnancy and infusion reaction (n = 1). These withdrawals complicated efficacy evaluation. However, at 1 year, six of the nine patients had no tender or swollen joints. Three of the four patients, who had achieved an ACR 70 response at week 10 and continued on therapy for a year, had an ACR 50 response at the end of the follow-up period.[101] Another year-long study included 21 patients with different subtypes of spondyloarthropathy, 9 of whom had PsA. Patients were given infliximab 5 mg/kg at weeks 0, 2, and 6. At 12 weeks, the PsA patients showed improvements in joint and skin symptoms.[102] The patients in this study were then allowed to go on a maintenance regimen of 5 mg/kg infliximab every 14 weeks. Although improvements were maintained over the 1-year follow-up period, the incidence of recurrence of symptoms prior to the next infusion increased over time, from 16% of patients at week 20 to 79% of patients at week 48, suggesting the need for a shorter interval between infusions. No separate data were given for PsA patients.[103]

Case studies also support the efficacy of infliximab in psoriasis[104–106] and PsA.[99,105,107,108] A larger controlled trial of infliximab in PsA is underway (C. Antoni, personal communication).

Other TNF inhibitors under development, such as adalimumab,[109] CDP870,[110] and onercept,[111] will also probably be employed in the treatment of psoriasis and PsA. Isis 104838, a topical TNF inhibitor, is in phase II clinical trials for psoriasis. This molecule is an antisense inhibitor that prevents the production of TNF.

Inhibitors of other proinflammatory cytokines

An antibody to IL-8, ABX-IL8, has been assessed in a double-blind, placebo-controlled phase IIa trial of 94 patients with psoriasis. Intravenous infusion of ABX-IL8 every 3 weeks for a total of five infusions resulted in statistically significant improvements in PASI scores for the 3 mg/kg dose, but not the 6 mg/kg dose.[112]

It is anticipated that, as inhibitors of specific proinflammatory cytokines implicated in the pathogenesis of inflammatory diseases are developed, future testing of the efficacy and safety of these compounds will occur not only in RA, but also PsA and the other spondyloarthropathies. Examples of such agents include other anti-TNF agents under development, the recently approved (for RA) anakinra, an IL-1 receptor antagonist, other IL-1 modulators, small molecules such as the p38 mitogen-activated protein (MAP) kinase and tumor necrosis factor converting enzyme (TACE) inhibitors, and ligand receptor antagonists.

Anti-inflammatory cytokines

Systemic therapy with cytokines that appear to downregulate the production of inflammatory cytokines is being investigated in psoriasis and

PsA. In an open-label, 7-week, phase II trial of recombinant IL-10 in 14 patients with chronic plaque-type psoriasis,[113,114] 10 patients (71%) had a reduction in PASI scores of >50%.[113] The number of activated T cells in the epidermis was reduced, and the cytokine pattern in responding patients shifted from a type 1 pattern to a type 2 pattern. No significant changes were observed in the production of TNF, IL-6, or IFN-γ.[114] Human recombinant IL-10 has also been tested in patients with PsA. In a double-blind, placebo-controlled study, IL-10 given subcutaneously for 28 days resulted in improvements in skin lesions, but not in articular disease activity scores. As in the psoriasis studies, type 1 cytokine production was suppressed, and decreased T-cell and macrophage infiltration into synovial tissues was observed.[115] IL-10 thus exerts immunomodulatory effects, but these effects may be more beneficial for the skin than for the joints.

Another anti-inflammatory cytokine, IL-11, has been tested in 12 patients with psoriasis. In an open-label trial of recombinant human IL-11 (2.5 or 5.0 mg/kg SC daily for 8 weeks), 11 patients (92%) showed improvements in PASI ranging from 20% to 80%. Examination of a prospectively defined target lesion indicated that seven patients (58%) had marked disease reduction as defined by decreased epidermal hyperplasia, reduced number of T cells in skin lesions, and decreased ICAM-1 production. Levels of inflammatory mediators were also reduced in responding patients.[116] No studies of recombinant human IL-11 have yet been reported in patients with PsA.

IL-2/IL-2 receptor blockade

Interactions between IL-2 and the IL-2 receptor play a critical role in the activation of T cells. One of the subunits of this receptor is CD25 (Tac antigen). A humanized monoclonal antibody to CD25, daclizumab, has been developed and tested in a dose-ranging trial in 19 patients with moderate-to-severe plaque-type psoriasis.[117] CD25 expression was blocked. Response in terms of clearing of plaques in this uncontrolled study appeared to be good up to week 8. Another anti-CD25 monoclonal antibody, the chimeric antibody basiliximab, has also been tested in psoriasis. In a case report, a single patient with treatment-refractory psoriasis was successfully treated with basiliximab.[118] In addition to antibodies, the IL-2 receptor has been targeted by a fusion protein consisting of IL-2 sequences coupled to diphtheria toxin fragments, denileukin diftitox. Intravenous administration of this agent at doses ranging from 0.5 to 5 mg/kg per day produced a 50% decrease in PASI scores in 8 of 35 patients (23%) with severe psoriasis.[119] Placebo-controlled studies with this agent have not yet been reported.

Agents that block T-cell interactions

Because of the role of T cells in psoriasis and PsA, intense interest has been focused on therapeutic agents that block T-cell interactions with other cell types involved in the inflammatory process. CD2 is a surface antigen expressed on all classes of T cells. It interacts with lymphocyte function-associated antigen-3 (LFA-3) on antigen-presenting cells, stimulating the proliferation of T lymphocytes. A recombinant LFA-3 fusion protein (alefacept) prevents cell–cell interaction between T lymphocytes and antigen-presenting cells, blocking T-cell activation. Alefacept, administered intravenously at doses of 0.025, 0.075 or 0.150 mg/kg once weekly, has been tested for efficacy in psoriasis in a multicenter, randomized, placebo-controlled, double-blind trial enrolling 229 patients with chronic psoriasis.[120] After 12 weeks, PASI scores were reduced by at least 75% in 33% of the patients receiving alefacept 0.025 mg/kg, 31% of those receiving alefacept 0.075 mg/kg, and 19% of those receiving alefacept 0.150 mg/kg, compared with 11% of patients in the placebo group (P = 0.02). Responses were observed within 2 weeks of treatment. In a subset of 26 patients who participated in subsequent studies of alefacept, responses were found to be sustained for a median period of 306 days before retreatment was required.[120] Patients who were treated with

alefacept had reduced levels of memory effector CD45RO⁺ T cells. A small study (n = 11) also suggests that alefacept may improve both joint and skin symptoms in PsA. After 12 weeks of treatment with alefacept 7.5 mg intravenously once weekly, seven (64%) patients achieved an ACR 20 response, and three (27%) achieved an ACR 50 response. Skin lesions, as assessed by PASI scores, improved in seven (64%) patients, with a mean improvement of 50%.[121] These studies clearly implicate T cells in the pathogenesis of psoriasis and possibly PsA.

Another agent, siplizumab, targets CD2, the molecule with which LFA-3 interacts. Siplizumab is a humanized monoclonal antibody. In phase I and phase I/II clinical trials, this agent mediated improvements in psoriasis and reduced lymphocyte populations in a dose-dependent manner. An intravenous formulation was shown to achieve a highly rapid and significant response, as judged by siplizumab serum levels and percentage CD2 receptor occupancy.[122] At the highest dosage (0.04 mg/kg IV or 5.0–7.0 mg SC weekly), more than one-third of the patients showed at least a 75% improvement in PASI scores.[123]

Blockade of LFA-1, the cell surface molecule that interacts with ICAM-1, has also been an attractive choice for psoriatic therapies. Efalizumab is a humanized monoclonal antibody to CD11a, a subunit of LFA-1. On the basis of clinical responses observed in a placebo-controlled phase II study,[124] a phase III trial in which 597 patients with moderate-to-severe plaque psoriasis were randomized to receive placebo or 1 or 2 mg/kg of efalizumab subcutaneously once weekly was initiated. After 12 weeks of treatment, 22% of patients in the 1 mg/kg group and 28% of patients in the 2 mg/kg group achieved PASI score improvements of 75% or greater, versus 5% for placebo. An additional 12 weeks of treatment and higher doses helped increase the number of responders.[125]

Disrupting interactions between B7 molecules on antigen-presenting cells and the T-cell surface antigens with which they interact, including CD28 and cytotoxic T-lymphocyte-associated antigen 4 (CTLA-4), may also be a useful strategy in psoriasis and PsA. A humanized antibody to B7, IDEC-114, has shown promising clinical activity in 35 patients with moderate-to-severe psoriasis, with a 50% or greater reduction in PASI scores observed in 40% of patients.[126] CTLA-4–Ig, a fusion protein of CTLA-4 and human immunoglobulin, has been assessed in a phase I open-label trial involving patients with psoriasis. Clinical improvement was associated with reduced cellular activation of T cells, keratinocytes and dendritic cells in the psoriatic lesions.[127]

An antibody to the CD3 antigen, a component of the T-cell receptor complex, may act by stimulating the proliferation of certain T cells rather than by preventing T-cell activation. A humanized, non-FcR-binding monoclonal antibody to CD3, huOKT3(1(ala-ala)), has been investigated for its ability to improve symptoms in patients with PsA. In vitro, this agent tolerizes type 1 T cells and induces the proliferation of type 2 T cells. In a phase I/II open-label trial, six of seven patients (86%) who received escalating doses of huOKT3(1(ala-ala) for 12–14 days had an ACR 70 or greater response at day 30. Transient T-cell depletion was noted, and one patient developed

mild cytokine-release syndrome symptoms. The effect of this agent on skin lesions was not reported.[128]

CONCLUSIONS

Though many traditional therapies for psoriasis and PsA have effects on cytokines that theoretically should make them clinically effective, few definitive clinical trials have been performed to establish their efficacy, and their problematic safety profile limits their acceptability as therapeutic agents. The potential for specific therapies that work through cytokine modulation is great. Therapies that interrupt the cytokine cascade (e.g. the TNF inhibitors) or block the cell–cell interactions required to activate T cells have now been proven effective and relatively safe in both psoriatic skin and joint disease. Because of their specificity, such agents are expected to be not only effective, but also better tolerated, than the systemic therapies traditionally used in psoriatic conditions. These agents may also provide new insights into the pathogenesis of psoriasis and PsA, and thus lead to even more novel and effective interventions.

REFERENCES

1. Centers for Disease Control and Prevention/National Center for Health Statistics. *Vital and Health Statistics: Current Estimates From the National Health Interview Survey, 1996.* Available at: http://www.cdc.gov/nchs/data/series/sr_10/sr10_200.pdf. Accessed 9 August, 1999.
2. Shbeeb M, Uramoto KM, Gibson LE et al. The epidemiology of psoriatic arthritis in Olmsted County, Minnesota, USA, 1982–1991. *J Rheumatol* 2000; **27**: 1247–50.
3. Brockbank J, Schentag CT, Rosen C, Gladman DD. Psoriatic arthritis (PsA) is common among patients with psoriasis and family medicine clinic attendees. *Arthritis Rheum* 2001; **44**(suppl): S94 (abstract).
4. Fleischer AB Jr, Feldman SR, Rapp SR et al. Disease severity measures in a population of psoriasis patients: the symptoms of psoriasis correlate with

self-administered psoriasis area severity index scores. *J Invest Dermatol* 1996; **107**: 26–9.
5. Kirby B, Richards HL, Woo P et al. Physical and psychologic measures are necessary to assess overall psoriasis severity. *J Am Acad Dermatol* 2001; **45**: 72–6.
6. Krueger GG, Feldman SR, Camisa C et al. Two considerations for patients with psoriasis and their clinicians: what defines mild, moderate, and severe psoriasis? What constitutes a clinically significant improvement when treating psoriasis? *J Am Acad Dermatol* 2000; **43**(2 Pt 1): 281–5.
7. McKenna KE, Stern RS. The impact of psoriasis on the quality of life of patients from the 16-center PUVA follow-up cohort. *J Am Acad Dermatol* 1997; **36**: 388–94.
8. Rapp SR, Feldman SR, Exum ML et al. Psoriasis causes as much disability as other major medical diseases. *J Am Acad Dermatol* 1999; **41**: 401–7.

9. Menter A, Barker JN. Psoriasis in practice. *Lancet* 1991; **338**: 231–4.

10. Gladman DD, Stafford-Brady F, Chang C-H et al. Longitudinal study of clinical and radiological progression in psoriatic arthritis. *J Rheumatol* 1990; **17**: 809–12.

11. Torre Alonso JC, Rodriguez Perez A, Arribas Castrillo JM et al. Psoriatic arthritis (PA): a clinical, immunological and radiological study of 180 patients. *Br J Rheumatol* 1991; **30**: 245–50.

12. Oriente CB, Scarpa R, Pucino A, Oriente P. Psoriasis and psoriatic arthritis: dermatological and rheumatological co-operative clinical report. *Acta Derm Venereol (Stockh)* 1989; **146**(suppl): 69–71.

13. Stern RS, Wu J. Psoriasis. In: Arndt KA, LeBoit PE, Robinson JK, Wintroub BU, eds. *Cutaneous Medicine and Surgery* (WB Saunders: Philadelphia, 1996) 295–321.

14. Bos JD, de Rie MA. The pathogenesis of psoriasis: immunological facts and speculations. *Immunol Today* 1999; **20**: 40–6.

15. Espinoza LR, Cuellar ML, Silveira LH. Psoriatic arthritis. *Curr Opin Rheumatol* 1992; **4**: 470–8.

16. De Keyser F, Mielants H, Veys EM. Current use of biologicals for the treatment of spondyloarthropathies. *Expert Opin Pharmacother* 2001; **2**: 85–93.

17. Scarpa R, Biondi OC, Oriente P. The classification of psoriatic arthritis: what will happen in the future? *J Am Acad Dermatol* 1997; **36**: 78–83.

18. Michet CJ, Conn DL. Psoriatic arthritis. In: Kelley WN, Harris ED, Ruddy S, Sledge CB, eds. *Textbook of Rheumatology*, 3rd edn (WB Saunders: Philadelphia, 1989) 1053–63.

19. Moll JMH, Wright V. Psoriatic arthritis. *Semin Arthritis Rheum* 1973; **3**: 55–78.

20. Sege-Peterson K, Winchester R. Psoriatic arthritis. In: Freedberg IM, Eisen AZ, Wolff K et al, eds. *Fitzpatrick's Dermatology in General Medicine*, 5th edn (McGraw Hill: New York, 1999) 522–3.

21. Roberts MET, Wright V, Hill AG, Mehra AC. Psoriatic arthritis: follow-up study. *Ann Rheum Dis* 1976; **35**: 206–12.

22. Gladman DD, Shuckett R, Russell ML et al. Psoriatic arthritis (PsA) – an analysis of 220 patients. *Q J Med* 1987; **62**: 127–41.

23. Fournié B, Crognier L, Arnaud C et al. Proposed classification criteria of psoriatic arthritis: a preliminary study in 260 patients. *Rev Rhum Engl Ed* 1999; **66**: 446–56.

24. Gladman DD, Farewell VT, Wong K, Husted J. Mortality studies in psoriatic arthritis: results from a single outpatient center. II. Prognostic indicators for death. *Arthritis Rheum* 1998; **41**: 1103–10.

25. Wong K, Gladman DD, Husted J et al. Mortality studies in psoriatic arthritis: results from a single outpatient clinic. I. Causes and risk of death. *Arthritis Rheum* 1997; **40**: 1868–72.

26. Nickoloff BJ, Wrone-Smith T. Injection of pre-psoriatic skin with CD4+ T cells induces psoriasis. *Am J Pathol* 1999; **155**: 145–58.

27. Chaudhari U, Romano P, Mulcahy LD et al. Efficacy and safety of infliximab monotherapy for plaque-type psoriasis: a randomised trial. *Lancet* 2001; **357**: 1842–7.

28. Asadullah K, Sterry W, Stephanek K et al. IL-10 is a key cytokine in psoriasis. Proof of principle by IL-10 therapy: a new therapeutic approach. *J Clin Invest* 1998; **101**: 783–94.

29. Bonifati C, Ameglio F. Cytokines in psoriasis. *Int J Dermatol* 1999; **38**: 241–51.

30. Ross EL, D'Cruz D, Morrow WJ. Localized monocyte chemotactic protein-1 production correlates with T cell infiltration of synovium in patients with psoriatic arthritis. *J Rheumatol* 2000; **27**: 2432–43.

31. Rottman JB, Smith TL, Ganley KG et al. Potential role of the chemokine receptors CXCR3, CCR4, and the integrin $\alpha E\beta 7$ in the pathogenesis of psoriasis vulgaris. *Lab Invest* 2001; **81**: 335–47.

32. Christophers E, Mrowietz U. Psoriasis. In: Freedberg IM, Eisen AZ, Wolff K et al, eds. *Fitzpatrick's Dermatology in General Medicine* 5th edn (McGraw Hill: New York, 1999) 495–521.

33. Uyemura K, Yamamura M, Fivenson DF et al. The cytokine network in lesional and lesion-free psoriatic skin is characterized by a T-helper type 1 cell-mediated response. *J Invest Dermatol* 1993; **101**: 701–5.

34. Schlaak JF, Buslau M, Jochum W et al. T cells involved in psoriasis vulgaris belong to the Th1 subset. *J Invest Dermatol* 1994; **102**: 145–9.

35. Giustizieri ML, Mascia F, Frezzolini A et al. Keratinocytes from patients with atopic dermatitis and psoriasis show a distinct chemokine production profile in response to T cell-derived cytokines. *J Allergy Clin Immunol* 2001; **107**: 871–7.

36. Duncan JI, Horrocks C, Ormerod AD et al. Soluble IL-2 receptor and CD25 cells in psoriasis: effects of cyclosporin A and PUVA therapy. *Clin Exp Immunol* 1991; **85**: 293–6.

37. Griffiths CE. Cutaneous leukocyte trafficking and psoriasis. *Arch Dermatol* 1994; **130**: 494–9.

38. Ortonne J-P. Recent developments in the understanding of the pathogenesis of psoriasis. *Br J Dermatol* 1999; **140**(suppl 54): 1–7.

39. Sigmundsdóttir H, Gudjónsson JE, Jónsdóttir I et al. The frequency of CLA+ CD8+ T cells in the blood of psoriasis patients correlates closely with the severity of their disease. *Clin Exp Immunol* 2001; **126**: 365–9.

40. Ritchlin C, Haas-Smith SA, Hicks D et al. Patterns of cytokine production in psoriatic synovium. *J Rheumatol* 1998; **25**: 1544–52.

41. Partsch G, Wagner E, Leeb BF et al. T cell derived cytokines in psoriatic arthritis synovial fluids. *Ann Rheum Dis* 1998; **57**: 691–3.

42. Costello PJ, Bresnihan B, O'Farrelly C, FitzGerald O. Predominance of CD8+ T lymphocytes in psoriatic arthritis. *J Rheumatol* 1999; **26**: 1117–24.

43. Kapp A. The role of cytokines in the psoriatic inflammation. *J Dermatol Sci* 1993; **5**: 133–42.

44. Mussi A, Bonifati C, Carducci M et al. Serum TNF-alpha levels correlate with disease severity and are reduced by effective therapy in plaque-type psoriasis. *J Biol Regul Homeost Agents* 1997; **11**: 115–18.

45. Chodorowska G. Plasma concentrations of IFN-γ and TNF-α in psoriatic patients before and after local treatment with dithranol ointment. *J Eur Acad Dermatol Venereol* 1998; **10**: 147–51.

46. Terajima S, Higaki M, Igarashi Y et al. An important role of tumor necrosis factor-α in the induction of adhesion molecules in psoriasis. *Arch Dermatol Res* 1998; **290**: 246–52.

47. Saklatvala J. Tumour necrosis factor alpha stimulates resorption and inhibits synthesis of proteoglycan in cartilage. *Nature* 1986; **322**: 547–9.

48. Bertolini DR, Nedwin GE, Bringman TS et al. Stimulation of bone resorption and inhibition of bone formation *in vitro* by human tumour necrosis factors. *Nature* 1986; **319**: 516–18.

49. Shinmei M, Masuda K, Kikuchi T, Shimomura Y. The role of cytokines in chondrocyte mediated cartilage degradation. *J Rheumatol* 1989; **6**(suppl. 18): 32–4.

50. Dayer JM, Beutler B, Cerami A. Cachectin/tumor necrosis factor stimulates collagenase and prostaglandin E_2 production by human synovial cells and dermal fibroblasts. *J Exp Med* 1985; **162**: 2163–8.

51. Prens E, van Joost T, Hegmans J et al. Effects of cyclosporine on cytokines and cytokine receptors in psoriasis. *J Am Acad Dermatol* 1995; **33**: 947–53.

52. Asadullah K, Döcke WD, Sabat RV et al. The treatment of psoriasis with IL-10: rationale and review of the first clinical trials. *Expert Opin Investig Drugs* 2000; **9**: 95–102.

53. Mussi A, Bonifati C, Carducci M et al. IL-10 levels are decreased in psoriatic lesional skin as compared to the psoriatic lesion-free and normal skin suction blister fluids. *J Biol Regul Homeost Agents* 1994; **8**: 117–20.

54. Danning CL, Illei GG, Hitchon C et al. Macrophage-derived cytokine and nuclear factor κB p65 expression in synovial membrane and skin of patients with psoriatic arthritis. *Arthritis Rheum* 2000; **43**: 1244–56.

55. ElKayam O, Yaron I, Shirazi I et al. Serum levels of IL-10, IL-6, IL-1ra, and sIL-2R in patients with psoriatic arthritis. *Rheumatol Int* 2000; **19**: 101–5.

56. Raychaudhuri SP, Jiang W-Y, Farber EM. Cellular localization of fractalkine at sites of inflammation: antigen-presenting cells in psoriasis express high levels of fractalkine. *Br J Dermatol* 2001; **144**: 1105–13.

57. Nickoloff BJ. The immunologic and genetic basis of psoriasis. *Arch Dermatol* 1999; **135**: 1104–10.

58. Pitzalis C, Pipitone N. Psoriatic arthritis. *J R Soc Med* 2000; **93**: 412–15.

59. Brockbank J, Gladman DD. Psoriatic arthritis. *Expert Opin Investig Drugs* 2000; **9** : 1511–22.

60. Espinoza LR, van Solingen R, Cuellar ML, Angulo J. Insights into the pathogenesis of psoriasis and psoriatic arthritis. *Am J Med Sci* 1998; **316**: 271–6.

61. Abu-Shakra M, Gladman DD. Aetiopathogenesis of psoriatic arthritis. *Rheumatol Rev* 1994; **3**: 1–7.

62. Wang Q, Vasey FB, Mahfood JP et al. V2 regions of 16S ribosomal RNA used as a molecular marker for the species identification of streptococci in peripheral blood and synovial fluid from patients with psoriatic arthritis. *Arthritis Rheum* 1999; **42**: 2055–9.

63. de Villiers EM, Ruhland A. Do specific human papillomavirus types cause psoriasis? *Arch Dermatol* 2001; **137**: 384–5.

64. Lebwohl M, Gelfand JM, Tan MH. Clinically significant therapeutic interactions for the practicing dermatologist. *Adv Dermatol* 1999; **14**: 1–26.

65. Lebwohl M, Ali S. Treatment of psoriasis. Part 1. Topical therapy and phototherapy. *J Am Acad Dermatol* 2001; **45**: 487–98.

66. Haustein UF, Rytter M. Methotrexate in psoria-

sis: 26 years' experience with low-dose long-term treatment. *J Eur Acad Dermatol Venereol* 2000; **14**: 382–8.

67. Ellis CN, Fradin MS, Messana JM et al. Cyclosporine for plaque-type psoriasis: results of a multidose, double-blind trial. *N Engl J Med* 1991; **324**: 277–84.

68. Faerber L, Braeutigam M, Weidinger G et al. Cyclosporine in severe psoriasis. Results of a meta-analysis in 579 patients. *Am J Clin Dermatol* 2001; **2**: 41–7.

69. Jegasothy BV, Ackerman CD, Todo S et al. Tacrolimus (FK 506) – a new therapeutic agent for severe recalcitrant psoriasis. *Arch Dermatol* 1992; **128**: 781–5.

70. Pringle F. A multidisciplinary approach to psoriatic arthropathy. *Community Nurse* 1999; **5**: 21–2.

71. Witman PM. Topical therapies for localized psoriasis. *Mayo Clin Proc* 2001; **76**: 943–9.

72. Jones G, Crotty M, Brooks P. Interventions for treating psoriatic arthritis (Cochrane Review). In: *The Cochrane Library*, Issue 1 (Update Software: Oxford, 2001).

73. Gallagher L, Gogarty M, Murphy E et al. Vascular endothelial growth factor and receptor expression in human inflammation joint disease. Presented at ACR 64th Annual Scientific Meeting and ARHP 35th Annual Scientific Meeting, Philadelphia, 2000 (abstract).

74. Kersley GD. Amethopterin (methotrexate) in connective tissue disease – psoriasis and polyarthritis. *Ann Rheum Dis* 1968; **27**: 64–6.

75. Chang DJ. A survey of drug effectiveness and treatment choices in psoriatic arthritis. *Arthritis Rheum* 1999; **42**(suppl): S372 (abstract).

76. Willkens RF, Williams HJ, Ward JR et al. Randomized, double-blind, placebo controlled trial of low-dose pulse methotrexate in psoriatic arthritis. *Arthritis Rheum* 1984; **27**: 376–81.

77. Spadaro A, Riccieri V, Sili-Scavalli A et al. Comparison of cyclosporin A and methotrexate in the treatment of psoriatic arthritis: a one-year prospective study. *Clin Exp Rheumatol* 1995; **13**: 589–93.

78. Farr M, Kitas GD, Waterhouse L et al. Sulphasalazine in psoriatic arthritis: a double-blind placebo-controlled study. *Br J Rheumatol* 1990; **29**: 46–9.

79. Combe B, Goupille P, Kuntz JL et al. Sulphasalazine in psoriatic arthritis: a randomized, multicentre, placebo-controlled study. *Br J Rheumatol* 1996; **35**: 664–8.

80. Clegg DO, Reda DJ, Mejias E et al. Comparison of sulfasalazine and placebo in the treatment of psoriatic arthritis: a Department of Veterans Affairs Cooperative Study. *Arthritis Rheum* 1996; **39**: 2013–20.

81. Clegg DO, Reda DJ, Abdellatif M. Comparison of sulfasalazine and placebo for the treatment of axial and peripheral articular manifestations of the seronegative spondylarthropathies: a Department of Veterans Affairs cooperative study. *Arthritis Rheum* 1999; **42**: 2325–9.

82. Salvarani C, Macchioni P, Olivieri I et al. A comparison of cyclosporine, sulfasalazine, and symptomatic therapy in the treatment of psoriatic arthritis. *J Rheumatol* 2001; **28**: 2274–82.

83. Palit J, Hill J, Capell HA et al. A multicentre double-blind comparison of auranofin, intramuscular gold thiomalate and placebo in patients with psoriatic arthritis. *Br J Rheumatol* 1990; **29**: 280–3.

84. Abu-Shakra M, Gladman DD, Thorne JC et al. Longterm methotrexate therapy in psoriatic arthritis: clinical and radiological outcome. *J Rheumatol* 1995; **22** : 241–5.

85. Moreland LW, Cohen SB, Baumgartner SW et al. Longterm safety and efficacy of etanercept in patients with rheumatoid arthritis. *J Rheumatol* 2001; **28**: 1238–44.

86. Bondeson J, Maini RN. Tumour necrosis factor as a therapeutic target in rheumatoid arthritis and other chronic inflammatory diseases: the clinical experience with infliximab (REMICADE). *Int J Clin Pract* 2001; **55**: 211–16.

87. Bathon JM, Martin RW, Fleischmann RM et al. A comparison of etanercept and methotrexate in patients with early rheumatoid arthritis [published errata appear in *N Engl J Med* 2001; **344**(1): 76 and *N Engl J Med* 2001; **344**(3): 240]. *N Engl J Med* 2000; **343**: 1586–93.

88. Mease PJ, Goffe BS, Metz J et al. Etanercept in the treatment of psoriatic arthritis and psoriasis: a randomised trial. *Lancet* 2000; **356**: 385–90.

89. Felson DT, Andersen JJ, Boers M et al. American College of Rheumatology preliminary definition of improvement in rheumatoid arthritis. *Arthritis Rheum* 1995; **38**: 727–35.

90. Fredriksson T, Pettersson U. Severe psoriasis – oral therapy with a new retinoid. *Dermatologica* 1978; **157**: 238–44.

91. Mease PJ, Goffe BS, Metz J et al. Enbrel® (etanercept) in patients with psoriatic arthritis and psoriasis. Presented at European League Against

Rheumatism (EULAR)/European Congress of Rheumatology, Prague, Czech Republic, 2002 (poster).

92. Mease P, Goffe B, Metz J, Vanderstoep A. Enbrel® (etanercept) in patients with psoriatic arthritis and psoriasis. *Arthritis Rheum* 1999; **42**(suppl): S377 (abstract).

93. Mease P, Kivitz A, Burch F et al. Improvement in disease activity in patients with psoriatic arthritis receiving etanercept (Enbrel®): results of a phase 3 multicenter clinical trial. Presented at European League Against Rheumatism (EULAR)/European Congress of Rheumatology, Prague, Czech Republic, 2002 (abstract).

94. Gottlieb AB, Lowe NJ, Matheson RT, Lebsack ME. Efficacy of etanercept in patients with psoriasis. Presented at American Academy of Dermatology, New Orleans, 2002 (poster).

95. ElKayam O, Yaron M, Caspi D. From wheels to feet: a dramatic response of severe chronic psoriatic arthritis to etanercept. *Ann Rheum Dis* 2000; **59**: 839.

96. Yazici Y, Erkan D, Lockshin MD. A preliminary study of etanercept in the treatment of severe, resistant psoriatic arthritis. *Clin Exp Rheumatol* 2000; **18**: 732–4.

97. Kurschat P, Rubbert A, Poswig A et al. Treatment of psoriatic arthritis with etanercept. *J Am Acad Dermatol* 2001; **44**: 1052.

98. Cuellar ML, Mendez EA, Collins RD et al. Efficacy of etanercept in refractory psoriatic arthritis (PsA). Presented at 64th Annual Scientific Meeting of the American College of Rheumatology and the 35th Annual Scientific Meeting of the Association of Rheumatology Health Professionals, Philadelphia, 2000 (abstract 235).

99. Antoni C, Dechant C, Lorenz H et al. Successful treatment of severe psoriatic arthritis with infliximab. *Arthritis Rheum* 1999; **42**(suppl): S371 (abstract).

100. Ogilvie AL, Antoni C, Dechant C et al. Treatment of psoriatic arthritis with antitumour necrosis factor-α antibody clears skin lesions of psoriasis resistant to treatment with methotrexate. *Br J Dermatol* 2001; **144**: 587–9.

101. Dechant C, Antoni C, Wendler J et al. One year outcome of patients with severe psoriatic arthritis treated with infliximab. Presented at 64th Annual Scientific Meeting of the American College of Rheumatology and the 35th Annual Scientific Meeting of the Association of Rheumatology

Health Professionals, Philadelphia, 2000 (abstract 212).

102. Van den Bosch F, Kruithof E, Baeten D et al. Effects of a loading dose regimen of three infusions of chimeric monoclonal antibody to tumour necrosis factor α (infliximab) in spondyloarthropathy: an open pilot study. *Ann Rheum Dis* 2000; **59**: 428–33.

103. Kruithof E, Van den Bosch F, Baeten D et al. TNF-alpha blockade with infliximab in patients with active spondyloarthropathy: follow-up of one year maintenance regimen. Presented at European League Against Rheumatism (EULAR)/European Congress of Rheumatology, Prague, Czech Republic, 2001 (abstract OP0056).

104. Gottlieb AB, Chaudhari U, Romano P et al. Infliximab monotherapy in the treatment of plaque-type psoriasis. *Arthritis Rheum* 2001; **44**(suppl): S383 (abstract).

105. Cauza EE, Spak MS, Cauza KC et al. Treatment of psoriatic arthritis and psoriasis vulgaris with the tumor necrosis factor blocker infliximab. Presented at European League Against Rheumatism (EULAR)/European Congress of Rheumatology, Prague, Czech Republic, 2001 (abstract SAT0014).

106. Kirby B, Marsland AM, Carmichael AJ, Griffiths CE. Successful treatment of severe recalcitrant psoriasis with combination infliximab and methotrexate. *Clin Exp Dermatol* 2001; **26**: 27–9.

107. Bolce RJ, Thompson J, Stevens MP. Treatment of psoriatic arthritis with infliximab in a small office-based rheumatology practice. *Arthritis Rheum* 2001; **44**(suppl): S121 (abstract).

108. Bray VJ, Huffstutter JE, Schwartzman S. Emerging role of infliximab (Remicade®) in psoriatic arthritis patients resistant to disease-modifying antirheumatic drugs: case studies. *Arthritis Rheum* 2001; **44**(suppl): S121 (abstract).

109. Kempeni J. Update on D2E7: a fully human anti-tumour necrosis factor α monoclonal antibody. *Ann Rheum Dis* 2000; **59**(suppl 1): i44–5.

110. Keystone E, Choy E, Kalden J et al. CDP870, a novel, pegylated, humanized TNF-α inhibitor, is effective in treating the signs and symptoms of rheumatoid arthritis (RA). Presented at 65th Annual Scientific Meeting of the American College of Rheumatology and the 36th Annual Scientific Meeting of the Association of Rheumatology Health Professionals, San Francisco, 2001 (abstract LB-3).

111. Trinchard-Lugan I, Ho-Nguyen Q, Bilham WM et

al. Safety, pharmacokinetics and pharmacodynamics of recombinant human tumour necrosis factor-binding protein-1 (Onercept) injected by intravenous, intramuscular and subcutaneous routes into healthy volunteers. *Eur Cytokine Netw* 2001; **12**: 391–8.

112. Abgenix. Abigenix's ABX-IL8 antibody associated with statistically significant improvement in psoriasis. Phase IIa trial also shows excellent safety profile. Available at: http://www.abgenix.com/Forms/press_release_detail.asp?pressID=114. Accessed 4 February, 2000.

113. Reich K, Garbe C, Blaschke V et al. Response of psoriasis to interleukin-10 is associated with suppression of cutaneous type 1 inflammation, downregulation of the epidermal interleukin-8/CXCR2 pathway and normalization of keratinocyte maturation. *J Invest Dermatol* 2001; **116**: 319–29.

114. Asadullah K, Friedrich M, Hanneken S et al. Effects of systemic interleukin-10 therapy on psoriatic skin lesions: histologic, immunohistologic, and molecular biology findings. *J Invest Dermatol* 2001; **116**: 721–7.

115. McInnes IB, Illei GG, Danning CL et al. IL-10 improves skin disease and modulates endothelial activation and leukocyte effector function in patients with psoriatic arthritis. *J Immunol* 2001; **167**: 4075–82.

116. Trepicchio WL, Ozawa M, Walters IB et al. Interleukin-11 therapy selectively downregulates type I cytokine proinflammatory pathways in psoriasis lesions. *J Clin Invest* 1999; **104**: 1527–37.

117. Krueger JG, Walters IB, Miyazawa M et al. Successful in vivo blockade of CD25 (high-affinity interleukin 2 receptor) on T cells by administration of humanized anti-Tac antibody to patients with psoriasis. *J Am Acad Dermatol* 2000; **43**: 448–58.

118. Owen CM, Harrison PV. Successful treatment of severe psoriasis with basiliximab, an interleukin-2 receptor monoclonal antibody. *Clin Exp Dermatol* 2000; **25**: 195–7.

119. Martin A, Gutierrez E, Muglia J et al. A multicenter dose-escalation trial with denileukin diftitox (ONTAK, DAB(389)IL-2) in patients with severe psoriasis. *J Am Acad Dermatol* 2001; **45**: 871–81.

120. Ellis CN, Krueger GG. Treatment of chronic plaque psoriasis by selective targeting of memory effector T lymphocytes. *N Engl J Med* 2001; **345**: 248–55.

121. Dinant HJ, van Kuijk AWR, Goedkoop AY et al. Alefacept (LFA3–IgG1 fusion protein, LFA3TIP) reduces synovial inflammatory infiltrate and improves outcome in psoriatic arthritis. *Arthritis Rheum* 2001; **44**(suppl): S91 (abstract).

122. Papp K, Langley R, Martinson R, Dingivan C. Safety, tolerance, and biological activity of MEDI-507 (siplizumab) for the treatment of moderate to severe psoriasis. Presented at Annual meeting of the American Academy of Dermatology, New Orleans, 2002 (poster).

123. BioTransplant Incorporated. Initial clinical results for MEDI-507 as psoriasis treatment presented at international psoriasis symposium [press release]. Available at: http://www.noonanrusso.com/news/biotransplant/01news/biotrans06.23.html. Accessed 4 February, 2002.

124. Papp K, Bissonnette R, Krueger JG et al. The treatment of moderate to severe psoriasis with a new anti-CD11a monoclonal antibody. *J Am Acad Dermatol* 2001; **45**: 665–74.

125. Genentech. Xanelim shows initial positive results in second pivotal phase III study [press release]. Available at: http://www.xoma.com/news/pressrel/01_07_31.html. Accessed 4 February, 2002.

126. IDEC Pharmaceuticals. Product candidate: IDEC-114 (anti-CD80). Available at: http://www.idecpharm.com/site/science/idec114.htm. Accessed 4 February, 2002.

127. Abrams JR, Kelley SL, Hayes E et al. Blockade of T lymphocyte costimulation with cytotoxic T lymphocyte-associated antigen 4-immunoglobulin (CTLA4Ig) reverses the cellular pathology of psoriatic plaques, including the activation of keratinocytes, dendritic cells, and endothelial cells. *J Exp Med* 2000; **192**: 681–94.

128. Utset TO, Auger JA, Peace D et al. Modified anti-CD3 therapy in psoriatic arthritis: a phase I/II clinical trial. *Arthritis Rheum* 2001; **44**(suppl): S92 (abstract).

129. Bhushan M, McLaughlin B, Weiss JB, Griffiths CEM. Levels of endothelial cell stimulating angiogenesis factor and vascular endothelial growth factor are elevated in psoriasis. *Br J Dermatol* 1999; **141**: 1054–60.

130. Bonifati C, Mussi A, Carducci M et al. Endothelin-1 levels are increased in sera and lesional skin extracts of psoriatic patients and correlate with disease severity. *Acta Derm Venereol* 1998; **78**: 22–6.

131. el Barnawi NY, Giasuddin ASM, Ziu MM, Singh

M. Serum cytokine levels in psoriasis vulgaris. *Br J Biomed Sci* 2001; **58**: 40–4.

132. Koga T, Duan H, Urabe K, Furue M. In situ localization of IFN-gamma-positive cells in psoriatic lesional epidermis. *Eur J Dermatol* 2002; **12**: 20–3.

133. Cuchacovich R, Japa S, Aris H et al. Cytokine profile in psoriatic arthritis (PsA): predominance of th-1 derived proinflammatory cytokines. Presented at 64th Annual Scientific Meeting of the American College of Rheumatology and the 35th Annual Scientific Meeting of the Association of Rheumatology Health Professionals, Philadelphia, 2000.

134. Riente L, Pratesi F, Frigelli S et al. Cytokine production by CD3+ t cell in synovial fluid from patients affected by psoriatic arthritis and rheumatoid arthritis. Presented at European League Against Rheumatism (EULAR)/European Congress of Rheumatology, Prague, Czech Republic, 2001 (abstract THU0035).

135. Romero LI, Ikejima T, Pincus SH. In situ localization of interleukin-1 in normal and psoriatic skin. *J Invest Dermatol* 1989; **93**: 518–22.

136. Cooper KD, Hammerberg C, Baadsgaard O et al. IL-1 activity is reduced in psoriatic skin. Decreased IL-1α and increased nonfunctional IL-1β. *J Immunol* 1990; **144**: 4593–603.

137. Bonifati C, Carducci M, Mussi A et al. IL-1 alpha, IL-1 beta and psoriasis: conflicting results in the literature. Opposite behaviour of the two cytokines in lesional or non-lesional extracts of whole skin. *J Biol Regul Homeost Agents* 1997; **11**: 133–6.

138. Mizutani H, Ohmoto Y, Mizutani T et al. Role of increased production of monocytes TNF-α, IL-1β and IL-6 in psoriasis: relation to focal infection, disease activity and responses to treatments. *J Dermatol Sci* 1997; **14**: 145–53.

139. Ameglio F, Bonifati C, Fazio M et al. Interleukin-11 production is increased in organ cultures of lesional skin of patients with active plaque-type psoriasis as compared with nonlesional and normal skin. Similarity to interleukin-1 beta, interleukin-6 and interleukin-8. *Arch Dermatol Res* 1997; **289**: 399–403.

140. Punzi L, Bertazzolo N, Pianon M et al. Value of synovial fluid interleukin-1β determination in predicting the outcome of psoriatic monoarthritis. *Ann Rheum Dis* 1996; **55**: 642–4.

141. Partsch G, Steiner G, Leeb BF et al. Highly increased levels of tumor necrosis factor-α and other proinflammatory cytokines in psoriatic

arthritis synovial fluid. *J Rheumatol* 1997; **24**: 518–23.

142. Nishibu A, Han GW, Iwatsuki K et al. Overexpression of monocyte-derived cytokines in active psoriasis: a relation to coexistent arthropathy. *J Dermatol Sci* 1999; **21**: 63–70.

143. Hammerberg C, Arend WP, Fisher GJ et al. Interleukin-1 receptor antagonist in normal and psoriatic epidermis. *J Clin Invest* 1992; **90**: 571–83.

144. Kristensen M, Deleuran B, Eedy DJ et al. Distribution of interleukin 1 receptor antagonist protein (IRAP), interleukin 1 receptor, and interleukin 1α in normal and psoriatic skin. Decreased expression of IRAP in psoriatic lesional epidermis. *Br J Dermatol* 1992; **127**: 305–11.

145. Wong WM, Howell WM, Coy SD et al. Interleukin-2 is found in the synovium of psoriatic arthritis and spondyloarthritis, not in rheumatoid arthritis. *Scand J Rheumatol* 1996; **25**: 239–45.

146. Bonifati C, Carducci M, Cordiali Fei P et al. Correlated increases of tumour necrosis factor-α, interleukin-6 and granulocyte monocyte-colony stimulating factor levels in suction blister fluids and sera of psoriatic patients – relationships with disease severity. *Clin Exp Dermatol* 1994; **19**: 383–7.

147. Bonifati C, Trento E, Cordiali-Fei P et al. Increased interleukin-7 concentrations in lesional skin and in the sera of patients with plaque-type psoriasis. *Clin Immunol Immunopathol* 1997; **83**: 41–4.

148. Szepietowski JC, Bielicka E, Nockowski P et al. Increased interleukin-7 levels in the sera of psoriatic patients: lack of correlations with interleukin-6 levels and disease intensity. *Clin Exp Dermatol* 2000; **25**: 643–7.

149. Sticherling M, Sautier W, Schroder JM, Christophers E. Interleukin-8 plays its role at local level in psoriasis vulgaris. *Acta Derm Venereol* 1999; **79**: 4–8.

150. Duan H, Koga T, Kohda F et al. Interleukin-8-positive neutrophils in psoriasis. *J Dermatol Sci* 2001; **26**: 119–24.

151. König A, Krenn V, Gillitzer R et al. Inflammatory infiltrate and interleukin-8 expression in the synovium of psoriatic arthritis – an immunohistochemical and mRNA analysis. *Rheumatol Int* 1997; **17**: 159–68.

152. Salvarani C, Olivieri I, Cantini F et al. Psoriatic arthritis. *Curr Opin Rheumatol* 1998; **10**: 299–305.

153. Ritchlin C, Haas-Smith SA. Expression of inter-

leukin 10 mRNA and protein by synovial fibroblastoid cells. *J Rheumatol* 2001; **28**: 698–705.

154. Yawalkar N, Karlen S, Hunger R et al. Expression of interleukin-12 is increased in psoriatic skin. *J Invest Dermatol* 1998; **111**: 1053–7.

155. Spadaro A, Rinaldi T, Riccieri V et al. Interleukin 13 in synovial fluid and serum of patients with psoriatic arthritis. *Ann Rheum Dis* 2002; **61**: 174–6.

156. Ruckert R, Asadullah K, Seifert M et al. Inhibition of keratinocyte apoptosis by IL-15: a new parameter in the pathogenesis of psoriasis? *J Immunol* 2000; **165**: 2240–50.

157. Deleuran M, Buhl L, Ellingsen T et al. Localization of monocyte chemotactic and activating factor (MCAF/MCP-1) in psoriasis. *J Dermatol Sci* 1996; **13**: 228–36.

158. Reilly DM, Parslew R, Sharpe GR et al. Inflammatory mediators in normal, sensitive and diseased skin types. *Acta Derm Venereol* 2000; **80**: 171–4.

159. Raychaudhuri SP, Jiang W-Y, Farber EM et al. Upregulation of RANTES in psoriatic keratinocytes: a possible pathogenic mechanism for psoriasis. *Acta Derm Venereol Suppl (Stockh)* 1999; **79**: 9–11.

160. Fukuoka M, Ogino Y, Sato H et al. RANTES expression in psoriatic skin, and regulation of RANTES and IL-8 production in cultured epidermal keratinocytes by active vitamin D_3 (tacalcitol). *Br J Dermatol* 1998; **138**: 63–70.

161. Konig A, Krenn V, Toksoy A et al. Mig, GRO alpha and RANTES messenger RNA expression in lining layer, infiltrates and different leucocyte populations of synovial tissue from patients with rheumatoid arthritis, psoriatic arthritis and osteoarthritis. *Virchows Arch* 2000; **436**: 449–58.

162. Economidou J, Barkis J, Demetriou Z et al. Effects of cyclosporin A on immune activation markers in patients with active psoriasis. *Dermatology* 1999; **199**: 144–8.

163. Partsch G, Wagner E, Leeb BF et al. Upregulation of cytokine receptors sTNF-R55, sTNF-R75, and sIL-2R in psoriatic arthritis synovial fluid. *J Rheumatol* 1998; **25**: 105–10.

164. Bonifati C, Trento E, Carducci M et al. Soluble E-selectin and soluble tumour necrosis factor receptor (60 kD) serum levels in patients with psoriasis. *Dermatology* 1995; **190**: 128–31.

165. Ettehadi P, Greaves MW, Wallach D et al. Elevated tumour necrosis factor-alpha (TNF-α) biological activity in psoriatic skin lesions. *Clin Exp Immunol* 1994; **96**: 146–51.

166. Fearon U, Reece R, Smith J et al. Synovial cytokine and growth factor regulation of MMPs/TIMPs: implications for erosions and angiogenesis in early rheumatoid and psoriatic arthritis patients. *Ann N Y Acad Sci* 1999; **878**: 619–21.

167. Pitzalis C, Cauli A, Pipitone N et al. Cutaneous lymphocyte antigen-positive T lymphocytes preferentially migrate to the skin but not to the joint in psoriatic arthritis. *Arthritis Rheum* 1996; **39**: 137–45.

168. Jones SM, Dixey J, Hall ND, McHugh NJ. Expression of the cutaneous lymphocyte antigen and its counter-receptor E-selectin in the skin and joints of patients with psoriatic arthritis. *Br J Rheumatol* 1997; **36**: 748–57.

169. Griffiths CEM, Voorhees JJ, Nickoloff BJ. Characterization of intercellular adhesion molecule-1 and HLA-DR expression in normal and inflamed skin: modulation by recombinant gamma interferon and tumor necrosis factor. *J Am Acad Dermatol* 1989; **20**: 617–29.

170. De Pita O, Ruffelli M, Cadoni S et al. Psoriasis: comparison of immunological markers in patients with acute and remission phase. *J Dermatol Sci* 1996; **13**: 118–24.

171. Gottlieb S, Hayes E, Gilleaudeau P et al. Cellular actions of etretinate in psoriasis: enhanced epidermal differentiation and reduced cell-mediated inflammation are unexpected outcomes. *J Cutan Pathol* 1996; **23**: 404–18.

172. Dunky A, Neumüller J, Menzel J. Interactions of lymphocytes from patients with psoriatic arthritis or healthy controls and cultured endothelial cells. *Clin Immunol Immunopathol* 1997; **85**: 297–314.

173. Baeten D, Kruithof E, Van den Bosch F et al. Immunomodulatory effects of anti-tumor necrosis factor alpha therapy on synovium in spondylarthropathy: histologic findings in eight patients from an open-label pilot study. *Arthritis Rheum* 2001; **44**: 186–95.

174. Veale D, Rogers S, FitzGerald O. Immunolocalization of adhesion molecules in psoriatic arthritis, psoriatic and normal skin. *Br J Dermatol* 1995; **132**: 32–8.

175. Prens E, Hooft-Benne K, Tank B et al. Adhesion molecules and IL-1 costimulate T lymphocytes in the autologous MECLR in psoriasis. *Arch Dermatol Res* 1996; **288**: 68–73.

176. Nickoloff BJ, Nestle FO, Zheng XG, Turka LA. T lymphocytes in skin lesions of psoriasis and

mycosis fungoides express B7-1: a ligand for CD28. *Blood* 1994; **83**: 2580–6.

177. Kang S, Yi S, Griffiths CE et al. Calcipotriene-induced improvement in psoriasis is associated with reduced interleukin-8 and increased interleukin-10 levels within lesions. *Br J Dermatol* 1998; **138**: 77–83.

178. Peters BP, Weissman FG, Gill MA. Pathophysiology and treatment of psoriasis. *Am J Health Syst Pharm* 2000; **57**: 645–62.

179. Cooper KD. Psoriasis. Leukocytes and cytokines. *Dermatol Clin* 1990; **8**: 737–45.

180. Teranishi Y, Mizutani H, Murata M et al. Increased spontaneous production of IL-8 in peripheral blood monocytes from the psoriatic patient: relation to focal infection and response to treatments. *J Dermatol Sci* 1995; **10**: 8–15.

181. Seitz M, Loetscher P, Dewald B et al. Interleukin 1 (IL-1) receptor antagonist, soluble tumor necrosis factor receptors, IL-1β, and IL-8 – markers of remission in rheumatoid arthritis during treatment with methotrexate. *J Rheumatol* 1996; **23**: 1512–16.

182. Shiohara T, Imanishi K, Sagawa Y, Nagashima M. Differential effects of cyclosporine and etretinate on serum cytokine levels in patients with psoriasis. *J Am Acad Dermatol* 1992; **27**: 568–74.

183. Macchioni P, Boiardi L, Meliconi R et al. Serum chemokines in patients with psoriatic arthritis treated with cyclosporin A. *J Rheumatol* 1998; **25**: 320–5.

184. Duvic M, Asano AT, Hager C, Mays S. The pathogenesis of psoriasis and the mechanism of action of tazarotene. *J Am Acad Dermatol* 1998; **39**: S129–33.

33

Spondyloarthropathies

Joachim Sieper and Jürgen Braun

Introduction • Treatment of ankylosing spondylitis with non-steroidal anti-inflammatory drugs • Treatment of ankylosing spondylitis with disease-modifying anti-inflammatory drugs • Treatment of ankylosing spondylitis with corticosteroids • Novel approaches in the treatment of ankylosing spondylitis • TNFα blockade in the treatment of ankylosing spondylitis • Efficacy of anti-TNF-α blockade in other spondyloarthropathies/other manifestations • Side-effects of anti-TNF therapy • Influence of anti-TNF therapy on biological parameters • Other potential targets for biologicals in spondyloarthropathies • Summary and conclusions • References

INTRODUCTION

The spondyloarthritides (SpA) comprise five subtypes: ankylosing spondylitis (AS), reactive arthritis (ReA), major parts of the arthritis/spondylitis spectrum associated with psoriasis (Psa) and inflammatory bowel disease (AIBD), and undifferentiated SpA (uSpA). AS is the most frequent subtype of SpA being slightly more prevalent than undifferentiated SpA, but psoriatic arthritis (PsA), based on the high prevalence of psoriasis, is also quite frequent,[1,2] while ReA and AIBD are relatively rare. The prevalence of the whole group of SpA has been recently estimated to be between 0.6% and 1.9%, with an implicated AS prevalence of 0.1–1.1%.[1–4] Thus, taken together, the SpA have a prevalence that is not much different from that of rheumatoid arthritis (RA).

AS is the subset with the most severe disease course. Only recently have researchers started to investigate the burden of disease in AS patients, both personally and economically. Apart from the inequality in the amount of available data (there are far more studies in RA), a direct comparison between RA and AS is difficult for a number of other reasons – one being that AS usually starts considerably earlier in life, in the third decade, which means that the burden of disease lasts longer. However, some comparisons on the basis of larger datasets from databases have been performed. When age- and sex-matched AS patients with severe disease were compared with severe RA patients, the grade of pain and disability was similar.[5] Furthermore, absence from work and work disability are clearly increased in AS patients compared to normals.[6,7] In a recent survey in the USA[8] the most prevalent quality-of-life concerns of AS patients included stiffness (90.2%), pain (83.1%), fatigue (62.4%), poor sleep (54.1%), concerns about appearance (50.6%), worry about the future (50.3%), and medication side-effects (41%). However, many AS patients cope better with their disease than RA patients. This might be due to the earlier onset in younger ages and the somewhat better education in AS patients. Also, affected hands might interfere more with daily life than a stiff and painful spine. In recent decades, patients, general practitioners and rheumatologists have accepted the current situation regarding AS because choice of treatments was limited.

Thus, SpA in general and AS especially are more prevalent than previously thought and there is a clear socio-economic impact on society. On this background, it becomes increasingly clear that more effective therapies are needed in this disease. This chapter concentrates on drug therapy, with a focus on biologicals, of AS – the most prevalent subtype and the most severe outcome of SpA. It also discusses the potential to treat patients with early AS effectively to prevent ankylosis. We will also briefly discuss available data for other SpA and uveitis. Treatment of PsA with biologicals is dealt with in more detail elsewhere in this book.

TREATMENT OF ANKYLOSING SPONDYLITIS WITH NON-STEROIDAL ANTI-INFLAMMATORY DRUGS

Non-steroidal anti-inflammatory drugs (NSAIDs) are accepted and frequently used drug treatments for AS.[9] NSAIDs are taken with variable efficacy by about 70–80% of AS patients. A good response to NSAID treatment has even been suggested as a criterion for the diagnosis of inflammatory back pain and SpA.[9] A bad or no response to NSAIDs of AS patients has been identified as a bad prognostic sign.[10] The patients' response to NSAIDs is generally similar, but individually often markedly different. Thus, several NSAIDs might need to be tried to identify the best one. Indomethacin, naproxene and diclofenac are among the most frequently used drugs in AS, but others clearly work as well. Finally, an almost historical but very effective agent, phenylbutazone, has been tried by experienced rheumatologists for severe patients. Up to 11% of AS patients enter remission during NSAID treatment.[11]

There is evidence that the novel, more COX-2-selective, drugs meloxicam and celecoxib[11,12] are no less effective in treating back pain of AS patients than conventional NSAIDs such as piroxicam and ketoprofen. This might be associated with there being less serious gastrointestinal events.

However, as in other rheumatic diseases, NSAIDs are valuable for improving the symptoms of spinal inflammation, but there is no evidence that permanent antiphlogistic treatment has an influence on the radiologic outcome or on function. It is widely believed that the amelioration of pain is associated with an improved ability to exercise daily – which, over time, supports the maintenance of function and helps to avoid stiffening. Nonetheless, a minority of AS patients are probably treated sufficiently with NSAIDs alone.

TREATMENT OF ANKYLOSING SPONDYLITIS WITH DISEASE-MODIFYING ANTI-INFLAMMATORY DRUGS

In great contrast to RA, there are no established disease modifying anti-rheumatic drugs (DMARDs) for AS. The best-investigated DMARD for the treatment of AS is sulfasalazine. In the two largest placebo-controlled studies, efficacy in peripheral arthritis but no clear effects on axial symptoms were reported.[13,14] However, mostly patients with long-standing disease (> 14 years disease duration) were treated in these studies. In an earlier placebo-controlled trial with 85 patients, 60% of whom had peripheral arthritis,[15] sulfasalazine had some effect also on the spinal symptoms of AS patients who had a relatively short disease duration of < 6 years. The peripheral arthritis of AS patients, as in other SpA, improved on treatment with sulfasalazine,[14] and there is also some evidence that sulfasalazine prevents attacks of AS-associated uveitis.[16] Taking all the evidence together, sulfasalazine is effective for peripheral arthritis in SpA, but there is no clear option for the axial manifestations. Presently, we are performing a placebo-controlled study in which 200 patients with early AS (duration of symptoms < 6 years) are being treated with sulfasalazine or placebo for 6 months. The results of this study will hopefully allow further evidence-based conclusions about the efficacy of sulfasalazine in early AS and uSpA.

Many fewer data are available on the efficacy of other DMARDs in AS. There have been a few small open studies with methotrexate, with controversial results. A recent placebo-controlled study with 15 patients in each arm[17] showed that methotrexate (MTX), in a dose of 10 mg once a week, was not superior to placebo. In contrast to the lack of efficacy thus demonstrated, MTX and sulfasalazine have been used by many AS patients,[18] which underlines the so far unmet need for an effective treatment.

There are no studies apart from case reports on the treatment of AS patients with other DMARDs which are effective in the treatment of RA, such as gold, azathioprine, cyclosporin A or leflunomide.

More therapies targeting the immune system have been tried in AS, with some positive effects, including lymphocyte-orientated apheresis.[19] There are recent reports on stem cell transplantation because of lymphoma in a patient who happened to also have AS.[20] However, in another case, SpA-like symptoms developed after stem cell transplantation.[21]

TREATMENT OF ANKYLOSING SPONDYLITIS WITH CORTICOSTEROIDS

AS patients are generally less responsive to corticosteroid therapy than RA patients. However, there is not even one controlled study to test the efficacy of systemic moderate- or low-dose corticosteroids in AS or other SpA. Differences in the expression of glucocorticoid receptors in the two diseases might constitute one explanation. Only single observations and open studies with high doses in a few patients[22] with AS are available. There is little doubt that intra-articular corticosteroids work quite well for short-term improvement in peripheral arthritis[23] and sacroiliitis.[24,25] In the sacroiliac joints, the effect of CT-guided injections probably lasts longer than that of the blind injection technique, which is also feasible.

NOVEL APPROACHES IN THE TREATMENT OF ANKYLOSING SPONDYLITIS

Bisphosphonates, which are active against osteoclasts and are used for the treatment of osteoporosis, have been tried in AS on the assumption that they inhibit bone turnover, which is probably increased in active AS. There have been two positive reports from small open studies on the treatment of AS with pamidronate. Both spinal and peripheral disease, including enthesitis, were successfully influenced by this intravenously applied drug. A gain in bone mass could be a positive side-effect in AS, where osteoporosis is associated with an increased risk of fractures. Preliminary results by the same group from a controlled study including 84 active AS patients in which a 60 mg dose was compared with a 10 mg dose of pamidronate in Canada suggest that the former is significantly more effective.[26] While clinical parameters clearly improved, there was no significant reduction in the erythrocyte sedimentation rate (ESR) or C-reactive protein (CRP) level. Adverse events were frequent, consisting primarily of transient arthralgias/ myalgias after the first intravenous infusion.

Thalidomide, on the basis of its tumour necrosis factor (TNF)-blocking potential, has been tried in an open study in France, but the toxicity and the side-effect of fatigue might prevent extensive use.[27] A recent study from China reported good efficacy (H. Feng, personal communication).

Radiation therapy for AS was successfully used in the past to improve spinal pain, but the risk of malignoma finally turned out to be increased too much. Refractory heel pain in SpA can still be treated by local radiation. With higher doses of intravenous radium-224 chloride used in the past, the risk of chronic myeloid leukemia was slightly increased. A rather pure application of radium-224 chloride at a dose of 10 MBq has recently been approved for the treatment of severe AS in Germany, mainly on the basis of older studies.[28] However, a controlled trial needs to be performed soon.

TNF-α BLOCKADE IN THE TREATMENT OF ANKYLOSING SPONDYLITIS

Today, there are two main biological agents targeting TNF-α: the chimeric monoclonal IgG$_1$ antibody infiximab (Remicade) and the 75 kDa IgG$_1$ fusion protein etanercept (Enbrel). Both catch soluble TNF-α in the plasma, etanercept also catches TNF-β. Infliximab also binds to cell membrane-bound TNF-α. As already cited, both clearly work in RA. Infliximab is approved in combination with methotrexate, because less antibodies against infliximab and somewhat fewer adverse events occurred with this regimen in RA, while etanercept is approved as monotherapy. Two other TNF-α-blockers, the fully humanized monoclonal antibody against TNF-α, adalimumab, and CDP870, an engineered human anti-TNF-α antibody Fab' fragment, are currently under active investigation in RA treatment trials but have not been tested so far in SpA.

The sacroiliac joint and the entheses are the most characteristic and almost pathognomonic sites involved in SpA.[29] Inflammation at the interphase of cartilage and bone has been convincingly demonstrated by MRI[30,31] and immunohistologic investigations on biopsies.[32–34] Especially in early cases of AS, dense mononuclear infiltrates can be seen which invade the cartilage.[34] We showed that T cells and macrophages present in these infiltrates produce plenty of TNF-α.[32]

On the basis of the early successful RA trials,[35] the decision to investigate the efficacy of the TNF-α-blocking monoclonal antibody infliximab in AS patients was the next logical step, although it has to be stressed that RA is pathogenetically clearly different from AS.

Further support for testing this drug in AS came from two other sets of data. First, AS and the whole group of SpA are associated with chronic inflammatory bowel diseases (IBD), since patients with IBD may develop AS and > 50% of patients with primary AS show histologic gut lesions similar to those of Crohn's disease.[36] Furthermore, TNF-α is strongly expressed in the inflamed gut of IBD patients,

and anti-TNF-α therapy with infliximab is effective and has been approved for Crohn's disease.[37] It might also be effective in ulcerative colitis, but further studies are needed. It is pathogenetically interesting that etanercept seems not to be effective in Crohn's disease, at least in the usual dosage,[38] although its efficacy in RA is similar to that seen in patients treated with infliximab.[39] Importantly, the joint symptoms of patients with Crohn's disease treated with infliximab improved on therapy.[40]

Second, anti-TNF-α therapy is effective in other SpA-related inflammatory rheumatic diseases, such as PsA.[41,42]

When we and others started our treatment trials, we used recently evaluated outcome parameters for AS treatment trials.[43–45] First, two open pilot studies were performed in patients with AS and other SpA. In the one performed in Berlin, infliximab improved the disease activity of severe AS patients with a mean disease duration of 5 years,[46] as measured by the 'Bath Ankylosing Spondylitis Disease Activity Index' (BASDAI).[43] Eleven patients received three infusions of infliximab 5 mg/kg at weeks 0, 2, and 6. Significant efficacy was already noted on the first day of therapy. In particular, spinal pain, fatigue and morning stiffness, but also peripheral arthritis, improved. Nine of 10 patients showed an improvement of > 50% in the BASDAI; the median improvement of the BASDAI after 4 weeks was 70%. Importantly, quality of life, as measured by the 'short form' (SF) 36 instrument, was significantly better after 4 weeks. In comparison to an age- and sex-matched normal healthy German population, the studied AS patients had clearly impaired initial assessments; in particular, physical functioning was very low. This could be significantly increased by anti-TNF-α therapy in the first 4 weeks. One patient, although an exception, remains in remission today, after the initial three infusions of infliximab. As major side-effects, three patients developed allergic reactions in this study and could not receive further treatment.

The same patients were then followed up for another 9 months. The next infusion of infliximab was not given before a relapse occurred, defined as 80% of the initial disease activity.[47] The first symptoms returned after a mean of 6 weeks, and a relapse occurred after a mean of 12 weeks. These patients were treated again three more times. Although all responded again, they did less well compared to the start of the study, probably due to the lack of the initial saturation phase.

There have been several open-label studies on infliximab in AS.[48–51] In a Belgian study, 21 SpA patients, including 11 with AS, were treated with infliximab with a similar dose regimen, but the patients had a longer disease duration (15 years) and the time intervals between the infusions were longer (14 weeks). The spinal and peripheral joint symptoms of all SpA patients improved significantly.[48] In Canada there were 24 AS patients,[49] in France 50 AS patients[50] and in Spain 42 SpA patients[51] who were successfully treated with infliximab; there was a similarly good response in about 80% of the patients. It is of interest that in the French study, the bone mineral density (BMD) of 31 patients (26 men, 5 women, mean age 40 years, mean disease duration 18 years) increased by $3.3 \pm 5.5\%$ (-6.1, 23.7) at the lumbar spine ($p < 0.002$), and $1.9 \pm 3.1\%$ (-4.9, 10.3) at the femoral neck ($p < 0.008$) after 6 months of infliximab therapy.[52]

We confirmed the good efficacy of infliximab in AS observed in these open studies in a randomized double-blind controlled trial in Germany.[53] In this placebo-controlled multicenter study conducted over 12 weeks, 70 AS patients with a BASDAI > 4 and spinal pain on a visual analogue scale (VAS) > 4 were included. A highly significant effect of infliximab treatment (5 mg/kg body weight given at weeks 0, 2, and 6) in the primary outcome parameter of a 50% improvement of disease activity (BASDAI) was achieved in the verum group compared to placebo. Fifty-three per cent of patients treated with infliximab versus 9% treated with placebo achieved this clinically highly relevant degree of improvement (Figure 33.1). Other parameters, such as the 'Bath Ankylosing Spondylitis Functional Index', measuring function, the 'Bath Ankylosing Spondylitis Metrology Index',

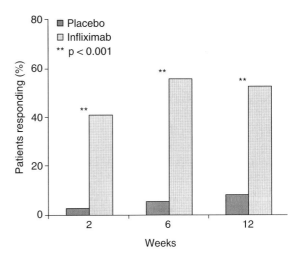

Figure 33.1   Percentage of patients responding by a 50% improvement of the Bath Ankylosis Spondylitis Disease Activity Index (BASDAI) during 3 months of treatment with infliximab compared to placebo. (Adapted from Braun et al. *Lancet* 2002; **359**: 1187–93.[53])

measuring spinal mobility, and the SF-36, measuring quality of life, showed a similar improvement. Although the numbers in the subgroups were small, patients with elevated CRP levels had a significantly greater benefit than those with low or normal levels.[53] Thus, an elevated CRP could identify good responders, a finding which has to be confirmed in future studies. Preliminary results from imaging follow-ups with spinal MRI, assessing both acute and chronic spinal changes, suggest a significant effect of infliximab on disease progression on this basis. Taken together, these data strongly suggest a major breakthrough in the short-term therapy of severe AS.

After the placebo phase of the study, these 70 patients are now being treated with infliximab at 5 mg/kg body weight every 6 weeks for 2 years. All placebo patients reached a similar level of improvement 6 weeks after the start of treatment with infliximab. Thus, the good results of the placebo-controlled phase were confirmed. After 54 weeks, about 75% of the patients are still on treatment. None of these patients stopped treatment because of loss of efficacy. Most importantly, the same level of response was maintained throughout the year. The study is still ongoing and will give more information about the long-term efficacy and safety of infliximab treatment in AS. During the placebo-controlled phase of the study, we observed three serious adverse events, including one case of lymph node tuberculosis, one of allergic granulomatosis of the lung, and one of transient leukopenia. Another eight serious adverse events occurred in the next 9 months during the open extension phase, among them three patients with symmetrical arthritis of their hands and positive anti-nuclear antbodies.

Regarding the optimal dosage of infliximab in SpA only limited data are available. In a small study we found the dose of 5 mg/kg to be superior to 3 mg/kg in patients with undifferentiated spondyloarthritis.[54] The optimal dosage needs to be investigated in future studies.

Treatment of AS with the soluble TNF-α receptor etanercept has not been studied extensively, but preliminary data from single cases,[55] an open study[56] and a recent double-blind study[57] treating 20 patients in each group for months, indicate a clearly favorable effect which seems to be very similar to that observed in the infliximab studies. Indeed, in our own small placebo-controlled etanercept study with 30 AS patients over 3 months, the level of improvement was very similar to that seen in AS patients treated with infliximab.[58] Currently, further studies with this drug are in progress or are planned.

EFFICACY OF ANTI-TNF-α BLOCKADE IN OTHER SPONDYLOARTHROPATHIES/OTHER MANIFESTATIONS

Psoriatic arthritis, arthritis associated with Crohn's disease and reactive arthritis

Etanercept is also highly effective in the treatment of PsA. In a double-blind placebo-controlled study over 3 months, a highly significant improvement compared to placebo

was found[41] (for more details, see elsewhere in this book). A similar level of improvement was seen in an open study of 10 PsA patients with infliximab.[42] Currently, a placebo-controlled study of infliximab treatment of PsA is underway. In a small trial including four patients with Crohn's-associated arthritis, the arthritic symptoms improved considerably in all patients treated with infliximab for gut symptoms.[40] There are no published data yet about TNF-α blockade in patients with chronic reactive arthritis. Because there is good evidence that the triggering bacteria such as *Chlamydia*, *Yersinia* and *Salmonella* persist in these patients, there exists the theoretical possibility that TNF-α blockers induce a reactivation of these persisting bacteria and thus worsen the disease. However, our own experiences with one patient with chronic *Yersinia*-induced reactive arthritis and reports from other investigators on *Chlamydia*-induced reactive arthritis (R. Schumacher, personal communication) suggest that treatment with infliximab is also favorable. However, larger studies are needed to answer this question.

Undifferentiated spondyloarthopathies

It has been known for some time that many patients have symptoms suggestive of spondyloarthropathies but do not fulfill the diagnostic criteria for any of the defined spondyloarthopathies. For these patients, a new term, undifferentiated SpA, has been suggested,[59] and criteria for diagnosing this subset have been discussed.[59] According to these criteria, patients with uSpA have to have at least the symptom of inflammatory back pain or of an asymmetrical peripheral arthritis predominantly of the lower limbs, plus one additional manifestation typical for the group of SpA. We showed that in these patients a sacroiliitis, which has not yet induced bony changes visible by normal X-rays, can be detected by MRI (Figure 33.2).[30] Among patients with uSpA, the majority have the leading symptom of inflammatory back pain.[1,2,59] Thus, many of these patients can be expected to develop the full picture of AS later on. Indeed, in

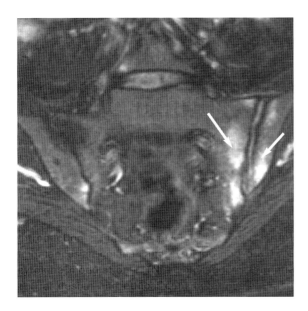

Figure 33.2 Acute inflammation of the left sacroiliac joint (arrows) as detected by MRI in a patient with an early form of ankylosing spondylitis.

a long-term follow-up study, 60% of these patients were diagnosed as having AS after 10 years.[60]

Again, while DMARDs such as sulfasalazine and possibly MTX seem to be effective for uSpA patients with peripheral arthritis,[13,14] there is currently no evidence that they work for the spinal symptoms. The data available at the moment suggest that infliximab is also highly effective in the treatment of these patients. In the open Belgian study, the patients with uSpA responded similarly to the other SpA patients to infliximab treatment,[48] and in a small open study we showed that infliximab works in uSpA and that a doses of 5 mg/kg body weight seems to be more effective than a doses of 3 mg/kg.[54] In another open study treating 10 uSpA patients with 2 × 25 mg etanercept given subcutaneously twice a week, we also observed a similar good response. Thus, both for the effective treatment of acute symptoms and for the prevention of long-term damage as seen in patients with AS,

TNF-α blockers seem to represent an interesting new treatment option for patients with uSpA, especially for those with spinal symptoms. An overview of the studies conducted so far in AS and uSpA is given in Table 33.1.

Uveitis

The response of patients with inflammatory eye disease to anti-TNF has been recently investigated in a limited number of patients. No clear picture can be formed. This subject is further complicated because there are different forms of uveitis with completely different pathogenesis. Both improvement and worsening of inflammatory eye disease upon treatment with infliximab may occur. In the first study,[61] 16 patients (4 males, 12 females, aged 7–78 years) who received etanercept ($n = 14$) or infliximab ($n = 2$) for either inflammatory eye disease or associated joint disease were studied retrospectively. Uveitis ($n = 9$) and scleritis ($n = 7$) of patients with RA ($n = 11$), AS ($n = 1$), psoriatic SpA ($n = 1$) and 3 patients with uveitis without systemic signs of disease were included. Although all 12 patients with active articular inflammation experienced improvement in joint disease (100%), in only 6 of 16 with ocular inflammation (38%) did the eye disease improve. Five patients even developed inflammatory eye disease for the first time while taking a TNF inhibitor.

In the other study,[62] which is more relevant to the discussion of TNF blockers in SpA, seven consecutive patients with acute onset of an HLA-B27-associated acute anterior uveitis were investigated. Infliximab at a dose of 10 mg/kg was given once intravenously. One patient received a second infusion 3 weeks after the first dosage, due to a relapse. The median duration (± SD) of uveitis was 8 ± 12 days. All patients responded to infliximab with a rapid improvement of clinical symptoms and a decrease of anterior chamber cells. Only one patient did not develop total resolution of the uveitis. On follow-up, three of seven patients relapsed after a median time of 120 days. In our own study,[53] anterior uveitis occurred in three patients in the

Table 33.1 Overview of clinical studies of anti-TNF-α agents in ankylosing spondylitis and undifferentiated spondyloarthropathies.

Study	Site	Study design	Patients (n)	Dose	Treatment duration
Infliximab					
Brandt et al[46,47]	Germany	OL	AS (n = 11)	5 mg/kg IV at weeks 0, 2, 6, and after relapse	3 months, plus 1-year follow-up
Van den Bosch et al[48]	Belgium	OL	SpA (n = 21), including 10 with AS	5 mg/kg IV at weeks 0, 2, 6, 20, 34, 48	84 days, plus 1-year follow-up
Stone et al[49]	Canada	OL	AS (n = 11)	5 mg/kg IV at weeks 0, 2, 6	14 weeks
Collantes et al[51]	Spain	OL	SpA (n = 26) including 18 with AS	5 mg/kg IV at weeks 0, 2, 6, 14, 22, 30	30 weeks
Brandt et al[54]	Germany	OL	uSpA (n = 6)	5 mg/kg IV at weeks 0, 2, 6	3 months
Breban et al[50]	France	OL	AS (n = 50)	5 mg/kg IV at weeks 0, 2, 6	6 months
Braun et al[53]	Germany	Randomized placebo-controlled trial; open-label extension phase	AS (n = 70)	5 mg/kg IV at weeks 0, 2, 6, then every 6 weeks	12 weeks RCT 48 weeks OL
Van den Bosch et al[68]	Belgium	Randomized placebo-controlled trial; open-label extension phase	SpA (n = 40) including 19 with AS	5 mg/kg IV at weeks 0, 2, 6	12 weeks RCT, plus 1-year follow-up
Etanercept					
Marzo-Ortega et al[56]	UK	OL	SpA (n = 10) including seven patients with AS	25 mg SC twice weekly	6 months
Gorman et al[57]	US	Randomized placebo-controlled trial; open-label extension phase	AS (n = 40)	25 mg SC twice weekly	4 months RCT 6 months OL
Brandt et al[58]	Germany	Randomized placebo-controlled trial; open-label extension phase	AS (n = 30)	25 mg SC twice weekly	6 weeks 3 months
Brandt et al (unpublished)	Germany	OL	uSpA (n = 10)	25 mg SC twice weekly	3 months

OL, open-label trial; RCT, randomized controlled trial; SpA, spondyloarthropathy; uSpA, undifferentiated spondyloarthropathy; AS, ankylosing spondylitis; IV, intravenous; SC, subcutaneous.

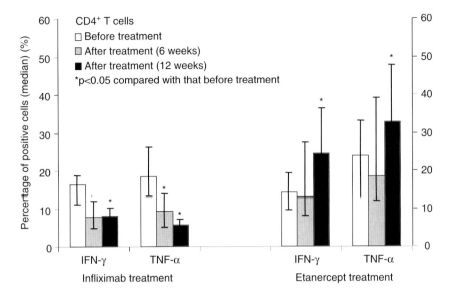

Figure 33.3 Percentage of CD4[+] T cells secreting IFN-γ or TNF-α after in vitro stimulation for 6 h with PMA/ionomycin. CD4[+] T cells, being double positive for one cytokine plus the activation marker CD69, were quantified by flow cytometry. During treatment of patients with ankylosing spondylitis with infliximab, the number of IFN-γ- and TNF-α-positive CD4[+] T cells decreased significantly, while, in contrast, during treatment with etanercept an increase was observed. PMA, phorbol myristate acetate.

placebo group but in only 1 patient in the infliximab group during the placebo-controlled phase. Thus, infliximab might be effective in HLA-B27-associated uveitis, but controlled studies and a systematic comparison with local and systemic steroid therapy is clearly needed.

SIDE-EFFECTS OF ANTI-TNF THERAPY

There are clearly side-effects to be considered in patients treated with anti-TNF agents. Three main types have occurred with infliximab (for details of our study, see above): (1) serious infections such as tuberculosis[63] (the prevalence for all infections in infliximab-treated patients was only slightly higher than in patients treated with placebo (51% versus 57%)); (2) allergic reactions, both acute and delayed, in one case leading to a self-limiting bronchocentric granulomatosis of the lung; and (3) autoimmune reactions in the form of arthritis symptoms and development of anti-nuclear antibodies. With etanercept there seem to be fewer problems with these three types of side-effect, but local injection reactions, cases of bone marrow suppression and multiple sclerosis-like diseases have been reported.

All patients who are treated with anti-TNF therapy should be carefully screened for infections and treated with antibiotics if there is a suspicion of bacterial infections. Prophylactic treatment with isoniazide (INH) for the first 6 months of therapy should be performed in patients for whom a decision is made to start infliximab treatment and who have a positive skin test for purified protein derivative (PPD), X-ray evidence of previous exposure to mycobacteria, or a recent history of confirmed tuberculosis contact.

It is not clear whether immunosuppressants such as MTX or azathioprin should or could be succesfully added to infliximab to prevent antibody formation and allergic side-effects. Until now, these kinds of studies have not been performed, because there is no indication that these drugs are effective in AS, and it seems problematic to give an immunosuppressive drug only to avoid the occurrence of side-effects.

INFLUENCE OF ANTI-TNF THERAPY ON BIOLOGICAL PARAMETERS

In our two placebo-controlled studies, which have already been mentioned above, we investigated cytokine secretion of T cells after antigen-specific and after non-specific stimulation in vitro during the 3 months of treatment with infliximab versus placebo and during treatment with etanercept versus placebo. In the infliximab study, we observed a clear decline of interferon (IFN)-γ and TNF-α secretion over 3 months after non-specific stimulation and after antigen-specific stimulation with the G1 domain of the cartilage proteoglycan aggrecan (data not shown), while no change in cytokine secretion was observed in the placebo group. However, a similar drop in cytokine secretion by T cells occurred after placebo patients were switched to infliximab.[64] In contrast, in the etanercept study, increases in TNF-α and IFN-γ secretion were observed during treatment, while again no changes were observed in the placebo group. Figure 33.3 compares the effect of infliximab and that of etanercept on cytokine secretion by T cells. Interestingly, when monocytes were stimulated in vitro with lipopolysaccharide (LPS), no change in the secretion of TNF-α was observed during either infliximab treatment or etanercept treatment (data not shown). Thus, infliximab seems to be effective, at least partly, through inhibition of T-helper 1 function which lasts for at least 6 weeks after the previous infusion, while etanercept seems to work preferentially by catching soluble TNF-α without suppression of T-cell function. The slight up-regulation of T-cell function observed in these patients can probably be seen as counter-regulation after neutralization of peripheral TNF-α. While the amounts of TNF-α produced by monocytes has been reported to decrease immediately after an infliximab infusion, this does not seem to play a role several weeks after the last infusion, despite the presence of a clinical effect. Our data therefore indicate that the T cells might represent a major target, at least for infliximab.

OTHER POTENTIAL TARGETS FOR BIOLOGICALS IN SPONDYLOARTHROPATHIES

Like TNF-α, we showed that IL-1 is also present in biopsies taken from the sacroiliac joint.[65] Thus,

the IL-1 receptor antagonist anakinra, which is effective in the treatment of RA, should be tested in AS and other SpA in the near future. The blockade of cytokines is relatively low in the hierachy of the immune response. We and others have argued in the past that AS is mainly a T-cell-driven disease[66] and have tried to identify peptides presented by the HLA-B27 molecule to CD8+ T cells;[67] more recently, we have described single peptides from the whole proteome of *Chlamydia trachomatis* presented to CD8+ T cells derived from HLA-B27-positive patients with *Chlamydia*-induced reactive arthritis by combining two computer programs for the prediction of peptide binding to HLA-B27 and for the creation of special peptides by the proteasome in the cytoplasm of cells with antigen-specific flow cytometry.[68] We hope that this approach will allow us to identify cross-reacting self-peptides, possibly derived from the cartilage,[29] and use these peptides for a new therapeutic approach to antigen-specific tolerance induction[69] by downregulation of the local immune response with few, if any, side-effects.

SUMMARY AND CONCLUSIONS

Especially for the spinal symptoms of the SpA, of which AS is the prototype, there is no effective disease-modifying treatment available. The new TNF-α blockers have been proven to be highly effective in improving the spinal symptoms and also the extraspinal manifestations of the SpA. Although a direct comparison between RA and AS has not been performed, there is good clinical evidence that TNF-α blockade is more effective in AS and other SpA compared to RA. This has to be seen on the background that 60–80% of patients with active RA can be sufficiently treated with currently available DMARDs, while this is not the case for AS. Side-effects, mainly infections and allergic reactions, are similar to those observed in RA treatment. Currently, there is no reason to combine TNF-α blockers with another DMARD for the treatment of AS, mostly because these DMARDs are not effective. Thus, TNF-α blockers seem to represent a major breakthrough in the treatment of AS and other SpA. Especially in the light of the high costs and the unknown long-term side-effects, the patients who are primary candidates for such a treatment need still to be defined. Furthermore, future studies have to show whether these biologicals not only suppress inflammation but also prevent long-term bony damage.

REFERENCES

1. Braun J, Bollow M, Remlinger G et al. Prevalence of spondylarthropathies in HLA B27-positive and -negative blood donors. *Arthritis Rheum* 1998; **41**: 58–67.

2. Brandt J, Bollow M, Haberle J et al. Studying patients with inflammatory back pain and arthritis of the lower limbs clinically and by magnetic resonance imaging: many, but not all patients with sacroiliitis have spondyloarthropathy. *Rheumatology (Oxford)* 1999; **38**: 831–6.

3. Gran JT, Husby G, Hordvik M. Prevalence of ankylosing spondylitis in males and females in a young middle-aged population of Tromso, northern Norway. *Ann Rheum Dis* 1985; **44**: 359–67.

4. Saraux A, Guedes C, Allain J et al. Prevalence of rheumatoid arthritis and spondyloarthropathy in Brittany, France. Societe de Rhumatologie de l'Ouest. *J Rheumatol* 1999; **26**: 2622–7.

5. Zink A, Braun J, Listing J, Wollenhaupt J. Disability and handicap in rheumatoid arthritis and ankylosing spondylitis – results from the German rheumatological database. German Collaborative Arthritis Centers. *J Rheumatol* 2000; **27**: 613–22.

6. Zink A, Listing J, Klindworth C, Zeidler H. The national database of the German Collaborative Arthritis Centres: I. Structure, aims, and patients. *Ann Rheum Dis* 2001; **60**(3): 199–206.

7. Boonen A, Chorus A, Miedema H, van Der Heijde D, van Der Tempel H, van der Linden S. Employment, work disability, and work days lost in patients with ankylosing spondylitis: a cross sectional study of Dutch patients. *Ann Rheum Dis* 2001; **60**: 353–8.

8. Ward MM. Health-related quality of life in ankylosing spondylitis: a survey of 175 patients. *Arthritis Care Res* 1999; **12**: 247–55.

9. Amor B, Dougados M, Mijiyawa M. Criteria for the classification of spondylarthropathies. *Rev Rhum Mal Osteoartic* 1990; **57**: 85–9.

10. Amor B, Santos RS, Nahal R, Listrat V, Dougados M. Predictive factors for the longterm outcome of spondyloarthropathies. *J Rheumatol* 1994; **21**: 1883–7.

11. Dougados M, Behier JM, Jolchine I et al. Efficacy of celecoxib, a cyclooxygenase 2-specific inhibitor, in the treatment of ankylosing spondylitis: a six-week controlled study with comparison against placebo and against a conventional nonsteroidal antiinflammatory drug. *Arthritis Rheum* 2001; **44**: 180–5.

12. Dougados M, Gueguen A, Nakache JP et al. Ankylosing spondylitis: what is the optimum duration of a clinical study? A one year versus a 6 weeks non-steroidal anti-inflammatory drug trial. *Rheumatology (Oxford)* 1999; **38**: 235–44.

13. Dougados M, van der Linden S, Leirisalo-Repo M et al. Sulfasalazine in the treatment of spondylarthropathy. A randomized, multicenter, double-blind, placebo-controlled study. *Arthritis Rheum* 1995; **38**: 618–27.

14. Clegg DO, Reda DJ, Abdellatif M. Comparison of sulfasalazine and placebo for the treatment of axial and peripheral articular manifestations of the seronegative spondylarthropathies: a Department of Veterans Affairs cooperative study. *Arthritis Rheum* 1999; **42**: 2325–9.

15. Nissila M, Lehtinen K, Leirisalo-Repo M, Luukkainen R, Mutru O, Yli-Kerttula U. Sulfasalazine in the treatment of ankylosing spondylitis. A twenty-six-week, placebo-controlled clinical trial. *Arthritis Rheum* 1988; **31**: 1111–6.

16. Benitez-Del-Castillo JM, Garcia-Sanchez J, Iradier T, Banares A. Sulfasalazine in the prevention of anterior uveitis associated with ankylosing spondylitis. *Eye* 2000; **14**: 340–3.

17. Roychowdhury B, Bintley-Bagot S, Hunt J, Tunn EJ. Methotrexate in severe ankylosing spondylitis: a randomised placebo controlled, double-blind observer study. *Rheumatology* 2001; **40**: 43.

18. Ward MM, Kuzis S. Treatment used by patients with with ankylosing spondylitis: comparison with treatment preferences by rheumatologists. *J Clin Rheumatol* 1999; **5**: 1–8.

19. Ueo T, Kobori K, Okumura H et al. Effectiveness

of lymphocytapheresis in a patient with ankylosing spondylitis. *Transfus Sci* 1990; **11**: 97–101.

20. Jantunen E, Myllykangas-Luosujarvi R, Kaipiainen-Seppanen O, Nousiainen T. Autologous stem cell transplantation in a lymphoma patient with a long history of ankylosing spondylitis. *Rheumatology (Oxford)* 2000; **39**(5): 563–4.

21. Koch B, Kranzhofer N, Pfreundschu M, Pees HW, Trumper L. First manifestations of seronegative spondylarthropathy following autologous stem cell transplantation in HLA-B27-positive patients. *Bone Marrow Transplant* 2000; **26**(6): 673–5.

22. Mercado U. The use of methylprednisolone pulse therapy in a severe case of HLA-B27 negative ankylosing spondylitis. *J Rheumatol* 1994; **21**(8): 1582–3.

23. Plant MJ, Borg AA, Dziedzic K, Saklatvala J, Dawes PT. Radiographic patterns and response to corticosteroid hip injection. *Ann Rheum Dis* 1997; **56**(8): 476–80.

24. Maugars Y, Mathis C, Berthelot JM, Charlier C, Prost A. Assessment of the efficacy of sacroiliac corticosteroid injections in spondylarthropathies: a double-blind study. *Br J Rheumatol* 1996; **35**(8): 767–70.

25. Braun J, Bollow M, Seyrekbasan F et al. Computed tomography guided corticosteroid injection of the sacroiliac joint in patients with spondyloarthropathy with sacroiliitis: clinical outcome and followup by dynamic magnetic resonance imaging. *J Rheumatol* 1996; **23**(4): 659–64.

26. Maksymowych WP, Fitzgerald A, LeClercq S et al. A 6 month randomized double-blinded dose response comparison of i.v. pamidronate (60mg vs 10mg) in the treatment of NSAID-refractory ankylosing spondylitis (AS). *Arthritis Rheum* 2001; **44**(9): S159.

27. Breban M, Gombert B, Amor B, Dougados M. Efficacy of thalidomide in the treatment of refractory ankylosing spondylitis. *Arthritis Rheum* 1999; **42**: 580–1.

28. Braun J, Lemmel M, Manger B, Rau R, Sörensen H, Sieper J. Therapy of ankylosing spondylitis with radiumchloride. *Z Rheumatol* 2001; **60**: 74–83.

29. Braun J, Khan MA, Sieper J. Enthesitis and ankylosis in spondyloarthropathy: what is the target of the immune response? *Ann Rheum Dis* 2000; **59**: 985–94.

30. Braun J, Bollow M, Eggens U, Konig H, Distler A, Sieper J. Use of dynamic magnetic resonance imaging with fast imaging in the detection of early and advanced sacroiliitis in spondylarthropathy patients. *Arthritis Rheum* 1994; **37**: 1039–45.

31. McGonagle D, Gibbon W, O'Connor P, Green M, Pease C, Emery P. Characteristic magnetic resonance imaging entheseal changes of knee synovitis in spondylarthropathy. *Arthritis Rheum* 1998; **41**: 694–700.

32. Braun J, Bollow M, Neure L et al. Use of immunohistologic and in situ hybridization techniques in the examination of sacroiliac joint biopsy specimens from patients with ankylosing spondylitis. *Arthritis Rheum* 1995; **38**: 499–505.

33. Francois RJ, Gardner DL, Degrave EJ, Bywaters EG. Histopathologic evidence that sacroiliitis in ankylosing spondylitis is not merely enthesitis. *Arthritis Rheum* 2000; **43**: 2011–24.

34. Bollow M, Fischer T, Reißhauer H, Sieper J, Hamm B, Braun J. T cells and macrophages predominate in early and active sacroiliitis as detected by magnetic resonance imaging in spondyloarthropathies. *Ann Rheum Dis* 2000; **59**(2): 135–40.

35. Elliott MJ, Maini RN, Feldmann M et al. Randomised double-blind comparison of chimeric monoclonal antibody to tumour necrosis factor alpha (cA2) versus placebo in rheumatoid arthritis. *Lancet* 1994; **344**: 1105–10.

36. Mielants H, Veys EM, Goemaere S, Cuvelier C, De Vos M. A prospective study of patients with spondyloarthropathy with special reference to HLA-B27 and to gut histology. *J Rheumatol* 1993; **20**: 1353–8.

37. Sandborn WJ. Anti-tumor necrosis factor therapy for inflammatory bowel disease: a review of agents, pharmacology, clinical results and safety. *Inflamm Bowel Dis* 1999; **5**: 119–33.

38. Sandborn WJ, Hanauer SB, Katz S et al. Etanercept for active Crohn's disease: a randomized, double-blind, placebo-controlled trial. *Gastroenterology* 2001; **121**: 1088–94.

39. Moreland LW, Baumgartner SW, Schiff MH et al. Treatment of rheumatoid arthritis with a recombinant human tumor necrosis factor receptor (p75)–Fc fusion protein. *N Engl J Med* 1997; **337**: 141–8.

40. Van den Bosch F, Kruithof E, De Vos M, De Keyser F, Mielants H. Crohn's disease associated with spondyloarthropathy: effect of TNF-alpha blockade with infliximab on articular symptoms. *Lancet* 2000; **356**(9244): 1821–2.

41. Mease PJ, Goffe BS, Metz J, VanderStoep A, Finck B, Burge DJ. Etanercept in the treatment of psoriatic arthritis and psoriasis: a randomised trial. *Lancet* 2000; **29**(356): 385–90.

42. Antoni C, Dechant C, Ogilvie A, Kalden-Nemeth D, Kalden JR, Manger B. Successful treatment of psoriatic arthritis with infliximab in an MRI controlled study. *J Rheumatol* 2000; **27**(suppl 59): 24.

43. Garrett S, Jenkinson TR, Kennedy LG, Whitelock HC, Gaisford P, Calin A. A new approach to defining disease status in ankylosing spondylitis. The Bath AS disease activity index. *J Rheumatol* 1994; **21**: 2286–91.

44. van der Heijde D, Bellamy N, Calin A, Dougados M, Khan MA, van der Linden S. Preliminary core sets for endpoints in ankylosing spondylitis. Assessments in Ankylosing Spondylitis Working Group. *J Rheumatol* 1997; **24**: 2225–9.

45. Anderson JJ, Baron G, van der Heijde D, Felson DT, Felson M. ASAS preliminary criteria for short term improvement in ankylosing spondylitis. *Arthritis Rheum*, 2001; **44**: 1878–86.

46. Brandt J, Haibel H, Cornely D et al. Successful treatment of active ankylosing spondylitis with the anti-tumor necrosis factor alpha monoclonal antibody infliximab. *Arthritis Rheum* 2000; **43**: 1346–52.

47. Brandt J, Haibel H, Reddig J, Sieper J, Braun J. Treatment of patients with severe ankylosing spondylitis with infliximab – a one year follow up. *Arthritis Rheum* 2001; **44**: 2936–7.

48. Van den Bosch F, Kruithof E, Baeten D, De Keyser F, Mielants H, Veys EM. Effects of a loading dose regimen of three infusions of chimeric monoclonal antibody to tumour necrosis factor alpha (infliximab) in spondyloarthropathy: an open pilot study. *Ann Rheum Dis* 2000; **59**: 428–33.

49. Stone M, Salonen D, Lax M, Payne U, Lapp V, Inman R. Clinical and imaging correlates of response to treatment with infliximab in patients with ankylosing spondylitis. *J Rheumatol* 2001; **28**: 1605–14.

50. Breban MA, Vignon E, Claudepierre P et al. Efficacy of infliximab in severe refractory ankylosing spondylitis (AS). Results of an open label study. *Ann Rheum Dis* 2001; **60**(suppl): 59.

51. Collantes E, Munoz-Villanueva MC, Sanmarti R et al. Infliximab in refractory spondyloarthropathies, preliminary results in Spanish population. *Ann Rheum Dis* 2001; **60**(suppl): 59–60.

52. Allali F, Roux C, Kolta S et al. Infliximab in the treatment of spondylarthropathy, bone mineral density effect. *Arthritis Rheum* 2001; **44**(9): S89.

53. Braun J, Brandt J, Listing J et al. Treatment of active ankylosing spondylitis with infliximab – a double-blind placebo controlled multicenter trial. *Lancet* 2002; **359**: 1187–93.

54. Brandt J, Haibel H, Reddig J, Sieper J, Braun J. Successful treatment of severe undifferentiated spondyloarthropathy with the anti-tumor necrosis factor α monoclonal antibody infliximab. *J Rheumatol* 2002, **29**: 118–22.

55. Barthel HR. Rapid remission of treatment-resistant ankylosing spondylitis with etanercept – a drug for refractory ankylosing spondylitis? *Arthritis Rheum* 2001; **45**: 404.

56. Marzo-Ortega H, McGonagle D, O'Connor P, Emery P. Efficacy of etanercept in the treatment of the entheseal pathology in resistant spondylarthropathy: a clinical and magnetic resonance imaging study. *Arthritis Rheum* 2001; **44**: 2112–17.

57. Gorman JD, Sack KE, Davis JC. Treatment of ankylosing spondylitis by inhibition of tumor necrosis factor. *N Engl J Med* 2002; **346**: 1349–56.

58. Brandt J, Kariouzov A, Listing J et al. Six months results of a German double-blind placebo controlled phase, phase-III clinical trial of etanercept in active ankylosing spondylitis. *Ann Rheum Dis* 2002; **61** (Suppl 1): 41.

59. Dougados M, van der Linden S, Juhlin R et al. The European Spondylarthropathy Study Group preliminary criteria for the classification of spondylarthropathy. *Arthritis Rheum* 1991; **34**: 1218–27.

60. Mau W, Zeidler H, Mau R et al. Clinical features and prognosis of patients with possible ankylosing spondylitis. Results of a 10–year followup. *J Rheumatol* 1988; **15**(7): 1109–14.

61. Smith JR, Levinson RD, Holland GN et al. Differential efficacy of tumor necrosis factor inhibition in the management of inflammatory eye disease and associated rheumatic disease. *Arthritis Rheum* 2001; **45**(3): 252–7.

62. El-Shabrawi Y, Hermann J. Anti-TNFa therapy with infliximab in the treatment of HLA B27 associated acute anterior uveitis – a one year follow up. *Arthritis Rheum* 2001; **44**(9): S425.

63. Keane J, Gershon S, Wise RP et al. Tuberculosis associated with infliximab, a tumor necrosis factor alpha-neutralizing agent. *N Engl J Med* 2001; **11**(15): 1098–104.

64. Zhou J, Rudwaleit M, Thiel A, Braun J, Sieper J. Downregulation of the nonspecific and the antigen-specific T cell cytokine response in ankylosing spondylitis after treatment with infliximab. *Arthritis Rheum* 2001; **44**: S236.

65. Braun J, Neure L, Francois R et al. Immuno-histologic examinations of sacroiliac inflammation in ankylosing spondylitis. *Arthritis Rheum* 1998; **41**: S112.

66. Sieper J, Braun J. Pathogenesis of spondylarthropathies. Persistent bacterial antigen, autoimmunity, or both? *Arthritis Rheum* 1995; **38**: 1547–54.

65. Ugrinovic S, Mertz A, Wu P, Braun J, Sieper J. A single nonamer from the Yersinia 60-kDa heat shock protein is the target of HLA-B27-restricted CTL response in Yersinia-induced reactive arthritis. *J Immunol* 1997; **159**: 5715–23.

66. Kuon W, Holzhutter HG, Appel H et al. Identification of HLA-B27-restricted peptides from the Chlamydia trachomatis proteome with possible relevance to HLA-B27-associated diseases. *J Immunol* 2001; **167**: 4738–46.

67. Sieper J, Kary S, Sorensen H et al. Oral type II collagen treatment in early rheumatoid arthritis. A double-blind, placebo-controlled, randomized trial. *Arthritis Rheum* 1996; **39**: 41–51.

68. Van Den Bosch F, Kruithof E, Baeten D et al. Randomized double-blind comparison of chimeric monoclonal antibody to tumor necrosis factor α (infliximab) versus placebo in active spondylarthropathy. *Arthritis Rheum* 2002; **46**: 755–65.

34

Systemic lupus erythematosus

George A Karpouzas and Bevra H Hahn

Overview • Biological therapies: non-specific targeting of T or B cells • Use of antigens to reduce quantities of antibodies to DNA and antibodies to phospholipids • Use of peptides to alter T cell interactions with anti-DNA-producing B cells: antigen-derived peptides • Targeting cell surface receptors that mediate second signals • Alteration of cytokine patterns as treatment for SLE • Therapeutic strategies employing cytokines • Therapeutic strategies involving complement proteins and inhibition of complement activation • References

OVERVIEW

Definition, patient characteristics and epidemiology

Systemic lupus erythematosus (SLE) is a multi-system disease caused by several autoantibodies and immune complexes. Disease manifestations depend upon the tissues targeted. Disease prevalence is approximately 8 females to 1 male in individuals aged 12–55 years (Table 34.1);[1] there is less female predominance in children and older adults – approximately 3 females to 1 male. SLE can begin at any age, but occur most frequently in females aged 16–45. SLE occurs in all ethnic groups; it is more prevalent and has a worse prognosis in African-American groups. Prevalence is estimated at 17–50 per 100 000 in American European Caucasian and European Caucasian females, compared to 60–280 per 100 000 in African American females.[1] Overall, the prevalence in the USA, northern Europe, New Zealand, Australia and Japan varies from 15 to 250 per 100 000.[1] Characteristics of SLE in a

cohort of patients gathered in the UCLA SLE Database are listed in Table 34.1.[2]

The clinical manifestations occurring in most patients include positive anti-nuclear antibodies (ANA), polyarthritis, dermatitis, hematologic manifestations (anemia/leukopenia/thrombocytopenia), and antibodies to double-stranded DNA (anti-dsDNA). Clinical nephritis varies from 20% to 50% in prevalence, depending upon the population characteristics of the patients described by different centers.

Disability, mortality and need for new therapies

Since SLE is a chronic incurable disease with substantial mortality, there is great interest in developing new therapeutic interventions. Chronic disability results partially from adverse effects of current non-specific anti-inflammatory and immunosuppressive therapies. These include obesity, hypertension, diabetes, infections, osteoporotic fractures and ischemic necrosis of bone related to chronic glucocorticoid

Table 34.1 Major clinical features of 473 SLE patients from the UCLA SLE database. Ethnicity is 57% Caucasian, 18% Asian, 12% Hispanic, 10% African-American, and 2% mixed.

Characteristics	Total
Age at diagnosis ± SD (years)	27 ± 10
Duration of Disease ± SD (years)	10 ± 7
Sex (F/M)	8:1
Clinical/laboratory features (%)	
ANA positive	98
Arthritis	82
Skin involvement	73
Hematologic disorders	61
Anti-dsDNA positive	70
Renal disease	45
Pleuritis	31
Pericarditis	16
Vasculitis	15
Psychosis/seizures	10
Secondary APS	8
Medication history (%)	
Corticosteroids	85
Antimalarials	72
Cytotoxic drugs	49
Anti-phospholipid syndrome	

ANA, anti-nuclear antibody.
APS, anti-phospholipid syndrome.

Table 34.2 The American College of Rheumatology 1982 revised criteria for classification of systemic lupus erythematosus.[3,84]

1. Malar rash
2. Discoid rash
3. Photosensitivity
4. Oral ulcers
5. Non-erosive arthritis
6. Pleuritis or pericarditis
7. Renal disorder
8. Seizures or psychosis
9. Hematologic disorder
10. Immunologic disorder
    (a) Anti-dsDNA
    (b) Anti-Sm
    (c) Anti-phospholipid
11. Positive anti-nuclear antibodies

Note: four or more criteria qualify the patient to be classified as having SLE.

Criteria for classification as SLE

The American College of Rheumatology has established classification criteria, facilitating communication between experts, updated in 1997,[3] and widely used internationally (Table 34.2). The specificity and sensitivity of these criteria are approximately 90% and 75%, respectively.

Measures of outcomes in patients with SLE

Approaches to measuring outcomes in SLE are critical to evaluating the validity of interventional trials in patients; however, the available methods are not ideal (Table 34.3). The most definitive outcome is death. Fortunately, mortality in all SLE patients in the first 10 years after diagnosis is only 7–30%. Ten-year mortality in this group is 7–15%. Since SLE is not a common disease, interventional studies cannot enroll enough patients, or follow them adequately

treatment, and infections, infertility and malignancies related to high cumulative doses of cytotoxic agents. Mortality ranges from 7% to 40% within 10 years of diagnosis.[1] Lower mortality rates are reported in Caucasian populations compared to African Americans, African Carribeans, and Latin Americans. Major causes of death in SLE are nephritis, vasculitis, central nervous system damage, infections, and thromboses. Thrombotic disease is related to antibodies to phospholipids and to accelerated atherosclerosis.[2]

Table 34.3   Outcome measures used to study SLE (most are reliable and valid).

Measure	Advantages	Disadvantages
Mortality	Definitive end point	Relatively infrequent
Renal function	Many features are definitive	Nephritis occurs in <50%

Disease activity:
  SLEDAI (SELENA modified)
  BILAG
  SLAM (revised)
  ECLAM
  Disease flare
	Combinations of clinical and laboratory disease manifestations, BILAG uses change in treatment as factor. Can be used in the absence of nephritis	Many components are somewhat subjective. Training of observers is required

Damage due to disease: SLICC/ACR	Defines irreversible organ damage. Nephritis not required	Does not distinguish damage produced from the disease from damage resulting from treatment
Health status: SF-36	Measures physical and emotional function, pain and general health	Cannot select factors specifically related to SLE
RIFLE	Measures change after introduction of intervention	Requires additional refinement and validation

SLEDAI, Systemic Lupus Erythematosus Disease Activity Index; BILAG, British Isles Lupus Assessment Group; SLAM, systemic lupus activity measure; ECLAM, European Consensus Lupus Activity Measure; SLICC, Systemic Lupus International Collaborating Clinics; ACR, American College of Rheumatology; SF-36, Short form-36; RIFLE, Responder Index for Lupus Erythematosus.

---

enough to use differences in mortality as a primary outcome. The effect of an intervention on renal disease, however, is a measurable outcome because of standard, widely accepted measures of renal function, such as serum levels of creatinine, glomerular filtration rates, and 24-h excretion of urinary protein. Since renal abnormalities are relatively easy to assess, and nephritis is a major cause of death, most of the studies setting the standard for treatment of all patients with SLE have been conducted in a subset of patients with nephritis. To address this problem, several instruments for evaluating extrarenal outcomes have been developed (Table 34.3). To date, there is no single laboratory or immunologic marker that alone is an accurate measure of disease activity, severity,

damage, or response to therapy. In 1998, an international group recommended that randomized controlled trials and longitudinal observational series for outcomes include a minimum of four domains: measures of disease activity, of health-related quality of life, of damage, and of toxicity/adverse events.[4,5]

Pathogenesis of SLE

SLE results from abnormally sustained immune responses occurring in an individual with genetic predisposition to SLE, probably in most cases after an environmental stimulus initiates an immune response. Female gender is an important predisposing factor, the basis of which is not understood.

Genetics

SLE is a multigenic disease,[6] with the possible exception of rare individuals who have homozygous deficiencies of a complement component, C1q, almost all of whom have developed SLE. Several groups have identified the same six chromosome regions in different cohorts of SLE patients containing gene(s) that increase risk for SLE. These regions are 1q22–24, 1q41–42, 2q37, 4p14–16, 6p11–22, and 16q12–13. In the HLA region on 6p11–22 are several susceptibility genes, including the complement components C2 and C4, the HLA antigens DR2 and DR3, and polymorphisms of tumor necrosis factor (TNF)-α. In the 1q22–24 region are FcγRIIIA and RIIA, which predispose primarily to lupus nephritis. Other genes known to increase risk are polymorphisms of IL-6 and of the promoter for IL-10; both cytokines increase B-cell maturation and antibody production.

Environmental factors

Environmental factors that may flare SLE or possibly cause it in some patients include ultraviolet light (UVB) and infections, particularly Epstein–Barr virus (EBV) infection.[7,8] In addition, female gender is permissive; sex hormones in women and men with lupus show increased metabolism of estrogenic compounds with sustained activity, and testosterone is metabolized to inactive forms. Such changes have multiple effects, probably including influences on the survival of immune cells.[9]

Autoantibodies of SLE and the source of antigens

Multiple autoantibodies are produced in patients and mice with SLE. Their targets include surface molecules on cells such as lymphocytes, erythrocytes and platelets, protein molecules that are altered and move from cytoplasm to surface during cell activation, and DNA–protein and RNA–protein complexes. DNA–protein and RNA–protein complexes in nuclei are 'hidden' from the immune system. However, during apoptosis they move to the cell surfaces encased in apoptotic blebs, which contain nucleosomes (probably the initial stimu-

lus resulting in antibodies to double-stranded DNA [dsDNA]), small nuclear spliceosomal ribonucleoproteins (RNPs) (recognized by antibodies to RNP and to Sm), and nuclear RNA–protein complexes recognized by antibodies to Ro (also called SSA, Sjögren's syndrome A antigen) and La (SSB, Sjögren's syndrome B antigen). During apoptosis, phospholipids 'flip' in the cell membrane so that antigenic portions of the molecule turn outwards towards the cell surface, thus presenting all these antigens to the immune system.[10] In SLE, apoptosis is enhanced and clearance of apoptotic cells impaired, abnormalities which probably enhance autoantibody production. In human SLE, anti-nuclear antibodies (ANAs) are the most prevalent autoantibodies (99%). However, ANAs occur in many inflammatory conditions, increase in prevalence with age, and have poor specificity for SLE. In contrast, certain autoantibodies are specific for the disease, such as IgG antibodies to Sm protein and to ds-DNA. Their prevalence is lower than that of ANAs – approximately 20% for anti-Sm and 70% for anti-dsDNA.[11] Others are pathogenic, such as subsets of antibodies to erythrocytes, to DNA, and to Ro-SSA. Probably, such antibodies are directly harmful to the tissues that they bind; in addition, immune complexes containing them can be trapped in tissues, fix complement, and initiate damage.[12] Antibodies to phospholipids, such as antibodies to cardiolipin, β2-glycoprotein1 (B2GP1), or lupus anticoagulant, are associated with increased risk of venous or arterial clotting and with fetal loss. As discussed below, some biologicals are targeted to reduce the quantities of specific autoantibodies of SLE, specifically anti-dsDNA and antiphospholipid.

B- and T-cell activation and regulation

Self-reactive B and T cells are present in the circulation of normal humans and mice. In normals, they are tightly regulated. The process of B- and T-lymphocyte activation has historically been described as a two-step phenomenon[13] (Figure 34.1). Optimal activation of antigen-specific lymphocytes requires antigen recognition by lymphocytes (signal 1) and additional or costim-

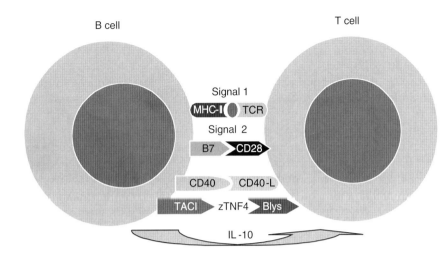

B cell

T cell

Signal 1

Signal 2

Figure 34.1 T-cell–B-cell cross-talk: the two-signal paradigm. Antigen presented to the T cell receptor (TCR) by the B cell receptor in the context of MHC antigen (signal 1). This causes upregulation of co-stimulatory molecules on the B cell surface (B.7 family molecules; CD40, TACI) that interact with their ligands (CD28, CD40-L and Blyss) on the T cell surface providing the signal 2 for full T cell activation. TACI, Transmembrane Activator and Calcium modulator and cyclophilin ligand Interactor.

ulatory signals (signal 2). Signal 1 is provided through the interaction of the B receptor with antigen, or T-cell receptor (TCR) with specific antigen, in the context of MHC molecules. Signal 2 is delivered to the T cell through upregulated surface expression of costimulatory molecules on the antigen-presenting cells (APCs), including B cells. This model actually oversimplifies the contribution of each signal, since the strength of the TCR signal has a quantitative influence on T-cell activation and differentiation. In fact, T-cell activation can occur in the absence of costimulation if the TCR signal is very strong.

Activation of B and T cells is generated after first signals by: (1) activation of CD28 on T cells linked to the B cell or other APC surface molecules B7.1 (CD80) or B7.2 (CD86); (2) interaction of CD40 on B or T cells with CD40 ligand (CD40L) on the opposite cell; and/or (3) interactions between Blys (also called BAFF, TALL or THANK) released by activated T cells with the TACI receptor on B cells.[14] When both signals are given, the B cell can either undergo activation and secrete immunoglobulin (Ig), or undergo activation-induced cell death (AICD) by apoptosis. Without the second signal, B and T cells are anergic.

In healthy individuals, B and T cells strongly reactive to self are deleted by AICD, following apoptotic signals via Fas and/or TNF receptors, or are rendered anergic.[15] Other autoreactive B

and T cells, probably those of low affinity, are quiescent due to lack of adequate antigenic stimulation or T-cell help.[15]

Autoreactive B cells are also subject to downregulation by CD4+CD25+ regulatory T cells[16] and cytotoxicity by CD8+ T cells.[17] Genetic defects in molecules that result in impaired functioning of these mechanisms of peripheral tolerance, i.e. Fas, TNF, cytotoxic T-lymphocyte antigen 4 (CTLA-4)/CD152, and transforming growth factor (TGF)-β, lead to autoimmunity.[18] There is evidence from transgenic mouse models[15] that the cells that initiate autoimmunity within the B-cell compartment are reactive to self, although generally of low affinity. They can be stimulated by self-antigen, or a cross-reactive epitope on an infecting or environmental agent, and then sustained by self-antigen. Provided that T-cell help is available, high-affinity B cells develop through somatic hypermutation and affinity maturation.

In mice and humans with SLE, genetic defects may result in heightened sensitivity of lymphocytes to stimulation by self-antigen[18] and heightened or prolonged response subsequent to activation.[19] Mapping studies in the NZM mouse model have identified chromosomal loci that segregate with enhanced T-cell activation and/or proliferation, and reduced AICD in the CD4+ compartment. Low-affinity ligands for TCR stimulate proliferation and enhance IL-2 production and activation marker expression in T cells of lupus-prone but not control mice. Moreover, T cells in SLE may not exhibit the same need for costimulation that is typical of immune responses to foreign antigen. Lupus-prone MRL/Fas[lpr] mice deficient in either B7-1 (CD80) or B7-2 (CD86) have similar phenotypes to B7[+/+] mice in terms of autoantibody production and nephritis.

Cognate T–B-cell interactions are a sine qua non of the positive-feedback autoimmune circuit in SLE. Anti-dsDNA antibody production in human and murine disease is heavily dependent on T-cell help.[20] Furthermore, studies of T-cell depletion by either antibodies or thymectomy[21] underscore the pivotal role of T cells in the initial expression and the natural course of the disease. Subsequent studies on genetic knockouts of T or B cells established the need for both subsets for the expression of disease.

BIOLOGICAL THERAPIES: NON-SPECIFIC TARGETING OF T OR B CELLS

Depletion or inactivation of CD4[+] T cells delays autoantibody production and nephritis, and prolongs survival in several mouse models of SLE. Wofsy et al[22] initially reported significant delays in autoantibody production and nephritis in (NZB × NZW) F1 mice, along with prolonged survival, when treated with a depleting monoclonal antibody (mAb) to Thy1.2. They reported similar results in MRL-Fas[lpr] and BXSB mice. Similarly, treatment of (NZW × BXSB) F1 mice with GK1.5, a cytotoxic mAb against CD4, resulted in survival rates at 6 months of age of 80%, compared to 30% in saline-treated controls. In contrast, administration of a depleting anti-CD8 mAb accelerated disease, with 0% survival.[23] Since mice can replace CD4[+] cells, even if thymectomized, they must be treated chronically with anti-CD4 to maintain survival.[21] Depleting or inactivating antibodies to CD4[+] cells are equally efficacious.

Okt3 is a humanized antibody similar to anti-Thy1: there is no published experience with this mAb in patients with SLE to date. Humanized monoclonal anti-lymphocyte antibodies against CD52 (e.g. Campath) have been administered to patients with rheumatoid arthritis.[24] CD52 is a glucose-6-phosphate isomerase (GPI)-anchored membrane glycolipid present on T and B lymphocytes, with weaker expression on monocytes. The arthritis in a proportion of patients improved measurably for varying periods (usually several weeks). CD4[+] cells were dramatically reduced in the peripheral blood, and a few serious infections occurred. However, CD4[+] cells in the target synovial tissues were not depleted. The substantial adverse effects of these antibodies outweigh their modest clinical benefits. No publications on the use of Campath or similar mAb in SLE have been found to date.

Depleting B cells with high, sustained weekly doses of anti-IgM prevented autoantibody production and glomerular and vascular immune complex-mediated lesions in (NZW × BXSB) F1 mice.[25] There has been interest in depleting B cells in humans as a therapy for SLE. A humanized monoclonal antibody to CD20 (Rituximab) – a surface molecule on mature B cells – has been approved for use in the treatment of B-cell lymphomas.[26] This mAb depletes peripheral blood mature CD19[+] CD20[+] B cells for up to 6 months. However, IgG levels and IgG antibody titers are usually not affected. The mAb probably does not affect long-lived plasma cells, which are probably the source of a substantial portion of pathogenic IgG autoantibodies in SLE. Nevertheless, there are case reports of substantial improvement in SLE patients after administration of Rituximab, particularly those with autoimmune cytopenias.[27] A phase I/II trial is in progress to determine the safety and potential efficacy of this treatment in SLE.

USE OF ANTIGENS TO REDUCE QUANTITIES OF ANTIBODIES TO DNA AND ANTIBODIES TO PHOSPHOLIPIDS

LJP394 – B-cell tolerogen for B cells making anti-DNA

Multivalent presentation of a B-cell epitope in the absence of T-cell epitopes can specifically tolerize

B cells (inducing anergy and/or apoptosis). Molecules presenting B cell epitopes in such a fashion, thus specifically suppressing antibody production, are called B-cell tolerogens. Antigen-specific suppression of antibody production after treatment with a tolerogen is specific B-cell tolerance. Potential therapeutic targets for such an approach are diseases characterized by autoantibodies with roles in the pathology, including SLE with nephritis (anti-dsDNA antibodies), clotting or fetal loss in individuals with antiphospholipid antibodies (primary or secondary antiphospholipid syndromes), myasthenia gravis (antiacetylcholine receptor antibodies), Graves' disease (anti-thyroid stimulating hormone receptor), and Rh hemolytic disease of the newborn (anti-Rh[D]).

LJP is a synthetic oligonucleotide conjugate[28–30] with four arms of synthetic double-stranded B-DNA, 20 base pairs each, attached through an aliphatic linker to a central branched platform of triethylene glycol. It was designed to promote B-cell anergy by providing a strong first signal, through crosslinking of surface anti-dsDNA receptors on the B cells, without a second signal (since it lacks T-cell epitopes).

Administration of LJP394 to male BSXB lupus mice suppressed anti-dsDNA-mediated pathologies. Premorbid mice treated with LJP394 300 µg intravenously or subcutaneously twice a week had significantly lower titers of serum anti-dsDNA, less proteinuria ($P < 0.05$), and milder renal pathology ($P < 0.05$), and lived significantly longer than saline-treated controls ($P < 0.05$). Based on the above observations, a phase I clinical trial of LJP394 was conducted in humans, establishing its safety and tolerability as an intravenously administered compound in healthy volunteers. It was well tolerated as a single (100 mg IV) or multiple infusions in lupus patients with high titers of anti-dsDNA. Treatment was associated with a rapid initial reduction of anti-DNA antibodies – within 1 h of infusion – suggesting that LJP394 formed immune complexes with anti-DNA antibodies, which were rapidly cleared.[29,30] After single infusions, recovery of the anti-DNA titers was observed between 14 and 28 days. Prolonged reduction was seen in some patients.

In a subsequent phase II, randomized, multicenter, double-blind, placebo-controlled study of 63 patients with stable disease, including nephritis, optimal dosing regimens for maximal suppression of anti-DNA antibodies were determined.[29] Once again, an immediate reduction in serum anti-dsDNA antibodies was observed. However, the effect was maintained for up to 8 weeks after the conclusion of the trial, suggesting an additional mechanism such as the B-cell tolerance observed in the BXSB mice. Additionally, it was shown that patients with pretreatment antibodies with high affinity for LJP394 exhibited greater serologic responses, as well as dose-dependent reduction in affinity, by the end of the study.[29] This information enables clinicians to prospectively define patients who are most likely to exhibit a desirable pharmacodynamic response to the drug, by using a pretreatment anti-DNA affinity assay. Subsequently, analysis of a multicenter, randomized, placebo-controlled, international, phase II/III clinical trial in patients with recent but stable lupus nephritis showed that patients with high-affinity IgG antibodies to LJP394 had clinical benefits, including increased time to and reduced number of renal flares, and increased time to institution of high-dose steroids and/or cyclophosphamide. An additional trial is in progress.

LJP993 – B-cell tolerogen for antibodies to phospholipids

Primary and secondary antiphospholipid antibody syndromes are characterized by venous and/or arterial thrombosis, thrombocytopenia, and fetal loss, with well-established roles of anti-cardiolipin (ACL) and anti-β_2GPI antibodies in the syndrome pathology. β_2GPI has been implicated as the natural antigen of what have been historically referred to as anti-cardiolipin antibodies. The discovery that domain 1 of β_2GPI was cross-reactive with patient anti-β_2GPI antibodies led to efforts aimed at developing a multivalent construct of this native polypeptide sequence as a tolerogen for autoimmune thrombosis. A tetravalent conjugate of the domain 1 of β_2GPI was synthesized (LJP993), and studies are in progress. To date, we have learned that LJP993 binds purified anti-B2GPI ACL in various assays. Furthermore, when used to immunize mice, LJP993 generates an immune response against domain 1 of GPI, and it induces peptide-specific tolerance in vivo. Phase I studies in humans are planned.

USE OF PEPTIDES TO ALTER T CELL INTERACTIONS WITH ANTI-DNA-PRODUCING B CELLS: ANTIGEN-DERIVED PEPTIDES

Peptides from nucleosomes

T cells of lupus-prone mice are primed very early in life to autoantigens, and respond to them in vitro by proliferation and by surface expression of CD40L. However, their capacity to provide help to B cells for antibody production is a maturational process and coincides temporally with the class switch from IgM to IgG anti-dsDNA antibodies. Nucleosomes are natural byproducts of apoptotic cell death. The normal immune system does not develop responses to nucleosomes. However, if they are presented in an inflammatory context, in excessive amounts, or if clearance of apoptotic materials is impaired, excessive quantities of antibodies to nucleosomes may arise.[31] Nucleosomal antigens are recognized by T cells in murine and human SLE, with antibodies to nucleosomes upon affinity maturation contributing to the IgG anti-dsDNA repertoire characteristic of clinical disease. Individuals predisposed to lupus undergo spontaneous expansion of nucleosome-reactive T cells, which have been identified in patients with SLE and in some B cells from apoptosis.[32] Immunodominant epitopes for murine T cells have been mapped in the core histones of nucleosomes at amino acid positions 1–33 of H2B, and 16–39 and 71–94 of H4, and in H1 in SNF1 (SWR × NZB) F1 mice.[31] Subcutaneous administration of these peptides in complete Freund's adjuvant (CFA) in young pre-nephritic mice activates predominantly Th1 cells, providing help for accelerated anti-DNA production and clinical

nephritis. If these peptides are administered tolerogenically (high doses given intravenously or intraperitoneally), there is a significant delay in appearance of multiple autoantibodies and clinical nephritis. Similarly in old nephritic mice, administration of a peptide from histone 4 (H4 16–39) results in a significant survival benefit over saline- or control peptide-treated mice. H4 16–39 is an efficient tolerogen for both T and B cells. The exact mechanisms are unknown. Most importantly, histone T-cell immunodominant determinants have been identified in patients with SLE. Human and murine histones are identical in sequence. Many SLE patients can recognize some of these determinants, even with the DR and DQ heterogeneity that occurs among these individuals. Remarkably, the determinants recognized by human T cells overlap the major determinants that stimulate T cells in SNF1 mice.[31]

There are several potential benefits of nucleosomal peptide tolerance. First, some of the peptides prolong survival in SNF1 mice. Second, tolerance apparently spreads to different Th subsets, so that antibodies to DNA and to other lupus-related autoantigens are suppressed. Third, glomerulonephritis is significantly delayed. The spreading of tolerance is due to both promiscuity and degeneracy in the TCR repertoire. Promiscuity refers to the ability of a single TCR to recognize a single epitope presented by different MHCs. Degeneracy refers to the ability of a single TCR to recognize multiple peptide epitopes presented by a single MHC. Promiscuity and degeneracy may be, at least in part, attributed to the charged residues present on both TCRs and peptides, accounting for the MHC-dependent, but unrestricted, recognition. Thus, either immune recognition or immune tolerance can spread from specificity of a clone of T cells for the initiating stimulus to multiple different T-cell subsets recognizing multiple different peptides. The utility of this result in managing autoimmune disease would depend on whether that engagement of additional T cells mediates stimulatory or inhibitory responses and how many different autoantibodies could be targeted. A single Th lupus clone can help either a dsDNA-specific, or a histone-specific, high-mobility protein (HMG, high mobility globin) specific or a nucleosome-specific B cell. This is probably because each of these individual B-cell subsets can bind intact chromatin with their individual surface receptors, and internalize, process and present the relevant peptide epitopes to the respective T cells. Therefore, inducing tolerance in a few T cells may affect help for many different B cells, and also prevent the determinant spreading that occurs as immune responses expand.

Many additional attempts to induce effective antigen-specific tolerizing therapies in lupus mouse models have been made and are reviewed below.

Peptides from Smith (Sm) antigen complex

Smith (Sm), is a well-characterized complex antigen consisting of nine different proteins based on patterns of electrophoretic mobility: B1, B2, B3, D1, D2, D3, D4, E, F, and G, representing the core proteins of the U1, U2, U4, U5, U6, U7, U11 and U12 small nuclear ribonucleoproteins (RNPs). Sm is highly conserved evolutionarily and is ubiquitously expressed. It is part of the spliceosomal complex, whose role is the splicing of the precursor mRNA to mature mRNA, and has an essential role in spliceosomal complex formation.[11,33] High-affinity anti-Sm antibodies are highly specific for SLE, with a prevalence of 5–25% in patients. They are usually of the IgG subclass, suggesting dependence on T cell help. T-cell immunity against Sm has been described in peripheral blood mononuclear cells (PBMCs) and lymphoid tissues of both SLE patients and mice.[34] Sm-reactive T cells demonstrate highly restricted TCR usage, characteristic of an antigen-driven response. Sm-reactive T clones exhibit the typical T-cell phenotype CD4[+], CD45RO[+], TCRab[+], and produce cytokines critical for T- and B-cell help and differentiation, including IL-2, interferon (IFN)-γ and IL-4 (Riemekasten, personal communication). SmD1 appears to be the most frequently

recognized peptide in the molecule. It is remarkably conserved and bears a 99% homology with the mouse D1 protein. The epitope $SmD1_{83-119}$ appears to be recognized with remarkable sensitivity and specificity by human SLE sera (70% in SLE versus 8.3% in healthy controls and other autoimmune diseases), possibly due to its highly positive charge and its conformation.[33]

In conclusion, $SmD1_{83-119}$ is very effective both as an immunogen and as a tolerogen in lupus-prone mice, is specifically recognized by T cells in both mice and humans, and provides B-cell help for both anti-dsDNA and anti-Sm antibody production. Therefore, it could represent a potential therapeutic target in human disease.

Peptides from autoantibody immunoglobulin (Ig peptides) as tolerogens

B cells can process their surface Ig and present Ig-derived peptides in surface MHC molecules.[35] Endogenous Ig peptides have been identified in MHC class I and II molecules of humans and mice.[36,37] Therefore, it is likely that both mice and humans with SLE help sustain production of autoantibodies by continuous T/B signalling via presentation of such processed peptides from Ig of the autoantibody itself. Several groups have shown that the VH regions of Ig molecules contain peptides that can induce T- and B-cell immune responses.[38–40] When administered as immunogens, such peptides can accelerate the appearance of autoantibodies and nephritis in lupus mice. When they are administered as tolerogens, significant delays in autoantibody production and in nephritis, with significant prolongation of survival, have been reported.[40,41] One group[38] has shown that administration of peptide from the CDR1 region of a murine mAb anti-dsDNA, or another from the CDR3 region, can delay disease in a murine lupus model induced by vaccination with the 16/6 idiotype, or in the spontaneous lupus of NZB/NZW F1 (BWF1) mice. Our group[39,40] has defined a group of 12-mer and 15-mer peptides located in the CDR1/FR2, FR2/CDR2 and FR3/CDR3 regions

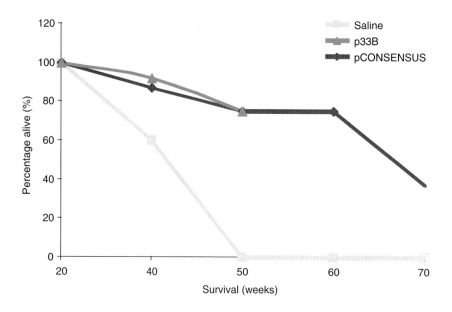

Figure 34.2 Effects of peptide-induced tolerance on survival. Ten-week old premorbid BWF1 female mice were tolerized with 1 mg IV of either pCONSENSUS, p33B or saline every month, and followed longitudinally for survival. Treatment with pCONSENSUS and p33B conferred a significant survival advantage, compared to saline-treated controls.

of several different murine mAb IgG anti-DNAs that are recognized spontaneously by T cells of young BWF1 females. Upon immunization with the peptides, disease is accelerated and mice die 6 weeks earlier than expected. In contrast, administration of 1000 µg intravenously once a month of several of the T-cell-stimulating Ig peptides delays disease significantly.[39,40] An artificial peptide derived from sequences of T-cell stimulatory peptides throughout the VH region of a mAb anti-DNA, labeled 'pConsensus', was even more effective, and prolonged survival by 30 weeks (Figure 34.2). Mechanisms by which these Ig peptides delay autoantibody production are under active investigation and are related in part to their ability to prevent the release of IFN-γ and IL-4, which herald the onset of clinical nephritis.[41]

The utility of Ig-peptide-induced tolerance in humans with SLE has been suggested by observations that SLE patients have T cells in their peripheral blood that are activated by peptides derived from Ig molecules of human antibodies to DNA.[41–43] Such T cells are more frequent in patients with SLE than in healthy controls, and they induce release of cytokines associated with

both human and murine lupus, such as IFN-γ, IL-4, and IL-10.

Prevention of murine lupus by administering peptides bound by anti-DNA

Several peptides have been identified that are mimotopes for anti-DNA.[42–44] That is, the peptides are members of a peptide library, which are bound by an anti-DNA mAb. The ability of one such mimotope, RLTSSLRYNPA, to bind mAb anti-dsDNA can be inhibited by ssDNA, dsDNA, and native RNA. It is possible that antibodies arising to these natural peptide epitopes use structural Ig genes that encode antibodies cross-reactive with DNA, or that are prone to develop anti-DNA reactivity after minimal somatic mutation. Some mimotopes administered as immunogens to mice can induce multiple lupus-like autoantibodies and clinical disease.[43] At least one has been administered in soluble form and has prevented deposition of pathogenic peptide-recognizing Ig in glomeruli, thus protecting lupus-prone mice from disease.[45] To date, treatment with peptide mimotopes of anti-DNA has not been tested clinically.

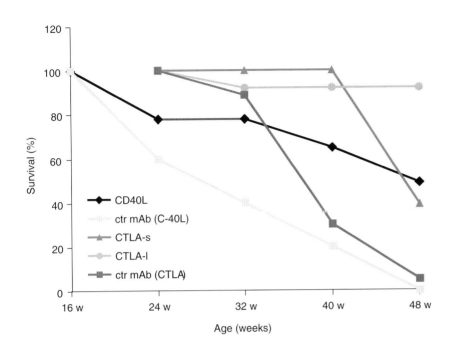

Figure 34.3 Effects of second signal blockade on disease survival in murine lupus. Data pooled from different studies not directly comparing all presented therapeutic approaches.

TARGETING CELL SURFACE RECEPTORS THAT MEDIATE SECOND SIGNALS

Other potential targets for biologicals to treat SLE include the signals between T and B cells which result in activation of either or both cell types.

Targeting CD28–B7 Interactions

CD28 interacting with B7.1 (CD80) and B7.2 (CD 86) provide second signals that result in T-cell activation and B-cell secretion of Ig (Figure 34.3). CD28 is a homodimeric glycoprotein on T cells. Antibodies to CD28 inhibit proliferative responses of CD4+ T cells to allogeneic cells and to soluble Ag-presenting non-T cells, and they inhibit T-helper-supported differentiation of B cells into Ig-secreting cells. Thus, interfering with CD28–B7 interactions should prevent autoantibody production and SLE. In the murine chronic graft-versus-host model of lupus, transfer of parental T spleen cells from CD28−/− donors protected F1 recipients from developing B-cell activation, autoantibodies, and immune glomerulonephritis.[46] Compared to genetically intact MRL/Fas[lpr] mice, CD28−/− MSRL/Fas[lpr] animals produced less IgG anti-DNA and rheumatoid factor and developed later immune glomerulonephritis, even though abnormal B220+ TCR-α/β T cells expanded and IgM autoantibody production was unchanged.[32] In the same MRL/Fas[lpr] model, animals deficient in B7-1 or B7-2 made IgG antibodies to snRNP and DNA. Compared to wild mice, the B7-1−/− mice developed more severe nephritis mediated by IgG and C3 complement deposition in glomeruli, but the B7-2−/− mice had less nephritis.[47] Overall, ligation of CD28 contributes to T-cell activation, whereas ligation of CTLA-4, which also binds B7-1 and B7-2, and with higher avidity than CD28, inactivates T cells. Therefore, all interventions must take this interplay into account. In murine lupus, delay of disease in young mice was achieved by administration of B-7-binding fusion protein, CTLA-4–Ig. The protein was generated by genetic fusion of the extracellular domain of murine CTLA-4 to the Fc portion of a mouse Ig_{2a} monoclonal antibody (muCTLA-4–Ig). In BWF1 mice, treatment with CTLA-4–Ig delayed autoantibody production and nephritis and significantly improved survival,[48] as it did in BXSB mice and in mice with chronic graft-versus-host disease (GVHD).[49] Expression of the fusion protein 'induced by gene delivery' is also effective in MRL/Fas[lpr] and BWF1 murine lupus.[50] The suppression of disease is more effective in mice with established nephritis if CTLA-4–Ig is given continuously, or combined with blockade of the CD40/CD40L second signal pathway, or combined with non-specific immunosuppression by cyclophosphamide.[51,52] Binding of B7-1 and B7-2 by CTLA-4–Ig probably prevents T-cell activation via CD28 and therefore reduces B-cell activation; however, reducing quantities of the ligand for CTLA-4 probably helps prevent T-cell downregulation – thus this therapeutic approach may be a two-edged sword.

A chimeric CTLA-4–Ig fusion protein (BMS-188667) is available and has been administered to patients with stable psoriasis vulgaris.[53] The skin lesions improved by approximately 50%, and this was associated with a reduction in the number of T cells infiltrating the skin. Immunologic tolerance to T-cell-dependent neo-antigens was not induced, but responses to the antigens were lower than expected. At least one controlled prospective trial of CTLA-4–Ig in patients with SLE has been planned but is not underway at the time of this writing.

Targeting CD40–CD40L interactions (gp39, CD154)

CD40–CD40L interaction provides a second signal that allows activation of both T and B cells. The interaction is of great importance in SLE. CD4+ and CD8+ T cells from SLE patients and mice express increased quantities of CD40L compared to healthy controls, and the expression of CD40L persists for longer, suggesting prolonged 'ready to be activated' status of the T cells.[54] Another effect of this sustained expression may be that apoptosis in multiple CD40-expressing cells (such as dendritic cells or endothelial cells) is potentiated (thus making more antigen available as well as damaging cells), while activation of B cells is promoted. In addition, B cells from murine and human SLE

individuals also express CD40L, which is considered aberrant. Normal mice modified by transgenes to express CD40L on B cells developed autoantibodies, and approximately 50% developed immune glomerulonephritis.

Treatment of SNF1 mice with monoclonal antibody to CD40L delayed the appearance of autoantibodies and nephritis. As with CTLA-4–Ig, long-term treatment is required to prevent disease or to suppress it, if treatment is started after clinical nephritis appears.[55]

Humanized monoclonal antibody to CD40L has been made. A phase I trial in patients with SLE indicated that repeated intravenous administration of one of these products (IDEC-131) is safe and that inactivating antibodies do not arise.[56] A later study compared responses of SLE patients to IDEC-131 against placebo; however, results have not been published.

Targeting BLyS–TACI interactions

Activated T cells express two additional members of the TNFR family that influence B-cell activation: APRIL and BLyS (also known as TALL-1, THANK and zTNF4), the latter of which is an abbreviation for 'B-lymphocyte stimulator'.[57] BLyS is released as a soluble factor and binds at least two receptors on B cells: BCMA ('B-cell maturation antigen') and TACI ('transmembrane activator and calcium modulator and cyclophilin ligand interactor'). BLyS seems to be critical to full B-cell activation. Mice transgenic for BLyS show B220+ B-cell accumulation in spleen, lymph nodes and Peyer's patches, and B-cell activation with increases in total IgM, IgG, IgA and IgE. They develop ANA and lupus-like nephritis.[58] TACI[-/-] mice also show increased B-cell accumulation and splenomegaly; their B cells produce increased quantities of Ig, both spontaneously and after immunization with specific antigen.[59] Circulating levels of BLys are elevated in BWF1 and MRL/Fas[lpr] mice, and in some patients with SLE, especially those with high titers of anti-DNA.[60]

BWF1 mice treated with a TACI–Ig fusion protein had significant delay in the appearance of proteinuria and significant prolongation of survival. A monoclonal antibody to BLys is under development and is likely to enter phase I trials soon.[61]

ALTERATION OF CYTOKINE PATTERNS AS TREATMENT FOR SLE

TNF-α

Whether TNF-α itself is safe to target in SLE patients is debatable. Lupus-prone mice derived from the NZW strain have an MHC haplotype that includes a TNF-α polymorphism, which encodes for production of unusually low quantities of TNF-α.[62] Furthermore, administration of TNF-α to young BWF1 mice delayed the development of SLE. An extended haplotype in humans (containing DR2 and/or DQw1) that predisposes some ethnic groups to SLE also contains polymorphisms of TNF-α associated with low production of the cytokine.

Knockout of TNF-α promotes autoimmunity on susceptible genetic backgrounds. Although NZB mice have milder autoimmune disease than BWF1 hybrids, F1 hybrids of NZB crossed with Tnf$^{-/-}$ mice developed enhanced autoimmunity and severe renal disease similar to BWF1 females.[63] On the other hand, serum levels of TNF-α and of soluble TNF receptors p55 and p75 are elevated in patients with SLE compared to healthy matched controls,[64] and may correlate with disease activity, anti-DNA, and other markers of inflammation such as C-reactive protein (CRP). TNF-α and interleukin (IL)-1β are both increased in renal lesions in murine and human SLE. Finally, some studies in murine lupus have shown that chronic administration of TNF-α accelerates lupus. Therefore, there may be some patients with SLE in whom downregulating TNF-α would be clinically beneficial.

IL-1 and IL-1ra

Data regarding IL-1 in murine and human SLE are confusing. Perhaps the clearest picture comes from sequential studies of MRL/Fas^{lpr} mice.[65] At an age when autoantibodies began to appear (14 weeks), serum levels of TNF-α increased; later, at 20 weeks, serum levels of IL-1α and IL-1β increased. Each cytokine in vivo upregulated expression of intercellular adhesion molecule-1 (ICAM-1) and vascular cellular adhesion molecule-1 (VCAM-1) on endothelial cells in lung, kidney, brain, and heart. By the time that disease was full-blown, administration of antibodies to both cytokines was required to suppress this activation of endothelial cells. This requirement for dual targeting may explain why treatment of BWF1 mice with IL-1 receptor antagonist (IL-1ra) reduced the degree of nephritis but did not prevent or reverse it. In patients with SLE, serum levels of IL-1ra may correlate with active disease, particularly extrarenal.[66] Low levels during nephritis flares suggest that IL-1/IL-1ra pathways may be activated in target tissue, which is supported by finding IL-1 in renal lesions in lupus mice. In summary, IL-1 and its regulators play a role in SLE.

Th1 and Th2 phenotypes: are they pertinent to SLE? IL-2, IFN-γ, IL-4, IL-6 and IL-10

Since Th1 cells generally support cell-mediated reactions, whereas Th2 cells give help to B cells for antibody production, there has been great interest in the possibility that skewing towards Th2 plays a major role in murine and human SLE. Such skewing has been suggested by the fact that T cells from BWF1 and MRL/Fas^{lpr} mice secrete less IL-2 as the mice age, with a decrease in IL-2 receptors on T-cell surfaces. However, most studies have shown that onset of disease is heralded by increases in IFN-γ, as well as IL-4,[40] suggesting involvement of both Th1 and Th2 cells. In our colonies of BWF1 mice, dramatic increases in plasma levels of IFN-γ and IL-4 occur at the time when high levels of IgG anti-DNA appear.[40] Since the dominant isotype eluted from glomerular lesions is IgG$_{2a}$, which depends on IFN-γ for its synthesis, Th1 cells (or Th0) may be important in inducing disease. In addition, our laboratory has accelerated disease in young BWF1 mice by the transfer of either Th1 or Th2 cell lines, implying that both subsets play important pathogenic roles. IL-6, secreted by Th2 and B cells, potentiates autoantibody formation. Administration of IL-6 accelerates disease, and antibodies to IL-6 delay it.[67] IL-10, made predominantly by monocyte–macrophages, is also important, is increased in sera and lymphoid tissues of mice and humans with SLE, and shifts repertoires from Th1 towards Th2, probably by suppressing IL-6. Indeed, administration of anti-IL-10 delays disease in BW mice.[68]

There is a large amount of data regarding levels of various Th1 and Th2 cytokines in serum, in mRNA of lymphoid cells, and secreted by peripheral blood cells in human SLE.[69] There is little agreement between studies, with the exception of IL-10; most have shown IL-10 levels to be elevated in serum from patients, as well as increased IL-10 mRNA and IL-10 secretion by PBMCs of these patients.[69,70] IL-10 is made by macrophages, T cells and B cells. It is a potent stimulator of B-cell differentiation and proliferation, attenuates production of Th1 cytokines and MHC class II expression, can induce anergy in CD4+ T cells, and can inhibit or stimulate CD8+ T cells. Serum levels of IL-10 correlate positively with disease activity and severity. It is the authors' opinion, based on recent studies in our UCLA cohort, that PBMNCs from SLE patients, when stimulated by specific self-antigens, are more likely than healthy matched controls to release IFN-γ and IL-10 in early disease, and to release IL-4 and IL-10 when disease has been present for 10 years or more.[71] These data are consistent with the widely held hypothesis that Th1 cells are important in induction and Th2 in maintenance of disease. On the other hand, it is likely that cells secreting these cytokines play regulatory roles, and responses measured after disease onset reflect both pathogenic and protective responses.

Defective regulatory cells in SLE and transforming growth factor beta (TGF-β)

TGF-β can mediate suppression, which is critical to controlling SLE-like immune responses. There is evidence that regulatory cells, which ordinar-

ily suppress activated T and/or B cells, are defective or missing in both murine and human SLE. These include CD8+, double-negative T cells, and natural killer (NK) T cells. CD8+ suppressor T cells behave abnormally.[72] In our colonies, total numbers of CD8+ cells in BWF1 mice decrease over time and are significantly reduced by the time that nephritis is full-blown. In SLE patients, the ability to produce TGF-β, both total and active, is impaired, and levels are lower than in matched healthy controls. Generation of cytotoxic CD8+ cells capable of downregulating B cells making autoantibodies requires priming of CD4+ precursors with IL-2 and TGF-β, the main source of which is NK cells.[73] Approximately 80% of patients with SLE are deficient in type I protein kinase A phosphotransferase activity in T lymphocytes related to a disorder of translation: correction of the PKA-RI deficiency in cells in vitro significantly increases IL-2 production.[74] It is possible that this subset of patients cannot generate appropriate CD8+ suppressor cells to control autoantibody production. The CD4+CD25+ regulatory T-cell subset mediates downregulation via membrane-fixed TGF-β.[75] There is recent evidence that double-negative NK T cells, which are non-HLA-specific killer T cells, are also reduced in number and function in patients with SLE. Some regulatory/suppressor cells exert their effects via TGF-β while others secrete IFN-γ or IL-10. It is possible that restoring the balance between these 'regulatory' cytokines and 'proinflammatory' cytokines will be helpful in the treatment of SLE.

THERAPEUTIC STRATEGIES EMPLOYING CYTOKINES

Manipulation of cytokines affecting T cells, B cells or target tissue alters murine lupus. Furthermore, gene therapies attempted in SLE were designed to manipulate cytokine levels in mouse models. As mentioned earlier, defects in IL-2 production and surface display of IL-2 receptors characterize many of the murine strains of spontaneous SLE and some patients. Replacing IL-2 might permit emergence of appropriate regulatory/suppressive cells and prevent emergence of Th2 cells that promote antibody production. Inoculation of MRL/Fas[lpr] mice with a live vaccinia recombinant virus expressing the human IL-2 gene prolonged survival and reduced autoantibody levels and nephritis.[76] In addition, oral administration of attenuated *Salmonella* carrying the gene for murine IL-2 to MRL/Fas[lpr] mice suppressed autoantibody production and nephritis.[77] However, in another study, gene therapy that provided IL-2 monthly, so that serum levels were elevated, worsened SLE in the same mouse lupus model. Treatment with drugs that inhibit IL-2, such as cyclosporin and FK506, is beneficial in murine and human lupus. Since some gene-carrying vectors are immunostimulatory, the benefits of manipulating IL-2 alone (in the absence of vector effects) as a treatment for SLE remain an open question.

In contrast, inhibition of IFN-γ has been successful for the most part in suppressing SLE in several murine strains. In BWF1 mice, most of the pathogenic anti-DNA are IgG$_{2a}$, an isotype depending on IFN-γ for its synthesis. There are high levels of mRNA for both IFN-γ and IL-10 in lymphoid tissues. Administration of IFN-γ worsens murine SLE in BW mice; administration of antibodies to IFN-γ or soluble IFN-γ receptors to BW mice before disease begins significantly prolongs survival and diminishes immunoglobulin deposition and lymphocytic infiltration of kidneys.[78,79] Gene therapy of MRL-Fas[lpr] mice with intramuscular injections of plasmids containing cDNA encoding IFN-γR–Fc molecules resulted in reduced serum levels of IFN-γ, autoantibodies, lymphoid hyperplasia, and glomerulonephritis, with prolonged survival.[80] Genetic deletion of IFN-γ receptor significantly delays nephritis in BW mice, although the mice developed lethal lymphomas at 1 year of age. On the other hand, one group administered plasmid encoding IL-12 to MRL-Fas[lpr] mice, resulting in elevated serum levels of IFN-γ; nevertheless, there was reduction in proteinuria and histologic glomerulonephritis.[81] This illustrates the complexity of cytokine networks.

Inhibition of IL-4 in mice transgenic for IL-4 prevented the glomerulosclerosis that occurs in these mice. There is at least one published study in which mAb anti-IL-10 was administered to patients with SLE. In a small, open-label trial, the disease activity index improved in all patients without major adverse effects. However, inactivating antibodies developed. A solution to this problem will probably trigger additional studies with anti-IL-10, since, by general agreement, its overexpression is characteristic of many patients with SLE.

As discussed above, the effects of TGF-β are complex and vary between suppressing and enhancing inflammatory responses. Administration of a gene encoding TGF-β to BWF1 mice increased serum levels of that cytokine and prolonged survival. On the other hand, administering the gene in *Salmonella typhimurium* to MRL/Fas[lpr] mice provided no improvement.

THERAPEUTIC STRATEGIES INVOLVING COMPLEMENT PROTEINS AND INHIBITION OF COMPLEMENT ACTIVATION

A predisposition to lupus in the face of genetic defects involving complement proteins, including C1q, C2, and C4, is well accepted. Previous reports showed that several C5-deficient NZB-derived inbred mouse strains, as well as C5-deficient SNF1 mice, develop immune complex nephritis, and this has been cited as evidence against a role for complement in BWF1 autoimmune disease. In an elegant study, Wang et al[82] demonstrated that complement inhibition with an anti-C5 monoclonal antibody, given biweekly, in the BWF1 mouse for 6 months significantly delayed proteinuria, improved kidney histology, reduced kidney disease, and increased survival, despite the ability of the mice to generate similar levels of anti-DNA antibodies. To our knowledge, there are no published data on anti-C5 mAb in clinical trials involving humans.

Primary and secondary antiphospholipid antibody syndromes are characterized by venous and/or arterial thrombosis, thrombocytopenia, and fetal loss, with well-established roles of ACL and anti-β$_2$GPI antibodies in the syndrome pathology. Holers et al[83] demonstrated in a mouse model that complement C3 activation is required for antiphospholipid antibody-induced fetal loss. They showed that mice injected intraperitoneally with affinity-purified human APL–IgG at days 8 and 12 of gestation exhibited evidence of significant fetal resorption and decreased fetal weight by day 15 of gestation, with significant deposition of C3 on the decidual layers and inflammatory infiltration, as compared to controls injected with an irrelevant hIgG. C3$^{-/-}$ mice were protected from the effects of the APL–IgG. Moreover, administration of Crry–Ig (fusion protein of C3 convertase inhibitor complement receptor 1-related gene/protein y with the Fc of a mouse IgG$_1$) intraperitoneally, concomitantly with APL–IgG, prevented complement activation and C3 deposition in the decidua, and inhibited fetal resorption and fetal loss. They also demonstrated that aPL–IgG-induced thrombophilia was inhibited by Crry–Ig by virtue of a decrease in the thrombus size in a mouse model of surgically induced thrombus formation. No data on Crry–Ig in human disease have been published to date.

ACKNOWLEDGMENTS

Dr Karpouzas is supported by the Mitchell Family Foundation. Portions of work discussed were supported by awards from the Public Health Service, R37 AI 46776, RO1 AR 43814, P60 AR 38834, and awards from the Arthritis Foundation Southern California Chapter and from the Paxson Family and the Dorough Foundation.

REFERENCES

1. Rus V, Hochberg MC. The epidemiology of systemic lupus erythematosus. In: Wallace DJ, Hahn BH, eds. *Dubois' Lupus Erythematosus*, 6th edn (Lippincott Williams & Wilkins: Philadelphia, 2002) 65–83.

2. Cervera R, Kamashta MA, Font J et al. Morbidity and mortality in systemic lupus erythematosus during a 5-year period. A multicenter prospective study of 1,000 patients. European Working Party on Systemic Lupus Erythematosus. *Medicine (Baltimore)* 1999; **78**: 167–75.

3. Hochberg MC. Updating the American College of Rheumatology revised criteria for the classification of systemic lupus erythematosus. *Arthritis Rheum* 1997; **40**: 1725.

4. Grossman JM, Kalunian KC. Definition, classification, activity, and damage indices. In: Wallace DJ, Hahn BH, eds. *Dubois' Lupus Erythematosus*, 6th edn (Lippincott Williams & Wilkins: Philadelphia, 2002) 19–31.

5. Smolen J, Strand V, Cardiel M et al. Randomized clinical trials and longitudinal observational studies in systemic lupus erythematosus: consensus on a preliminary core set of outcome domains. *J Rheumatol* 1999; **26**: 504–7.

6. Tsao BP, Hahn BH. Systemic lupus erythematosus. In: Rimoin DL, Connor JM, Pyeritz RE, Korf BR, eds. *Emery and Rimoin's Principles and Practice of Medical Genetics*, 4th edn (Churchill Livingsone: London, 2002) 2012–27.

7. Wysenbeck AJ, Block DA, Fries JF. Prevalence and expression of photosensitivity in SLE. *Rheum Dis* 1989; **48**: 461.

8. James JA, Neas BR, Moser KL et al. Systemic lupus erythematosus in adults is associated with previous Epstein–Barr virus exposure. *Arthritis Rheum* 2001; **44**(5): 1122–6.

9. Lahita RG. Emerging concepts for sexual predilection in the disease systemic lupus erythematosus. *Ann NY Acad Sci* 1999; **876**: 64–9.

10. Pickering MC, Botto M, Taylor PR, Lachmann PJ, Walport MJ. Systemic lupus erythematosus, complement deficiency, and apoptosis. *Adv Immunol* 2000; **76**: 227–324.

11. Tan EM. Autoantibodies and autoimmunity: a three-decade perspective. A tribute to Henry G. Kunkel. *Ann NY Acad Sci.* 1997 **5**(815): 1–14.

12. Hahn BH. Antibodies to DNA. *N Engl J Med* 1998; **338**(19): 1359–68.

13. Bernard A, Lamy And L, Alberti I. The two-signal model of T-cell activation after 30 years. *Transplantation* 2002; **7**(1 Suppl.): S31–5.

14. Mackay F, Mackay CR. The role of BAFF in B-cell maturation, T-cell activation and autoimmunity. *Trends Immunol* 2002; **23**(3): 113–5.

15. Goodnow CC, Glynne R, Akkaraju S et al.

Autoimmunity, self-tolerance and immune homeostasis: from whole animal phenotypes to molecular pathways. *Adv Exp Med Biol* 2001; **490**: 33–40.

16. Nakamura K, Kitani A, Strober W. Cell contact-dependent immunosuppression by CD4(+) CD25(+) regulatory T cells is mediated by cell surface-bound transforming growth factor beta. *J Exp Med* 2001; **194**(5): 629–44.

17. Linker-Israeli M, Quismorio FP Jr, Horwitz DA. CD8+ lymphocytes from patients with systemic lupus erythematosus sustain, rather than suppress, spontaneous polyclonal IgG production and synergize with CD4+ cells to support autoantibody synthesis. *Arthritis Rheum.* 1990; **33**(8): 1216–25.

18. Morel L, Croker BP, Blenman KR et al. Genetic reconstitution of systemic lupus erythematosus immunopathology with polycongenic murine strains. *Proc Natl Acad Sci USA* 2000; **97**(12): 6670–5.

19. Vratsanos GS, Jung S, Park YM, Craft J. CD4(+) T cells from lupus-prone mice are hyperresponsive to T cell receptor engagement with low and high affinity peptide antigens: a model to explain spontaneous T cell activation in lupus. *J Exp Med* 2001; **193**(3): 329–37.

20. Datta SK, Patel H, Berry D. Induction of a cationic shift in IgG anti-DNA autoantibodies. Role of T helper cells with classical and novel phenotypes in three murine models of lupus nephritis. *J Exp Med* 1987; **165**(5): 1252–68.

21. Connolly K, Roubinian JR, Wofsy D. Development of murine lupus in CD4-depleted NZB/NZW mice. Sustained inhibition of residual CD4+ T cells is required to suppress autoimmunity. *J Immunol* 1992; **149**(9): 3083–8.

22. Wofsy D, Ledbetter JA, Hendler PL. Treatment of murine lupus with monoclonal anti-T cell antibody. *J Immunol* 1985; **134**: 852.

23. Adachi Y, Inaba M, Sugihara A et al. Effects of administration of monoclonal antibodies (anti-CD4 or anti-CD8) on the development of autoimmune diseases in (NZW × BXSB)F1 mice. *Immunobiology* 1998; **198**(4): 451–64.

24. Weinblatt ME, Maddison PJ, Bulpitt KJ et al. CAMPATH-1H, a humanized monoclonal antibody, in refractory rheumatoid arthritis. An intravenous dose-escalation study. *Arthritis Rheum* 1995; **38**: 1589–94.

25. Ceerny A, Starobinski M, Hugin AW et al. Treatment with high doses of anti-IgM prevents, but with lower doses accelerates autoimmune disease in (NZW × BXSB)F1 hubrid mice. *J Immunol* 1987; **138**: 4222–8.

26. Coiffier B. Rituximab in the treatment of diffuse large B-cell lymphomas. *Semin Oncol* 2002; **29**(suppl): 30–5.

27. Perrotta S, Locatell F, La Manna A et al. Anti-CD20 monoclonal antibody (Rituximab) for life-threatening autoimmune haemolytic anaemia in a patient with systemic lupus erythematosus. *Br J Haematol* 2002; **116**: 465–7

28. Furie RA, Cash JM, Cronin ME et al. Treatment of systemic lupus erythematosus with LJP 394. *J Rheumatol.* 2001; **28**(2): 257–65.

29. Wallace DJ. Clinical and pharmacological experience with LJP-394. *Expert Opin Investig Drugs* 2001; **10**(1): 111–7.

30. Weisman MH, Bluestein HG, Berner CM, de Haan HA. Reduction in circulating dsDNA antibody titer after administration of LJP 394. *J Rheumatol* 1997; **24**(2): 314–8

31. Kaliyaperumal A, Michaels MA, Datta SK. Naturally processed chromatin peptides reveal a major autoepitope that primes pathogenic T and B cells of lupus. *J Immunol* 2002; **168**(5): 2530–7.

32. Tada Y, Nagasawa K, Ho A et al. Role of the costimulatory molecule CD28 in the development of lupus in MRL/lpr mice. *J Immunol* 1999; **163**: 3153–9.

33. Riemekasten G, Marell J, Trebeljahr G et al. A novel epitope on the C-terminus of SmD1 is recognized by the majority of sera from patients with systemic lupus erythematosus. *J Clin Invest* 1998; **102**(4): 754–63

34. Riemekasten G, Kawald A, Weiss C et al. Strong acceleration of murine lupus by injection of the SmD1(83–119) peptide. *Arthritis Rheum* 2001; **44**(10): 2435–45.

35. Yurin VL, Rudensky AY, Mazel SM et al. Immuoglobulin-specific T–B cell interaction. II. T cell clones recognize the processed form of B cells' own surface immunoglobulin in the context of the major histocompatibility complex class II molecule. *Eur J Immunol* 1989; **19**: 1903–9.

36. Singh RR, Kumar V, Ebling FM et al. T cell determinants from autoantibodies to DNA can up-regulate autoimmunity in murine systemic lupus erythematosus. *J Exp Med* 1995; **181**: 2017–27

37. Jouanne C, Avrameas S, Payelle-Brogard B. A peptide derived from a polyreactive monoclonal anti-DNA natural antibody can modulate lupus development in (NZB × NZW)F1 mice. *Immunology* 1999; **96**: 333–9.

38. Eilat E, Zinger H, Nyskaa A, Mozes E. Prevention of systemic lupus erythematosus-like disease in (NZB × NZW)F1 mice by treating with CDR1- and CDR3-based peptides of a pathogenic autoantibody. *J Clin Immunol* 2000; **20**: 268–78.

39. Singh RR, Ebling FM, Sercarz EE, Hahn BH. Immune tolerance to autoantibody-derived peptides delays development of autoimmunity in murine lupus. *J Clin Invest* 1995; **96**: 2990–6.

40. Hahn BH, Singh RR, Wong WK et al. Treatment with a consensus peptide based on amino acid sequences in autoantibodies prevents T cell activation by autoantigens and delays disease onset in murine lupus. *Arthritis Rheum* 2001; **44**: 432–41.

41. Williams WM, Staines NA, Muller S, Isenberg DA. Human T cell responses to autoantibody variable region peptides. *Lupus* 1995; **4**: 464–71.

42. Sibille P, Ternynck T, Nato F et al. Mimotopes of polyreactive anti-DNA antibodies identified using phage-display peptide libraries. *Eur J Immunol* 1997; **27**: 1221–8.

43. Putterman C, Diamond B. Immunization with a peptide surrogate for double-stranded DNA (dsDNA) induces autoantibody production and renal immunoglobulin deposition. *J Exp Med* 1998; **188**: 29–38.

44. Sun Y, Fong KY, Chung MC, Yao ZJ. Peptide mimicking antigenic and immunogenic epitope of double-stranded DNA in systemic lupus erythematosus. *Int Immunol* 2002; **13**: 223–32.

45. Gaynor B, Putterman C, Valadon P et al. Peptide inhibition of glomerular deposition of an anti-DNA antibody. *Proc Natl Acad Sci USA* 1997; **94**: 1955–60.

46. Ogawa S, Nitta K, Hara Y et al. CD28 knockout mice as a useful clue to examine the pathogenesis of chronic graft-versus-host reaction. *Kidney Int* 2000; **58**: 2215–20.

47. Liang B, Kashgarian MJ, Sharpe AH, Mamula MJ. Autoantibody responses and pathology regulated by B7-1 and B7-2 costimulation in MRL/lpr lupus. *J Immunol* 2000; **165**: 3436–43.

48. Finck BK, Linsley PS, Wofsy D. Treatment of murine lupus with CTLA4Ig. *Science* 1994; **26**: 1225–7.

49. Via CS, Rus V, Nguyen P et al. Differential effect of CTLA4Ig on murine graft-versus-host disease (GVHD) development: CTLA4Ig prevents both acute and chronic GVHD development but reverses only chronic GVHD. *J Immunol* 1996; **157**: 4258–67.

50. Takiguchi M, Muakami M, Nakagawa I et al. CTLA4Ig gene delivery prevents autoantibody production and lupus nephritis in MRL/lpr mice. *Life Sci* 2000; **66**: 991–1001.

51. Daikh DI, Wofsy D. Cutting edge: reversal of murine lupus nephritis with CTLA4Ig and cyclophosphamide. *J Immunol* 2001; **166**: 2913–16.

52. Wang X, Huang W, Mihara M et al. Mechanism of action of combined short-term CTLA4Ig and anti-CD40 ligand in murine systemic lupus erythematosus. *J Immunol* 2002; **168**: 2046–53.

53. Abrams JR, Lebwohl mg, Guzzo CA et al. CTLA4Ig-mediated blockade of T-cell costimulation in patients with psoriasis vulgaris. *J Clin Invest* 1999; **103**: 1243–52.

54. Desai-Mehta A, Lu L, Ramsey-Goldman R, Datta SK. Hyperexpression of CD40 ligand by B and T cells in human lupus and its role in pathogenic autoantibody production. *J Clin Invest* 1996; **97**: 2063–73.

55. Kalled, SL, Cutler AH, Datta SK, Thomas DW. Anti-CD40 ligand antibody treatment of SNF1 mice with established nephritis: preservation of kidney function. *J Immunol* 1998; **160**: 2158–65.

56. Davis JC Jr, Totoritis MC, Rosenberg J et al. Phase I clinical trial of a monoclonal antibody against CD40-ligand (IDEC-131) in patients with systemic lupus erythematosus. *J Rheumatol* 2001; **28**: 95–101.

57. Xu S, Lam KP. B-cell maturation protein, which binds the tumor necrosis factor family members BAFF and APRIL, is dispensable for humoral immune responses. *Mol Cell Biol* 2001; **21**: 4067–74.

58. Khare SD, Sarosi I, Xia XZ et al. Severe B cell hyperplasia and autoimmune disease in TALL-1 transgenic mice. *Proc Natl Acad Sci USA* 2000; **97**: 3370–5.

59. Yan M, Wang H, Chan B et al. Activation and accumulation of B cells in TACI-deficient mice. *Nat Immunol* 2001; **2**: 638–43.

60. Cheema GS, Roschke V, Hilbert DM, Stohl W. Elevated serum B lymphocyte stimulator levels in patients with systemic immune-based rheumatic diseases. *Arthritis Rheum* 2001; **44**: 1313–19.

61. Haseltine WA. Genomics and drug discovery. *J Am Acad Dermatol* 2001; **45**: 473–5.

62. Jacob CO, Fronek Z, Lewis GD et al. Heritable major histocompatibility complex class II-associated differences in production of tumor necrosis factor alpha: relevance to genetic predisposition

to systemic lupus erythematosus. *Proc Natl Acad Sci USA* 1990; **87**: 1233–7.

63. Kontoyiannis D, Kollias G. Accelerated autoimmunity and lupus nephritis in NZB mice with an engineered heterozygous deficiency in tumor necrosis factor. *Eur J Immunol* 2000; **30**: 2038–47.

64. Studnicka-Benke A, Steiner G, Petera PK, Smolen JS. Tumour necrosis factor alpha and its soluble receptors parallel clinical disease and autoimmune activity in systemic lupus erythematosus. *Br J Rheumatol* 1996; **35**: 1067–74.

65. McHale JF, Harari OA, Marshall D, Haskard DO. TNF-alpha and IL-1 sequentially induce endothelial ICAM-1 and VCAM-1 expression in MRL/lpr lupus-prone mice. *J Immunol* 1999; **163**: 3993–4000.

66. Sturfelt G, Roux-Lombard FA, Dayer JM. Low levels of interleukin-1 receptor antagonist coincide with kidney involvement in systemic lupus erythematosus. *Br J Rheumatol* 1997; **36**: 1283–9.

67. Finck BK, Chan B, Wofsy D. Interleukin 6 promotes murine lupus in NZB/NZW F1 mice. *J Clin Invest* 1994; **94**: 585–91.

68. Ishida H, Muchamuel T, Sakaguchi S et al. Continuous administration of anti-interleukin 10 antibodies delays onset of autoimmunity in NZB/W mice. *J Exp Med* 1994; **179**: 305–10.

69. Froncek MJ, Horwitz DA. Cytokines in the pathogenesis of systemic lupus erythematosus. In: Wallace DJ, Hahn BH, eds. *Dubois' Lupus Erythematosus*, 6th edn. (Lippincott, Williams and Wilkins: Philadelphia, 2002) 187–204.

70. Houssiau FA, Lefebvre C, Berghe MV et al. Serum interleukin 10-titres in systemic lupus erythematosus reflect disease activity. *Lupus* 1995; **4**: 393–5.

71. Kalsi J, Grossman JM, Kim J et al. Proinflammatory cytokines are produced by PBL of SLE patients stimulated by selected Ig derived peptides. *Arthritis Rheum* 2001; **44**: S98.

72. Filaci G, Bacilieri S, Frvega M et al. Impairment of CD8+ T suppressor cell function in patients with active systemic lupus erythematosus. *J Immunol* 2001; **166**: 6452–7.

73. Ohtsuka K, Gray JD, Quismorio FP Jr et al. Cytokine-mediated down-regulation of B cell activity in SLE: effects of interleukin-2 and transforming growth factor-beta. *Lupus* 1999; **8**: 95–102.

74. Khan IU, Laxminarayana D, Kammer GM. Protein kinase A RI beta subunit deficiency in lupus T lymphocytes: bypassing a block in RI beta translation reconstitutes protein kinase A activity and augments IL-2 production. *J Immunol* 2001; **166**: 7600–5.

75. Nakamura K, Kitani A, Strober W. Cell contact-dependent immunosuppression by CD4+CD25+ regulatory T cells is mediated by cell surface-bound transforming growth factor beta. *J Exp Med* 2001; **194**: 629–44.

76. Gutierrez-Ramos JC, Andreu JL, Reveilla Y et al. Recovery from autoimmunity of MRL/lpr mice after infection with an interleukin-2/vaccinia recombination virus. *Nature* 1990; **346**: 271–4.

77. Huggins ML, Huang FP, Xu D et al. Modulation of autoimmune disease in the MRL-lpr/lpr mouse by IL-2 and TGF-beta-1 gene therapy using attenuated Salmonella typhimurium as gene carrier. *Lupus* 1999; **8**: 29–38.

78. Jacob CO, van der Meide PH, McDevitt HO. In vivo treatment of (NZB × NZW)F1 lupus-like nephritis with monoclonal antibody to γ interferon. *J Exp Med* 1987; **166**: 798.

79. Haas C, Ryffel B,. Le Hir M. IFN-gamma receptor deletion prevents autoantibody production and glomerulonephritis in lupus-prone (NZB × NZW)F1 mice. *J Immunol* 1998; **160**: 3713–18.

80. Lawson BR, Prud'Homme GJ, Chang Y et al. Treatment of murine lupus with cDNA encoding IFNgamma-R/Fc. *J Clin Invest* 2000; **106**: 207–15.

81. Hagiwara E, Okubo T, Ohno I et al. IL-12-encoding plasmid has a beneficial effect on spontaneous autoimmune disease in MRL/MP-lpr/lpr mice. *Cytokine* 2000; **12**: 1035–41.

82. Wang Y, Hu Q, Madri JA et al. Amelioration of lupus-like autoimmune disease in NZB/WF1 mice after treatment with a blocking monoclonal antibody specific for complement component C5. *Proc Natl Acad Sci USA* 1996; **93**(16): 8563–8.

83. Holers VM, Girardi G, Mo L et al. Complement C3 activation is required for antiphospholipid antibody-induced fetal loss. *J Exp Med* 2002; **195**(2): 211–20.

84. Tan EM, Cohen AS, Fries JF et al. The 1982 revised criteria for the classification of systemic lupus erythematosus. *Arthritis Rheum* 1982: **25**: 1271–7.

35

Vasculitis

Gary S Hoffman, Leonard H Calabrese and Patrick Liang

Introduction • Giant cell (temporal) arteritis • Takayasu's arteritis • Wegener's granulomatosis and microscopic polyangiitis • Churg–Strauss syndrome • Vasculitis associated with chronic viral infection • References

INTRODUCTION

The systemic vasculitides are heterogeneous in regard to clinical phenotype, prognosis and etiology. In only a few instances is the cause of a specific form of vasculitis well established. For severe forms of disease, treatment has been frustratingly familiar, incorporating corticosteroids (CS), and, in special cases, cytotoxic therapies. It is important for the practitioner to not become prematurely jaded about these broadbased immunosuppressive/anti-inflammatory agents. While such crude measures may be intellectually unfulfilling, when used judiciously they undoubtedly reduce disease morbidity and may be life-saving. The provision of more disease-specific treatments will emerge as our understanding of pathogenesis improves. This, in fact, is already occurring. In this chapter, we will focus primarily on new insights into the pathogenesis of certain vasculitides and how those insights are changing approaches to patient care.

GIANT CELL (TEMPORAL) ARTERITIS

Giant cell arteritis (GCA) is a disease of unknown cause, affecting large and medium-sized arteries, in patients generally older than 50 years. Women are affected at least twice as often as men.[1,2] In the USA, the annual incidence is approximately 2.5/100 000 population, and 18/100 000 among persons >50 years old. The prevalence of GCA in this age group has been estimated to be 223/100 000 population[1-4] and the approximate total number of prevalent cases in the USA alone is 162 340.

Characteristic features of GCA are provided in Table 35.1.[3-9] Morbidity from GCA itself is substantial. In the era preceding the availability of CS, 30–60% of patients experienced visual loss, compared to 5–20% of CS-treated patients in more recent series.[10-15] In one population-based study, 17% of GCA patients developed aortic aneurysms that were sometimes associated with dissection or vessel rupture.[16] Aortic branch vessel stenoses may cause extremity (upper > lower) claudication (15%).[17,18] Patients may also experience polymyalgia rheumatica (PMR) (~50%), constitutional symptoms (~50%), and stroke (0–5%).[3-9,19-22]

Conventional medical therapy for giant cell arteritis

There is general agreement that once a convincing diagnosis of GCA is assumed, treatment

Table 35.1   Giant cell arteritis: clinical features (% frequency).

	Author (no. of cases)				
	Hunder (94)	Liozan (147)	Gonzalez-Gay (239)	Chevalet (164)	Hoffman (98)[a]
Headache	77	NS	83	67	93
Abnormal temporal artery	53	55	72	21	NS
Jaw claudication/pain	51	38	39	16	60
Constitutional symptoms	48	65	70	NS	NS
Polymyalgia rheumatica	34	27	47	49	55
Fever	27	NS	11	46	5
Diploplia	12	NS	7	NS	NS
Amaurosis	5	NS	17	NS	NS
Blindness	13	13	14	NS	18
Stroke	NS	NS	3.5	NS	0
Mean age (years)	75	75	73	73	74
Percentage female	74	63	56	71	71

[a]At presentation; NS, not stated.

with CS should begin immediately. This sense of urgency is conveyed because of the knowledge that in the pre-CS era, GCA was frequently complicated by blindness. Prednisone is the most common form of CS therapy employed.

How much prednisone?

How long should the initial dose be maintained before it is tapered? How long should one expect to treat a patient with GCA? The answers to such questions are as numerous as the authorities who have studied GCA. Comparative studies have not been performed that would clearly recommend any one approach above others.

Whereas some early reports of GCA suggested that treatment may only be necessary for 6–12 months, in 1973 Beevers et al[23] recognized the chronic nature of this illness and noted that in many cases CS therapy may be required for several years. Indeed, this is now a widely accepted perception. Relapse rates in the course

of CS tapering have been reportedly ~30% to >80% over 1–4 years of follow-up.[20–27]

It is apparent that GCA is not readily controlled in many patients once CS therapy is reduced to low or moderate doses (i.e. prednisone 5–15 mg/day). Even after 2–3 years of therapy, about 50% of patients remain CS-dependent, a situation that has led to substantial morbidity in an already fragile elderly population. The risks of fractures and cataracts are five and three times greater, respectively, in patients with GCA compared to age-matched controls not treated with CS.[19] Nesher et al[28,29] found that among 43 patients followed for a mean period of 3 years, 35% had fractures and 21% had severe infections, which in two-thirds of cases led to death. An important role for CS could be implicated in 37% of all deaths. The need for prolonged CS therapy to control GCA, and the goal of reducing disease- and treatment-related morbidity and mortality, has led investigators to explore the use of adjunctive agents to improve outcomes.

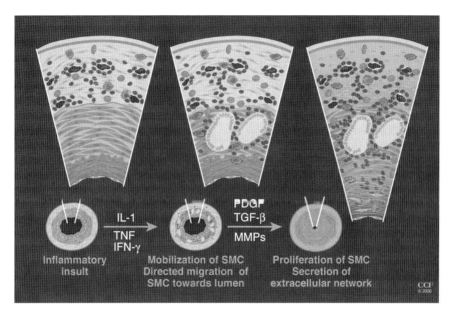

Figure 35.1   GCA: proposed pathogenesis. The earliest sign of disease in vessels appears to be activation of dendritic cells and Th 1 lymphocytes (that produce TNF and IFNγ). About 2–5% of these cells are clonally expanded in the adventitia of vessels, but not in the circulation, suggesting that antigen presentation may occur in the vascular adventitia. In turn, macrophages are activated (and produce IL-1, IL-6, TNF). As macrophages migrate into the media, they assume a different phenotype, producing matrix metalloproteinases (MMPs), toxic oxygen radicals, and toxic nitration of proteins that damages the media. Subsequently, synthetic products include growth factors [platelet derived growth factor (PDGF), transforming growth factor β (TGFβ)] and vascular endothelial growth factor (VEGF), that leads to microvascular neoangiogenesis within the vessel wall. Eventually myointimal proliferation, including smooth muscle cells (SMCs), leads to vascular stenosis and ischemia. (Adapted from Weyand and Goronzy.[30,34–36])

Adjunctive therapy to corticosteroids in giant cell arteritis

Numerous studies have explored the utility of either methotrexate or azathioprine as a means of achieving improved disease control and less dependence on CS therapy. Two recent randomized, double-blind, placebo-controlled studies of weekly methotrexate (MTX) have been completed. In both, the rate of CS taper was rapid, so that in the absence of relapse, CS withdrawal could be accomplished in 4 months[24] or 6 months.[9] In both studies, relapses were frequent, and the first relapse occurred with equal frequency in the CS-only and CS + MTX groups. However, the frequency of more than one relapse differed between groups in one study and not in the other. Jover et al[24] found

that MTX diminished second relapses and cumulative CS use, whereas Hoffman et al[9] did not find MTX to be beneficial. The reason for these different conclusions is uncertain. Consequently, what role MTX or other adjunctive therapies may play in GCA remains unsettled.

New insights into pathogenesis, new opportunities for treatment

Our inability to control GCA, without producing CS-related morbidity, may not be at an impasse. Although the pathogenesis of GCA has not been completely elucidated, our understanding of the disease has grown substantially. Biopsy specimens obtained at different stages in the evolution of vascular lesions have revealed that

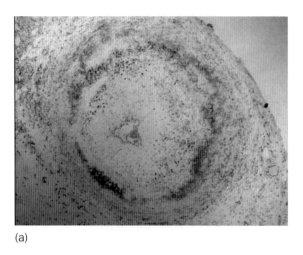

(a)

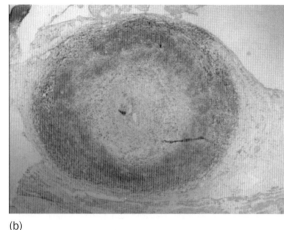

(b)

Figure 35.2 GCA: temporal artery biopsies. Immunohistochemistry, utilizing monospecific stains, demonstrates IL-1 (a) and TNF (b) in the media of the vessel wall. (Courtesy of Dr Maria Cid, Barcelona.)

inflammatory cells are initially concentrated in the adventitia and are absent or sparse in the intima, with an intermediate presence in the media. Mononuclear cells migrate into the vessel wall from the adventitia.[30–36] Slow flow of blood in the adventitial microcirculation (vasa vasorum) compared to the larger vessel lumen favors initial vessel wall inflammation in this location. CD4+ T cells, dendritic cells and CD68+ macrophages are more commonly found in the adventitia than in the media. Giant cells appear to be formed from macrophages and dendritic cells are recruited from the adventitia and traverse the media, later also appearing in the intima of the large vessel lumen (Figure 35.1).[30,34–36] CD4+ T cells are prevalent in this infiltrate, and may play a key role in driving the inflammatory attack. Production of interleukin (IL)-2, tumor necrosis factor (TNF)-α and interferon (IFN)-γ by CD4+ T cells indicates a predominant Th1 response.[30,33–36] Products of activated macrophages include IL-1 and TNF-α (Figure 35.2),[33] which are proinflammatory cytokines that further stimulate the Th1 response. Granuloma formation depends on Th1 cytokines, and, in animal models, anti-TNF-α therapy has been shown to block granuloma

formation. Blockade of these cytokines could theoretically play an important role in selective interference with disease progression.

TNF-α inhibitors such as infliximab and eternacept, and IL-1 receptor antagonist (IL-1ra), have been shown to abrogate inflammatory responses and limit tissue damage in patients with rheumatoid arthritis and are being studied in other illnesses in which macrophage- and Th1-mediated responses may be important. Our new understanding of the pathogenesis of GCA suggests that interfering with vascular injury due to the products of activated macrophages and Th1 lymphocytes would be worthy of investigation.

TAKAYASU'S ARTERITIS

Takayasu's arteritis (TA) is an idiopathic systemic inflammatory disease that may lead to segmental stenosis, occlusion, dilatation and/or aneurysm formation of the aorta and/or its main branches. Coronary and/or pulmonary arteries may also be affected. A significant number of patients fail to achieve and sustain remission despite prolonged treatment with CS and cytotoxic agents.

As is true for GCA, granuloma formation is a characteristic feature in the inflammatory lesions of TA. Granuloma formation is in part dependent on TNF-α. TNF-α production occurs primarily in macrophages, T cells and natural killer (NK) cells. TNF-α induces macrophage production of IL-12 and IL-18, which are potent cytokines that bias CD4 T cells to differentiate as Th1 cells, and activate NK cells. IL-18-influenced Th 1 lymphocyte production of IFN-γ leads to enhanced recruitment and activation of macrophages, a critical feature of granuloma formation. The pathogenesis of TA includes vessel injury due to activated T cells, NK cells, γδ cells and macrophages. Therefore, it is logical to consider that TNF-α inhibition, as was noted for GCA, might enhance control of the inflammatory process in TA.

We have performed a preliminary study of anti-TNF therapy in five patients with treatment refractory TA (Hoffman et al, unpublished observations). Patients had previously failed to maintain remission on tapering courses of CS and concurrent therapy with methotrexate, azathioprine, cyclosporin, mycophenolate mofetil and/or tacrolimus. Mean duration of disease prior to anti-TNF therapy was 5.2 years. Patients had previously experienced multiple relapses. Prior to trials of anti-TNF therapy, relapses had occurred when the mean prednisone dose was less than 21 mg of prednisone (range 10–40) a day. At lower doses, relapses occurred that led to starting anti-TNF therapy. Prior to anti-TNF therapy (etanercept in four and infliximab in one), no patient had previously sustained remission after discontinuation of prednisone. After anti-TNF therapy was begun, time to achieving a degree of unprecedented improvement was less than 2 months in all patients. The duration of follow-up on anti-TNF therapy has been 23.6 (mean, range 18–27) months. Four patients were able to discontinue prednisone after starting anti-TNF therapy, and the fifth patient continues to be in remission while taking 10 mg prednisone daily. The mean period of continued disease remission, while receiving anti-TNF therapy, has been 13.4 months. The mean period of remission, without

CS, on anti-TNF therapy alone has been 6.8 (range 1–18) months. Although these results must be regarded as preliminary, they do suggest that anti-TNF therapy is a useful adjunct to CS in the treatment of TA. Anti-TNF therapy for TA should be evaluated in a larger study to determine its potential utility in achieving disease control, while minimizing the use of CS.

WEGENER'S GRANULOMATOSIS AND MICROSCOPIC POLYANGIITIS

Wegener's granulomatosis (WG) is a systemic inflammatory disease of unknown etiology characterized by necrotizing granulomatous inflammation of the upper and lower airways, necrotizing crescentic glomerulonephritis (NCGN), and systemic vasculitis of small and medium vessels. Manifestations may be limited to the respiratory tract, or be more generalized.[37,38]

Microscopic polyangiitis (MPA) is also a form of small- and medium-sized vessel vasculitis, and is distinguished histologically from WG by not having granuloma formation. MPA manifests most often as necrotizing crescentic glomerulonephritis (NCGN), pulmonary hemorrhage, constitutional symptoms, and skin and peripheral nervous system involvement. Like WG, it can present as a pulmonary–renal syndrome.[39] If granulomas are not found on a biopsy, because either they are truly not present or the biopsy sample was inadequate for detection, the vasculitic component of WG may not be histologically distinguishable from MPA. In the absence of destructive upper airway disease, these two syndromes may also be clinically indistinguishable.[40]

Both WG and MPA have been transformed by the use of CS plus cytotoxic agents (e.g. cyclophosphamide (CP)) from being usually fatal illnesses to being chronic diseases. CS plus CP is the mainstay of treatment for severe systemic vasculitis. CS plus CP has been shown to induce remission in a majority of patients.[37] Significant morbidity, however, may result from long-term administration of these agents. It is encouraging that, once remission is obtained,

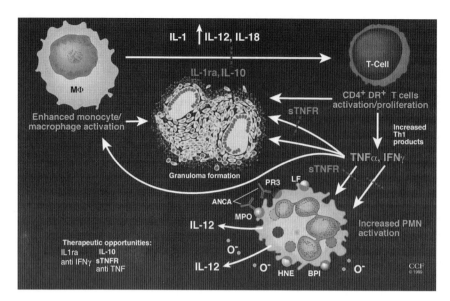

Figure 35.3 Immune dysfunction in Wegener's granulomatosis. BPI, bacteriocidal permeability increasing protein; HNE, human neutrophil elastase; LF, lactoferrin; MΦ, macrophage; MPO, myeloperoxidase.

maintenance of remission can be achieved with less toxic alternatives to CP, e.g. methotrexate and azathioprine. Unfortunately, failure to achieve remission, relapse of disease and drug-related adverse events still plague a substantial proportion of patients, underscoring the need for better therapy. As pathogenic mechanisms of vasculitis become better understood, newer, more selective and, hopefully, less toxic agents are becoming available.

Evolving concepts in pathogenesis

Classical histopathologic features of diseased tissues in WG comprise multifocal lesions that include a mixed inflammatory infiltrate, areas of dense polymorphonuclear neutrophil (PMN) accumulations (microabcesses), geographic necrosis surrounded by palisading histiocytes and giant cells, granuloma formation, and vasculitis.[41-43] Most investigators have noted that immune complexes (ICs) are conspicuously rare to absent. Collectively, these findings suggest dominance of cell-mediated immune responses. However, a recent study of biopsies from acute skin lesions has demonstrated the presence of ICs and has raised questions about their transient presence and possible role in triggering

chronic disease.[44] In addition, in vitro evidence points to an important role for anti-neutrophil cytoplasmic antibodies (ANCAs) in the pathogenesis of WG. Overall, the pathogenesis of WG appears to involve both interactive humoral and cellular immune-mediated injury.

Granuloma formation may result from an inability or reduced capabilities of activated macrophages to eradicate an antigen, be it exogenous (e.g. mycobacteria, or non-infectious, particulate materials, such as silica) or endogenous (e.g. self-antigens, elastic fibers).[45] A typical granuloma consists of a focal accumulation of macrophages, macrophage-derived epithelioid cells, multinucleated giant cells and lymphocytes. Other cells that may also be present include B cells, plasma cells, NK cells, fibroblasts and neutrophils. As noted in discussions of GCA and Takayasu's arteritis (see above), TNF-α and IFN-γ have been shown to be important in the process of giant cell and granuloma formation.[46,47]

In active WG, macrophages are activated, as reflected by increased expression of surface markers and production of neopterin, a monocyte-specific protein.[48,49] Peripheral blood monocytes from WG patients produce increased IL-12 and IL-18, thereby favoring a Th1 pattern

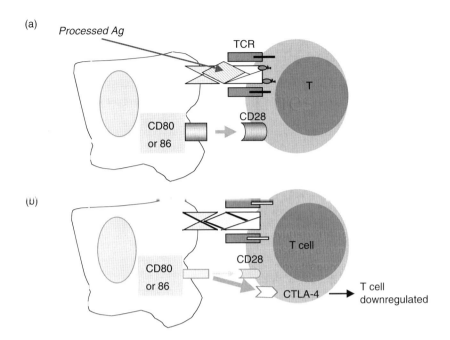

(a) *Processed Ag*

Figure 35.4 (a) Ag processing and T-cell activation: second signal. (b) Downregulation of T cells by CTLA-4. CTLA-4 resembles CD28 and binds CD80 and CD86 more avidly than CD28, but CTLA-4 provides an inhibitory signal.

of cytokine secretion (Figure 35.3).[50] TNF-α, INF-γ, IL-12 and IL-18 have been identified in diseased tissues, consistent with a Th1-mediated process.[50–52] Dysregulated secretion of Th1 cytokines may be important in granulomatous inflammation.

The selective expansion of certain T-cell receptor (TCR) Vβ chains[53,54] lends support to a pathogenic role for activated T cells being antigen-driven. Furthermore, T cells reactive to proteinase 3 (PR3), the main antigen for ANCAs in WG, have been identified in higher quantities in patients with active WG compared to those in remission and normal controls.[55,56]

Genetic influences

Genetic polymorphisms of costimulatory molecules may be of importance in the pathogenesis of WG. Under normal circumstances, a naive T cell, after being presented with an antigen by an antigen-presenting cell (APC), must receive further positive signals to become activated.[57] Such signals are provided by interactions between costimulatory molecules on the APC (such as CD80, CD86) and their ligands on the T cell, such as CD28. Once activated, the T cell will express another surface molecule, cytotoxic T-lymphocyte antigen 4 (CTLA-4), which competes with CD28 for the CD80/CD86 sites on the APC. However, unlike the action of CD28, CTLA-4 sends an inhibitory signal, thus providing negative feedback to downregulate the T-cell immune response. Polymorphisms in the CTLA-4 gene have been identified and are associated with various autoimmune diseases, including WG.[58] In both Swedish and American cohorts, significant differences were found to exist in a microsatellite polymorphism, (AT)n, located in the 3′-untranslated region of exon 3 in WG patients and normal controls. The shortest microsatellite allele (86 AT base pairs) was markedly underrepresented in WG patients compared to normal controls.[58,59] The shorter CTLA-4 alleles are associated with a more stable form of messenger RNA and, consequently, greater CTLA-4 protein production. Underrepresentation of these alleles in WG patients could then translate into less cell surface CTLA-4 expression, with the end result being enhanced T-cell activation (Figure 35.4).

In another study, CD4+ T-cell surface expression of CTLA-4 was found to be increased in

WG,[60] reflecting an activated state. However, upon stimulation by mitogen, these T cells failed to upregulate CTLA-4, again suggesting an impairment of T-cell function in WG.

Polymorphisms in the genes for IL-1, IL-6, TNF-α and TNF receptors have not been shown to differ when comparing normal controls and WG patients, although these cytokines and receptors are abundantly produced in WG. Their elevated levels might be due to events that alter post-transcriptional regulation or to exogenous factors (such as infections) rather than to genetic polymorphisms.[61]

Role of ANCAs

ANCAs are directed against enzymes located within the cytoplasmic granules of neutrophils and the lysosomes of monocytes.[62] In WG patients, specificity of ANCA is usually to PR3 (~70%), and less often to MPO (~20%), whereas in MPA, ANCAs most often target MPO. ANCAs can be detected in the majority of patients with active generalized WG and MPA. Substantial in vitro evidence points to a significant pathogenic role for these antibodies.[62-65] One proposed sequence of events leading to vessel injury suggests an interaction between activated endothelial cells, PMNs and monocytes that have been attracted by chemokines and are bound by adhesion molecules. When primed by inflammatory stimuli, PMNs and monocytes express PR3 and MPO on their surface.[66,67] ANCAs can bind either PR3 or MPO, and fully activate the PMN, with resultant degranulation and enhanced respiratory burst.[62,68] When they are in proximity to endothelial cells, cytotoxity from proteolytic enzymes and reactive oxygen intermediates (ROI) may result.[68] In addition, free PR3 may also become bound to endothelial cells. In vitro, ANCAs binding to PR3 present on endothelial surface have been shown to induce neutrophil-mediated antibody-dependent cell cytotoxicity (ADCC).[69] Thus, vessel damage may result from the combined effects of proteolytic enzymes, ROI and ADCC. One limitation of this model is its inability to account for selection of targeted organs in these diseases.

Developing new therapies from new insights

Because tissue injury in WG is associated with increased quantities of TNF, blocking the effects of this cytokine is a feasible target for treatment. To date, promising results from small, open-label studies in WG have been reported for two agents: etanercept and infliximab.

In a study aimed at evaluating the safety of etanercept in WG, 20 patients received the drug at a dose of 25 mg subcutaneously, twice a week, together with conventional therapy. During the 6-month period of the trial, 16 patients (80%) achieved remission at some point, although mild-to-moderate flares were reported in 12 patients. Three patients had severe flares.[70]

These encouraging results led to the ongoing WG Etanercept Trial (WGET), a multicenter, double-blind, placebo-controlled, randomized trial in which the objective is to test the efficacy of etanercept in maintaining disease remission when added to conventional therapies.[71]

In another study, infliximab was evaluated in six patients with biopsy-proven, active WG that was refractory to high-dose CS and CP. Five patients achieved significant improvement following infliximab treatment.[72] Similar findings were reported in another study, where 10 patients with systemic vasculitis, including 7 with WG, rapidly improved following addition of infliximab (5 mg/kg).[73]

Suppression of ANCA-producing cells might also constitute an attractive alternative to conventional therapies. B-cell depletion can be achieved with rituximab, a humanized monoclonal antibody directed against CD20, a B-cell-restricted differentiation antigen. Positive results with this agent have been obtained in B-cell malignancies as well as in autoimmune diseases associated with pathogenic antibodies, such as myasthenia gravis and autoimmune thrombocytopenia.[74] In a study of one patient who suffered from a chronic relapsing course of WG (antibody positive for PR3), rituximab was able to produce a long-lasting remission. Insofar as ANCAs could still be detected after remission, it is likely that the exact mechanism of action of this drug is more complex than merely decreasing levels of this antibody.[75] Because these results are preliminary, they will need to be confirmed in a prospective standardized trial.

IL-1 is a potent proinflammatory cytokine. It is secreted by several cell populations, including monocytes–macrophages, PMNs and endothelial cells. It can be detected in kidney tissue from patients with ANCA-associated vasculitis.[76] In vitro, ANCAs can stimulate PMN and human umbilical vein endothelial cells (HUVEC) to produce IL 1,[77] which in turn leads to further activation of inflammatory cells and endothelial cells. In cultures, this reaction can be prevented by the addition of rIL-1ra (IL-1 receptor antagonist).[78] IL-1ra is a naturally occurring competitive inhibitor of IL-1. Its important physiologic role can be inferred from knockout animal models. In one strain of IL-1ra knockout mice, erosive arthritis developed, whereas in another strain, large-vessel necrotizing vasculitis developed.[79,80] These observations emphasize the multifactorial nature of vasculitis. Clinical trials of IL-1ra in vasculitis have not yet been conducted.

IFN-γ is a cytokine produced by CD4+ T lymphocytes. IFN-γ biases T-cell differentiation towards a Th1 pathway. IFN-γ is also produced by NK cells. It activates mononuclear phagocytes, increases expression of class II MHC molecules on APCs and endothelial cells,[81,82] activates neutrophils and endothelial cells, potentiates many of the actions of TNF, and is important in granuloma formation. In WG, increased concentrations of IFN-γ have been detected in lesions as well as in peripheral blood mononuclear cells (PBMC) from patients.[50,51] At present, there is no specific commercially available antagonist to IFN-γ. Nonetheless, blocking this cytokine may theoretically be useful in granulomatous vasculitides.

Using CTLA-4 to block the interaction of CD80/CD86 and CD28 (and therefore blocking the second signal) could be an interesting way to achieve immune tolerance. A soluble fusion protein made of a CTLA-4 molecule linked to the Fc portion of a human IgG$_1$ antibody (CTLA-4–Ig) has been designed and has been studied in psoriasis: in a 26-week phase I dose-escalation study, >50% improvement in clinical parameters was observed in 19 of 43 patients. Improvement correlated with a decrease of T cells in skin lesions.[83] In addition, a multicenter randomized, controlled trial of CTLA-4–Ig in rheumatoid arthritis is underway.

As mentioned previously, WG patients have genetic polymorphisms of CTLA-4 that may hypothetically lead to decreased expression of the gene product on the cell surface, thus favoring unregulated activation of the T cell. If this finding can be confirmed in functional studies, it would provide further support for a therapeutic role of CTLA-4–Ig.

CHURG–STRAUSS SYNDROME

Churg–Strauss syndrome (CSS) is a rare vasculitic disorder, occurring in 2.4 patients/million population.[84] The full-blown syndrome is typically preceded by a prodromal phase of asthma and eosinophilia. Chronic sinusitis, non-cavitating pulmonary infiltrates, peripheral neuropathy, gastrointestinal symptoms, cardiomyopathy and extravascular granulomas are the distinguishing features of CSS. Clinically and histopathologically, CSS may resemble WG. CS used as the sole agent may be able to achieve remission for patients without organ- or life-threatening disease.[84,85] For more serious or refractory disease, another immunosuppressive agent, usually CP, is added and can be changed to a less toxic drug as the disease enters remission.[84]

Evolving concepts in pathogenesis

ANCA positivity has been reported with variable frequency, ranging from approximately one-third to two-thirds of patients.[86,87] Given the large proportion of patients with CSS who are ANCA negative, it appears unlikely that ANCAs play a major or essential role in pathogenesis. Evidence suggests that CSS may predominantly be a T-cell-mediated process. Activated T cells (CD4+ and CD8+) are present in diseased tissues and in peripheral blood.[88,89] The cytokine profile in peripheral blood (IL-13, IL-4 and IL-10) suggests a Th2 process.[90]

The prominent eosinophilia and eosinophil-rich infiltrates that are found in CSS have been suggested to result from a hypersensitivity reaction to an exogenous antigen, as disease onset has been linked to prior vaccination, desensitization, drugs[91,92] and inhalation of allergens.[93] Proteins stored within the eosinophils' granules may be responsible for the tissue damage seen in CSS. In the hypereosinophilic syndrome, the eosinophilic cationic protein is thought to be responsible for the observed cardiotoxicity and could also be important in CSS.[87] Another protein, the eosinophil-derived neurotoxin, could participate in causing neuropathy.

Eotaxin, a chemokine specific for eosinophils,[94] has been shown to induce the expression of the adhesion molecules intercellular adhesion molecule 1 (ICAM-1) and vascular cellular adhesion molecule-1 (VCAM-1) on endothelial cells.[95]

Cysteinyl leukotriene receptor antagonists

Cases of CSS occurring during treatment of asthma with cysteinyl leukotriene receptor antagonists have been described.[91,96,97] In the majority of patients, systemic CS were employed prior to use of these agents. CS may have masked underlying CSS.[91,96,98] CS taper, rendered possible by improvement after leukotriene antagonists could then have allowed overt expression of CSS.[98] On the other hand, CSS has been reported in patients using leukotriene antagonists, who have not been receiving CS. Thus, although the true role of leukotriene antagonists in pathogenesis of CSS is unresolved, withdrawal of these agents in asthmatic patients who develop CSS is recommended.

CSS: developing new therapies from new insights

To the extent that eosinophils may be prominent factors in CSS, therapies that block their recruitment and activation may be useful. IFN-α, an inhibitor of eosinophilopoiesis[99] and degranulation,[94] has been studied in a small, open-label trial.[100] Four patients with CSS partially respon-

sive to high doses of CS and cytotoxic agents were treated with varying doses of IFN-α. Improvement was dose-dependent and correlated with a decrease in eosinophil counts.[100] Rapid improvements in pulmonary function and skin lesions in one patient were also reported in another publication.[101]

Other anti-eosinophil agents that may hold promise in the treatment of CSS are anti-IL-5 monoclonal antibodies and antagonists of CCR3. IL-5 is a cytokine necessary for the development, differentiation, recruitment, activation and survival of eosinophils.[94,102] Blocking IL-5 with monoclonal antibodies has been shown to prevent onset of allergic airway diseases in animal models[102] and might be of use in CSS, although trials have not been conducted yet. Most chemokines interacting with eosinophils bind to a chemokine receptor that is relatively restricted to eosinophils: CCR3.[94,103] In future trials, blocking this interaction may also be an interesting therapeutic option.

VASCULITIS ASSOCIATED WITH CHRONIC VIRAL INFECTION

There is perhaps no area of vascular inflammatory disease where the rationale for a biological approach is more inviting than for those vasculitic syndromes associated with chronic viral infections.

Traditional therapies for vasculitis rely on broad-based immunosuppression, which is clearly not favorable from the perspective of controlling underlying infectious diseases, and thus a more selective approach to controlling both infection and inflammation is highly desirable. Advances in our understanding of viral pathogenesis, including the role of cytokines, and the development of new and more effective antiviral agents offer new therapeutic approaches to many of these disorders.

The pathogenesis of virus-associated vasculitis is heterogeneous. At least two major mechanisms are involved. First, viral replication within the vessel itself may induce direct injury (e.g. equine viral arteritis). Second, vascular inflammation and damage might result from immune mechanisms, humoral and/or cellular, directed against the virus itself. While vasculitis has been implicated in the setting of numerous viral pathogens, the epidemiologic evidence is strongest linking three pathogens as having a direct role in pathogenesis, namely hepatis B virus (HBV), hepatitis C virus (HCV) and the human immunodeficiency virus type 1 (HIV-1).[104]

Hepatitis B virus

There are two types of vasculitic syndromes associated with HBV infection. A self-limiting small-vessel vasculitis affecting mainly the skin has been described in the early stages of the infection. This condition is generally self-limiting and subsides with the appearance of jaundice. Circulating ICs appear to play a critical role in this syndrome, having been detected in the circulation, synovium and vessel wall.[105]

The other form of vascular inflammatory disease, namely a polyarteritis nodosa-like vasculitis, is far more serious. The term 'polyarteritis nodosa (PAN)-like' is used because primary PAN is not associated with a known infectious agent. HBV with a medium-sized vessel arteritis is chacterized by multisystem involvement. It usually occurs in the early stages of chronic HBV infection,[106] generally the first 6–12 months following acute HBV infection. The clinical manifestations are similar to those of the idiopathic form of the disease. Despite its explosive nature, HBV arteritis usually lasts for only a few months. In successfully treated patients, relapses are rare.

Conventional therapy of HBV-associated vasculitis

The standard therapy of idiopathic PAN with high-dose CS and CP is also effective in controlling the vascular inflammatory phase of HBV-associated arteritis in the short term, but long-term results demonstrate near-universal viral persistence, virus-associated complications and relapse.[107,108] More recent strategies for HBV-associated arteritis have focused on control of both vascular inflammation and viral infection.

New insights into pathogenesis, new opportunities for therapy

The pathogenesis of this syndrome appears to involve both viral and host elements, with the formation and deposition of viral-specific ICs.[108] A number of studies have provided evidence for a role of ICs in both the early occurring small-vessel vasculitis form of disease and the more severe systemic arteritis phenotype.[109] Evidence includes the presence of circulating ICs containing HBV-specific antibody and complement, hypocomplementemia, and vascular deposition of virus and host-derived immune products. It is not clear whether the pathogenic antigen is actually HbsAg, as originally thought, or HbeAg, based on its molecular size and distribution.[108] Other immune factors such as cytokine production and immune activation may also play a role.

Despite the lack of controlled data, Guillevin and Trepo have demonstrated the efficacy of a combination of therapies for HBV-associated systemic arteritis.[108] Each of their trials has applied four principles: (1) initial use of CS to rapidly control vascular inflammation; (2) discontinuation of CS after about 2 weeks, so as not to compromise immunologic clearance of HBV; (3) concurrent best available antiviral therapy; and (4) plasma exchange to facilitate clearance of ICs. This strategy has appeared to improve outcomes and favor HbeAg to HbeAb seroconversion.

This approach was initially employed with the relatively weak antiviral agent vidarabin, subsequently with IFN-α and most recently with the antiviral nucleoside analog lamivudine. Response rates have improved to 90%, with HbeAg to HbeAb seroconversion noted in 70% of patients. Because the vascular inflammation is linked to HBV replication, prospects for improved therapy for vasculitis are tied to new and more effective antiviral drugs.

Unresolved questions include the following. What is the relative importance of CS therapy and plamapheresis in this treatment regimen? Is it possible that only antiviral therapy may be adequate for certain patients with milder forms of HBV-associated arteritis? It is unlikely that

Table 35.2 Clinical findings in essential mixed cryoglobulinemia.	
	Prevalence (%)
Purpura	90–100
Arthralgias	50–90
Weakness	70–100
Peripheral neuropathy	3–70
Renal involvement	10–55
Hepatic involvement	60–70
Splenomegaly	50
Lymphadenopathy	Rare–15
Lung involvement	Rare
Sjögren's syndrome	20–40
Raynaud's phenomenon	10–35
Skin ulcers	10–30

large-scale controlled trials of this rare illness will ever be performed.

Heptitis C virus

HCV has most frequently been associated with small-vessel vasculitis resulting from deposition of IC-containing cryoglobulins in the vessel wall (HCV-associated mixed cryoglobulinemia or HCV-MC). Small studies and scattered case reports have indicated the occasional association of HCV with medium-sized (PAN-like) or large-vessel vasculitides.

In the more common form of HCV vasculitis, HCV-MC, the clinical findings can range from a pure cutaneous leukocytoclastic vasculitis to a multisystem disorder including neruropathies and membranoproliferative glomerulonephritis. The clinical features of HCV-MC are outlined in Table 35.2.[110] The clinical features of the PAN-like disorder associated with HCV are more reminiscent of idiopathic PAN with larger-caliber vessel involvement.[111] It should be emphasized that such cases of PAN-like HCV are quite rare.

Conventional therapy of HCV-associated vasculitis

Prior to the molecular discovery of HCV in 1989 the standard therapy of 'essential' MC was a combination of CS, CP and plasmapheresis.[112] Such therapy appeared to be effective in the short term but for the most part was palliative and rarely led to long-term remission. In addition, past literature about 'essential' cryoglobulinemia described an increased incidence of lymphomas among CS/CP-treated patients. This gave further pause to the chronic use of alkylating agents in the treatment of HCV vasculitis. Given that >90% of 'essential MC' cases have been found to be associated with chronic HCV infection, treatment strategies have been reconsidered.

New insights into pathogenesis, new opportunities for therapy

The pathogenesis of this disorder also appears to involve both viral and host-associated factors. Clear evidence of both virus and specific antibody deposition in ICs has been found in skin lesions.[113] Similar evidence in other organs such as nerve and kidney has been less compelling. A role for virus-specific ICs is also supported by the high concentration of virus and specific antibodies within the cryoprecipitates.[110] A clear correlation exists between the effectiveness of antiviral therapy, reductions in cryoglobulin concentrations and improvements in vasculitis, all of which supports a direct role of HCV as a cause of small-vessel vasculitis in certain predisposed individuals.[110] In the far less common, medium-sized artery form of illness, data on pathogenesis are quite limited. Viral-associated ICs are also presumed to play a critical role in this phenotype, but the reasons for differences in selection of vessel types and the more fulminate course of illness remain unknown.

In addition to IC-mediated vasculitis, HCV infection is associated with a spectrum of lymphoproliferative disorders. These range from monoclonal gammopathies of undetermined origin (MGUS), generally of the IgG class, to low-grade lymphoproliferative disorders

Table 35.3 Treatment approach to vasculitis in the setting of HCV infection.[115]

	Therapy
Mild disease	
Isolated purpura without ulceration, mild sensory neuropathy	Best antiviral regimen, i.e. INF-α plus ribavirin, or PEG INF-α plus ribavirin, no glucocorticoids or cytotoxic agents
Moderate to severe disease	
Severe skin disease, motor neuropathy, glomerulonephritis	Initial therapy with glucocorticoids to control inflammatory phase with or without cyclophosphamide followed by best antiviral therapy
Catastrophic disease	
Ischemic necrosis of extremities, rapidly progressive glomerulonephritis or neuropathy	Same regimen as for moderate to severe disease combined with plasmapheresis

resulting in the elaboration of monoclonal immunoglobulins of the IgM class that have rheumatoid factor (RF) activity.[114] Rarely, patients may also develop de novo high-grade lymphomas of the non-Hodgkin's disease type.[114] The RF produced in the setting of chronic HCV infection appears to arise from a limited set of genes of germline origin. The precise stimuli for these monoclonal RFs are still ill-defined. They may arise as a polyspecific response to an HCV-related stimulus and gradually evolve into a monoclonal response, in a stepwise fashion. Alternatively, they may arise clonally in a de novo fashion. There is evidence that limited somatic mutations may then lead to the acquisition of RF activity, suggesting that some element of antibody formation is HCV antigen driven. At this stage, the disorder becomes less dependent on viral stimulation and may pose a further challenge for designing therapy.

The current therapeutic approach to vasculitis in the setting of chronic HCV infection is directed at both the vascular inflammatory state and the underlying viral infection. Data are limited, but there have been three controlled trials of IFN-α in the setting of HCV-associated MC, and all have shown transient benefit in those patients who have had a good antiviral response.[115] Unfortunately, the rate of relapse was nearly 100% following discontinuation of therapy. This high relapse rate reflects the recognized ineffectiveness of IFN monotherapy for treating chronic HCV infection. More recently, newer therapies, including combinations of IFN-α and the nucleoside analog ribavirin, have significantly increased the enduring viral response rate in HCV infection. Newer versions of IFN-α incorporating polyethylene glycol (PEG) also appear to have improved pharmacokinetic properties of this agent as well as the viral response rate. There are only limited reports, which are uncontrolled, of combination therapy (i.e. standard IFN-α and ribavirin). They describe encouraging results in small numbers of patients with HCV-MC.[116]

Unfortunately, even with an improved antiviral armamentarium, there appears to be a need for concomitant immunosuppressive therapy in HCV-MC and HCV arteritis patients.[115] This is especially true of those patients with more severe forms of disease, e.g. severe skin involvement, motor neuropathies and progressive renal disease. The use of antiviral agents alone, in such patients, is often inadequate and has led to exacerbations and even death in rare cases. Although there are no controlled studies of different therapeutic regimens for such patients, a stepwise algorithm has been recently proposed[115] and is summarized in Table 35.3.

The role of cytokine inhibition in the treatment of HCV-associated vasculitis remains untested. Anecdotal reports have described both the safe use of TNF inhibitors and significant toxicity when TNF inhibitors have been used for other rheumatic conditions (e.g. rheumatoid arthritis) associated with HCV infection.[115] Prospective trials to further define both the efficacy and safety of these and other biological agents are needed.

HIV-associated vasculitis

Unlike the vasculitic syndromes associated with HBV and HCV, the vascular inflammatory disorders described in the setting of HIV disease are highly heterogeneous.[104] The most frequently described syndrome is a PAN-like illness with involvement of muscles and nerves, and extremity gangrene. Another more unique vasculitic syndrome has been reported nearly exclusively from Africa and is characterized by large-vessel involvement with occlusion and aneurysm formation. Histopathologic assessment of large vessels revealed leukocyctoclastic vasculitis of the vasonervosum. This phenotype occurred principally in patients with advanced HIV disease. As is the case in most forms of vasculitis, the reasons for differences in selection of affected vessels and organs remain unclear.[117]

There are no controlled trials of therapy in any form of HIV-associated vasculitis, and there is perhaps no other form of vasculitis where the potential for adverse effects of immunosuppressive therapy exists.

A recent report by French investigators[118] described the use of a combination of vasodilators, antiviral therapy and plasma exchange in eight patients with the PAN-like form of the disease. This is the first published series documenting successful therapy of this disorder with adjunctive immunosuppressive agents.

Non-HCV-associated cryoglobulinemia

Cryoglobulins containing a monoclonal immunoglobulin component (types I and II) may arise in a variety of settings aside from chronic HCV infection. These include lymphoproliferative disorders such as Waldenstrom's macroglobulinemia, non-Hodgkin's lymphoma, and, rarely, 'autoimmune' diseases, especially Sjögren's syndrome.[119] The clinical manifestations of cryoglobulinemic vasculitis in these settings may be particularly severe. In addition to visceral target organ involvement, cold-induced ischemic changes in the extremities may lead to occlusive vasculopathy and gangrene.

Traditional therapy of non-HCV-associated cryoglobulinemia has generally been directed at the underlying condition. Idiopathic or 'essential cases' have been treated with combinations of plasmapheresis, high-dose CS and CP, and other cytotoxic agents.[119] The knowledge that all type I and type II cryoglobulins are associated de facto with clonal B-cell expansions provides a theoretical basis for treatment with more specific therapies such as the anti-CD20 chimeric monoclonal antibody (rituximab). Rituximab has recently been reported to be successful in treating several other autoimmune disorders, including WG[75] and immune-mediated thrombocytopenia.[120] To date, there are no published reports of the use of this agent in essential MC.

REFERENCES

1. Salvarani C, Gabriel SE, O'Fallon WM, Hunder GG. The incidence of giant cell arteritis in Olmsted County, Minnesota: apparent fluctuations in a cyclic pattern. *Ann Intern Med* 1995; **123**: 192–4.

2. Matteson EL, Gold KN, Block DA, Hunder GG. Long-term survival of patients with giant cell arteritis in the American College of Rheumatology giant cell arteritis classification criteria cohort. *Am J Med* 1996; **100**: 193–6.

3. Hunder GG. Giant cell (temporal) arteritis. *Rheum Dis Clin North Am* 1990; **16**: 399–409.

4. Hunder GG, Valente RM, Hoffman GS, Weyand CM. Giant cell arteritis: clinical aspects. In: Hoffman GS, Weyand CM, eds. *Inflammatory Diseases of Blood Vessels* (Marcel Dekker: New York, 2002) 425–41.

5. Liozon E, Herrmann F, Ly K et al. Risk factors for visual loss in giant cell (temporal) arteritis: a prospective study of 174 patients. *Am J Med* 2001; **111**: 211–17.

6. Gonzáles-Gay MA, García-Porrúa C, Vázquez-Caruncho M et al. The spectrum of polymyalgia rheumatica in northwestern Spain: incidence and analysis of variables associated with relapse in a 10 year study. *J Rheumatol* 1999; **26**: 1326–32.

7. Gonzalez-Gay MA, Blanco R, Rodriguez-Valverde V et al. Permanent visual loss and cerebrovascular accidents in giant cell arteritis – predictors and response to treatment. *Arthritis Rheum* 1998; **41**: 1497–504.

8. Chevalet P, Barrier JH, Pottier P et al. A randomized, multicenter, controlled trial using intravenous pulses of methylprednisolone in the initial treatment of simple forms of giant cell arteritis: a one year followup study of 164 patients. *J Rheumatol* 2000; **27**: 1484–91.

9. Hoffman GS, Cid MC, Hellmann DB et al. A multicenter, randomized, double-blind, placebo-controlled trial of adjuvant methotrexate treatment for giant cell arteritis. *Arthritis Rheum* 2002; **46**: 1309–18.

10. Gordon LK, Levin LA. Visual loss in giant cell arteritis. *JAMA* 1998; **280**: 385–6.

11. Myklebust G, Gran JT. A prospective study of 287 patients with polymyalgia rheumatica and temporal arteritis: clinical and laboratory manifestations at onset of disease and at the time of diagnosis. *Br J Rheumatol* 1996; **35**: 1161–8.

12. Bengtsson B-A, Malmvall B-E. The epidemiology of giant cell arteritis including temporal arteritis and polymyalgia rheumatica. *Arthritis Rheum* 1981; **24**: 899–904.

13. Font C, Cid MC, Coll-Vincent B, Lopez-Soto A, Grau JM. Clinical features in patients with permanent visual loss due to biopsy-proven giant cell arteritis. *Br J Rheumatol* 1997; **36**: 251–4.

14. Cid MC, Font C, Oristrell J et al. Association between strong inflammatory response and low risk of developing visual loss and other cranial ischemic complications in giant cell (temporal) arteritis. *Arthritis Rheum* 1998; **41**: 26–32.

15. Aillo PD, Trantmann JC, McPhee TJ et al. Visual prognosis in giant cell arteritis. *Ophthalmology* 1993; **100**: 550–5.

16. Evans JM, O'Fallen WM, Hunder GG. Increased incidence of aortic aneurysm and dissection in giant cell (temporal) arteritis. *Ann Intern Med* 1995; **122**: 502–7.

17. Greene GM, Lain D, Sherwin RM et al. Giant cell arteritis of the legs. *Am J Med* 1986; **81**: 727–33.

18. Ninet JP, Bachet P, Dumontet CM et al. Subclavian and axillary involvement in temporal arteritis and polymyalgia rheumatica. *Am J Med* 1990; **88**: 13–20.

19. Rob-Nicholson C, Chang RW, Anderson S et al. Diagnostic value of the history and examination in giant cell arteritis: a clinical pathological study of 81 temporal artery biopsies. *J Rheumatol* 1988; **15**: 1793–6.

20. Delecoeuillerie G, Joly P, DeLara AC, Paolaggi JB. Polymyalgia rheumatica and temporal arteritis: a retrospective analysis of prognostic features and different corticosteroid regimens (11 year survey of 210 patients). *Ann Rheum Dis* 1988; **47**: 733–9.

21. Graham E, Holland A, Avery A, Russel RWR. Prognosis in giant cell arteritis. *BMJ* 1981; **282**: 269–71.

22. Hachulla E, Boivin V, Pasturel-Michon U et al. Prognosis factors and long term evolution in a cohort of 133 patients with giant cell arteritis. *Clin Exp Rheumatol* 2001; **19**: 171–6.

23. Beevers DG, Harpur JE, Turk, KAD. Giant cell arteritis – the need for prolonged treatment. *J Chron Dis* 1973; **26**: 571–84.

24. Jover JA, Hernández-García C, Morado IC et al. Combined treatment of giant-cell arteritis with methotrexate and prednisone. A randomized, double-blind, placebo-controlled trial. *Ann Intern Med* 2001; **134**: 106–14.

25. Kyle V, Hazleman BL. Treatment of polymyalgia rheumatica and giant cell arteritis. I. Steroid regimens in the first two months. *Ann Rheum Dis* 1989; **48**: 658–61.

26. Kyle V, Hazleman BL. Treatment of polymyalgia rheumatica and giant cell arteritis. II. Relation between steroid dose and steroid associated diseases. *Ann Rheum Dis* 1989; **48**: 662–6.

27. Lundberg I, Hedfors E. Restricted dose and duration of corticosteroid treatment in patients with polymyalgia rheumatica and temporal arteritis. *J Rheumatol* 1990; **17**: 1340–5.

28. Nesher G, Sonnenblick M, Friedlander Y. Analysis of steroid related complications and mortality in temporal arteritis: a 15-year survey of 43 patients. *J Rheumatol* 1994; **21**: 1283–6.

29. Nesher G, Rubinow A, Sonnenblick M. Efficacy and adverse effects of different corticosteroid dose regimens in temporal arteritis: a retrospective study. *Clin Exp Rheumatol* 1997; **15**: 303–6.

30. Weyand CM. The pathogenesis of giant cell arteritis. *J Rheumatol.* 2000; **27**: 517–22.

31. Nordborg E, Nordborg C. The inflammatory reaction in giant cell arteritis: an immunohistochemical investigation. *Clin Exp Rheumatol* 1998; 165–8.

32. Nordborg C, Nordborg E, Petursdottir V. The pathogenesis of giant cell arteritis: morphological aspects. *Clin Exp Rheumatol.* 2000; **18**(suppl. 20): 18–21.

33. Cid MC, Hernandez-Rodriguez J, Sanchez M et al. Tissue expression of pro-inflammatory cytokines (IL-1β, IL-6, TNF-α) in giant cell arteritis patients. Correlation with intensity of systemic inflammatory response. *Arthritis Rheum.* 2001; **44**(S): 341.

34. Brack A, Geisler A, Martinez-Taboada VM et al. Giant cell arteritis is a T cell-dependent disease. *Mol Med* 1997; **3**: 530–43.

35. Weyand CM, Goronzy JJ. Arterial wall injury in giant cell arteritis. *Arthritis Rheum.* 1999; **42**: 844–53.

36. Weyand CM, Wagner AD, Bjornsson J, Goronzy JJ. Correlation of topographical arrangement and functional pattern of tissue-infiltrating macrophages in giant cell arteritis. *J Clin Invest* 1996; **98**: 1642–9.

37. Hoffman GS, Kerr GS, Leavitt RY, et al. Wegener granulomatosis: an analysis of 158 patients. *Ann Intern Med.* 1992; **116**: 488–98.

38. Reinhold-Keller E, Beuge N, Latza U et al. An interdisciplinary approach to the care of patients with Wegener's granulomatosis. Long term outcome in 155 patients. *Arthritis Rheum.* 2000; **43**: 1021–32.

39. Guillevin L, Durand-Gasselin B, Cevallos R et al. Microscopic polyangiitis. Clinical and laboratory findings in eighty-five patients. *Arthritis Rheum.* 1999; **42**: 421–30.

40. Falk RJ, Jennette JC. ANCA small-vessel vasculitis. *J Am Soc Nephrol* 1997; **XX**: 314–22.

41. Devaney KO, Travis WD, Hoffman G et al. Interpretation of head and neck biopsies in Wegener's granulomatosis. A pathologic study of 126 biopsies in 70 patients. *Am J Surg Pathol* 1990; **14**: 555–64.

42. Jennette JC. Antineutrophil cytoplasmic autoantibody-associated diseases; a pathologist's perspective. *Am J Kidney Dis* 1991; **18**: 164–70.

43. Travis WD, Hoffman GS, Leavitt RY et al. Surgical pathology of the lung in Wegener's granulomatosis. Review of 87 open lung biopsies from 67 patients. *Am J Surg Pathol* 1991; **15**: 315–33.

44. Brons RH, de Jong MCJM, de Boer NK et al. Detection of immune deposits in skin lesions of patients with Wegener's granulomatosis. *Ann Rheum Dis.* 2001; **60**: 1097–102.

45. Williams GT, Williams WJ. Granulomatous inflammation – a review. *J Clin Pathol* 1983; **36**: 723–33.

46. Kindler V, Sappino AP, Grau GE et al. The inducing role of tumor necrosis factor in the development of bactericidal granulomas during BCG infection. *Cell* 1989; **56**: 731–40.

47. Vignery A. Osteoclasts and giant cells: macrophage–macrophage fusion mechanism. *Int J Exp Pathol* 2000; **81**: 291–304.

48. Nassonov E, Samsonov M, Beketova T et al. Serum neopterin concentrations in Wegener's granulomatosis correlate with vasculitis activity. *Clin Exp Rheum* 1995; **13**: 353–6.

49. Muller Kobold AC, Kallenberg CGM, Cohen Tervaert JW. Monocyte activation in patients with Wegener's granulomatosis. *Ann Rheum Dis* 1999; **58**: 237–45.

50. Ludviksson BR, Sneller MC, Chua KS et al. Active Wegener's granulomatosis is associated with HLA-DR+ CD4+ T cells exhibiting an unbalanced Th1-type T cell cytokine pattern: reversal with IL-10. *J Immunol* 1998; **160**: 3602–9.

51. Csernok E, Trabandt A, Müller A et al. Cytokine profile in Wegener's granulomatosis. Predominance of type 1 (Th1) in the granuloma-

tous inflammation. *Arthritis Rheum* 1999; **42**: 742–50.

52. Müller A, Trabandt A, Gloeckner-Hofmann K et al. Localized Wegener's granulomatosis: predominance of CD26 and IFN-γ expression. *J Pathol* 2000; **192**: 113–20.

53. Grunewald J, Halapi E, Wahlström J et al. T-cell expansions with conserved T-cell receptor β chain motifs in the peripheral blood of HLA-DRB1 0401 positive patients with necrotizing vasculitis. *Blood* 1998; **92**: 3737–44.

54. Giscombe R, Grunewald J, Nityanand S, Lefvert AK. T cell receptor (TCR) V gene usage in patients with systemic necrotizing vasculitis. *Clin Exp Immunol* 1995; **101**: 213–19.

55. Brouwer E, Stegeman A, Huitema MG et al. T cell reactivity to proteinase 3 and myeloperoxidase in patients with Wegener's granulomatosis (WG). *Clin Exp Immunol* 1994; **98**: 448–53.

56. Van Der Geld YM, Huitema MG, Franssen CFM et al. In vitro T lymphocyte responses to proteinase 3 (PR3) and linear peptides of PR3 in patients with Wegener's granulomatosis (WG). *Clin Exp Immunol* 2000; **122**: 504–13.

57. Reiser H, Stadecker MJ. Costimulatory B7 molecules in the pathogenesis of infectious and autoimmune diseases. *N Engl J Med* 1996; **355**: 1369–77.

58. Huang D, Giscombe R, Zhou Y, Lefvert AK. Polymorphisms in CTLA-4 but not tumor necrosis factor-α or interleukin 1β genes are associated with Wegener's granulomatosis. *J Rheumatol.* 2000; **27**: 397–401.

59. Zhou Y, Huang D, Hoffman GS. Genetic polymorphisms in the TNF, IL-1, IL-6 and cytotoxic lymphocyte-associated antigen 4 (CTLA-4) in Wegener's granulomatosis (WG). *Arthritis Rheum* 2001; **44**(suppl): S344.

60. Steiner K, Moosig F, Csernok E et al. Increased expression of CTLA-4 (CD152) by T and B lymphocytes in Wegener's granulomatosis. *Clin Exp Immunol* 2001; **126**: 143–50.

61. Huang D, Zhou Y, Hoffman GS. Pathogenesis: immunogenetic factors. *Best Pract Res Clin Rheum* 2001; **15**: 239–58.

62. Jennette JC, Ewert BH, Falk RJ. Do antineutrophil cytoplasmic autoantibodies cause Wegener's granulomatosis and other forms of necrotizing vasculitis? *Rheum Dis Clin North Am* 1993; **19**: 1–14.

63. Russel KA, Specks U. Are antineutrophil cytoplasmic antibodies pathogenic? Experimental

approaches to understand the antineutrophil cytoplasmic antibody phenomenon. *Rheum Dis Clin North Am* 2001; **27**: 815–32.

64. Harper L, Savage CO. Pathogenesis of ANCA-associated systemic vasculitis. *J Pathol* 2000; **190**: 349–59.

65. Heeringa P, Jennette JC, Falk RJ. Microscopic polyangiitis: pathogenesis. In: Hoffman GS, Weyand CM, eds. *Inflammatory Diseases of Blood Vessels* (Marcel Dekker: New York, 2001) 339–53.

66. Harper L, Cockwell P, Dwoma A, Savage COS. Neutrophil priming and apoptosis in anti-neutrophil cytoplasmic autoantibody-associated vasculitis. *Kidney Int* 2001; **59**: 1729–38.

67. Csernok E, Ernst M, Schmitt W et al. Activated neutrophils express proteinase 3 on their plasma membrane in vitro and in vivo. *Clin Exp Immunol* 1994; **95**: 244–50.

68. Savage COS, Pottinger BE, Gaskin G et al. Autoantibodies developing to myeloperoxidase and proteinase 3 in systemic vasculitis stimulate neutrophil cytotoxicity toward cultured endothelial cells. *Am J Pathol* 1992; **141**: 335–42.

69. Mayet WJ, Schwarting A, Meyer Zum Büschenfelde KH. Cytotoxic effects of antibodies to proteinase 3 (C-ANCA) on human endothelial cells. *Clin Exp Immunol* 1994; **97**: 458–65.

70. Stone JH, Uhlfelder ML, Hellman DB et al. Etanercept combined with conventional treatment in Wegener's granulomatosis. A six-month open-label trial to evaluate safety. *Arthritis Rheum* 2001; **44**: 1149–54.

71. Stone JH, Etanercept in Wegener's granulomatosis (WG): design of a randomized multi-center trial. *Clin Exp Immunol* 2000; **120**: 72.

72. Lamprecht P, Voswinkel J, Lilienthal T et al. Successful treament of refractory Wegener's granulomatosis with infliximab. *Arthritis Rheum* 2001; **44**(suppl): S56.

73. Bartolucci P, Ramanoelina J, Cohen P et al. Pilot study on infliximab for 10 patients with systemic vasculitis not reponding to steroids and immunosuppressants. *Arthritis Rheum* 2001; **44**(suppl): S56.

74. Stasi R, Pagano A, Stipa E, Amadori S. Ribuximab chimeric anti-CD20 monoclonal antibody treatment for adults with chronic idiopathic thrombocytopenic purpura. *Blood* 2001; **98**: 952–7.

75. Specks U, Fervenza FC, McDonald TJ, Hogan MCE. Response of Wegener's granulomatosis to anti-CD20 chimeric monoclonal antibody therapy. *Arthritis Rheum* 2001; **44**: 2836–40.

76. Rastaldi MP, Ferrario F, Tunesi S et al. Intraglomerular and interstitial leukocyte infiltration, adhesion molecules, and interleukin-1α expression in 15 cases of antineutrophil cytoplasmic autoantibody-associated renal vasculitis. *Am J Kidney Dis* 1996; **27**: 48–57.

77. Brooks CJ, King WJ, Radford DJ et al. IL-1beta production by human polymorphonuclear leucocytes stimulated by antineutrophil cytoplasmic autoantibodies: relevance to systemic vasculitis. *Clin Exp Immunol* 1996; **106**: 273–9.

78. De Bandt M, Ollivier V, Meyer O et al. Induction of interleukin-1 and subsequent tissue factor expression by anti-proteinase 3 antibodies in human umbilical vein endothelial cells. *Arthritis Rheum* 1997; **40**: 2030–8.

79. Dinarello C. The role of the interleukin-1 receptor antagonist in blocking inflammation mediated by interleukin-1. *N Eng J Med* 2000; **343**: 732–4.

80. Nicklin M, Hughes D, Barton J et al. Arterial inflammation in mice lacking the interleukin 1 receptor antagonist gene. *J Exp Med* 2000; **191**: 303–12.

81. Abbas AK, Lichtman AH, Pober JS. Saunders *Cellular and Molecular Immunology*, 3rd edn (WB Saunders: Philadelphia, 1997) 249–77.

82. Pober JS. Endothelial–lymphocyte interactions: lessons for vasculitis. *Clin Exp Immunol* 2000; **120**(suppl 10): 1.

83. Abrams JR, Lebwohl mg, Guzzo CA et al. CTLA4Ig-mediated blockade of T-cell costimulation in patients with psoriasis vulgaris. *J Clin Invest* 1999; **103**: 1243–52.

84. Guillevin L, Lhote F, Cohen P. Churg–Strauss syndrome: clinical aspects. In: *Inflammatory Diseases of Blood Vessels* (Marcel Dekker: New York, 2001) 399–412.

85. Cohen P, Mouthon L, Godmer P et al. Corticosteroids (CS) alone for Churg–Strauss syndrome (CSS) without initial poor prognostic factor (Five factor score (FFS) = 0): preliminary results at 4 years of a French multicenter prospective study. *Arthritis Rheum* 2001; **44**(suppl): S56.

86. Cohen P, Mouthon L, Godmer P et al. Corticosteroids (CS) and 6 vs 12 cyclophosphamide (CY) pulses for Churg–Strauss syndrome (CSS) with initial poor-prognostic factors (five factor score (FFS) ≥1): preliminary results at 4 years of a French multicenter prospective randomized trial. *Arthritis Rheum* 2001; **44**(suppl): S271.

87. Eustace JA, Nadasdy T, Choi M. The Churg Strauss syndrome. *J Am Soc Nephrol* 1999; **10**: 2048–55.

88. Hattori N, Ichimura M, Nagamatsu M et al. Clinicopathological features of Churg–Strauss syndrome-associated neuropathy. *Brain* 1999; **122**: 427–39.

89. Schmitt WH, Csernok E, Kobayashi S et al. Churg–Strauss syndrome. Serum markers of lymphocyte activation and endothelial damage. *Arthritis Rheum* 1998; **41**: 445–52.

90. Kiene M Csernok E, Muller A et al. Predominant Th2 cytokine profile in Churg–Strauss syndrome. *Clin Exp Immunol* 2000; **120**(suppl 1): 49.

91. Weller PF, Plaut M, Taggart V, Trontell A. The relationship of asthma therapy and Churg–Strauss syndrome: NIH workshop summary report. *J Allergy Clin Immunol* 2001; **108**: 175–83.

92. D'Cruz DP, Barnes NC, Lockwood CM. Difficult asthma or Churg–Strauss syndrome? *BMJ* 1999; **318**: 475–6.

93. Mouthon L, Khaled M, Cohen P et al. Antigen inhalation as triggering factor in systemic small-sized-vessel vasculitis. *Ann Med Interne* 2001; **152**: 152–6.

94. Rothenberg ME. Eosinophilia. *N Engl J Med* 1998; **338**: 1592–600.

95. Hohki G, Terada N, Hamano N et al. The effects of eotaxin on the surface adhesion molecules of endothelial cells and on eosinophil adhesion to microvascular endothelial cells. *Biochem Biophys Res Commun* 1997; **241**: 136–41.

96. Wechsler ME, Finn D, Gunawardena D et al. Churg–Strauss syndrome in patients receiving montelukast as treatment of asthma. *Chest* 2000; **117**: 708–13.

97. Hashimoto M, Fujishima T, Tanaka H et al. Churg–Strauss syndrome after reduction of inhaled corticosteroid in a patient treated with pranlukast for asthma. *Intern Med* 2001; **40**: 432–4.

98. Conron M, Beynon HLC. Churg–Strauss syndrome. *Thorax* 2000; **55**: 870–7.

99. Weller PF, Bubley GJ. The idiopathic hypereosinophilic syndrome. *Blood* 1994; **83**: 2759–79.

100. Tatsis E, Schnabel A, Gross W. Interferon-α treatment of four patients with the Churg–Strauss syndrome. *Ann Intern Med* 1998; **129**: 370–4.

101. Termeer CC, Simon J, Schopf E. Low-dose interferon alfa-2b for the treatment of Churg–Strauss syndrome with prominent skin involvement. *Arch Dermatol* 2001; **137**: 136–8.

102. O'Byrne PM, Inman MD, Parameswaran K. The trials and tribulations of IL-5, eosinophils, and

allergic asthma. *J Allergy Clin Immunol* 2001; **108**: 503–8.

103. Heath H, Qin SX, Rao P et al. Chemokine receptor usage by human eosinohils: the importance of CCR3 demonstrated using an antagonistic monoclonal antibody. *J Clin Invest* 1997; **99**: 178–84.

104. Vassilopoulos D, Calabrese LH Viral associated vasculitides: clinical aspects. In: Hoffman GS, Weyand CM, eds. *Inflammatory Diseases of the Blood Vessels.* (Marcel Dekker: New York, 2002) 553–64.

105. Dienstag JL. Immunopathogenesis of the extrahepatic manifestations of hepatitis B virus infection. *Springer Semin Immunopathol* 1981; **3**: 461–72.

106. Guillevin L, Lhote F, Cohen P et al. Polyarteritis nodosa related to hepatitis B virus. A prospective study with long-term observation of 41 patients. *Medicine (Baltimore)* 1995; **74**: 238–53.

107. McMahon BJ, Heyward WL, Templin DW et al. Hepatitis B-associated polyarteritis nodosa in Alaskan Eskimos: clinical and epidemiologic features and long-term follow-up. *Hepatology* 1989; **9**: 97–101.

108. Trepo C, Guillevin L. Polyarteritis nodosa and extrahepatic manifestations of HBV I infection: the case against autoimmune intervention. *J Autoimmun* 2001; **16**: 269–74.

109. Misiani R, Viral associated vasculitides: basic aspects. In: Hoffman GS, Weyand CM, eds. *Inflammatory Diseases of the Blood Vessels* (Marcel Dekker: New York, 2002) 553–64.

110. Agnello V. The etiology and pathophysiology of mixed cryoglobulinemia secondary to hepatitis C virus infection. *Springer Semin Immunopathol* 1997; **19**: 111–29.

111. Cacoub P, Maisonobe T, Thibault V et al. Systemic vasculitis in patients with hepatitis C. *J Rheumatol* 2001; **28**: 109–18.

112. Gorevic PD, Kassab HJ, Levo Y et al. Mixed cryoglobulinemia: clinical aspects and long-term follow-up of 40 patients. *Am J Med* 1980; **69**: 287–308.

113. Agnello V, Abel G. Localization of hepatitis C virus in cutaneous vasculitic lesions in patients with type II cryoglobulinemia. *Arthritis Rheum* 1997; **40**: 2007–15.

114. Dammacco F, Sansonno D, Piccoli C et al. The lymphoid system in HCV infection: autoimmunity, mixed cryoglobulinemia and overt B-cell malignancy. *Semin Liver Dis* 2000; **20**: 143–57.

115. Vassilopoulos D, Calabrese LH. Hepatitis C virus infection and vasculitis: implications of antiviral and immunosuppressive therapies. *Arthritis Rheum* 2002; **46**: 585–97.

116. Zuckerman E, Keren D, Slobodin G et al. Treatment of refractory, symptomatic, hepatitis C virus related mixed cryoglobulinemia with ribavirin and interferon-alpha. *J Rheumatol.* 2000; **27**: 2172–8.

117. Nair R, Robbs JV, Chetty R et al. Occlusive arterial disease in HIV infected patients: a preliminary report. *Eur J Endovasc Surg* 2000; **20**: 353–7.

118. Gisselbrecht M, Cohen P, Lortholary O et al. Human immunodeficiency virus-related vasculitis. Clinical presentation of and therapeutic approach to eight cases. *Ann Med Interne* 1998; **149**: 398–405.

119. Lamprecht P, Gause A, Gross W. Cryoglobulinemic vasculitis. *Arthritis Rheum* 1999; **42**: 2507–16,.

120. Ratanatharathorn V, Carson E, Reynolds C et al. Anti D20 monoclonal antibody treatment of immune mediated thrombocytopenia in a patient with chronic graft-versus-host disease. *Ann Intern Med* 2000; **133**: 275–9.

36

Myositis

Frederick W Miller

Introduction • Pathology and immune abnormalities • Possible pathogenic mechanisms • Biological therapy of myositis • Synthesis • Acknowledgments • References

INTRODUCTION

The myositis syndromes, or idiopathic inflammatory myopathies (IIM), constitute a diverse group of rare, acquired, systemic disorders, which share the primary feature of chronic muscle inflammation of unknown cause. The main forms of these juvenile and adult-onset diseases are polymyositis (PM), dermatomyositis (DM) and inclusion body myositis (IBM), but less common variants include cancer-associated forms and those in which myositis is seen as an overlap syndrome with other disorders such as lupus or scleroderma. Given that the pathogeneses are unknown, but that inflammation in affected tissues is the primary pathologic finding associated with muscle weakness and other symptoms, the treatment of these conditions has been directed at inhibiting immune responses via immunosuppressive agents and at strengthening remaining muscles via exercise and physical therapy. In the past, most immunosuppressive therapies have been non-specific in terms of cellular targets, but recently, clinical trials have attempted to utilize new information, which suggests possible immune-mediated pathogenetic mechanisms, to more finely focus therapy to the relevant molecular targets. This chapter summarizes current evidence support-

ing this more targeted molecular biological approach in myositis and the preliminary clinical findings that have resulted from it.

PATHOLOGY AND IMMUNE ABNORMALITIES

Whatever mechanisms are hypothesized to result in the IIM must be consistent with the pathology that is seen. The pathology in the muscle, skin and other affected tissues is characterized by collections of mononuclear cells.[1] This inflammation is often focal and inhomogeneous.[2] Thus, essentially normal tissue can be present next to active inflammatory lesions, which can juxtapose areas characterized by nearly complete fibrosis from prior inflammation. In skeletal muscle, the muscle cells (myocytes) show evidence of focal necrosis with degeneration and regeneration, and there is often increased connective tissue or fibrosis in the interstitial areas around the myocytes.

Immunohistochemical and other investigations implicate different pathogeneses in the various forms of myositis.[3,4] In PM and IBM, the weight of evidence suggests a predominant cytotoxic T-lymphocyte-mediated process with CD8+ T cells surrounding and invading otherwise normal-appearing myocytes in endomysial areas. In DM, on the other hand, the infiltrate mainly comprises B lymphocytes and CD4+ helper T cells in perimysial areas around the muscle fascicles and small blood vessels. Blood vessel pathology with endothelial cell damage from complement deposition and atrophy of the myofibers at the periphery of the fascicle due to the more tenuous blood supply in this area – called perifascicular atrophy – is also character-istic of DM, as is a decrease in the overall vascu-lature in muscle.[5] It is of interest that the same cellular infiltrates and vasculopathy found in muscle are also present in the skin and other target organs in DM.[6,7] IBM differs pathologi-cally from PM and DM by the presence in myocytes of characteristic reddish inclusions and vacuoles rimmed by purple granules on trichrome staining, as well as by amyloid β-protein deposition and nuclear or cytoplasmic 15–18-nm tubulofilamentous inclusions as demonstrated by electron microscopy.[8]

The immunopathology in the IIM consists of a wide variety of cellular and humoral abnormali-ties (Table 36.1). Cellular findings include T- and B-lymphocyte activation in the circulation and infiltrating target tissues. Several other lines of evidence are consistent with the working hypothesis that cell-mediated myotoxicity is operative, especially in PM and IBM.[7] Humoral abnormalities include autoantibodies, which are found in over 90% of PM and DM patients.[9] Although it remains unclear what role, if any, autoantibodies play in IIM pathogenesis, in some cases the serum levels of autoantibodies do correlate highly with myositis disease activ-ity and can become negative after prolonged remission.[10–12] The most frequent autoantibodies in IIM are antinuclear antibodies (ANAs), but many others are commonly seen, including rheumatoid factor, anti-La, anti-Ro and those known as myositis-associated autoantibodies (anti-U1RNP, anti-PM/Scl and anti-Ku autoanti-bodies).[13] None of these are diagnostic for PM or DM, but, if present, they do assist in distinguish-ing the IIM from other non-inflammatory forms of myopathy. About one-third of IIM patients have autoantibodies that are diagnostic for IIM, known as myositis-specific autoantibodies.[14] The most common of these are anti-synthetase

---

Table 36.1 Summary of immune abnormalities in the myositis syndromes.[7]

Cellular abnormalities
- Activated CD8+ lymphocytes in the periphery and target tissues in PM and IBM
- Activated CD4+ T and B lymphocytes in the periphery and target tissues in DM and JDM
- Soluble circulating T-cell activation markers including sIL-2R, sCD4 and sCD8
- Elevated cytokine and chemokine levels in circulation and increased expression in target tissues
- Abnormal trafficking of peripheral blood mononuclear cells to muscle
- T-cell stimulatory responses to autologous cultured muscle cells
- T-cell cytotoxicity to allogeneic and autologous cultured muscle cells
- Restricted T-cell receptor expression by circulating and muscle-infiltrating T-cells
- Perforin release and granule orientation towards target tissues in PM
- Oligoclonal expansion of CD8+ T cells in PM

Humoral abnormalities
- Myositis-associated autoantibodies (anti-U1RNP, anti-Ku, anti-PM/Scl)
- Myositis-specific autoantibodies (anti-synthetase, anti-Mi-2, anti-SRP)
- Circulating immune complexes in DM
- C3 and immune complex deposition in endothelium and muscle in DM
- Membranolytic attack complex of complement on microvascular endothelium in muscle and in skin in DM

PM, polymyositis; DM, dermatomyositis; JDM, juvenile DM; IBM, inclusion body myositis; sIL-2R, soluble interleukin-2 receptors; sCD4, soluble CD4; sCD8, soluble CD8; SRP, signal recognition particle.

(including anti-Jo-1) autoantibodies, anti-signal recognition particle (SRP) autoantibodies, and anti-Mi-2 autoantibodies. Each of these autoanti-bodies is strongly associated with a distinct clinical presentation, immunogenetic risk factor, response to therapy and prognosis, suggesting that each may represent a truly different myositis syndrome.[15]

POSSIBLE PATHOGENIC MECHANISMS

The inflammatory pathology,[3] the frequent finding of autoantibodies and other immune abnormalities,[16] the overlap of myositis with autoimmune diseases such as systemic lupus erythematosus and rheumatoid arthritis in some patients,[17] the immunogenetic risk factors,[18] and the clinical response to anti-inflammatory agents[19] all suggest an immune-mediated component to the pathogenesis of the myositis syndromes. As is the case with other autoimmune conditions, however, the IIM are probably complex disorders resulting from chronic immune activation and dysregulation following selected environmental exposures in genetically susceptible individuals.[20] As summarized above, current evidence also suggests that the mechanisms differ for different forms of myositis and possibly differ at different stages of disease.[3,7,21]

Immune-mediated mechanisms

Given the pathology seen in the IIM, a number of investigations have focused on understanding possible immunoregulatory control mechanisms that could account for the inflammation seen. Abnormalities in the expression of immunologic synapse components, cytokines, chemokines and their receptors, costimulatory molecules, cell migration regulators, matrix metalloproteinases and complement components have all been associated with immune effector and/or target cells in IIM (Table 36.2). Further evidence for the relevance of many of these findings to the disease process comes from investigations that suggest strong correlations between the immune abnormalities noted and the severity of disease.[7] Some of these studies also suggest that myocytes, myoblasts or endothelial cells themselves may serve as antigen-presenting cells, but the finding of CD86/CD40 and CD86/MHC class II antigens and cells with

dendritic cell morphologies in myositis muscle biopsies implies that some professional antigen-presenting cells may also be present in the inflamed muscle tissue.[22] These findings, taken together, strongly suggest intimate cell–cell interactions, cell–cell communication and immune activation as necessary, but probably not sufficient, activities prior to cell migration and other effector functions in IIM. Despite the impressive pathologic changes in the different forms of IIM, it is somewhat surprising that many studies suggest that the same molecular abnormalities are universal in all forms of myositis.[21] Nonetheless, it remains unclear as to whether these are primary events or possibly secondary non-specific changes induced by whatever primary events are actually triggering these diseases.

Complement

Complement has been hypothesized to play a role in the pathogenesis of myositis in a number of possible ways. The first evidence for this came from early studies demonstrating deposition of immunoglobulin and complement (C3) in the microvasculature, particularly in DM and juvenile DM (JDM).[23] Since that time, others have confirmed these findings and suggested the possible role of infectious agents,[24,25] cryoglobulins[26] or other mechanisms to explain these deposits.[27] Circulating immune complexes or abnormal complement levels have also been found in DM[28] and PM[29] cases and in a spontaneous familial canine dermatomyositis syndrome that closely mimics human DM.[30,31] More recently, the C5b–C9 membrane attack complex has been implicated in the pathology of DM vessels and myocytes.[32]

Hypoxia or oxidative stress

Primary processes – which could be myotrophic infections, or myotoxic or immune-activating environmental exposures – may result in secondary inflammatory responses or altered physiology in muscle, skin or other target organs.[7,33] These or other changes could affect

Table 36.2   Possible targets for biological therapy of idiopathic inflammatory myopathies (IIM).

Target	Increased expression in IIM groups	Comments	References
Immunological synapse components			
HLA class I	PM, DM, JDM, IBM	Classical HLA A, B and C antigens on myocytes	79,80
HLA-G	PM, DM, IBM	Non-classical HLA class I protein co-expressed on all HLA class I+ myocytes	81
HLA class II	PM, DM, JDM, IBM	Increased expression by PBLs and myocytes	80,82,83
TCR	PM, IBM, anti-Jo-1 autoantibody+	Restricted α/β families found in the periphery and muscle-infiltrating T cells	84–87
ICAM-1	PM, DM, IBM	Expressed on muscle microvessel (arteriole, capillary and venuole) endothelium	88–91
LFA-1a	PM, DM	Expressed on muscle-infiltrating T cells	91,92
Cytokines			
Il-1α	PM, DM, JDM, IBM	Expressed by endothelial cells > inflammatory cells, may be directly myotoxic	79,93
IL-1RA	PM, DM, JDM	Increased circulating levels, polymorphisms in gene a risk factor for JDM	94–96
IL-1β	PM, DM, IBM	Expressed on inflammatory cells	92,93
IL-6	Possibly in PM, DM, IBM	Constitutive expression by myoblasts	97
TNF-α	PM, DM, JDM, IBM	Expressed on CD8+ T cells and myocytes and increased in serum; may be directly myotoxic	98–100
sTNFR	PM, DM, JDM	Elevated in serum	94,101
TGFβ1–3	PM, DM, IBM	Antigen and mRNA both upregulated in muscle	92,93
Chemokines/receptors			
MIP-1α	PM, DM, IBM	Both message and protein increased	93,102
MIP-1β	PM, DM, IBM	Both message and protein increased	102
RANTES	PM, DM, IBM	Expressed on inflammatory cells	102
MCP-1	DM > PM, IBM	Expressed on myocytes, binds to CCR2	103
CCR2	PM, IBM > DM	Expressed on vessel walls and mononuclear cells, the primary receptor for MCP-1	103
Costimulators			
BB-1 (CD80, B7 family)		Expressed on MHC-I+ cells and makes contact with CD28 or CTLA-4	104
CD40	PM, DM	Expressed on myocytes	105
CD40L	PM, DM	Expressed on muscle-infiltrating T cells	105
CTLA-4	PM, DM	Expressed on muscle and infiltrating T cells	106
CD28	PM, DM	Expressed on muscle cells	106
Cell migration regulators			
VCAM-1	PM, DM, IBM	Some studies suggest DM > PM	88–90

Table 36.2 Continued

Target	Increased expression in IIM groups	Comments	References
VLA-4	PM, DM, IBM	Upregulated on infiltrating leukocytes; interacts with VCAM-1 expressed on endothelial cells	107
Metalloproteinases			
MMP-9/ MMP-2	PM, IBM	MMP-9 and -2 on non-necrotic and MHC-1-expressing myofibers; MMP-9 on CD8$^+$ T cells	108
Complement factors			
C3, C5β-9 membrane attack complex	DM, JDM	C3 and the membranolytic attack complex on capillary endothelium and myocytes	32,109

PM, polymyositis; DM, dermatomyositis; IBM, inclusion body myositis; CD, complementary determining; MNC, mononuclear cell; ICAM-1, intercellular adhesion molecule-1; VCAM-1, vascular cellular adhesion molecule-1; LFA-1, leukocyte function-associated antigen-1; VLA-4, very late antigen-4; TCR, T-cell receptor; HLA, human leukocyte antigen; IL-1, interleukin-1; IL-1RA, IL-1 receptor antagonist; PBL, peripheral blood lymphocytes; TNF-α, tumor necrosis factor alpha; TGFβ, transforming growth factor beta; MIP-1, macrophage inflammatory protein-1; RANTES, regulated on activation, normal T-cell expressed and secreted; MCP 1, monocyte chemoattractant protein-1; CCR2, chemokine receptor-2; CTLA-4, cytotoxic T-lymphocyte antigen-4; MMP, matrix metalloproteinase; C3, third component of complement.

blood supply to muscles and induce subsequent hypoxia. This has been hypothesized in DM, in which decreased capillary density and increased markers of hypoxia, including IL-1 and transforming growth factor (TGF)-β, are prominent,[21] and one study has actually documented hypoxia in the muscle tissue of myositis patients.[34] Hypoxia may also alter endothelial cell function by increasing interleukin-1 (IL-1) and intercellular adhesion molecule-1 (ICAM-1) expression.[35] Another pathologic finding in IIM is that of occasional ragged red fibers and cytochrome *c* oxidase (COX) negative fibers in muscle biopsies.[36] This may be further evidence for ischemic changes in IIM, since animal models show similar ischemia-induced mitochondrial changes and ragged red fibers in skeletal muscle.[37] Alternatively, oxidative stress may also play a role in IIM, as has been specifically suggested in IBM based upon the finding of excess intracellular nitric oxide, which can combine with superoxide to produce highly toxic peroxynitrite that can nitrate tyrosines of proteins.[8,38] Additional evidence for metabolic disturbances in myositis comes from magnetic resonance spectroscopy studies, suggesting both decreased energy production[39] and altered choline/lipid and creatine/lipid ratios,[40] and from a Coxsackie B virus-induced animal model, in which muscle lactate and CO_2 are significantly elevated.[41] Again, the major uncertainty regarding the implications of these metabolic studies concerns whether they represent primary etiopathogenic events or secondary processes resulting from the complex physiologic changes that accompany chronic inflammatory changes in muscle and other target tissues.

Direct myotoxic effects from cytokines

The cytokines present in the muscle and endothelium of myositis biopsies may be involved in the regulation of immune responses but may also have diverse direct effects on muscle and other target tissues.[21] This is true for TNF-α, which has been shown to directly induce a wide array of changes in muscle, from accelerated catabolism to contractile dysfunction to inhibition of myogenic differentiation through nuclear factor kappaB (NFκB).[42,43] Il-1α also may play a role in direct myotoxicity via its influence on insulin-like growth factor, leading to metabolic disturbances in nutrition supply[44] and by suppressing myoblast proliferation as well as myoblast fusion, leading to poor muscle regeneration.[45]

Inhibitors of apoptosis

Although apoptosis of multinucleated muscle fibers could be an expected outcome – given the muscle pathology, the many inflammatory processes described above, and the fact that Fas/FasL are expressed in some muscle tissue – convincing evidence for myocyte apoptosis has not been produced in IIM.[22] This somewhat surprising fact has resulted in several investigations that have attempted to define the mechanisms that may block muscle cell apoptosis. Using laser capture microscopy, it has recently been shown that Fas-associated death domain-like IL-1-converting enzyme-inhibitory protein (FLIP) is expressed in the muscle fibers and on infiltrating lymphocytes of myositis biopsies.[46] Other apoptotic inhibitors also appear to be expressed in myositis biopsies, including an inhibitor of apoptosis (IAP)-like protein (hILP)[47] as well as Bcl-2 on Fas+ muscle fibers and Bcl-XL and cyclin-dependent kinase inhibitory proteins (CdkIs, p16 and p57) on Fas+ inflammatory cells.[48] Therefore, both the effector cells and the target cells in the muscle of IIM patients may have separate mechanisms for inhibiting apoptotic events. Whether this relates to the syncitial nature of skeletal muscle myocytes remains unclear.

BIOLOGICAL THERAPY OF MYOSITIS

The rarity and heterogeneity of the IIM have limited therapeutic studies in these diseases. Additionally, it has been difficult to interpret or compare the results of the few studies that have been performed due to the lack of validated outcome measures, little consistency in the use of classification criteria, and no consistency in clinical trial designs. Only recently have international consortia of experts been organized to define and validate outcome measures and standardize the conduct of clinical trials in juvenile and adult myositis.[49,50]

No proven treatments exist for myositis, and those in use often result in serious toxic and other complications. Standard therapy has focused on inhibiting immune responses with immunosuppressive agents and on strengthening muscles through exercise and physical therapy. The usual therapeutic approach is to begin treatment with corticosteroids alone in less severe cases with good prognostic factors, or corticosteroids in addition to azathioprine, methotrexate or similar non-specific immunomodulatory drugs in severe cases with poor prognostic factors, using drug doses proportionate to the degree of disease activity present.[7] Although many patients respond to such therapies to some extent, the IIM remain serious diseases, with high morbidity and mortality, in need of safer and more effective therapies.[19] The molecular immunopathologic findings described above have generated interest in developing targeted therapies for DM/JDM and PM/IBM, using similar approaches as have been successfully employed in other rheumatic diseases. Over the last decade, a variety of biological agents have been reported to possibly benefit IIM patients on the basis of case reports, case series or controlled trials (Table 36.3). For the most part, these data represent preliminary, and sometimes conflicting, clinical observations, often not controlled, without validated endpoints, and from which conclusions are unable to be firmly drawn. Thus, compared to some other rheumatic diseases, the biological therapy of myositis is in its infancy.

Intravenous immunoglobulin

Intravenous immunoglobulin (IVIg) is the best-studied biological agent in the treatment of myositis.[51] Based upon empirical IVIg therapy in a patient with X-linked agammaglobulinemia who developed echovirus meningoencephalitis and myositis–fasciitis that resulted in dramatic clinical response[52] and anecdotal responses in other immune-mediated diseases, controlled and uncontrolled trials have been reported in PM, DM and IBM, and uncontrolled studies have been performed in JDM and retrovirus-associated PM (Table 36.3).

The strongest evidence for the effectiveness of IVIg in IIM comes from a double-blind, placebo-controlled, crossover protocol of 1 g/kg per day for 2 consecutive days each month in DM, which demonstrated an improvement in strength in 11 of 12 patients who received IVIg compared to 3 of 11 in the placebo group.[53] These patients also had significant improvements in a neuromuscular symptoms score and in their skin rashes. These clinical changes were accompanied by significant histologic improvements in muscle biopsies, including decreases in the expression of MHC class I and ICAM-1, and significant increases in muscle fiber diameter and capillary density. The limitations of this study include the fact that many patients were also receiving corticosteroids and other immunomodulatory agents that may have influenced these responses and that each treatment period was only 3 months long, with little follow-up after the end of the protocol to assess adverse events and response durability.

Juvenile-onset DM, which shares many clinical, immunologic and pathologic features with adult-onset DM,[54] has also been reported to be responsive to IVIg therapy in uncontrolled studies.[55] In several small open-label or retrospective case series, the majority of patients had some response; however, it was often short-lived, and, because most patients were also taking other immunosuppressive therapy, it remains unclear what role the IVIg truly played in the responses.[56,57]

Studies of IVIg therapy in PM and IBM, which are thought to be cytotoxic T-cell-mediated diseases rather than involving complement activation and immunoglobulin deposition as in the case of DM, have been inconclusive (Table 36.3). An attempt to use IVIg as first-line therapy in PM and DM, as proposed by some investigators, failed to show any benefit.[58] Although open-label studies in which PM patients received IVIg with other immunosuppressive therapy suggest short- and long-term responses in some patients,[59] results from an ongoing controlled trial have not been reported.[60] And, despite encouraging responses from an open-label study in IBM patients,[61] two subsequent double-blind, placebo-controlled trials in IBM have failed to demonstrate significant benefit from IVIg.[62,63]

The mechanism of action of IVIg in most diseases for which it is prescribed remains unknown, and it is likely that different mechanisms may be at work in different diseases. Possible effects of IVIg include Fc receptor blockade, inactivation of complement effector functions, inhibition of lymphocyte activation and cytokine release, increased catabolism of IgG, immunomodulation by anti-idiotype antibodies, or diverse immunologic effects from the non-IgG components present in IVIg.[51,64] In both DM and animal model (experimental autoimmune myositis) studies, however, it appears that IVIg may exert its positive effects via blocking complement activation and inhibiting the deposition of the membranolytic attack complex of complement on myocytes and vascular endothelium.[65,66]

The problems associated with IVIg are numerous and include: high cost, as measured by both the cost of preparations and extensive time commitments of patients and healthcare providers; intermittent product shortages; variable composition and effectiveness from manufacturer to manufacturer and from lot to lot; few data on frequencies, risk factors, and rates of adverse events at the doses being used for myositis; uncertain long-term risks; the need for repeated administration; and, of greatest importance, the lack of response or tachyphylaxis in most patients.[67] Other difficulties with IVIg are: anaphylaxis, especially as a result of

Table 36.3 Published and ongoing biological therapy of myositis.

Agent	Clinical experience	Subgroup	Outcome	Reference
IVIg	Open-label trial (n = 6 DM of 20 IIM)	DM	5 of 6 pts improved in strength on 2 g/kg/month for 4 months	110
IVIg	Double-blind, placebo-controlled crossover trial (n = 12)	DM	Significant clinical (in 11/12 pts on IVIg versus 3/11 pts on placebo), laboratory and muscle biopsy improvement after 3 months of 2 g/kg/month treatment	111
IVIg	Open-label trial (n = 19)	DM	7 of 19 pts (with severe skin disease, no cancer or antibodies) improved in strength and rash	112
IVIg	Open-label trial (n = 5)	JDM	5 of 5 refractory pts improved in strength and rash	113
IVIg	Retrospective clinical review (n = 9)	JDM	9 of 9 pts showed evidence of clinical improvement, but most were on other therapies	114
IVIg	Open-label trial (n = 7)	JDM	6 of 7 pts showed evidence of clinical strength improvement, but few maintained responses	56
IVIg	Retrospective chart review (n = 18)	JDM	12 of 18 pts showed evidence of clinical strength improvement, but many pts were on other immunosuppressive therapies	57
IVIg	Open-label trial (n = 14 PM of 20 IIM)	PM	10 of 14 pts improved in strength on 2 g/kg/month for 4 months	110
IVIg	Open-label trial (n = 35)	PM	Clinical and laboratory improvement in 25 of 35 pts after 6 months of 2 g/kg/month treatment, 7 relapsed in 4–23 months, but the rest were stable	59
IVIg	Open-label case series (n = 3)	HIV-1+ or HTLV-1+ PM	No improvement	60
IVIg	Open-label (n = 4)	IBM	Improvement in 3 of 4 pts after 2 g/kg/month for 2 months	115
IVIg	Double-blind, placebo-controlled, crossover trial (n = 19)	IBM	No significant improvement in strength in 9 pts on 2 g/kg/month treatment	62

Agent	Study type	Disease	Outcome	Reference
IVIg	Double-blind, placebo-controlled trial (n = 36)	IBM	No significant improvement in strength in 19 pts on 2 g/kg/month treatment with prednisone versus 17 on placebo and prednisone for 3 months	63
Etanercept	Open-label (n = 4)	JDM	Little response, little toxicity, trial just completed	68
Etanercept	Open-label (n = 4)	PM, DM, JDM	Improvements in all pts; all had been refractory to prior therapies	116
Etanercept	Open-label	DM	Trial ongoing	Personal communication Dr Kumar Sivakumar
Infliximab	Open-label (n = 2)	PM, DM	Clinical, laboratory and pathologic improvement in both pts	70
Infliximab	Case report (n = 1)	JDM	Dramatic clinical and laboratory improvement in a refractory case	71
Anti-C5 mAb	Randomized, double-blind, placebo-controlled phase 1 trial (n = 12)	DM	Little toxicity noted, trial ongoing	Personal communication Dr Chris Mojcik
Rituximab (anti-CD20)	Phase 1, open-label, dose-escalation trial (n = 10)	DM	Initial improvements in all DM patients, including 2 JDM pts treated out of protocol; trial ongoing	Personal communication Dr Todd Levine
Stem cell therapy	Case reports (n = 2)	Anti-Jo-1 + PM	Improved myositis and pulmonary disease, but toxicity in both pts; experience accumulating in ongoing European and US studies	117,118
IFN-β	Phase 1 randomized, placebo-controlled trial (n = 30)	IBM	Little toxicity, little evidence of improvement; phase 2 trial underway	78

IVIg, intravenous immunoglobulin; anti-Jo-1, autoantibodies to Jo-1 antigen (histidyl-tRNA synthetase) present; pts, patients; CK, creatine kinase; mAb, monoclonal antibody; IFN, interferon. For other abbreviations see footnote to Table 36.2.

preformed IgE anti-IgA antibodies in IgA-deficient persons; infusion-related back pain, nausea, vomiting, abdominal pain, myalgias and fevers; possible interference with responses to live vaccines (measles, mumps, rubella) resulting in the recommendation that vaccinations should be deferred for 6 months after IVIg if possible; aseptic meningitis, in which a risk factor in DM appears to be a history of migraine headaches; false-positive laboratory tests for hepatitis B and C and other assays relating to the presence of infused immunoglobulin; occasional transmission of infectious agents, including hepatitis C virus, in the past; thromboembolic events in patients with high serum viscosity; and rare hemolysis, wheezing, pulmonary edema, congestive heart failure, arthralgias, rashes and renal and immune complex disease in patients with high-titer rheumatoid factors.[67]

In summary, despite numerous studies of IVIg in IIM, there remains inadequate information to determine the optimal dose or schedule to use for treatment, and which groups of myositis patients, under what circumstances, and for how long, respond to IVIg. At present, given the many limitations of the product and its questionable cost-effectiveness, it would seem reasonable to reserve IVIg treatment for short-term therapy in those patients, especially with DM and JDM, who have failed methotrexate and/or azathioprine, are severely ill, or are so immunocompromised or infected that other agents would not be advisable.

Anti-tumor necrosis factor agents

As outlined above, data from a number of studies suggest the central role of tumor necrosis factor alpha (TNF-α) in the pathogenesis of myositis (Table 36.2). Therefore, the blocking of TNF-α effects by the use of etanercept (a dimeric fusion protein consisting of the extracellular ligand-binding portion of the soluble human 75-kDa TNF-α receptor linked to the Fc portion of human IgG$_1$) or infliximab (a chimeric IgG$_{1k}$ monoclonal antibody composed of human constant and murine variable regions directed against TNF-α) has been clinically assessed.

Anti-TNF-α therapy in phase I studies or case series has been reported to result in improvements in strength and the capacity to taper other medications in some patients with IIM (Table 36.3). An open-label trial in JDM of etanercept has not resulted in improvements to date.[68] Other reports, however, claim substantial clinical, laboratory and pathologic improvement from open-label experience with etanercept and infliximab in PM or DM patients who were particularly difficult to manage and had failed multiple prior agents.[69,70] A single case of dramatic improvement in a refractory JDM patient with infliximab has also been reported.[71] Several phase I/II studies in children and adults are ongoing and should give a more complete understanding of the benefit/risk ratios when they are completed.

Other biological therapies

Several other biological therapies have been studied in small numbers of IIM patients. Based on the hypothesized important role of complement in the pathogenesis of DM, a randomized, double-blind, placebo-controlled pilot study of the effect of h5G1.1-mAb (a monoclonal antibody which binds C5, the fifth component of complement, preventing cleavage into C5a and C5b) is undergoing multicenter phase I/II trials in DM patients. Another monoclonal antibody, rituximab, which is directed against the B-lymphocyte marker CD20 and is approved for use in B-cell lymphoma, is also undergoing pilot investigations in DM, given the strong evidence that B cells play a pathologic role in that disease.

The intriguing concept that one might be able to reset the 'immunostat' by depleting a patient's current immune system of activated cells and replenishing them with autologous stem cells, which would be expected to undergo differentiation to different effector cells in a new environment, has resulted in a wide range of investigations of stem cell therapy (SCT) in many pediatric and adult autoimmune diseases.[72,73] Case reports of muscle and lung improvement in two PM subjects with the anti-synthetase syndrome (interstitial lung disease with anti-Jo-1 autoantibodies) have provided a basis for the several ongoing SCT investigations in adult and juvenile IIM.

Although treatment of malignancies and infections with interferon (IFN)-α has been associated with the development of myositis in case reports,[74-77] the positive response in multiple sclerosis to INF-β1a has prompted a phase I, randomized, placebo-controlled trial of 30 IBM patients.[78] This was a 24-week, multicenter, clinical trial of 30 mg IFN-β1a administered intramuscularly once a week. Twenty-nine of the 30 subjects enrolled completed the study; however, two subjects (one in the placebo group, one in the INF-β1a group) experienced severe adverse events. No subjects required dosage reductions, and the adverse-event profile was similar for the placebo and INF-β1a groups. Unfortunately, there were no significant differences in the changes in muscle strength and muscle mass between the placebo and INF-β1a groups at 6 months. Nonetheless, this study has demonstrated little evidence of toxicity, and a phase II trial is now underway.

SYNTHESIS

Dramatic strides in understanding the molecular immunopathologic abnormalities in the myositis syndromes have been made in the last decade. The upregulation of a number of cell surface or soluble proteins – critical to the function of the immunologic synapse, the activation, recruitment and trafficking of effector cells into target tissues, the complement system, and the breakdown of extracellular matrix components via matrix metalloproteinases – has now been documented and confirmed. While it remains unclear whether these abnormal expressions are primary or secondary events, they have served as the basis for the initiation of a number of clinical observations and trials of novel biological agents that specifically inhibit or block the action of these proteins. Although we must temper the early optimism that often accompanies positive case reports and other uncontrolled experiences when a new agent is introduced, it is likely that one or more biological therapies directed against targets summarized in this chapter will find a role in the armamentarium of physicians who treat myositis in the future. Novel biological and cellular therapies – coupled with the recent establishment of international multidisciplinary consortia that are developing guidelines on outcome measures and clinical trial design issues in IIM to increase the efficiency and reliability of trials – will probably play an increasing role in understanding the best management of myositis disease activity and damage and will hopefully result in safer and more effective treatments in the near future.

ACKNOWLEDGMENTS

The author thanks Dr Lisa Rider for constructive comments on the manuscript and useful discussions.

REFERENCES

1. Engel AG, Hohlfeld R, Banker BQ. The polymyositis and dermatomyositis syndromes. In: Engel AG, Franzini-Armstrong C, eds. *Myology* (McGraw-Hill: New York, 1994) 1335–83.
2. Dalakas MC, Sivakumar K. The immunopathologic and inflammatory differences between dermatomyositis, polymyositis and sporadic inclusion body myositis. *Curr Opin Neurol* 1996; **9**: 235–9.
3. Engel AG, Arahata K, Emslie-Smith A. Immune effector mechanisms in inflammatory myopathies. *Res Publ Assoc Res Nerv Ment Dis* 1990; **68**: 141–57.
4. Hohlfeld R, Engel AG, Goebels N, Behrens L. Cellular immune mechanisms in inflammatory myopathies. *Curr Opin Rheumatol* 1997; **9**: 520–6.
5. Emslie-Smith AM, Engel AG. Microvascular changes in early and advanced dermatomyositis: a quantitative study. *Ann Neurol* 1997; **27**: 343–56.

6. Crowson AN, Magro CM. The role of microvascular injury in the pathogenesis of cutaneous lesions of dermatomyositis. *Hum Pathol* 1996; **27**: 15–19.

7. Miller FW. Inflammatory myopathies: polymyositis, dermatomyositis, and related conditions. In: Koopman WJ, ed. *Arthritis and Allied Conditions, A Textbook of Rheumatology* (Lippincott, Williams and Wilkens: Philadelphia, 2000) 1562–89.

8. Askanas V, Engel WK. Sporadic inclusion-body myositis and hereditary inclusion-body myopathies: current concepts of diagnosis and pathogenesis. *Curr Opin Rheumatol* 1998; **10**: 530–42.

9. Targoff IN. Update on myositis-specific and myositis-associated autoantibodies. *Curr Opin Rheumatol* 2000; **12**: 475–81.

10. Miller FW. Humoral immunity and immunogenetics in the idiopathic inflammatory myopathies. *Curr Opin Rheumatol* 1991; **3**: 902–10.

11. Miller FW, Waite KA, Biswas T, Plotz PH. The role of an autoantigen, histidyl-tRNA synthetase, in the induction and maintenance of autoimmunity. *Proc Natl Acad Sci USA* 1990; **87**: 9933–7.

12. Miller FW, Twitty SA, Biswas T, Plotz PH. Origin and regulation of a disease-specific autoantibody response. Antigenic epitopes, spectrotype stability, and isotype restriction of anti-Jo-1 autoantibodies. *J Clin Invest* 1990; **85**: 468–75.

13. Targoff IN. Immune manifestations of inflammatory muscle disease. *Rheum Dis Clin North Am* 1994; **20**: 857–80.

14. Love LA, Leff RL, Fraser DD et al. A new approach to the classification of idiopathic inflammatory myopathy: myositis-specific autoantibodies define useful homogeneous patient groups. *Medicine (Baltimore)* 1991; **70**: 360–74.

15. Miller FW. Myositis-specific autoantibodies. Touchstones for understanding the inflammatory myopathies. *JAMA* 1993; **270**: 1846–9.

16. Plotz PH, Rider LG, Targoff IN et al. Myositis: immunologic contributions to understanding cause, pathogenesis, and therapy. *Annals Int Med* 1995; **122**: 715–24.

17. Jury EC, D'Cruz D, Morrow WJ. Autoantibodies and overlap syndromes in autoimmune rheumatic disease. *J Clin Pathol* 2001; **54**: 340–7.

18. Shamim EA, Rider LG, Miller FW. Update on the genetics of the idiopathic inflammatory myopathies. *Curr Opin Rheumatol* 2000; **12**: 482–91.

19. Oddis CV. Current approach to the treatment of polymyositis and dermatomyositis. *Curr Opin Rheumatol* 2000; **12**: 492–7.

20. Shamim EA, Miller FW. Familial autoimmunity and the idiopathic inflammatory myopathies. *Curr Rheumatol Rep* 2000; **2**: 201–11.

21. Lundberg IE. The physiology of inflammatory myopathies: an overview. *Acta Physiol Scand* 2001; **171**: 207–13.

22. Nagaraju K. Update on immunopathogenesis in inflammatory myopathies. *Curr Opin Rheumatol* 2001; **13**: 461–8.

23. Whitaker JN, Engel WK. Vascular deposits of immunoglobulin and complement in idiopathic inflammatory myopathy. *N Engl J Med* 1972; **286**: 333–8.

24. Roig QM, Damjanov I. Dermatomyositis as an immunologic complication of toxoplasmosis. *Acta Neuropathol (Berl)* 1982; **58**: 183–6.

25. Damjanov I, Moser RL, Katz SM, Lyons P. Immune complex myositis associated with viral hepatitis. *Hum Pathol* 1980; **11**: 478–81.

26. Lambie PB, Quismorio FP Jr. Interstitial lung disease and cryoglobulinemia in polymyositis. *J Rheumatol* 1991; **18**: 468–9.

27. Shimada K, Koh CS, Tsukada N, Shoji S, Yanagisawa N. Detection of immune complexes in the sera and around the muscle fibers in a case of myasthenia gravis and polymyositis. *Rinsho Shinkeigaku* 1989; **29**: 432–5.

28. Solling J, Solling K, Jacobsen KU. Circulating immune complexes in lupus erythematosus, scleroderma and dermatomyositis. *Acta Derm Venereol* 1979; **59**: 421–6.

29. Behan WM, Barkas T, Behan PO. Detection of immune complexes in polymyositis. *Acta Neurol Scand* 1982; **65**: 320–34.

30. Hargis AM, Winkelstein JA, Moore MP et al. Complement levels in dogs with familial canine dermatomyositis. *Vet Immunol Immunopathol* 1988; **20**: 95–100.

31. Hargis AM, Prieur DJ, Haupt KH et al. Prospective study of familial canine dermatomyositis. Correlation of the severity of dermatomyositis and circulating immune complex levels. *Am J Pathol* 1986; **123**: 465–79.

32. Kissel JT, Mendell JR, Rammohan KW. Microvascular deposition of complement membrane attack complex in dermatomyositis. *N Engl J Med* 1986; **314**: 329–34.

33. Love LA, Miller FW. Noninfectious environmental agents associated with myopathies. *Curr Opin Rheumatol* 1993; **5**: 712–18.

34. Niinikoski J, Paljarvi L, Laato M, Lang H, Panelius M. Muscle hypoxia in myositis. *J Neurol Neurosurg Psychiatry* 1986; **49**: 1455.

35. Shreeniwas R, Koga S, Karakurum M et al. Hypoxia-mediated induction of endothelial cell interleukin-1 alpha. An autocrine mechanism promoting expression of leukocyte adhesion molecules on the vessel surface. *J Clin Invest* 1992; **90**: 2333–9.

36. Chariot P, Ruet E, Authier FJ, Labes D, Poron F, Gherardi R. Cytochrome c oxidase deficiencies in the muscle of patients with inflammatory myopathies. *Acta Neuropathol (Berl)* 1996; **91**: 530–6.

37. Heffner RR, Barron SA. The early effects of ischemia upon skeletal muscle mitochondria. *J Neurol Sci* 1978; **38**: 295–315.

38. Yang CC, Alvarez RB, Engel WK et al. Nitric oxide-induced oxidative stress in autosomal recessive and dominant inclusion-body myopathies. *Brain* 1998; **121**(Pt 6): 1089–97.

39. Park JH, Vital TL, Ryder NM et al. Magnetic resonance imaging and P-31 magnetic resonance spectroscopy provide unique quantitative data useful in the longitudinal management of patients with dermatomyositis. *Arthritis Rheum* 1994; **37**: 736–46.

40. Chung YL, Smith EC, Williams SC et al. In vivo proton magnetic resonance spectroscopy in polymyositis and dermatomyositis: a preliminary study. *Eur J Med Res* 1997; **2**: 483–7.

41. Chowdhury SA, Ytterberg SR, Wortmann RL. Abnormal energy metabolism in murine polymyositis. *Arthritis Rheum* 1989; **32**: S125.

42. Li YP, Reid MB. Effect of tumor necrosis factor-alpha on skeletal muscle metabolism. *Curr Opin Rheumatol* 2001; **13**: 483–7.

43. Langen RC, Schols AM, Kelders MC et al. Inflammatory cytokines inhibit myogenic differentiation through activation of nuclear factor-kappaB. *FASEB J* 2001; **15**: 1169–80.

44. Fang CH, Li BG, James JH et al. Cytokines block the effects of insulin-like growth factor-I (IGF-I) on glucose uptake and lactate production in skeletal muscle but do not influence IGF-I-induced changes in protein turnover. *Shock* 1997; **8**: 362–7.

45. Ji SQ, Neustrom S, Willis GM, Spurlock ME. Proinflammatory cytokines regulate myogenic cell proliferation and fusion but have no impact on myotube protein metabolism or stress protein expression. *J Interferon Cytokine Res* 1998; **18**: 879–88.

46. Nagaraju K, Casciola-Rosen L, Rosen A et al. The inhibition of apoptosis in myositis and in normal muscle cells. *J Immunol* 2000; **164**: 5459–65.

47. Li M, Dalakas MC. Expression of human IAP-like protein in skeletal muscle: a possible explanation for the rare incidence of muscle fiber apoptosis in T-cell mediated inflammatory myopathies. *J Neuroimmunol* 2000; **106**: 1–5.

48. Vattemi G, Tonin P, Filosto M et al. T-cell anti-apoptotic mechanisms in inflammatory myopathies. *J Neuroimmunol* 2000; **111**: 146–51.

49. Rider LG, Feldman BM, Perez MD et al. Development of validated disease activity and damage indices for the juvenile idiopathic inflammatory myopathies: I. Physician, parent, and patient global assessments. Juvenile Dermatomyositis Disease Activity Collaborative Study Group. *Arthritis Rheum* 1997; **40**: 1976–83.

50. Miller FW, Rider LG, Chung YL et al for the International Myositis Outcome Assessment Collaborative Study Group. Proposed preliminary core set measures for disease outcome assessment in adult and juvenile idiopathic inflammatory myopathies. *Rheumatology (Oxford)* 2001; **40**: 1262–73.

51. Patel SY, Kumararatne DS. From black magic to science: understanding the rationale for the use of intravenous immunoglobulin to treat inflammatory myopathies. *Clin Exp Immunol* 2001; **124**: 169–71.

52. Mease PJ, Ochs HD, Wedgwood RJ. Successful treatment of echovirus meningoencephalitis and myositis–fasciitis with intravenous immune globulin therapy in a patient with X-linked agammaglobulinemia. *N Engl J Med* 1981; **304**: 1278–81.

53. Dalakas MC, Illa I, Dambrosia JM et al. A controlled trial of high-dose intravenous immune globulin infusions as treatment for dermatomyositis. *N Engl J Med* 1993; **329**: 1993–2000.

54. Rider LG, Miller FW. Idiopathic inflammatory muscle disease: clinical aspects. *Baillieres Best Pract Res Clin Rheumatol* 2000; **14**: 37–54.

55. Rider LG, Miller FW. Classification and treatment of the juvenile idiopathic inflammatory myopathies. *Rheum Dis Clin North Am* 1997; **23**: 619–55.

56. Tsai MJ, Lai CC, LIn SC et al. Intravenous immunoglobulin therapy in juvenile dermatomyositis. *Zhonghua Min Guo Xiao Er Ke Yi Xue Hui Za Zhi* 1997; **38**: 111–15.

57. Al Mayouf SM, Laxer RM, Schneider R et al. Intravenous immunoglobulin therapy for juvenile dermatomyositis: efficacy and safety. *J Rheumatol* 2000; **27**: 2498–503.

58. Cherin P, Piette JC, Wechsler B et al. Intravenous gamma globulin as first line therapy in polymyositis and dermatomyositis: an open study in 11 adult patients. *J Rheumatol* 1994; **21**: 1092–7.

59. Cherin P, Pelletier S, Teixeira A et al. Results and long-term followup of intravenous immunoglobulin infusions in chronic, refractory polymyositis: an open study with thirty-five adult patients. *Arthritis Rheum* 2002; **46**: 467–74.

60. Dalakas MC. Controlled studies with high-dose intravenous immunoglobulin in the treatment of dermatomyositis, inclusion body myositis, and polymyositis. *Neurology* 1998; **51**: S37–S45.

61. Soueidan SA, Dalakas MC. Treatment of inclusion-body myositis with high-dose intravenous immunoglobulin. *Neurology* 1993; **43**: 876–9.

62. Dalakas MC, Sonies B, Dambrosia J et al. Treatment of inclusion-body myositis with IVIg: a double-blind, placebo-controlled study. *Neurology* 1997; **48**: 712–16.

63. Dalakas MC, Koffman B, Fujii M et al. A controlled study of intravenous immunoglobulin combined with prednisone in the treatment of IBM. *Neurology* 2001; **56**: 323–7.

64. Miller FW. Inflammatory Myopathies: Polymyositis, dermatomyositis and related conditions. In: Koopman W, ed. *Arthritis and Allied Conditions, A Textbook of Rheumatology*, 14th edn (Williams and Wilkins: Baltimore, 1996) 1562–89.

65. Basta M, Dalakas MC. High-dose intravenous immunoglobulin exerts its beneficial effect in patients with dermatomyositis by blocking endomysial deposition of activated complement fragments. *J Clin Invest* 1994; **94**: 1729–35.

66. Wada J, Shintani N, Kikutani K et al. Intravenous immunoglobulin prevents experimental autoimmune myositis in SJL mice by reducing anti-myosin antibody and by blocking complement deposition. *Clin Exp Immunol* 2001; **124**: 282–9.

67. Miller FW. Intravenous immunoglobulin in polymyositis/dermatomyositis. In: Strand V, ed. *Proceedings: Early Decisions in DMARD Development IV. Biologic Agents in Autoimmune Disease* (Arthritis Foundation: Atlanta, 1996) 205–12.

68. Miller ML, Mendez E, Klein-Gitelman, M, Pachman LM. Experience with etanercept in chronic juvenile dermatomyositis: preliminary results. *Arthritis Rheum Suppl* 2000.

69. Saadeh CK. Etanercept is effective in the treatment of polymyositis/dermatomyositis which is refractory to conventional therapy. *Arthritis Rheum* 2001; **43**(9 suppl): S193.

70. Hengstman GJ, van den Hoogen FH, van Engelen BG et al. Anti-TNF-blockade with infliximab (Remicade) in polymyositis and dermatomyositis. *Arthritis Rheum* 2000; **43**(9 suppl): S193.

71. Nzeusseau A, Durez P, Houssiau FA. Devogelaer JP. Successful use of infliximab in a case of refractory juvenile dermatomyositis. *Arthritis Rheum* 2001; **39**(suppl): S90.

72. Barron KS, Wallace C, Woolfrey CEA et al. Autologous stem cell transplantation for pediatric rheumatic diseases. *J Rheumatol* 2001; **28**: 2337–58.

73. Furst DE. The status of stem cell transplantation for rheumatoid arthritis: a rheumatologist's view. *J Rheumatol* 2001; **28**(suppl 64): 60–1.

74. Matsuya M, Abe T, Tosaka M et al. The first case of polymyositis associated with interferon therapy. *Intern Med* 1994; **33**: 806–8.

75. Cirigliano G, Della RA, Tavoni A et al. Polymyositis occurring during alpha-interferon treatment for malignant melanoma: a case report and review of the literature. *Rheumatol Int* 1999; **19**: 65–7.

76. Hengstman GJ, Vogels OJ, ter Laak HJ et al. Myositis during long-term interferon-alpha treatment. *Neurology* 2000; **54**: 2186.

77. Dietrich LL, Bridges AJ, Albertini MR. Dermatomyositis after interferon alpha treatment. *Med Oncol* 2000; **17**: 64–9.

78. Muscle Study Group. Randomized pilot trial of betaINF1a (Avonex) in patients with inclusion body myositis. *Neurology* 2001; **57**: 1566–70.

79. Nyberg P, Wikman AL, Nennesmo I, Lundberg I. Increased expression of interleukin 1alpha and MHC class I in muscle tissue of patients with chronic, inactive polymyositis and dermatomyositis. *J Rheumatol* 2000; **27**: 940–8.

80. Zhou X, Filemon KT, Xion M et al. Gene expression profile of muscle biopsies from patients with inflammatory myopathies. *Arthritis Rheum* 2000; (suppl): S275.

81. Wiendl H, Behrens L, Maier S et al. Muscle fibers in inflammatory myopathies and cultured myoblasts express the nonclassical major histocompatibility antigen HLA-G. *Ann Neurol* 2000; **48**: 679–84.

82. Inukai A, Kuru S, Liang Y et al. Expression of HLA-DR and its enhancing molecules in muscle fibers in polymyositis. *Muscle Nerve* 2000; **23**: 385–92.

83. Miller FW, Love LA, Barbieri SA et al. Lymphocyte activation markers in idiopathic myositis: changes with disease activity and differences among clinical and autoantibody subgroups. *Clin Exp Immunol* 1990; **81**: 373–9.

84. O'Hanlon T, Miller FW. T cell-mediated immune mechanisms in myositis. *Curr Opin Rheumatol* 1995; **7**: 503–9.

85. Fyhr IM, Moslemi AR, Tarkowski A et al. Limited T-cell receptor V gene usage in inclusion body myositis. *Scand J Immunol* 1996; **43**: 109–14.

86. Lindberg C, Oldfors A, Tarkowski A. Restricted use of T cell receptor V genes in endomysial infiltrates of patients with inflammatory myopathies. *Eur J Immunol* 1994; **24**: 2659–63.

87. Amemiya K, Granger RP, Dalakas MC. Clonal restriction of T-cell receptor expression by infiltrating lymphocytes in inclusion body myositis persists over time: studies in repeated muscle biopsies. *Brain* 2000; **123**: 2030–9.

88. De Bleecker JL, Engel AG. Expression of cell adhesion molecules in inflammatory myopathies and Duchenne dystrophy. *J Neuropathol Exp Neurol* 1994; **53**: 369–76.

89. Tews DS, Goebel HH. Expression of cell adhesion molecules in inflammatory myopathies. *J Neuroimmunol* 1995; **59**: 185–94.

90. Lundberg IE. The role of cytokines, chemokines, and adhesion molecules in the pathogenesis of idiopathic inflammatory myopathies. *Curr Rheumatol Rep* 2000; **2**: 216–24.

91. Iannone F, Cauli A, Yanni G et al. T-lymphocyte immunophenotyping in polymyositis and dermatomyositis. *Br J Rheumatol* 1996; **35**: 839–45.

92. Lundberg I, Ulfgren AK, Nyberg P et al. Cytokine production in muscle tissue of patients with idiopathic inflammatory myopathies. *Arthritis Rheum* 1997; **40**: 865–74.

93. Lundberg IE, Nyberg P. New developments in the role of cytokines and chemokines in inflammatory myopathies. *Curr Opin Rheumatol* 1998; **10**: 521–9.

94. Rider L, Ahmed A, Beausang L et al. Elevations of interleukin-1 receptor antagonist (IL-1RA), sTNFR, sIL2R, and IL-10 in juvenile idiopathic inflammatory myopathies suggest a role for monocyte/macrophage and B lymphocyte activation. *Arthritis Rheum* 1998; **41**(suppl): S265.

95. Son K, Tomita Y, Shimizu T et al. Abnormal IL-1 receptor antagonist production in patients with polymyositis and dermatomyositis. *Intern Med* 2000; **39**: 128–35.

96. Rider LG, Artlett CM, Foster CB et al. Polymorphisms in the IL-1 receptor antagonist gene VNTR are possible risk factors for juvenile idiopathic inflammatory myopathies. *Clin Exp Immunol* 2000; **121**: 47–52.

97. De Rossi M, Bernasconi P, Baggi F et al. Cytokines and chemokines are both expressed by human myoblasts: possible relevance for the immune pathogenesis of muscle inflammation. *Int Immunol* 2000; **12**: 1329–35.

98. Kuru S, Inukai A, Liang Y et al. Tumor necrosis factor-alpha expression in muscles of polymyositis and dermatomyositis. *Acta Neuropathol (Berl)* 2000; **99**: 585–8.

99. Fedczyna TO, Lutz J, Pachman LM. Expression of TNF-αlpha by muscle fibers in biopsies from children with untreated juvenile dermatomyositis: association with the TNF-αlpha-308A allele. *Clin Immunol* 2001; **100**: 236–9.

100. De Bleecker JL, Meire VI, Declercq W, Van Aken EH. Immunolocalization of tumor necrosis factor-alpha and its receptors in inflammatory myopathies. *Neuromuscul Disord* 1999; **9**: 239–46.

101. Shimizu T, Tomita Y, Son K et al. Elevation of serum soluble tumour necrosis factor receptors in patients with polymyositis and dermatomyositis. *Clin Rheumatol* 2000; **19**: 352–9.

102. Adams EM, Kirkley J, Eidelman G et al. The predominance of beta (CC) chemokine transcripts in idiopathic inflammatory muscle diseases. *Proc Assoc Am Physicians* 1997; **109**: 275–85.

103. Bartoli C, Civatte M, Pellissier JF, Figarella-Branger D. CCR2A and CCR2B, the two isoforms of the monocyte chemoattractant protein-1 receptor are up-regulated and expressed by different cell subsets in idiopathic inflammatory myopathies. *Acta Neuropathol (Berl)* 2001; **102**: 385–92.

104. Murata K, Dalakas MC. Expression of the costimulatory molecule BB-1, the ligands CTLA-4 and CD28, and their mRNA in inflammatory myopathies. *Am J Pathol* 1999; **155**: 453–60.

105. Sugiura T, Kawaguchi Y, Harigai M et al. Increased CD40 expression on muscle cells of polymyositis and dermatomyositis: role of CD40–CD40 ligand interaction in IL-6, IL-8, IL-15, and monocyte chemoattractant protein-1 production. *J Immunol* 2000; **164**: 6593–600.

106. Nagaraju K, Raben N, Villalba ML et al. Costimulatory markers in muscle of patients with idiopathic inflammatory myopathies and in cultured muscle cells. *Clin Immunol* 1999; **92**: 161–9.

107. Cid MC, Grau JM, Casademont J et al. Leucocyte/endothelial cell adhesion receptors in muscle biopsies from patients with idiopathic inflammatory myopathies (IIM). *Clin Exp Immunol* 1996; **104**: 467–73.

108. Choi YC, Dalakas MC. Expression of matrix metalloproteinases in the muscle of patients with inflammatory myopathies. *Neurology* 2000; **54**: 65–71.

109. Whitaker JN, Engel WK. Vascular deposits of immunoglobulin and complement in inflammatory myopathy. *Trans Am Neurol Assoc* 1971; **96**: 24–8.

110. Cherin P, Herson S, Wechsler B et al. Efficacy of intravenous gammaglobulin therapy in chronic refractory polymyositis and dermatomyositis: an open study with 20 adult patients. *Am J Med* 1991; **91**: 162–8.

111. Dalakas MC, Illa I, Dambrosia JM et al. A controlled trial of high-dose intravenous immune globulin infusions as treatment for dermatomyositis. *N Engl J Med* 1993; **329**: 1993–2000.

112. Gottfried I, Seeber A, Anegg B et al. High dose intravenous immunoglobulin (IVIg) in dermatomyositis: clinical responses and effect on sIL-2R levels. *Eur J Dermatol* 2000; **10**: 29–35.

113. Lang BA, Laxer RM, Murphy G et al. Treatment of dermatomyositis with intravenous gammaglobulin. *Am J Med* 1991; **91**: 169–72.

114. Sansome A, Dubowitz V. Intravenous immunoglobulin in juvenile dermatomyositis – four year review of nine cases. *Arch Dis Child* 1995; **72**: 25–8.

115. Soueidan SA, Dalakas MC. Treatment of inclusion-body myositis with high-dose intravenous immunoglobulin. *Neurology* 1993; **43**: 876–9.

116. Saadeh, C. K. Etanercept is effective in the treatment of polymyositis/dermatomyositis which is refractory to conventional therapy including steroids and other disease modifying agents. *Arthritis Rheum* 2000; (suppl): S193.

117. Bingham S, Griffiths B, McGonagle D et al. Autologous stem cell transplantation for rapidly progressive Jo-1-positive polymyositis with long-term follow-up. *Br J Haematol* 2001; **113**: 840–1.

118. Baron F, Ribbens C, Kaye O et al. Effective treatment of Jo-1-associated polymyositis with T-cell-depleted autologous peripheral blood stem cell transplantation. *Br J Haematol* 2000; **110**: 339–42.

Section VII

Immunoglobulin manipulation

37

Intravenous immunoglobulin as therapy for RA

Yaniv Sherer and Yehuda Shoenfeld

Introduction • IVIg in RA • Mechanisms of IVIg activity in RA • Conclusions • References

INTRODUCTION

Intravenous immunoglobulin (IVIg) is an immunomodulatory therapeutic option in various autoimmune diseases such as immune thrombocytopenic purpura, systemic lupus erythematosus and vasculitides.[1,2] IVIg use in rheumatoid arthritis (RA) is less established and still regarded as controversial. However, given the inflammatory nature of RA, and the good results obtained with the use of new biological therapies (such as monoclonal antibodies), IVIg seems a more feasible option in RA.

IVIg IN RA

Negative results

Several negative results have been reported regarding antibodies and IVIg use in RA. The safety and efficacy of a murine anti-CD4 monoclonal antibody has been evaluated in 58 patients with RA compared to treatment with placebo.[3] All patients were in an active state of the disease, and the treatment was randomized between murine anti-CD4 or placebo intravenously for 10 consecutive days. There was no difference between groups regarding global 20%

or 50% response. However, C-reactive protein (CRP) levels decreased in the anti-CD4 group. In another study, four patients with severe refractory RA who had failed at least four second-line drugs were given IVIg at a dose of 1 g/day for 2 days once a month for 3 months.[4] None of them improved or worsened, but tumor necrosis factor (TNF)-α production in lipopolysaccharide (LPS)-stimulated whole blood assays was enhanced in three out of the four patients during therapy. Twenty other patients with active RA were recruited to a study aiming to examine whether low-dose IVIg is beneficial in RA.[5] Ten patients were given six courses of IVIg (5 mg/kg) and another 10 patients received albumin (5 mg/kg) once every 3 weeks. There were no significant differences between treatment groups during the 18-week trial in terms of global activity indices (patient or physician assessment), joint swelling, joint pain or tenderness, erythrocyte sedimentation rate (ESR), CRP level, or rheumatoid factor. Another study failed to demonstrate any role of intra-articular administration of IgG.[6]

Beneficial effect of IVIg in RA

As opposed to these failures, most studies indicate that IVIg is justified in RA. In 6 of 11 patients treated with IVIg, there was an impressive clinical response.[7] However, this response was only transient in three patients. The IVIg therapy was associated with a decrease in T-cell ratio (CD4/CD8) caused by a reduction in CD4-positive cells in vivo. Additional findings were suppression of early B-cell activation, and reduction in the levels of polyethyleneglycol-precipitated circulating immune complexes.[7] In another study, seven patients with severe RA (in whom previous treatment with non-steroidal anti-inflammatory drugs (NSAIDs), corticosteroids and, in some cases, also with other disease-modifying anti-rheumatic drugs (DMARDs) was unsuccessful) received monthly courses of 400 mg/kg IVIg for 6 months. In six of these seven patients, there was a 50% improvement in the Ritchie index, and morning stiffness was reduced from greater than 2 h to less than 30 min.[8] Additionally, swollen joints and Lee index improved in all patients. There was no change in CD4/CD8 ratio in these patients. Tumiati et al[9] treated 10 patients with active, severe RA that was unresponsive to first- and second-line agents with monthly IVIg courses for 6 months. Nine patients completed the therapeutic protocol, and all showed significant improvement in both subjective and objective parameters of disease activity that were noted to occur as early as after the second infusion of IVIg. There was also a decrease in the CD4$^+$CDw29$^+$ to CD4$^+$CD45RA$^+$ cell ratio. Nonetheless, the patients had a relapse of the disease within a few weeks after discontinuation of treatment.[9]

The efficacy of longer-term IVIg therapy was evaluated in another 10 patients with active RA and prior unsuccessful treatment with at least one slow-acting anti-rheumatic drug.[10] Their treatment protocol included 400 mg/kg of IVIg for the first 3 days and then once a month for 12 months. The authors reported a late but significant clinical improvement that was observed after 6 months with regard to both symptoms and functional capability. There was also a rapid and persistent decrease in serum TNF-α and a late and significant reduction in soluble interleukin (sIL)-2R concentrations, the latter corre-

lating with the late decrease in disease activity.[10] Levels of other cytokines, such as IL-1α, IL-1β, IL-6 and interferon (IFN)-γ, were unaffected. In another study, the response of systemic-onset juvenile RA was evaluated in 27 patients treated with IVIg monthly for 3–54 months.[11] Five patients were unresponsive to IVIg therapy, and two dropped out of the study, whereas 6 months post-IVIg 20 patients had a least a 50% decrease in at least one of the following: number of days with fever; prednisone dose; or the number of active joints. In a follow-up visit (mean 37.6 ± 18 months), 11 of the 20 responders were in remission, 3 significantly improved but still had active arthritis, and 6 were unresponsive.[11] Others have reported on a comparison between methylprednisolone pulse therapy and IVIg in 20 patients with polyarticular or systemic juvenile chronic arthritis in combination with methotrexate and low-dose steroids.[12] Both treatment protocols resulted in regression of inflammatory activity, decreases in CD4 and CD8 cells, and normalization of the CD4/CD8 ratio. Whereas methylprednisolone pulses decreased the number of B cells, IVIg treatment increased their numbers. Opposite effects were noted regarding natural killer cells.

The use of IVIg has also been evaluated in seven patients having adult Still's disease.[13] They were treated with one to eight courses of 1 g/kg per day of IVIg for 2 consecutive days. All of them had a beneficial response to the treatment, which lasted between 1 and 90 days in three patients, who subsequently relapsed, but lasted for an average of 13 months (2–24 months) in the other four patients. The authors could not identify any clinical features that could aid in distinguishing who among the patients could respond more beneficially to IVIg therapy.[13] Another seven patients with adult Still's disease who were unresponsive or poorly responsive to NSAIDs were treated with monthly courses of IVIg.[14] Two patients were unresponsive, and five were initially considered to have a positive response, defined as disappearance of fever and arthritis within 2 weeks after the first IVIg infusion. They were given four to six IVIg infusions; one of them relapsed at the time of the fourth IVIg infusion, while the others had a favorable clinical and biological course.[14] Other authors also reported a 50% long-term remission rate in patients treated with monthly courses of IVIg 2 g/kg for 6 months, and suggested IVIg use in patients refractory to NSAIDs before the use of steroids.[15]

Several controlled trials also support the beneficial role of IVIg in RA. Patients with polyarticular juvenile RA resistant to other forms of therapy received infusions of IVIg at a dose between 1.5 and 2.0 g/kg per infusion (100 g maximum) bimonthly for the first 2 months, and then monthly for up to 6 months.[16] Beginning at month 3, those who met the criteria for clinically important improvement were randomized to receive monthly infusions for 4 months of either placebo or IVIg in a double-blind phase. Patients were permitted NSAIDs, slow-acting anti-rheumatic drugs, and low-dose (<10 mg/day) prednisone at constant doses. Nineteen of 25 (76%) children who entered the trial met the criteria for clinically important improvement during the open phase and entered the double-blind study.[16] IVIg resulted in a beneficial effect in the open phase, and patients who continued IVIg in the double-blind phase continued to show improvement over that achieved in the open phase. On the other hand, those given placebo showed a rapid loss of efficacy, suggesting that IVIg has a limited duration of effect after discontinuation. Thirty-one children with active, refractory, systemic juvenile RA were randomized into a multicenter, double-blind, placebo-controlled trial. Patients received infusions of 1.5 g/kg of IVIg or placebo (0.1% albumin) every 2 weeks for 2 months, and then monthly for 4 months.[17] A higher proportion of patients in the IVIg group improved (50% versus 27%) as assessed by the physician's global assessment, but, due to the small number of patients, this difference did not reach statistical significance.

Other conditions have been reported to be treated with IVIg. Three of eight patients with undifferentiated mono- and oligoarthritis whose synovial tissue tested positive for parvovirus B19 DNA by PCR suffered from progressive inflammatory arthritis disease despite conventional therapy and repeated synovectomy.[18] They received 0.4 g/kg body weight of IVIg over 5 days, and in two of them there was a marked improvement. Thus these patients did not need repeated synovectomy during follow-up periods of 7 and 10 months.[18] Another interesting case report described the dramatic improvement of thrombotic microangiopathy in a patient with adult Still's disease following IVIg administration.[19] On the other hand, there is a case report of arthritis which developed following IVIg treatment and was associated with elevated circulating immune complex level.[20]

MECHANISMS OF IVIg ACTIVITY IN RA

The mechanisms of action of IVIg in the treatment of RA are diverse but certainly include modulation of cytokine levels. In one study, 14 patients with highly active RA (at least five swollen joints, more than 2 h of morning stiffness, ESR > 40 mm/h) were treated with 0.4 g/kg body weight of IVIg for 5 consecutive days.[21] There was a 38% reduction in the Lansbury joint count, a 50% reduction in morning stiffness and a 53% decrease in pain levels following IVIg therapy. This treatment also resulted in decreases in CRP, α_2-globulin and IL-6 levels, whereas TNF-α levels increased during the infusion.[21] The levels of soluble receptor of TNF-α also increased post-IVIg therapy, as well as the ratio between TNF-α and its receptor. However, it seems that TNF-α blockade is beneficial in RA. Ten RA patients received a single 10 mg/kg infusion of anti-TNF-α monoclonal antibody.[22] This therapy significantly reduced granulocyte migration into affected joints, and there were simultaneous and significant reductions in the numbers of infiltrating synovial CD3+ T cells, CD22+ B cells, and CD68+ macrophages, and in the expression of IL-8 and monocyte chemotactic protein 1.[22] Animal models also support this assumption: IVIg treatment inhibited the active induction of two experimentally induced T-cell autoimmune diseases in rats (experimental autoimmune encephalomyelitis and adjuvant arthritis).[23] IVIg treatment led to decreased production of TNF-α, while it did not decrease T-cell recognition of self-antigens. Hence, IVIg treatment may exert its beneficial effect by inhibition of the biological consequences of T-cell recognition, rather than T-cell recognition per se.[23]

However, modulation of other cytokine levels is also associated with the beneficial effect of IVIg in RA. Kekow et al[24] reported that the immunosuppressive cytokine transforming growth factor (TGF)-β is present in substantial amounts in commercially available IVIg preparations. IVIg treatment of 15 patients with RA resulted in increases in both latent and bioactive TGF-β levels, thus supporting the latter's role in the clinical response of RA patients to IVIg. We also tested the levels of several cytokines in five commercially available IVIg products. These included: IL-1 receptor antagonist, IL-2, sIL-2R, IL-4, IL-5, IL-6, IL-8, IL-10, IL-12, TNF-α, TNF receptor, IFN-α and IFN-β.[25] None of the measured cytokines in any of the IVIg preparations tested were above the reference range of a given test. It should also be noted that IVIg exerts its beneficial effects in RA via other mechanisms, such as enhancement of circulating immune complex clearance, and downregulation of activation of B lymphocytes and their differentiation.[26] Another possible mechanism of action of IVIg in RA is its anti-infectious activity. Recently, we have reported antiviral and antibacterial activity of several commercial IVIg preparations directed to a wide range of infec-tious agents.[27] As infection is presumed to be involved in the pathogenesis of RA, this property of IVIg could represent another possible mechanism of action. Regarding the safety of IVIg, although there was an adverse effect rate of about 36% in our cohort of 56 patients with autoimmune diseases, most were mild and transient.[28] These include, for example headache, low-grade fever, chills, transient hypotension and nausea. There are also rare adverse effects reported in the literature, such as acute renal failure and hypercoagulability resulting in thrombosis, but as a general rule IVIg is quite safe.

CONCLUSIONS

There are enough data to support a beneficial role of IVIg in RA, even though some studies contradict this assumption. The earlier the treatment is administered, the more beneficial it probably is, as it affects the early phase of RA associated with inflammation without irreversible changes. Modes of action of IVIg in RA are diverse, as in other autoimmune diseases, but include mainly modulation of the cytokine network. More data from clinical studies are required with respect to the preferred dosage of IVIg, its mode of administration, number of treatment courses, factors predicting beneficial patients' outcome, etc. Nonetheless, it now seems that IVIg provides a relatively safe therapeutic agent in RA that will be used more in the future as its costs decline.

REFERENCES

1. Levy Y, Sherer Y, Ahmed A et al. A study of 20 SLE patients with intravenous immunoglobulin – clinical and serologic response. *Lupus* 1999; **8**: 705–12.
2. Levy Y, Sherer Y, Ahmed A et al. Serologic and clinical response to treatment of systemic vasculitis and associated autoimmune disease with intravenous immunoglobulin. *Int Arch Allergy Immunol* 1999; **119**: 231–8.
3. Wendling D, Racadot E, Wijdenes J et al. A randomized, double blind, placebo controlled multicenter trial of murine anti-CD4 monoclonal antibody therapy in rheumatoid arthritis. *J Rheumatol* 1998; **25**: 1457–61.
4. Maksymowych WP, Avina-Zubieta A, Luong M, Russell AS. High dose intravenous immunoglobulin (IVIg) in severe refractory rheumatoid arthritis: no evidence for efficacy. *Clin Exp Rheumatol* 1996; **14**: 657–60.
5. Kanik KS, Yarboro CH, Naparstek Y et al. Failure of low-dose intravenous immunoglobulin

therapy to suppress disease activity in patients with treatment-refractory rheumatoid arthritis. *Arthritis Rheum* 1996; **39**: 1027–9.

6. Bagge E, Geijer M, Tarkowski A. Intra-articular administration of polyclonal immunoglobulin G in rheumatoid arthritis. A double-blind, placebo-controlled pilot study. *Scand J Rheumatol* 1996; **25**: 174–6.

7. Becker H, Mitropoulou G, Helmke K. Immunomodulating therapy of rheumatoid arthritis by high-dose intravenous immunoglobulin. *Klin Wochenschr* 1989; **67**: 286–90.

8. Tumiati B, Veneziani M, Castellini G, Belelli A. High-dose immunoglobulins for the treatment of rheumatoid arthritis: pilot study of 7 cases. *Medicina* 1990; **10**: 398–401.

9. Tumiati B, Casoli P, Veneziani M, Rinaldi G. High-dose immunoglobulin therapy as an immunomodulatory treatment of rheumatoid arthritis. *Arthritis Rheum* 1992; **35**: 1126–33.

10. Muscat C, Bertotto A, Ercolani R et al. Long term treatment of rheumatoid arthritis with high doses of intravenous immunoglobulins: effects on disease activity and serum cytokines. *Ann Rheum Dis* 1995; **54**: 382–5.

11. Uziel Y, Laxer RM, Schneider R, Silverman ED. Intravenous immunoglobulin therapy in systemic onset juvenile rheumatoid arthritis: a followup study. *J Rheumatol* 1996; **23**: 910–18.

12. Oppermann J, Mobius D. Therapeutical and immunological effects of methylprednisolone pulse therapy in comparison with intravenous immunoglobulin. Treatment in patients with juvenile chronic arthritis. *Acta Univ Carol* 1994; **40**: 117–21.

13. Permal S, Wechsler B, Cabane J et al. Treatment of Still disease in adults with intravenous immunoglobulins. *Rev Med Interne* 1995; **16**: 250–4.

14. Vignes S, Wechsler B, Amoura Z et al. Intravenous immunoglobulin in adult Still's disease refractory to non-steroidal anti-inflammatory drugs. *Clin Exp Rheumatol* 1998; **16**: 295–8.

15. Vignes S, Wechsler B. Still's disease in adults: treatment with intravenous immunoglobulins. *Rev Med Interne* 1999; **20** (Suppl 4): 419–22.

16. Giannini EH, Lovell DJ, Silverman ED et al. Intravenous immunoglobulin in the treatment of polyarticular juvenile rheumatoid arthritis: a phase I/II study. Pediatric Rheumatology Collaborative Study Group. *J Rheumatol* 1996; **23**: 919–24.

17. Silverman ED, Cawkwell GD, Lovell DJ et al. Intravenous immunoglobulin in the treatment of systemic juvenile rheumatoid arthritis: a randomized placebo controlled trial. Pediatric Rheumatology Collaborative Study Group. *Ind J Rheumatol* 1994; **21**: 2353–8.

18. Stahl HD, Pfeiffer R, Emmrich F. Intravenous treatment with immunoglobulins may improve chronic undifferentiated mono- and oligoarthritis. *Clin Exp Rheumatol* 2000; **18**: 515–17.

19. Diamond JR. Hemolytic uremic syndrome/thrombotic thrombocytopenic purpura (HUS/TTP) complicating adult Still's disease: remission induced with intravenous immunoglobulin G. *J Nephrol* 1998; **10**: 253–7.

20. Lisak RP. Arthritis associated with circulating immune complexes following administration of intravenous immunoglobulin therapy in a patient with chronic inflammatory demyelinating polyneuropathy. *J Neurol Sci* 1996; **135**: 85–8.

21. Pap T, Reinhold D, Kekow J. Effects of intravenous immunoglobulins on disease activity and cytokine plasma levels in rheumatoid arthritis. *Scand J Rheumatol* 1998; **27**: 157–9

22. Taylor PC, Peters AM, Paleolog E et al. Reduction of chemokine levels and leukocyte traffic to joints by tumor necrosis factor alpha blockade in patients with rheumatoid arthritis. *Arthritis Rheum* 2000; **43**: 38–47.

23. Achiron A, Margalit R, Hershkoviz R et al. Intravenous immunoglobulin treatment of experimental T cell-mediated autoimmune disease. Upregulation of T cell proliferation and downregulation of tumor necrosis factor alpha secretion. *J Clin Invest* 1994; **93**: 600–5.

24. Kekow J, Reinhold D, Pap T, Ansorge S. Intravenous immunoglobulins and transforming growth factor beta. *Lancet* 1998; **351**: 184–5.

25. Sherer Y, Wu R, Krause I et al. Cytokine levels in various intravenous immunoglobulin (IVIg) preparations. *Human Antibodies* 2001; **10**: 51–3.

26. Delire M. Different modes of action of high-dose immunoglobulins in rheumatoid arthritis. *Acta Univ Carol* 1994; **40**: 95–9.

27. Krause I, Wu R, Sherer Y et al. In vitro antiviral and antibacterial activity of commercial intravenous immunoglobulin preparations – a potential role for adjuvant intravenous immunoglobulin therapy in infectious diseases. *Tranfus Med* 2002; **12**: 133–9.

28. Sherer Y, Levy Y, Langevitz P et al. Adverse effects of intravenous immunoglobulin therapy in 56 patients with autoimmune diseases. *Pharmacology* 2001; **62**: 133–7.

38

Apheresis

Winfried B Graninger

Conceptual background • Clinical effectivity • Conclusion • References

CONCEPTUAL BACKGROUND

Historical perspective

The removal of pathogenic constituents from blood by various methods has been critizived as 'an ancient medical remedy used in the management of diseases whose pathophysiology is poorly understood and whose effective treatment modalities are lacking'.[1,2] Nevertheless, the association of abnormalities in the cellular and humoral immune system with various autoimmune diseases still serves as a rationale for the use of apheresis technologies in desperate patients with systemic inflammatory rheumatic conditions. After centuries of blood letting and leeching, advances in the technology of extracorporeal blood separation and isolation of the culprit plasma fractions have made apheresis a relatively safe, albeit still very costly, procedure.

Technical definitions

Numerous devices are available for the continuous separation of cellular blood components and plasma from peripheral venous access.

Plasma exchange was defined as replacement of the patient's plasma with plasma from healthy donors. Plasmapheresis also involves the removal of whole patient plasma; it leads to non-

specific loss of plasma constituents and requires volume and electrolyte repletion and, in the majority of cases, the substitution of non-autologous protein (human albumin or, quite often, fresh-frozen plasma). The terms plasma exchange and plasmapheresis are often erroneously used synonymously; however, the kind of protein replacement is pharmacologically and biologically relevant. Accepted indications for this procedure include hyperviscosity syndromes, Goodpasture's syndrome, acquired myasthenia gravis, hemolytic–uremic syndrome, thrombotic thrombocytopenic purpura, and hyperlipidemia.

Within the field of autoimmune diseases and, in particular, in rheumatological disorders, plasmapheresis has recently been considered obsolete since the development of more antibody-specific adsorption devices.

Immunapheresis or immunoadsorption uses extracorporeal contact of separated plasma with a variety of immunoglobulin-binding ligands which are bound to a fixed matrix (Table 38.1). Immunoadsorption devices can be subdivided into non-selective, semi-selective and highly selective adsorbers. While non-selective adsorbers (dextran sulfate, tryptophan, and phenylalanine) reduce the plasma levels of many different substances, such as fibrinogen, albumin, lipids and immunoglobulins, semi-

Table 38.1   Commonly used absorber devices for immunapheresis in autoimmune diseases.

	Selesorb	IM-TR 350	Prosorba	Immunosorba	Ig-Therasorb	Miro
Company (Germany)	Kaneka	Diamed	Fresenius	Fresenius	Plasmaselect	Fresenius
Ligand	Dextran sulfate	Tryptophan, phenylalanine	Protein A	Protein A	Polyclonal sheep anti-human Ig	C1q
Matrix		Polyvinylalcohol	Silica	Sepharose	Sepharose	Polyacrylate
Specificity	Anti-DNA antibodies, lipids, fibrinogen	Immunoglobulin, fibrinogen	IgG, IgA, IgM	IgG, IgA, IgM	IgG, IgA, IgM	C1qCIC, C1qAb, Antiphospholipid Ab

selective adsorbers (staphylococcal protein A, anti-human Ig adsorber) show affinity for only one group of plasma proteins. Highly selective adsorbers eliminate specific substances without changing the blood levels of other plasma components.[3–5]

Modern blood-banking equipment allows the removal of leukocytes; this experimental therapeutic approach to immune-mediated diseases is called cytapheresis or leukapheresis.[6–9]

A related technique which actually does not remove anything from patient blood is photopheresis, whereby extracorporeal irradiation of leukocytes with ultraviolet light after treatment with 8-methoxypsoralen is followed by reinfusion of plasma and autologous blood cells. The mechanisms of this intervention are subject to interesting hypotheses;[10] uncontrolled reports of its efficacy in rheumatoid arthritis and systemic lupus erythematosus (SLE) have been published.[11,12]

Proposed mechanisms of (immun)-apheresis therapy

The concept of circulating pathogenic autoantibodies lies at the heart of the immunoadsorption approach. In addition to elimination of such autoantibodies, circulating immune complexes can be extracted or modified in their composition, a 'deblocking effect' on the reticuloendothelial system has been postulated, and the influence of the procedure on the composition of lymphocyte subsets and the change in cytokine network activity (last, but not least, by the extracorporeal circulation), as well as the effects of the anticoagulants used, cannot be excluded.[13,14] A novel suggestion for the mechanism of protein A columns is the release of the staphylococcal protein into the circulation.

The quantitative capacity for extraction of immunoglobulins differs considerably between the absorption devices.[15–17] Ligands for the specific purging of defined (auto)antibodies as well as for the purging of circulating DNA from the plasma have been devised. The amount of protein to be withdrawn for maximum therapeutic benefit, the frequency and time intervals of apheresis procedures, and the disputable need to countervene possible rebound immunoglobulin synthesis, have not yet been fully explored.

Substitution of intravenous immunoglobulin preparations after immunapheresis is practiced in many centers and possibly has a strong immunomodulatory effect on its own.[18,19]

It is not clear whether the therapeutic effects of apheresis in autoimmune diseases are due to the actual elimination process or rather due to an ill-defined complex of events called immunomodulation.

Immunological laboratory sequelae of immunapheresis

After successful immunoglobulin depletion from circulating blood by a consecutive series of apheresis sessions, redistribution of immunoglobulin from the interstitium is observed. The rate of resynthesis depends on B-cell activity, which quite often is the target of concomitant pharmacological immunosuppression. The effect of complement activation by the extracorporeal circulation has to be considered.[20] In addition, effects of blood cell separation and extracorporeal surface exposition on leukocyte and lymphocyte activity[21] and phenotype[13,22–24] as well as cytokine production[14] have been reported.

CLINICAL EFFECTIVITY

Difficulties in the evaluation of therapeutic power

The great majority of reported studies of apheresis in SLE and other rare rheumatological diseases are case reports without any conclusive control groups. Ethical and practical problems have hindered the implementation of randomized clinical trials. The assessment of individual treatments is difficult, because apheresis procedures are often used in combination with drug therapy. Outcome measures vary enormously, and sometimes are not well defined. In addition, therapeutic despair is often the main motivation for performing apheresis in cases refractory to conventional treatment. The term 'adjunctive treatment', which is sometimes used for the 'immunomodulatory' effects of such an invasive and expensive procedure, further illustrates the limitations in the understanding of the published research evidence.

In contrast to many other therapeutic interventions targeting the immune system, apheresis procedures appear to be relatively safe in the short term, with rates of serious adverse events of 0.5–0.8%.[25–27]

Systemic lupus erythematosus

Plasmapheresis

SLE can be seen as the prototype candidate indication for apheresis therapy, since it is considered to be an immune complex disease with impaired clearance of circulating immune complexes, and the pathogenic role of autoantibodies is at least reasonable. The removal of immune complexes lessens the damage to blood vessels and organs triggered by immune complex deposition.[28,29] The first report of beneficial clinical effects of plasma removal in four SLE patients was published in 1976;[30] improvements in splenic function and the clearance function of the reticuloendothelial system were observed after the procedure.[31,32] The numerous case reports and uncontrolled studies which followed mostly described positive short-term effects of plasmapheresis in lupus patients;[33] they have been compiled by Euler et al.[34]

The first controlled study of plasmapheresis in SLE included only 20 patients: the frequency and degree of clinical improvement were the same in both the plasma exchange and control groups.[35] While short-term clinical and serological benefit was observed in similarly designed studies,[36] larger studies of plasmapheresis alone or as an adjunct to oral cyclophosphamide in lupus nephritis did not find any long-term benefit.[37] In contrast, the side-effects of lupus treatment, such as life-threatening bacterial and viral infections and mortality, occur more frequently in patients undergoing plasmapheresis and cyclophosphamide bolus therapy than among patients with similarly active SLE treated with cyclophosphamide alone.[38]

The concept of synchronization of plasma exchange and high-dose intravenous cyclophosphamide involves the clonal deletion of the pathogenic B cells produced as a rebound mechanism after therapeutic depletion of immunoglobulins. The large international trial of the Lupus Plasmapheresis Study Group included 147 patients from 45 centers. No therapeutic advantage of adding plasmapheresis to high-dose intravenous cyclophosphamide was found.[39,40] While some of the authors of this study switched to a high-dose cyclophosphamide (2 g/m² body surface) protocol without plasma exchange, the concept of plasmapheresis for the treatment of lupus nephritis was abandoned in most centers.

Nevertheless, individual SLE patients with life-threatening manifestations refractory to steroids and immunosuppressive drugs are still considered candidates for plasmapheresis if the technically more demanding equipment for selective immunoadsorption is not available. Case descriptions of clinical success in such situations continue to appear in the literature.[41–47]

Immunoadsorption (immunapheresis)

With technical progress in engineering, absorbing devices with selective binding capacities for immunoglobulin became available and were used for the treatment of patients with SLE.[48] It still has to be considered, however, that multiple cycles of apheresis sessions are necessary to achieve a quantitative removal of immunoglobulins and that redistribution of immunoglobulins from the 50% extravascular compartment will occur.[49,50]

After the first reports using rather simple approaches towards selective immunapheresis in SLE,[51,52] a variety of absorbers were tested (Table 38.1).

Dextran sulfate cellulose has a high affinity for anti-DNA antibodies, anti-cardiolipin antibodies and complement factors. In uncontrolled series, a decline in anti-DNA titers in lupus patients was found in addition to some anecdotal improvement in clinical signs.[53–58] Although dextran sulfate absorbers hold promise, especially for patients with antiphospholipid syndrome, in whom immunosuppressive therapy should be avoided, no controlled clinical studies are available for this device.

Phenylalanine and tryptophan absorbers were studied in an open study with 50 SLE patients, and a significant improvement in lupus activity was sustained for up to 6 months.[59,60] Moreover, a prospective randomized trial compared tryptophan absorbers and a sheep anti-human immunoglobulin device, and found both methods to produce a clinical response with a decrease in lupus activity in 20 SLE patients.[61] With intensified treatment, a 58–75% reduction in anti-DNA antibodies was achieved.

Staphylococcal protein A bound to either silica or sepharose is also marketed for immunapheresis absorbers. In an open series, remission of severe, treatment-resistant lupus was reported to have occurred in seven of eight patients,[62] but no controlled studies are available yet. The leakage of protein A was reported to be almost undetectable; however, side-effects were observed when protein A was bound to silica.[63]

A regenerable immunoglobulin-absorbing column was created using sheep anti-human antibodies covalently bound to sepharose.[64] It was used for rapid elimination of factor VIII inhibitors,[65] and in patients with severe manifestations of SLE in small, uncontrolled series.[66] A comparison with phenylalanine absorbers was performed in a controlled prospective study,[61] but unfortunately no control group without immunoadsorption was included in this study.

The complement factor C1q immobilized on an acrylate matrix is used as a ligand for complexed immunoglobulins, anti-C1q autoantibodies, DNA, and nucleosomes. Immunoadsorption with such an absorber was reported to be safe and effective in SLE patients in a preliminary study.[3,67] Although this approach sounds very promising, confirmational controlled studies have to be awaited.

While the place of immunoadsorption in the treatment of SLE patients in general is not yet defined clearly, due to the lack of conclusive controlled studies, the indication to use immunapheresis is attractive in the situation where immunosuppressive treatment is contraindicated, as in pregnancy[68–70] or in cases with severe bone marrow failure. In lupus nephritis, chronic nephrotic syndrome may be an interesting oppportunity for immunoadsorption, since it was shown to decrease proteinuria significantly, albeit by unknown mechanisms.[71,72]

Systemic vasculitis

Regarding the serious prognosis in patients with systemic vasculitides, plasmapheresis has been applied sucessfully in anecdotal patients.[73] A more systematic approach in France found that combined treatment with prednisone and plasma exchange is not superior to treatment with prednisone alone and must not be systematically employed for the initial treatment of panarteritis nodosa (PAN) and Churg–Strauss syndrome (CSS). In most cases, cyclophosphamide alone was effective and well tolerated.[74,75]

In addition to a Swedish report finding a similar outcome when comparing plasma exchange with immunoadsorption in rapidly progressive crescentic glomerulonephritis,[76] immunoadsorption was reported as being clinically effective in three cases of c-ANCA-positive vasculitis (ANCA, antineutrophil cytoplasma antibodies; C, cytoplasmic).[77] With the use of a protein A absorber in primary systemic vasculitis, histologically proven inactivation of renal involvement was demonstrated, but the patients were also treated with immunosuppressive drugs.[60]

Rheumatoid arthritis

Extracorporeal immunoadsorption with a protein A–silica column has been suggested for use in patients with rheumatoid arthritis who have failed conventional treatments.[78–80] While the rationale for using immunapheresis in rheumatoid arthritis is not easily understood, the mechanisms of the therapeutic action of this column are entirely unclear. It was shown that the procedure did not alter the concentrations of albumin, IgG, IgM, and IgA, and that mean values of circulating immune complexes were not significantly decreased.[17] Thus, instead of removing something, the procedure was supposed to add protein A to the circulation or to modify complement or circulating immune complex composition. Very interesting for explaining the mechanisms of action is the finding that the oligovalent structure of protein A induces apoptotic cell death that results in immunomodulation of B-cell responses.[81]

Regardless of the mechanism of action, randomized clinical trials in treatment-refractory patients with rheumatoid arthritis have shown statistical superiority of this protein A 'pheresis' over sham extracorporeal treatment, with response rates of 41%.[80,82]

CONCLUSION

In the past two decades, the medical community has increasingly used therapeutic apheresis. Technically, a patient's plasma and/or the cellular parts of blood are separated and then removed from the circulation. It was believed that abnormal or harmful substances are thereby removed, leading to a cure or arrest of the disease. The high costs of apheresis and the fact that entirely different conditions (from cancer to arthritis) are being treated with these procedures have evoked a critical attitude and strong debates.

In the area of autoimmune diseases, which sometimes have a detrimental prognosis, the evaluation of effectiveness and effectivity is hindered by the rare occurrence of the diseases themselves and even more by the rarity of life- or organ-threatening situations. Nevertheless, controlled trials have been funded and performed, and they have shown, for instance, that plasmapheresis is not effective for the treatment of most patients with SLE or systemic vasculitides. The personal experience of physicians who have seen dramatic beneficial (sometimes life-saving) effects of apheresis procedures stands in contrast to the systematic approaches of cost-effectiveness investigations.

The advances in absorber technology will allow us to target almost any molecule which is recognized as harmful and remove it from the circulation. While this approach certainly will always have the character of a short-term intervention, a better understanding of the mechanisms of action of some of the apheresis procedures will possibly lead towards ways of genuinely rational immunological intervention and thus hopefully will make expensive extracorporeal procedures obsolete in the treatment of autoimmune diseases.

REFERENCES

1. Campion EW. Desperate diseases and plasmapheresis. *N Engl J Med* 1992; **326**(21): 1425–7.
2. Illei GG, Klippel JH. Apheresis. *Rheum Dis Clin North Am* 2000; **26**(1): 63–73, viii.
3. Hiepe F, Pfuller B, Wolbart K et al. A multifunctional ligand for a new immunoadsorption treatment. *Ther Apher* 1999; **3**(3): 246–51.
4. Hiepe F, Wolbart K, Schossler W et al. Development of a DNA-adsorbent for the specific removal of anti-DNA autoantibodies in systemic lupus erythematosus (SLE). *Biomater Artif Cells Artif Organs* 1990; **18**(5): 683–8.
5. Kong DL, Schuett W, Boeden HF et al. Development of a DNA immunoadsorbent: coupling DNA on sepharose 4FF by an efficient activation method. *Artif Organs* 2000; **24**(11): 845–51.
6. Hidaka T, Suzuki K. Efficacy of filtration leukocytapheresis on rheumatoid arthritis with vasculitis. *Ther Apher* 1997; **1**(3): 212–14.
7. Hidaka T, Suzuki K, Matsuki Y et al. Filtration leukocytapheresis therapy in rheumatoid arthritis: a randomized, double-blind, placebo-controlled trial. *Arthritis Rheum* 1999; **42**(3): 431–7.
8. Hidaka T, Suzuki K, Kawakami M et al. Dynamic changes in cytokine levels in serum and synovial fluid following filtration leukocytapheresis therapy in patients with rheumatoid arthritis. *J Clin Apher* 2001; **16**(2): 74–81.
9. Ueki Y, Yamasaki S, Kanamoto Y et al. Evaluation of filtration leucocytapheresis for use in the treatment of patients with rheumatoid arthritis. *Rheumatology* 2000; **39**(2): 165–71.
10. Aringer M, Graninger WB, Smolen JS et al. Photopheresis treatment enhances CD95 (fas) expression in circulating lymphocytes of patients with systemic sclerosis and induces apoptosis. *Br J Rheumatol* 1997; **36**(12): 1276–82.
11. Malawista SE, Trock D, Edelson RL. Photopheresis for rheumatoid arthritis. *Ann NY Acad Sci* 1991; **636**: 217–26.
12. Knobler RM, Graninger W, Graninger W et al. Extracorporeal photochemotherapy for the treatment of systemic lupus erythematosus. A pilot study. *Arthritis Rheum* 1992; **35**(3): 319–24.
13. Goto H, Matsuo H, Nakane S et al. Plasmapheresis affects T helper type-1/T helper type-2 balance of circulating peripheral lymphocytes. *Ther Apher* 2001; **5**(6): 494–6.
14. Hehmke B, Salzsieder E, Matic GB et al. Immunoadsorption of immunoglobulins alters intracytoplasmic type 1 and type 2 T cell cytokine production in patients with refractory autoimmune diseases. *Ther Apher* 2000; **4**(4): 296–302.
15. Matic G, Hofmann D, Winkler R et al. Removal of immunoglobulins by a protein A versus an antihuman immunoglobulin G-based system: evaluation of 602 sessions of extracorporeal immunoadsorption. *Artif Organs* 2000; **24**(2): 103–7.
16. Ikonomov V, Samtleben W, Schmidt B et al. Adsorption profile of commercially available adsorbents: an in vitro evaluation. *Int J Artif Organs* 1992; **15**(5): 312–19.
17. Sasso EH, Merrill C, Furst TE. Immunoglobulin binding properties of the Prosorba immunadsorption column in treatment of rheumatoid arthritis. *Ther Apher* 2001; **5**(2): 84–91.
18. Schmaldienst S, Mullner M, Goldammer A et al. Intravenous immunoglobulin application following immunoadsorption: benefit or risk in patients with autoimmune diseases? *Rheumatology* 2001; **40**(5): 513–21.
19. Wolf HM, Eibl MM. Immunomodulatory effect of immunoglobulins. *Clin Exp Rheumatol* 1996; **14**(suppl 15): S17–S25.
20. Alarabi AA, Nilsson B, Nilsson U et al. Complement activation during tryptophan immunoadsorption treatment. *Artif Organs* 1993; **17**(9): 782–6.
21. Ijichi S, Mishima M, Matsuda T et al. Concentration of activated T lymphocytes in extracorporeal blood circulation for plasma separation. *J Clin Apher* 1991; **6**(2): 88–9.
22. Csipo I, Kiss E, Soltesz P et al. Effect of plasmapheresis on ligand binding capacity and expression of erythrocyte complement receptor type 1 (CR1) of patients with systemic lupus erythematosus (SLE). *Clin Exp Immunol* 1999; **118**(3): 458–64.
23. Paglieroni T, Caggiano V, MacKenzie MR. Effects of plasmapheresis on peripheral blood mononuclear cell populations from patients with macroglobulinemia. *J Clin Apher* 1987; **3**(4): 202–8.
24. Snyder HW Jr, Balint JP Jr, Jones FR. Modulation of immunity in patients with autoimmune disease and cancer treated by extracorporeal immunoadsorption with PROSORBA columns. *Semin Hematol* 1989; **26**(2 Suppl 1): 31–41.
25. Bussel A, Pourrat J, Elkharrat D, Gajdos P. The

French registry for plasma exchange: a four year experience. *Int J Artif Organs* 1991; **14**(7): 393–7.

26. McLeod BC, Sniecinski I, Ciavarella D et al. Frequency of immediate adverse effects associated with therapeutic apheresis. *Transfusion* 1999; **39**(3): 282–8.

27. Sutton DM, Nair RC, Rock G. Complications of plasma exchange. *Transfusion* 1989; **29**(2): 124–7.

28. Wallace DJ. Apheresis for lupus erythematosus. *Lupus* 1999; **8**(3): 174–80.

29. Wallace DJ. Apheresis for lupus erythematosus: state of the art. *Lupus* 2001; **10**(3): 193–6.

30. Jones JV, Cumming RH, Bucknall RC, Asplin CM. Plasmapheresis in the management of acute systemic lupus erythematosus? *Lancet* 1976; **1**(7962): 709–11.

31. Lockwood CM, Worlledge S, Nicholas A et al. Reversal of impaired splenic function in patients with nephritis or vasculitis (or both) by plasma exchange. *N Engl J Med* 1979; **300**(10): 524–30.

32. Low A, Hotze A, Krapf F et al. The nonspecific clearance function of the reticuloendothelial system in patients with immune complex mediated diseases before and after therapeutic plasmapheresis. *Rheumatol Int* 1985; **5**(2): 69–72.

33. Zielinski C, Muller C, Smolen J. Use of plasmapheresis in therapy of systemic lupus erythematosus: a controlled study. *Acta Med Austriaca* 1988; **15**(5): 155–8.

34. Euler HH, Zeuner RA, Schroeder JO. Plasma exchange in systemic lupus erythematosus. *Transfus Sci* 1996; **17**(2): 245–65.

35. Wei N, Klippel JH, Huston DP et al. Randomised trial of plasma exchange in mild systemic lupus erythematosus. *Lancet* 1983; **1**(8314–15): 17–22.

36. Derksen RH, Hene RJ, Kallenberg CG et al. Prospective multicentre trial on the short-term effects of plasma exchange versus cytotoxic drugs in steroid-resistant lupus nephritis. *Neth J Med* 1988; **33**(3–4): 168–77.

37. Lewis EJ, Hunsicker LG, Lan SP et al. A controlled trial of plasmapheresis therapy in severe lupus nephritis. The Lupus Nephritis Collaborative Study Group. *N Engl J Med* 1992; **326**(21): 1373–9.

38. Aringer M, Smolen JS, Graninger WB. Severe infections in plasmapheresis-treated systemic lupus erythematosus. *Arthritis Rheum* 1998; **41**(3): 414–20.

39. Clark WF, Dau PC, Euler HH et al. Plasmapheresis and subsequent pulse cyclophosphamide versus pulse cyclophosphamide alone in severe lupus: design of the LPSG trial. Lupus Plasmapheresis Study Group (LPSG). *J Clin Apher* 1991; **6**(1): 40–7.

40. Wallace DJ, Goldfinger D, Pepkowitz SH et al. Randomized controlled trial of pulse/synchronization cyclophosphamide/apheresis for proliferative lupus nephritis. *J Clin Apher* 1998; **13**(4): 163–6.

41. Fukuda M, Kamiyama Y, Kawahara K et al. The favourable effect of cyclophosphamide pulse therapy in the treatment of massive pulmonary haemorrhage in systemic lupus erythematosus. *Eur J Pediatr* 1994; **153**(3): 167–70.

42. Shiraishi H, Migita K, Honda S. Successful plasmapheresis in alveolar hemorrhage associated with systemic lupus erythematosus. *Modern Rheumatol* 2001; **11**(4): 340–3.

43. Bonnet F, Mercie P, Morlat P et al. Devic's neuromyelitis optica during pregnancy in a patient with systemic lupus erythematosus. *Lupus* 1999; **8**(3): 244–7.

44. Erickson RW, Franklin WA, Emlen W. Treatment of hemorrhagic lupus pneumonitis with plasmapheresis. *Semin Arthritis Rheum* 1994; **24**(2): 114–23.

45. Fukui W, Sano H, Tanabe T et al. A case of severe neuropsychiatric lupus erythematosus treated by plasmapheresis: diagnostic values of serum antiribosomal P protein antibodies and interleukin-6 in cerebrospinal fluid. *Nihon Rinsho Meneki Gakkai Kaishi* 1998; **21**(4): 172–9.

46. Huang DF, Tsai ST, Wang SR. Recovery of both acute massive pulmonary hemorrhage and acute renal failure in a systemic lupus erythematosus patient with lupus anticoagulant by the combined therapy of plasmapheresis plus cyclophosphamide. *Transfus Sci* 1994; **15**(3): 283–8.

47. Santos-Ocampo AS, Mandell BF, Fessler BJ. Alveolar hemorrhage in systemic lupus erythematosus: presentation and management. *Chest* 2000; **118**(4): 1083–90.

48. Mistry-Burchardi N, Schonermarck U, Samtleben W. Apheresis in lupus nephritis. *Ther Apher* 2001; **5**(3): 161–70.

49. Braun N, Gutenberger S, Erley CM, Risler T. Immunoglobulin and circulating immune complex kinetics during immunoadsorption onto protein A sepharose. *Transfus Sci* 1998; **19** (Suppl): 25–31.

50. Braun N, Risler T. Immunoadsorption as a tool for the immunomodulation of the humoral and cellular immune system in autoimmune disease. *Ther Apher* 1999; **3**(3): 240–5.

51. Palmer A, Gjorstrup P, Severn A et al. Treatment of systemic lupus erythematosus by extracorporeal immunoadsorption. *Lancet* 1988; **2**(8605): 272.

52. Terman DS, Buffaloe G, Mattioli C et al. Extracorporeal immunoadsorption: initial experience in human systemic lupus erythematosus. *Lancet* 1979; **2**(8147): 824–7.

53. Matsuki Y, Suzuki K, Kawakami M et al. High-avidity anti-DNA antibody removal from the serum of systemic lupus erythematosus patients by adsorption using dextran sulfate cellulose columns. *J Clin Apher* 1996; **11**(1): 30–5.

54. Suzuki K, Taman J, Matsuki Y et al. Anti-dsDNA antibody kinetics during in vivo apheresis in systemic lupus erythematosus patients and in an in vitro apheresis model. *J Clin Apher* 1996; **11**(4): 211–16.

55. Matsuki Y, Suzuki K, Kawakami M et al. Adsorption of anaphylatoxins from the plasma of systemic lupus erythematosus patients using dextran sulfate cellulose columns. *J Clin Apher* 1998; **13**(3): 108–13.

56. Kinoshita M, Aotsuka S, Funahashi T et al. Selective removal of anti-double-stranded DNA antibodies by immunoadsorption with dextran sulphate in a patient with systemic lupus erythematosus. *Ann Rheum Dis* 1989; **48**(10): 856–60.

57. Hashimoto H, Tsuda H, Kanai Y et al. Selective removal of anti-DNA and anticardiolipin antibodies by adsorbent plasmapheresis using dextran sulfate columns in patients with systemic lupus erythematosus. *J Rheumatol* 1991; **18**(4): 545–51.

58. Suzuki K. The role of immunoadsorption using dextran-sulfate cellulose columns in the treatment of systemic lupus erythematosus. *Ther Apher* 2000; **4**(3): 239–43.

59. Schneider M, Berning T, Waldendorf M et al. Immunoadsorbent plasma perfusion in patients with systemic lupus erythematosus . *J Rheumatol* 1990; **17**(7): 900–7.

60. Schneider M, Gaubitz M, Perniok A. Immunoadsorption in systemic connective tissue diseases and primary vasculitis. *Ther Apher* 1997; **1**(2): 117–20.

61. Gaubitz M, Seidel M, Kummer S et al. Prospective randomized trial of two different immunoadsorbers in severe systemic lupus erythematosus. *J Autoimmun* 1998; **11**(5): 495–501.

62. Braun N, Erley C, Klein R et al. Immunoadsorption onto protein A induces remission in severe systemic lupus erythematosus. *Nephrol Dial Transplant* 2000; **15**(9): 1367–72.

63. Samtleben W, Schmidt B, Gurland HJ. Ex vivo and in vivo protein A perfusion: background, basic investigations, and first clinical experiences. *Blood Purif* 1987; **5**(2–3): 179–92.

64. Koll RA. Ig-Therasorb immunoadsorption for selective removal of human immunoglobulins in diseases associated with pathogenic antibodies of all classes and IgG subclasses, immune complexes, and fragments of immunoglobulins. *Ther Apher* 1998; **2**(2): 147–52.

65. Knoebl P, Derfler K, Korninger L et al. Elimination of acquired factor VIII antibodies by extracorporeal antibody-based immunoadsorption (Ig-Therasorb). *Thromb Haemost* 1995; **74**(4): 1035–8.

66. Graninger M, Schmaldienst S, Derfler K, Graninger W. Immunoadsorption therapy in patients with severe lupus erythematosus. *Acta Med Austriaca* 2002; **29**: 26–9.

67. Pfueller B, Wolbart K, Bruns A et al. Successful treatment of patients with systemic lupus erythematosus by immunoadsorption with a C1q column: a pilot study. *Arthritis Rheum* 2001; **44**(8): 1962–3.

68. Nakamura Y, Yoshida K, Itoh S et al. Immunoadsorption plasmapheresis as a treatment for pregnancy complicated by systemic lupus erythematosus with positive antiphospholipid antibodies. *Am J Reprod Immunol* 1999; **41**(5): 307–11.

69. Takeshita Y, Turumi Y, Touma S, Takagi N. Successful delivery in a pregnant woman with lupus anticoagulant positive systemic lupus erythematosus treated with double filtration plasmapheresis. *Ther Apher* 2001; **5**(1): 22–4.

70. Toyama M, Oozono S, Uruta Y et al. Effective treatment with double filtration plasmapheresis (DFPP) and high dose intravenous gammaglobulin therapy in a pregnant patient with systemic lupus erythematosus. *Nippon Naika Gakkai Zasshi* 1989; **78**(11): 1601–2.

71. Dantal J, Godfrin Y, Koll R et al. Antihuman immunoglobulin affinity immunoadsorption strongly decreases proteinuria in patients with relapsing nephrotic syndrome. *J Am Soc Nephrol* 1998; **9**(9): 1709–15.

72. Wallace DJ, Goldfinger D, Bluestone R, Klinenberg JR. Plasmapheresis in lupus nephritis with nephrotic syndrome: a long-term followup. *J Clin Apher* 1982; **1**(1): 42–5.

73. Lewis EJ. Plasmapheresis in collagen vascular diseases. *Ther Apher* 1999; **3**(2): 172–7.

74. Guillevin L, Fain O, Lhote F et al. Lack of superiority of steroids plus plasma exchange to steroids alone in the treatment of polyarteritis nodosa and Churg–Strauss syndrome. A prospective, randomized trial in 78 patients. *Arthritis Rheum* 1992; **35**(2): 208–15.

75. Guillevin L, Jarrousse B, Lok C et al. Longterm followup after treatment of polyarteritis nodosa and Churg–Strauss angiitis with comparison of steroids, plasma exchange and cyclophosphamide to steroids and plasma exchange. A prospective randomized trial of 71 patients. The Cooperative Study Group for Polyarteritis Nodosa. *J Rheumatol* 1991; **18**(4): 567–74.

76. Stegmayr BG, Almroth G, Berlin G et al. Plasma exchange or immunoadsorption in patients with rapidly progressive crescentic glomerulonephritis. A Swedish multi-center study. *Int J Artif Organs* 1999; **22**(2): 81–7.

77. Matic G, Michelsen A, Hofmann D et al. Three cases of C-ANCA-positive vasculitis treated with immunoadsorption: possible benefit in early treatment. *Ther Apher* 2001; **5**(1): 68–72.

78. Caldwell J, Gendreau RM, Furst D et al. A pilot study using a staph protein A column (Prosorba) to treat refractory rheumatoid arthritis. *J Rheumatol* 1999; **26**(8): 1657–62.

79. Wiesenhutter CW, Irish BL, Bertram JH. Treatment of patients with refractory rheumatoid arthritis with extracorporeal protein A immunoadsorption columns: a pilot trial. *J Rheumatol* 1994; **21**(5): 804–12.

80. Felson DT, LaValley MP, Baldassare AR et al. The Prosorba column for treatment of refractory rheumatoid arthritis: a randomized, double-blind, sham-controlled trial. *Arthritis Rheum* 1999; **42**(10): 2153–9.

81. Goodyear C, Silverman G. Evidence of a novel immunomodulatory mechanism of action of Prosorba therapy: release of staphylococcal protein A induces a VH region targeted apoptotic death of B lymphocytes. *Arthritis Rheum* 2001; **44**(9)(suppl): S296.

82. Gendreau RM. A randomized double-blind sham-controlled trial of the Prosorba column for treatment of refractory rheumatoid arthritis. *Ther Apher* 2001; **5**(2): 79–83.

Section VIII

Ethics and study design

39

Ethical issues in rheumatologic investigation and practice

Richard S Panush, Arthur Kavanaugh and Paul L Romain

Introduction • Historical considerations • Principles of biomedical ethics • Ethical issues, clinical trials, and biologicals in rheumatology • Relationships with the biotechnology and pharmaceutical industry • Ethics and professionalism • Closing comments • Acknowledgments • References

Progress in biomedical science and technology has made available novel biological therapies for the rheumatic diseases. These have resulted in meaningful advances in the treatment of patients suffering from these disorders. This is emphatically reflected by the publication of this volume and in its breadth and depth. Increasing attention to ethical issues in bioscience and medicine in the face of such progress is not coincidental. Concerns surrounding these and other issues have helped focus public and academic interest in the ethical dimensions of these advances and current clinical care. This chapter will address general medical ethical principles, human experimentation, uncertainties regarding risk and costs of new technologies, the increasing interactions between academia, clinicians and the biotechnology and pharmaceutical research industry, and matters of professionalism.

INTRODUCTION

Historically, biomedical science and clinical medicine mirrored the societies in which they existed. They were paternalistic enterprises in which the government had only a modest role. The public had little knowledge or influence and trusted their doctors, although it could be argued that they had little choice to do otherwise. Medical ethics, even as recently as the 1960s, has been described as 'a mixture of religion, whimsy, exhortation, legal precedents, various traditions, philosophies of life, miscellaneous moral rules, and epithets'.[1] A number of events during the mid-twentieth century provided the background to the scholarly work which led to the current generally accepted consensus on the principles and the resultant vocabulary of discourse of modern biomedical ethics.

HISTORICAL CONSIDERATIONS

Several seminal events occurring over the past half-century have had a profound impact on ethical concerns related to clinical research. Prior to this time, the predominant ethical principles guiding physicians conducting experiments with humans were the tenets of the Hippocratic oath. Accordingly, physicians were obliged to act with 'φρονησις', or wise and considered judgment, in the care of their patients. Two key components of this are beneficence, or acting for the good of the patient, and non-maleficence, or avoiding harm. It is of note that this paternalistic viewpoint largely excluded the viewpoints of patients, including those participating in clinical research.

The horrors of the Nazi medical atrocities[2,3] led to the 'Doctors' Trial' and the development of the Nuremberg code. This formally articulated the doctrine and components of voluntary informed consent to be exercised by human subjects. This principle of autonomous decision-making on the part of the patient was viewed as 'absolutely essential' for human experimentation.[3] Other key requirements were that an experiment should be terminated if there was likelihood of injury or disability of the subject and that efforts should be taken to minimize risk. Beecher's influential 1966 publication critically examined a number of research studies and found them strikingly deficient with regard to respect for the rights of research subjects in numerous instances. He appealed to the medical profession and medical journal editors to require authors to indicate how the consent of subjects for research was obtained as a condition for publication.[4] These and related events (taking place in the social context of the growth of the rights-based movements of the 1950s and 1960s[5]) and reports about the infamous Tuskegee syphilis study (perpetrated on African-Americans in the USA, in which effective treatment was withheld from the research subjects once available[2]) eventually led to the formation of the National Commission for the Protection of Human Subjects of Biomedical and Behavioral Research in the United States. In 1978 the Commission issued *The Belmont Report: Ethical Principles and Guidelines for the Protection of Human Subjects*.[6] This report articulated three core principles – respect for persons, beneficence, and justice. This and the influential text by Beauchamp and Childress first published in 1979[7] helped reframe the view of human research ethics and clinical ethics. They informed the public about science and medicine's understanding of biomedical ethics and offered a common language in which to critically view these concerns.

The Declarations of Helsinki from the World Medical Association have been among the most referenced documents concerning the ethics of clinical trials.[8] First created in 1964, this document has undergone extensive revision; the fifth version was approved in 2000 (available at www.wma.net). This document has codified many principles intrinsic to the ethical conduct of clinical research, including the necessity for an independent committee empowered to review and oversee the design and implementation of clinical studies (e.g. institutional review board (IRB) or ethics committee). While frequently referenced, the declaration of Helsinki also highlights one of the difficulties in consideration of ethical issues in clinical research – namely that there is no universally agreed upon set of ethical guidelines. Interestingly, the creators of the most recent version have raised some controversy in that regard by asserting the primacy of the Declaration of Helsinki over any potentially competing national, judicial, institutional or other regulatory requirements.[8]

Other forces shaped our current understandings. These included technological advances, such as mechanical ventilation with its implications for increasing the options and also the difficulties of end-of-life decision-making, and the advent of hemodialysis and subsequently organ transplantation, which raised difficult questions about not only end-of-life issues but also about just distribution of resources. Pharmaceutical advances led to increasing numbers of new, effective and more costly drugs; these and the costs of the other new technologies (and other factors) created more powerful tools for patient care and also contributed to substantial increases in the cost of healthcare. The economic impact of these changes has been largely responsible for a reshaping of the private insurance industry and government programs in efforts to control costs in the USA. This has resulted in limited availability of some therapies. The high production costs of the newer biologicals and their higher prices have paradoxically resulted in some physicians and healthcare organizations being at financial risk for these costs, while others have found opportunities to reap large financial rewards (e.g. by provision of these medications in profitable 'infusion centers' or through close relationships with pharmaceutical companies who seek to especially influence the physicians they identify as 'thought leaders').

PRINCIPLES OF BIOMEDICAL ETHICS

As a means of addressing ethical issues relevant to clinical trials, we will frame several key concerns according to relevant ethical principles. As already noted, there are four fundamental principles that represent a common ground on which ethical questions in biomedicine can be effectively analyzed. These include respect for autonomy, non-maleficence, beneficence, and justice.[6,7]

Autonomy

Respect for autonomy, analogous in political thought to the liberty rights of an individual, is expressed clearly in the early modern bioethics movement. The Nuremberg code and later commissions asserted that voluntary informed consent was the keystone to ethical research on human subjects. Research consent and its ethical underpinnings quickly made their way into clinical medicine. The rights of the patient to participate centrally in decisions regarding their own healthcare are now widely recognized. The doctrine of voluntary informed consent in clinical decision-making includes among its important requirements the communication of all pertinent available information regarding potential risks and benefits of therapeutic options. It ideally is characterized by an ongoing dialog by which physicians and patients can form a therapeutic alliance or, as exemplified by a research trial, a reciprocal collaboration. Respect for autonomy means that the ultimate decision-makers will be the patients themselves; this obligates the clinician or researcher to provide the appropriate information that a reasonable person would need to make that decision.

Many ethicists feel that patient autonomy may be the most important ethical principle. The tangible expression of patient autonomy as it pertains to clinical research is this process of informed consent. There are several key components to adequate informed consent in addition to information on risks, benefits, and alternatives and their consequences. The reader is referred to several helpful sources for a fuller discussion and practical guidance on these important issues.[9–13]

First, the patient must have a level of decision-making capacity necessary to make a meaningful choice. Decision-making capacity is similar to the legal concept of 'competence'. It includes the ability to understand the information disclosed, demonstrate appreciation of the potential risks and benefits of participation, engage in a reasoning process to include alternatives, and express a choice. The conduct of clinical research studies among vulnerable populations, including children and persons incapable of making sound decisions about their healthcare, has been an area of increasing interest, as more studies are conducted in such groups.[14]

A second component of informed consent is that the patient or potential research subject must be provided with all of the information necessary to make a decision whether or not to participate in language that they understand.[15] This seemingly simple requirement may be one of the more challenging current issues in rheumatology. For example, in the USA, a common guideline is that informed consent documents must be understandable to someone who has completed only 8 years of primary school education. As the science and technology enabling novel therapeutics have become ever more complex, adequately providing full informed consent has become more challenging. For example, how does one adequately explain at an eighth-grade level a novel treatment consisting of a fragment of a putative antigen linked to an HLA molecule in order to induce immunologic tolerance? How much knowledge does a person reasonably need to assess whether they wish to participate in an experiment trial?

Similarly, the complexity of adverse events potentially associated with newer agents has increased substantially. How can information concerning a potentially increased risk of developing certain types of cancer many years hence be adequately presented to patients when experts in the area disagree as about the extent or even the existence of such a risk? Two approaches sometimes used to respond to these problems are themselves potentially troubling. A common approach in informed consent documents is to provide an encyclopedic list of any and all potential adverse events, making the documents appear more like legal disclaimers than information pieces. Rather than providing clarity, this type of 'information overload' makes consent documents lengthy and potentially incomprehensible, and may obfuscate common understandable risks. On the other hand, paternalistically oversimplifying these complex issues runs the risk of impinging on patient autonomy. Striking a balance for the necessary documentation, while ensuring that informed consent is based on an ongoing process of communication, rather than a piece of paper alone, is central to this effort's success.

The third key component of informed consent is that it must be given free of coercion or duress. In years past, practices contrary to this principle included research on prisoners and other egregious violations. Currently, difficulties adhering to this may be much more subtle. For example, because of the relatively high acquisition costs of tumor necrosis factor (TNF) inhibitors, these agents have not been available to patients in some countries outside of participation in clinical trials. With worldwide dissemination of knowledge via the internet and other outlets, patients can be aware of the most up-to-date results in clinical trials of novel treatments. Even in countries where newer drugs are available, access may not be universal. After the introduction of inhibitors of TNF in the USA, recruitment of patients into further studies became more difficult in some areas, as some patients chose to receive medication 'open label' and not risk receiving placebo.[16] For patients who do not have access to newer medications,

could the potential for receiving these agents in a study be considered coercive? If so, does the promise of continued 'open-label' therapy with the agent after the study mollify this consideration or make it even more problematic?

Finally, how much information regarding potential conflicts of interest should the patient be given? Patients often assume that their physicians would not recommend therapy, even in this context of a clinical trial, that is not in their interest. But the goals of a physician as the patient's clinician and advocate are distinct from the goals and responsibilities of a clinical investigator. The best strategy to protect the patients from this confusion and its potential for mistaken assumptions on entering a trial is the same strategy which would protect the clinician and investigator. It is for the clinical trialist and the treating clinician to be different individuals. The trialist protects the integrity of research and the community of patients, while the treating clinician is the advocate and advisor for the individual patient. Should the patient be informed of the financial benefits to the trialist or their physician's practice or department? This question remains a matter of debate.

Distributive justice

The principle of justice also supports the individual by expecting provision of a decent minimum of healthcare to all and fair distribution of resources; however, this can also represent a counter-weight to unlimited autonomy. Debate over the fair distribution of resources (some of them scarce) addresses the issue of distributive justice. Budgetary and other resource constraints at the levels of practitioners, healthcare groups and institutions and governments create strain on how we define and exercise the fair distribution of goods, rights, and services. The cost of some highly effective agents, such as the TNF inhibitors, raises issues both in those countries where they are available commercially (for example, are patients who cannot afford these therapies coerced into participating in trials?) and in those countries where they are not (for example, what is the responsibility of the company to continue to provide medication to study patients after a study is done but before it is commercially available?).[17,18]

Non-maleficence

Non-maleficence derives from the ancient principle to do no harm. This remains an important test for our medical decisions and research protocols. It represents our effort to minimize risk. It is a familiar principle to clinicians that is part of the usual calculus in clinical care. However, this seemingly straightforward principle sometimes leads to difficult questions over, for example, when or even if placebo should be employed in a research study.[16–19]

A number of ethical considerations in rheumatology surround the definition of the best controls for trials. While few would argue that patients should be allowed to receive no treatment other than placebo, there is disagreement about what the comparator treatment(s) should be. The proven clinical efficacy of cytokine inhibitors has made this debate all the more acute. The optimal duration of clinical trials is also a matter of debate; the ethical considerations of minimizing patient exposure to ineffective placebos or less effective treatments while damage may occur is often pitted against regulatory demands for longer-duration trials to establish specific outcome claims.

Because clinical studies should be predicated on the concept of equipoise (i.e. it is not known whether or not a new treatment assessed in a study is superior to the comparator), the tremendous clinical efficacy of biological agents in rheumatology has had profound implications concerning optimal study design, including the use of placebos and other controls. As clinical studies have increasingly become multinational, this has added complexity to ethical considerations. Importantly the use of novel agents in clinical trials and the subsequent clinical use of biological agents has also been an area of debate.[18,20–23]

Beneficence

Beneficence, also an ancient principle and the underpinning of the paternalistic (or parentalistic) mode of medical practice for centuries, is also quite familiar to physicians. This is the benefit part of the 'risk–benefit' (or non-maleficence versus beneficence) analysis. Apparent or real conflicts may arise between beneficence and autonomy because of its roots in the physician's paternalistic concern, rather than deriving from or depending on the patient's own values and goals to define what is 'good'.

The declarations of Helsinki have affirmed that, while obtaining knowledge to advance science is an important goal of research, consideration of the wellbeing of the human subject takes precedence. In the past, research projects invoking a utilitarian philosophy were performed that ignored the individual in favor of the potential overall benefit to society. While hopefully this is no longer an issue, other potential conflicts may still interfere with the goal of achieving a good outcome for the patient. One example is the potential for financial gain and conflicts of interest related to conduct of studies.

Although it may not have always been so, contemporary clinical research is unmistakably big business. The introduction of a new therapeutic agent has profound economic consequences, consideration of which underscores the potential for ethical concerns. It has been estimated that at the turn of the last century, approximately 6 billion dollars (USA) per year were being spent on clinical trials worldwide. This reflected not only tremendous advances and discoveries of myriad new therapies, but also greater complexity and cost of bringing new drugs to market. Indeed, the cost of introducing a new drug has increased approximately 10-fold from the 1970s to the present; in the year 2000, the cost of developing a single drug was estimated to be 500 million dollars (USA). However, financial rewards can be substantial for a drug successfully brought to market. Retail pharmaceutical sales in the world's 12 leading markets were estimated at 207 billion dollars (USA) in 1999, with musculoskeletal drugs constituting the fastest growing of the main therapeutic categories. Estimated sales for the two currently marketed TNF inhibitors, etanercept and infliximab, rose from 1.026 billion dollars in 2000 to 1.565 billion dollars (USA) in 2001. With such large sales at stake, it has been estimated that for each day that a new 'blockbuster' drug is delayed from approval to market, a company could lose 1 million dollars. It can therefore be readily appreciated that there is tremendous pressure at various levels to conduct research studies as quickly as possible. These financial considerations raise the potential for bias and conflict of interest in addition to those alluded to in the discussion of informed consent above. Potential areas where these might arise include clinical trial design, study conduct, and interpretation and publication of trial results. Other pertinent confounding ethical dilemmas are for-profit IRBs and direct patient recruitment, advertising for studies, and liability of IRBs for suits.

Principles, values, and context

Further support for the utility of these moral principles for modern biomedical ethics evolves from the need for a description of the shared values that underlie our practical decision-making about what the 'right' thing to do is in a given situation. The weight given to each of these principles depends on the individual situation at hand and the individual stakeholders in a particular conflict. Often there is a tension between principles, as noted. It is important to recognize that there are other issues and values that may inform analysis in a given situation. They may shape how these principles are applied and their relationship to one another. Religious, cultural and social factors, institutional practices, and other contextual issues, as well as a fundamental respect for human dignity, all influence determination of what is the right decision.

ETHICAL ISSUES, CLINICAL TRIALS, AND BIOLOGICALS IN RHEUMATOLOGY

Issues related to the conduct of clinical research may be the most directly linked with ethical considerations among the various areas of medicine. Indeed, many of the milestones in ethical principles have come from deliberations surrounding infamous historical events in clinical research. In rheumatology, the intimate association of ethics and clinical research is illustrated well in the case of novel biological agents. The introduction of these powerful new therapeutics was predicated upon results from clinical trials. Their substantial clinical efficacy has not only spawned numerous other research studies but has also raised questions concerning ethical trial design. The success of biological agents has initiated ethical discussions heretofore unnecessary in rheumatology. Indeed, ethical issues and clinical research have been and almost certainly will be inexorably intertwined.[17] For example, now that these powerful new agents are available, what are the most appropriate comparators for future studies of novel agents? Under what circumstances, if any, should the use of placebos be permitted? What is the responsibility of the sponsor and/or the healthcare payor in continuing to provide expensive therapies to patients after they have participated in clinical studies? In phase I studies, where no benefit is likely, has this been made sufficiently clear to the subject? Is there risk in phase I and later-phase clinical studies of the 'therapeutic misconception' common in clinical trials that both physicians and their patients expect greater likelihood of benefit than available data might suggest? Has the researcher clearly distinguished him- or herself from the clinician in the eyes of the patient, or is there room left for confusion based on a dual role and the belief that 'my doctor wouldn't suggest something if it wasn't good for me'? Is there a financial conflict of interest for the physician or researcher due to the mechanism by which studies are reimbursed, such as a higher payment for completers, or due, for example, to consulting or other financial arrangements? Have these been disclosed in research reports, at educational forums, or to patients in clinical trials? Is there conflict of interest not from financial lures, but from the goal of academic promotion? Does the investigator in a trial 'own' the rights to publish the data, regardless of study outcome, or can certain data be hidden from the scrutiny of the research community? How do insurance and other reimbursement issues affect clinical choices? What are the consequences for other patients of limited resources being expended on expensive drugs, sometimes only with marginal benefits over other less expensive medications? How should pharmacogenomic information be used, and who should have access to it? How should it influence who gets studied? Can non-local human subject research committees, such as IRBs, be truly accountable? Are local, institutionally based IRBs unduly influenced by a desire to support one's colleagues? Are IRBs tainted by institutional and financial conflicts of interest? Are their processes adequate?

As in ethical discussions in other disciplines, the issues in rheumatology are increasingly complex. It seems that there are more questions than answers. The continuous dramatic progress in basic immunology and biopharmaceutical technology will demand ongoing ethical appraisal in this area in the setting of evolving pharmacoeconomic and sociopolitical concerns. Some may assert that most of the answers are self-evident, and that we are honorable and honest, caring and respectful clinicians. How could we go wrong? Two issues provide important examples that merit serious reflection and force us to question these assumptions. One example is how we are affected by the pervasive influence of the pharmaceutical industry throughout medicine and the financial influences of industry striving to meet its fiduciary responsibilities to its shareholders. The other example connects rheumatology and its lexicon to the Nazi doctors and points out how easily we may unknowingly honor someone whose moral positions we reject.

As we will illustrate by these two examples, it is imperative that physicians remain as vigilant in matters of ethics as in all other matters essential to practicing the highest level of medical care for our patients. Jeremiah Barondess persuasively argues that history has demonstrated that the medical ethos – comprising our core values

of healing, relief of suffering, and compassion – is not immutable, being shaped not only by financial forces and other conflicts, but also by larger political, social, and cultural forces as well.[24]

Ethical issues are therefore critical not only to the optimal deliberative and ongoing assessment and use of novel therapeutic agents but also to the clinical practice of rheumatology.

RELATIONSHIPS WITH THE BIOTECHNOLOGY AND PHARMACEUTICAL INDUSTRY

The relevant medical ethics

Medicine is humane science inextricably bound to an ethical lattice. It is a moral enterprise.[24–27] Individual physicians and their professional association(s) are committed to promote the welfare of those they serve. They should affirm the moral imperatives from which derive authenticity and integrity by demanding the highest possible standards. Opportunities for professional associations and their individual members to accept monetary support and/or gifts, to generate income, and to 'partner' with industry in order to promote their interests, perceived privileges, and sense of entitlement, challenge our ability to recognize moral dilemmas and to subordinate self-interest to the interests of our patients. Medicine, however, is not about physicians and our practices, institutions, organizations or individual organization, needs, research, careers, prerequisites, prerogatives, agendas, or perceived entitlements. It is about dedication and devotion to our patients and to their welfare even at personal and professional risk to profit, pride, and position.[25–31]

About gifts

It is necessary to understand 'gifts' and 'gift' giving in order to derive individual and professional ethics for these and related activities.[26,27,32,33] Gift giving and receiving exemplify the potentially problematic individual and professional relationships with industry. 'Gifts' in this context is used to reflect relationships from which personal or organizational benefit may accrue. Individuals are confronted with the allure of widely available 'gifts'. There is now a growing literature pertaining to 'gifts'. There is general recognition that professional and personal gift giving and receiving pose ethical conflicts to physicians and organizations, and that there must be codes of conduct to govern this. Indeed the American College of Rheumatology (ACR) was one of the first professional societies to realize this, and developed and has long had a set of standards higher than those of many other professional organizations.[26,27,34,35] There is less guidance relating to broader relationships with industry and other commercial sources, but the professional and ethical issues are essentially the same as for 'gifts'. 'Gifts' and industry/commercial relationships are pervasive.

Readers of this chapter will probably be familiar with many pertinent aspects of the historical relationships between medicine and industry, and growing government and public scrutiny. These are presented elsewhere in detail.[26,27]

Positions of professional organizations

Many professional societies have adopted positions about this.[36–40] The Royal College of Physicians, in 1986,[36] wrote that physicians should not accept excessive or inordinate hospitality, that hospitality should not extend to spouses, and that the criterion of acceptability may be 'would you be willing to have these arrangements generally known?' The American Surgical Association (ASA) in 1989 was among the first professional societies to develop a position statement. The ASA stated 'that it is unethical for a surgeon to accept remuneration or material reward for participating in the advertising or other product promotional activity of a health care related industry with no relationship to professional service rendered'.[37] It did not object to small gifts, sponsorship of educational lunches, or complimentary coffee and donuts for operating room teams. The ACR, also in 1989, established stringent policies for corporate sponsorship at its meetings, limited

the value of gifts distributed, prohibited brand names at meeting venues, banned social and competing events from scientific meetings, and supported social events with members' fees.[34,35] In 1990, the American College of Physicians published its policies. These have recently been affirmed and updated.[38]

> 'The acceptance of individual gifts, hospitality, trips, and subsidies of all types from industry by an individual physician is discouraged. Physicians should not accept gifts, hospitality, services, and subsidies from industry if acceptance might diminish, or appear to others to diminish, the objectivity of professional judgment. Helpful questions for gauging whether a gift relationship is ethically appropriate include 1) What would my patients think about this arrangement? What would the public think? How would I feel if the relationship was disclosed through the media? 2) What is the purpose of the industry offer? 3) What would my colleagues think about this arrangement? What would I think if my own physician accepted this offer?'

Also

> 'physicians who have financial relationships with industry, whether as researchers, speakers, consultants, investigators, owners, partners, employees, or otherwise, must not in any way compromise their objective clinical judgment or the best interests of patients or research subjects. Physicians must disclose their financial interest in any medical facilities or office-based research to which they refer or recruit patients.'

Those who accept industry sponsorship for continuing medical education (CME) should have and enforce explicit policies to maintain programmatic control. Professional societies should have similar guidelines and discourage excessive gifts, amenities, and hospitality. Clinical trials should conform with scientific methodology. The American Medical

---

Quotes reproduced with permission from Coyle SL et al. *Ann Intern Med* 2002; **136**: 396–402.

Association's policy, from its council and from its ethical and judicial affairs committee, followed in 1991.[39] This stated that gifts should not be of substantial value, that education subsidies should be funneled through sponsors, that gifts should not be conditional, and that travel, lodging and expenses should not be accepted for the purpose of attending conferences and meetings. The Canadian Medical Association's policies were the most restrictive.[40] Among their 33 principles were recommendations to accept no gifts except patient teaching aids and those with no product logos. There is an extensive array of additional opinions in the literature regarding this. They make interesting reading.[26,27]

Gifts

Gifts are powerful symbols throughout cultures used to initiate and sustain relationships.[26,27,32] This must be understood to appreciate a discussion of their potential influence. Gifts are used ubiquitously to seduce and influence physicians. Companies are motivated by profit, not altruism. Gifts cost money. Costs are ultimately passed on to patients without their explicit knowledge or consent. Accepting a gift may contribute to erosion of the perception that the medical profession serves patients' best interests. Acceptance of a gift establishes a relationship between the donor and recipient with a vague but real obligation. Contemporary society has lost sight of the importance of gifts as regulators of human relationships. Offering a gift proffers friendship. Acceptance of a gift initiates or reinforces a relationship. Acceptance of a gift involves the assumption of social obligations of grateful conduct, grateful use, reciprocation, and response. While gift giving is an act of apparent generosity, it serves the self-interest of the giver. A special relationship is formed between people who share food and a fine meal in an atmosphere of conviviality and agreement. Formal contracts can be dissolved but gift relationships are subtle and less well defined. Companies' ultimate goals are to increase profit to shareholders.

Table 39.1   Can physicians be bought, rented, or influenced?
• Physicians' prescribing habits reflected a preponderance of commercial over scientific influence
• Physicians' requests to add drugs to formularies were strongly and specifically associated with physicians' interactions with companies manufacturing the drugs
• Of articles published in the literature, more with drug company support than without were likely to favor the drug of interest
• Authors supporting calcium channel blockers, during a recent controversy, were much more likely to have financial relationships to the manufacturers than other authors
• Significant increases in physicians' prescribing followed all-expenses paid 'educational' meetings at luxurious resorts
• Faculty and residents who were surveyed changed their prescribing habits and recommended formulary additions based on contacts with drug representatives
• Funding sources introduced bias into CME programs favoring sponsors
• Some chief residents considered the reliability of drug representatives to be superior to the medical literature
• Not all drug representatives' statements were accurate or complied with FDA requirements
Reproduced from Panush R, *J Rheum* 2002; **29**: 1049–57.[27]

Three ethical problems arise for individual physicians with regard to gifts. One concerns 'unjust' practices – spending patients' money without their knowledge to benefit physicians and industry. Another threatens the physician–patient relationship, eroding the physician's fiduciary role of trustee of the patient's welfare above all. The last is the potential to affect the physician's character, disturbing the delicate balance between self-interest and altruism.

Can physicians be bought, rented, or influenced?

Yes. These data are briefly summarized in Table 39.1, and have been reviewed extensively elsewhere.[26,27]

What then is the problem?

The problem for physicians is considered to be the following: (1) we may be learning much about drug (product) prescribing – our most common activity – from sources which stand to profit from our choices; (2) we may be abdicating our responsibility to educate ourselves impartially; (3) we may be selling access to our young (students, residents, and fellows) when they are most impressionable in exchange for institutional and personal perquisites; (4) we may risk losing the trust of society and our patients through ethically inappropriate relationships that other fiduciaries (i.e. bankers, judges, journalists, or purchasing agents) would not accept; and (5) we may risk inviting outside regulation to curb perceived excesses and costs if we do not do this ourselves.

Organizational ethics

While there is a growing literature about the ethical behavior of individual physicians, there is substantially less pertaining to the ethics of professional societies. Guidelines for medical organizations have been suggested.[25] These include the following. (1) The organization's mission should be consonant with that of the medical profession generally and should be responsive to patients' welfare, public needs, and high standards of professionalism. Associations should be aware of the dangers of focusing unduly on the economic concerns of members to the detriment of transcendent obligations to patients and the public. (2) Associations should not be unions. Unions become self-serving and subordinate patients' interests to those of union members. They are probably incompatible with a true professional association. (3) Professional organizations should derive financial support from members' dues. Support from or deals with the healthcare industry inevitably risk and create unacceptable conflicts of interest. (4) Associations must ensure the editorial independence of their publications and journals. (5) Scientific meetings sponsored by professional associations should abide by the preceding guidelines and be free of industry sponsorship, even if offered as unrestricted and for general education purposes. (6) Associations should be governed by bylaws adopted by members, and association leaderships should be fully accountable to members. All association activities and policies should be publicly disclosed.

Summary

Medicine and industry have a special relationship. In many instances, our interests are concordant and our interactions mutually beneficial. There are areas, however, where potential ethical and professional conflicts arise. Such an area is industry gifts and relationships. Gifts and relationships obligate. Acceptance of 'gifts' or industry/commercial benefit(s) involves the assumption of obligations of grateful conduct, grateful use, reciprocation, and response. Increasing and compelling data document that industry support, gifts, hospitality, generosity and other contributions clearly influence physicians. Physicians aspiring to the highest standards of professionalism, physicians with leadership responsibilities, and the organizations they serve, will consider these issues in their personal and organizational conduct.

There is no ethically intrinsically 'right' or 'correct' course of conduct regarding acceptance of 'gifts' or other industry-related largesse, their disclosure, and conflicts of interest. As with virtually all ethical decisions, individuals and organizations must make choices based on their own belief systems, character, integrity, sense of morality, and professionalism. Gifts create or enhance social relationships and obligate the recipient. Physicians, however, have duties of non-malfeasance, fidelity, justice, and self-improvement. Physicians should adhere to professional standards of altruism, accountability, excellence, duty, honor and integrity, and respect for others. Organizational behavior should mirror that of its member physicians.

ETHICS AND PROFESSIONALISM

We conclude this chapter with brief consideration of certain aspects of ethics and professionalism. The ACR recently developed a code of ethics to address many aspects of individual and organizational conduct.[27,41] The authors of this chapter are proud to have been members of the committee which prepared this.

What should be the consequences of unprecedented, extraordinary unprofessional conduct or ethical misbehavior? An extreme example merits discussion. Compelling evidence has been offered that Hans Reiter, whose name has been linked with a rheumatologic syndrome, was complicit with atrocities in Nazi Germany. He was president of the Reich health office and responsible for heinous violations of ethical, humanitarian, professional and medical precepts.[42–45] How should Reiter be remembered? Does he merit eponymous distinction? The difficulty of this issue has been reflected by the inability of respected and thoughtful rheumatologists to arrive at a consensus on this subject. This was discussed separately at meetings of the ACR Board of Directors and of rheumatology editors, without resolution. Rheumatology editors declined to take a position. The ACR board drafted a general statement about 'principles of patient care', which as of this writing had not yet been disseminated.[46]

The ethical issues include the following.[2,4,45,47–49] Should Reiter's record as a Nazi reflect how rheumatologic and medical history regard him? Were Nazi atrocities different from other 'ordinary' crimes? Should science ignore ethics or morality? Does it matter that Reiter thought his actions 'right'? Is a 'greater good' served by ignoring Reiter's Nazi activities and recognizing his legitimate medical report(s)? Were ethical standards and expectations different in his time than now? Can we trust the science of a man who would permit and justify 'experiments' that were nothing less than bestial abominations? Of a man who even later did not acknowledge or repent those acts but defended them? Who has – or takes – responsibility for making these judgments? What are the thresholds for acceptable behavior and for condemnation? Is Reiter's Nazi complicity clear? Can this be investigated further and documented with greater certainty? Does it matter that Reiter was never tried or convicted of crimes? Should ethical or other issues affect the legacy of creative artists – like painters, writers, or musicians? Is there a transcendent ethical principle?

There are also historical and clinical issues.[43,44,50] Was Reiter's the original description of the syndrome that bears his name? Was his report of overriding significance? Is there a better name for that syndrome? Is 'Reiter's syndrome' a necessary, useful and irreplaceable term in our rheumatologic vocabulary?

An issue of *Seminars in Arthritis and Rheumatism* will be devoted to this topic and include our own[45] and others'[41,42] views.

CLOSING COMMENTS

Ethical issues are inextricably intertwined with rheumatologic investigation and practice. We hope that this explication has illustrated this truism and offered some measure of greater perspective and understanding to our colleagues.

> There are 3 'crowns' (symbols of earthly accomplishment, stature, dignity and respect): that of learning, that of priesthood, and that of royalty; but the 'crown' of a good name is the most exalted of all. Talmud Avot 4:17.

ACKNOWLEDGMENTS

The authors appreciated the excellent assistance of Romaine Colter in the preparation of this manuscript. Dr Romain was a Visiting Research Fellow in the Division of Medical Ethics, Harvard Medical School, Boston, MA, during the manuscript's preparation.

REFERENCES

1. Evans JH. A sociological account of the growth of principlism. *Hastings Center Rep* 2000; **30**: 31–8.
2. Panush RS. Upon finding a Nazi anatomy atlas: the lessons of Nazi medicine. *The Pharos* 1996; Fall: 18–22.
3. Shuster E. Fifty years later: the significance of the Nuremberg code. *N Engl J Med* 1997; **337**: 1436–40.
4. Beecher HK. Ethics and clinical research. *N Engl J Med* 1966; **274**: 1354–60.
5. Brandt A. Bioethics: then and now. *Medical Ethics: the Lahey Clinic Medical Ethics Newsletter.* 2000; Spring: 1–2. (www.lahey.org/ethics)
6. National Commission for the Protection of Human Subjects in Biomedical and Behavioral Research. *The Belmont Report: Ethical Principles and Guidelines for the Protection of Human Subjects of Research* (GPO: Washington, DC, 1978).
7. Beauchamp TL, Childress JF. *Principles of Biomedical Ethics*, 4th edn (Oxford University Press: New York, 1994).
8. Forester H, Emanuel E, Grady C. The 2000 revision of the Declaration of Helsinki: a step forward or more confusion? *Lancet* 2001; **358**: 1449–53.
9. Applebaum PS, Lidz CW, Meisel A. *Informed Consent: Legal Theory and Clinical Practice* (Oxford University Press: New York, 1987).
10. Faden R, Beauchamp T. *A History and Theory of Informed Consent* (Oxford University Press: New York, 1986).
11. Meisel A, Kuczewski M. Legal and ethical myths about informed consent. *Arch Intern Med* 1996; **156**: 2521–6.
12. Braddock CH, Edwards KA, Hasenberg NM, Laidley TL, Levinson W. Informed decision making in outpatient practice. Time to get back to basics. *JAMA* 1999; **282**: 2313–20.
13. Barry MJ. Involving patients in medical decisions. *JAMA* 1999; **282**: 2356–7.
14. Zion D, Gillam L, Loff B. The declaration of Helsinki, CIOMS, and the ethics of research on vulnerable populations. *Nat Med* 2000; **6**: 615–17.
15. Lantos J. Informed consent: the whole truth for patients? *Cancer* 1993; **72**: 2811–15.
16. Stein CM, Pincus T. Placebo-controlled studies in rheumatoid arthritis: ethical issues. *Lancet* 1999; **353**: 400–3.
17. Rothman KJ, Michels KB. The continuing unethical use of placebo controls. *N Engl J Med* 1994; **331**: 394–8.
18. Shapiro H, Meslin E. Ethical issues in the design and conduct of clinical trials in developing countries. *N Engl J Med* 2001; **345**: 139–42.
19. Kleijnen J, de Craen AJ, van Everdingen J, Krol L. Placebo effect in double-blind clinical trials: a review of interactions with medications. *Lancet* 1994; **344**: 1347–9.
20. Montaner J, O'Shaughnessy M, Schechter M. Industry- sponsored clinical research: a double-edged sword. *Lancet* 2001; **358**: 1893–5.
21. Bodenheimer T. Uneasy alliance: clinical investigators and the pharmaceutical industry. *N Engl J Med* 2000; **342**: 1539–44.
22. Kahn J, Mastroianni A. Moving from compliance to conscience; why we can and should improve the ethics of clinical research. *Arch Intern Med* 2001; **161**: 925–8.
23. Ramsay S. Johns Hopkins takes responsibility for volunteer's death. *Lancet* 2001; **358**: 213.
24. Barondess JA. Care of the medical ethos: reflections on social Darwinism, racial hygiene, and the Holocaust. *Ann Intern Med* 1998; **129**: 891–8.
25. Pellegrino ED, Relman AS. Professional medical associations. Ethical and practical guidelines. *JAMA* 1999; **282**: 984–6.
26. Panush RS. Introduction to miscellaneous topics, In: Panush RS, ed. *Yearbook of Rheumatology, Arthritis, and Musculoskeletal Diseases* (Mosby: St Louis, 2001) 349–59
27. Panush RS. Not for sale, not even for rent: just say no. Thoughts about the American College of Rheumatology adopting a code of ethics viewpoint. *J Rheumatol* 2002; **29**: 1049–57.
28. Relman AS. Separating continuing medical education from pharmaceutical marketing. *JAMA* 2001; **285**: 2009–12.
29. Angell M. Is academic medicine for sale? *N Engl J Med* 2000; **342**: 1516–18.
30. Kassirer JP. Financial indigestion. *JAMA* 2000; **284**: 2156–7.
31. Korn D. Conflicts of interest in biomedical research. *JAMA* 2000; **284**: 2234–6.
32. Chren M, Landefeld S, Murray TH. Doctors, drug companies and gifts. *JAMA* 1989; **262**: 3448–51.
33. DeAngelis CD. Conflict of interest and the public trust. *JAMA* 2000; **284**: 2237–8.
34. Stobo JD. From the president. *ACR News* 1989; **8**(5): 3.
35. ACR adopts new guidelines on industry relations. *ACR News* 1991; **10**(4): 1, 5, 8.

36. The relationship between physicians and the pharmaceutical industry. A report of the Royal College of Physicians. *J R Coll Physicians Lond* 1986; **20**(4): 235–42.

37. Bricker EM. Sounding board: industrial marketing and medical ethics. *N Engl J Med* 1989; **320**: 1690–2.

38. Coyle SL, for the Ethics and Human Rights Committee, American College of Physicians–American Society of Internal Medicine. Physician–industry relations. Part 1: Individual physicians, and Part 2: Organizational issues. *Ann Intern Med* 2002; **136**: 396–402, 403–6.

39. American Medical Association. Gifts to physicians from industry. *JAMA* 1991; **265**: 501.

40. Canadian Medical Association. Physicians and the pharmaceutical industry. *Can Med Assoc J* 1994; **150**: 256A–C.

41. American College of Rheumatology. *Code of Ethics* (ACR: Atlanta, GA).

42. Wallace D, Weisman M. The physician Hans Reiter as prisoner of war in Nuremberg: a contextual review of his interrogation (1945–1947). *Semin Arthritis Rheum* (in press).

43. Wallace DJ, Weisman M. Should a war criminal be rewarded with eponymous distinction? The double life of Hans Reiter (1881–1969). *J Clin Rheumatol* 2000; **6**: 49–54.

44. Wallace DJ, Weisman M. Comments regarding Hans Reiter's role in Nazi Germany. *J Clin Rheumatol* 2001; **7**: 127–30.

45. Panush RS, Paraschiv D, Dorff E. Reiter wrong? The tainted legacy of Hans Reiter. *Seminars Arthritis Rheum* (in press).

46. American College of Rheumatology. Principles of patient care. *Semin Arthritis Rheum* (in press).

47. Panush RS, Briggs RM. The exodus of a medical school. *Ann Intern Med* 1996; **123**: 963.

48. Panush RS. About a Nazi anatomy atlas. *JAMA* 1996; **276**: 1633–4.

49. Panush RS. Reply to origins of the Pernkopf anatomy atlas. *JAMA* 1997; **277**: 1122.

50. Inman RD. Classification criteria for reactive arthritis. *J Rheumatol* 1999; **26**: 1219–21.

40

Randomized controlled trials

Vibeke Strand and Lee S Simon

Introduction • Issues specific to biological agents • Confounding characteristics of biological therapies • Randomized controlled trials • Conduct of the randomized controlled trial • Outcome measures • The stages of product development: phases 1–3 • Conclusions • References

INTRODUCTION

The recent addition of biological agents to our therapeutic armamentarium has rejuvenated the practice of rheumatology. Many more products are expected to be developed for the treatment of rheumatoid arthritis (RA) and other clinical indications, including seronegative spondyloarthropathies and systemic lupus erythematosus (SLE). Designing randomized controlled trials to demonstrate the safety and efficacy of these new products will require progressively more innovative and unique approaches.

ISSUES SPECIFIC TO BIOLOGICAL AGENTS

Randomized controlled trials (RCTs) with biological agents must take into account many issues which distinguish them from traditional pharmaceutical products (Table 40.1). These products are designed to achieve sustained or maximal alteration of a relevant immune response or target, yet it remains difficult to administer these agents without concomitant downregulation of other immune functions, possibly compromising immune surveillance. Despite rational design and hypothesized

Table 40.1 Issues specific to biological agents.

- Immunologically active, may downregulate other immune functions
- Mechanism of action may be altered by redundant cytokine cascades and cell circuitry
- In vitro or ex vivo tests may not predict in vivo responses
- Interference with other immune effector functions may lead to infections, autoimmune manifestations and/or lymphoproliferative disorders
- Parenteral administration; systemic rather than targeted delivery
- 'Industrial strength' rather than pharmacologic or physiologic doses
- Limited preclinical and toxicology data

mechanism of action, these therapeutic interventions may more closely resemble manipulation of a black box, given the redundant cytokine cascades and cell circuitry which characterize the immune system. Naturally occurring autoantibodies to cytokines are more prevalent in patients with autoimmune disease, and may prolong the activity of cytokines or prevent their degradation, as well as downregulating their effects.[1] In vitro tests may not predict in vivo responses; sampling of the target at the site of disease may be difficult; and serum sampling may not reflect biologically active levels of cytokines or other important mediators. Finally, the toxicity of many of these biological agents may be limited to interference with other immune effector functions, leading to an increased incidence of infections, autoimmune manifestations and lymphoproliferative disorders. These types of rare adverse event may not be observed during clinical development of the product, as exposure of a large number of patients will be required for them to emerge. Recently, regulatory agencies have emphasized the importance of a large safety database prior to approval, including studies designed to assess the safety of the product in patients receiving usual care. Large post-marketing surveillance studies have also been requested in an effort to identify potential rare adverse events.

Most biological agents are parenterally administered, resulting in systemic exposure rather than targeted delivery to the site of activity. They are immunologically active, and should only be studied in patients. Dose schedules are frequently empirically determined, and doses often approximate maximally tolerated doses (MTD), leading to administration of 'industrial strength' rather than pharmacologic or physiologic levels of product. As they are foreign proteins, they will eventually stimulate an immune response.

Preclinical toxicology and efficacy data for biological agents are often limited by species specificity, precluding administration beyond 14–21 days when an immune response develops in the animal. Even when sufficient structural homology is conserved across species to allow long-term administration in animal models of established disease, they offer 'proof of concept' but do not closely predict responses in humans.[2] Alternative approaches include studying the analogous recombinant murine product, especially for reproductive toxicology, or transplantation of human tissue into SCID-hu mice.[3] These are expensive and still may not closely predict clinical responses.

Clinical development programs for biological agents could be more efficient than those for traditional pharmaceutical products if biological markers indicating their successful delivery and resultant effects of administration were available. Although they may not correlate directly with clinical responses, these markers would be utilized to predict on and off effects of the experimental agent. They may be utilized with sparse pharmacokinetic data to yield important pharmacodynamic information. They may help in understanding effects which persist beyond the measurable half-life of the administered agent, due to upregulation of cell surface receptors, prolongation of receptor binding, secretion of an active mediator in latent form, or alterations in autocrine and/or paracrine regulation of cytokine networks. Transient or prolonged decreases in specific circulating cell populations may distinguish sequestration or depletion, particularly in adult patients with little remaining thymic function.[4–6] Ideally, one or more of these biological markers will predict clinical responses and can therefore serve as surrogate markers. Unfortunately this has not yet been proven – even rapid and profound decreases in C-reactive protein (CRP) levels following administration of a tumor necrosis factor (TNF)-α inhibitor in RA do not always identify patients who achieve clinical benefit, nor were restored lysozyme levels following interferon (IFN)-γ administration predictive of responses in chronic granulomatous disease.[7]

CONFOUNDING CHARACTERISTICS OF BIOLOGICAL THERAPIES

Parenteral administration, first-dose and infusion reactions and rapid onset of effect all may contribute to unblinding in clinical trials of biological agents (Table 40.2). First-dose reactions are related to proinflammatory cytokine (TNF-α, IFN-γ, interleukin-6 (IL-6)) release

Table 40.2 Confounding characteristics of biological agents.
Potential unblinding due to rapid onset of action, and first dose and infusion reactions
Immunogenicity
Injection-site reactions
Concomitant effects of background therapy
Expectation bias

from T cells and/or accessory cells, are dependent upon immunoglobulin–FcγR interactions, and can be abrogated by developing aglycosyl or mutated Fc portions of monoclonal antibodies or soluble receptor fusion proteins.[8] Infusion reactions can be decreased by avoiding bolus injections and slowing the infusion rate, as well as premedication with antihistamines, antiemetics, hydrocortisone and/or methylprednisolone.[9]

Immunogenicity depends upon the product, route of administration, dose, and dose schedule. Administration of monoclonal antibodies results in anti-idiotypic and isotypic responses, both of which are T cell dependent and are increased if the biological agent binds to cells.[10] Humanized and fully human monoclonal antibodies and soluble receptors still elicit antiglobulin responses.[11,12] Although all foreign proteins are potentially immunogenic, many recombinant products can be administered repetitively over the long term, such as insulin. Once an immune response develops, the pharmacokinetic profile is altered due to more rapid clearance of the product; tachyphylaxis occurs less frequently, and allergic or anaphylactic reactions are rare. Development of neutralizing antibodies in some patients may attenuate or abrogate clinical responses. Injection-site reactions may reflect immunogenicity and/or formulation of the product. Concomitant administration of low-dose methotrexate appears to prolong the half-life of several biological agents, presumably by altering FcγR clearance mechanisms. This increased half-life may lead to increased overall exposure to the therapy, 'the area under the curve', potentially leading to more efficacy as well as an increased risk for toxicity.

Expectation bias, on the part of physicians and patients, has traditionally been higher in RCTs with promising new biological agents.[13] These products are 'sexy'; rapid onset of effect and infusion reactions may result in early unblinding of the RCT. To minimize this possibility, separate blinded assessors of safety and efficacy are frequently employed, as well as premedication and slowing of infusion rates to reduce treatment-associated reactions.[14]

RANDOMIZED CONTROLLED TRIALS

RCTs represent an essential component of the clinical development program for new biological agents. Open-label trials are usually positive, especially in diseases such as RA and SLE, where therapeutic options are limited, the natural course of the disease is difficult to predict, and underlying disease activity is variable. Placebo responses are regularly observed, even in patients with long-standing active disease. Because treatment effects may be small, use of an appropriate control group is essential, whether placebo or active comparator.[14] Random assignment to active or placebo treatment should be allocated on a 'by-patient' basis and must be concealed from all study personnel.[15] Separate blinded assessors for safety and efficacy should be utilized to minimize unblinding due to rapid response, infusion or injection-site reactions. Other pitfalls include failure to clearly define the hypothesis to be addressed by the RCT and/or attempting to answer too many questions in a single protocol (Table 40.3).

Over the past 5 years, guidance documents issued by the US Food and Drug Administration (FDA) and the European Agency for the Evaluation of Medicinal Products (EMEA) have facilitated new product development, especially in RA.[16,17] Defined regulatory pathways and recent approvals are helping to define 'roadmaps' for the development of new treatments in other disease indications, including seronegative spondyloarthro- pathies, osteoarthritis (OA) and SLE. The importance of guidance documents

Table 40.3 Essential components of an RCT for a new biological agent.
Appropriate control treatment group
Adequate sample size
Selection of appropriate patient population
Sufficient duration of treatment to demonstrate effect
Prospectively defined outcome measure assessed on a by-patient basis
Prospectively defined statistical analysis plan
Central randomization on a by-patient basis, concealed from all study personnel
Separate blinded assessors for safety and efficacy
Means to reduce treatment-associated toxicities
Clearly defined hypothesis

Table 40.4 Alternatives to placebo-controlled RCTs.
Equivalence to an active comparator previously demonstrated to be effective versus placebo
Superiority to a standard of care
Non-equivalence between 'gold standard', experimental therapy and combination of the two

cannot be overestimated. The 'roadmap' provided allows companies to perceive what a regulatory approval hurdle will require. Iterative approaches to achieving levels of labeling approval allow increased interest in new drug development. From a marketing perspective, this allows the new therapy to achieve clinical indications that differentiate it from other products.

Trial design

Ideally, regulatory approval of a new therapeutic product in a given clinical indication requires the demonstration of its superiorities to placebo and its equivalence to the current standard of care. The use of placebo is controversial, especially in diseases where irreversible morbidity may occur if active treatment is withheld and effective therapies exist. However, placebo controls are essential early in the clinical development process for accurate assessment of safety. Until the experimental agent has been shown to have efficacy, there is no ethical dilemma in comparing it with placebo. Later in the development process, placebo may be used

if superimposed upon 'background therapy' in patients with persistently active disease, provided that early exit from the study for documented lack of efficacy then allows them to receive the experimental therapy.

Now that three new disease-modifying antirheumatic drugs (DMARDs) have been approved in RA, and more are expected, use of placebo controls beyond initial introduction into the clinic, even with background therapy, is increasingly questioned (Table 40.4). Active controlled trials using a gold standard such as methotrexate or even one of the newly approved biological agents are considered more ethically appropriate and may yield information more relevant to day-to-day practice. Even in the context of an RCT, collection of data allowing a cost-effectiveness comparison of the experimental agent with an existing therapy will offer additional information important to clinicians, payors and healthcare regulators.

Proving equivalence to presently available therapies presents unique problems. Equivalence trials require much larger sample sizes; a good estimate is roughly six times those required for a placebo RCT. Equivalence is best defined using confidence intervals, where the null hypothesis of non-equivalence is rejected.[18] Unfortunately, demonstration of equivalence between two treatments does not necessarily indicate that they are effective; each therapy may be equally ineffective.[19,20] It is therefore preferable to select an active comparator approved for use in the specified clinical indication which, more importantly, has previously been demonstrated to be efficacious versus placebo. Ideally, an equivalence RCT should mimic the earlier placebo-controlled trial, so that the active comparator can again be shown to be effective to a similar degree as when it was compared with placebo. This may not be easy to accomplish: clinical practice may have evolved, utilizing different doses or dosing schedules than what is specified in the product label; and concomitant use of medications, patient populations eligible for treatment with the agent and even outcome measures may have changed. Choosing methotrexate as the active comparator provides an excellent example of how much clinical practice has changed since this DMARD was approved for the treatment of active RA in 1986, based on a total of 126 patients enrolled in two RCTs treated for a maximum of 24 weeks.[21] RCTs in RA are now expected to be 6–24 months in duration and employ composite outcomes such as the American College of Rheumatology (ACR) response criteria or the Disease Activity Index (DAS). Methotrexate dosing schedules, escalation for lack of efficacy, even maximum doses, administered subcutaneously or intramuscularly as well as orally, have changed considerably, including concomitant administration of folate.

RCTs designed to demonstrate superiority of the experimental agent to the standard of care may be preferable, as they will require smaller sample sizes. However, we are treating heterogeneous populations with variable disease courses where no 'cures' exist. We lack sufficient individual therapies in all of our patient populations – and require multiple effective drugs, as none behaves in the same way in all patients. It is therefore difficult to demonstrate statistical superiority of an experimental treatment over an accepted therapy, and such designs are often risky.

Comparing the addition to background treatment of a new therapy versus placebo has successfully demonstrated the efficacy of several TNF-α inhibitors.[22,23] However, superimposing certain other biological agents designed to alter T-cell function in patients who were partial responders to methotrexate resulted in more

treatment-associated toxicity, increasing the degree and duration of cell depletion.[24–27]

Another alternative is a three-way comparison of monotherapy with a 'gold standard of care' or the experimental agent versus combination of the two. This design may satisfy obvious questions on the part of treating physicians and care providers once the product is approved, but may prove risky to the sponsor. By what criterion should non-equivalence be defined? Despite more rapid onset of benefit and resulting differences in area under the curve of 'response', so far it has been difficult to show statistical differences using our accepted outcome criteria.

Crossover designs may constitute an option, but traditionally have been rejected in rheumatic diseases because of their vulnerability to carryover effects of the previous treatment. Recently such a design very successfully demonstrated the superiority of a traditional non-steroidal anti-inflammatory drug (NSAID) over acetaminophen for the treatment of OA.[28] Biological agents with rapid onset of effect, as well as rapid loss of effect when they are withdrawn, may be ideally suited to such a design, provided that a brief washout and new baselines are established at the time of crossover. In fact, a crossover design is employed when patients are allowed to exit initial treatment assignment for documented lack of efficacy in placebo RCTs, on the supposition that they were randomized to placebo, and then receive active treatment. Comparison of clinical responses in these crossover populations facilitates understanding individualization of treatment, as occurs in day-to-day practice.

Crucial to the success of a well-designed RCT is enrollment of a sufficient number of patients to demonstrate a true treatment difference. Placebo responses are uniformly observed; disease populations are heterogeneous; small pilot studies rarely accurately reflect clinical responses. This poses a significant problem when treating orphan indications, such as vasculitis or SLE patients with nephritis. Additionally, data from a variety of RCTs in RA have shown that placebo responses tend to be higher when the active comparators are less potent, although effective nonetheless.[29] A good rule of thumb is to remember that when treatment differences between the experimental agent and the control decrease by 50%, the required sample size increases four-fold.

Similarly, placebo responses are not uniformly predictable. They tend to occur early, but may be of long duration in some patients. Placebo responses have been shown to exceed active treatment at all time points in some failed trials of biological agents.[30] In another 2-year RCT with blinded continuation treatment, placebo responses of 3 years' duration were documented in a small number of patients.[31] These have been ascribed to the increased interest in the clinical welfare of their patients on the part of physicians participating in RCTs as well as enthusiasm for the experimental agent, which may affect the patient's response to its administration.

Selection of an appropriate patient population

Selection of the appropriate patient population is crucial. Typically, clinical development programs of biological agents have sought to enroll patients who would be predicted to be most responsive to the product, based on its mechanism of action. To date, however, we have not succeeded in identifying characteristics which distinguish these patients. Further, exclusion of patients who have previously failed a product with a similar mechanism of action may not be prudent. Not only can this result in restrictive labeling of the product, but it will fail to answer an important question in day-to-day practice, perpetuate a false assumption, and deny treatment to patients who most need it. To avoid overspecification of a protocol population, it is often best to define the members of this population as those who would receive the active comparator in day-to-day practice. The choice of different active comparators in each RCT will then select patients with different disease characteristics and facilitate broad labeling by regulatory agencies. It will also make results from these RCTs more generalizable to everyday practice.

It is equally important to enroll patients with active disease, in whom improvement can be demonstrated. Interestingly, typical definitions of disease activity used in recent RCTs have been broadly applicable to populations with early as well as late disease, and improvement has been demonstrated in patients with long-standing disease, previously considered 'refractory'. However, the broad use of methotrexate has made it difficult to include elevated CRP levels in definitions of active disease, despite other manifestations, including multiple tender and/or swollen joints and prolonged morning stiffness.

RA, SLE and other musculoskeletal autoimmune diseases are most frequently diagnosed in individuals 30–40 years of age, and although they may result in significant morbidity, they are typically associated with a long life expectancy. Realistically, selection of therapies for these conditions must be considered in the perspective of 30–50 years of treatment. RCTs to determine the safety and efficacy of new, experimental therapies are of limited duration. Despite recent recommendations and regulatory approvals which have encouraged long-term RCTs to assess safety and efficacy in these disease populations, discontinuation rates for protocol participation typically approach 40–50% in protocols of 3, 6, 12 and 24 months.[31,32] Interestingly, dropouts are not only due to adverse events or lack of efficacy, but also occur for 'other' reasons, including convenience, change of healthcare provider, and/or geographic relocation, regardless of interference with work activities within or outside the home.

These dropout rates argue that long-term assessments of efficacy in RCTs may only be inferred using detailed sensitivity analyses, which demonstrated the robustness of X-ray analyses for recently approved biological and synthetic DMARDs in RA.[22,32] Alternatively, randomized open-label trials designed to mimic regular clinical practice may yield more valid information regarding long-term safety and efficacy, as well as offering more accurate assessments of the economic costs of the promising new therapy.

CONDUCT OF THE RANDOMIZED CONTROLLED TRIAL

Just as design of an RCT requires careful attention to detail, so must its conduct be carefully regulated. Statistical analysis plans are critical, and must be prospectively defined. Certain rules apply and are, in a regulatory sense, immutable. These include appropriate methods to ensure randomization, equal distribution of baseline demographic and disease characteristics, and maximum effort to avoid selection bias.

As previously discussed, central randomization is strongly recommended. Use of an analysis model which accounts for multiple potential parameters of variability is typically preferable to stratification of enrollment based on fewer predefined characteristics. Not only is it difficult to predict clinical responses in heterogeneous rheumatic disease populations, but stratification often precludes rapid protocol enrollment and will probably reduce statistical significance. If necessary, balanced enrollment by one, or at best two, parameters should be utilized, and other potential covariates included in the model analyzing efficacy according to enrollment site, geographic distribution, baseline disease characteristics, and prior treatment.

In clinical indications where treatment options are limited and rarely result in cures (or remissions), definitions of accepted or best standard therapy may change, even during the conduct of an RCT with limited duration. Recently true in RA, this is likely to occur more frequently in seronegative spondyloarthropathies and SLE, as promising new therapies are studied. The statistical analysis plan must therefore include appropriate rules for modification based on clinical information, even changes in therapeutic practice, which may become available only after protocol treatment is initiated.[33] These changes must be identified prospectively such that statistical analyses remain robust and retain their relevance to day-to-day clinical practice.

Clinical indications with limited available treatments and no definitive cures make it difficult to calculate sample sizes to identify statistically significant and/or clinically meaningful efficacy of an experimental therapy compared with a placebo and/or active control therapy. Data from phase 1 and 2 trials offer important information, but these trials are frequently conducted in patient populations of insufficient size and/or limited to a small number of clinical practices which may not reflect accepted day-to-day realities. Based on imperfect estimates of required sample size, blinded interim analyses can ensure protocol populations of sufficient size and/or treatments of sufficient duration to demonstrate statistical significance. Nonetheless, these blinded analyses alter conduct of the protocol, even when a blinded adjudication committee is utilized – although they offer no additional clinical information to the sponsor, they include recommendations on whether the RCT should continue either enrollment and/or treatment or be stopped. Conduct of these interim analyses will therefore require adjustment of the P-value.[34,35]

However, full disclosure and informed consent educate both patients and investigators to expect the worst and potentially unblind RCTs more frequently than any of the above considerations. Informed consents require that a variety of signs and symptoms, attributable to the disease as well as allowed background therapy, are explained in detail to patients, who may be tolerant of these effects. Such information may suggest that addition of a new (active and/or placebo) treatment may result in new or worsened symptoms, yet omits discussion of potential benefits that may be observed with the experimental agent. Although clinical investigators and monitors have been carefully trained to avoid soliciting specific adverse-event reports based on previous signs and symptoms reported in RCTs with the experimental agent, it is difficult to exclude physician (and patient) biases based on previous clinical experiences.

OUTCOME MEASURES

Particularly in rheumatology clinical indications, early RCTs used multiple outcome measures which did not offer a single, comprehensible assessment of clinical improvement. In

RA and OA, a variety of physician and patient reported outcome measures were utilized, requiring large sample size populations to differentiate small differences between potentially active and placebo therapies.

In RA, the Outcome Measures in Rheumatology Clinical Trials (OMERACT) consensus process, initiated in 1991, identified a minimum number (core set) of outcome measures to be used in RCTs; subsequent efforts to develop consensus resulted in validation and use of two 'responder indices' in RCTs in patients with active RA: ACR > 20% response (ACR > 20) and Disease Activity Score (DAS).[21,30] Use of both criteria facilitated US and EU regulatory approvals of new biological and pharmaceutical therapies for the treatment of RA, and, more importantly, established precedents for subsequent development and approval strategies. Similar efforts are underway to develop composite indices for clinical responses in SLE, OA, and seronegative spondyloarthropathies.[36,37]

Composite responder indices used in RA have included patient- and physician-reported outcomes, to assess both disease activity at baseline (DAS) and change over time (ACR ≥ 20 responses; DAS good and moderate responses).[38–40] Data from recent RCTs in RA have demonstrated several points:

- Utilization of DAS can 'stratify' patient populations at baseline, and help to identify those responding to treatment; yet it and ACR response criteria fail to identify 'clinical remissions', nor do they emphasize outcomes important to patients.
- Although the ACR ≥ 20/50/70 definition of response is not a continuous measure, its components are continuous measures. Recent RCTs of newly approved therapies in RA have demonstrated that improvement, by ACR ≥ 20 or DAS definitions of 'good and moderate' responses, are closely correlated, identifying ±10% of the same population.

Biological therapies specifically targeted against proinflammatory cytokines have resulted in significant clinical responses with rapid onset, and sustained improvements in physical function and radiographic measures of disease progression. Nonetheless, use of these biological agents, even in combination with standard DMARD therapies, has resulted in relatively few disease remissions, most of which are treatment dependent.

Increasingly, there has been recognition of the importance of 'patient-reported' outcome measures. These differ according to patient expectations, including comprehension, reasignment and acquiescence to a chronic disease which affects not only performance of required daily activities but also perception of self, within the home and in accepted social situations, as well as work-related and/or public activities. Now that new therapies in RA have demonstrated statistically as well as clinically significant improvements in performance of physical and psychosocial activities important to patients, we better comprehend the multiple ways in which diseases such as RA, SLE, seronegative spondyloarthropathies and OA impact on everyday living and its associated activities – health-related quality of life.

When assessing experimental versus control treatments, patient-reported outcomes are gaining increasing value among physicians, healthcare evaluators and economists. This is evident in RA, where responder analyses, by ACR ≥ 20 responses and/or DAS, have correlated with individual patient assessments of global disease activity (by visual analog scale or VAS), pain (by VAS) and, importantly, physical function (using validated instruments such as Health Assessment Questionnaire Disability Index (HAQ DI), Modified Health Assessment Questionnaire (MHAQ), Multidimensional Health Assessment Questionnaire (MDHAQ), Arthritis Impact Measurement Scale (AIMS), Arthritis Impact Measurement Scale-2 (AIMS-2), Problem Elicitation Technique (PET) and/or McMaster Toronto Arthritis patient preference questionnaire (MACTAR)). Although typically reported using mean changes across treatment groups, multiple analyses have identified minimal clinically important differences/ improvements (MCID) in patient-reported outcomes assessing physical function and health-related quality of life that identify changes perceptible to patients which result in clinically meaningful change.[39–42] These definitions allow physicians and other healthcare workers to better comprehend and compare changes in outcome measures in RCTs evaluating specific treatment regimens in a specific clinical indication. Although it is difficult to extrapolate mean and/or median score with active compared with control treatment, mean and/or median improvements of >50% with active treatment which exceed control can be taken to indicate that a majority of patients in that group are reporting clinically meaningful improvements.

Definitions of MCID in patient-reported outcomes facilitate physician assessments of clinical benefits reported in various RCTs, comparing treatments across disease populations. They can also be utilized to identify the 'number needed to treat' (patients) with an experimental therapy resulting in clinically meaningful improvement (compared with a 'gold standard' such as methotrexate). Improvements in physical function, assessed using rheumatology-specific measures such as HAQ DI and AIMS 2, can be compared with improvements in generic measures of health-related quality of life, such as Medical Outcomes Survey Short Form-36 (SF-36) or EuroQOL 5 Dimensional (EQ5D), instruments validated in many disease states (including hypertension, diabetes, OA, dialysis patients) and cross-culturally in multiple languages and populations.

Recent RCTs in RA have demonstrated a close correlation between treatment-associated improvements in physical function and changes in domains of health-related quality of life, in addition to those reflecting physical activities. A broad assessment of changes in health-related quality of life includes the impacts of other comorbid conditions, which occur frequently in RA populations but less so in those with SLE. Furthermore, baseline decrements and improvements with protocol treatment can be correlated with other age-, gender- and culture-matched populations, and facilitate comparisons of patient populations with musculoskeletal disease to those with other chronic, debilitating conditions.

The use of generic measures of health-related quality of life and health utilities facilitates economic evaluations of new therapies. Analysis of SF-36 responses can be used to derive health utility measures, and EQ5D includes a health utility measure; either can be utilized alone, or responses can be correlated with health utilities elicited by feeling thermometer or direct queries utilizing time trade-off or standard gamble techniques. The economic costs of diseases such as RA or SLE have traditionally been underestimated; indirect costs saved or gained by new treatments which maintain physical function and work capacity are crucial to their approval and adoption in clinical use. Increasingly, inclusion of new therapies in rheumatic diseases is dependent on collection of direct and indirect costs during RCTs as well as disease-specific and generic measures of health-related quality of life. However, RCTs typically identify the potential efficacy and toxicity of a new treatment under ideal or maximized conditions of use, where inclusion and exclusion criteria defining the protocol population are clearly defined, and potential adverse events, even if symptomatic, are prospectively defined and treated according to a protocol-specified algorithm.

THE STAGES OF PRODUCT DEVELOPMENT: PHASES 1–3

Phase 1 trials

Although phase 1 trials are traditionally safety studies, they can provide early signs of therapeutic effect if appropriate pharmacodynamic or biological markers are utilized (Table 40.5). As they are performed in patients, it is important to include a control group for accurate assessment of safety. It is also important to minimize the number of patients who must be exposed to product without potential therapeutic benefit. Use of biological markers may therefore allow repetitive dosing after single-dose administration within the same protocol. Following an

Table 40.5 Phase 1 development.

Predominantly safety trials
Usually requires a placebo treatment arm to assess safety and potential efficacy
Usually dose-ranging
Use of biological markers may predict more important clinical response
May provide useful information about pharmacokinetic or pharmacodynamic properties

recently approved biological agents have demonstrated significant clinical benefits even in these RA patient populations. If the product has already been studied in another clinical indication, it is still important to recognize that patients with rheumatic diseases, especially RA, may be more sensitive to treatment effects and manifest specific safety signals, due to either the underlying disease, associated comorbidities, and/or use of background therapies.

It is increasingly difficult to enroll patients in even short-term phase 1 trials without the use of background therapy which may alter the tolerability, immunogenicity or pharmacokinetic profile of the experimental product. Cell depletion following administration of several T-cell-targeted monoclonal antibodies (anti-CD4 and CAMPATH 1-H) was greater in magnitude and longer in duration than expected when patients were receiving background methotrexate. When infliximab is co-administered with methotrexate, the serum half-life is prolonged and immunogencity decreased.[43]

appropriate washout period after the single dose and ascertainment that all pharmacokinetic, laboratory and immune parameters have normalized, weekly, biweekly or monthly dosing at the same dose level may be administered in the same cohort. In other circumstances, treatment may be initiated with an intravenous dose followed by multiple subcutaneous doses after an appropriate washout period.

These dose-escalation trials should include at least one placebo control at each dose level; data in patients receiving placebo may be combined as a single group for comparison with the other active-treatment groups. Ideally, phase 1 trials will identify both a 'no-effect' dose and the MTD. However, dose–response curves with many biological agents are relatively flat, and short-term treatment may not elicit an adverse-event profile sufficient to identify a maximum dose level. Alternatively, dose escalation may be limited by the amount of protein that can be delivered intravenously or subcutaneously.

If this is the first time that the product has been in humans, it will be necessary to start with very low doses, 10–100 times less than the estimated MTD. It may be difficult to predict a product's tolerability profile from short-term animal studies or with species-specific products.[42] Therefore, a patient population with refractory disease is typically selected for these early trials, comprising patients who have failed all currently available treatments, or have active disease despite background therapy. Nonetheless,

Phase 2 trials

Phase 2 trials are pilot efficacy trials which should result in a 'go/no go decision' regarding further clinical development of the product. Ideally, high versus moderate versus no effect doses are selected for dosing, based on data from phase 1 trials, including the pharmacokinetic/pharmacodynamic profile of the product

Table 40.6 Phase 2 development.

Early studies, but clear signals of efficacy should be required
Should define minimally effective dose and maximally effective dose
Should determine the dose and dose schedule for phase 3 RCTs
Begin to establish a long-term safety database by offering continued treatment to those patients who respond to and tolerate therapy

and its effects on biological markers (Table 40.6). As these are short-term trials, it is important to select a responsive patient population and outcome measures sensitive to change. In RA, both the ACR response criteria and DAS have reflected clinical improvement within days to weeks of initiating treatment (depending on the agent studied). Patient-reported measures of physical function and health-related quality of life also reflect early clinical improvement. Biological or pharmacodynamic measures from phase 1 studies may be included, if practical, to see if they serve as 'leading indicators' of response. Potential sources of unblinding must be avoided: separate assessors for safety and efficacy and premedication to avoid infusion reactions may be necessary.

It is ethically important to offer patients continued treatment after the protocol is completed, particularly if they have shown improvement with an acceptable tolerability profile. This will also provide information regarding long-term safety of the product, duration of benefit, and potential retreatment regimens when clinical responses are lost. The ultimate goal of the phase 2 trials should be a well-characterized product whose times of onset and offset of clinical effect and appropriate dose and dose schedules are known. A practical dose schedule amenable to patients and physicians must be utilized, but it should be based on data and not empirically selected. Too often, phase 2 trials with biological agents are shortened in an effort to make the clinical development program more efficient. At best, this will require inclusion of more than one dose or dose schedule in the phase 3 trials; at worst, it may preclude identification of the best efficacy/tolerability profile of the product.

Phase 3 trials

Ideally, these are multicenter RCTs designed to confirm the safety and efficacy of the product in a significantly larger number of patients than has been studied in either of the previous phases of development. From a regulatory point of view, although a single 6-month RCT may be

---

Table 40.7 Phase 3 development.

Multicenter RCTs to recruit sufficient numbers of patients to ensure achieving adequate safety exposure

Multiple trials to confirm efficacy in different patient populations

Patients to be recruited should reflect the heterogeneity of the real-world population with regard to the targeted disease

Should consider strongly 12-month RCTs with extensions to 24 months, for adequate safety and efficacy assessments in long-term treatment of a chronic disease

If placebo is considered, typically used for a short period of time, with defined 'rescue'

Active background therapy reflecting accepted standard of care is usually provided

---

sufficient to demonstrate efficacy in improving the signs and symptoms of disease in the USA, these data offer limited information in clinical indications, where regular treatment for many years is expected. Both FDA and EMEA documents regarding product development in RA now require at least 12- or 24-month RCTs to gain specific labeling regarding benefit on radiographic progression or sustained improvement in physical function and health-related quality of life. In the context of diseases that will require treatment for many years, long-term trials to assess safety and efficacy are crucial.

Patient populations for enrollment in phase 3 trials should be broadly selected (Table 40.7). Ideally, patients with early, moderate and, later, more severe disease will be recruited according to the active comparator employed in the trial, or the background therapy selected. It is important to avoid overly restrictive inclusion and exclusion criteria. Selection of active or placebo controls determines the size of the protocol and the time required to complete enrollment. Placebo treatment may be limited to 3 or 6 months, although increasingly it is thought unethical to utilize placebo in indications such as RA, because irreversible deterioration in physical function can occur over this relatively short period of time. If utilized, even in the presence of background therapy, active treatment must be offered to patients upon completion of the controlled trial, or following discontinuation of protocol participation due to lack of efficacy. If there exist stringent criteria for defining lack of efficacy, then patients receiving active as well as placebo treatment may switch to an alternative therapy, while still retaining the blind. Whether active or placebo comparators are utilized, it is crucial to avoid excessive dropouts in any treatment arm. These include allowing limited changes in supportive therapies, and bridging with short-duration treatments, including joint injections.

Creative treatment regimens may be explored, particularly with biological agents with rapid onsets of effect. Induction treatment and sequential or combination regimens may be studied in phase 3 RCTs, provided the agent is well characterized and is utilized with other broadly prescribed products. A comparison of the new therapy versus an accepted treatment versus the combination of the two is a popular design that can yield useful information for clinical practice, and may demonstrate clinical superiority of the combination and non-equivalence of the two monotherapies.

CONCLUSIONS

RCTs are the only way to determine true response when developing new therapies. In studying treatment effects in patients with rheumatic diseases, significant placebo responses are expected. The introduction of biological therapies has ushered in a new era of product development in rheumatology. These therapies provide early responses, frequently after the first or second dose, whereas previously, at least 3 months of DMARD administration was required before confirming treatment failure. Adherence to careful trial design will be required to minimize some of the confounding effects of these newer therapies.

REFERENCES

1. Bendtzen K, Hansen MB, Ross C et al. Cytokines and autoantibodies to cytokines. *Stem Cells* 1995; **13**: 206–22

2. Fishwild DM, Hudson DV, Deshpande U, Kung AHC. Differential effects of administration of a human anti-CD4 monoclonal antibody, HM6G, in nonhuman primates. *Clin Immunol* 1999; **92**: 138–52.

3. Hencke JW, Hilbish KG, Serabian MA et al. Reproductive toxicity testing of therapeutic biotechnology agents. *Teratology* 1996; **53**: 185–95.

4. Strand V. Are there special considerations relevant to trials of biological agents? *J Rheumatol* 1994; **21**(suppl 41): 41–9

5. Mackall CL, Hakim FT, Gress RE. T cell regeneration: all repertoires are not created equal. *Immunol Today* 1997; **18**: 245–51.

6. Jendro MC, Ganten T, Matteson EL et al. Emergence of oligoclonal T cell populations following therapeutic T cell depletion in rheumatoid arthritis. *Arthritis Rheum* 1995; **38**: 1242–51.

7. Mouy R, Seger R, Bourquin JP et al. Interferon for chronic granulomatous disease. *N Engl J Med* 1991; **324**: 509–16

8. Wing MG, Moreau T, Greenwood J et al. Mechanism of first dose cytokine release syndrome by CAMPATH 1H: involvement of CD16 and CD11a/CD18 on NK cells. *J Clin Invest* 1996; **98**: 2819–26

9. Alegre M-L, Vandenabeele P, Depierreux M et al. Cytokine release syndrome induced by the 145–2C11 anti CD3 monoclonal antibody in mice: prevention by high doses of methylprednisolone. *J Immunol* 1991; **146**: 1184–91.

10. Isaacs JD. From bench to bedside: discovering rules for antibody design and improving serotherapy with monoclonal antibodies. *Rheumatology* 2001; **40**: 724–8.

11. Kneer J, Luedin E, Lesslauer W et al. An assessment of the effect of anti drug antibody formation on the pharmacokinetics and pharmacodynamics of sTNFr55–IgG in patients with rheumatoid arthritis. *Arthritis Rheum* 1988; **41**: S58

12. Christen U, Theurkauf R, Stevens R et al. Immunogenicity of a human TNFR55–IgG1 fusion protein in rheumatoid arthritis and multiple sclerosis *Arthritis Rheum* 1988; **41**: S58

13. Epstein WV. Expectation bias in rheumatoid arthritis clinical trials. The anti CD4 monoclonal antibody experience. *Arthritis Rheum* 1996; **39**: 1773–9.

14. Strand V, Scott DL, Panayi GS. Evaluating biological agents in rheumatoid arthritis: a framework for clinical trials. *J Rheumatol* 1994; **21**: 1390–2.

15. Schulz KF. Assessing allocation concealment and blinding in randomized controlled trials: why bother? *ACP J Club* 2000; **132**: A11–12

16. Clinical Development Programs for Drugs, Devices, and Biological Products for the Treatment of Rheumatoid Arthritis (RA). http://www.fda.gov/cder/guidance/1208fnl.htm.

17. Points to consider on clinical investigation of slow-acting anti-rheumatic medicinal products in rheumatoid arthritis, December 1998. http://www.eudra.org/emea.html

18. Jones B, Jarvis P, Lewis JA, Ebbutt AF. Trials to assess equivalence: the importance of rigorous methods. *BMJ* 1996; **313**: 36–9.

19. Temple R, Ellenberg SS. Placebo controlled trials and active control trials in the evaluation of new treatments. Part 1: ethical and scientific issues *Ann Intern Med* 2000; **133**: 455–63

20. Temple R, Ellenberg SS. Placebo controlled trials and active control trials in the evaluation of new treatments. Part 2: practical issues and specific cases. *Ann Intern Med* 2000; **133**: 464–70.

21. Weinblatt ME, Coblyn JS, Fox DA et al. Efficacy of low-dose methotrexate in rheumatoid arthritis. *N Engl J Med* 1985; **312**: 818–22

22. Lipsky PE, van der Heijde DM, St Clair EW et al. Infliximab and methotrexate in the treatment of rheumatoid arthritis. Anti-Tumor Necrosis Factor Trial in rheumatoid arthritis with concomitant therapy study group. *N Engl J Med* 2000; **343**: 1594–602

23. Weinblatt ME, Kremer JM, Bankhurst AD et al. A trial of etanercept, a recombinant tumor necrosis factor receptor–Fc fusion protein, in patients with rheumatoid arthritis receiving methotrexate. *New Engl J Med* 1999; **340**: 253–9.

24. Moreland L, Bucy RP, Tilden A et al. Use of a chimeric monoclonal anti-CD4 antibody in patients with refractory rheumatoid arthritis. *Arthritis Rheum* 1993: 36: 307–18.

25. Strand V, Lipsky PE, Cannon GW et al. Effects of administration of an anti-CD5 immunoconjugate in rheumatoid arthritis. *Arthritis Rheum* 1993; **36**: 620–30.

26. Mason U, Aldrich J, Breedveld F et al. CD4 coating, but not CD4 depletion, is a predictor of efficacy with primatized monoclonal anti CD4 treatment of active rheumatoid arthritis. *J Rheumatol* 2002: 29: 220–9.

27. Jorgensen C, Mason U, Baton F. Eleven month clinical safety follow up in RA patients with CD4 lymphopenia following treatment with the primatized anti-CD4 monoclonal antibody, keliximab. *Arthritis Rheum* 1998; **41**: S56.

28. Pincus T, Koch GG, Sokka T et al. A randomized, double-blind, crossover clinical trial of diclofenac plus misoprostol versus acetaminophen in patients with osteoarthritis of the hip or knee. *Arthritis Rheum* 2001; **44**: 1477–80.

29. Paulus HE, Egger MJ, Ward JR et al. Analysis of improvement in individual rheumatoid arthritis patients treated with disease modifying antirheumatic drugs, based on the findings in patients treated with placebo. *Arthritis Rheum* 1990; **33**: 477–91.

30. Olsen NJ, Brooks RH, Cush JJ et al. A double blind placebo controlled study of anti-CD5 immunoconjugate in patients with rheumatoid arthritis. *Arthritis Rheum* 1996; **39**: 1102–8

31. Cohen S, Cannon G, Schiff M et al. Two year treatment of active rheumatoid arthritis with leflunomide compared with methotrexate. *Arthritis Rheum* 2001; **40**: 1984–92.

32. Sharp JT, Strand V, Leung H et al. Treatment with leflunomide slows radiographic progression of RA – results from three randomized controlled trials of leflunomide in patients with active rheumatoid arthritis. *Arthritis Rheum* 2000; **43**: 495–505.

33. Wittes J. On changing a long term clinical trial midstream. *Statistics in Medicine* 2002 (in press).

34. O'Brien PC, Fleming TR. A multiple testing procedure for clinical trials. *Biometrics* 1979; **35**: 549–56

35. Lan KKG, DeMets DL, Halperin M. More flexible sequential and non-sequential designs in long-term clinical trials. *Commun Stat A Theory Methods* 1984; **13**: 2339 –53.

36. Smolen JS, Strand V, Cardiel M et al. Randomized clinical trials and longitudinal observational studies in systemic lupus erythematosus: consensus on a preliminary core set of outcome domains. *J Rheumatol* 1999; **26**: 504–7

37. Calin A, Nakache JP, Gueguen A et al. Defining disease activity in ankylosing spondylitis: is a combination of variables (Bath Ankylosing Spondylitis Disease Activity Index) an appropriate instrument? *Rheumatology (Oxford)* 1999; **38**: 878–82

38. Goldsmith C, Boers M, Bombardier C et al. Criteria for clinically important changes in outcomes: development, scoring and evaluation of rheumatoid arthritis patient and trial profiles. *J Rheumatol* 1993; **20**: 561–5.

39. Wells GA, Tugwell P, Kraag GR et al. Minimum important differences between patients with rheumatoid arthritis: the patient's perspective. *J Rheumatol* 1993; **20**: 557–60.

40. Kosinski M, Zhao SZ, Didhiya S et al. Determining minimum clinically important changes in generic and disease-specific health-related quality of life questionnaires in clinical trials of rheumatoid arthritis. *Arthritis Rheum* 2000; **43**: 1478–87.

41. Kujawski SC, Kosinski M, Martin R et al. Determining meaningful improvement in SF-36 scale scores for treatment studies of early, active RA. *Arthritis Rheum* 2000; **43**: S140.

42. Black LE, Bendele AM, Bendele RA et al. Regulatory decision strategy for entry of a novel biological therapeutic with a clinically unmonitorable toxicity into clinical trials: pre IND meetings and a case example. *Toxicol Pathol* 1999; **27**: 22–6.

43. Kavanaugh A, St Clair EW, McCune WJ et al. Chimeric anti TNFa monoclonal antibody treatment of patients with rheumatoid arthritis receiving methotrexate therapy. *J Rheumatol* 2000; **27**: 841–2.

41

Long-term observational studies

Eswar Krishnan, Gurkirpal Singh and Peter Tugwell

Introduction • Definitions • Role of long-term observational studies in biologicals • Types of observational study • Interpretation of data from observational studies • References

INTRODUCTION

The common denominators of rheumatic diseases comprise; autoimmune etiology, unknown precipitating factors, relentless progression of disease activity, and consequent damage to the tissues. Rheumatoid arthritis (RA) is a prototypic rheumatic disease characterized by progressive disability and sometimes premature mortality. Over the past 50 years, observational studies have contributed to our understanding of the natural history (Framingham study and heart failure), causation (e.g. smoking and lung cancer), risk factors (hypertension and congestive heart failure), and rare drug toxicities (thalidomide and phocomelia). This chapter focuses on the relevance and importance of long-term observational studies in the evaluation of medications for rheumatic diseases, especially biologicals. The use of biologicals in rheumatology is a relatively recent advance, and the medications have primarily been used in the treatment of RA. Although this chapter will discuss the role of observational studies of biologicals, using the medications used for RA as an example, the concepts delineated here are applicable to all rheumatic diseases.

DEFINITIONS

The branch of epidemiology that deals with studies on the use of drugs is known as pharmacoepidemiology. There are two types of pharmacoepidemiologic studies: experimental studies and observational studies. In experimental studies, the investigator controls which treatment subjects receive. This is not possible in observational studies, where the assignment, e.g. the decision to treat with a biological, is done by the individual physician based on individual circumstances of the patient, taking into account the balance between potential benefit and harm. The investigator in the observational study, however, has control over the selection of study subjects. There are two types of observational studies. The strongest pharmacoepidemiologic observational design is a cohort study (also called follow-up study or incidence study), which is similar to an experimental study in that the patients are identified before the outcome is known and followed prospectively, and the outcomes are compared across different exposure groups, i.e. different doses of the drug and the control groups not receiving the biological.

Three types of studies may be conducted within a cohort design: case–cohort studies, nested case–control studies, and surveillance studies. A case–cohort study may be defined as a case–control study where every person has an equal chance of being chosen as a control regardless of the person-time they have contributed to the cohort. Let us say that in a cohort of RA patients, where some are treated with etanercept and some are not, we wish to assess the risk of leukemia among those treated with etanercept. In the case–cohort method, patients who develop the cancer are the cases, and all patients in the cohort, irrespective of whether they have been in the cohort for weeks or years, have an equal chance of being selected as a control. On the other hand, in a nested case–control study, the controls are selected from among those who are at risk for outcome at the instant the event of interest happened – in this case a diagnosis of leukemia. The advantage of a nested case–control study over a case–cohort study is that it selects the controls with the same person-time of exposure as the controls. Post-marketing surveillance (PMS) is the term given for long-term longitudinal study of drugs in the general population. It is defined as a continuous and systematic process of collection, analysis, interpretation and dissemination of descriptive information for monitoring health problems associated with the use of medications. PMS aims to monitor the population for increased incidence of rare adverse events as well as to monitor effectiveness. In that sense, a PMS program is not necessarily hypothesis driven; the many individual studies nested within are.

The second type of observational study is the case–control study (also known as the incident case–control study), which involves sampling study subjects in terms of their outcome and subsequently determining the exposure status, i.e. treatment/no treatment. With the available information on the probability of exposure given the outcome, one can compute the probability of outcome given the probability of exposure.

Another axis of classification of observational studies is prospective versus retrospective data collection. The definition of whether a study is prospective or retrospective strictly refers to the timing of the outcome occurrence with exposure measurement. Thus, a case–control and a cohort study can use either prospective or retrospective data collection. A prospective case–control study uses exposure measurements taken prior to the occurrence of the outcome, while a retrospective case–control study uses exposure measurement taken after the occurrence of the event. Both case–control and cohort studies may employ a mixture of prospective and retrospective measurements using data collected after and before the disease occurrence.

ROLE OF LONG-TERM OBSERVATIONAL STUDIES IN BIOLOGICALS

The treatment options in RA have evolved from high-dose aspirin, a panoply of non-steroidal anti-inflammatory drugs (NSAIDs), disease modifiers such as methotrexate and leflunomide, and, recently, molecules tailored to have specific targets in the inflammation cascade. The biologicals such as etanercept, infliximab and anakinra have all shown efficacy comparable to or even superior to the current standard of therapy, i.e. methotrexate.

There are two specific concerns about the biologicals that cannot be answered in clinical trial settings. The first is the issue of effectiveness versus efficacy. While the randomized control trial is the gold standard to evaluate efficacy, these trials tend to be of relatively short duration (less than 2 years) and very expensive to conduct. In addition, the long duration of RA, strict exclusion and inclusion criteria that reduce the generalizeability of the data, and rigid dosing schedules, make the results from clinical trials less applicable to day-to-day clinical decision-making. As an example, although an overview of the published clinical trials suggested equivalent efficacies for sulfasalazine, D-penicillamine, methotrexate and parenteral gold,[1] long-term observational studies have shown that all disease-modifying anti-rheumatic drugs (DMARDs) except methotrexate have high 5-year discontinuation rates.[2-5] This clinic-based observation is confirmed by population-based data.[6] The chief causes of discontinuation are loss of efficacy and toxicity in that order. Thus, although an agent may be shown to be efficacious in well-performed short-term clinical trials with substantive improvement in the clinical picture, its utility in day-to-day clinical practice, i.e. the 'street value', is much less. The relationship between effectiveness and efficacy is summarized as follows;[7]

Effectiveness =

$$\frac{\text{Access to health care} \times \text{diagnosis of RA} \times}{\text{recommendation of therapy} \times \text{efficacy} \times \text{adherence}}$$

Probability of adverse events

Using this model, the excellent efficacy of etanercept (48% reduction in ACR 20 compared to placebo[8]) translates into a mediocre effectiveness (23% reduction) even if all the patients with RA in the community who will benefit from the drug have access to it. Similarly, the effectiveness of anakinra is estimated at about 9%, as opposed to an efficacy of 16%.[9] Thus, efficacy is important but not sufficient to deliver benefit to patients in day-to-day clinical care. Observational studies can answer the question – is this drug effective in reducing outcomes in day-to-day clinical care? To this end, a core set of domains of outcomes (Table 41.1) and reporting requirements for longitudinal studies (Table 41.2) have been defined.[10]

Table 41.1 Outcome measurement in long-term observational studies.

Core domains
   Health status
   Disease process
   Damage
   Mortality
   Toxicity/adverse reactions
Optional domains
   Work disability
   Costs

Table 41.2 Minimum reporting requirements for longitudinal observational studies in rheumatology.

- Study design type: true prospective, retrospective, or mixed
- Source of cases: true population-based, catchment population, consecutive series (specify clinic type), or other
- Timing of patient recruitment in relation to disease onset: cases followed from disease onset, cases followed from first presentation, or prevalent cases
- Inclusion criteria: classification criteria, age, range, sex
- Demographic data: sex, age, socio-economic factors, ethnicity
- Baseline clinical data: specify individual items of data collected at baseline; distinguish between items ascertained from medical records and those collected prospectively using a standard pro forma; specify number of observers, training requirements, and any measures of observer variability
- Follow-up data: specify frequency of follow-up and decision rules about timing of each assessment; provide information on proportion of patients with missing follow-up information at each time point and estimate potential for loss to follow-up bias; indicate means of follow-up data collection (interview, questionnaire, mail, or telephone); report number of observers involved in prospective data collection and nature of training, and report on observer variability; report on principal and subsidiary outcome measures chosen; comment on observer blindness to baseline variables
- Analysis: specify strategies used for missing data and loss to follow-up; indicate, in relation to person-years of follow-up, the power to detect clinically meaningful differences for the major outcomes analyzed; if a statistical model is generated, indicate performance in a validation sample

Reproduced from Silman and Symmons. *J Rheumatol* 1999; **26**: 481–3.[11]

The second major concern about biologicals is long-term safety. Men with RA are thought to be at higher risk for lymphoproliferative disorders (LPDs).[12] In comparison with the general population, a 3–8-fold increase in patients with moderate or severe disease has been reported,[13] with additional increments in those treated with azathioprine[14,15] and possibly cyclosporin A. Overall, a conservative estimate of about 5000 new cases of LPD in about 500 000 RA patients treated with methotrexate has been reported – a crude incidence proportion of 0.01%.[16]

In the case of biologicals, to date two cases of non-Hodgkin's lymphoma (NHL) and one case of Hodgkin's lymphoma (HL) have been reported in a study of 159 patients given anti-tumor necrosis factor (TNF)-α antibodies.[16] Two cases of NHL were diagnosed after administration of anti-CHD52 monoclonal antibody to 140 patients. One case was reported after treatment of about 200 patients with primatized anti-CD4 antibodies. Are these observations chance occurrences or do they portend an increased incidence of LPDs caused by the biological therapies? Will the combination therapy with methotrexate increase the risk further? Are there teratogenic effects of these medications?

TNF-α is a very important cytokine in maintaining homeostasis. The TNF-α antagonists appear to be produced not only by the activated macrophages in the synovial tissues but also by T lymphocytes and mononuclear phagocytes. Blockade of TNF-α can theoretically lead to an unintended reduction in cell-mediated immunity to intracellular pathogens such as *Mycobacterium tuberculosis*, as well as reduced tumor surveillance leading to an increased incidence of neoplasia. There are emerging data for the former.[17] Although no increase in the incidence of neoplasia has been reported so far with TNF-α antagonists, it is conceivable that cancers whose risk is increased by these agents have a long preclinical period, and therefore an excess incidence will not be obvious until much later. These two issues dominate the long-term safety concerns with any targeted, highly efficacious biological molecule and can only be addressed by long-term observational studies.

EXAMPLES OF OBSERVATIONAL STUDIES

The ARAMIS-PMS example

A cohort study is the most straightforward type of pharmacoepidemiologic study. Cohort studies on the effectiveness on medications, including the biologicals, begin with assembling a single group of patients (called the cohort – from the Latin word for one of the 10 divisions of a Roman Legion) who are heterogeneous with respect to exposure to medications. Typically, patients are recruited from the physician's office or by advertising in the local media. Additionally, there is always an attempt to recruit all the patients from within a well-defined population (e.g. Olmsted County, MN, USA) or a country (e.g. National Databank of Rheumatic Diseases[18]) and include them in a registry for follow-up. Arthritis, Rheumatism and Aging Medical Information System–Post Marketing Surveillance Program (ARAMIS-PMS) is the prototypical pharmacoepidemiologic program thatd aims to answer the questions such as: Does this drug work when used outside of clinical trials? Are there new toxicities? Are patients satisfied with this drug? What is the cost-effectiveness of this drug in a real-life setting?

ARAMIS is the US National Arthritis Data Resource, enabled under the Arthritis Act of 1974, and funded by the National Center for Health Services Research in 1975 and 1976, and from 1977 to the present day by the National Institute of Health (NIH). ARAMIS includes multiple databank centers in the USA and Canada, and follows about 17 000 patients with specific arthritis conditions and normal populations of aging people. ARAMIS initiated the concept of the chronic disease databank,[19] in which consecutive patients are enrolled, followed for life, and regularly assessed for multiple factors including demographics, socioeconomic status, the biology of disease, the influence of comorbidities, the mechanics and setting of care, specific medical and surgical treatments, and associated costs. Over 800 peer-reviewed publications have emanated from the ARAMIS program. An experienced multidisci-

Table 41.3 Data collected by ARAMIS.	

11 databanks

9 centers

Average of 10 observations for RA patients and 5 for OA patients

10 databanks approach patients at the usual point of clinical care

95% patients consent to enter the study

Successive data collection cycles each 6 months

    Mailed questionnaires

    Clinic visits

    Telephone interviews

Variables

    Background information questionnaire

    Full clinical data

    Health Assessment Questionnaire

        Pain

        Disability

        Global self-assessment

        Medications

            35 rheumatic disease-specific medications

            15 classes of other medications

            The list of medications are updated

        Symptom checklist

        Drug side-effects

        Hospitalizations and emergency room visits

        Comorbid conditions

        Health behaviors

    Mortality data

    Databank specific questions

Patients enrolled in studies are coded as such; later, when the randomization code is opened, the correct medication code is entered retrospectively

Strict data quality checks; error rates <1%

The earliest contributions of the ARAMIS program to outcomes research relevant to observational studies were the development of the HAQ[20,21] and the Childhood Health Assessment Questionnaire (CHAQ)[22] (Table 41.4). The HAQ as an instrument has been extensively studied, with over 500 publications on its validity, reliability and application. The HAQ has been validated in over 25 languages. The CHAQ has been translated into nine different languages. The HAQ has been employed in ARAMIS studies regularly since 1979, with over 200 000 assessments to date, and provides up to 21 years of longitudinal cost and utilization data through this study period.[23]

In recent years, ARAMIS has systematically recruited and followed the Rheumatoid Arthritis National Inception Cohort. This cohort consists of 950 patients with RA seen within the first year of disease, with disease onset between 1 July 1995 and 30 June 1997, recruited by clinical members of the American College of Rheumatology. Clinical data are collected from the respective clinicians annually, and disability is measured semi-annually using the HAQ with standard ARAMIS protocols. A serum and DNA databank on these patients is also maintained.

The ARAMIS-PMS program was started in 1992 with the specific mission of following up patients on arthritis medications with a view to identifying rare adverse events as well as to assessing long-term effectiveness. The ARAMIS-PMS program is uniquely related to yet distinct from the ARAMIS program, in that both share the same data collection strategies, but the latter focuses entirely on the pharmacoepidemiology of drugs.

The ARAMIS-PMS is a collaborative effort between several centers around the USA and Canada, with about 17 000 patient enrollees, of whom about 6400 have RA.[24,25] In this program, patients are enrolled continuously, and followed up regularly by semi-annual questionnaires (Table 41.3), which include the Health Assessment Questionnaire (HAQ), prescription and over-the-counter medication data, and adverse events, including those that patients attribute to any medication. In addition, data are

plinary team includes biostatisticians, epidemiologists, health economists, health service researchers, clinical investigators, and support staff from Stanford and other institutions.

Table 41.4   Some of the notable contributions of the ARAMIS-PMS program.

The Health Assessment Questionnaire
NSAID Toxicity Index
Inversion of therapeutic pyramid
Sawtooth strategy in treatment of RA
The childhood Health Assessment Questionnaire
Excess mortality in RA
Magnitude of NSAID gastropathy epidemic
Cost models for treatment of RA
Models of cost-effectiveness for the biologicals

collected on hospitalizations, and verified by periodic audits and death information from the National Death Index database.[26]

An important contribution of the ARAMIS-PMS program to the pharmacoepidemiology of DMARDs is the documentation that early and persistent use of DMARDs is superior to NSAID-based strategies in reducing long-term disability by one-third to one-half.[27,28] This approach will be extended to the biologicals as the data become available. The PMS studies revealed the long-term toxicity profiles of various DMARDs and prolonged immunosuppression, which is again highly relevant to the biologicals.[29,30] Together, the pharmacoepidemiologic studies from the PMS have contributed substantially to our knowledge of major adverse effects of medications and costs.[31,32] The gastrointestinal toxicity of NSAIDs was grossly underestimated until 1980–90. A series of ARAMIS-PMS studies have quantitated the magnitude of the epidemic of NSAID gastropathy, documenting the patient and societal costs.[33,34] The use of the observational data has permitted quantitation of the frequencies of hospitalizations and deaths and differential risks of NSAIDs. In addition, the data were successfully used to develop and validate a

quantitative model called SCORE (standardized calculator for risk events) for prediction of individual risks of serious gastrointestinal toxicities.[35,36] The use of long-term observational data will help us to identify and quantitate models of infection and malignancy risks with biologicals.

Another use of the data from the PMS program was for the development of toxicity indices for DMARDs and NSAIDs that take into account adverse events, laboratory tests and hospitalizations.[37–39] A separate gastrointestinal toxicity index has also been developed.[40] By use of this toxicity index, DMARDs were shown to have similar toxicity to NSAIDs, without there being a clear safety advantage for either group; a fact that supports aggressive use of DMARDs instead of NSAIDs. These data provided the strategic depth in the newer paradigm of early, consistent use of DMARDs. Longitudinal data will help assess the toxicity–efficacy trade-offs and help establish similar strategic depth in the use of biologicals in RA, spondylarthropathies and lupus.

International Rheumatoid Arthritis Database (IRAD)

The World Health Organization has designated the decade 2000–2010 as the 'Bone and Joint Decade'. One of the strategic research objectives during this decade is to foster a close working relationship between epidemiologic data and bench research. As a part of this international strategy, the IRAD is being set up as a highly collaborative and consultative organization which will help to pool data from various ongoing epidemiologic studies across the world, thereby bringing a much wanted global perspective to the epidemiology of RA. The logic underlying the core database, the structure of the research agenda, and its rendering into IRAD, were conceived and are being implemented by Marissa Lassere and Kent Johnson. The objectives of the database are given in Table 41.5. The initiative described here is the first formal global study of chronic disease, and will serve as a model for internationally coordinated study of other chronic disorders which impact on public

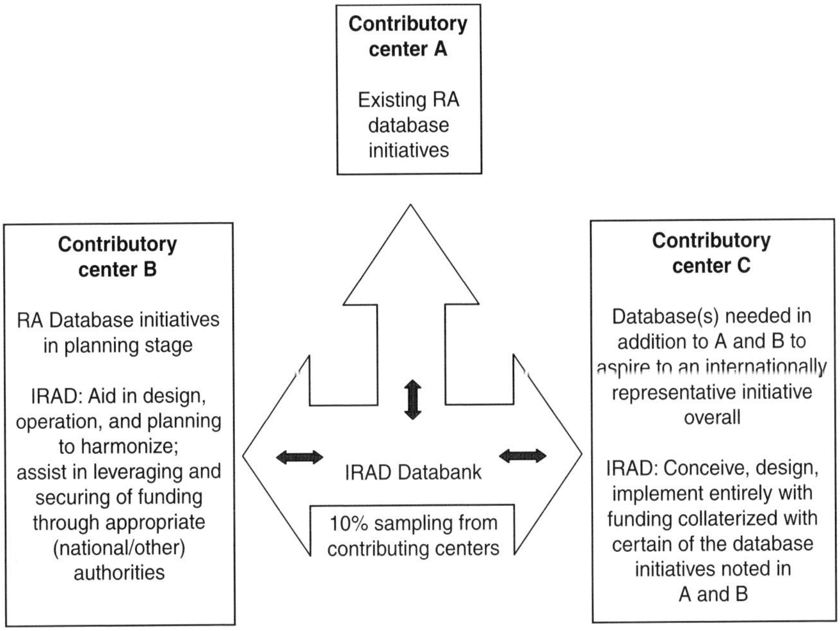

Figure 41.1 IRAD fundamental structure and operations.

Table 41.5 International Rheumatoid Arthritis Database (IRAD).

IRAD has five objectives:

- An umbrella function as a repository of information on design and operation of RA databases

- A communication and instruction function as a worldwide forum for coordination of database designs and operations

- A leveraging function by assisting under-resourced emerging or planned RA databases

- A practical research function in outcomes and health policy by making available its worldwide representative database (IRAD Core Databank) to all participants for descriptive and hypothesis-testing uses

- A methodological research function to optimally understand existing databases, and systematically elucidate (for the first time) the validity of formal pooling across databases

health (Figure 41.1). IRAD is intended to supplement and strengthen the existing databases, help develop new databases, and foster a culture of shared research objectives.

RAPOLO

Recently, a new cohort study has been established to follow long-term outcomes in patients with RA treated with etanercept – the Rheumatoid Arthritis Prospective Observational Longitudinal Outcomes Study (RAPOLO). This study, based at the University of California at San Francisco, recruited and followed 700 RA patients who were originally enrolled in clinical trials of etanercept. Irrespective of their initial allocation to receive active drug, most patients in the trials subsequently received etanercept, given the impressive efficacy shown in those clinical trials. Patients underwent a baseline telephone interview at the time of entry into the study and then quarterly interviews for four cycles. The frequency of interviews subsequent to this is annual. RAPOLO is an example how clinical trials can be extended into a cohort

Table 41.6 Factors influencing the quality of an observational study.

Quality of the study	Factors influencing the quality	Ways to improve quality
Precision	Sampling error	Increasing the size of the study population
	Measurement error	More accurate ascertainment of exposure and outcomes
		Sensitivity analysis
		Use of case–cohort and nested case–control studies
		Statistically efficient apportionment of subjects into study groups
		Matching
Internal validity	Selection bias	Choice of reference groups
	Self-selection bias	Internal versus external
	Diagnosis bias	Verification of exposure and diagnosis
		Medical records
		Pathologic or radiologic reports
	Confounding	Restriction of admission criteria
		Matching
	Information bias	
	Misclassification of effects and outcomes	Validation studies
	– Differential	
	– Non-differential	
	– Misclassification of confounders	
Generalizability	Choice of subjects	Selection of subjects for characteristics that enable distinction between competing risk factors

study, thereby saving considerable amounts of money. Similar efforts are underway in Europe to develop a surveillance program for adverse events related to the use of biologicals.[41]

INTERPRETATION OF DATA FROM OBSERVATIONAL STUDIES

Overall, the goal in observational studies is to accurately estimate the effectiveness, toxicity and costs associated with treatment. The estimates derived from observational study data can be erroneous if one is not careful. The sources of error in estimation can be either random or systematic. The design, conduct, analysis and interpretation of observational studies, therefore, must be such that these errors are anticipated and minimized. Precision is defined as the degree of lack of random error, while validity is defined as the lack of both systematic and random error. When the measurements are accurate and not attributable to random error, the inference is said to be internally valid or valid within the study group. An inference from a study is generalizable or externally valid when it is thought that it can be applied universally to populations not sampled in the study. The term confounding may simply be considered as meaning confusion or distortion of effects. The measured or unmeasured factors responsible for the relationship between exposure and outcome are known as external confounders. External confounders are associated with both the exposure under study and the outcome. The factors determining precision and validity are given in Table 41.6.

Two important major factors affecting inferences from observational studies are attrition bias and confounding by indication. In long-term studies, it is inevitable that some patients drop out of the study due to death or are lost to follow-up. This subject attrition is not necessarily random and may often be informative, i.e.

related to the exposure and/or outcomes under study. There have been fewer published studies on attrition in rheumatologic cohorts[42,43] than there have been on clinical trials.[44,45]

Therefore, results from observational studies should be examined for the effect of inferences from the dropped-out patients separately from the overall analysis. Another significant problem in interpreting the results of drug data from observational studies is that the observer does not assign treatment. Thus, patients receiving a specific therapy may be receiving it specifically because they have milder (e.g. single-agent hydroxychloroquine) or more severe (e.g. biologicals) disease. Although statistical tools such as propensity scoring[46] have been proposed as a solution to this problem, and their usefulness has been examined in longitudinal studies in RA,[47] it is unclear how well they can identify and adjust for confounders.

REFERENCES

1. Felson DT, Anderson JJ, Meenan RF. The comparative efficacy and toxicity of second-line drugs in rheumatoid arthritis. Results of two metaanalyses. *Arthritis Rheum* 1990; **33**(10): 1449–61.
2. Papadopoulos NG, Alamanos Y, Papadopoulos IA et al. Disease modifying antirheumatic drugs in early rheumatoid arthritis: a longterm observational study. *J Rheumatol* 2002; **29**(2): 261–6.
3. Pincus T. The paradox of effective therapies but poor long-term outcomes in rheumatoid arthritis. *Semin Arthritis Rheum* 1992; **21**(6 Suppl 3): 2–15.
4. Sany J, Anaya JM, Lussiez V et al. Treatment of rheumatoid arthritis with methotrexate: a prospective open longterm study of 191 cases. *J Rheumatol* 1991; **18**(9): 1323–7.
5. Wolfe F, Hawley DJ, Cathey MA. Termination of slow acting antirheumatic therapy in rheumatoid arthritis: a 14-year prospective evaluation of 1017 consecutive starts. *J Rheumatol* 1990; **17**(8): 994–1002.
6. Berard A, Solomon DH, Avorn J. Patterns of drug use in rheumatoid arthritis. *J Rheumatol* 2000; **27**(7): 1648–55.
7. Suarez-Almazor ME. In quest of the holy grail: efficacy versus effectiveness in rheumatoid arthritis. *J Rheumatol* 2002; **29**(2): 209–11.

8. Moreland LW, Schiff MH, Baumgartner SW et al. Etanercept therapy in rheumatoid arthritis. A randomized, controlled trial. *Ann Intern Med* 1999; **130**(6): 478–86.
9. Cohen S, Cannon GW, Schiff M et al. Two-year, blinded, randomized, controlled trial of treatment of active rheumatoid arthritis with leflunomide compared with methotrexate. Utilization of Leflunomide in the Treatment of Rheumatoid Arthritis Trial Investigator Group. *Arthritis Rheum* 2001; **44**(9): 1984–92.
10. Wolfe F, Lassere M, van der Heijde D et al. Preliminary core set of domains and reporting requirements for longitudinal observational studies in rheumatology. *J Rheumatol* 1999; **26**(2): 484–9.
11. Silman A, Symmons D. Reporting requirements for longitudinal observational studies in rheumatology. *J Rheumatol* 1999; **26**(2): 481–3.
12. Baecklund E, Ekbom A, Sparen P et al. Disease activity and risk of lymphoma in patients with rheumatoid arthritis: nested case-control study. *BMJ* 1998; **317**(7152): 180–1.
13. Kamel OW, van de Rijn M, LeBrun DP et al. Lymphoid neoplasms in patients with rheumatoid arthritis and dermatomyositis: frequency of

Epstein-Barr virus and other features associated with immunosuppression. *Hum Pathol* 1994; **25**(7): 638–43.

14. Silman AJ, Petrie J, Hazleman B et al. Lymphoproliferative cancer and other malignancy in patients with rheumatoid arthritis treated with azathioprine: a 20 year follow up study. *Ann Rheum Dis* 1988; **47**(12): 988–92.

15. Kinlen LJ. Incidence of cancer in rheumatoid arthritis and other disorders after immunosuppressive treatment. *Am J Med* 1985; **78**(1A): 44–9.

16. Lipani JA, Strand V, Johnson K et al. A proposal for developing a large patient population cohort for longterm safety monitoring in rheumatoid arthritis. OMERACT Drug Safety Working Party. *J Rheumatol* 2001; **28**(5): 1170–3.

17. Keane J, Gershon S, Wise RP et al. Tuberculosis associated with infliximab, a tumor necrosis factor alpha-neutralizing agent. *N Engl J Med* 2001; **345**(15): 1098–104.

18. Arthritis Research Center Foundation. www.arthritis-research.org; Accessed February 23, 2002.

19. Fries JF. The chronic disease data bank: first principles to future directions. *J Med Philos* 1984; **9**(2): 161–80.

20. Fries JF, Spitz P, Kraines RG et al. Measurement of patient outcome in arthritis. *Arthritis Rheum* 1980; **23**(2): 137–45.

21. Fries JF, Spitz PW, Young DY. The dimensions of health outcomes: the health assessment questionnaire, disability and pain scales. *J Rheumatol* 1982; **9**(5): 789–93.

22. Singh G, Athreya BH, Fries JF et al. Measurement of health status in children with juvenile rheumatoid arthritis. *Arthritis Rheum* 1994; **37**(12): 1761–9.

23. Ramey DR, Fries, J.F, Singh, G. The Health Assessment Questionnaire 1995 - status and review. Chapter 25. In: Spiker B, ed. *Pharmacoeconomics and quality of life in clinical trials* (New York: Raven Press, 1995).

24. Singh G. Arthritis, Rheumatism and Aging Medical Information System Post- Marketing Surveillance Program. *J Rheumatol* 2001; **28**(5): 1174–9.

25. ARAMIS: Arthritis, Rheumatism and Aging Medical Information Systems. http://aramis. stanford.edu/; Accessed February 23,2002.

26. NCHS- Research and Development: National Death Index. http://www.cdc.gov/nchs/r&d/ ndi.htm; Accessed February 23, 2002.

27. Fries JF, Williams CA, Morfeld D et al. Reduction in long-term disability in patients with rheumatoid arthritis by disease-modifying antirheumatic drug-based treatment strategies. *Arthritis Rheum* 1996; **39**(4): 616–22.

28. Fries JF. Safety, cost and effectiveness issues with disease modifying anti-rheumatic drugs in rheumatoid arthritis. *Ann Rheum Dis* 1999; **58** Suppl 1: I86–9.

29. Singh G, Fries JF, Williams CA et al. Toxicity profiles of disease modifying antirheumatic drugs in rheumatoid arthritis. *J Rheumatol* 1991; **18**(2): 188–94.

30. Fries JF. Safety issues related to DMARD therapy. *J Rheumatol Suppl* 1990; **25**: 14–17.

31. Lubeck DP, Spitz PW, Fries JF et al. A multicenter study of annual health service utilization and costs in rheumatoid arthritis. *Arthritis Rheum* 1986; **29**(4): 488–93.

32. Lubeck DP. The economic impact of arthritis. *Arthritis Care Res.* 1995; **8**(4): 304–10.

33. Singh G, Ramey DR, Morfeld D et al. Gastrointestinal tract complications of nonsteroidal anti-inflammatory drug treatment in rheumatoid arthritis. A prospective observational cohort study. *Arch Intern Med* 1996; **156**(14): 1530–6.

34. Singh G, Ramey DR. NSAID induced gastrointestinal complications: the ARAMIS perspective-1997. Arthritis, Rheumatism, and Aging Medical Information System. *J Rheumatol* 1998; **S**(51): 8–16.

35. Singh G, Ramey DR, Triadafilopoulos G et al. GI score: A simple self-assessment instrument to quantify the risk of serious NSAID-related complications in RA and OA. *Arthritis Rheum* 1996; **39**(S): 75.

36. Singh G, Triadafilopoulos G. Epidemiology of NSAID induced gastrointestinal complications. *J Rheumatol* 1999; **26**(Suppl 56): 18–24.

37. Fries JF, Spitz PW, Williams CA et al. A toxicity index for comparison of side effects among different drugs. *Arthritis Rheum* 1990; **33**(1): 121–30.

38. Fries JF, Williams CA, Bloch DA. The relative toxicity of nonsteroidal antiinflammatory drugs. *Arthritis Rheum* 1991; **34**(11): 1353–60.

39. Fries JF, Williams CA, Ramey DR et al. The relative toxicity of alternative therapies for rheumatoid arthritis: implications for the therapeutic progression. *Semin Arthritis Rheum* 1993; **23**(2 Suppl 1): 68–73.

40. Singh G, Williams C, Ramey DR et al. A toxicity index for comparison of gastrointestinal toxicity of non-steroidal antiinflammatory drugs. *Arthritis Rheum* 1996; **39**: S178.

41. Silman A, Klareskog L, Breedveld F et al. Proposal to establish a register for the long term surveillance of adverse events in patients with rheumatic diseases exposed to biological agents: the EULAR Surveillance Register for Biological Compounds. *Ann Rheum Dis* 2000; **59**(6): 419–20.

42. Reisine S, Fifield J, Winkelman DK. Characteristics of rheumatoid arthritis patients: who participates in long-term research and who drops out? *Arthritis Care Res* 2000; **13**(1): 3–10.

43. Leigh JP, Ward MM, Fries JF. Reducing attrition bias with an instrumental variable in a regression model: results from a panel of rheumatoid arthritis patients. *Stat Med* 1993; **12**(11): 1005–18.

44. Maetzel A, Wong A, Strand V et al. Meta-analysis of treatment termination rates among rheuma-toid arthritis patients receiving disease-modifying anti-rheumatic drugs. *Rheumatology (Oxford)* 2000; **39**(9): 975–81.

45. Goldman AI, Holcomb R, Perry HM Jr et al. Can dropout and other noncompliance be minimized in a clinical trial? Report from the Veterans Administrative National Heart, Lung and Blood Institute cooperative study on antihypertensive therapy: mild hypertension. *Control Clin Trials* 1982; **3**(2): 75–89.

46. Rubin DB, Thomas N. Matching using estimated propensity scores: relating theory to practice. *Biometrics* 1996; **52**(1): 249–64.

47. Wiles NJ, Lunt M, Barrett EM et al. Reduced disability at five years with early treatment of inflammatory polyarthritis: results from a large observational cohort, using propensity models to adjust for disease severity. *Arthritis Rheum* 2001; **44**(5): 1033–42.

42

Long-term monitoring of novel therapies

Arthur Kavanaugh, John J Cush and Christian Antoni

Introduction • Sources of data • Pharmacovigilance • Long-term monitoring of novel therapies: experience with TNF inhibitors • Conclusions • References

INTRODUCTION

Recent years have witnessed tremendous progress in the development of novel therapeutic agents for the treatment of various autoimmune disorders. This has been made possible by the confluence of several factors. First, there has been a growing recognition of the severity and consequences of autoimmune diseases. Greater appreciation of the tremendous morbidity associated with these pernicious, chronic conditions has resulted in alteration of treatment paradigms towards more widespread and earlier utilization of aggressive therapeutic regimens. Second has been the progress in delineating the immunologic abnormalities underlying these conditions; this provides relevant therapeutic targets for novel immunomodulatory therapies. Third, there has been extraordinary progress in biotechnology. Over the past decade, several specific biological agents, including monoclonal antibodies and soluble receptor constructs, have been developed.

A tangible example of the successful development of novel therapeutic agents for autoimmune diseases has been the introduction of inhibitors of the key proinflammatory cytokine tumor necrosis factor (TNF) for rheumatoid arthritis (RA). As of 2000, two TNF inhibitors had been approved for clinical use worldwide: the soluble TNF receptor construct etanercept, and the anti-TNF-α monoclonal antibody infliximab. Several other TNF inhibitors are currently in development. Etanercept and infliximab received regulatory approval on the basis of their considerable clinical efficacy and favorable tolerability, as demonstrated in a number of controlled clinical trials. Accompanying the excitement surrounding the introduction of these agents into the clinic, and the impressive efficacy subsequently seen in clinical practice, has been a sense of watchfulness regarding the potential safety profile of these agents. In the past, several traditional synthetic agents that had been brought to the clinic for rheumatologic indications (e.g. benoxaprofen, zomepirac) were subsequently withdrawn based upon safety concerns that came to light post-approval. The biological agents not only represent potent novel agents, but their introduction from clinical trials to the clinic was relatively expedited.

The ultimate utility of any novel agent is predicated on its long-term effectiveness and safety in real-world practice. This can only be addressed by the kind of comprehensive, long-term data that are typically unavailable from relatively short clinical trials. In autoimmune diseases, the alteration of treatment paradigms toward more

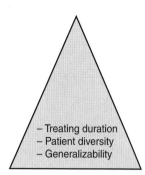

Sources of data
- DBPCRCT
- Long-term follow-up of patients in DBPCRCT
- Cohort studies
- Mandatory post-marketing surveillance
- Spontaneous post-marketing surveillance
- Case–control studies
- Case series, anecdotes

– Treating duration
– Patient diversity
– Generalizability

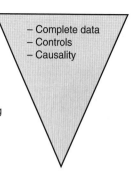

– Complete data
– Controls
– Causality

Figure 42.1 Data concerning the safety of new medications have inherent strengths and weaknesses depending on their source. DBPCRCT, double-blind, placebo-controlled, randomized clinical trials.

aggressive therapy earlier in the disease and for longer duration has elevated the relevance and significance of the issue of long-term safety. Will the long-term safety profile of the new agents warrant treating more patients and treating them earlier? In addition, because many of the novel agents are potent modulators of the immune response, and because this can impact on factors such as host resistance to infection and immuno-surveillance, consideration of long-term safety has become all the more important. In the foreseeable future, the trend towards more aggressive therapy might be expected to expand. The use of combinations of novel immunomodu-latory agents, which is currently under investiga-tion, may become more commonplace. Such an approach to treatment would heighten concerns about long-term safety and hence the need for monitoring. Finally, because the agents used are truly novel types of therapeutic agents (e.g. biological agents, gene therapy), long-term monitoring for previously unseen or even unanticipated adverse effects is required.

While, at first glance, assessment of long-term safety might appear straightforward, it is a quite complex and difficult issue. Consideration of long-term safety requires critical assessment of different sources of data and various reporting and monitoring techniques.

SOURCES OF DATA

Simply stated, there is no single perfect source of data for assessing the long-term safety of novel therapeutic agents. Potential sources that might provide relevant information include: (1) double-blind, placebo-controlled, randomized clinical trials (DBPCRCTs) and other clinical trials; (2) long-term open-label follow-up of patients from DBPCRCTs; (3) cohort studies; (4) mandated or regulated post-marketing surveil-lance (e.g. registries); (5) spontaneous post-marketing surveillance; (6) case–control studies; and (7) case series and individual anecdotes. For each source of data, there are certain biases that critically affect factors such as the reliability and extrapolability of the data (Figure 42.1). Periodic reviews of the medical literature can synthesize information from these varied sources.

For many clinicians, it has become somewhat of an aphorism that the 'best' clinical data are derived from DBPCRCTs. Because of the completeness of the data collection and the presence of a comparison or control population, data from controlled trials do indeed have the greatest internal validity, and offer several distinct advantages. Completeness of the data permits true estimation of the frequency of adverse events. This is a distinct advantage over less rigorous avenues for data collection, where the 'denominator' of patients exposed may not be readily known, making the actual incidence difficult to determine. In addition, because of the completeness with which adverse effects are generally collected during a clinical trial, unexpected adverse events that might be overlooked in less formal analyses may be identi-fied, provided they occurred commonly. Because patients with various rheumatic diseases suffer certain outcomes at a greater frequency than the general population, the presence of a control group may be the most important advantage of data from controlled clinical trials. This is particularly true for immunomodulatory therapies, where pertinent adverse effects would be those potentially resulting from suppression of the immune response, including increased risk of infection or malignancy. Confounding assessment of the long-term safety of immunomodulatory therapies for patients with rheumatic diseases is the increased risk of events including infections and malignancy inherent to the diseases, apart from any effect of treatment. For example, patients with RA develop infectious complications and certain malignancies at a greater rate than age-matched controls.[1–4] This is not limited to RA, as it is true for patients with different systemic inflammatory conditions, including psoriasis, systemic lupus erythematosus (SLE) and others.[5] Moreover, the risk of developing infection and malignancy for patients with rheumatic disease often varies with the severity and activity of the disease itself. For example, the RA patients most susceptible to infections are those with the most severe disease. Of note then, it is common for newer agents to be initially used primarily for patients with the most severe and refractory disease. Therefore, whether a therapeutic agent increases the risk of a particular adverse effect in a given condition can only be determined using appropriate controls.[6] In addition, the presence of a control group offers the best chance of demonstrating causality for adverse events noted among patients receiving therapy with novel therapeutics. Data from controlled clinical trials typically form the basis for regulatory approval and licensure of therapies. While animal studies and small preclinical analyses can detect major toxicities that would preclude further drug development, they may miss much relevant safety data. Therefore, at the time of initial approval and introduction to the clinic, almost all that is known concerning an agent's safety is derived from the results of clinical trials.

However, some information concerning the ultimate real-world safety and efficacy of new therapies is best obtained not from clinical trials but from other sources of data. Part of the reason for this is that there is the substantial potential for ascertainment bias inherent to the selection of patients enrolling in research studies.[7,8] Patients in rheumatology clinical trials tend to be similar as regards not only diagnoses, but also stage of disease, level of activity of disease, and other characteristics. Moreover, patients enrolling in research trials may be more genetically homogeneous, have less comorbidity, generally achieve greater compliance with visits and treatments, and use fewer concomitant medications as compared with unselected groups of patients with the same disease. Thus, they may not necessarily be representative of the more heterogeneous overall population of patients. This could have a substantial impact on the occurrence and/or the severity of certain side-effects related to a given therapy. For example, patients with comorbid conditions such as diabetes or pulmonary disease, who would typically be excluded from rheumatology clinical trials, could be expected to suffer infectious complications more commonly than other patients. Another critical consideration regarding assessment of safety is that clinical trials tend to be relatively short in duration and limited in size. Important but uncommon toxicities may not be seen to develop for the group of patients enrolled, during the course of the research study. For example, if a particular adverse event occurred at an incidence of 1 in 1000 patients, a study would need to include data from several thousand patients to reliably detect such an event. Clinical trials in rheumatology are rarely so large. For these reasons, data other than those generated in controlled clinical trials may have greater generalizability or external validity. Such data are therefore crucial for long-term assessment and monitoring of the safety of novel therapies after their release. Typically, this type of data is obtained after a drug is approved for use in the clinic. Various mechanisms allow the collection of long-term safety data, including spontaneous and regulated post-marketing surveillance, cohort studies, case series and published anecdotal clinical experience (see above; also Figure 42.1). The collection of data on therapies after they have been marketed is often referred to as 'pharmacovigilance'.

PHARMACOVIGILANCE

The main goal of pharmacovigilance is the accurate assessment of the real-world safety of new therapeutic agents over time. Along with assessments of efficacy, this allows optimal determination of the risk/benefit ratio for newly approved drugs. As noted, pharmacovigilance requires data other than those available from controlled clinical trials. Importantly, it will provide information about long-term safety of a drug in heterogeneous patient populations over long time periods. In addition, pharmacovigilance often uncovers other clinically relevant data. For example, therapeutic agents receive regulatory approval for use in specific conditions, based upon the results of research studies conducted on patients with those diseases. However, once they are introduced to the market, these same agents are likely to be used in patients unlike those in clinical trials and for diseases different from those for which they received approval. This is of particular relevance in rheumatology. Many drugs that were initially studied and approved for use in RA came to be utilized in the treatment of patients with various other, less common, types of inflammatory arthritis, such as psoriatic arthritis, ankylosing spondylitis, and SLE. Pharmacovigilance may uncover adverse effects that were not detected in the initial studies on one condition, but that may occur when the same agent is used for other diseases. For example, the hepatotoxicity potentially associated with methotrexate appears to be much more of an issue among patients with psoriasis as compared to those with RA. In addition, pharmacovigilance may also detect toxicity associated with unapproved or even improper use of novel therapies, such as variations in the dose or dosing schedule.

Consideration of the implications of pharmacovigilance involves several caveats. Pharmacovigilance is, in essence, the study of long-term adverse effects. However, even the definition of what constitutes an adverse effect

Table 42.1 FDA MedWatch definition of a serious adverse event.

A serious adverse event is any event that:
- is fatal
- is life-threatening
- is permanently/significantly disabling
- requires or prolongs hospitalization
- is a congenital anomaly
- requires intervention to prevent permanent impairment or damage

can be an area of contention.[9] According to World Health Organization definitions, an adverse drug reaction refers to any noxious, unintended and undesired effect of a drug which occurs at doses used in humans for prophylaxis, diagnosis, or therapy.[10] Such a strict definition would exclude events related to inappropriate dosing of a drug. While operationally stringent, exclusion of adverse effects derived from such circumstances might restrict potentially useful information. Of course, among possible adverse events there is greatest concern about those that could be serious. Whether a particular adverse event is serious may be somewhat subjective; it can depend not only on the specific characteristics and outcome of the event, but also potentially upon the opinion and experience of both the patient and provider. One widely used definition comes from the MedWatch program of the Food and Drug Administration (FDA) of the USA (Table 42.1).[11] A serious adverse event is any event that is fatal, life-threatening, permanently/significantly disabling, requires or prolongs hospitalization, is a congenital anomaly, or requires intervention to prevent permanent impairment or damage. Nonetheless, the estimation and study of serious adverse events is an important objective of pharmacovigilance.

Inherent in any consideration of the clinical implications of potential adverse events is the issue of causality. Determination of the likeli-

Table 42.2 Determining a causal relationship between events and agents.[a]

Primary elements	Secondary elements
Temporal association	Analogy
Lack of likely alternative	Dose responsiveness
Dechallenge	Specificity
Rechallenge	
Biological plausibility	

[a]For a relationship to be causal, at least three of five primary elements (including temporal association and lack of likely alternative) and four of eight total elements should be present.

hood that there is a cause-and-effect relationship between an adverse event and exposure to a drug is referred to as attribution analysis. Important characteristics that would help implicate a causal relationship include chronology of administration and event, response to discontinuation (de-challenge) and repeat exposure (re-challenge), and biological plausibility based on mechanism of action or previously known toxicity. Criteria using these and some other characteristics have been proposed (Table 42.2).[12] However, the area is not without its ambiguities. Of note, for adverse events reported to the FDA MedWatch program, causality is not a prerequisite; only suspicion that an event might possibly be related to the use of an agent is required. As noted above, a particular problem with definitive attribution of causality for adverse effects of therapeutic agents used for patients with rheumatic diseases is the increased propensity for certain events, including infection and malignancy, intrinsic to many of the autoimmune diseases.

The history of pharmacovigilance

Consideration of the history of pharmacovigilance is relevant to contemporary consideration of long-term monitoring of novel therapies.

Pharmacovigilance may have begun at the end of the 19th century in Britain, with the establishment by the *Lancet* of a commission to collect information concerning deaths related to the use of the newly introduced general anesthetic agents.[13] Ever since, the impetus for developments in this area has continued to consist most often of therapeutic misadventures that are either egregious or politically charged. Developments in pharmacovigilance are often marked by the imprimatur of legislation. In 1906 in the USA, in response to adverse events caused by several dubious 'remedies', the Federal Pure Food and Drug Act was passed. This required drugs to be free from contaminants. Probably the seminal event in pharmacovigilance was the realization in the early 1960s that severe congenital abnormalities were associated with the use of the drug thalidomide, which was marketed in several countries as an anti-emetic for pregnant women and as a sedative.[14] In the USA, the Food and Drug Act was amended to require that efficacy and safety data be reported to the FDA prior to marketing. The fact that the FDA had not yet approved thalidomide for use in the USA enhanced public support for and, ultimately, the authority of the FDA. The thalidomide controversy stimulated development of mechanisms for the spontaneous reporting of adverse events worldwide. In the UK, the 'yellow card' system for spontaneous reporting was introduced in 1964. Over the years, often in response to unsuspected toxicities related to new therapies, there have been calls for wider awareness of and greater participation in such programs. In some instances, these systems have worked efficiently. Data from spontaneous reports have led to the identification of many important unsuspected toxicities. More importantly, such information has resulted in decisive actions that have enhanced patient safety. These actions have included increasing the level of awareness of potential adverse events. Mechanisms for achieving this have included changing the labeling or package insert information, such as the 'black box' warning in the USA and the 'black triangle' designation in the UK. Also, practitioners have been alerted by mailings, such as the 'Dear Doctor', 'Dear Healthcare

Provider' or 'Dear Pharmacist' letters. Provisions have been made for disseminating information to patients in the form of medication guides. In instances where severe adverse events have been noted, withdrawal of the causal agent from the market, either by voluntary suspension or regulatory requirement, has resulted. As is the case with approval of new agents, actions taken as a result of pharmacovigilance data are not necessarily uniform worldwide. Based on the same safety information, drugs may be restricted in one country yet withdrawn in another. In addition to thalidomide, some other widely used medications that were removed from the market based on pharmacovigilance data derived largely from spontaneous reporting of adverse events include benoxaprofen (due to hepatotoxicity), zomepirac (due to severe allergic reactions), dexfenfluramine (due to pulmonary hypertension), nomifensine (due to hemolytic anemia), troglitazone (due to hepatotoxicity), and alosetron (due to ischemic colitis).

Reporting of adverse events

The success of pharmacovigilance in highlighting important adverse events has resulted in the establishment of formal procedures for accruing such data in a number of countries.[15] Various agencies have used resources, including the Internet, to collect and disseminate information regarding drug safety (Table 42.3). Information obtained as part of post-marketing surveillance may be obtained by voluntary reporting or may be mandated by law or regulation. The distinction has relevance as regards the interpretation of the data obtained, as different requirements for reporting may affect the types of bias to which the data may be subject. Also, regulations in different countries affect who may or must report data, and how they need to be reported, another potential source of bias. In general, reporting by individual practitioners tends to be voluntary, although in some countries (e.g. Germany) it is required. Of course, assiduous reporting of adverse effects may be considered a responsibility of the medical profession, and many professional medical organizations

Table 42.3 Pharmacovigilance: selected Internet sites[a].

USA: Food and Drug Administration, www.fda.gov/medwatch
Europe: EMEA (European Agency for the Evaluation of Medicinal Products), www.emea.eu.int/ See also EudraWatch (EMEA pharmacovigilance database), www.eudra.org
Canada: Health Canada Therapeutic Products Directorate, www.hc-sc.gc.ca/english/index.htm
Sweden: Medicinal Products Agency, www.mpa.se
United Kingdom: Medicine Control Agency, www.mca.gov.uk

[a]Accessed February 2002.

strongly advocate this obligation. However, practitioners may overlook this responsibility, due in part to disincentives such as uncompensated time and effort, unwanted peer review, and breech of confidentiality. Regulations for reporting of adverse effects by healthcare organizations, e.g. hospitals, may be more stringent than those for individual practitioners, although in some countries it remains the obligation of the treating doctor. For manufacturers and distributors of therapeutic agents, reporting of adverse effects is typically mandatory or legislated. Thus, for most agencies, reporting from the pharmaceutical industry is more common and more complete than information derived from physicians or patients. The specific requirements for reporting of adverse events, e.g. the time frame in which a report must be filed with a regulatory agency and the extent of requisite information, often vary with the severity of the event. In some countries, the establishment of formal procedures for post-marketing surveillance is part of the process for new drug applications.[15] Thus, registries of all patients receiving treatment with certain novel medicines or classes or medicine

Table 42.4 Spontaneous post-marketing surveillance: strengths and limitations.

Strengths
  Rapid identification of adverse events
  Detection of rare events
  Long-term follow-up
  Identification of risk factors for adverse events
  Assessment of safety in large, diverse populations

Limitations
  Underreporting
  Unverifiable data (diagnoses, duplicate reports)
  Incomplete data (comorbidity, concomitant medications)
  Ascertainment bias
  Causality difficult to establish

may be required. While such regulated reporting contributes to the overall knowledge about therapeutic agents, a great deal of information is still gleaned from spontaneous reports of adverse effects.

Success of spontaneous adverse-event reporting

Inherent in spontaneous reports of adverse events are both strengths and limitations that impact on their ultimate utility (Table 42.4). Much of the value of spontaneous reporting relates to the ease with which information can be obtained concerning large numbers of patient exposures in heterogeneous populations. This optimizes the generalizability of the data. Ideally, such reports represent a rapid yet inexpensive source of information regarding the long-term safety of a drug as used in varied practice settings. In this way, information concerning rare adverse events can be detected. Also, by collecting information over the whole

lifetime of an agent's use, uncommon adverse events that might be seen only in particular clinical circumstances can be detected. Information obtained from spontaneous reports can quickly highlight important toxicities that were unidentified or unexpected from clinical trials, allowing swift action that might obviate greater exposure and harm. However, there are several factors that may affect the quality of the data and hence tend to limit the utility of spontaneous adverse-event reports. By their very nature, as well as statutes and regulations established to enhance patient privacy, information in the reports may be unverifiable. Diagnoses may be inaccurate, and the nature or extent of the adverse event may be erroneous. Moreover, the presence of relevant comorbidities or concomitant medications may not be revealed. Clearly such considerations can affect the data, and limit the ability to directly attribute causality. While the potential for individual reports to be duplicated (e.g. being reported independently by manufacturer, physician, and patient) exists, a more important problem with spontaneous reporting of adverse events is the issue of underreporting.[16] It has been estimated that less than 1% of serious adverse drug reactions have been directly reported to the FDA.[17] Moreover, spontaneous reporting is not homogeneous. A number of factors affect the likelihood of whether an adverse event will be reported, thereby introducing ascertainment bias in the accrual of reports. An important factor affecting reporting is whether an adverse effect is deemed serious. In the UK spontaneous reporting system, it has been estimated that approximately 2–4% of non-serious adverse events are reported, compared to 10% of serious events.[18] When this was assessed more formally in an observational study, the percentages of adverse events reported in the UK was somewhat higher: 9% of non-serious adverse events, and 23% of serious adverse events were reported.[19] Interestingly, another formal study of reporting performed several years later showed consistent levels of reporting of non-serious adverse events (9%) but greater reporting of serious adverse events (53%), suggesting that reporting behavior may vary.[20] Two other factors that affect the likelihood that an adverse drug reaction will be reported are the time for which a medication has been on the market, and the type of adverse reaction that occurred. A peak in the number of adverse events reported has been shown to occur near the end of the second year that a drug has been on the market; this is followed by a sharp decline in reporting.[21] Sometimes called the 'Weber effect', it has been suggested that this may relate to physicians' growing familiarity with a medication, and the medication's expected toxicities. Indeed, physicians are more likely to report unanticipated adverse events, such as those not included on the package labeling for the medication.[15,20] Thus the type of adverse event can also result in ascertainment bias. Another factor that can affect reporting of adverse events, popular opinion, is harder to quantify, but may nevertheless be quite powerful. An example of this was the widespread impression that calcium channel blockers caused various adverse events such as cancers, bleeding, and suicide.[22] Subsequent systematic analyses contradicted preliminary suspicions that had been derived from spontaneous post-marketing surveillance and were subsequently widely disseminated in the press. Other examples of suspicions raised by spontaneous reports that were subsequently disproven by more rigorous analyses have also occurred in recent years. A type of post-marketing study that provides more rigorous controlled data than spontaneous reporting would be a cohort study. Such studies, because they include a denominator, can provide actual incidence information about adverse events. Such data can be used to make comparisons among agents with regard to particular toxicities, such as gastrointestinal toxicities related to non-steroidal anti-inflammatory drugs (NSAIDs).[23] However, the adverse events assessed in such a trial must occur with an incidence high enough to be detected, given the size of the population studied and the time frame of the analysis. Thus, such rigorous studies are subject to some of the same limitations as clinical trials, including substantial costs.

LONG-TERM MONITORING OF NOVEL THERAPIES: EXPERIENCE WITH TNF INHIBITORS

Biological agents have become increasingly established as therapeutic agents for patients with autoimmune disease. Important experience is currently accruing with longer term monitoring of the two currently available TNF inhibitors, etanercept and infliximab. During the clinical trials of these agents, a number of toxicities were noted; these have been published, and are reviewed elsewhere in this book. In this chapter, we will focus on the growing body of data concerning longer-term safety with these agents. The information accumulated to date has been instructive, in that it highlights both the capabilities as well as the limitations of data derived from different sources. A number of key questions concerning the safety of these agents remain to be answered. Nonetheless, knowledge and experience gained with the two TNF inhibitors will aid in the establishment of paradigms for the optimal long-term monitoring of other biological agents in the future.

As one method to extend safety information gathered during controlled trials with etanercept and infliximab, the manufacturers of both agents established registries to gather longer-term safety information on patients who participated in these trials.[24–27] By extending the time of observation, these studies provide some assurance that important adverse events related to the treatment could still be detected. Among potential adverse events related to the use of immunosuppressive medications, the development of malignancy is of particular concern. For solid tumors (exclusive of non-melanoma skin cancers), data for both etanercept and infliximab reveal an incidence of approximately 0.007 cases per patient-year of follow-up.[24–27] To provide a frame of reference, the number of solid organ malignancies that would be expected during follow-up of an aged matched cohort can be obtained from the Surveillance, Epidemiology, and End Results (SEER) database of the National Cancer Institute of the United States.[28] Solid organ tumors observed during follow-up of patients treated in clinical trials with etanercept and infliximab closely approximate the number expected from the SEER database. Analysis of the risks of developing lymphoproliferative tumors is made somewhat more complex in studies of RA, because the incidence of tumors such as lymphoma is increased from 2- to 20-fold among RA patients.[29–31] Moreover, the risk of developing lymphoma has been shown to correlate with the severity and activity of disease, as well as with exposure to immuno-suppressive medications. It is of note that the RA patients enrolled in many of the trials of TNF inhibitors were patients with severe active disease that was typically refractory to other treatments, including immunosuppressants. For both etanercept and infliximab, the incidence of lymphoma is approximately 0.002 cases per patient-year.[24–27] Moreover, development of lymphoma did not appear to relate to the dose or the duration of treatment. Thus far, it does not appear, based on these data, that treatment with TNF inhibitors is associated with an increased risk of developing cancer. Another important potential risk of treatment with TNF inhibitors is infection. Assessing data from longer-term follow-up of patients treated in clinical trials of etanercept and infliximab, the incidence of developing serious infection approximated that in other controlled trials, and did not exceed the incidence observed among patients who had received placebo in the earlier clinical trials.

Longer-term follow-up of patients from clinical trials provides useful information, particularly as regards the potential for adverse events that might not be observed during the shorter time frame of the original controlled clinical trials. However, such data are still subject to some of the limitations of the original study, including the potential for homogeneity and lack of comorbidity among the patient population. Therefore, data from post-marketing surveillance are also quite relevant to the assessment of the long-term safety of these agents. Pharmacovigilance data concerning etanercept and infliximab have constituted an area of great interest among clinicians. They have highlighted both the potential and the difficulties with infor-

mation gained in this manner. Soon after giving etanercept initial approval for use in RA in November 1998, the FDA began receiving reports of infections among treated patients. In the first 6 months after release, with an estimated 25 000 prescriptions having been written, 30 serious infections, including 6 deaths, were reported. As a result of this post-marketing surveillance information, a 'Dear Doctor' letter was sent, informing practitioners of the infections, and the package insert was modified. While initially there was a great deal of concern, analysis of the facts surrounding the individual cases provided some reassurance. Thus, all patients had advanced severe RA, and many had significant comorbidities and used other immunosuppressive medications that could also be expected to increase susceptibility to infection. For example, of the six patients who died, four had pre-existing infections, two had diabetes, three had congestive heart failure, and one had renal failure. Further, when examined against the background of infections that had been reported in the literature and in clinical trials, the numbers of infections observed appeared to approximate what might have been expected among patients with severe active RA. In this case, pharmacovigilance served to highlight the potential for serious infections in patients treated with a TNF inhibitor, and also delineated some risk factors that might further increase the risk of infection (i.e. diabetes mellitus, active infection, history of chronic infection). In summary, this underscores the need for assiduous follow-up of treated patients, looking for this type of adverse event.

In January of 2001, after a number of reports of *Mycobacterium tuberculosis* infection among patients treated with infliximab had been received by the FDA, the manufacturer issued a 'Dear Doctor' letter alerting clinicians to this outcome, and urging that appropriate care be taken.[32] In large measure driven by considerations of infectious and other adverse events related to the use of TNF inhibitors, the FDA convened a meeting of the Arthritis Advisory Committee in August 2001. At this meeting, in addition to FDA panel members, representatives

Table 42.5   Adverse events and selected infections related to the use of TNF inhibitors reported at an FDA advisory committee meeting 17 August 2001.

Infectious agent or adverse event	Infliximab ($n \sim$ 170 000)[a]	Etanercept ($n \sim$ 104 000)[a]	Historic population incidence rate[b]
Mean age (years)	53	56	–
Mycobacterium tuberculosis	84	11	USA 8.2/100 000 pt-yrs[c]
			Spain 27/100 000 pt-yrs[d]
			USA RA 6/100 000[36]
			Spain RA 117/100 000 pt-yrs[37]
Atypical mycobacterium[e]	0	8	NA
Histoplasmosis	9	1	NA
Listeria monocytogenes	11	1	NA
Pneumocystis carinii	12	5	NA
Aspergillosis	6	2	NA
Candiasis	7	3	NA
Cryptococcosis	2	3	NA
Coccidioidomycosis	2	0	NA
Pancytopenia	15	12	NA
Aplastic anemia	0	4	RA 5.7–8.2/100 000 pt-yrs
Multiple sclerosis: total	6	14	NA
Multiple sclerosis: new diagnosis	3	6	4/100 000 pt-yrs
Optic neuritis	4	3	5/100 000 pt-yrs
Seizures	29	26	35/100 000 pt-yrs
Lupus-like disease	4	4	NA
Colonic perforations	NA	13	NA
Lymphoma	10	18	NA

Adapted from American College of Rheumatology (ACR) Hotline, available at: www.rheumatology.org/research/hotline/0901tnf.html (accessed February 2002).
[a]Number exposed to drug worldwide; all data are as of August 2001.
[b]Reference incident rates are historic and derived from the literature.
[c]US age-adjusted incidence rate, American Thoracic Society.
[d]Spanish age-adjusted incidence rate, Spanish Thoracic Society.
[e]Includes six cases of M. avium intracellulare and one each of M. kansansii and M. marinarum.
NA, not available; pt-yrs, patient-years.

of the manufacturers of etanercept and infliximab presented data relevant to the safety of these agents (Table 42.5). A great deal of interest centered on tuberculosis (TB). It is of note that among infliximab-treated patients developing TB, 75% developed infection within the first 3 months of treatment, and 97% within the first 6 months, suggesting that this represented reactivation of latent TB. About 25% of patients presented with features of disseminated TB, and more than half had extrapulmonary involvement; these are much higher percentages than those seen among the general population. Considering the specific role of TNF in limiting TB infections in animal models,[33,34] it might be anticipated that inhibition of TNF in patients could be associated with increased risk of infection. To what extent patients with RA may have an increased risk of developing TB apart from treatment with TNF inhibitors is uncertain (Table 42.5); it probably relates to the risk of developing TB in various populations. It is of note that even though more than two-thirds of all patients receiving treatment with infliximab worldwide reside in the USA, roughly 80% of the cases of TB occurred outside of the USA, mostly in countries with a higher rate of TB among the general population. In addition to TB, other opportunistic infections have been observed. Finally, other adverse events, including demyelinating disorders, have been observed during post-marketing surveillance of TNF inhibitors (Table 42.5).[35] The association between treatment and development of adverse events, and whether these events occur at a greater frequency than would be expected among the general population with RA, remain to be fully delineated.

CONCLUSIONS

The introduction of biological agents may well mark the beginning of a new therapeutic paradigm for autoimmune diseases. There has been tremendous excitement surrounding not only the clinical efficacy of these agents, but also the potential ability of such therapies to attenuate structural damage and improve functional status for patients. Accompanying the enthusiasm that has surrounded the introduction of biological agents into the clinic has been vigilance regarding the long-term safety of these potent immunomodulators. Indeed, the introduction of biological agents into the clinic has highlighted the necessity for long-term monitoring of novel therapies. Discussions related to the various methods of accruing relevant data, as well as the factors that affect the interpretation of the data, are proceeding. In addition to ushering in the era of biological agents, experience being gained with the TNF inhibitors etanercept and infliximab will hopefully pave the way for defining optimal approaches for the accumulation of long-term safety data for novel agents. As treatment evolves, e.g. with the use of combinations of biologicals or gene therapy, this experience should prove invaluable.

REFERENCES

1. Doran M, Gabriel S. Infections in rheumatoid arthritis – a new phenomenon? *J Rheumatol* 2001; **28**: 1942–3.
2. Hernandez-Cruz B, Sifuentes-Osornio J, Rosales P, Diaz-Jouanen E. Mycobacterium tuberculosis infection in patients with systemic rheumatic diseases. A case series. *Clin Exp Rheumatol* 1999; **17**: 289–96.
3. Matteson E, Hickey AM, Maguire A et al. Occurrence of neoplasia in patients with rheumatoid arthritis enrolled in a DMARD registry. *J Rheumatol* 1991; **18**: 809–14.
4. Gridley G, Mclaughlin J, Ekbom A et al. Incidence of cancer among patients with rheumatoid arthritis. *J Natl Cancer Inst* 1993; **85**: 307–11.
5. Stern R, Thibodeau L, Kleinerman R, Parrish J, Fitzpatrick T. Risk of cutaneous carcinoma in patients treated with oral methoxsalen photochemotherapy for psoriasis. *N Engl J Med* 1979; **300**: 809–13.
6. van den Borne B, Landewe R, Houkes I et al. No increased risk of malignancies and mortality in cyclosporin A-treated patients with rheumatoid arthritis. *Arthritis Rheum* 1998; **41**: 1930–7.
7. Robinson D, Woerner M, Pollack S, Lerner G. Subject selection biases in clinical trials: data from a multicenter schizophrenia treatment study. *J Clin Psychopharmacol* 1996; **16**: 170–6.
8. Tejeda H, Green S, Trimble E et al. Representation of African-Americans, Hispanics and whites in National Cancer Institute cancer treatment trials. *J Natl Cancer Inst* 1996; **88**: 812–16.
9. Ross SD. Drug-related adverse events: a readers' guide to assessing literature reviews and meta-analyses. *Arch Intern Med* 2001; **161**: 1041–6.

10. World Health Organization. *International Drug Monitoring: The Role of the Hospital* (World Health Organization: Geneva, 1966). Technical Reports Series, no. 425.

11. Kessler D. Introducing MedWatch: a new approach to reporting medication and device adverse effects and product problems. *JAMA* 1993; **269**: 2765–8.

12. Miller FW, Hess EV, Clauw DJ et al. Approaches for identifying and defining environmentally associated rheumatic disorders. *Arthritis Rheum* 2000; **43**: 243–9.

13. Routledge P. 150 years of pharmacovigilance. *Lancet* 1998; **351**: 1200–1.

14. Taussig HB. A study of the German outbreak of phocomelia. *JAMA* 1963; **180**: 1106–14.

15. Meyboom R, Egberts A, Gribnau F, Hekster Y. Pharmacovigilance in perspective. *Drug Safety* 1999; **21**: 429–47.

16. Eland IA, Belton KJ, van Grootheest AC, Meiners AP, Rawlins MD, Stricker BH. Attitudinal survey of voluntary reporting of adverse drug reactions. *Br J Clin Pharmacol* 1999; **48**: 623–7.

17. Scott H, Rosenbaum S, Waters W et al. Rhode Island physicians' recognition and reporting of adverse drug reactions. *R I Med J* 1987; **70**: 311–16.

18. Rawlins MD. Pharmacovigilance: paradise lost, regained, or postponed? *J R Coll Physicians Lond* 1995; **29**: 41–9.

19. Martin RM, Kapoor KV, Wilton LV, Mann RD. Underreporting of suspected adverse drug reactions to newly marketed ('black triangle') drugs in general practice: observational study. *BMJ* 1998; **317**: 119–20.

20. Heeley E, Riley J, Layton D, Wilton L, Shakir S. Prescription-event monitoring and reporting of adverse drug reactions. *Lancet* 2001; **358**: 1872–3.

21. Weber J. Epidemiology of adverse reactions to nonsteroidal antiinflammatory drugs. *Adv Inflam Res* 1984; **6**: 1–7.

22. Kizer JR, Kimmel SE. Epidemiologic review of the calcium channel blocker drugs: an up-to-date perspective on the proposed hazards. *Arch Intern Med* 2001; **161**: 1145–58.

23. MacDonals T, Morant S, Robinson G et al. Association of upper gastrointestinal toxicity of non-steroidal anti-inflammatory drugs with continued exposure: a cohort study. *BMJ* 1997; **315**: 1333–7

24. Schaible T. Long term safety of infliximab. *Can J Gastroenterol* 2000; **14**(suppl C): 29C–32C.

25. Kavanaugh A, Keenan G, Dewoody K et al. Long-term follow-up of patients treated with Remicade (infliximab) in clinical trials. *Arthritis Rheum* 2001; **44**(suppl): S81.

26. Klareskog L, Moreland L, Cohen S et al. Global safety and efficacy of up to five years of etanercept (Enbrel) therapy. *Arthritis Rheum* 2001; **44**(suppl): S77.

27. Moreland L, Cohen S, Baumgartner S et al. Longterm safety and efficacy of etanercept in patients with rheumatoid arthritis. *J Rheumatol* 2001; **28**: 1238–44.

28. National Cancer Institute. Surveillance, Epidemiology, and End Results (SEER) database. SEER Stat for Windows 95/NT, 1997.

29. Becklund E, Ekbom A, Sparen P et al. Disease activity and risk of lymphoma in patients with rheumatoid arthritis: nested case–control study. *BMJ* 1998; **317**: 180–1.

30. Gridley G, McLaughlin JK, Ekbom A et al. Incidence of cancer among patients with rheumatoid arthritis. *J Natl Cancer* Inst 1993; **85**: 307–11.

31. Asten P, Barrett J, Symmons D. Risk of developing certain malignancies is related to duration of immunosuppressive drug exposure in patients with rheumatic diseases. *J Rheumatol* 1999; **26**: 1705–14.

32. Keane J, Gershon S, Wise R et al. Tuberculosis associated with infliximab, a tumor necrosis factor α-neutralizing agent. *N Engl J Med* 2001; **345**: 1098–104.

33. Mohan V, Scanga C, Yu K et al. Effects of tumor necrosis factor alpha on host immune responses in chronic persistent tuberculosis: possible role for limiting pathology. *Infect Immun* 2001; **69**: 1847–55.

34. Senaldi G, Yin S, Shaklee CL, Piguet PF, Mak TW, Ulich TR. Corynebacterium parvum- and Mycobacterium bovis bacillus Calmette–Guerin-induced granuloma formation is inhibited in TNF receptor I (TNF-RI) knockout mice by treatment with soluble TNF-RI. *J Immunol* 1996; **157**: 5022–6.

35. Mohan N, Edwards E, Cupps et al. Demyelination occurring during anti-tumor necrosis factor α therapy for inflammatory arthritides. *Arthritis Rheum* 2001; **44**: 2862–9.

36. Wolfe F, Flowers N, Anderson J, Urbansky K. Tuberculosis rates are not increased in rheumatoid arthritis. *Arthritis Rheum* 2001; **44**(suppl): S105

37. Carmona L, Gonzalez-Alvaro I, Sanmarti R et al. Rheumatoid arthritis is associated with a four-fold increase in tuberculosis infection incidence in the pre-biologicals era. *Arthritis Rheum* 2001; **44**(suppl): S173.

43

Regulatory issues

Jeffrey N Siegel

Introduction • RA guidance document • Issues in clinical trial design • Safety assessment • Drug development for other rheumatic diseases • References

INTRODUCTION

The last few years have witnessed the approval of the first biological agents for the treatment of rheumatic disease. The first such agents approved for rheumatoid arthritis (RA) were the TNF-α blockers. Subsequently, the first IL-1 blocker, anakinra, was licensed for improvement in signs and symptoms of RA. Clinical trials of TNF-blocking agents have demonstrated high levels of efficacy in RA, even in patients refractory to treatment with conventional disease-modifying anti-rheumatic drugs (DMARDs). Data to date suggest that the TNF blockers are well tolerated even for use up to two years. However, there are reports of serious adverse events in a minority of treated patients. The high levels of efficacy and generally favorable safety profile of the TNF blockers have led to their widespread use, and suggest that the next few years may see the development of a large number of new biological agents, both novel molecules targeting TNF-α and IL-1 as well as agents with novel mechanisms of action.

The development of novel therapeutic agents involves interactions at many different stages between the developer and regulatory agencies. In the United States, developers of novel products need to submit an investigational new drug (IND) application to the US Food and Drug Administration (FDA) in order to initiate clinical trials. The FDA reviews the initial IND application and additional trials submitted. After the pivotal trials have been completed and the sponsor submits a marketing application, the FDA reviews all the data on the product to determine whether there is adequate information for an approval. The US Code and the Code of Federal Regulations set forth the specific legal requirements. The purpose of the regulations is to ensure the safety and efficacy of new products.

In this chapter we review the ways that the clinical development process can be carried out in a manner that enhances safety for patients participating in clinical trials and allows for a characterization of the safety and efficacy of new agents. We focus on RA since regulatory guidance is more fully established for that indication and because that is one of the major areas for development of biologicals for rheumatic disease at the present time. The term sponsor is intended to describe the group responsible for carrying out clinical trials and would include pharmaceutical company or biotechnology company sponsors as well as sponsor-investigators.

Table 43.1   FDA guidance on design and conduct for RA trials.

Claim	Duration	Endpoint
Reduction in signs and symptoms of RA	≥ 6 months unless product belongs to an already well-characterized pharmacologic class (e.g. NSAIDs)	Composite endpoints, such as ACR or Paulus criteria, or well-accepted signs/symptoms measures
Major clinical response	≥ 6 months	ACR70 for 6 consecutive months
Complete clinical response	≥ 6 months	Remission by ACR criteria and no radiographic progression for 6 consecutive months
Remission	≥ 6 months	Remission by ACR criteria and no radiographic progression for 6 consecutive months while off all anti-rheumatic therapy
Improvement in physical function	2–5 years	HAQ or AIMS and SF-36
Inhibition of progression of structural damage	≥ 1 year	Slowing x-ray progression using Larsen or Modified Sharp score or other validated radiographic index

AIMS, Arthritis Impact Measure Scales; ACR, American College of Rheumatology; HAQ, Health Assessment Questionnaire; NSAID, non-steroidal anti-inflammatory drug.

RA GUIDANCE DOCUMENT

During the 1990s, the FDA reviewed its approach to the development of new products for the treatment of RA. In a collaborative effort, the FDA centers that review drugs (CDER), biologicals (CBER) and devices (CDRH) consulted with members of the academic community, pharmaceutical industry representatives and members of the general public to formulate guidelines for the best approach to developing new products. These efforts resulted in the publication of an FDA guidance document[1] that articulated current agency thinking on the conduct of clinical trials in RA. The RA guidance document defines a series of claims that represent distinct benefits that may be achieved by treatment of patients with RA

(Table 43.1). The document begins with a claim of improvement in signs and symptoms of RA, but goes on to define enhanced claims that represent benefits in other aspects of the disease process.

Reduction in the signs and symptoms of RA

The basic claim for products for use in treating RA is improvement in signs and symptoms. A clinical trial demonstrating improvement in signs and symptoms should be of at least 6 months in duration, except for new products in a class with a well-established mechanism of action such as non-steroidal anti-inflammatory drugs (NSAIDs) where trials of shorter duration may be adequate. Acceptable outcome measures would include validated composite endpoints, such as the ACR20[2,3] or the DAS,[4] or well-accepted sets of signs and symptom measures. There are several reasons for the recommendation of a clinical trial duration of 6 months. First, since RA is a chronic disease often lasting a lifetime, a longer trial duration is important to establish that benefits are sustained. Second, since many biological agents are foreign proteins, they may be immunogenic. Longer studies of potentially immunogenic products are important to determine whether antibodies to the product diminish the clinical activity over time and whether adverse events develop related to the antibodies. Finally, some adverse drug reactions are only observed with longer duration of exposure.

Major clinical response

When the RA guidance document was being developed some clinicians expressed a concern that while there were products available that improved signs and symptoms, the level of response was often modest. To define a response that was larger in magnitude, the FDA used data indicating that an ACR70 response was rarely seen among patients receiving placebo in randomized clinical trials. Based on this information, the RA guidance document defined a major clinical response as an ACR70 response lasting for 6 consecutive months. A trial demonstrating a major clinical response would be one where a greater proportion of patients in the treatment arm achieved a major clinical response during the study than in the control arm. Although some skepticism was expressed at the time the guidance was being developed that a major clinical response was a realistic goal for treatment of RA, major clinical responses have subsequently been documented in clinical trials of etanercept[5] (23% of patients) and of infliximab[6] (10% of patients).

Complete clinical response/remission

Although it is uncommon to achieve a response with a complete absence of signs and symptoms of RA with currently available therapies, the RA guidance document defines a claim for a product capable of reducing measurable disease activity to zero for a sustained period. A complete clinical response is defined as a response with both remission by ACR criteria and no progression in radiographic changes for a continuous 6-month period. A trial demonstrating a complete clinical response would be one where a greater proportion of patients in the treatment arm achieve a complete clinical response during the study than in the control arm. Remission is defined identically to complete clinical response, except that patients must be off all anti-rheumatic medications to be considered to be in remission.

Improvement in physical function/prevention of disability

Clinicians have long recognized that some patients develop progressive disability despite receiving treatment that appears to be effective at reducing signs and symptoms. The claim of improvement in physical function/prevention of disability was intended to encourage longer-term trials of therapeutic products for RA to determine whether the long-term crippling changes could be reduced or prevented. Trials to achieve this claim should use a validated measure of disability, such as the Arthritis Impact Measure Scales (AIMS)[7] or the Health Assessment Questionnaire (HAQ),[8] and be 2–5 years in duration. The study should also include a more general health-related quality of life measure, such as the SF-36, and patients should not show a worsening during the trial. Sponsors seeking this claim should plan to have demonstrated previously, or to demonstrate concomitantly, improvement in signs and symptoms.

Underlying the claim in the RA guidance document was the assumption that disability as measured by the HAQ accumulated slowly over time and was by and large irreversible. However, recent short-term studies of TNF-blocking agents have demonstrated that treatment can substantially reduce HAQ scores even in a 3-month time frame, suggesting that much of the disability may be related to synovitis rather than to irreversible joint damage. Moreover, longitudinal studies of the natural history of RA indicate that the disability that is related to structural damage to joints may take longer than a 5-year time frame to develop.[9] Thus, it may not be possible in a 2–5-year study to demonstrate prevention of development of disability because HAQ scores may not increase in the control arm. Clinical trials of therapeutic agents that produce a decrease in HAQ scores in the treatment arm and stable scores in the control arm may more accurately be described as improving physical function, rather than preventing disability. Infliximab is the first product to demonstrate improvement in physical function in a 2-year trial.

Inhibition of progression of structural damage

Severe damage to joints from RA has been clearly associated with joint dysfunction. In addition, there are reports that some patients develop progressive structural damage to joints even though signs and symptoms of RA have appeared to be in control. Thus, the RA guidance document included inhibition of progression of structural damage as one of the claims. Studies supporting a claim of inhibition of progression of structural damage should be of at least 1 year in duration and show a decrease in the rate of progression compared to control utilizing a validated index of radiographic damage, such as the total Sharp score or the Larsen score. At the present time, leflunomide, etanercept and infliximab have attained a structural damage claim based on 12-month studies.

While endpoints that do not directly measure signs and symptoms are important in assessing the efficacy of new products, the FDA generally approves new products based on a demonstration that the product produces some clinical benefit to the patient. Since structural damage is, strictly speaking, a non-clinical endpoint, a demonstration of inhibition in progression of structural damage alone would not ordinarily be sufficient for a product to be approved.

Evidence of clinical benefit – e.g. improvement in signs and symptoms or improvement in physical function – should be provided as well.

In some situations a product may be expected to have significant effects on radiographic progression but clinical effects may not be measurable for many years. This may be the case for products that inhibit the processes that mediate joint destruction, but do not inhibit inflammation. Degradative enzyme inhibitors, such as the metalloproteinase inhibitors, and inhibitors of osteoclast activation may be examples of this type of product. The RA guidance document states that federal regulations could allow an approval based on a demonstration of significant slowing of radiographic progression in a seriously affected population of RA patients under some circumstances. Sponsors should consult with the relevant FDA staff before embarking on a clinical program based on these regulations.

ISSUES IN CLINICAL TRIAL DESIGN

Designing clinical trials in RA to provide definitive evidence of safety and efficacy can present a number of challenges. For example, when is a placebo control appropriate and what are the alternatives to the placebo-controlled trial? How can you make conclusions about safety and efficacy in long-term trials if large numbers of patients drop out? If a therapeutic product is associated with characteristic adverse effects, how can you be sure that the results of a clinical trial are not biased by unblinding? These issues, and others, can give rise to significant uncertainties in the analysis of clinical trials, but careful thought in planning the trial may allow these issues to be addressed. Sponsors should consult with FDA staff to discuss optimal clinical trial design for their clinical development plans.

Choice of control

Before there were products available that were highly effective for RA, pharmaceutical company sponsors carried out clinical trials in which patients were withdrawn from their DMARDs and randomized to receive study drug or placebo for the 6 months or longer of the trial. With the advent of marketed products that induce ACR20 responses of 50% or more with proven efficacy in inhibiting the progression of structural damage, some individuals have raised concerns that leaving patients on no DMARD for 6 months or longer in the presence of active disease is unethical because it may produce irreversible damage to the joints. There are several ways this concern can be addressed. First, if there is evidence that the new product is safe in combination with a DMARD, e.g. methotrexate (MTX), then the study can be designed as add-on to standard of care. For example, patients with active disease despite MTX could be randomized to add either study drug or placebo to background MTX. Second, early escape provisions can be included so patients who do not respond by a certain time (e.g. 3 months) would be declared a treatment failure and be free to receive other treatments, or to receive the study drug open-label.

Investigators and pharmaceutical company sponsors should give careful thought to the objectives of the trial in deciding the appropriate control treatment. If the study is intended to simply determine whether the product has efficacy, then a placebo control may be appropriate, but to find out whether the new product is better or safer than alternative products, an active control trial would be more informative.

Investigators and sponsors may carry out active control trials with the aim of demonstrating superiority of the new product to the comparator product or to demonstrate efficacy by showing comparable results to the active control. The latter trials are termed equivalence trials or non-inferiority trials. One approach to analyzing non-inferiority trials is to assess the difference in the results in the two study arms, which should be small if the two products are similar in efficacy. The data would demonstrate non-inferiority if the lower bound of the confidence interval around the difference rules out some predetermined acceptable margin of inferiority of the new product to the old. Obviously, the allowed margin of inferiority should not be larger than the effect size that the active comparator can reliably be expected to have in the setting of the planned trial. In some cases, the allowed margin of inferiority should be considerably less than the effect size of the active comparator to be able to conclude that most of the efficacy is retained.

Non-inferiority trials pose several major challenges, of which a few are highlighted.[10] If there is no placebo arm, there is no internal confirmation that the active comparator had the expected level of efficacy. The expected level of efficacy of the active control is usually estimated from the results of previous placebo-controlled trials. Unfortunately, sometimes trials of even proven efficacious agents have given results no different from the placebo control.[11,12] When trials of therapeutic agents using a particular design and clinical setting have consistently produced a given level of efficacy then those trials are said to exhibit historical sensitivity to drug effects. If similarly designed trials have not regularly distinguished the active control treatment from ineffective treatments, then the sensitivity to drug effects is low and a non-inferiority trial may produce misleading results. Another difficulty with non-inferiority trials is that they may require a very large sample size to reach conclusions. Even if the point estimates (e.g. the proportion of patients achieving an ACR20) are identical between the study arms, it may require a large number of patients for the confidence interval to be small enough to exclude the maximum tolerable difference, e.g. a loss of 50% of the efficacy of the active control.

Alternative clinical trial designs

In addition to the randomized, placebo-controlled superiority trial and the active-control non-inferiority trial, sponsors may consider several other study designs under certain circumstances to provide efficacy data for a new product. A dose–response trial can be utilized where efficacy is inferred from a statistically significant increase in responses with higher doses than lower doses. Sponsors must take care to choose doses that differ in their activity because a trial with similar results in the different study arms may not be able to distinguish between the possibility that all doses are equally efficacious or are equally lacking in efficacy.

Another alternative study design is the randomized withdrawal trial. In situations where the efficacy of a product has been established in one patient population but it is unclear whether another patient population would benefit, a randomized withdrawal trial may provide evidence of efficacy. In a randomized withdrawal trial of this type, all subjects would initially receive the product open-label. Then the patients who achieve a response would be randomized to continue the product or be blindly withdrawn to placebo. Efficacy is inferred based on a higher relapse (or flare) rate in the placebo group than in those remaining on the study drug. Immunex used a randomized withdrawal design successfully to establish the efficacy of etanercept for children with juvenile RA.[13] Unfortunately, randomized withdrawal studies do not provide blinded data on initial response rates so they may not provide as much information as a placebo-controlled parallel-arm study. Randomized withdrawal trials also do not provide as much comparative safety information as the standard parallel-arm study. Among the advantages of randomized withdrawal studies are that they allow all subjects to receive study treatment and no subject receives placebo unless they have already benefited from their participation in the trial.

Design of studies to show improvement in physical function

Studies intended to show improvement in physical function may use the change from baseline in a measure of disability, such as the HAQ at 2 years, as the primary outcome measure. Unfortunately, long-term studies are often plagued by large numbers of dropouts. To reach conclusions from a study that has a substantial amount of missing data, it is necessary to make assumptions about how patients would have done had they stayed in the study until the end. Such determinations are not always easy to make accurately because patient data are not usually missing at random. For example, one source of missing data is patients experiencing drug toxicity, for whom imputation techniques such as last value carried forward may not be the most valid method. Therefore it is critical to minimize the amount of missing data. One way to design a study that may decrease dropouts would be to study superiority of a new product to a known effective control. In this way, patients in the control arm would not receive ineffective therapy and dropouts due to lack of efficacy may be avoided. Ultimately, sensitivity analyses exploring various ways of imputing the missing data should be carried out to determine the robustness of the conclusions of the trial.

Another way to collect data on improvement in function over 2 years would be to use a categorical endpoint of success-or-failure that takes into account how the patient responds during the course of the trial and not just at the final time point. For example, suppose a certain level of improvement in HAQ had been identified as a difference that patients perceive as clinically meaningful (e.g. 0.22 units).[14] Then success could be defined as exceeding that level. For a therapeutic agent that is expected to have a substantial benefit, the study could define success as an improvement in HAQ of at least 0.3 units at month 3, month 6, month 12 and month 24. A subject who did not have at least an improvement of 0.3 units at month 3 or month 6 could be considered a non-responder for purposes of the primary endpoint. To the extent that patients who drop out due to lack of efficacy would not have a large improvement in HAQ scores, such patients could be captured as failures for the primary endpoint, rather than as missing data. Hopefully, with careful thought to appropriate study design, it will be possible to capture long-term treatment data in studies while minimizing uncertainty due to missing data.

Design of studies to show inhibition in progression of structural damage

It is important to conduct studies of structural damage in a rigorous manner to avoid confounding factors that can raise questions about the robustness of the results. Studies should specify how films should be taken and the quality of the x-rays to be obtained. Quality control measures, e.g. assessing the adequacy of films before patients leave the radiology suite, may increase the proportion of high-quality films.

The completeness of datasets is a key to ensuring that the conclusions stand up to scrutiny. There are many ways to improve the completeness of data collection. Using an active control, rather than a placebo control, may help ensure that the majority of patients stay in the study because they are experiencing a clinical benefit from their participation in the study. One way this can be accomplished is to study DMARD-naive patients with early RA randomized to study drug or standard or care, e.g. MTX. Superiority to the active control could be interpreted as evidence of efficacy. Another way to minimize dropouts in a 1-year x-ray study is to allow adjustments in DMARDs (e.g. addition of hydroxychloroquine or sulfasalazine or dose adjustments of medications the patient is already taking) during the second 6 months of the trial for patients who fail to experience a clinical response, e.g. an ACR20 response. Of course, care must to taken not to allow patients in the control arm to take medications that would prevent the trial from demonstrating a drug effect. In addition, imbalances in concomitant DMARDs would need to be taken into account in analyzing the study results.

Obtaining a relatively complete dataset in radiographic studies in RA is a practical goal. Inclusion of provisions to maximize collection of x-rays, such as those described above, has led to substantial improvements in data completeness. In contrast to earlier radiographic studies where one-third or more of the data was not available at 1 year, more recent studies of biological agents have demonstrated high levels of completeness. For the etanercept ERA study in early RA, over 90% of films were available at 1 year and 72% at 24 months.[5] For the infliximab ATTRACT study, 80% of films were available at 1 year.[6]

SAFETY ASSESSMENT

When the FDA considers a new product for approval for marketing, information is available about the safety of the product in the population that was studied in the clinical trials. The available safety data are carefully scrutinized to determine whether the clinical benefits to the patient population outweigh the potential risks. Unfortunately, the safety profile observed during clinical trials may not fully reflect the safety of new products after they are marketed. Among the important factors accounting for this are the limited size of the safety database at the time of approval and differences between the patients studied in clinical development and the population that receives the product after it is marketed.

Size of the safety database

One of the main reasons that new safety concerns emerge after marketing is that rare, but serious, adverse events may occur at a frequency that is too small to detect with the limited number of patients treated during clinical development. The 'Rule of Three' provides an estimate of how confidently we can rule out that a product is associated with a serious adverse event (SAE) if that event is not observed in clinical trials. If no SAE is seen in a trial of 100 subjects, using the upper bound of the 95% confidence interval allows us to state that it is unlikely the SAE would go unobserved if the true incidence were 3% or greater. Similarly, an SAE with a true incidence of 3 in 1000 is unlikely to go unobserved in a trial of 1000 stubjects. Since marketed products used in RA can be used in hundreds of thousands of people, it would take a study of over 100,000 patients to assess all the rare but serious adverse events that may occur. Clearly this is impractical since the number of patients exposed to new products prior to approval never approaches the numbers who may receive the product when it is marketed. Also of note, very rare events may have a limited impact on the desirability of using a therapy with substantial efficacy in a serious disease such as RA.

The E1A document of the International Conference on Harmonization, which is also an FDA guidance document, provides recommendations for the safety information that should be available for new drugs and biological products intended for chronic use.[15] Overall, the E1A document recommends safety data on at least 1000–1500 patients treated for any duration. To assess short-term safety, the E1A document recommends collecting safety information on 300–600 patients treated for 6 months. The E1A document recommends longer-term data collection to assess adverse events (AEs) that increase in frequency or severity with time and to measure AEs that occur only with longer-term use. The E1A document states that data collection on 100 patients treated for 1 year may be adequate if no SAEs are observed. However, more or longer-term data may be required if late-developing AEs are observed or if AEs are observed that increase in severity or frequency over time. In addition, more data may be required if there are concerns based on preclinical toxicity testing, pharmacology or inferences from similar agents.

The recent experience with safety concerns arising following the approval of the TNF antagonists illustrates some of these principles.[16] Despite the fact that their mechanism of action is to inhibit an important arm of host defenses, clinical trial data from etanercept and infliximab did not clearly show an increase in infections at the time of their approvals. Nonetheless, the product labels did include precautions about the possibility of increased propensity to infections based on their mechanism of action and other considerations. After approval, reports of serious infections with both etanercept and infliximab led to the addition of bold warnings of rare but serious infections that were occasionally fatal. Later still, reports of reactivation of latent tuberculosis infection led to revisions to both labels. A boxed warning was added to the infliximab label recommending screening of all patients for latent tuberculosis infection prior to initiating treatment and treatment with antituberculous medications for any patient testing positive. In addition, the FDA became aware of

cases of multiple sclerosis (MS) and other demyelinating syndromes in patients treated with TNF blockers, leading to the addition of warnings to both the Enbrel and Remicade labels. Because these SAEs are uncommon, the risk/benefit ratio is still favorable for both these agents in selected patients with RA. Nonetheless, these events demonstrate how incomplete the safety database may be at the time a product is approved.

How many patients should be exposed to a new product for RA prior to approval? The appropriate size of the safety database depends on a number of factors, including the mechanism of action of the product and the size of the intended patient population. For products that are expected to be immunosuppressive or immunomodulatory, a safety database that meets the minimum recommendations of the E1A document may not be adequate. A larger database with more long-term exposure may be better suited to assessing the frequency of uncommon SAEs in potentially immunosuppressive agents.

Long-term safety

Some adverse events are observed only after prolonged exposure to therapeutic agents. Unfortunately, even studies of 1 or 2 years in duration may not reveal adverse events that appear only with long-term use. One recent example is the issue of whether the use of azathioprine and methotrexate is associated with an increase in the risk of lymphoma. Reports of lymphoma in RA patients receiving chronic treatment with these agents suggested that the risk might be increased. However, careful epidemiological studies revealed that the background rate of lymphoma may be increased in RA patients.[17,18] Furthermore, two recent studies have suggested that the risk of lymphoma is particularly increased in RA patients with high levels of inflammation, suggesting that the association with azathioprine and methotrexate may be related to the severe nature of the disease rather than to the drugs themselves.[19,20] This example illustrates how difficult it may be to determine accurately the safety of long-term use of therapeutic agents. It also illustrates how critical it is to systematically collect data to address long-term safety issues.

Since immune surveillance against tumors is an important role of the immune system, immunomodulatory and immunosuppressive agents could increase the risk of malignancy. Clinical trial data from the etanercept, infliximab and anakinra studies did not clearly reveal an increase in the incidence of malignancies. However, longer-term data are required to reach firm conclusions. The agency encourages sponsors to collect long-term safety data over a span of at least 3–5 years in a sufficient number of patients to evaluate the risk of malignancies, serious infections and the induction of new autoimmune diseases.

Other safety concerns

Clinical trials of novel therapeutic agents are more restrictive compared to usual clinical practice with respect to the patients who are included in trials and the concomitant medications that are allowed. The strict rules followed in clinical trials provide a relatively homogeneous patient population that maximizes the ability to discern the treatment effect of a new agent and to assess adverse events that are associated with use of the product. Unfortunately, because of the way these strict rules define the patient population in clinical trials, the safety data may not be fully generalizable to patients in usual clinical practice.[21] For example, there may be important interactions between the novel product and other antirheumatic medications and with concomitant medical conditions that are missed during drug development.

Unexpected SAEs associated with specific concomitant medical conditions have been observed in several recent examples. Studies in pre-clinical models suggested that TNF-α blockade may be beneficial for MS. Based on this information, studies of lenercept (a soluble TNF receptor) and infliximab were carried out in patients with MS.[22,23] Surprisingly, both studies observed a worsening of disease activity. These studies, along with post-marketing adverse event reports, led to a warning in the package insert for both etanercept and infliximab to avoid use in patients with pre-existing MS. A second example is the use of TNF antagonists in patients with CHF. Again, pre-clinical models suggested that TNF-α was harmful in CHF and that TNF blockade may ameliorate disease. However, instead of seeing benefit, two clinical trials of etanercept in patients with CHF were stopped early because of futility and one study showed a suggestion of possible worsening. A clinical trial of infliximab in patients with class III and IV CHF was also stopped early because of evidence of worsening of CHF and increased mortality in infliximab-treated patients.

How can we ensure that the safety data available at the time of approval of new agents more fully reflect the safety of the products when they are marketed? One way to address this issue is to carry out randomized safety studies prior to approval with flexible inclusion and exclusion criteria that enroll a patient population closer to typical clinical practice. For a product for RA, such a study could include any patient with active disease with liberal inclusion and exclusion criteria. Unless there are specific, known safety concerns, any medication and combination of medications could be allowed. Patients with concomitant medical conditions could be enrolled so long as there were no specific contraindications. Finally, while complete adverse event data would be collected, other data collection could be kept to a minimum to encourage enrollment of patients who might not otherwise participate in clinical trials because of the inconvenience factor.

Amgen carried out a randomized safety study of anakinra as part of their clinical development program prior to its approval. In addition to phase 2 studies that enrolled a total of 892 patients and a 506-patient phase 3 trial, Amgen carried out a randomized, placebo-controlled safety study with 1414 subjects.[24] The study included patients receiving a wide range of concomitant DMARDs, including methotrexate, hydroxychloroquine, sulfasalazine, leflunomide and others, alone and in combination. A significant proportion (5–10% each) had a variety of common concomitant medical conditions, including COPD, asthma, coronary artery disease and diabetes. The study demonstrated a higher incidence of serious infection among anakinra-treated patients, a result that had not been apparent from earlier studies. The data did not indicate any association between serious infections and either concomitant DMARDs or concomitant medical conditions, with the exception of a higher incidence of serious infections in patients with underlying asthma.

Data from the usual types of clinical trials conducted during drug development may not fully reflect the safety of new products when they are marketed. The experience with the anakinra safety trial demonstrates that it is feasible to gather safety data on the use of new agents in a patient population more similar to that seen in usual clinical practice. Safety studies of this type would provide additional data on the safety of new products in a variety of clinical settings, may pinpoint subsets of patients who should avoid the new agent and may decrease the frequency of occurrence of unexpected SAEs in the post-marketing experience.

DRUG DEVELOPMENT FOR OTHER RHEUMATIC DISEASES

While much of the focus of drug development for the new biological agents has been on RA during the last few years, clinical trials of biological agents have been carried out in other, less common rheumatic diseases, including systemic lupus erythematosus (SLE) and scleroderma. Some of the reasons for the intense interest in RA are that RA represents a considerably larger market and that the pathogenic mechanisms are better understood than for some other diseases. However, development of new treatments for SLE, scleroderma, Wegener's granulomatosis, Behcet's and certain other rheumatic diseases represents an unmet medical need so that development of promising new therapies should be encouraged. At the current time, regulatory

guidance is most developed for RA and osteoarthritis.[25] Regulatory guidance is also available for clinical development programs for osteoporosis.[26] For other rheumatic conditions, decisions may be made on a case-by-case basis.

There has been considerable interest in developing a guidance document for clinical trials in SLE.[27] One of the challenges of measuring improvement of disease activity in SLE in therapeutic trials is that the disease presents in such varied ways. Fortunately, there has been a great deal of work on developing indices that provide a common metric for measuring disease activity in patients exhibiting differing manifestations of disease. Responder indices that are currently under development may also prove useful for measuring responses in clinical trials. Currently there is a consensus that clinical trials in SLE should address a minimum set of domains of disease, including disease activity, health-related quality of life and, for longer-term trials, damage.[28]

The spondylarthropathies are another area where there is growing interest in treatment with biological agents. Etanercept was recently approved for the treatment of active peripheral arthritis in patients with psoriatic arthritis based on a clinical trial design that was quite similar to that used commonly in RA.[5] In addition, there is growing interest in the use of both infliximab and etanercept in ankylosing spondylitis (AS). Consensus panels have recently proposed endpoints that could be used in short-term trials in AS.[29] These proposed outcome measures address the signs and symptoms and impaired physical function associated with the disease. Unfortunately, assessing whether new therapies impact the slowly accumulating disability and structural damage seen in AS will require considerable thought because they will involve long-term studies that may lack adequate control groups.

Development of new therapies for scleroderma is especially urgent because of the considerable morbidity and mortality associated with this disease and the lack of proven disease-modifying therapeutic agents. The design of clinical trials for scleroderma would be dependent on the mechanism of action of the product and the targeted patient population. For example, a clinical trial testing the efficacy of a product that is focused on ameliorating signs and symptoms in one organ system, such as the recently approved epoprostenol sodium for pulmonary hypertension, might use a primary endpoint focused on the organ system in question. In contrast, another therapy undergoing testing in scleroderma is high dose immunosuppression plus autologous stem cell rescue, which is hoped to have more generalized beneficial effects on disease activity but also carries significant short-term toxicity associated with the conditioning regimen and transplantation.[30] Studies to show a benefit for this therapy would need to use outcome measures that could demonstrate benefits for a variety of major organ system manifestations and be long enough to assess the impact of the therapy on survival. Because of the complexities of risk/benefit assessment in scleroderma, sponsors should consult with the FDA early on optimal study design.[31]

REFERENCES

1. FDA. Guidance for industry: clinical development programs for drugs, devices, and biological products for the treatment of rheumatoid arthritis (RA). FDA guidance document, issued February 1999 <http: //www.fda.gov/cder/guidance/1208fnl.htm>
2. Felson DT, Anderson JJ, Boers M et al. The American College of Rheumatology preliminary core set of disease activity measures for rheumatoid arthritis clinical trials. *Arthritis Rheum* 1993; **36**(6): 729–40.
3. Felson DT, Anderson JJ, Boers M et al. American College of Rheumatology preliminary definition of improvement in rheumatoid arthritis. *Arthritis Rheum.* 1995; **38**(40): 1–9.
4. van der Heijde DM, van 't Hof MA, van Riel PL et al. Judging disease activity in clinical practice in rheumatoid arthritis: first step in the development of a disease activity score. *Ann Rheum Dis* 1990; **49**: 916–20.
5. Etanercept (Enbrel) package insert.
6. Infliximab (Remicade) package insert.
7. Meenan RF, Gertman PM, Mason JH, Dunaif R. The Arthritis Impact Measurement Scales: further investigations of health status measure. *Arthritis Rheum* 1982; **25**: 1048–53.
8. Fries JF, Spitz PW, Young DY. The Dimensions of Health Outcomes: the Health Assessment Questionnaire, Disability, and Pain Scales. *J Rheumatol* 1982; **9**: 789–93.
9. Scott DL, Pugner K, Kaarela K et al. The links between joint damage and disability in rheumatoid arthritis. *Rheumatol (Oxford)* 2000; **39**(2): 122–32.
10. ICH E10. Choice of control group and related issues in clinical trials. FDA guidance document, issued May 2001 <http: //www.fda.gov/CDER/guidance/4155fnl.htm>.
11. Temple R, Ellenberg SS. Placebo-controlled trials and active-control trials in the evaluation of new treatments. Part 1: ethical and scientific issues. *Ann Intern Med* 2000; **133**(6): 455–63.
12. Ellenberg SS, Temple R. Placebo-controlled trials and active-control trials in the evaluation of new treatments. Part 2: practical issues and specific cases. *Ann Intern Med* 2000; **133**(6): 464–70.
13. Lovell DJ, Giannini EH, Reiff A et al. Etanercept in children with polyarticular juvenile rheumatoid arthritis. Pediatric Rheumatology Collaborative Study Group. *N Engl J Med* 2000; **342**(11): 763–9.
14. Redelmeier DA, Lorig K. Assessing the clinical importance of symptomatic improvements. An illustration in rheumatology. *Arch Intern Med* 1993; **153**(11): 1337–42.
15. ICH E1A. The extent of population exposure to assess clinical safety: for drugs intended for long-term treatment of non-life-threatening conditions. FDA guidance document. Reference for E1A document <http: //www.FDA.gov/CDER/guidance/index.htm>.
16. Safety update on TNF-α antagonists: infliximab and etanercept. FDA briefing document, issued August 2001 <http: //www.fda.gov/ohrms/dockets/ac/01/briefing/3779b2.htm>.
17. Beauparlant P, Papp K, Haraoui B. The incidence of cancer associated with the treatment of rheumatoid arthritis. *Semin Arthritis Rheum* 1999; **29**(3): 148–58.

18. Thomas E, Brewster DH, Black RJ, Macfarlane GJ. Risk of malignancy among patients with rheumatic conditions. *Int J Cancer* 2000; **88**(3): 497–502.

19. Baecklund E, Ekbom A, Sparen P et al. Disease activity and risk of lymphoma in patients with rheumatoid arthritis: nested case-control study. *BMJ* 1998; **317**(7152): 180–1.

20. Wolfe F. Inflammatory activity, but not methotrexate or prednisone use predicts non-Hodgkin's lymphoma in rheumatoid arthritis: a 25-year study of 1,767 RA patients. *Arthritis Rheum* 1998; **41**(9S): S188.

21. Suarez-Almazor ME. In quest of the holy grail: efficacy versus effectiveness in rheumatoid arthritis. *J Rheumatol* 2002; **29**(2): 209–11.

22. TNF neutralization in MS: results of a randomized, placebo-controlled multicenter study. The Lenercept MS study group and the University of British Columbia MS/MRI Analysis Group. *Neurology* 1999; **53**(3): 457–65.

23. van Oosten BW, Barkhof F, Truyen L et al. Increased MRI activity and immune activation in two multiple sclerosis patients treated with the monoclonal anti-tumor necrosis factor antibody cA2. *Neurology* 1996; **47**: 1531–4.

24. Clinical review, Amgen, Biologic licensing application, STN 103950, anakinra for use in the treatment of rheumatoid arthritis. FDA briefing document, issued July 2001 <http: //www. fda.gov/ohrms/dockets/ac/01/briefing/3779b 1.htm>.

25. FDA. Guidance for industry: clinical development programs for drugs, devices, and biological products intended for the treatment of osteoarthritis (OA). FDA draft guidance document, issued July 1999 <http: //www. fda.gov/cder/guidance/2199dft.doc>.

26. FDA. Guidelines for preclinical and clinical evaluation of agents used in the prevention or treatment of postmenopausal osteoporosis. FDA guidance document, issued April 1994 <http: //www.fda.gov/cder/guidance/osteo.pdf>.

27. Siegel JN. Development of an FDA guidance document for clinical trials in SLE. *Lupus* 1999; **8**(8): 581–5.

28. Strand V, Gladman D, Isenberg D et al. Outcome measures to be used in clinical trials in systemic lupus erythematosus. *J Rheumatol* 1999; **26**(2): 490–7.

29. Anderson JJ, Baron G, van der Heijde D et al. Ankylosing spondylitis assessment group preliminary definition of short-term improvement in ankylosing spondylitis. *Arthritis Rheum* 2001; **44**(8): 1876–86.

30. Binks M, Passweg JR, Furst D et al. Phase I/II trial of autologous stem cell transplantation in systemic sclerosis: procedure related mortality and impact on skin disease. *Ann Rheum Dis* 2001; **60**(6): 577–84.

31. Woolfrey A, Laxer RM, Hirsch R, Horwitz M. Autologous stem cell transplantation for pediatric rheumatic diseases. *J Rheumatol* 2001; **28**(10): 2337–58.

Index